Craniomaxillofacial Reconstructive and Corrective Bone Surgery

Alex M. Greenberg, DDS

Assistant Clinical Professor, Division of Oral and Maxillofacial Surgery, Columbia University
School of Dental and Oral Surgery; Clinical Instructor, Division of Oral and Maxillofacial
Surgery, Mount Sinai School of Medicine; and Assistant Attending, Division of Oral and
Maxillofacial Surgery, Beth Israel Medical Center, and Associate Attending, Division of Oral
and Maxillofacial Surgery, St. Luke's/Roosevelt Hospital, New York, New York, USA

Joachim Prein, MD, DDS

Professor of Maxillofacial Surgery; and Head, Clinic for Reconstructive Surgery,
Kantonsspital Basel, Basel, Switzerland

Editors

Craniomaxillofacial Reconstructive and Corrective Bone Surgery

Principles of Internal Fixation Using the AO/ASIF Technique

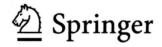 Springer

Alex M. Greenberg, DDS
Assistant Clinical Professor
Division of Oral and Maxillofacial
    Surgery
Columbia University School of Dental
    and Oral Surgery
and
Clinical Instructor
Division of Oral and Maxillofacial
    Surgery
Mount Sinai School of Medicine
and
Assistant Attending
Division of Oral and Maxillofacial
    Surgery
Beth Israel Medical Center
and
Associate Attending
Division of Oral and Maxillofacial
    Surgery
St. Luke's/Roosevelt Hospital
New York, NY, USA

Joachim Prein, MD, DDS
Professor of Maxillofacial Surgery
and
Head, Clinic for Reconstructive Surgery
Kantonsspital Basel
CH-4031 Basel, Switzerland

Library of Congress Cataloging-in-Publication Data

Craniomaxillofacial reconstructive and corrective bone surgery : principles of internal fixation
using the AO/ASIF technique / edited by Alex M. Greenberg, Joachim Prein.
    p. cm.
    Includes bibliographical references and index.
    ISBN 0-387-94686-1 (hardcover : alk. paper)
    1. Facial bones—Surgery. 2. Jaw—Surgery. 3. Skull—Surgery. 4. Internal fixation
in fractures. I. Greenberg, Alex M. II. Prein, J. (Joachim), 1938–
    [DNLM: 1. Facial Bones—surgery. 2. Bone Diseases—surgery. 3. Surgery,
Plastic—methods. 4. Internal Fixators. 5. Bone Plates. 6. Skull—surgery.
WE 705 C8909 1997]
RD523 .C73 1997
617.5′2059—dc20   96-035162

ISBN 0-387-94686-1   Printed on acid-free paper.
ISBN 978-0-387-94686-1

10 9 8 7 6 5

springer.com

To my wife, Sigal Greenberg,
and
my daughter, Aurie Greenberg,
for their special love, support, and inspiration

To my father, Rubin Greenberg,
for his love and devotion to his family

In loving memory of my mother, Nancy Greenberg

AMG

This book represents my tribute and thanks to so many surgical
colleagues worldwide for their help, collaboration, fellowship, and
lifelong friendship over my professional career.

JP

Preface

These are exciting times for the diverse group of surgeons who perform craniomaxillofacial surgery. The AO/ASIF (Swiss Association of Internal Fixation) has played a crucial role in the growth of this field through its leadership in research, teaching, and cooperation with industry. As clinicians fascinated by the extraordinary progress in the field, the goal is to advance this new knowledge by teaching AO/ASIF courses and writing textbooks that supplement these courses and related workshops.

This textbook adopts the case presentation format used in *Craniomaxillofacial Fractures: Principles of Internal Fixation Using the AO/ASIF Technique*. The breadth of the subject meant that a coeditor was advisable and, fortunately, Joachim Prein accepted that role. To make this a comprehensive textbook, 75 international authorities wrote chapters in the areas of oral and maxillofacial surgery, plastic and reconstructive surgery, and otolaryngology and head and neck surgery.

This textbook presents progress in craniomaxillofacial surgery through the technical and scientific advances in biomaterials, microvascular surgery, dental implantology, and surgical techniques. Section I covers basic considerations in the diagnosis of craniomaxillofacial defects and disorders. Section II comprises chapters on the biomechanics and biocompatability of internal fixation and dental osseointegration implantology. These developments have helped to revolutionize craniomaxillofacial bone surgery by providing the structural support that also meets the functional needs of the patient. Section III is the first of three sections on specific considerations in craniomaxillofacial reconstructive and bone surgery. This first section includes the AO/ASIF mandibular hardware system and basic aesthetic considerations. Section IV provides a regional approach to each section of the midface and mandible that may require reconstruction because of defects resulting from trauma, infections, and tumors. Section V reviews elective osteotomies of the skull and facial bones, including the maxilla, mandible, upper midface, and skull. The two appendices present updated material on the ITI dental implant system and distraction osteogenesis of the mandible. Chapters 22 and 41, in particular, also present up-to-date information on the AO/ASIF hardware systems of instrumentation and implants separate and distinct from the other chapters to allow easier understanding of these biomaterials.

The editors hope that this textbook will be an indispensable reference for medical students, residents in training, and attending surgeons in the diverse fields of craniomaxillofacial surgery. Surgery cannot develop without honoring the achievements of the past and the assimilation of current knowledge; this textbook is intended to assist in this process.

Alex M. Greenberg, DDS
New York, New York, USA

Joachim Prein, MD, DDS
Basel, Switzerland

January 2002

Acknowledgments

The editors would like to acknowledge the many individuals who have contributed to this book. First are the many chapter authors from Europe, Asia, North America, and South America who represent all aspects of the discipline. They are a truly outstanding group of surgeons, who have contributed greatly to the progress evident in this book. Many have been AO/ASIF (Swiss Association for Internal Fixation) faculty members and have been active in teaching courses all over the world.

We also thank Synthes Maxillofacial, Paoli, Pennsylvania; the Institut Strauman, Waldenburg, Switzerland; and Professor Tomas Albrektsson, Department of Biomaterials/Handicap Research, Gothenburg University, Gothenburg, Sweden, for providing financial support to reproduce the many color figures in this textbook.

We are also appreciative of the assistance of Fr. Inge Jundt, Secretary, Clinic for Reconstrucitve Surgery, at Kantonsspital Basel, Basel, Switzerland, for her role in the preparation of the manuscript; Synthes Maxillofacial, Paoli, Pennsylvania; and STRATEC, Oberdorf, Switzerland, for advice concerning technical aspects of AO/ASIF hardware and instrumentation, and Ms. Laurel Lhowe for her outstanding illustrations.

Alex M. Greenberg, DDS
New York, New York, USA

Joachim Prein, MD, DDS
Basel, Switzerland

Contents

Preface vii

Acknowledgments ix

Contributors xvii

1   Introduction 1
Alex M. Greenberg and Joachim Prein

**Section I   Basic Considerations in the Diagnosis of Craniomaxillofacial Bone
Defects and Disorders**

2   Evaluation of the Craniomaxillofacial Deformity Patient 5
Jackson P. Morgan, III and Richard H. Haug

3   Craniofacial Deformities: Review of Etiologies, Distribution,
and Their Classification 22
Craig R. Dufresne

4   Etiology of Skeletal Malocclusion 38
Bruce L. Greenberg

5   Etiology, Distribution, and Classification of Craniomaxillofacial
Deformities: Traumatic Defects 43
Richard H. Haug and Jackson P. Morgan, III

6   Etiology, Distribution, and Classification of Craniomaxillofacial
Deformities: Review of Nasal Deformities 49
John G. Hunter

7   Review of Benign Tumors of the Maxillofacial Region and Considerations
for Bone Invasion 59
Joachim Prein

8   Oral Malignancies: Etiology, Distribution, and Basic Treatment Considerations 65
Anna-Lisa Söderholm

9   Craniomaxillofacial Bone Infections: Etiologies, Distributions,
and Associated Defects 76
Darin L. Wright and Robert M. Kellman

10   A New Classification System for Craniomaxillofacial Deformities 90
      Richard H. Haug and Alex M. Greenberg

Section II   Biomechanics of Internal Fixation and Dental Osseointegration Implantology

11   Craniomaxillofacial Bone Healing, Biomechanics, and Rigid Internal Fixation 101
      Frederick J. Kummer

12   Metal for Craniomaxillofacial Internal Fixation Implants
      and Its Physiological Implications 107
      Samuel G. Steinemann

13   Bioresorbable Materials for Bone Fixation: Review of
      Biological Concepts and Mechanical Aspects 113
      Riitta Suuronen and Christian Lindqvist

14   Advanced Bone Healing Concepts in Craniomaxillofacial Reconstructive
      and Corrective Bone Surgery 124
      Tomas Albrektsson, Lars Sennerby, and Anders Tjellström

15   The ITI Dental Implant System 138
      Hans-Peter Weber, Daniel A. Buser, and Dieter Weingart

16   Localized Ridge Augmentation Using Guided Bone Regeneration in
      Deficient Implant Sites 155
      Daniel A. Buser, Dieter Weingart, and Hans-Peter Weber

17   The ITI Dental Implant System in Maxillofacial Applications 164
      Dieter Weingart, Daniel A. Buser, and Hans-Peter Weber

18   Maxillary Sinus Grafting and Osseointegration Surgery 174
      Jeffrey I. Stein and Alex M. Greenberg

19   Computerized Tomography and Its Use for Craniomaxillofacial
      Dental Implantology 198
      Morton Jacobs

20A   Radiographic Evaluation of the Craniomaxillofacial Region 210
      Dorrit Hallikainen, Christian Lindqvist, and Anna-Lisa Söderholm

20B   Atlas of Cases 220
      Christian Lindqvist, Dorrit Hallikainen, and Anna-Lisa Söderholm

21A   Prosthodontic Considerations in Dental Implant Restoration 232
      James H. Abjanich and Ira H. Orenstein

21B   Overdenture Case Reports 262
      Alex M. Greenberg

Section III   Craniomaxillofacial Reconstructive and Corrective Bone Surgery

22   AO/ASIF Mandibular Hardware 269
      Joachim Prein and Alex M. Greenberg

23   Aesthetic Considerations in Reconstructive and
      Corrective Craniomaxillofacial Bone Surgery   280
      R. Gregory Smith and Luc M. Cesteleyn

Section IV   Craniomaxillofacial Reconstructive Bone Surgery

24   Considerations for Reconstruction of the Head and Neck Oncologic Patient   289
      Douglas W. Klotch and Neal D. Futran

25   Autogenous Bone Grafts in Maxillofacial Reconstruction   295
      Michael Ehrenfeld and Christine Hagenmaier

26   Current Practice and Future Trends in Craniomaxillofacial Reconstructive
      and Corrective Microvascular Bone Surgery   310
      Hubert Weinberg, Lester Silver, and Jin K. Chun

27   Considerations in the Fixation of Bone Grafts for the Reconstruction
      of Mandibular Continuity Defects   317
      Peter Stoll, Joachim Prein, Wolfgang Bähr, and Rüdiger Wächter

28   Indications and Technical Considerations of Different Fibula Grafts   327
      Peter Stoll

29   Soft Tissue Flaps for Coverage of Craniomaxillofacial Osseous Continuity
      Defects with or Without Bone Graft and Rigid Fixation   335
      Barry L. Wenig

30   Mandibular Condyle Reconstruction with Free Costochondral Grafting   343
      Christian Lindqvist

31   Microsurgical Reconstruction of Large Defects of the Maxilla, Midface,
      and Cranial Base   356
      Rainer Schmelzeisen

32   Condylar Prosthesis for the Replacement of the Mandibular Condyle   372
      Joachim Prein

33   Problems Related to Mandibular Condylar Prosthesis   377
      Christian Lindqvist, Anna-Lisa Söderholm, and Dorrit Hallikainen

34   Reconstruction of Defects of the Mandibular Angle   389
      Mark A. Schusterman and Elisabeth K. Beahm

35   Mandibular Body Reconstruction   395
      Anna-Lisa Söderholm, Dorrit Hallikainen, and Christian Lindqvist

36   Marginal Mandibulectomy   411
      Sanford Dubner and Keith S. Heller

37   Reconstruction of Extensive Anterior Defects of the Mandible   414
      Joachim Prein and Beat Hammer

38   Radiation Therapy and Considerations for Internal Fixation Devices   419
      Peter Stoll and Rüdiger Wächter

39 Management of Posttraumatic Osteomyelitis of the Mandible 433
    Robert M. Kellman and Darin L. Wright

40 Bilateral Maxillary Defects: THORP Plate Reconstruction with
    Removable Prosthesis. Technique/Atlas Case Reports 439
    Christian Lindqvist, Lars Sjövall, Anna-Lisa Söderholm, and Dorrit Hallikainen

41 AO/ASIF Craniofacial Fixation System Hardware 445
    Alex M. Greenberg and Joachim Prein

42 Microvascular Reconstruction of the Condyle and the Ascending Ramus 462
    Rainer Schmelzeisen and Friedrich Wilhelm Neukam

43 Orbital Reconstruction 478
    Beat Hammer

44 Nasal Reconstruction Using Bone Grafts and Rigid Internal Fixation 483
    Patrick K. Sullivan, Mika Varma, and Arlene A. Rozzelle

45 Transfacial Access Osteotomies to the Central and
    Anterolateral Skull Base 489
    Robert B. Stanley, Jr.

Section V Craniomaxillofacial Corrective Bone Surgery

46 Orthognathic Examination 497
    Peter Ward-Booth

47 Considerations in Planning for Bimaxillary Surgery and the Implications
    of Rigid Internal Fixation 522
    Brian Alpert, George M. Kushner, and Gerald D. Verdi

48 Reconstruction of Cleft Lip and Palate Osseous Defects and Deformities 539
    Klaus Honigmann and Adrian Sugar

49 Maxillary Osteotomies and Considerations for Rigid Internal Fixation 581
    Alex M. Greenberg

50 Mandibular Osteotomies and Considerations for Rigid Internal Fixation 606
    Victor Escobar, Alex M. Greenberg, and Alan Schwimmer

51 Genioplasty Techniques and Considerations for Rigid Internal Fixation 623
    Frans H.M. Kroon

52 Long-Term Stability of Maxillary and Mandibular Osteotomies with
    Rigid Internal Fixation 639
    Joseph E. Van Sickels, Paul Casmedes, and Thomas Weil

53 Le Fort II and Le Fort III Osteotomies for Midface Reconstruction and
    Considerations for Internal Fixation 660
    Keith Jones

Section VI Craniofacial Surgery

54   Craniofacial Deformities: Introduction and Principles of Management 671
      G.E. Ghali, Wichit Tharanon, and Douglas P. Sinn

55   The Effects of Plate and Screw Fixation on the Growing Craniofacial Skeleton 693
      Michael J. Yaremchuk

56   Calvarial Bone Graft Harvesting Techniques: Considerations for Their Use
      with Rigid Fixation Techniques in the Craniomaxillofacial Region 700
      John L. Frodel, Jr.

57   Crouzon Syndrome: Basic Dysmorphology and Staging of Reconstruction 713
      Jeffrey C. Posnick

58   Hemifacial Microsomia 727
      John H. Phillips, Kevin Bush, and R. Bruce Ross

59   Orbital Hypertelorism: Surgical Management 738
      Antonio Fuente del Campo

60   Surgical Correction of the Apert Craniofacial Deformities 749
      E. Clyde Smoot, III and William L. Hickerson

Appendix A1   Distraction Osteogenesis of the Mandible 757
Alex M. Greenberg and Joachim Prein

Appendix A2   ITI Strauman Dental Implant System 765
Alex M. Greenberg

Index 769

Contributors

James H. Abjanich, DDS
Assistant Clinical Professor, Division of Postgraduate Prosthodontics, Columbia University School of Dental and Oral Surgery, New York, NY 10022, USA

Tomas Albrektsson, MD, PHD, ODhc
Professor and Head of Biomaterials/Handicap Research, Department of Surgical Sciences, Gothenburg University, S-413 12 Gothenburg, Sweden

Brian Alpert, DDS
Professor and Chair, Department of Oral and Maxillofacial Surgery, School of Dentistry, Louisville, KY 40292, USA

Wolfgang Bähr, MD, DDS, PhD
Oral and Maxillofacial Surgeon, Plastic Surgeon, Christoph-Mang-Strasse 18-20, 79100 Freiburg, Germany

Elisabeth K. Beahm, MD
Assistant Professor, Department of Plastic Surgery, MD Anderson Cancer Center, University of Texas Medical Center, Houston, TX 77030-4095, USA

Daniel A. Buser, DMD
Professor, Department of Oral Surgery and Stomatology, School of Dental Medicine, University of Bern, CH-3010 Bern, Switzerland

Kevin Bush, MD
Assistant Clinical Professor of Surgery, Division of Plastic Surgery, University of British Columbia, Vancouver, British Columbia V67 2C7, Canada

Paul Casmedes, MD, DDS
Oral and Maxillofacial Surgery, Austin Surgical Arts, Austin, TX 78731, USA

Luc M. Cesteleyn, MD, DDS
Assistant Adjunct Clinical Professor, University of Michigan, Department of Maxillofacial Surgery, University of Ghent, 9000 Ghent, Belgium

Jin K. Chun, MD
Clinical Associate Professor of Surgery, Division of Plastic Surgery, Mount Sinai Hospital, New York, NY 10029, USA

Sanford Dubner, MD
Assistant Clinical Professor of Plastic Surgery, Albert Einstein College of Medicine, Lake Success, NY 11042, USA

Craig R. Dufresne, MD, FACS, FICS
Clinical Professor of Plastic Surgery, Georgetown University, Director, Center for Facial Rehabilitation, Fairfax Hospital, Chevy Chase, MD 20815, USA

Michael Ehrenfeld, MD, DDS, PhD
Chair, Department of Oral and Maxillofacial Surgery, Ludwidg-Maximillians-University, 80337 Munich, Germany

Victor Escobar, DDS, PhD
Staff Oral and Maxillofacial Surgeon, Department of Oral and Maxillofacial Surgery, Christie Clinic Association, Champaign, IL 61822, USA

John L. Frodel, Jr., MD, FACS
Associate Professor, Division of Otolaryngology and Plastic Surgery, University of New Mexico Health Science Center, Albuquerque, NM 87131-5341, USA

Antonio Fuente del Campo, MD
Associate Professor of Plastic and Craniomaxillofacial Surgery, Universidad National Autonoma de Mexico, Mexico City DF 53830, Mexico

Neal D. Futran, MD, DMD
Associate Professor, Department of Otolaryngology—Head and Neck Surgery, University of Washington School of Medicine, Seattle, WA 98195, USA

G.E. Ghali, MD, DDS, FACS
Associate Professor of Surgery, Chief, Division of Oral and Maxillofacial Surgery/Head and Neck Surgery, Department of Surgery, Louisiana State University Health Sciences Center, Shreveport, LA 71130-6101, USA

Alex M. Greenberg, DDS
Assistant Clinical Professor, Division of Oral and Maxillofacial Surgery, Columbia University School of Dental and Oral Surgery; Clinical Instructor, Division of Oral and Maxillofacial Surgery, Mount Sinai School of Medicine; Assistant Attending, Division of Oral and Maxillofacial Surgery, Beth Israel Medical Center; Associate Attending, Division of Oral and Maxillofacial Surgery, St. Luke's Roosevelt Hospital, New York, NY, USA

Bruce L. Greenberg, DDS
Orthodontist, 30 East 60 Street, New York, NY 10022, USA

Christine Hagenmaier, MD, DDS
Assistant Clinical Professor, Department of Oral and Maxillofacial Surgery, Ludwig-Maximillians-University, 80337 Munich, Germany

Dorrit Hallikainen, MD, PhD, Docent
Turku University, Institute of Dentistry, Senior Radiologist (Retired), Department of Diagnostic Radiology, Helsinki University Central Hospital, 00610 Helsinki, Finland

Beat Hammer, MD, DDS
Associate Professor of Maxillofacial Surgery, Clinic for Plastic and Reconstructive Surgery, Kantonsspital Basel, CH-4031 Basel, Switzerland

Richard H. Haug, DDS
Professor and Division Chief, Division of Oral and Maxillofacial Surgery, Head, Department of Hospital Dentistry, Assistant Dean for Hospital Affairs, University of Kentucky College of Dentistry, Lexington, KY 40536-0297, USA

Keith S. Heller, MD
Chief, Head and Neck Surgery, Long Island Jewish Medical Center, Clinical Professor of Surgery, Albert Einstein College of Medicine, Lake Success, NY 11042, USA

William L. Hickerson, MD, FACS
Associate Director, Plastic and Reconstructive Surgery, Joseph M. Still Burn Center, Augusta, GA 30909, USA

Klaus Honigmann, MD, DDS
Associate Professor of Maxillofacial Surgery, University Clinic for Plastic and Reconstructive Surgery, Kantonsspital Basel, CH-4031 Basel, Switzerland

John G. Hunter, MD, FACS
Chief, Division of Plastic Surgery, New York Methodist Hospital; Assistant Attending, New York Presbyterian Hospital; Clinical Assistant Professor of Surgery, Weill Medical College of Cornell University, New York, NY 10021, USA

Morton Jacobs, MD
Chairman of Radiology, Manhattan Eye, Ear, and Throat Hospital, Manhattan Diagnostic Radiology, New York, NY 10022, USA

Keith Jones, FDSRCS (Eng.)
Consultant Oral and Maxillofacial Surgeon, Maxillofacial Unit, Derbyshire Royal Infirmary NHS Trust, Derby DE1 2GY, UK

Robert M. Kellman, MD
Professor and Chairman, Department of Otolaryngology, State University of New York Health Science Center, Syracuse, NY 13210, USA

Douglas W. Klotch, MD, FACS
Clinical Professor of Surgery, Department of Otolaryngology—Head and Neck Surgery, University of South Florida College of Medicine, Tampa, FL 33613, USA

Frans H.M. Kroon, DMD, PhD
Department of Oral and Maxillofacial Surgery, Academic Medical Center, University of Amsterdam, NL-1105 A2 Amsterdam, The Netherlands

Frederick J. Kummer, PhD
Associate Director and Research Professor, Department of Bioengineering, Hospital for Joint Diseases, Orthopedic Institute, New York, NY 10003, USA

George M. Kushner, MD, DMD
Associate Professor of Oral and Maxillofacial Surgery, Director, Advanced Educational Program in Oral and Maxillofacial Surgery, University of Louisville School of Dentistry, Louisville, KY 40290, USA

Christian Lindqvist, MD, DDS, PhD, FDSRCS (Eng.)
Professor, Departments of Oral and Maxillofacial Surgery, Institute of Dentistry, Helsinki University and Surgical Hospital, Helsinki University Central Hospital, 00114 Helsinki, Finland

Jackson P. Morgan, III, DDS
Oral and Maxillofacial Surgery, 5202 Waters Avenue, Savannah, GA 31404, USA

Friedrich Wilhelm Neukam, MD, DDS, PhD
Professor and Chairman, Department of Oral and Maxillofacial Surgery,
Friedrich-Alexander-Universität Erlangen-Nuremberg, 91054 Erlangen, Germany

Ira H. Orenstein, DDS
Assistant Clinical Professor, Division of Postgraduate Prosthodontics, Columbia University
School of Dental and Oral Surgery; Staff Dentist, Department of Veterans Affairs, Bronx, NY
10468, USA

John H. Phillips, MD, FRCS(C)
Associate Surgeon, Center for Craniofacial Care and Research, Department of Plastic Surgery,
Hospital for Sick Children, Toronto Institute of Aesthetic Surgery, Toronto, Ontario M5R 2J3,
Canada

Jeffrey C. Posnick, MD, DMD, FRCS(C), FACS
Clinical Professor of Plastic Surgery, Departments of Otolaryngology/Head and Neck Surgery,
Oral and Maxillofacial Surgery, and Pediatrics, Georgetown University School of Medicine,
Chevy Chase, MD 20815, USA

Joachim Prein, MD, DDS
Professor of Maxillofacial Surgery, Head, Clinic for Reconstructive Surgery, Kantonsspital
Basel, CH-4031 Basel, Switzerland

R. Bruce Ross, DDS, MSc
Department of Dentistry, Hospital for Sick Children, University of Toronto, Toronto,
Ontario M5F 1X8, Canada

Arlene A. Rozzelle, MD, FACS, FAAP
Assistant Professor, Wayne State University; Chief, Plastic and Reconstructive Surgery,
Children's Hospital of Michigan, Detroit, MI 48230, USA

Rainer Schmelzeisen, MD, DDS, PhD
Professor and Chairman, Department of Oral and Maxillofacial Surgery and Plastic Surgery,
Freiburg University, D-79106 Freiburg, Germany

Mark A. Schusterman, MD
Clinical Professor, Division of Plastic Surgery, Baylor College of Medicine, Houston, TX
77030, USA

Alan Schwimmer, DDS
Associate Professor of Dentistry, Albert Einstein College of Medicine, Division of Dental
Medicine, Beth Israel Medical Center, New York, NY 10003, USA

Lars Sennerby, DDS, PhD
Professor of Biomaterials/Handicap Research, Department of Surgical Sciences, Gothenburg
University, 413 90 Gothenburg, Sweden

Lester Silver, MD
Professor of Surgery, Chief, Division of Plastic Surgery, Mount Sinai Hospital, New York,
NY 10029, USA

Douglas P. Sinn, DDS
Professor and Chairman, Division of Oral and Maxillofacial Surgery, Department of Surgery, University of Texas Southwestern Medical Center, Dallas, TX 75390-9109, USA

Lars Sjövall, DDS
Specialist, Fixed and Removable Prothodontics, Jarvenpaan Hammaslaakarikeskus, 04400 Jarvenpaa, Finland

R. Gregory Smith, MD, DDS
Assistant Adjunct Clinical Professor, Department of Oral and Maxillofacial Surgery, University of Florida; Assistant Adjunct Professor, Department of Oral and Maxillofacial Surgery, Case Western Reserve University, Cleveland, OH; PonteVedra Cosmetic Surgery, Ponte Verdra Beach, FL 32082, USA

E. Clyde Smoot, III, MD, FACS
Plastic Surgery, Lake Charles Medical and Surgical Center, Lake Charles, LA 70601, USA

Anna-Lisa Söderholm, MD, DDS, PhD, Docent
Senior Maxillofacial Surgeon, Department of Oral and Maxillofacial Surgery, Surgical Hospital, Helsinki University Central Hospital, 00029 Helsinki, Finland

Robert B. Stanley, Jr., MD, DDS
Professor, Department of Otolaryngology—Head and Neck Surgery, University of Washington School of Medicine, Chief, Department of Otolaryngology—Head and Neck Surgery, Harborview Medical Center, Seattle, WA 98104-2499, USA

Jeffrey I. Stein, DDS
Chief, Oral and Maxillofacial Surgery, White Plains Hospital Center, White Plains, NY 10601-4710, USA

Samuel G. Steinemann, DrPhil
Professor Emeritus, Faculty of Science, Institute of Experimental Physics, University of Lausanne, CH-1015 Lausanne, CH-4054 Basel, Switzerland

Peter Stoll, MD, DDS, PhD
Professor, formerly, Department of Oral and Maxillofacial Surgery, University Hospital, D-79106 Freiburg, Germany, and Oral and Maxillofacial Surgeon, Plastic Surgeon, D-79098, Freiburg, Germany.

Adrian Sugar, BChD, FDSRCS (Eng.)
Consultant, Oral and Maxillofacial Surgery, Maxillofacial Unit, The Welsh Centre for Burns, Plastic Surgery and Maxillofacial Surgery, Morriston Hospital NHS Trust, Swansea SA6 6NL, UK

Patrick K. Sullivan, MD
Associate Professor, Department of Plastic Surgery, Director, Craniofacial Service, Brown University School of Medicine, Providence, RI 02905, USA

Riitta Suuronen, MD, DDS, PhD, Docent
Lecturer, Department of Oral and Maxillofacial Surgery, Helsinki University; Consultant, Department of Oral and Maxillofacial Surgery, 00-14 Helsinki, Finland

Wichit Tharanon, DDS
Head, Cranio-Maxillofacial Reconstruction Unit, Director, Dental and Craniofacial Implant Center, Faculty of Dentistry, Thommasat University, Klong Luang, Pathum-Thani, 12121 Thailand

Anders Tjellström, MD, PhD
Associate Professor of ENT Surgery, ENT Clinic of Sahlgren's University Hospital, SE
413 45 Gothenburg, Sweden

Joseph E. Van Sickels, DDS
Professor and Director of Residency Education, Division of Oral and Maxillofacial Surgery,
University of Kentucky College of Dentistry, Lexington, KY 40536, USA

Mika Varma, MD
Assistant Professor of Surgery, Department of Surgery, University of California, San Francisco,
San Francisco, CA 94143, USA

Gerald D. Verdi, MD, DDS
Clinical Professor, Division of Plastic and Reconstructive Surgery, Department of Surgery,
Adjunct Clinical Professor, School of Dentistry, University of Louisville, Louisville, KY 40202,
USA

Rüdiger Wächter, MD, DDS
Oral and Maxillofacial Surgery, D036937 Fulda, Germany, and formerly, Department of Oral
and Maxillofacial Surgery, Freiburg University, Freiburg, Germany

Peter Ward-Booth, FDSRCS (Eng.)
Consultant Maxillofacial Surgeon, Queen Victorial Hospital NHS Trust, East Grinstead,
West Sussex RH19 3DZ, UK

Hans-Peter Weber, DMD
Associate Professor and Chairman, Department of Restorative Dentistry, Harvard School of
Dental Medicine, Boston, MA 02115-5888, USA

Thomas Weil, MD, DDS
Oral and Maxillofacial Surgery, Austin, TX 78759, USA

Hubert Weinberg, MD
Clinical Professor of Surgery, Division of Plastic Surgery, Mount Sinai Hospital, New York,
NY 10029, USA

Dieter Weingart, MD, DMD
Professor and Chairman, Department of Oral and Maxillofacial Surgery and Plastic Surgery,
Katharinenhospital, D-70174 Stuttgart, Germany

Barry L. Wenig, MD, MPH, FACS
Professor, Northwestern University Medical School, Director, Division of Head and Neck
Surgery, Department of Otolaryngology, Evanston Northwestern Health Care, Chicago, IL
60612, USA

Darin L. Wright, MD
Spokane Ear, Nose, and Throat Clinic, Spokane, WA 99201, USA

Michael J. Yaremchuk, MD
Clinical Professor of Surgery, Harvard Medical School; Chief, Craniofacial Surgery,
Department of Plastic and Reconstructive Surgery, Massachusetts General Hospital, Boston,
MA 02114, USA

1
Introduction

Alex M. Greenberg and Joachim Prein

From the observation by Danis that bone healing was promoted by stabilization, even in the presence of compression, instrumentation and hardware were developed to allow functionally stable internal fixation by AO/ASIF pioneers Allgöwer, Müller, Schneider, and Willenegger, and were introduced to the field of orthopedics in the 1950s.[1] The maxillofacial surgeons were exposed to these fixation concepts as a result of their close cooperation with the orthopedic surgeons and traumatologists over 30 years ago. Within the AO Group, this was seized and further adapted into the field of maxillofacial surgery by Spiessl and Schilli among others, who performed a series of clinical and laboratory research experiences that dealt with biomechanical and metallurgical problems, resulting in the development of a variety of stainless steel implants to provide stable internal fixation of the mandible. These implants provided rigid internal fixation of fracture and osteotomy segments via absolute stability supplemented by compression. The introduction of a reconstruction plate allowed for the bridging of defects. In his textbooks *New Concepts in Maxillofacial Bone Surgery* (1976) and *Internal Fixation of the Mandible: A Manual of AO/ASIF Techniques* (1989), Spiessl documented this development.[2,3]

Following these early successful experiences with functionally stable internal fixation of the mandible, the field of application was widened and finally included the entire craniomaxillofacial region. With the development of lighter and more biocompatible titanium implants, the concepts of internal hardware–supported osteosynthesis were able to evolve from the conceptual need for "rigid or absolutely stable internal fixation" to a "functionally stable internal fixation," which is based on the surgeon's judgment and experience to provide adequate protection from functional forces of the maturing callus and bone healing in each individual situation. Resorbable plates and screws are now able to provide adequate functionally stable internal fixation in selected circumstances without the need for possible hardware removal, and is an advance from purely metallic implants. These new AO/ASIF techniques for the application of internal fixation

to fractures of the entire craniomaxillofacial skeleton were reviewed in Greenberg's 1993 textbook, *Craniomaxillofacial Fractures: Principles of Internal Fixation Using the AO/ASIF Technique*.[4]

This edition presents a complete representation of the progression of the field of craniomaxillofacial surgery as it has evolved from these earlier works. It represents the entire field as it has developed from traumatology and advanced into the entire range of craniomaxillofacial reconstructive and corrective bone surgery. By eliminating the sole focus on the biomechanical requirements of internal fixation and examining considerations regarding the surgical methods for operating on all these problems, the field of craniomaxillofacial surgery has matured as a result of these technical accomplishments. However, the continued importance of hardware in this evolution is evident through the development of rigid fixation applications for bone lengthening through the principles of distraction osteogenesis.

With the concurrent publication in 1998 of Prein's *Manual of Internal Fixation in the Cranio-Facial Skeleton: Techniques Recommended by the AO/ASIF Maxillofacial Group*[5], a concise presentation of the AO/ASIF surgical techniques in an atlas format is now available. These two new texts permit a clear understanding of craniomaxillofacial surgical techniques and clinical experience in a complementary manner.

It has always been the fundamental policy of the AO Group to develop a faculty to provide the education to use the implant materials prior to clinical application, which has brought considerable advantages for patients through the refinement of new surgical procedures, whether for treatment of trauma, tumors, or malformations. Regardless of the problem, there are major advantages for the management of them all.

This policy has impacted the educational process from internal pressures within the surgical community and increased public awareness because the use of these implants requires greater responsibility and improved accuracy in the performance of these techniques. When used correctly, through the appropriate learning of techniques, the benefit to the patient's care is immeasurable. Whether it is greater comfort and safety

1

gained from immediate function or decreased danger from infection, greater security is achieved by the stability of these methods.

From an economic point of view, there is a reduced burden on the public, which has gained from these developments in internal fixation, with decreased morbidity, disability, and mortality. The medical community, however, suffers because of longer operating time, decreased use of facilities, reduction in procedures, direct cost of equipment and implants, and the costs of continuing education. The question of what the future holds remains. Who will make the decisions regarding the availability of these highly effective, technically demanding techniques? Will this be guided directly and indirectly by national governments, municipalities, local hospitals, staff, or industrial establishments? Will the great advances of the past 25 years in the evolution of craniomaxillofacial surgery from issues related mainly to the mandible, with the progression to the entire skull, continue in an environment in which the ability of doctors to make decisions is impacted by the concern of others? In the future, who will develop new techniques? In the current environment, can there be a similar process as it related to metallurgically based implants, in the search of a superior material (e.g., bioresorbable ones)? The correct relationship between industry, medical and research personnel, and government, based on appropriate economic models, is necessary to permit the continued research and development that has until today brought the field of craniomaxillofacial surgery to its present state.

The chapters in this book will permit the reader to gain a complete appreciation of the broad spectrum of problems in the craniomaxillofacial region that may be addressed by a variety of clinicians with subanatomic specializations. This is further demonstrated by the international array of representative colleagues from these various disciplines. We hope that with this inclusion of all of these specialists we can promote the necessary close cooperation between the disciplines, by showing that there cannot be any boundaries between these different groups. Rather, we hope for continued progress in the level of communication among these different specialties that has been of benefit to all concerned, especially the patients, through the continued availability of the resources necessary to advance the art and science of this evolving surgical subspecialty.

References

1. Müller ME, Allgöwer M, Schneider R, Willenegger H. *Manual of Internal Fixation*. New York: Springer-Verlag; 1990.
2. Spiessl B, ed. *New Concepts in Maxillofacial Bone Surgery*. New York: Springer-Verlag; 1976.
3. Spiessl B. *Internal Fixation of the Mandible: A Manual of AO/ASIF Principles*. New York: Springer-Verlag; 1989.
4. Greenberg AM, ed. *Craniomaxillofacial Fractures: Principles of Internal Fixation Using the AO/ASIF Technique*. New York: Springer-Verlag; 1993.
5. Prein J, ed. *Manual of Internal Fixation in the Cranio-Facial Skeleton: Techniques Recommended by the AO/ASIF Maxillofacial Group*. New York: Springer-Verlag; 1998.

Section I
Basic Considerations in the Diagnosis of Craniomaxillofacial Bone Defects and Disorders

2
Evaluation of the Craniomaxillofacial Deformity Patient

Jackson P. Morgan, III and Richard H. Haug

Few procedures are more challenging than the surgical repair of patients with craniomaxillofacial deformities. These deformities are the end results of the effects of trauma, cancer, infection, or congenital anomalies. Experience has shown us that these defects involve both bone and overlying soft tissue. Regardless of the etiology, surgeons must direct their repair toward the correction of the aesthetic defect with the restoration of function. When treating patients who have undergone tumor resection or suffered severe facial trauma, both the surgeon and the patient must understand that the patient most likely will never function or appear as they did prior to their trauma or tumor surgery. Unlike those with facial trauma and maxillofacial tumors, patients who suffer congenital defects are able, for the most part, to have their facial aesthetics and function improved over their preoperative state. Craniomaxillofacial defects are the direct response to trauma, disease, development, and/or the undesirable response to treatment or nontreatment. Undesirable postsurgical results can arise when fractures are misdiagnosed, unrecognized, or the initial surgical treatment is inadequate. When concurrent life-threatening complications interfere with or cause the delay of proper initial treatment, less than optimal results may also occur. No matter how subtle a deformity is, it will more than likely be quite obvious when involving the craniomaxillofacial region.

While much is known about the epidemiology of craniomaxillofacial fractures and congenital defects, it is impossible to truly identify the incidence of craniomaxillofacial defects due to trauma, cancer, or infection; this is because of the large number of local and systemic variables that contribute to the formation of these deformities.

The difficult task for the craniomaxillofacial surgeon is not the surgical correction of the deformity, but the basic understanding of the deformity's nature. Information obtained in an organized preoperative evaluation is the first step in the diagnosis of craniomaxillofacial deformities.[1] The mechanisms that create these deformities can be summarized into three groups: congenital, developmental, and acquired.[2]

The congenital deformity may be unilateral or bilateral. Examples of these deformities include clefts, craniofacial dysostosis, hemifacial microsomia, as well as deformities associated with branchial arch syndromes, to name just a few. Developmental deformities, on the other hand, are influenced by a multitude of factors such as the involvement of specialized structures, trauma, infection, nutritional deficiencies, endocrine imbalances, and arthritis. Congenital anomalies that involve specialized structures such as hemifacial microsomia with associated facial nerve defects are frequent occurrences. Trauma's role in developmental deformities usually occurs early in life, interrupting and limiting normal development. Infection, such as with trauma, has the potential to cause developmental deformities if it occurs early in life. If it occurs during adulthood, it will most likely lead to an acquired deformity such as bone loss from osteomyelitis as compared to excessive scar tissue formation that restricts bony development in the child. Nutritional disorders, such as vitamin D deficiencies, can influence development but are extremely rare. The more common endocrine disorders are capable of causing deformities that involve bone and/or soft tissue. Mandibular prognathism associated with adult growth hormone disorders and exophthalmus and associated ophthalmopathy, which is usually associated with hyperthyroidism, are examples of endocrine-influenced deformities. Finally, arthritic and autoimmune disorders, such as adult and juvenile rheumatoid arthritis, can also influence deformities. These deformities can range from a mandibular asymmetry and malocclusion due to condylar degeneration in the adult to ankylosis and associated micrognathia in juvenile patients.

The purpose of this chapter is to describe an organized and accurate means of comprehensively assessing the craniomaxillofacial deformity patient regardless of the deformity's etiology. Not only is this essential for the proper diagnosis of underlying problems, but this evaluation will be helpful when communicating between specialists as well as providing a medical-legal document.[3]

Initial Assessment

As with all patient interviews and examinations, the information obtained during the initial assessment will be the first insight into the patient's general health and mental readiness regarding their surgical treatment. This information should be clearly recorded and readily accessible to all those involved with the patient's treatment. Legally, this is a public document that should be available to other physicians, insurance companies with the patient's permission, and the court system by subpoena.

The first part of the initial assessment should consist of basic identification information such as the date and time of the examination, name, age, race, marital status, and telephone number of the patient. The informant should also be identified regarding from whom the history was obtained. At this point, the surgeon's feelings toward the accuracy and reliability of the history and information obtained should be stated. Was the patient or informant confused, cooperative, and was there a language barrier? Psychosocial problems that may pose potential problems regarding the surgery and its final outcome should be identified early in the patient interview if possible.

The patient's chief complaint should be identified and recorded using the patient's own words. This should not be his or her diagnosis, but rather their complaint. In the craniomaxillofacial deformity patient, the chief complaint is usually multiple and lengthy. In the adolescent and adult patient, the surgeon should try to identify who is the driving force regarding the chief complaint (i.e., the patient, family members, or friends). This information will again reflect the psychosocial status of the patient and family and should be noted because missed signals at this point may cause problems for the treating surgeon when patients enter treatment with unrealistic or misconceived expectations.[4] When indicated, patients should be referred for psychological evaluation and counseling. Also remember that the patient's perceived needs may be totally different than what the surgeon sees and must be addressed.

A detailed history of the deformity is an important part of the evaluation. Traumatic defects should be investigated to identify the etiology of the initial injury and associated concomitant injury in the acute setting. Acquired medical problems such as blindness, preexisting hardware, and seizures should be documented preoperatively.

Deformities secondary to ablated tumor resection should be investigated to determine the type of tumor resected. Some surgeons feel comfortable using a planned primary reconstructive technique immediately following their ablated tumor resection, while other surgeons prefer the delayed secondary reconstructive approach. Regardless of which reconstructive technique has been used, the surgical correction of deformities in these patients should proceed only after it has been es-tablished that there is no recurrence of tumor, which must be verified both clinically and radiographically. A detailed history of radiation therapy must also be known, and therapy should begin as indicated.

Medical/Dental History

A variety of medical conditions are commonly associated with craniomaxillofacial syndromes. In planning for the surgical correction of craniomaxillofacial deformities, medical risk factors that contraindicate general anesthesia and surgical reconstruction must be identified.[5] Proper evaluation of the patient's general health requires a comprehensive review of all medical records and a general physical examination such as done on all patients undergoing elective surgery and general anesthesia. Common disease entities such as diabetes mellitus, asthma, and congenital heart defects, just to name a few, can pose little additional risk when appropriately managed in the preoperative setting. Spine and extremity deformities are often associated with craniomaxillofacial syndrome patients as well as patients with acquired deformities. Situations such as these make intubation procedures difficult and can complicate surgery by limiting and interfering with patient positioning during the procedure. No matter how grotesque a deformity is, surgical correction is still considered an elective procedure in which the risks and benefits must be clearly evaluated. In the record, a statement of the patient's appraisal of his or her general health should be recorded. Previous examinations and treatments should also be noted. A chronologic summary of all hospital admissions, diagnoses, and previous surgical procedures should be recorded as well. This information is of great value and can greatly affect the surgical outcome. A list of medications that the patient takes regularly should be included along with medications that led to untoward reactions in the past. Any other allergies, sensitivities, and blood product transfusions should also be recorded in this section.

The dental history is important. Periodontal disease may indicate poor oral hygiene and compliance, which may slow healing, predisposing the patient to infection and other postoperative complications. When possible, it is best to preoperatively treat all periodontal disease, periapical pathology, and carious lesions when providing optimal comprehensive treatment.

Patients who exhibit or have a history of temporomandibular joint dysfunction must be closely investigated to establish their current joint status. The temporomandibular joint will be directly or indirectly affected in many patients with craniomaxillofacial deformities. Patients with acquired deformities and no history of temporomandibular joint dysfunction in the past may now demonstrate some form of dysfunction, especially if the acquired deformity is secondary to

TABLE 2.1 Common signs of temporomandibular joint dysfunction.

Joint pain
Preauricular pain
Muscle pain
Joint clicking
Joint crepitus
Tinnitus
Vertigo
Decreased motion/function
Deviation upon opening
Muscular spasm
Persistent headaches

trauma. Common joint signs that must be closely evaluated are shown in Table 2.1.

Much controversy exists regarding when to sequence the treatment of symptomatic temporomandibular joints and craniomaxillofacial deformities. Regardless of when symptomatic joints are managed, it is commonly agreed that the correction of craniomaxillofacial deformities may improve the symptoms or potentially create or aggravate joint symptoms in patients with little or no history when correction of the jaws is required. Therefore, it is imperative to accurately document any joint signs or symptoms preoperatively and whether the joint problems will be addressed with concurrent surgical treatment or separately.[6,7]

Surgical-orthodontic therapy must be considered when planned procedures include the jaws. Early discussion and review of dental casts, bite registrations, and diagnostic mountings with an orthodontist may initially delay the surgery but will greatly reduce the amount of operating time by uncomplicating diagnosis and eliminating unfavorable postoperative results in most cases.

Finally, the services provided by a maxillofacial prosthodontist when dealing with patients who have large acquired deformities can overcome many problems associated with the crippled craniomaxillofacial patient.

Clinical Evaluation

Over the past two-and-a-half decades, there has been an increasing awareness of the vast variations of anomalies and classic syndromes seen in the patient population today.[8] Anthropologists, artists, and facial surgeons have studied normal and abnormal facial relationships extensively.[9–14] Radiographs, CT scans, dental study models, and photographic measurements can give accurate information regarding large bony movements but should never be substituted for the facial clinical examination. This examination is the surgeon's most useful diagnostic tool in treating craniomaxillofacial deformities.[15]

Anatomic Soft Tissue Landmarks

Clinically, the face is easily and readily examined, but to know what to look for and understand this information, certain repeatable landmarks should be analyzed to compare observations regarding the normal and abnormal. These landmarks should be noted in the frontal and lateral views. During evaluation, the patient should be sitting comfortably upright and the head should be in the neutral position. For examination purposes the neutral position is achieved when a line that passes through the tragus and infraorbital rim of the patient is parallel to the floor. This reference point is called the Frankfort horizontal plane (FH).

The following anatomic landmarks in the frontal and lateral view may be absent or distorted in the craniomaxillofacial deformity patient. Trichion (Tr) is the point at the most superior portion of the forehead that meets the midpoint of the hairline. Proceeding inferiorily, the next landmark is the soft tissue glabella (G), the most anterior point of the forehead in the midline between the eyebrows. Soft tissue nasion (N) is the most posterior point of the contour of the nasal bridge and is formed by the soft tissue overlying the most anterior portion of the frontonasal suture. Orbitale (Or) is the lowest point of the inferior orbital rim. Subnasale (Sn) is the inferior junction of the columella or base of the nose with the upper lip. The superior (Vs) and inferior (Vi) vermilion borders are the junctions between the skin and the mucous membranes on the upper and lower lips. Stomion (St) represents the distance between the upper and lower lips at rest. Stomion superioris (Ss) represents the most inferior portion of the upper lip in the midsagittal plane, in which the stomion inferioris (Si) is the most superior portion of the lower lip in the midsagittal plane. Tragion (Tg) represents the supratragus notch of the ear. Rhinion (Rh) represents the junction between the most inferior extent of the nasal bones where they join the cartilaginous nasal dorsum. Tip-defining point (Tp) is the most anterior portion of the nasal tip. The alar crease (A) represents the most posterior portion of the nasal base on the right and left side. The mentolabial sulcus (MLS) is the deepest depression between the chin and the lower lip. Soft tissue pogonion (Pg) is the most anterior point of the soft tissue chin. Soft tissue menton (M) is the most inferior point of contour on the chin at the midline. Gnathion (Gn) is a point in space formed by the intersection of tangents of pogonion and menton. Finally, the throat point (C) is the intersection of tangents drawn vertically along the anterior neck and horizontally through the soft tissue menton, creating a specific soft tissue point in the neck-mandibular region. These anatomic landmarks are shown in Figure 2.1.

Continuing with the specific anatomic landmarks, four common facial angles are used to evaluate facial relationships in the lateral view. These angles are the nasofrontal angle (NFA), which is formed by tangents following the nasodor-

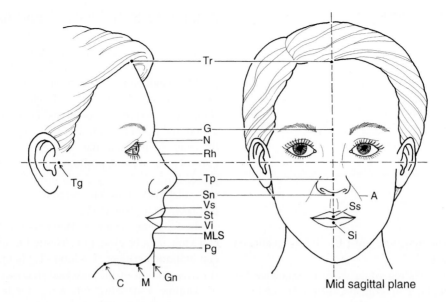

FIGURE 2.1 Anatomic landmarks in the profile and frontal views. FH, Frankfort horizontal plane; Tr, trichion; G, soft tissue glabella; Sn, subnasale; Vs, superior vermilion border; Vi, inferior vermilion border; St, stomion; Ss, stomion superioris; Si, stomion inferioris; Tg, tragion; Rh, rhinion; Tp, tip-defining point; A, alar crease; MLS, mentolabial sulcus; Pg, soft tissue pogonion; M, soft tissue menton; Gn, gnathion; C, throat point.

sum, passing through the soft tissue nasion and a tangent extending from nasion through the soft tissue glabella. The nasolabial angle (NLA) is formed by the intersection of tangents paralleling the columella and parelleling the upper lip passing through the vermilion border. The facial contour angle (FCA) is the angle formed by the upper facial plane (glabella to subnasale) and the lower facial plane (subnasale to soft tissue mention). The mentocervical angle (MCA) is formed by a tangent extending from pogonion to gnathion and gnathion through menton.

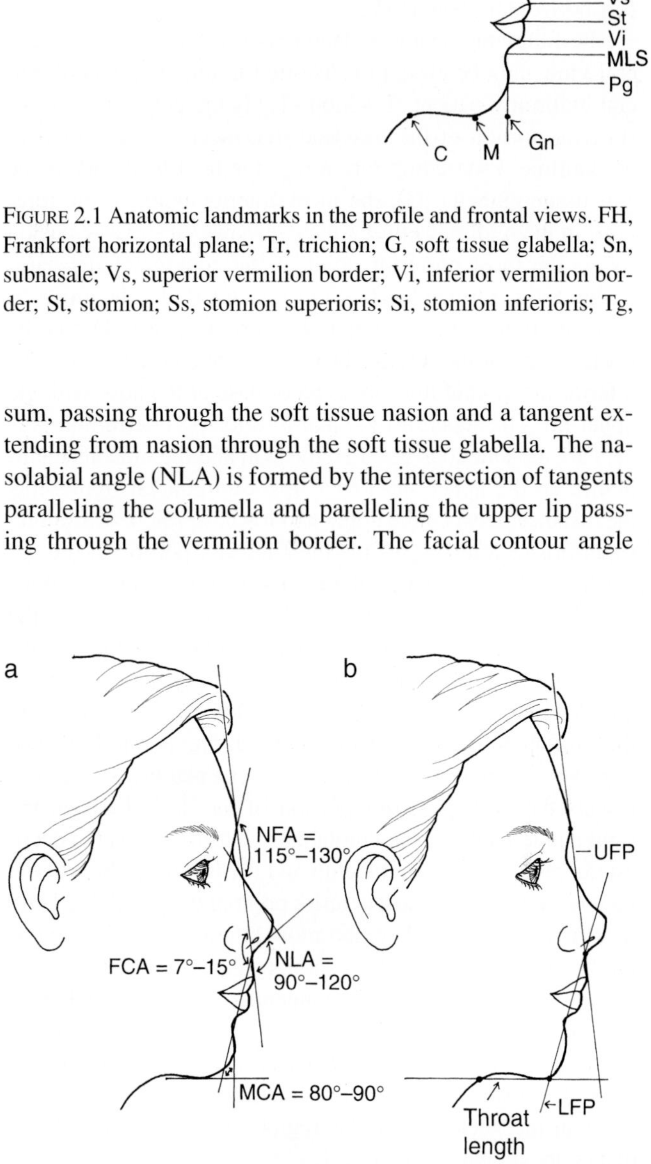

The most common facial planes are the upper and lower facial plane and the throat plane, or length. The upper facial plane (UFP) follows a line that passes through the soft tissue glabella and subnasale. A line passing from subnasale through soft tissue menton creates the lower facial plane (LFP). Throat length is the distance along a line extending from the throat point (C) through menton. The common facial planes and angles are shown in Figure 2.2a,b.

General Asymmetry Assessment

Dating back to ancient civilizations, many attempts have been made to establish a set of standards for facial beauty.[13] Mathematicians have also attempted to calculate and quantify facial measurements to distinguish what is beautiful and what is not, but these calculations can be complex and difficult to interpret.[14–17] However, it was Leonardo da Vinci who felt that anatomic relationships were more valuable than absolute numerical values and divided the face into equal thirds.[18] He noted that these divisions should be relatively equal and symmetric.[18] Therefore, the clinical examination should begin with the general assessment of symmetry and deformity in the frontal and profile views.

FIGURE 2.2 (a) Common facial angles used in the profile evaluation. NFA, nasofrontal angle; NLA, nasolabial angle; FCA, facial contour angle; MCA, mentocervical angle. (b) Common facial planes. UFP, upper facial plane; LFP lower facial plane; throat length, the distance between point C and M.

Frontal View

The symmetry assessment is accomplished by dividing the face vertically in half at the midline. This is accomplished by having an assistant hold a silk suture vertically with one hand above the trichion and the other hand below the soft tissue menton with the suture passing through a point between the eyebrows and extending in front of the nasal tip. This allows for the general assessment of right- and left-sided symmetry as well as the relationships between the upper and lower dental midlines. If the deformity or defect is subtle, the frontal profile can be further divided into fifths. Each fifth should approximate one eye's width beginning at the lateralmost aspect of the ears and extending to the lateral canthus on the right and left sides. Each eye should then be measured from its lateral to medial canthus, and finally, the medial canthal distance should be measured and recorded. This evaluation can also be performed and reviewed at a later date by using a 5 × 8 frontal photograph. With lines paralleling the midline reference, each fifth should be equal to one eye's width or the medial canthal distance, thus identifying the region in which subtle asymmetries or deformities are located. During this assessment one should keep in mind that the ideal frontal facial appearance is oval with a width-to-height ratio of three to four.[19]

Knowing that deformities exist in all three planes of space, the frontal assessment should also be reviewed in relation to horizontal divisions to appreciate the facial balance. This is accomplished by horizontal measurements or lines dividing the face into thirds. The upper third represents the distance between the trichion and soft tissue glabella. The middle third is the space from the soft tissue glabella to subnasale, and the lower third is from the subnasale to soft tissue menton. Again, these clinical measurements can be compared and checked with measurements performed on photographs. The lower facial third is also commonly divided into an upper third from the subnasale to stomion and a lower two-thirds from the stomion to soft tissue menton. It should also be noted that upper-facial-third measurements and relations can be misleading due to the varying, and possibly absent, hairlines in some individuals.

The Profile Examination

The profile examination is performed in a similar fashion using the same horizontal landmarks as in the frontal exam. The common facial angles and planes should also be evaluated at this time, assessing the degree of facial convexity or concavity. The Gonzalez-Ulloa line is a reference line that is perpendicular to the Frankfurt horizontal line and passes through the soft tissue nasion. This line helps to establish profiles and the proper chin position.[20]

At this time all general asymmetries, defects, and deformities should be recorded. Remember that a perfectly symmetric face is an uncommon finding even in the aesthetically beautiful individual. Frontal and profile facial divisions are shown in Figure 2.3a–c.

Cranial Circumference

Absolute measurements of cranial circumference vary with normal adult individuals of the same age and opposite sex. The circumference is approximately 9 mm greater in males

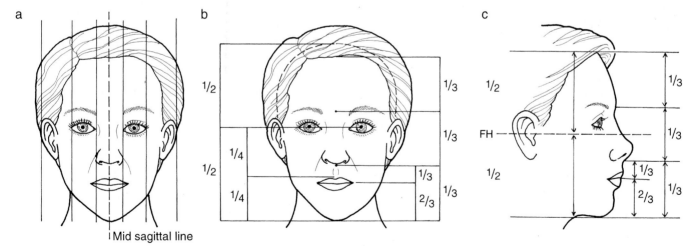

FIGURE 2.3 (a) The face is divided into vertical fifths. Each fifth is approximately equal to one eye's width, beginning at the most lateral aspect of the ear continuing across to the lateral aspect of the opposite ear. (b) Horizontal divisions in the frontal view. The upper third is from trichion to glabella, the middle third is from glabella to subnasale, and the lower third is from subnasale to soft tissue menton. The lower third can also be subdivided into an upper third and lower two-thirds. The face can also be divided into halves with the distance between the vertex and the midpupillary point being the upper half and the distance from the midpupillary point to menton being the lower half. (c) The facial thirds in the profile view. FH, Frankfort horizontal plane.

than in females of the same age.[21,22] In males, cranial growth is rapid during the first 2 years of life with a second growth spurt between ages 12 and 16, whereas females demonstrate their growth spurt between ages 12 and 14 years.[21,22] Cranial circumference is not important in adults except when a craniofacial syndrome exists. This measurement is most useful in infants and is a good indication of the size of the intercranial contents as well as of thoracic circumference and body weight.[22] The cranial circumference should be measured in centimeters with a measuring tape placed just above the supraorbital rim and encompassing the occiput posteriorly.

Cranial Sutures and Fontanelles

Numerous conditions exist that involve the cranial sutures and fontanelles in infants. This examination should not be overlooked, especially if a syndrome or cranial circumference abnormality is suspected.

The tension and size of the fontanelles[23] are used to estimate intracranial pressure such as that which occurs with meningitis, and it is also used to estimate the degree of brain development. The anterior fontanelle is the largest and is usually obliterated by 2 years of age and replaced by the bregma in the adult skull. During the examination, the area of the fontanelle can be calculated using the formula for the area of a quadrilateral, which is:[24]

$$\text{Area of } ABCD = \frac{AC \times BX}{2}$$

These reference points are made by placing the examiner's index finger into the right, left, superior, and inferior corners of the fontanelle while using a felt tip pen to mark a point just distal to the examiner's fingertip.[24] The marks are then transferred to a piece of paper by placing the paper directly over the freshly made marks. The points are labeled as in Figure 2.4. Points A and C are connected with a straight line. Then a line parallel to line AC that passes through point D is drawn. A perpendicular line is drawn from line D extending through point B.[24] The area is then calculated using the aforementioned formula for the area of a quadrilateral, and compared to the mean values shown in Table 2.2.

Cranial deformities are uncommon and occur when cranial sutures close prematurely. Scaphocephaly occurs when the sagittal suture closes too soon causing the skull to become narrow and elongated. Turrincephaly occurs when the coronal and lambdoid sutures prematurely close giving the skull a tower-like appearance. When the skull becomes even more pointed this condition is called acrocephaly. Complicating matters further, plagiocephaly is caused by an asymmetric premature closure of the coronal or lambdoid sutures resulting in a plethora of asymmetries. The area of the fontanelles and the closure of sutures should be noted and recorded when appropriate.

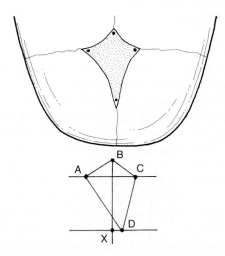

FIGURE 2.4 The examiner's index finger being placed into the right, left, superior, and inferior corners of the anterior fontanelle, demonstrating the technique for examining and determining the area of a fontanelle. Each mark is made with a felt tip pen and transferred to a separate piece of paper by gently pressing the paper on top of the freshly made marks. Points A, B, C, and D are labeled, creating a quadrilateral. The area is then calculated using the formula.

Of the fontanelles, the anterior is the best indicator of brain growth. A small frontal fontanelle for a specific age may indicate abnormally slow brain growth. A third fontanelle, when present, is approximately 2 cm anterior to the posterior fontanelle and occurs in approximately 10% of normal infants and 60% of Down's syndrome infants.[25,26] Figure 2.5a,b shows the fontanelles and their connecting sutures.

Forehead

The forehead composes the upper third of the face, extending from trichion to soft tissue glabella and laterally to the supraorbital rims.

The majority of patients who require surgical correction of the bony forehead usually suffer from craniostenosis, the effects of trauma, or ablative tumor resection. Although the forehead rarely requires surgical correction in normal adults and is commonly overlooked, it does provide important landmarks that are used to evaluate deformities and aesthetics of the rest of the face. In the profile examination, the forehead should exhibit a slight convexity as it extends from trichion to the soft tissue glabella.

TABLE 2.2 Mean areas of the infant's anterior fontanelle (mm²).

Age	Mean (mm²)
Preterm (28–32 weeks)	113
Preterm (33–36 weeks)	162
Term (37–42 weeks)	220
Small-for-dates	540

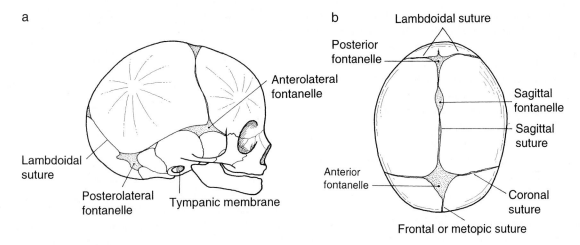

FIGURE 2.5 (a) Superior view of the infant cranium showing its common fontanelles and connecting sutures. (b) Lateral view of infant cranium with its associated lateral fontanelles.

Structures along the periphery of the forehead that must be evaluated include the hairline, soft tissue glabella, supraorbital rims, and eyebrows. In men, the hairline is generally positioned more superiorly than in females. A history of male pattern baldness must be reviewed, and this information may influence the decision as to the type and design of the surgical incision when gaining access to this region. Characteristics of shape, contour, and thickness of the hairline must be noted. Proper investigation and planning here will possibly eliminate unsightly scars along the scalp from a bitemporal incision that was placed too anteriorly.

The eyebrows and underlying supraorbital rims should be evaluated for symmetry, shape, and height. Defects in this region may be bony or soft tissue, and their etiology must be identified. The supraorbital rim should be approximately 5 to 8 mm anterior to the cornea when viewed laterally, thus shadowing and protecting the eyes. Glabella should be viewed as a separate projection that lies between the eyebrows. Its position should be in the midline and is more pronounced in males.[27]

Finally, the nasofrontal angle (G-n-Tp) is another means of assessing the forehead. The nasofrontal angle should range between 115° and 130°. Deformities that deepen this angle will shorten the appearance of the nose and increase the appearance of the nasal tip. Surgical correction that makes the angle more obtuse will give a lengthening appearance to the nose.

Remember, the profile and contour of the forehead vary among normal men and women. Regardless of its shape, it is the greatest contributor to the overall profile of the entire face.

Temporal Region

The temporal region extends from the superior nuchal line to the depth of the infratemporal fossa and back up to the zygomatic arch. Although the bony contour of this region is grossly concave, the clinical appearance is usually convex when a normal temporalis muscle is present. The convexity of this region should be subtle.

Concavities of this region are abnormal and unattractive. Malnutrition, acquired loss of the temporalis muscle (temporal wasting), or excessive temporal bossing (as in Apert's syndrome) are major contributors to concavities in this region. The inferior portion of the temporal convexity should smoothly blend into the zygomatic arch and lateral orbital rim. Hairstyles may hide defects or deformities in this region; therefore, the area must be inspected by palpation. Inadequately treated zygomatic complex fractures resulting in an overcontoured arch also give a concave appearance to the inferior portion of the temporal region or cause the same area to be excessively convex. The temporal convexity should be evaluated from the frontal and superior views.

Periorbital Region and Eye

Physical examination of the periorbital and orbital region should include the orbital rims, upper and lower eyelids, and the globe. A detailed history regarding all associated structures should be obtained. Determination of the preoperative visual status should be of major concern when planning for the surgical correction of deformities or defects in this region. Preservation of the visual status must be achieved regardless of how the defect was obtained.

The Eye

A history of ocular trauma, visual acuity disorders, and blindness must be documented. Pain, photophobia, tearing with a purulent discharge, enophthalmus, proptosis, exophthalmus, and diplopia must also be documented. When possible, the patient's visual acuity should be established. In most cases, this can easily be done using a Snelling chart or a Rosenbaum pocket chart. When a patient is not able to read the largest letter on a Snelling chart, which reveals a visual acuity of 20/400, the examiner should then try to identify the greatest distance at which the patient can count fingers (CF).[28] If the patient cannot see the examiner's fingers, one should try to establish at what distance the patient can note hand motion (HM) by the examiner.[28] If HM cannot be established, one must determine if light perception (LP) or no light perception (NLP) exists.[28] Other tests that must be considered are determination of extraocular movements, visual fields, and color perception.

Examination of the pupils should not be overlooked and is best performed in a darkened room using the bright light of an ophthalmoscope. The size, shape, and reactivity of each pupil should be evaluated. At this time, a funduscopic examination of each eye should be done evaluating the optic media, disc, and any abnormal pathology. When abnormalities in vision or the ocular examination are noted, a detailed evaluation by an ophthalmologist is recommended.

The Orbit

The clinical evaluation of the interocular distance must be assessed by an actual measurement because clinically the appearance of the distance between the eyes is greatly influenced by the overall height and width of the face, glabellar

TABLE 2.3 Mean palpebral widths and lengths in Caucasians.

Age (yrs)	Width (mm)		Length (mm)	
	Range	Mean	Range	Mean
1	8.0–8.5	8.2	18–21	19
2–10	8.5–9.0	8.7	19–29	25
11–Adult	8.0–11.2	9.0	23–33	28

prominence or absence, the shape of the nasal bridge, or the presence or absence of epicanthal folds. Many formulas and methods for evaluating the intercanthal and interpupillary distances appear in the literature.[29] A firm distinction between intercanthal distance and interpupillary distance should be made. This is because in patients with anomalies such as Waardenburg syndrome, the outward appearance of ocular hypertelorism is actually a primary telecanthus caused by the lateral displacement of the medial canthus and punctum. Interpupillary and intercanthal measurements are commonly used to assess the position of the orbit and globe.[30] The intercanthal distance should be between 30 and 35 mm as compared to the interpupillary distance of 60 to 70 mm.[29,30] The interpupillary distance on average should be twice the intercanthal distance and the alar-to-alar nasal base width should be approximately equal to the intercanthal distance in normal Caucasian patients.[30]

Radiographic measurements can also be used to assess orbital position in children and adults by measuring the distance between the right and left medial orbital walls on an anteroposterior skull radiograph.[31] This method has also been used to measure the distance between lateral orbital walls but is shown to have little clinical importance.[29] Figure 2.6 demonstrates the relationship between intercanthal and interpupillary measurements as well as their relationship to other facial structures.

If an abnormality is noted in the intercanthal distance, one should also examine the palpebral length and width. In normal infants, the palpebral fissure is extremely narrow and rapidly widens in the first several weeks of life.[32,33] In normal infants, children, and adults, measurements of palpebral length will differ between the right and left side 30% of the time.[33] Differences greater than 1 mm are usually considered abnormal.[33] Table 2.3 demonstrates palpebral lengths and widths.

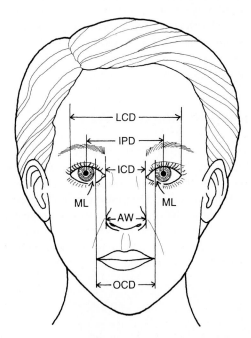

FIGURE 2.6 The relationship between the intercanthal and interpupillary distances. LCD, lateral canthal distance; IPD, interpupillary distance; ICD, intercanthal distance; AW, alar width; OCD, oral commissure distance; ML, medial limbus tangent to oral commissure.

The Eyebrows

Eyebrow position can be readily evaluated from the frontal view. Abnormalities can obviously be created by soft tissue defects or underlying deformities of the supraorbital rims. The normal eyebrow should begin medially at a point where a vertical line extends up from the medial canthus. It ends laterally at a point along an oblique line that begins at the alar base and extends up through the lateral canthus.[34] The medial and lateral extent of the eyebrow should lie on a horizontal line. The eyebrow's point of maximum height should be positioned at a point where a vertical line extends up from the lateral limbus of the eye and crosses the brow.[34] One must also consider that the integrity of the frontal branch of the facial nerve may also affect brow position. Finally, the brow in men lies on top of the supraorbital rim, while in women it lies above the rim.[34]

The Eyelids

The upper and lower eyelids should be evaluated for symmetry, shape, and function. The larger and generally more rounded upper eyelid should cover approximately 2 to 3 mm of the iris. The lower eyelid is straight and lies at the margin of the inferior limbus. This assessment should be made with the patient in a primary gaze. No sclera should be noted below the inferior limbus. Excessive anterior position of the globe and/or a poorly supported lower lid will cause excessive sclera to show. Entropion, ectropion, ptosis, elasticity, and function of the lower eyelid should be noted as well as the presence or absence of inferior scleral show.

Globe Position

The anterior, posterior, and superior position of the globe must not be overlooked. The etiology of exorbitism, exophthalmus, and enophthalmus must be identified and noted. Globe position is usually compared to orbital rim projection with the supraorbital rim being approximately 5 to 8 mm anterior to the cornea. The inferior orbital rim should be approximately 2 mm anterior to the cornea. The lateral orbital rims should be approximately 10 to 12 mm posterior to the cornea. These measurements are easily made using a clear ruler and examining the patient from the lateral view with the patient in primary gaze.

Ocular Mobility

Assessment of ocular mobility can be difficult in children and patients who have suffered acute trauma. We suggest that the examiner sit in front of the patient while asking the patient to follow a pen light or the examiner's fingers. The finger or light should be moved into the six cardinal directions of gaze.[35] After the six directions of gaze have been examined, one should ask the patient to follow the light or the examiner's finger as it is moved toward the nasal bridge. The eyes should converge. This is sustained to within 5 to 8 cm.[35] This examination should detect most mobility disorders. If the patient complains of pain or visual disturbances, the exact eye position at which this happens should be documented. If there is a question of entrapment, a forced duction test performed after a local anesthetic is administered will usually differentiate between true entrapment and muscular weakness.

The Nose

The nose is one of the most aesthetic and functional structures on the face. Its midline position is best examined in the frontal view, and its anterior projection from the profile view. Aesthetically, the nose is not considered as an isolated structure unless it is deformed. The nose is examined in relation to the forehead, orbital rims, eyes, maxilla, lips, and chin. It has been suggested that an aesthetically pleasing nose should flow into the underlying craniomaxillofacial skeleton, represented by smooth interconnecting lines and curves on the topography of the face.[36] For traditional examination purposes, the nose is divided into thirds relative to their underlying supporting structures. The proximal third is supported by the nasal bones. The middle third is supported by the upper lateral nasal cartilages. The distal third is supported by the lower lateral cartilages medially and the sesamoid cartilages and dermis laterally.

The nasal septum provides support for both aesthetics and function by separating the bony and cartilaginous vault of the nose. The nasal septum also aids airflow and supports the tip and columella. Owing to trauma, heredity, and developmental changes, the nasal septum is rarely straight.

The mobile portion of the nose includes the membranous septum, columella, and lobule, which contains the tip and alae. The nasal sill and soft triangle make up and support the opening into the nasal vestibule. Figure 2.7a,b shows the common anterior landmarks of the nose.

Congenital, developmental, and acquired deformities of the nose are extremely complex and challenging. Examination of the nose should include inspection from the lateral, frontal, and submental vertex views, as well as a complete intranasal examination.

Because of the vast amount of detailed information concerning the aesthetic evaluation and surgical correction of nasal deformities, the purpose of this section is to provide basic information that describes the normal nose.[37–39] When a nasal deformity is identified, obviously a more detailed and specific nasal evaluation is in order. This examination focuses on the characteristics of symmetry, width, projection, and function.

In the frontal view, the nose should be in the midline. A silk suture extending from the glabella to the pogonion should pass through the center of the nasal tip. This divides the nose into equal halves and identifies asymmetries of the nasal bridge and tip. The alar-to-alar width has been described as being approximately 70% of the distance between nasion and the tip-defining point.[19,39] This region should be slightly wider in the black and Asian population.[19]

The area in which the nasal bones and nasal process of the frontal bone blend into the frontal bone makes up the *radix*, or root, of the nose.[39] A normal radix should possess a curvilinear line that begins at the supraorbital ridges and follows the nasal dorsum on the right and left sides of the nose.[36,39] Figure 2.8 demonstrates the curvilinear lines of the radix. The

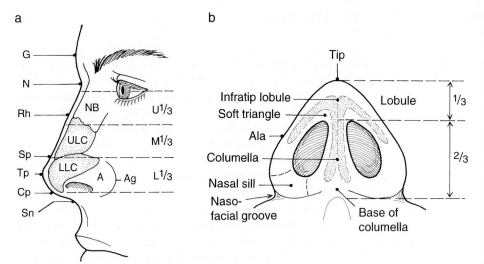

FIGURE 2.7 (a) Common landmarks and divisions of the nose in the lateral view. G, soft tissue glabella; N, soft tissue nasion; Rh, rhinion; Sp, supra-tip-break; Tp, tip-defining point; Cp, columella point; Sn, subnasale; A, ala; Ag, alar groove. The nose is divided into thirds according to its underlying support. The upper third is supported by the nasal bones (NB), the middle third is supported by the upper lateral cartilages (ULC), and the lower third is supported by the lower lateral cartilages (LLC). (b) The basilar view of the nose and its anatomic landmarks and divisions. The lobule should be one third of the total height of the base of the nose.

nasal frontal angle (G-N-Tp) should range between 125° and 135°, with the nasal bridge extending approximately 5 to 8 mm anterior to a normally positioned globe.[39]

The profile view allows one to evaluate nasal length, projection, and rotation of the nasal tip. Projection is defined as the anterior position of the tip relative to the anterior facial plane. Rotation is defined as the inclination of the tip and is indicated by the nasolabial angle. The nasofacial angle assesses the degree of nasal projection and is created by the intersection of facial and nasal planes. For measurement purposes, the angle is represented by a line passing from the soft tissue glabella to the soft tissue nasion and is intersected by a tangent that parallels the nasal dorsum. An angle of between 30° and 35° represents a normal nasal projection.[39,40] It has been suggested that nasal projection can easily be assessed where the distance between tip-defining point and subnasial (Tp-Sn) should equal the distance between subnasale and the vermilion border (Sn-Vs) in a normal nose.[41] Situations that alter upper lip length, such as a cleft lip and mentolabial posturing, can make this assessment unpredictable. The nasolabial angle, as described earlier, also evaluates nasal tip projection. Although there are several other techniques used to assess tip projection, the methods that were discussed here are quick, easy, and commonly used.[42–44]

In the submental vertex view, the nasal base and nostrils are evaluated by merely having the patient tip their head back. A normal base resembles an equilateral triangle.[45] The columella should be straight and in the midline. The lobule–nasal base width ratio should be 3:4 in a normal nose. The nostrils should take on a gentle pear shape with the top part of the pear pointing toward the lobule.[39,45]

When a nasal deformity is present, the nature of the overlying skin should be closely evaluated because superficial scars may distort the mobile portion of the nose and thus make it appear that an underlying defect exists when in reality it does not. Thick skin can make significant bony movements less noticeable and should be considered in the treatment plan, while thin skin may reveal dramatic changes after only subtle bony movements.

The internal nasal exam should identify abnormalities in the septum, turbinates, and/or pathology such as polyps and synechiae. Findings such as these should be documented and investigated as indicated prior to any reconstruction attempts.

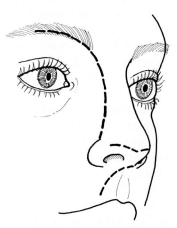

FIGURE 2.8 The topographical curves of the nose. The radix extends from the supraorbital ridges to the lateral dorsal region; the lobular-alar rim should be a wide V shape at the tip; the nasolabial junction follows the contour of the upper lip passing through the subnasale extending along the columella.

The Cheeks

Subtle deformities that affect malar prominence can be difficult to assess when the overlying skin, underlying bone, and amount of buccal fat mask the true etiology of the deformity. It is agreed that prominent malar bones and arches are generally considered aesthetic and represent a youthful facial appearance. Normally, the zygomatic arches make up the widest part of the face when viewed frontally. Temporal convexity, buccal fat, and the position of the orbit and auricle influence the interpretation of arch prominence and facial width. When evaluating cheek prominence, one must assess symmetry, projection, and height.

For examination purposes, the cheek can be divided into three regions: suborbital (zone 1), preauricular (zone 2), and the buccal mandibular (zone 3).[46] Figure 2.9 shows the zones of the cheek.

Zone 1 extends along the lateral border of the nose medially, the inferior orbital rim and eyelid/cheek junction superiorly, slightly above the gingival sulcus inferiorly, and anterior to the sideburn posteriorly. The underlying bony support in this region is mainly the malar bone and the zygomatic arch. Additional support comes from the anterior maxillary wall and the piriform aperture. Zone 2 extends anteriorly to the anterior border of the masseter muscle and overlaps zone 1 at the malar prominence. Superiorly, it extends above the zygomatic arch to the helix of the ear. Posteriorly, it follows the posterior border of the mandible in the preauricular region and extends all the way to the angle. The inferior border of the mandible makes up its inferior boundary. Bony supporting structures in this region include the zygomatic arch, mandibular ramus, and angle. Other supporting structures in this region include the masseter muscle as well as the parotid gland. The anterior boundary of zone 3 extends from the oral commissure and terminates at the chin midpoint. The superior border meets the inferior border of zone 1, which is su-

perior to the gingival sulcus. The posterior border extends back to the masseter muscle and the inferior boundary is made by the remaining inferior border of the mandible. Underlying bony support in this region is made by the mandibular body and symphysis. Significant underlying structures that also provide support and influence the aesthetic appearance of the malar bone are the muscles of facial expression and mastication, which are commonly overlooked.

All three zones overlap at the region of the buccal fat pad. Deformities or defects in any of these regions may affect the overall appearance of the malar bone in zone 1. Thus an apparent malar bone deformity may in reality be normal, while the actual deformity is hidden in zones 2 or 3. Although there are technically three zones for evaluation, the zygomatic arch and malar prominence in zone 1 is where the most attention is directed when evaluating cheek or malar deformities. Close inspection of the other zones must be performed to truly understand the defects' etiology. Facial nerve palsy, parotid pathology, and the absence of dentoalveolar structures also play a significant role in the interpretation of deformities in this region.

The aesthetic position of the malar region is more dependent on an overall feel for symmetry and balance than an actual measurement. When examining the malar region, the examiner must view the patient from the frontal, profile, oblique, and submental vertex views.[47]

On frontal view, the examiner must visually inspect and palpate both malar bones and their defects as well as the zygomatic arch and orbital rims for orientation purposes. Deformities in the cheeks, paranasal, and buccal areas must be noted.[47] Zygomaticus, the point of maximum prominence of the zygomatic arch, should be identified and compared to the opposite side. Symmetry is of importance here. The most prominent portion of the malar bone should be located approximately 1 cm lateral and 1.5 to 2.0 cm inferior to the normal lateral canthus with the patient in the repose position. Deviations from this point should be documented.

Zone 1 can be further divided into the cheek, paranasal, and buccal areas as described by Zide and Epker to specifically evaluate malar bone position.[47] The buccal, cheek, masseter muscle, and intraoral malar buttress region should be palpated to assess the overall thickness of this region. Extraorally, this portion of the cheek should be flat in appearance and should not extend beyond a tangent that extends from the lateral aspect of the malar bone and angle of the mandible.[46] Tissue that extends lateral to this line on frontal view is considered to be unaesthetic and abnormal.

The same landmarks should be evaluated when viewing the patient in the profile, oblique, and submental vertex views. When viewing the patient in the profile position for malar deficiencies, one must not overlook globe position and its relation to the supraorbital and infraorbital rims. Exorbitism is a common finding in the non-Caucasian population and usually presents as a malar deficiency.[48]

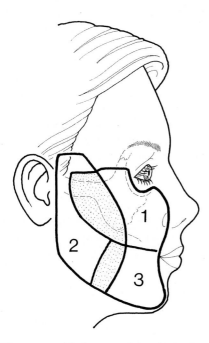

FIGURE 2.9 The topographical zones of the cheek. Suborbital (zone 1), preauricular (zone 2), oral buccomandibular (zone 3). The shaded region represents the area of overlap.

The Auricle

The auricle is an extremely intricate structure made up of convoluted cartilage that is covered by very thin skin except in the lobe region, which is composed of primarily fibrofatty tissue. Figure 2.10 depicts the normal anatomy of the ear. The underlying contour of the cartilage depicts the actual shape of the auricle, making surgical reconstruction difficult. Repair or correction of auricle deformities is one of the greatest challenges a craniomaxillofacial surgeon may be faced with.

The ear is a rich vascular structure that receives its blood supply from the superficial temporal and posterior auricular vessels. The ear has a relatively narrow base when compared to its overall surface area; therefore, any abnormality, previous surgery, or trauma that may involve one of these vessels must be evaluated prior to any reconstruction attempts.

Microtic, constricted, and protruding ear deformities have been shown to have many anatomic and genetic relationships.[49] Ear deformities are frequently expressed among families with a history of mandibulofacial dysostosis.[50] Studies have also shown that ear deformities may be present in up to 10% of patients or family members of patients with cleft or high-arched palates.[50] Possibly up to 25% of patients who present with microtia have family members who demonstrate some evidence of craniofacial microsomia.[51] Damage to the stapedial artery causing ischemia has been postulated to be a possible cause of congenital ear deformities as well.[52]

Congenital ear deformities are evident from birth through adulthood. Traumatic avulsions or loss of ear structure from tumor surgery are dependent on the nature of the injury or location of the tumor and can be acquired at any age. When an ear has been avulsed or amputated and reimplantation attempts have failed, consultation with a maxillofacial prosthodontist is strongly suggested.

The purpose of this section is to give a brief background on the etiology of congenital ear deformities and review the shape and position of the normal ear for examination purposes. Generalities and averages will be discussed, and one should remember that normal ears are as distinctive as normal fingerprints.

Although the auricle continues to grow throughout adulthood, it reaches approximately 85% to 90% of its total length by age three and changes very little after the first decade of life.[53] The ear grows between 40 and 60 mm until puberty and then continues to enlarge minimally throughout life.[53,54] Table 2.4 shows average ear heights and widths associated at various ages for Caucasians.

The width of the ear should be measured from the base of the tragus to the posterior margin of the helical rim. Height is measured from the superior margin of the helical rim to the tip of the earlobe. Ear projection, the amount or degree the ear is elevated off the head, is assessed by measuring the greatest distance the helix is from the mastoid prominence. Although specific numerical values are achieved by measurements, the projection and position of the ear is still considered subjective.[55] Actually, ear position should also be related to the position of the external auditory meatus.[55] Neck length, cranial vault height, mandibular ramus height, and axial rotation of the auricle all affect the subjective interpretation of ear position.

Preauricular pits, sinuses, appendages, and acquired deformities should be documented. Evaluation of the external auditory canal and tympanic membrane should be performed in a routine fashion in which canal caliber, ossicular function, and integrity of the tympanic membrane should be noted and documented. When external ear deformities exist or when a decrease in hearing acuity is noted, a complete otologic and audiologic evaluation is indicated because middle ear deformities are usually associated with auricle deformities.

If a deformity is present, the surgeon must fully and completely explain the technical limitations involved in the surgical correction or reconstruction of the auricle. The age at which the reconstruction should proceed is determined by both physical and psychologic considerations specific to each individual. Correlation with other necessary facial surgery must be considered.

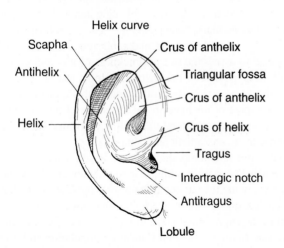

FIGURE 2.10 The topographical anatomy of the auricle.

TABLE 2.4 Average ear widths and heights for males and females.

Age (yrs)	Ear width (mm)	Ear height (mm)
0–9 months	26	42.5
1	29.5	48.5
4	32	51.5
8	33.5	56
10	34	57.5
16	34.5	60
18	34.5	62.5
30–40	34.5	63.5
50–60	34.5	66.5
70–80	35	71

The Lips

For clinical purposes, the lips should be viewed as they relate to the base of the nose, chin, maxilla, and upper and lower anterior dentition. Much has been written on the physical dimensions of the lips and perioral structures. Unfortunately, most of it is of little clinical importance. With oral competence being the major function of the lips, they are generally viewed as being normal or abnormal by their position and aesthetic value.

The lips should be examined from the facial and profile view where symmetry and balance are of importance. Obvious deformities such as clefts, scars, lesions, and asymmetric regions should be documented. Clefts that involve the lips usually occur once in every 800 to 900 births. The craniofacial and lateralfacial clefts as described by Tessier that can involve the lips are categorized as No. 0 (median craniofacial dysraphia), No. 1 (paramedian craniofacial cleft), No. 2 (similar to No. 1 but more lateral), No. 3 (occlusonasal cleft), No. 4 (occlusofacial cleft I), No. 5 (occlusofacial cleft II), and No. 7 (temporozygomatic cleft).[56] Figure 2.11 shows the position of the craniofacial clefts that may involve the lips according to Tessier.

The normal anatomy of the lips should present with two philtral columns along the paramidline of the upper lip. Between the philtral columns, a philtral groove or dimple should be present. Just inferior to the philtral groove should lie the symmetric Cupid's bow that follows the vermilion border of the upper lip in the midline. The white roll of the upper lip should follow the vermilion border lateral to the Cupid's bow. The tubercle occupies the mucosal portion of the upper lip, inferior to the Cupid's bow, and is in the midline. Both the

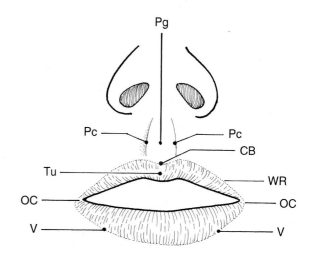

FIGURE 2.12 The topographical anatomy of the normal lips. Pg, philtral groove; Pc, philtral column; Cb, Cupid's bow; Tu, tubercle; Wr, white roll; Oc, oral commissure; V, vermilion.

right and left commissures should be symmetric in repose and the vermilion identifies the vermilion border of the lower lip. Figure 2.12 shows the topographical anatomy of normal lips.

Much has been written about the length of the upper lip. It is measured from subnasale to the stomion. On average, it has been shown to be approximately 11 mm in infants, 16 mm at age one, and 20 to 22 mm in the adult (which is reached by 6 years of age).[57] Because its borders are poorly defined in many normal individuals, the width of the philtrum is of little concern. The commissure width is measured with the lips in their repose position.[58] Table 2.5 shows normal intercommissural widths in Caucasians.

Normal lip fullness is extremely variable, especially in ethnic individuals. Measurements can be made from the middle of the lip to the stomions of the upper or lower lip.

In the repose position, the upper and lower lips should be apart, creating a gap of 3.0 to 3.5 mm. In this position, the amount of upper tooth that is exposed should be approximately 2 to 5 mm from the incisal edge to the bottom of the upper lip. The lower dentition is usually not exposed while the lips are in the reposed position. On full smile, the entire maxillary anterior teeth should be exposed and only 1 to 2 mm of gingival exposure is desirable.[59] Abnormal tooth show may be due to jaw or tooth abnormalities, not just lip position.

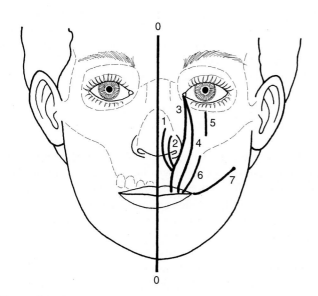

FIGURE 2.11 The position and numbering of craniofacial clefts that involve the lips using Tessier's classification system.

TABLE 2.5 Mean intercommissural width in Caucasians.

Age (yrs)	Females (mm)	Males (mm)
0–1	27	32
2–3	30	35
8–9	42	44
12–13	45	48
14–15	47	50
16–Adult	50	52

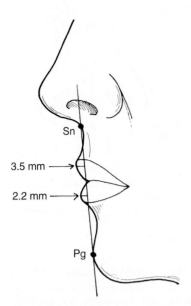

On profile view, the upper lip should be fuller than the lower lip. Using a clear plastic ruler, a reference line can be established, which extends from the subnasale to the soft tissue pogonion. This can also be accomplished on a lateral photograph or cephalometric x-ray. The upper lip should be 3.5 mm anterior to the line as compared to the lower lip, which should be 2.2 mm anterior to this line.[60] Figure 2.13 shows the protrusion of the normal upper and lower lip.

Finally, the function of the upper and lower lips should be evaluated with the patient in full smile, repose, and the pucker position. Any weaknesses or asymmetries during function may suggest damage to the motor innervation, which is supplied by the buccal and marginal mandibular rami of cranial nerve VII. The locations of these deficiencies should be documented.

Chin-Neck Contour

Generally, the chin and neck contours are evaluated in the frontal and profile views. Clinically, the chin begins at soft tissue menton and extends superiorly into the mentolabial sulcus. The depth of the mentolabial sulcus can give a false interpretation of lower facial height in the frontal view as well as a false interpretation of the protrusion or retrusion of the chin point in the profile view. The correct depth of the mentolabial sulcus is subjective and can be influenced by the actual chin position, lower lip length and position, and the lower anterior dental alveolar structures. Its depth should lie approximately 3 to 4 mm posterior to a line that passes from the vermilion border of the lower lip and extends through soft

tissue pogonion.[61] Excessive anterior flare of the mandibular anterior dentition or mandibular prognathism will usually present with a deficient mentolabial sulcus giving the lower facial third a rather flat appearance. A short lower facial height and a retrognathic mandible will usually be associated with an excessive mentolabial sulcus. The aging face is also associated with an excessive mentolabial sulcus.

Soft tissue chin projection is evaluated in the profile view, in which the distance from the soft tissue pogonion to the Gonzales line (a line extending interiorly from soft tissue nasion and is perpendicular to the Frankfort horizontal plane) is measured. A soft tissue pogonion that falls within 3 mm anterior or posterior to the Gonzales line is considered a normal chin position.

Frontally, the most important clinical aspect of the chin is symmetry and balance. Any abnormality should be documented, remembering that the relative position of the nose, dentition, lips, and neck contour or deformities of these structures will affect the overall appearance and position of the chin.

The neck contour should be evaluated in the frontal, profile, and basilar views. When examining the patient in a frontal and profile position, the patient's head should be in the neutral position with the facial muscles and lips in the repose position. In the frontal view, a definite line should be easily followed outlining the inferior border of the mandible. Bilateral and symmetric contour concavities should be noted when following the lateral border of the mandibular angle and lateral neck, which should feather out inferiorily and laterally along the trapezius muscle. The sternocleidomastoid muscle should be subtly visible just medial to the mandibular angle and extending inferior and medially as it approaches the sterno-clavicular region. Any abnormalities in facial width, mandibular (chin) position, and/or excessive laxity of the overlying skin will obviously affect neck contour and appearance. The examiner should palpate the skin in this region to determine its laxity and adherence to underlying structures as well as any hidden mass or defects.

In the profile view, there should be a subtle but definite outline of the inferior border of the mandible as it extends from the chin to the posterior ramus region. The right and left sides should be evaluated and compared where gross asymmetries and defects should be recorded. The chin-neck angle is also evaluated in this position and should be compared to the overall chin projection, lower lip position, and mentolabial sulcus depth. The chin-neck angle is formed by the anterior border of the neck and the submental region extending from point C through soft tissue menton. Normal chin-neck angles are usually between 110° and 120°. Also in the normal neck, one should be able to identify the anterior border and body of the sternocleidomastoid muscle.

Finally, the chin-neck region should be evaluated in the basilar position. One should appreciate symmetry and the amount of redundant tissue in the submental region as well as the skin's adherence to the underlying structures.

With all of this in mind, the chin-neck area can be classified according to the amount of redundant tissue, platysmal development, and the relative chin position.[62] For examination purposes, there are six classes with specific characteristics. Class I presents with a normal chin-neck angle and normal skin tone. Class II shows an increased laxity of the skin with a relatively normal platysma muscle tone. Class III shows a definite accumulation of submental fat. Class IV has obvious banding of the platysma muscle. Class V is seen when the mandible is moderately retrognathic. Class IV presents with an excessively obtuse chin-neck angle and may be due to an inferiorly positioned hyoid bone.[62]

Oral Cavity and Occlusion

Before any attempts are made to surgically correct any craniomaxillofacial deformity, whether congenital, developmental, or acquired, a complete examination of the oral cavity and occlusion must be performed and not overlooked. While it is easy to focus one's attention on the very obvious and dramatic aesthetic craniomaxillofacial deformities that a patient may have, the examining surgeon must keep in mind that facial asymmetry and imbalance may be due to poor dentoalveolar structures and relationships. The examination should include a close survey of the lips, labial mucosa, buccal mucosa, mucobuccal fold, hard palate, soft palate and uvula, oropharynx, nasopharynx, tongue, floor of the mouth, muscles of mastication, periodontium, teeth, and occlusion.

While examining the lips and labial mucosa, the overall muscular control of the lips can be evaluated during normal conversation. Visual inspection of the lips will reveal most abnormalities and enlargements. The color and texture of the vermilion border should be noted, and the lips should also be examined for fissuring. Any submucosal nodules or other abnormalities of the lips and labial mucosa can be identified by using bidigital palpation.

The buccal mucosa can easily be evaluated when the patient's mouth is partially opened using a mouth mirror to retract the cheek laterally. This will allow direct visualization of the area hidden by the maxillary tuberosity. The mucosa of the buccal cheek should be dried using a gauze sponge, and with the aid of bimanual palpation, the parotid gland can be milked, thus evaluating its function and the integrity of Stenson's duct. Foul-smelling and discolored saliva should be noted.

The mucobuccal fold is usually hidden but should be examined visually and by palpation. This is easily done by retracting the buccal mucosa laterally at its vestibular depth and palpating its depth and alveolar bone using one's index finger. Contour abnormalities, excessive scar bands, fistulas, and painful regions as well as clefts should be documented.

The hard and soft palate and uvula can be examined by direct vision. The mucosa overlying the hard palate is extremely keratinized and firmly attached. It should be pale pink in color as compared to the soft palate, which sometimes may appear more yellow in color due to its increased amount of adipose tissue and its thin mucosal covering. This region should be palpated and any abnormality should be documented. The patient's gag reflex should also be noted and appreciated.

The oropharynx and nasopharynx should be inspected by direct and indirect vision. The entire anterior tonsillar pillar should be examined for symmetry and palpated to identify any submucosal masses. Using a gauze sponge to grip the tip of the tongue, retracting it anteriorly, while placing a warmed mouth mirror at its base and having the patient say "ahh," one can easily and clearly visualize the oropharynx. The nasopharynx can be personally viewed by just rotating this mirror to reflect superiorly. A flexible fiberoptic scope should be used if available. Regardless of the technique used, patient compliance is imperative when examining these regions. The use of topical local anesthetics may decrease the tendency to gag when using the mirror technique and must be used intranasally along with a vasoconstrictive spray when advancing a flexible fiberoptic scope through the nose.

The tongue should be examined. The use of a gauze sponge will aid in retracting the tongue forward, upward, and to the right and left. The entire tongue should be palpated and its shape, size, fissural pattern, color, deformities, and unusual tremors noted.

The floor of the mouth is evaluated by having the patient raise the tongue, enabling the examiner to visually inspect this region. Bimanual palpation of this region is mandatory and is accomplished by placing the index finger along the floor while the other hand supports the submandibular region extraorally. The entire floor should be examined in this fashion. The lingual aspect of the mandible should also be palpated, noting any irregularities. The function and quality of the saliva from the submandibular gland should be evaluated as was performed when examining the parotid gland.

The muscles of mastication should be palpated extraorally and intraorally when possible. Hypertrophy, function, and tenderness should be noted and may indicate possible temporomandibular joint dysfunction.

The periodontium, when visually inspected, is a good indicator of the overall oral hygiene. Poor oral hygiene and inflammation should be noted. The quality, health, and amount of attached gingiva should also be recorded. Selective periodontal probing is recommended in areas where inflammation is noted or where segmental osteotomies may be planned. Patients who present with obvious periodontal disease should be evaluated and treated by a dentist or periodontist to achieve the best gingival health possible prior to any procedure that involves the dentoalveolar structures. This should decrease the chance of postoperative complications such as wound dehiscence and infection.

Finally, the teeth are examined both clinically and radiographically. Missing teeth should be noted. Decayed, symptomatic, and mobile teeth should be restored if at all possible. The occlusion should be examined clinically and by the

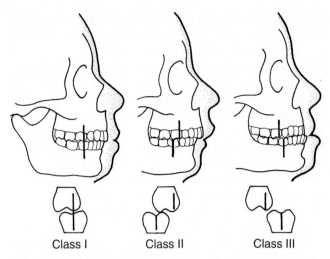

Class I   Class II   Class III

FIGURE 2.14 Angle's classification of occlusion is based on the position of maxillary and mandibular permanent first molars. Class I is considered normal; the mesiobuccal cusp of the maxillary first permanent molar should rest in the mesiobuccal groove of the mandibular first permanent molar. Class II is considered retrognathic with the mesiobuccal cusp of the maxillary first permanent molar resting anterior to the mesiobuccal groove of the mandibular first permanent molar. Class III is considered prognathic, with the mesiobuccal cusp of the maxillary first permanent molar resting posterior to the mesiobuccal groove of the mandibular first permanent molar.

use of dental study models. Angle's classification is most commonly used to describe the occlusion. It is based on the position of the maxillary and mandibular first permanent molars. Figure 2.14 shows Angle's classification of occlusion. The general arch shape and transverse width must also be noted. Other techniques such as transillumination, percussion, and pulp testing should be used as specifically indicated.

Conclusion

When treating craniomaxillofacial deformity patients, it is extremely important that the examining surgeon develop a comprehensive, stepwise system for examining and documenting the complex deformities with which these patients may present. Only through a systematic approach can information and data be collected, reviewed, and interpreted, thus diagnosing the true etiology of the craniomaxillofacial deformity. The examination provides only part of the information that is required to make the diagnosis. Dental study models, radiographs, cephalometric analysis, CT scans, and photo documentation must also be used in conjunction with the clinical examination to both diagnose and document the patient's preoperative state. These study aids can also be shown to the patient and family members to demonstrate the etiology of their deformity. In today's litigious society, accurate and organized documentation of the patient's preoperative state is mandatory, thus providing a complete medical record and good risk management.

Today, third-party payers will often request supplemental information, such as study models, x-rays, and photographs that support your diagnosis and indication for surgery before approval can be granted. Knowing that the information obtained and treatment plan is different for each patient, additional information pertaining to more specific deformities or problems may be needed.

The information obtained in this examination should allow one to accurately diagnose and formulate a treatment that will provide a predictable, functional, and aesthetic result.

References

1. Wood NK. *Treatment Planning: A Pragmatic Approach*. St. Louis, MO: C.V. Mosby; 1978: ch 2, 29.
2. McCarthy JG. *Plastic Surgery, The Face*, vol. 2. Philadelphia: W.B. Saunders; 1990: ch 29, 1188.
3. Weed LL. Medical records that guide and teach. *N Engl J Med* 1968;278(11):593.
4. Peterson LJ, Frost DE. *Database Collections. Principles of Oral and Maxillofacial Surgery*, vol. 3. Philadelphia: J.B. Lippincott Company; 1992, ch 49.
5. Proffit WR, Epker BN, Ackerman JL. Systematic description of dentofacial deformities: the data base. In: Bell WE, Proffit WR, White RW, eds. *Surgical Correction of Dentofacial Deformities*. St. Louis, MO: C.V. Mosby; 1980: ch 5, 105.
6. Tucker MR, Thomas PM. Temporomandibular pain and dysfunction in the orthodontic surgical patient: Rationale for evaluation and treatment sequencing. *Int J Adult Orthop Orthogn Surg.* 1986;1:11.
7. Karabouta I, Mantis C. The TMJ dysfunction syndrome before and after sagittal split osteotomy of the rami. *J Oral Maxillofac Surg.* 1989;13:185.
8. Gorney M, Harries T. The preoperative and postoperative considerations of natural facial asymmetry. *Plast Reconstr Surg.* 1974;54:187.
9. Gonzalez-Ulloa M. A quantum method for the appreciation of the morphology of the face. *Plast Reconstr Surg.* 1964;34:241.
10. Baer MJ. Dimensional changes in the human head and face in the third decade of life. *Am J Phys Anthropol.* 1956;14:557.
11. Whitaker LA, LaRossa, D, Randall P. Structural goals in craniofacial surgery. *Cleft Palate J.* 1975;12:23.
12. Farkas LG, Katic MJ, Hreczko Ta, et al. Anthropometric proportions in the upper lip–lower lip–chin area of the lower face in young white adults. *Am J Orthol.* 1984;86:52.
13. Peck H, Peck S. A concept of facial aesthetics. *Angle Orthod.* 1970;40:284.
14. Tolleth H. Concepts for the plastic surgeon from art and sculpture. *Clin Plast Surg.* 1987;14:585.
15. Showfety KJ, Vig PS, Matteson S. A simplified method for taking neutral-head-position cephalograms. *Am J Orthod.* 1983;83:495.
16. Romm S. Art, love and facial beauty. *Clin Plast Surg.* 1987;14:579.
17. Ricketts RM. Divine proportions in facial esthetics. *Clin Plast Surg.* 1982;9:401.
18. Larrabee WF. Facial analysis for rhinoplasty. *Otolaryngol Clin North Am.* 1987;20:653.

19. McGraw-Wall B. Facial analysis. In: Bailey BJ, ed. *Head and Neck Surgery—Otolaryngology*. Philadelphia: J.B. Lippincott Company; 1993: ch 158, 2070.

20. Gonzalez-Ulloa M. Quantitative principles in cosmetic surgery of the face (profile-plasty). *Plast Reconstr Surg.* 1962;29:186.

21. Westropp CK, Barber CR. Growth of the skull in young children: I. Standards of head circumference. *J Neurol Neurosurg Psychiatry.* 1956;29:52.

22. Illingworth RS, Eid EE. The head circumference in infants and other measurements to which it may be related. *Acta Pediatr Scand.* 1971;333:60.

23. Popich GA, Smith DW. Fontanelles: range of normal size. *J Pediatr.* 1972;80:749.

24. Davies DP, Ansari BM, Cooke TJ. Anterior fontanelle size in the neonate. *Arch Dis Child.* 1975;50:81.

25. Chemke J, Robinson A. The third fontanelle. *J Pediatr.* 1969;75:617.

26. Tan KL. The third fontanelle. *Acta Paediatr Scand.* 1971;60:329.

27. Ousterhout DK. Feminization of the forehead: contour changing to improve female aesthetics. *Plast Reconstr Surg.* 1987;79:701.

28. Jelks GW, Jelks EB, Ruff G. Clinical and radiographic evaluation of the orbit. *Otolaryngol Clin North Am.* 1988;21:13.

29. Laestadius N, Aase JM, Smith DW. Normal canthal and outer orbital dimensions. *J Pediatr* 1969;74:465.

30. Holt GR, Holt JE. Nasoethmoid complex fractures. *Otolaryngol Clin North Am.* 1985;18:89.

31. Hansman CF. Growth of interorbital distance and skull thickness as observed in roentgenographic measurements. *Radiology.* 1966;86:87.

32. Chouke KS. The epicanthus or mongolian folds in caucasian children. *Am J Phys Anthropol.* 1929;13:255.

33. Fox SA. The palpebral fissure. *Am J Opthalmol* 1966;62:73.

34. Brennan GH. Correction of the ptotic brow. *Otolaryngol Clin North Am.* 1980;13:265.

35. Bates B. *A Guide to Physical Examination and History Taking.* 4th ed. Philadelphia: J.B. Lippincott Company; 1982: ch 7, 170.

36. Sheen JH. Secondary rhinoplasty. *Plast Reconstr Surg.* 1975; 56:137.

37. Rollin DK, Leslie FG. Rhinoplasty: image and reality. *Clin Plast Surg.* 1988;15(1):1–10.

38. Larrabee WF. Facial analysis for rhinoplasty. *Otolaryngol Clin North Am.* 1987;20(4):653.

39. Stella JP, Epker BN. Systematic aesthetic evaluation of the nose for cosmetic surgery. *Oral Maxillofac Surg Clin of North Am.* 1990;2(2):273.

40. Brown JB, McDowell F. *Plastic Surgery of the Nose.* St. Louis, MO: C.V. Mosby; 1951: ch 2, 30.

41. Simons RL. Nasal tip projection, ptosis and supratip thickening. *J Ear Nose Throat.* 1982;61:452.

42. Baum SJ. Introduction. *J Ear Nose Throat.* 1982;61:426.

43. Powell N, Humphries B. *Proportions of the Esthetic Face.* New York: Thieme-Stratton; 1984.

44. Crumley RL, Lancer R. Quantitative analysis of nasal tip projection. *Laryngoscope.* 1988;98:202.

45. Bernstein L. Esthetics in rhinoplasty. *Otolaryngol Clin North Am.* 1975;8:705.

46. Zide BM. Deformities of the lips and cheeks. In: McCarthy JG, ed. *The Face*, vol. 2. Philadelphia: W.B. Saunders; 1990: ch 38, 2037.

47. Zide MF, Epker BN. Systematic aesthetic evaluation of the cheeks for cosmetic surgery. *Oral Maxillofac Surg Clin North Am.* 1990;2(2):351.

48. Block MS, Zide MF. Orbital decompression by midfacial osteotomy. *Oral Surg Oral Med Oral Pathol.* 1984;57:479–484.

49. Rogers B. Microtia, lop, cup and protruding ears: four directly inherited deformities? *Plast Reconstr Surg.* 1968;41:208.

50. Rogers B. Berry-Treacher Collins syndrome: a review of 200 cases. *Br J Plast Surg.* 1964;17:109.

51. Tanzer RC. Total reconstruction of the auricle. The evaluation of a plan of treatment. *Plast Reconstr Surg.* 1971;47:523.

52. McKenzie J, Craig J. Mandibulo-facial dysostosis (Treacher-Collins syndrome). *Arch Dis Child* 1955;30:391.

53. Lucas WP, Pryor HB. Range and standard deviations of certain physical measurements in healthy children. *J Pediatr.* 1935;6:533.

54. Rubin LR, Bromberg BE, Walden RH, et al. An anatomic approach to the obtrusive ear. *Plast Reconstr Surg.* 1962;29:360.

55. Robinow M, Roche AF. Low-set ears. *Am J Dis Child.* 1973;125:482.

56. Tessier P. Anatomical classification of facial, cranio-facial and latero-facial clefts. *J Maxillofac Surg.* 1976;4:69.

57. Feingold M, Bossert WH. Normal values for selected physical parameters: An aid to syndrome delineation. *Birth Defects.* 1974;10(13):1.

58. Cervenka J, Figalová P, Gorlin RJ. Oral intercommissural distance in children. *Am J Dis Child.* 1969;117:434.

59. Vig KD, Ellis E. Diagnosis and treatment planning for the surgical-orthodontic patient. *Clin Plast Surg.* 1989;16:645.

60. Burstone CJ. Lip posture and its significance in treatment planning. *Am J Orthod.* 1967;53:262.

61. Simons RL. Adjunctive measures in rhinoplasty. *Otolaryngol Clin North Am.* 1975;8:717.

62. Dedo DD. A preoperative classification of the neck for cervicofacial rhytidectomy. *Laryngoscope* 1980;90:1984.

3
Craniofacial Deformities: Review of Etiologies, Distribution, and Their Classification

Craig R. Dufresne

Clinicians who study or treat individuals with congenital malformations of the head and neck realize that the spectrum of craniofacial malformations represents a relatively rare set of conditions that exist in a multitude of patterns and in varying degrees of severity. Over several years, many groupings of classifications have been put forth in an attempt to organize these conditions.[1,2] Most either had been arbitrary or could not be standardized enough to be widely accepted because of extreme or bizarre distortions of the anatomy.[3,4] Further confusion has arisen because there has not been any unanimity of terminology or satisfactory standardization of the classification of the innumerable craniofacial syndromes. At present, there are over 150 craniofacial syndromes, with new syndromes being described and published at the rate of 25 to 50 per year.[5,6] Many specialties within the health profession have taken an interest in this task as the study of craniofacial malformations has developed into a multidisciplinary science. This diversity of focus and interest contributes to the difficulty in creating a generalized and acceptable approach to classifications.[2] What appears to be an acceptable designation of a particular anomaly or anatomic defect for a geneticist or syndromologist may fall short for the craniofacial anatomist or surgeon.[5–10] As human genetics and embryology become better defined and the etiologic factors at the gene and molecular level are studied, it is possible that a more exacting classification system will be devised.

Section A—Facial Clefting Incidence

The most common congenital facial anomaly is the cleft lip and palate. The frequency of its occurrence ranges from 0.60 to 2.13 per 1000 births.[11,12] Sex, ethnic, and racial backgrounds influence the incidence of these anomalies. Blacks have been found to have the lowest incidence of cleft lip and palate, Caucasians are noted to have a higher incidence, and Asians have the highest incidence. Cleft lips with or without an associated cleft palate are seen more commonly in males.

Females, however, have a higher incidence of isolated clefts of the palate.[5,6,10]

Hemifacial or craniofacial microsomia (also known as the *first and second branchial arch syndrome*) is the next most frequent congenital facial anomaly. The frequency of this anomaly is estimated to be between 0.18 and 0.33 per 1000 births.[5,10,13]

The incidence of the remaining craniofacial anomalies is not well documented because of the very low rate of occurrence. A rough approximation of their frequency is in the range of 0.014 to 0.048 per 1000 births.[5,6,14,15]

Classified Schemas

The earliest classification schemas of the craniofacial malformations are often identified according to the names of the authors who first described them, such as Goldenhar, Pierre Robin, Treacher Collins, and Pfeiffer syndromes.[3,4,15–18] Other malformations are identified by their descriptive appearance and have been given names such as hemifacial microsomia, retromandibulism, and hypertelorism without regard to their various causes. Other classifications are based on anatomic topography, with some authors dividing the face into various regions and others grouping the defects around the brain, sensory organs, or the branchial arch system. Ambiguities in terminology and multiple areas of overlap will be simplified to present an orderly development and working knowledge of this complex subject.[1,4,5,9,10,15]

Morian Classification

Morian is credited with the first attempt to classify craniofacial anomalies. In 1886, he described three types of facial clefts. The type I, or oronasal cleft, described a maxillary cleft located between the central and the lateral incisors extending into the nasal region. The type II, an *oro-ocular* cleft, described a maxillary cleft located between the incisor and the canine teeth that extends toward the orbit. The type III, also an oro-ocular cleft, described a maxillary cleft located behind the canine teeth that extends toward the orbit.[5,6,14,15]

Degenhardt Classification

Several subsequent classifications were attempted by such authors as Sanvenero-Rosselli, Burian, and others, but it was not until Degenhardt (in 1961) that a more complete, general category of craniofacial dysplasias were defined.[5,6,14,16,18]

Degenhardt describes four major groups of defects: (1) dysplasias in the region of the first and second branchial arches; (2) dysplasias in the region of the premaxilla and the maxilla; (3) dysplasias of the soft tissues; and (4) craniofacial syndromes.[5,14]

Degenhardt's first group of dysplasias of the first and second branchial archs contains two subgroups: (1) hypoplasias (including mandibular dysostosis, oculoauricular dysplasia, mandibulofacial dysostosis, oculomandibulofacial dysmorphia, oculomandibulofacial dyscephaly, and oculovertebral dysplasia); and (2) fusion anomalies (synechiae and syngnathia).[5,6]

In the second group, Degenhardt categorizes dysplasias of the premaxillary and maxillary regions, which are subdivided into hypoplasias and cleft formations. The hypoplasias included premaxillary hypoplasia (ankyloglossia superior syndrome) and premaxillary hypoplasias with other anomalies (anecephaly and anophthalmia). The cleft malformation subgroup includes cleft lip and palate with and without associated malformations, such as frontal encephalocele and arrhinia.[5,6]

Dysplasias of the soft tissue make up Degenhardt's third major grouping. This is subdivided into lateral facial clefts, macrostomia, and astomia malformations.[5]

The fourth and last group under Degenhardt's classification is a broad classification of craniofacial syndromes. This is subdivided into hypoplastic alterations in one region of the neural and visceral cranium (holoprosencephaly and aprosopia) and other characteristic syndromes, such as acrofacial dysostosis, dyscraniopygophalangy, and Crouzon's disease.[5,17,18]

Lund Classification

The next major classification was presented by Lund in 1966. Lund attempted a more comprehensive approach to classify several craniofacial syndromes, particularly the ocular and cerebral syndromes. He developed five categories, attempting to separate cranial dysplasias from facial dysplasias, including several transitional forms, reduplications of the head region, and phakomatoses. The cranial dysplasias, Lund felt, are primary malformations at the base of the skull, occurring at the fifth to seventh week of embryological development. Facial dysplasias were considered to result from disturbances in the first and/or second visceral arches and their derivatives at the seventh week in utero.[5,6,19]

Lund's theory considered most craniofacial dysplasias to be multifactorial in origin, with single gene expression playing an insignificant role. He relied on the concept that specific "head organizers" located in the prosencephalic and rhombencephalic brain developmental regions explained the diverse combinations of eye, ear, face, skull, and brain abnormalities.[15,19–21]

American Association of Cleft Palate Rehabilitation—Harkens Classification

In 1962, the American Association of Cleft Palate Rehabilitation (AACPR) attempted to standardize a classification for facial syndromes and clefts by endorsing a system proposed by Harkens and associates. These clefting syndromes are divided into four major groups: (1) mandibular process clefts; (2) naso-ocular clefts; (3) oro-ocular clefts; and (4) oroaural clefts. The clefts of the mandibular process include clefts of the lip, mandible, and lip pits. The naso-ocular clefts extend from the alar region toward the medial canthus. The clefts of the oro-ocular group extend externally from the mouth toward the palpebral fissures and are subdivided into the oromedial canthal and orolateral canthal clefts. The latter group is on the temporal extension of the cleft from the lateral canthus. The last group of clefts, the oroaural clefts, extend from the mouth toward the ear.[5,12,15]

The classification, however, has several deficiencies, primarily because it is based on the surface anatomy and does not integrate the underlying craniofacial skeletal defects. It also fails to include major midline facial clefts or Treacher Collins syndrome.[5,6,12–15,17,18]

Boo-Chai Classification

Boo-Chai noted the deficiencies of the AACPR classification. In particular, Boo-Chai subdivided the description of the oro-ocular cleft into types I and II. The Boo-Chai types I and II clefts both bypass the nose and leave the piriform aperture intact, in contrast to the naso-ocular cleft. The infraorbital foramen was used to separate the two types of clefts.[5,7,8,11,13,14,21] Morian was the first to distinguish and further describe the anatomic difference between the clefts and to note the importance of the infraorbital foramen.[5,14]

In the type I cleft, the soft tissue aspect of the upper lip differs from a common cleft lip in that it begins lateral to the Cupid's bow. The cleft then courses lateral to the nasal alae into the nasoalar groove and ends as a coloboma in the midportion of the lower eyelid or, alternatively, at the lateral canthus. The bony element starts in the region of the bicuspids and courses lateral to the infraorbital foramen on its way to the inferolateral portion of the orbit.[5]

Tessier Classification

It was not until 1976 that Paul Tessier was able to present the first orderly anatomic classification system for all the established craniofacial clefting malformations.[17] To simplify the nomenclature of the clefts, Tessier devised a system in which a number is assigned to the site of each malformation, based on its relationship to the sagittal midline. The classification system is purely descriptive, however, and not related to the embryological development of the malformation or the underlying pathology. Nevertheless, this system has become widely accepted because of the ease of recording and simplicity of communicating the various malformations. It also has been found to correlate clinical appearance with practical surgical anatomy.[17,18,22]

The facial clefts, according to Tessier, are basically orbitocentric in nature, distributing the involvement through the soft tissues of the face as well as the skeletal tissues of the maxilla, mandible, and neurocranium[17] (see Figures 3.1 and 3.2) Clefts of the soft tissues and clefts of the craniofacial skeleton may not always exactly coincide; however, there exists an intimate relationship between the two structures. The orbit is the key structure for this classification schema. Its strategic location separates the cranial skeleton from the facial skeleton. A horizontal line can then be drawn through the canthi as an equator to divide the cranial and facial portions of the cleft. Tessier describes the clefting syndromes as developing according to constant axes, which are divided into 15 regions, or "time zones," numbered 0 to 14 across and around the orbit. The facial clefts numbered 0 to 7 are found caudal to the orbital equator, and the clefts numbered 9 to 14 are found cephalad to the orbital equator. The No. 8 cleft coincides with the equator and passes laterally from the lateral canthus.[17,18]

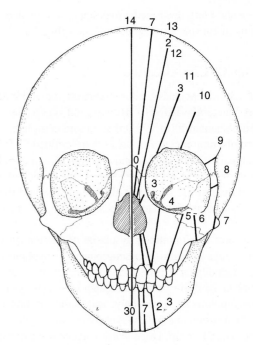

FIGURE 3.1 The Tessier classification of craniofacial clefts are represented here as they appear through the bony framework of the skull. The system is based on an orbitocentric pattern with the facial component numbered from 0 to 7, with the exception of the mandible (midline mandibular cleft is designated as a No. 30 cleft). The cranial component of the clefts are numbered from 14 to 7 in a clockwise pattern. The axial pattern when added together totals 14 for the complete form of the cleft as it traverses through the facial to the cranial area.

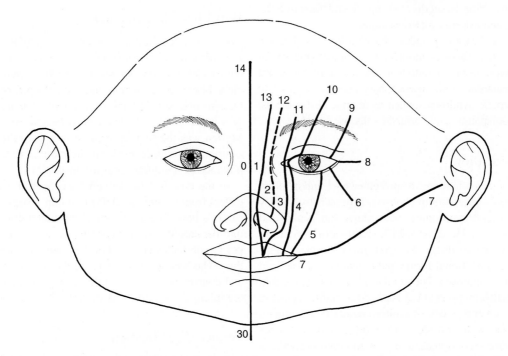

FIGURE 3.2 The Tessier classification of craniofacial clefts is shown here as they appear through the soft tissues of the face. They follow the same patterns as that of the bony clefts with the same designation and numbering.

The facial clefts and the cranial clefts can occur independently of each other or in combination to form a craniofacial cleft. Although bilateral representatives of craniofacial clefts occur, unilateral forms are more common. Multiple craniofacial clefts are also seen in the same individual and have long been associated with certain syndromes. They need not be symmetric or of equal severity. Because the cranial and facial clefts tend to follow the same axis, Tessier incorporated this concept as the keystone of his classification. Its importance lies in the analysis and examination of the patient. This concept forces the clinician to look up and down the axis and neighboring zones, resulting in the possible discovery of unexpected or overlooked malformations.

Clefts of the soft tissues and clefts of the craniofacial skeleton may not always coincide in severity. The extent of involvement of each component is often quite variable, and as a rule, the bony deformation is greater in the facial clefts. Conversely, in clefts medial to the infraorbital foramen, the defect of the soft tissue tends to be generally greater (with the exception of cleft No. 3).[17,18]

The Nos. 0 to 14 clefts of Tessier are median craniofacial dysraphia (Figure 3.3). This is probably secondary to a defect of closure of the anterior neuropore. The cleft involves the frontal bone resulting in a median encephalocele, the ethmoid region (creating a duplication of the crista galli), the nose (resulting in duplication of the septum and columella), and finally, the maxilla and lip. Intraorally, a diastema separates the central incisors, whereas the palate itself can be cleft through the midline. The No. 0 cleft usually results in hypertelorism, whereas if agenesis or hypoplasia is the predominant malformation, a partial or total absence of the philtrum and the premaxilla can occur. The nose can be flat, side, small, and lacking a columella. The nostrils are intact and laterally displaced. A midline groove in the columella and nasal tip, resulting in a bifid nose, is seen. At the other extreme, a proboscis or arrhinencephaly can be seen with the resultant orbital hypotelorism, cebocephaly, or cyclopia.[17,18]

Prolongation of the No. 0 cleft or No. 30 cleft of Tessier onto the mandible could be represented in its most minor form as a notch in the lower lip, and it can become progressively more severe by involving the mandible, tongue, chin, neck, hyoid bone, and even the sternum. The tongue is frequently bifid and bound to the mandible by a dense band of tissue. The cleft of the alveolus is located in the midline passing between the central incisors.

The Tessier No. 1 cleft is a paramedian, craniofacial cleft that traverses through the soft tissues from the cupid's bow region to the dome of the alar cartilage, resulting in a notch in the dome of the nostril extending to the medial aspect of the eyebrow. If the No. 1 cleft extends more superiorly onto the frontal bone, it is referred to as the No. 13 cleft. The olfactory groove of the cribiform plate becomes widened, resulting in hypertelorism. The groove or cleft then passes between the nasal bone and the frontal process of the maxilla.

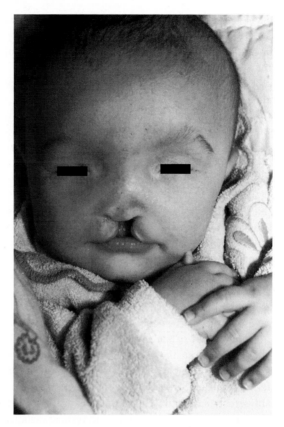

FIGURE 3.3 An example of a infant with a Tessier No. 0 to 14 facial cleft with the midline cleft lip and palate, hypertelorism, agenesis of the midline nasal structures, absence of the premaxilla and philtrum, underlying cranial base defect, and encephalocele.

Inferiorly, the No. 1 cleft continues through the alveolus between the central and lateral incisors.[14,17,18]

The Tessier No. 2 appears identical to the No. 1 cleft, but it is actually more lateral in a paranasal location. There is some question of whether this a true entity of a transitional form between clefts No. 1 and No. 3. It traverses the soft tissue of the nose between the summit and the base of the alar cartilage and then onto the lip. The palpebral fissure is not involved in this cleft. Distortion of the eyebrow occurs just lateral to its medial end point as the cleft continues into the frontal region as a No. 12 cleft of Tessier. The location of the eyebrow coloboma distinguishes this cleft from neighboring clefts. The bony facial skeletal component of this cleft crosses the alveolus in the region of the lateral incisor. The nasal septum remains intact, but it may be distorted by surrounding malformations. Septation is present between the nasal cavity and the maxillary sinus, and notching is seen near the junction of the nasal bone with the frontal process of the maxilla. The nasolacrimal system is not disturbed as in the No. 3 cleft. Enlargement of the ethmoidal labyrinth results in orbital hypertelorism. Usually, the glabella is flattened and the frontal sinus is enlarged. The Tessier No. 12 cleft is the cranial equivalent of the Tessier No. 2 facial cleft.[14,17,18]

Tessier believes that nasal hemiatrophy, supernumerary nostrils, and proboscis lateralis are probably different degrees and forms of the same paracentral defect. These malformations may be associated with clefts No. 2 and No. 3 because of malformations in the ethmoidal labyrinth and the lacrimal apparatus.

The Tessier No. 3 cleft is a medial orbitomaxillary cleft that extends through the bony skeleton as a paranasal cleft traversing obliquely across the lacrimal groove. The frontal process of the maxilla as well as the medial wall of the maxillary sinus is often completely absent. The cleft lies in the area of the embryological union of the medial nasal, lateral nasal, and maxillary processes. The cleft is believed to result from a lack of fusion, insufficient mesodermal penetration, or failure of the nasolacrimal system. Through the soft tissue, the cleft passes across the lacrimal segment of the lower eyelid around the alar base into the nasolabial fold and traverses the lip and alveolar ridge (Figures 3.4a,b).[17,18]

The lip and palate deformities associated with the Tessier No. 3 cleft are located in the same region as the common clefts of the lip and palate in the Tessier No. 1 and No. 2 clefts. In the nasal area, the Tessier No. 3 cleft changes course and passes through the base of nasal ala. The mildest form of this cleft is represented by a coloboma of the nasal ala. The resultant defect can manifest itself as a distortion or absence of the frontal process of the maxilla. The vertical distance between the alar base and the medial canthus is disturbed, and the nasolacrimal duct is obliterated. Malformations of the oc-

ular region are usually characteristic of this cleft and include dystopia of the medial canthus, colobomas of the lower eyelid medial to the punctum, and hypoplasic, inferiorly displaced medial canthal tendons. Ocular involvement is variable and may be represented as microphthalmia in its severest forms. The Tessier No. 11 cleft represents the more superior, or "northbound," extension of the cleft into the medial third of the upper eyelid and eyebrow and then onto the forehead.[14,17,18]

The Tessier No. 4 cleft is a median orbitomaxillary cleft that traverses through the soft tissue Tessier No. 4 cleft almost vertically to involve the inferior eyelid; medial to the punctum, the infraorbital rim; and the floor of the orbit, medial to the infraorbital nerve. The cleft continues onto the lip between the philtral crest and the commissure. Superiorly, the superior portion continues into the medial third of the eyelid and eyebrow. As a result of the lateral location of the cleft, the nasolacrimal canal and lacrimal sac remain intact. The medial canthal tendon appears almost normal with respect to its direction and insertion. In the most severe forms, the range of anomalies can culminate in the development of anophthalmia. The cleft on the anterior surface of the maxilla passes medial to the infraorbital foramen and produces a bony defect in the medial portion of the inferior orbital rim and floor. The contents of the orbit may tend to settle into this fissure, resulting in orbital dystopia. In the complete form of the cleft, the orbital cavity, maxillary sinus, and oral cavity are all confluent. Posterior nasal choanal atresia is often associated with the defor-

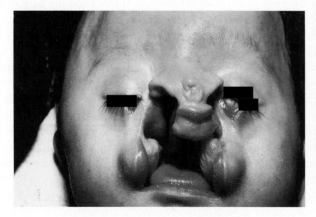

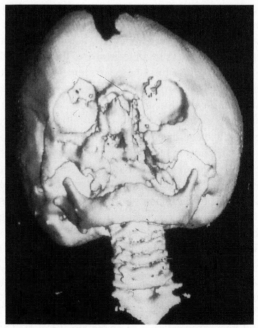

a   b

FIGURE 3.4 (a) This young Asian child exhibits a bilateral form of a Tessier No. 3 to 11 cleft with skin bridges along the lower eyelids, but with evidence of medial eyelid hypoplasia, lacrimal system involve- ment, and medial maxillary hypoplasia. (b) The skeletal involvement runs parallel to the soft tissue clefts and is evident as bony defects along the medial maxilla, palate, orbital floors, and cranial base.

mity. In bilateral cases, the nose appears smaller than normal, and the premaxilla is protruded. On the upper facial bony skeleton, the Tessier No. 10 cleft corresponds to the superior extension of the Tessier No. 4 facial cleft (Figures 3.5a,b).[17,18]

The Tessier No. 5 cleft is the rarest of the oblique facial clefts. This cleft also corresponds to the oculofacial II cleft and Morian III cleft. The cleft of the lip is found just medial to the angle of the mouth but not at the commissure itself. It courses upward across the lateral cheek to and between the medial and lateral thirds of the eyelid. The vertical distance between the mouth and the lower eyelid is decreased, resulting in a pulling of the upper lid and lower eyelid toward each other. Microphthalmia is infrequently present. The bony skeletal malformation parallels the path of the cleft. The alveolar portion of the cleft now begins posterior to the cuspid, and it is found in the premolar region. Passing lateral to the infraorbital foramen, the cleft enters the orbit through the inferolateral part of the orbital rim and floor. The orbital contents may prolapse into this gap and, therefore, into the maxillary sinus.[17,18]

Tessier No. 6 cleft is characteristically recognized as the incomplete form of the Treacher Collins' syndrome. The external ears can be normal or almost normal, but a hearing deficit is often present. The antimongoloid slant of the palpebral fissures is milder, but the coloboma of the lower eyelid

occurs at the usual medial third locations. The bony malformations of this cleft has set it apart from the complete form of the syndrome. In this cleft, the malar bone is present, but hypoplastic with an intact zygomatic arch. The cleft runs between the hypoplastic malar bone and the maxilla in the region of the zygomaticomaxillary suture.[17,18]

The Tessier No. 7 cleft is the most common and probably the earliest recorded craniofacial cleft, having been found in the cuneiform inscriptions by the Chaldeans of Mesopotamia in 2000 B.C. The No. 7 cleft is also synonymous with multiple other anomalies, including necrotic facial dysplasia, hemifacial microsomia and microtia, otomandibular dysostosis, unilateral facial agenesis, auriculobranchiogenic dysplasia, intrauterine facial necrosis, hemignathia and microtia syndrome, lateral facial clefts, transverse facial clefts, and oromandibular-auricular syndrome. Goldenhar's syndrome is also comparable in many of its features, but it also involves epibulbar cysts and vertebral anomalies.[17,18]

The clinical expression of this cleft varies from a slight facial asymmetry with minimal auricular malformations to severe malformations of the external auditory canal and the middle ear ossicles. Tessier believes the cleft is centered in the region of the zygomaticotemporal suture.[14,17,18] Hypoplasia of the maxilla, temporal bone, soft palate, and tongue has been seen. The parotid gland and duct can be absent, along with

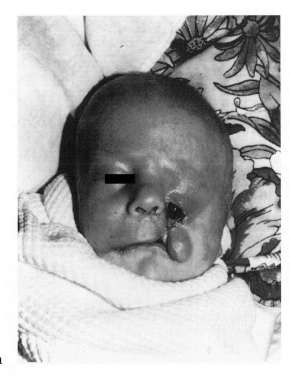

a

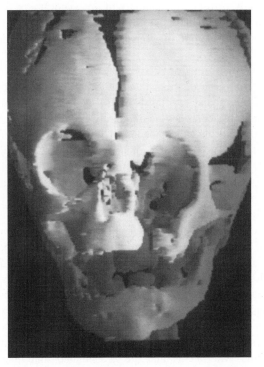

b

FIGURE 3.5 (a) A newborn infant with a Tessier No. 4 to 10 cleft on the left and Tessier No. 7 cleft on the right side of the facial structures. (b) The facial and lower eyelid tissues are very hypoplastic on the left, and the palate is cleft in line with the soft tissue cleft. There is widening of the right commissure and a soft tissue deficiency running along the axis of the facial cleft to the right ear. There is a left vertical dystopia and flattening of the frontal bone and hypoplasia of the cranial base noted on the CT scan corresponding to the bony skeletal cleft.

portions of the mandible and zygoma. The fifth and seventh nerves can be involved along with their innervated musculature, represented by weakness of the muscles of mastication (first branchial arch structures and trigeminal nerve) and muscles of facial expression (second branchial arch structures and facial nerve). As a result of the hypoplastic maxilla and the reduced height of the mandible ramus, there is a cephalad cant to the occlusal plane on the affected side. In the complete form, the mandibular condyle and ramus can be missing. There may only be a soft tissue ear tag or a soft tissue cleft extending from the corner of the mouth toward the ear. As a result of the hypoplasia of the zygoma, there may be drooping of the superolateral angle of the orbit with lateral canthal dystopia.

The Tessier No. 8 cleft corresponds to the temporal continuation of the orolateral canthus cleft of the AACPR classification and the commissural clefts of the ophthalmo-orbital malformation of Karfik.[20] The isolated form of the No. 8 cleft is rarely seen. The soft tissue cleft begins at the lateral commissure of the palpebral fissure and extends toward the temporal region. The lateral coloboma can be occupied by a dermatocele. The bony elements of the cleft lie in the region of the frontozygomatic suture. When combined with the No. 6 and No. 7 clefts, the zygoma is absent.[5,14,16–18]

Tessier has noted a unique bilateral combination of clefts No. 6, No. 7, and No. 8.[5,14,15,17,18] This combination is best demonstrated by the malformation known as Treacher Collins syndrome, Franceschetti-Zwahlen-Klein syndrome, or mandibulofacial dysostosis. The hallmark of this syndrome is the absent malar bone, which is the result of these clefts of the maxillozygomatic, temporozygomatic, and frontozygomatic sutures.

Soft tissue malformations associated with the No. 6 cleft result in a coloboma of the lower eyelid and deficiency or absence of the medial two thirds of the eyelashes. The infraorbital neurovascular bundle frequently exits the orbit and goes directly into the subcutaneous tissues. The No. 7 cleft results in the absence of the zygomatic arch, fusion and hypoplasia of the masseter and temporalis muscles, otic malformation (resulting in conductive hearing loss), medial displacement of sideburns, microtia, and mandibular deficiencies. Since the characteristic underlying deformity of the complete form of the syndrome is the absence of the zygoma, the lack of bony support results in the eyelid coloboma and the antimongoloid slant of the palpebral fissure. The No. 8 cleft results in the absence of the lateral orbital rim with associated lateral canthal dystopia. The abnormal configuration of the masseter muscle and temporalis muscle results in changes in the mandible. The vertical dimension of the ramus is foreshortened, producing a retrognathic mandible with an open bite. Microgenia and the accentuated mandiblar notch represents the lower third of the facial deficit. This complex of malformations completes the typical facies of the syndrome.[5,17,18]

The Tessier No. 9 cleft is a superolateral orbital cranial cleft traversing the lateral third of the upper eyelid and superolateral angle of the orbit. It is the first of the "northbound" cranial counterparts of the facial clefts. This cranial cleft (No. 9) seems to correspond to facial cleft No. 5, but both are rare. The cleft is centered in the superolateral angle of the orbit. This disrupts the orbital rim as the cleft continues into the frontotemporal cranium.[17,18]

The Tessier No. 10 cleft is a central superior orbital cleft located at the medial third of the supraorbital rim, lateral to the supraorbital nerve. It extends across the roof of the orbit and the frontal bone. The midportion of the bony orbital rim and the adjacent orbital roof and frontal bone are cleaved. A fronto-orbital encephalocele is often found in this area and results in a laterally and inferiorly rotated orbit. The soft tissue deformity is characterized by the coloboma of the medial third of the upper eyelid and can occur as a total lack of eyelids in its severest form. The eyelid and eyebrow are divided into two portions, the lateral portion being vertical and joining the scalp hairline and the medial portion being atrophic or occasionally absent. The No. 10 cleft appears to be the more superior cranial equivalent of facial cleft No. 4 with both clefts possibly having a coloboma of the iris.[17,18]

The Tessier No. 11 cleft is a superomedial orbital cleft. The coloboma of the medial third of the upper eyelid sometimes extends to the eyebrow and can extend into the frontal hairline. The skeletal malformations of this cleft have not been identified but seem to be the cranial equivalent of facial cleft No. 3. The cleft can pass lateral to the ethmoid bone and result in a cleft in the medial third of the eyebrow and orbital rim, or it can take an alternative pathway through the ethmoid labyrinth, resulting in orbital hypertelorism.[17,18]

The Tessier No. 12 cleft is located medial to the medial canthus passing through the frontal process of the maxilla and the nasal bone. This flattening results in telecanthus. The ethmoidal labyrinth is increased in transverse dimensions, resulting in orbital hypertelorism. The cleft passes across the lateral mass of the ethmoid and frontal bone lateral to the cribriform plate and olfactory groove. The cleft in the soft tissues extends from the root of the eyebrows and into the frontal hairline. The cranial equivalent of the No. 12 cleft is facial cleft No. 2.[17,18]

The Tessier No. 13 cleft corresponds to the cranial extension of the No. 1 cleft of the face. The distinctive feature of this malformation is the widening of the olfactory grooves and cribriform plate, resulting in hypertelorism. The cribriform plate can be displaced inferiorly by the paramedian frontal encephalocele. The severest forms of orbital hypertelorism can result from the bilateral forms of this cleft, when the ethmoid labyrinth is enlarged and extensive pneumatization of the frontal sinus exists. The eyelids and eyebrows are displaced laterally by the cleft. Another distinct feature of the cleft is an omega-shaped disruption of the hairline away from the midline.[17,18]

The Tessier No. 14 cleft, unlike the No. 0 cleft, is always associated with hypertelorism. The embryological malformation is attributed to the formation of the nasal capsule. As a result of the morphokinetic arrest of the movement of the eyes, the orbits tend to remain in the widespread fetal position. The result is a cranium bifidum or displacement by a large medial frontal encephalocoele. The crista galli is widened or duplicated, and the distance between the olfactory grooves is increased. The ethmoid bone prolapses caudally because of the increased intraorbital space. The frontal bone flattens and the glabella appears indistinct.[17,18]

This completes the axial dysplasias of the craniofacial syndromes proposed by Tessier. At present, this is the most widely accepted and used classification among craniofacial surgeons.

Van der Meulen et al. Classification

In recent years, a group of European plastic surgeons proposed a redefinition of terms and a new classification to facilitate communication among specialties. This schema also attempted to avoid confusion among the craniofacial syndromes and embryological pathophysiology. Their classification respresents the collective experience of five craniofacial surgeons (van der Meulen, Mazzola, Vermey-Keers, Stricker, and Raphael) working in three different countries (Netherlands, France, and Italy) (Table 3.1).[23]

The van der Meulen et al. schema proposes that instead of a clefting syndrome in the area of the malformation, there is actually a form of "dysplasia." Embryologically, regardless of the cause, an arrest of tissue (skin, muscle, or bone development) manifests itself as a "focal fetal dysplasia." The ultimate appearance and severity of the dysplasia depends on the localization of the area(s) involved and the time at which the disturbance of developmental arrest occurs (Figure 3.6).[24]

The van der Meulen et al. classification, the most recent of the new classifications, attempts to associate the clinical presentations of the craniofacial anomalies with the pathology arising from the maldevelopment at the embryological level. Their proposed craniofacial developmental helix is useful in relating the clinical and embryological anomalies. New terminology has also been introduced to explain the morpholopathogenesis, but at present, this has only begun to be analyzed and standardized.[5,6,23]

Section B—Craniosynostosis

A second major group of congenital malformations that has been alluded to several times during the discussion of previous craniofacial classifications is the craniosynostosis anomalies. These deformities are not the result of a cleft but a premature closure of one or more of the cranial sutures. The severity of the resultant deformity is directly proportional to the area of suture involved (Figures 3.7–3.10). The range of facial deformation can be minimal, as a ridge along the sagittal suture or as in a mild trigonocephaly deformity, with the premature closure of the metopic suture, to severe, as in the

TABLE 3.1 Van Der Meulen et al. classification.

Cerebral Craniofacial Dysplasia
Interophthalmic dysplasia
Ophthalmic dysplasia
Craniofacial Dysplasia
Dysostoses
Frontosphenoid dysplasia
Frontal dysplasia
Frontofrontal dysplasia
Frontonasoethmoid dysplasia
Internasal dysplasia
Nasal dysplasia
Type 1—nasal aplasia
Type 2—nasal aplasia with proboscis
Type 3—nasoschizis
Type 4—nasal duplication
Nasomaxillary dysplasia
Maxillary dysplasia
Medial maxillary dysplasia
Lateral maxillary dysplasia
Maxillozygomatic dysplasia
Zygomatic dysplasia
Zygofrontal dysplasia
Zygotemporal dysplasia
Temporoaural dysplasia
Zygotemporoauromandibular dysplasia
Temporoauromandibular dysplasia
Maxillomandibular dysplasia
Mandibular dysplasia
Intermandibular dysplasia
Craniofacial Synostoses

craniofacial dysostosis syndromes as in Crouzon's syndrome or Kleeblattschädel deformity in which multiple sutures are involved (Figure 3.11).[1–5,7,8,25,26]

Virchow, in 1851, was the first to coin the term *craniosynostosis* and presented an attempt to develop an organized classification system.[4] The word *craniosynostosis* has been used recently to describe the process of premature fusion, with *craniostenosis* being the result. At present, the terms are interchangeable. There are several different types of craniosynostosis (Table 3.2). Craniosynostosis may be either simple or compound. The simple form refers to the involvement of the suture being prematurely fused, whereas the compound form involves synostosis of two or more sutures.[1,3–5]

Craniosynostosis may also be designated as either a primary or secondary type. In primary craniosynostosis, the sutures prematurely fuse as a result of a genetic predisposition. In secondary craniosynostosis, suture closure is secondary to a known disorder, such as one of certain hematologic disorders (thalassemic), metabolic disorders (hyperthyroidism), and/or malformations (e.g., microcephaly).[4]

The last category defining craniosynostosis involves separation into isolated or syndromic forms. The isolated craniosynostosis form is present in patients who have no other abnormalites except those that occur secondarily to premature suture obliteration, such as neurologic or ophthalmologic manifestations. Syndromic craniosynostosis occurs in patients with other primary defects of morphogenesis (as in Carpen-

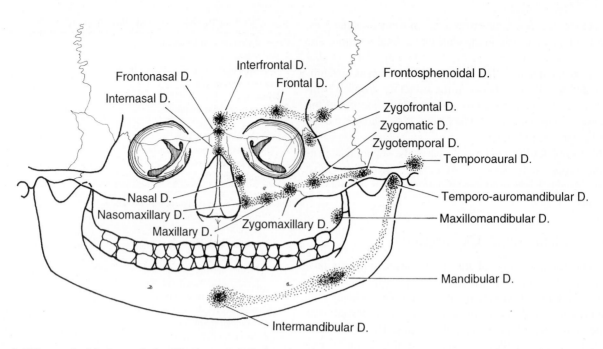

FIGURE 3.6 The van der Meulen et al. classification uses an S-shaped configuration to represent the embryological development and malformations in the craniofacial helix starting at the lateroposterior wall of the orbit to the lower face. The upper half of the helix encircles the orbit while the lower half encircles the mouth. The dysplasias in the upper half of the S may be associated with ocular and periocular malformations, clefts, or hypoplasias, while dysplasias of the lower helix are associated with clefts, malformations, preauricular tags, pits, and fistulas.

ter's syndrome, where polysyndactyly and congenital heart defects accompany the craniosynostosis).[4,5]

Three theories have been proposed for the pathogenesis of craniosynostosis. The first theory, proposed by Virchow, maintained that craniosynostosis was the primary event and the associated cranial base deformity was secondary to the craniosynostosis. The converse of this theory was proposed by Moss, who postulated that the cranial base malformation was the primary anomaly, resulting in secondary premature closure of the cranial sutures. A third theory postulates a primary defect in the mesenchymal blastema that results in both craniosynostosis and an abnormal cranial base.[4,21,25,27]

Regardless of the primary event, the calvarium reflects the results of a rapidly expanding brain. With a prematurely closed suture, the calvarial growth becomes inhibited in a perpendicular direction to the closed suture. This results in a compensatory overexpansion and growth in the areas of the normal sutures to accomodate the growth of the brain. Since the midfacial structures are attached to the undersurface of the cranial vault, alterations in the growth of the anterior cranium will be reflected on the developing face. The alterations can be unilateral, as in the distortion seen by the premature closure of a hemicoronal suture (plagiocephaly), or bilateral malformations, such as craniosynostosis of the metopic or sagittal sutures or coronal sutures that can also result in severe midfacial retrusion (Crouzon's syndrome).

Various estimates of the incidence of simple craniosynostosis have been made in the literature. The range extends from 0.4/1000 births to 1.6/1000 births. The former value is considered the most accurate estimation.[1,2,5,10]

Virchow's Classification

Historically, as in attempts at facial clefting classification, many attempts have been made to group various characteristics into an organized pattern. These categorizations have reflected the current knowledge, interests, and experience of the classifier. Virchow, in 1851, was the first to classify head shape based on specific sites of cranial suture synostosis as he observed from the examination and measurement of preserved skulls and not on clinical experience (Table 3.3). He also made an attempt to deal with partial synostosis as well as with involvement of the cranial base. This anatomic classification was abandoned in time because of the numerous narrow categories and as more was learned about the dynamics of craniosynostosis.[4–6]

Simmons-Peyton Classification

Another proposed classification was put forth by Simmons and Peyton in 1947, in an attempt to present a simple and useful system for the clinician (Table 3.4). Their objective was to establish important groupings, minimize duplicated terminology and disregard insignificant narrow or minor variations.[5,14,15]

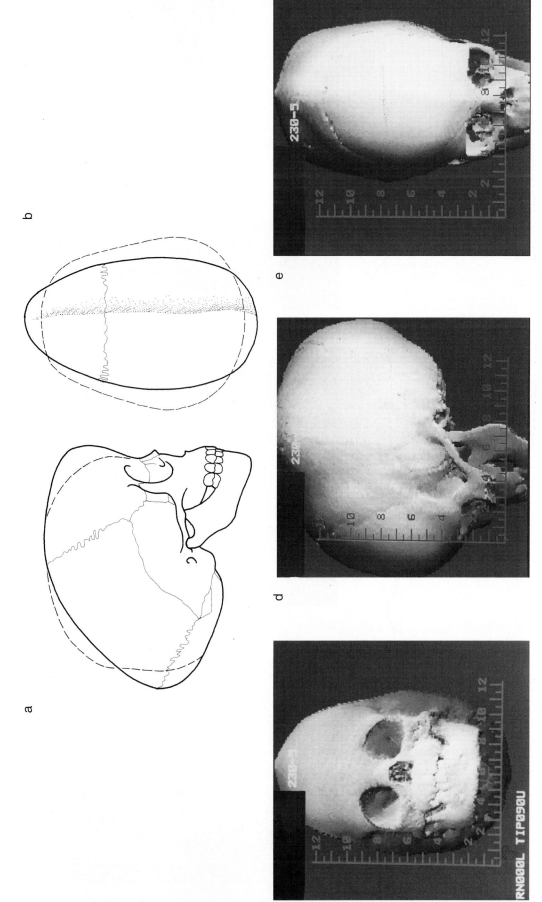

FIGURE 3.7 (a,b) The scaphocephaly deformity can arise secondary to sagittal craniosynostosis. This presents as generalized elongation and narrowing of the cranium. This also results in a temporal constriction and often a ridging that occurs along the involved sagittal suture. Bossing is noted both anteriorly and posteriorly in the cranium beyond the normal configuration of the cranium noted by the dotted line. (c,d,e) CT scans demonstrate the three-dimensional cranial contour of the skull with ridging along the course of the obliterated sagittal suture.

31

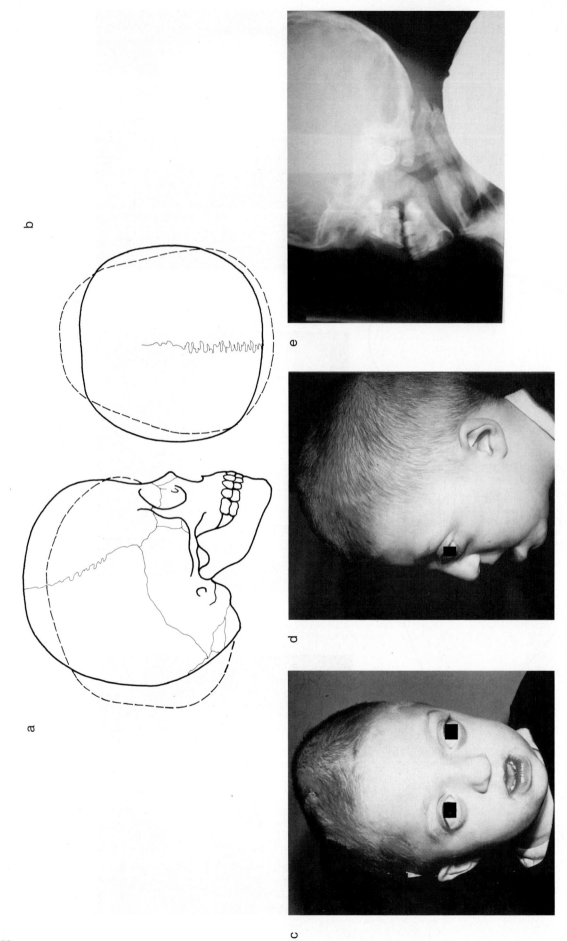

FIGURE 3.8 (a,b) Bicoronal craniosynostosis can be seen in Crouzon's disease and cranio-cephalic disorders of Karfik-Group D. This represents a typical patient with bilateral coronal synostosis and a "tower skull" deformity with increased cranial height and overincrease in the width of the skull. (c,d,e) Severe midfacial retrusion is also often evident in these pa-tients since the cranial base is often involved. The head is often wide with a decreased anterior posterior dimension (brachycephaly) as in this young child with Crouzon's syndrome demonstrating intracranial "thumbprinting" and class III malocclusion.

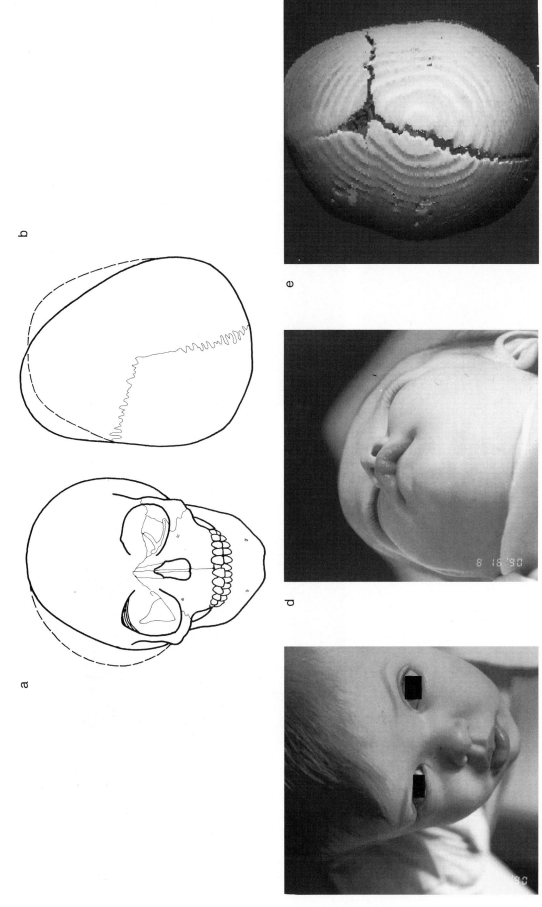

FIGURE 3.9 (a,b) Unilateral coronal synostosis results in a plagiocephaly deformity. In this figure, the affected right frontal area is foreshortened, the contralateral frontal area is bossed anteriorly. There is periorbital distortion along the right roof of the orbit and asymmetry around the orbital walls, sphenoid wing, and anterior cranium. (c,d) This clinical example is a young girl with left coronal craniosynostosis. Note the flattening of the left frontal area and supra-orbital rim. (e) The CT scan reveals the underlying bone deformity with patency of all the cranial sutures except for the left coronal.

33

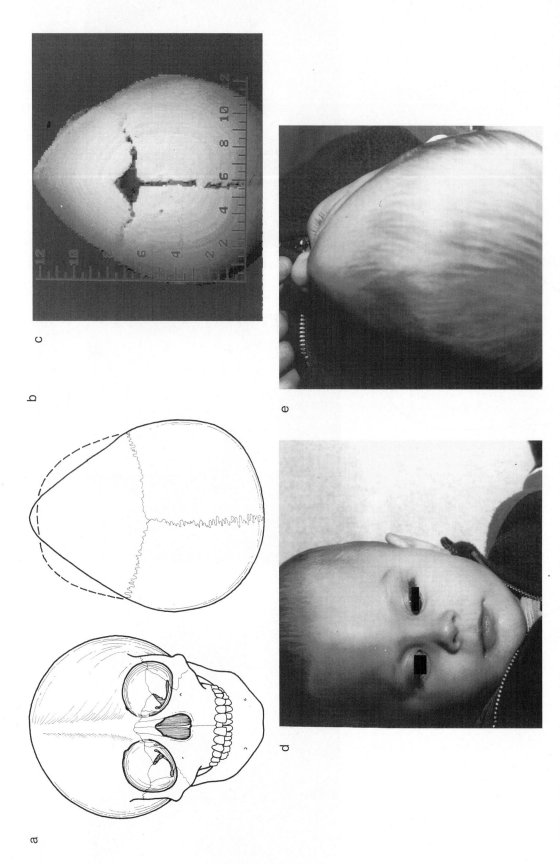

FIGURE 3.10 (a,b) Premature closure of the metopic suture results in a secondary trigono-cephaly deformity. This results in a triangular deformity of the frontal bone with central frontal bossing (keel) and constriction of the temporal areas. (c,d) The young boy reveals the same deformity as well as a degree of orbital hypotelorism. (e) The CT scan reveals the patency of the other cranial sutures with the anterior triangular cranial deformity.

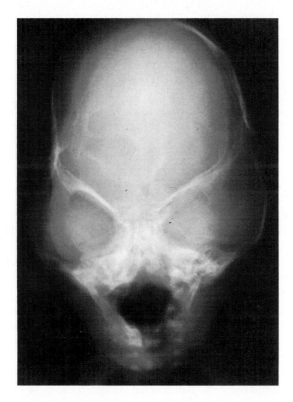

FIGURE 3.11 The Kleeblatschädel deformity is characteristically a trilobed cranial deformity as reflected in this case. Multiple cranial sutures are involved and severely increased intracranial pressure is evidenced by the cranial "thumbprinting."

Cohen Classification

As with the complex variety of clefting syndromes, the craniosynostosis syndromes present a formidable challenge to the embryologist, geneticist, anatomist, and the surgeon. Cohen, in an effort to categorize and describe these anomalies, proposed three specific classifications based on clinical similarities, anatomy, pathogenesis, and genetic transmission (Tables 3.5–3.7).[1–5]

Tessier Classification

Tessier, in 1981, because of his vast clinical experience put forth a classification based on involved anatomy and topography related to the craniosynostosis as well as other associated facial anomalies (Table 3.8).[25,26] This classification is practical for the clinician and surgeon because the craniofacial conditions are grouped for surgical purposes. Even though their genetic classification and ethiology may be different, their pathogenesis and phenotypes may be very similar. Due to the limitation of this text, a brief discussion of some of the common types of craniosynostosis syndromes will be presented.

Crouzon's syndrome is one of the most common and best known malformations characterized by premature synostosis of the coronal suture and, at times, the sagittal-lambdoidal sutures. The deformity results in a foreshortened cranial base

TABLE 3.2 Types of craniosynostosis.

Type	Definition
Simple	One suture involved with craniosynostosis
Compound	Two or more sutures are involved with craniosynostosis
Primary	Craniosynostosis of cranial sutures being the isolated problem or process
Secondary	Craniosynostosis secondary to a known metabolic or hematologic disorder
Isolated	Craniosynostosis is the principal problem or deformity
Syndromic	Craniosynostosis associated with other primary defects of morphogenesis

and a retropositioned frontal bone. The midface is hypoplastic and retruded, and the orbits are shallow, resulting in exorbitism. Mild hypertelorism is also part of the syndrome. Clinically, the appearance is one of psuedomandibular prognathism. If the exorbitism is severe, exposure keratitis can result. The retropositioned soft palate fills the oral and nasal pharynx and may result in airway obstruction. Intelligence is usually normal; however, if the malformation is severe, an increase in intracranial pressure can result, with concomitant secondary effect on cerebration and vision.[25,26]

Apert's syndrome, or acrocephalosyndactyly, is an anomaly in which the calvarium has a short, broad, tower-like appearance (turribrachycephaly). The coronal sutures are prematurely synostosed, but the sagittal and lambdoidal sutures can contribute to the deformity. The face has a high, flat forehead with a transverse ridge in the supraorbital region. The occipital bone is flattened, which contributes to the brachycephalic appearance. The exorbitism is milder than that seen in Crouzon's syndrome, although there is a greater degree of hypertelorism. Divergent strabismus and exophoria are also present along with some degree of mental retardation. The

TABLE 3.3 Virchow's classification.

  I. Simple macrocephaly (hydrocephaly)
 II. Simple microcephaly
III. Dolichocephaly (long-headedness)
    A. Upper central synostosis
       1. Dolichocephaly (sagittal synostosis)
       2. Sphenocephaly (sagittal synostosis with protruding bregma)
    B. Lower lateral synostosis
       1. Leptocephaly (sphenofrontal synostosis)
       2. Clinocephaly (sphenoparietal or temporal synostosis)
    C. Fetal synostosis of the frontal suture
       1. Trigonocephaly (metopic synostosis)
IV. Brachycephaly (short-headedness)
    A. Posterior synostosis
       1. Pachycephaly (lambdoidal synostosis)
       2. Oxycephaly (lambdoidal and temporoparietal synostosis with protruding bregma)
    B. Upper anterior and lateral synostosis
       1. Platycephaly (coronal synostosis)
       2. Trochocephaly (partial coronal synostosis)
       3. Plagiocephaly (unilateral coronal synostosis)
    C. Lower central synostosis
       1. Simple brachycephaly (cranial base synostosis)

TABLE 3.4 Simmons-Peyton classification.

A. Complete, early premature synostosis of the cranial sutures (oxycephaly, turricephaly)
　　1. Oxycephaly without facial deformity
　　2. Craniofacial dysostosis of Crouzon
　　3. Acrocephalosyndactylism
　　4. Delayed oxycephaly (onset after birth)
B. Incomplete early synostosis of the cranial sutures
　　1. Scaphocephaly (premature closure of the sagittal suture)
　　2. Brachycephaly (premature closure of the coronal sutures or to the coronal and lambdoidal sutures)
　　3. Plagiocephaly (asymmetric premature sutural closure)
　　4. Mixed
C. Late premature synostosis of cranial sutures after skull has reached nearly adult size so that no deformities and no symptoms result (i.e., nonpathologic requiring no surgical intervention).

TABLE 3.6 Cohen's anatomic/genetic perspectives.

Anatomic perspective	Genetic perspective
Specific suture synostosed of primary importance	Specific suture synostosed of secondary importance
Clinical description	Overall pattern of anomalies
Growth and development	Which family members are affected
Surgical management	

midface, again, is hypoplastic with the resultant pseudo-mandibular prognathism. Clefts of the soft palate occur in approximately one third of the patients, but invariably, a high-arched constricted palate is present. The anomaly of the hands and the feet in Apert's syndrome is symmetric syndactyly of both the hands and the feet, particularly in the middle three digits.[24,25]

The facial features of the Pfeiffer syndrome resemble those of the previously described craniosynostosis syndromes. The coronal suture is the primary site of premature synostosis, resulting in the typical hypoplastic midface with a turri-brachycephalic calvarium. The hypertelorism and exorbitism are mild, and the intelligence is normal. The hallmark of the syndrome is manifested by the digitial anomalies, again with

the thumb and the great toe being broad and directed in a varus direction.

In the Saethre-Chotzen syndrome, again, an acrocephalic configuration of the cranium is present as a result of premature synostosis of the coronal suture. However, the midfacial hypoplasia is not a feature of this anomaly. The face is asymmetric with deviation of the nasal septum and with the orbits at unequal levels. The frontal hairline is low set with upper eyelid ptosis often present. The nose appears beaked, or there appears to be an absence of the frontonasal angle. The extremity anomalies associated with this syndrome result in foreshortened digits with a partial cutaneous syndactyly between the index and middle digits.[25,26]

In Carpenter's syndrome, the anomaly results from premature synostosis of the coronal suture, causing an acrocephalopolysyndactyly deformity. When unequal sutural closures are present, there is an asymmetric tower-shaped skull deformity. This craniosynostosis disorder is characterized again by the anomalies present, and there is a tendency to have congenital heart malformations.[5,25,26]

The clover-leaf skull, or Kleeblattschädel anomaly, results in a trilobed skull. This results from premature synostosis of varying combinations of the temporoparietal, coronal, lambdoidal, and metopic sutures. Hydrocephalus is associated with this deformity, in addition to a hypoplastic midface with exorbitism. There is a high mortality with this anomaly.

TABLE 3.5 Cohen's anatomic classification of craniosynostosis.

Name	Premature sutural synostosis
Simple synostosis	
Brachycephaly	Coronal suture
Dolichocephaly	Sagittal suture
(scaphocephaly is also used interchangeably)	
Trigonocephaly	Metopic suture
Pachycephaly	Lambdoidal sutures
(this term is neither well known nor well accepted)	
Plagiocephaly	Unilateral coronal or unilateral lambdoidal
(some associate this term only with unilateral coronal synostosis)	
Compound synostosis	
Acrocephaly	All sutures
(oxycephaly is also used interchangeably with this term; some define acrocephaly as synostosis of the coronal suture plus one other suture)	
Kleeblattschädel, and other terms	Clover-leaf skull deformity and other combinations of suture involvement that lead to characteristic shapes

TABLE 3.7 Conditions with secondary craniosynostosis.

Metabolic disorders
　Hyperthyroidism
　Rickets (various forms)
Mucopolysaccharidoses and related disorders
　Hurler's syndrome
　Morquio's syndrome
　Beta-glucuronidase deficiency
　Mucolipidosis III
Hematologic disorders
　Thalassemia
　Sickle cell anemia
　Polycythemia vera
　Congenital hemolytic icterus
Malformations
　Holoprosencephaly
　Microcephaly
　Encephalocele
Iatrogenic disorders
　Hydrocephaly with shunt
　Malformation secondary to shunt malfunction

TABLE 3.8 Tessier classification.

A. Isolated cranial vault dysmorphism
B. Symmetric orbitocranial dysmorphism (with or without telorbitism)
    1. Trigonocephaly
    2. Acro-oxycephaly
    3. Brachycephaly without telorbitism
    4. Brachycephaly with euryprosopia and telorbitism
C. Asymmetric orbitocranial dysmorphism (plagiocephaly)
    1. Pure vertical discrepancy of orbital cavities
    2. Plagiocephaly without telorbitism
    3. Plagiocephaly with telorbitism
D. Saethre-Chotzen syndrome group
E. Crouzon syndrome group
    1. Regular Crouzon syndrome
    2. Top Crouzon syndrome
    3. Bottom Crouzon syndrome
    4. Trilobular Crouzon syndrome
F. Apert's syndrome group
    1. Hyperacrocephalic Apert's syndrome
    2. Hyperbrachycephalic Apert's syndrome
    3. Pfeiffer syndrome
    4. Trilobular Apert's syndrome
    5. Carpenter syndrome

The remainder of the anomalies classified and categorized by Tessier's schema are extremely rare, and complex malformations and are not within the scope of this discussion.[5,24,25]

Summary

At present, no single classification satisfactorily explains all of the various craniofacial malformations, nor is one universally applicable to all specialties. The better known, more recent, and more widely accepted classifications have been briefly presented and discussed. Better classifications have evolved and are continuing to evolve through communication, standardization of terminology, and the advancement of the science of embryology and genetics. It still remains to develop an all-encompassing classification that will clarify the complex morphopathogenesis of craniofacial malformations.

References

1. Cohen MM Jr. Perspectives on craniosynostosis. *West J Med.* 1980;132:507.
2. Cohen MM Jr. Craniosynostosis and syndromes with craniosynostosis: incidence, genetics, penetrance, variability and new syndrome updating. *Birth Defects.* 1979;15:13.
3. Cohen MM Jr. An etiologic and nosologic overview of craniosynostosis syndromes. *Birth Defects.* 1975;11:137.
4. Cohen MM Jr., ed. *Craniosynostosis—Diagnosis, Evaluation, and Management.* New York: Raven Press; 1986.
5. Dufresne C, Jelks G. Classification of craniofacial anomalies. In: Smith B, ed. *Ophthalmic Plastic and Reconstructive Surgery.* Philadelphia: C.V. Mosby; 1987:1185–1207.
6. Dufresne C. Classifications of craniofacial anomalies. In: Dufresne C, Carson B, Zinreich SJ, eds. *Complex Craniofacial Problems.* New York: Churchill Livingstone, 1992:43–74.
7. DeMeyer W, Zemen W, Palmer CA. The face predicts the brain: diagnostic significance of median facial anomalies for holoprosencephaly (arrhinencephaly). *Pediatrics.* 1964;34:256.
8. DeMeyer W. Median facial malformations and their implications for brain malformations. *Brain Defects.* 1975;11:155.
9. Dufresne CR, Corner B, Richtsmeier J. Categorization of craniofacial dysmorphology for the prediction of surgical outcome. In: Montoya AG, ed. *Craniofacial Surgery: Proceedings of the Fourth Meeting of the International Society of Cranio-Maxillo-Facial Surgery.* Monduzzi, Italy: 1991:41–43.
10. Gorlin RJ, Cohen MM, Levin SL, eds. *Syndromes of the Head and Neck.* 3rd ed. New York: Oxford University Press; 1990.
11. Gorlin RJ, Cervanka J, Pruzansky S. Facial clefting and its syndromes. *Birth Defects.* 1971;7:3.
12. Harkins CS, Berlin A, Hardings RL, Longacre JJ, Snodgrass RM. A classification of cleft lip and cleft palate. *Plast Reconstr Surg.* 1962;29:31.
13. Poswillo D. The pathogenesis of the first and second branchial arch syndrome. *Oral Surg.* 1973;35:302.
14. Kawamoto HK, David JD. Rare craniofacial clefts. In: McCarthy JG, ed. *Plastic Surgery.* Philadelphia: W.B. Saunders; 1990: 2922–2973.
15. Rogers BO. Rare craniofacial deformities. In: Converse JM, ed. *Reconstructive Plastic Surgery.* Philadelphia: W.B. Saunders; 1964.
16. Sanvenero-Rosselli G. Developmental pathology of the face and the dysraphia syndromes—an essay of interpretation based on experimentally produced congenital defects. *Plast Reconstr Surg.* 1953;11:36.
17. Tessier P. Anatomic classification of facial, craniofacial and latero-facial clefts. *J Maxillofac Surg.* 1976;4:69.
18. Tessier P, Rougier J, Hervouet F, Woillez M, Lekieffre M, Derome P, eds. A new anatomical classification of facial clefts, craniofacial and lateralateral clefts and their distribution around the orbit. In: *Plastic Surgery of the Orbit and Eyelids.* New York: Masson; 1981:118–134.
19. Lund OE. Combination of ocular and cranial malformations with craniofacial dysplasia. *Ophthalmologica.* 1966;152:13.
20. Karfik V. Proposed classification of rare congenital cleft malformation in the face. *Acta Chir Plast.* 1966;8:163.
21. Moss ML. The pathogenesis of premature cranial synostosis in man. *Acta Anat.* 1959;37:351.
22. Poswillo D. Orofacial malformation. *Proc R Soc Med.* 1974;67:13.
23. Tessier P. Orbital hypertelorism successive surgical attempts, material and methods causes and mechanisms. *Scand J Plast Reconstr Surg.* 1972;6:135.
24. Van der Meulen JC, Mazzola R, Vermey-Keers C, Sticker M, Raphael B. A morphogenetic classification of craniofacial malformations. *Plast Reconstr Surg.* 1983;71:560.
25. Tessier P, Rougier J, Hervouet F, Woillez M, Lekieffre M, Derome P, eds. The craniofaciostenoses (CFS): the Crouzon and Apert diseases: the plagiocephalies. In: *Plastic Surgery of the Orbit and Eyelids.* New York: Masson; 1981:200–223.
26. Tessier P. Relationship of craniostenoses to craniofacial dysostoses and to faciostenoses. A study with therapeutic implications. *Plast Reconstr Surg.* 1971;48:224.
27. Moss ML. The primacy of functional matrices in orofacial growth. *Dent Pract Rec.* 1968;19:65.

4
Etiology of Skeletal Malocclusion

Bruce L. Greenberg

Malocclusion is a developmental deformity which may vary from minor to major deformities of dental or skeletal origin, including systemic syndromic anomalies. It may be limited to the maxillofacial bones or encompass the entire craniomaxillofacial region. Because this book is devoted to surgical reconstruction of the craniomaxillofacial skeleton with the goals of achieving normality of health, function, and facial aesthetics, it is important to review how these skeletal malocclusions arise and are classified. Skeletal malocclusion is a set of human craniofacial morphologic characteristics that either exceed or exhibit deficiency of volume and proportion. It results in an improper relationship of the jaws—a relationship that distorts the normal balance of the face, because of difficulties with dental occlusion and the temporomandibular joints. Conceptually this book focuses on the aggregate effect of abnormal growth and development of the distinct skeletal units of the craniofacial anatomy as they relate to function and physical appearance. When considering this problem theoretically, however, the problems of growth and development break down into the interrelationship between human genetics and the response of the genome to the environmental factors that influence its phenotypic expression.

Genetic and functional factors are responsible for skeletal malocclusions and underlie the problems of vertical, sagittal, and transverse interrelationships. The human genome specifies the blueprint for the biochemical components that make up cells, and indeed the aggregate formation of cells as tissues with specialized functions. Genetic expression is the basis for human craniofacial development and represents the responsible mechanisms for how this developmental process may go awry.[1] During the process of craniofacial development, neural crest cells play an important role. They migrate into the mesodermal cell layer, becoming the neurovascular bundles, and the head mesenchyme, from which the craniofacial skeleton will form. Fundamentally, the quality and quantity of neural crest cell migration and the distribution of vascular networks during embryogenesis may directly impact favorably or unfavorably on the facial skeletal endowment.[2,3] At this early stage of human growth and development, genetic factors signal tissue differentiation. These genetic factors play the most direct role in setting the stage for the skeleton's formation. The differentiation of tissues into functional units relates to how the genetic qualities of the major functional cranial components interact physiologically with the functional environment to cause developmental changes and balance of the skeletal units.[4]

This type of genetic and environmental analysis can result in a greater appreciation of the skeletal malocclusions encountered in clinical practice. Physicians can also provide patients with a better prospective understanding of their condition. This has many benefits during diagnosis, treatment planning, treatment, and the posttreatment phases. A patient and or parent who grasps the etiologic causality of the problem will have a more accurate understanding of the condition and hopefully a more realistic set of expectations when assessing treatment outcome. Therefore, each type of skeletal malocclusion will be considered, with a discussion of the genetic and functional aspects of its development.

Most basically, all malocclusions may be categorized as Class I, Class II, or Class III, based upon Angle's classification (Figure 4.1). However, skeletal malocclusion must be considered in terms of the three dimensions of craniofacial anatomy—defined as the vertical, sagittal, and transverse planes of space. These parameters serve as the basis for the assessment of skeletal malocclusions and allow clinicians to understand that from a genetic and functional perspective, these three dimensions are clearly interrelated. An isolated distortion in one of these dimensions will impact upon the others to result in a clinical abnormality.[5]

Sagittal Interrelationships

Sagittal problems will exhibit either a skeletal open bite or a skeletal deep bite, with retrognathic or prognathic jaw relationships. Transverse problems may result in asymmetry, open bite, deep bite, retrognathia, or prognathism. The dimensions of skeletal anatomy are, as well, intimately interrelated.

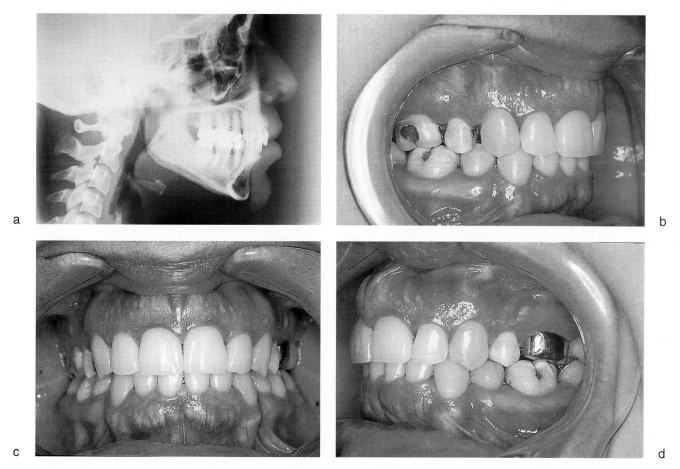

FIGURE 4.1 (a) Lateral cephalometric radiograph demonstrating Class I occlusion. (b) Intraoral view of right lateral aspect of Class I occlusion. (c) Intraoral view of frontal aspect of Class I occlusion. (d) Intraoral view of left lateral aspect of Class I occlusion.

Because of the interrelationships among the skeletal dimensions, a severe mandibular retrognathia can imply a transverse problem. The narrow part of the mandibular arch may occlude with the wider aspect of the maxillary arch (Figure 4.2). Similarly a prognathic mandible relates the wider part of the mandibular arch to the narrower part of the maxillary arch (Figure 4.3). Both of these situations imply a transverse occlusal problem resulting from either a Class II or Class III skeletal relationship. The Class II maxillomandibular relationship may also result in a vertical deficiency because of the geometric overclosure of the jaws that accompanies a severe overjet. The Class III will tend toward a vertical excess because of the underclosure that accompanies underjet and its inherent lengthening of the lower third of the face.

Vertical Interrelationships

Vertical and sagittal dimensions are closely interrelated. As the vertical dimension increases, the mandible will rotate distally, accentuating a retrognathia. On the other hand, a decreased vertical dimension will result in a mesial mandibular rotation accentuating a prognathia. Pure vertical problems usually do not impact on the transverse dimension greatly.

Transverse Interrelationships

The transverse dimension impacts on both the vertical and the sagittal dimensions because of the role of dental anatomy on skeletal jaw positions, which is also related to direct skeletal incompatibilities. A jaw width mixmatch, with its associated containment of the maxillary dental arch within the mandibular dental arch, will cause distal mandibular rotation and a resultant retrognathia with anterior open bite. In contradistinction, containment of the mandibular dental arch within the maxillary dental arch, a much more infrequent condition, will lead to mesial mandibular rotation and mandibular prognathism as well as deep bite. Asymmetric relationships of the jaws tend to result in unilateral crossbites, chin point deviation, and midfacial asymmetry, and will vary in their sagittal and vertical effects depending on such factors as dental compensations and condylar positioning.[6]

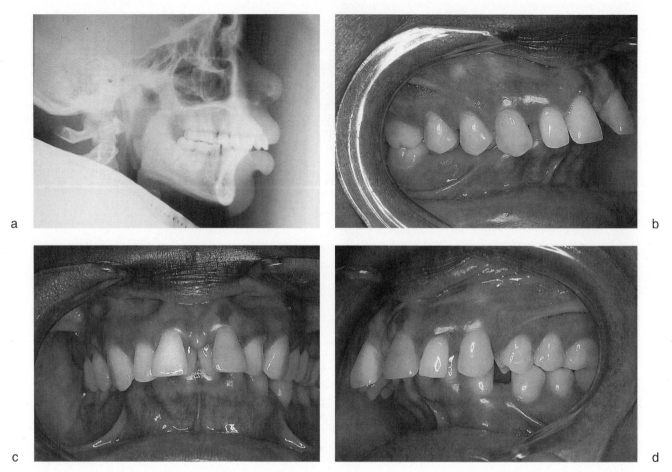

FIGURE 4.2 (a) Lateral cephalometric radiograph demonstrating Class II occlusion. (b) Intraoral view of right lateral aspect of Class II occlusion. (c) Intraoral view of frontal aspect of Class II occlusion. (d) Intraoral view of left lateral aspect of Class II occlusion.

Specific examples of how these genetic and environmental factors affect the craniofacial skeleton can be appreciated in ways that permit interpretation of skeletal malocclusion. Consider facial asymmetries such as the hemifacial microsomias. This is a good example of how early vascular imbalance may fail to adequately support the neural crest derived head mesenchyme leading to a quantitative tissue deficit. The reduced tissue endowment ultimately means a reduced volume of connective tissue mass and musculoskeletal formation. For bone as with adipose tissue, it is the cell count that is most important. The osteogenic potential that is derived from these early developmental processes ultimately contributes to cell numbers. Although the genetic factors seem to override the embryonic events of neural crest migration as a primitive influence, the later phenotypic expression of cell morphologic type and number plays a significant role in understanding the functional cranial components. Functions of the craniofacial skeleton include vision, olfaction, respiration, deglutition, speech, and hearing. Clearly there is tremendous sensory input and motor output occurring throughout the craniofacial complex. To the extent that, for example, the lining tissues composing these functional cranial components exhibit their genetic phenotype in a normal way, skeletal units will tend to follow suit.

If the genetics are unfavorable in terms of the quality and quantity of secretions following an immunohistochemical mechanism, the functional cranial component may be disturbed. The result may be abnormal, although obligatory and compensatory, skeletal morphologic changes that may have an unfavorable impact on skeletal development.[7] Perhaps the clearest application of this phenomenon is in the adenoid faces in which tonsillar and adenoid tissue masses along with the lining respiratory epithelium contribute to an altered pattern of breathing, jaw posture, tongue posture, and muscle tone. This leads to excessive vertical skeletal growth, distal mandibular rotation, mandibular retrognathia, and apertognathia.

The timing of craniofacial sutural closure and fusion will also be a result of the genomic expression and may significantly affect the symmetry of the entire upper, middle, and lower facial thirds, quite often demonstrating a significant torsion of the facial skeleton. This may often be seen as a significant deviation of the nasal septum toward the longer side of the face and of the chin to the shorter side of the face. For example, if the right side of the face grows for a longer period of time than the left side, the right eye will be observed to be higher than the left, the nasal septum will deviate to the right side with a bowing of the nasal complex around a cen-

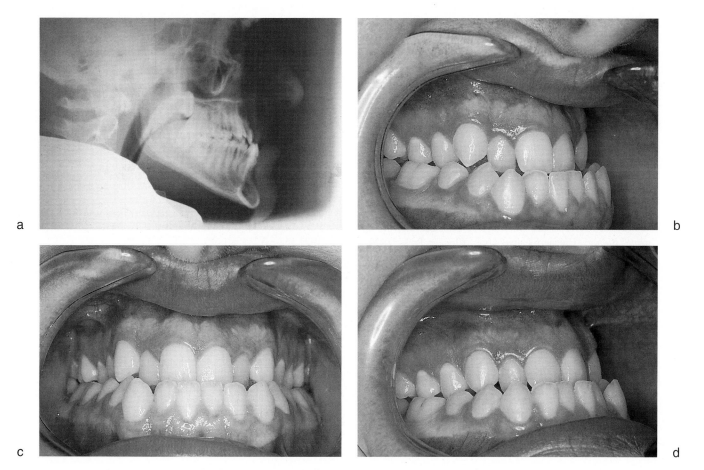

FIGURE 4.3 (a) Lateral cephalometric radiograph demonstrating Class III occlusion. (b) Intraoral view of right lateral aspect of Class III occlusion. (c) Intraoral view of frontal aspect of Class III occlusion. (d) Intraoral view of left lateral aspect of Class III occlusion.

ter of rotation being to the left of the midline, and the right mandible will be longer with the chin deviated to the left side.[8] All too often, deviation of the chin point with a resultant mandibular asymmetry is attributed to condylar dysgenesis, which is often incorrectly diagnosed. Bone scans later reveal normal metabolism. However, this does not mean to exclude the cases of actual condylar hyperplasia. The condyle may be considered one of the multifocal mandibular growth centers, which are characterized by epiphyseal bone formation. Genetic regulation of endochondral ossification in these structures may be unilaterally flawed to result in an asymmetric Class III malocclusion. Head and neck osteogenesis is also influenced by intramembranous ossification, which in the case of disruption of the growth potential of the orbital contents will lead to a consequent maxillary deformity. This may also be associated with potential overgrowth of the maxillary sinus without the balancing functional limitation of the orbit, resulting in maxillary hypertrophy and consequent changes in the dental occlusion. So we can see that there is an underlying interrelationship between what the genome programs and the environment may influence, which aids in our understanding the phenomenon of craniofacial growth and development.[9] For example, analysis of the cranial base angle pro-

vides another determinant of the jaw relationship and may be a contributing factor to skeletal malocclusion. A highly deflected cranial base will tend to position the craniomandibular articulation more anteriorly and inferiorly. This would contribute to the Class III as well as the brachyfacial pattern. The minimally deflected cranial base will tend to position the articulation more posterosuperiorly, favoring the Class II as well as dolichofacial pattern.[10] Clearly abnormal jaw growth and development may be rooted in fundamental genetic and long-term environmental influences, which more often than not are refractory to modification with functional orthopedic appliances and dentofacial orthopedics. Ultimately, the combined approaches of orthodontics and orthognathic surgery are the only means of correcting the skeletal malocclusion upon completion of growth.

Reconstructive craniomaxillofacial surgery requires the operating surgeon and other members of the team to restore the patient to the correct functional and cosmetic skeletal jaw, occlusal, and facial relationships and dimensions. Whatever the patient's preexisting occlusal relationship, it should be restored in the most optimal way. Corrective craniomaxillofacial surgery differs in its approach—selective surgical, orthodontic, and restorative dental procedures alter the skeletal jaw relationship to the cranial base, ultimately achieving the goals of a Class I occlusion with optimal facial esthetics and temporomandibular joint function. Utilizing diagnostic tests and skills to establish objective criteria based on a thorough grasp of the etiology of skeletal malocclusion allows for proper treatment planning for reconstructive and corrective craniomaxillofacial surgery.

References

1. Enlow DH, Hans MG. *Essentials of Facial Growth*. Philadelphia: W.B. Saunders; 1996.
2. Monroy A, Moscona AA. *Introductory Concepts in Developmental Biology*. Chicago: University of Chicago Press; 1979.
3. Moss ML. Neurotropic processes in orofacial growth. *J Dent Res*. 1971;50:1492.
4. Moss ML. Genetics, epigenetics, and causation. *Am J Orthod*. 1950;36:481.
5. Arnett GW, Bergman RT. Facial keys to orthodontic diagnosis and treatment planning, Part I. *Am J Orthod*. 1993;103:299.
6. Arnett GW, Bergman RT. Facial keys to orthodontic diadnosis and treatment planning, Part II. *Am J Orthod*. 1993;103:395.
7. Moss ML. The primary role of functional matrices in facial growth. *Am J Orthod*. 1969;55:566.
8. Dr. Robert L. Williams. Personal communication.
9. Moss ML, Salentijn L. The capsular matrix. *Am J Orthod*. 1969B;56:474.
10. Jarabak JR, Fizzell JA. *Technique and Treatment with Light-Wire Edgewise Appliances*, Vol. II, 2d ed. St. Louis: C.V. Mosby; 1972.

5
Etiology, Distribution, and Classification of Craniomaxillofacial Deformities: Traumatic Defects

Richard H. Haug and Jackson P. Morgan, III

Perhaps no defect is as emotionally devastating as a deformity of the face caused by trauma.[1] An individual who even minutes before led a normal life may have the focal point of their self-image permanently disfigured. This can leave enormous psychological as well as physical scars, even beyond those associated with congenital deformities whose victims have never known a different life. Yet posttraumatic defects have rarely been the focus of epidemiologic or demographic investigations. Their description has been relegated to individual case reports, anecdotal experiences, or review articles that discuss avulsion defects in general terms. Thus a description of the etiology, distribution, and classification of the traumatic deformity becomes a difficult endeavor based only upon intuitive reasoning and individual institutional experiences.

Classification

No uniform or universal classification system exists for the description of traumatic defects. They are usually described in general anatomic terms or by the mechanism of the injury. Generally, craniomaxillofacial avulsion injuries are described as mandibular, midfacial, or cranial. These are then subclassified as those with or without soft tissue loss.

Virtually every type of mandibular osseous defect is possible (Figures 5.1–5.3). The classification of each anatomic area follows the classification system devised for fractures by Ivy and Curtis as condyle, coronoid, ramus, angle, body, and symphysis.[2] These may or may not be associated with the loss of cutaneous or mucosal soft tissues (Figure 5.4).

The next major category of craniomaxillofacial defects is the midface. Because of the amount of energy required to avulse hard tissues, midfacial avulsion injuries are rarely isolated defects but tend to have damage involving multiple anatomic regions (Figures 5.3 and 5.5). These may involve any combination of the bones of the maxilla, palate, naso-orbital-ethmoid region, zygoma, or orbits. As with mandibu-

lar injury, these may also be associated with or without soft tissue loss (Figure 5.6). Additionally, considerations in the midface are the loss of such specialized structures as the nose, eyes, or ears.

The last major area in the classification of craniomaxillofacial avulsion injuries is the cranium (Figure 5.7). These include the frontal bone (and sinus), temporal bones, parietal bones, occipital bones, and base of skull. They may also be associated with or without loss of soft tissues. Consideration of neurologic injury is of paramount concern in cranial avulsion injuries (Figure 5.8).[3,4]

The other common system for classification of traumatic defects is by the etiology. Virtually all of the mechanisms of these types of injuries are of high energy with variations of the wounding mechanism's parameters. Kinetic energy is described as

$$\frac{1}{2}(Mass)(Velocity)^2$$

Handgun injuries are produced by low caliber, low velocity projectiles and are usually considered to be low- to moderate-energy injuries. Yet if a handgun is held close to the victim (Figures 5.9 and 5.10), all of the energy is absorbed by the patient. Rifle injuries are produced by low or high caliber projectiles fired at high velocity and thus are high-energy injuries. Shotgun injuries are caused by multiple low velocity, low caliber projectiles. When a single pellet injures the victim, it is usually innocuous. However, hundreds of pellets act collectively to increase the total mass and thus produce high-energy injuries, particularly at close range. Explosions are considered ultra-high-energy injuries. Occupational and industrial accidents are caused by machinery or large pieces of equipment. Although traveling at low velocity, they are so large that the mass is increased to a point that the energy transferred is that of a high-energy wound (or crush). The only other types of avulsion injuries are those caused by tearing (as in animal bites) or abrasion (as in a victim dragged by a motor vehicle).

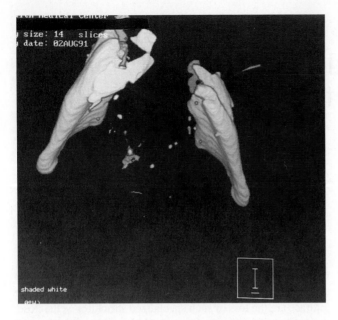

FIGURE 5.1 Note the loss of the entire symphysis region in this computed tomographic three-dimensional reconstruction of a close-range handgun injury.

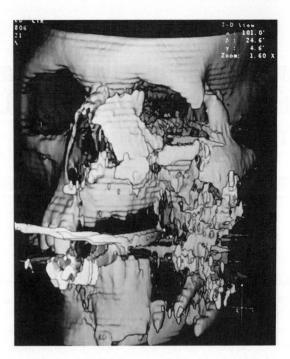

FIGURE 5.3 This three-dimensional computed tomographic image reveals a gross avulsion injury of the patient's mandibular body, ramus, left maxilla, orbital floor, and nose.

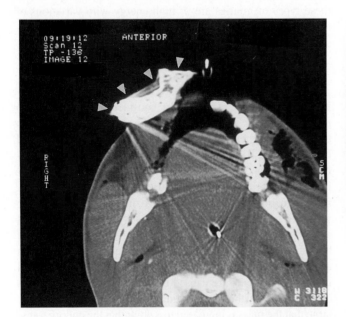

FIGURE 5.2 Note in this two-dimensional computed tomographic image that the patient's mandibular symphysis and body regions have been avulsed. They are found external to the patient (arrows).

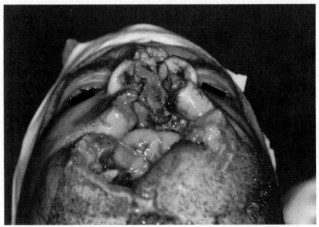

FIGURE 5.4 The soft tissues overlying the mandible (patient seen in Figure 5.1) have been avulsed along with the bone. Note that the skin and mucosa of the lower lip, upper lip, and portions of the nose were lost by this suicide attempt with a handgun at close range. (This case courtesy of Drs. Roderick Jordan and Anthony Smith of the MetroHealth Medical Center of Cleveland, Ohio)

FIGURE 5.5 This computed tomographic image of a self-inflicted gunshot wound demonstrates that the amount of energy produced will damage or avulse multiple midfacial structures. Note that the left globe along with the nasal bones, nasoethmoid region, orbit, and zygoma are absent.

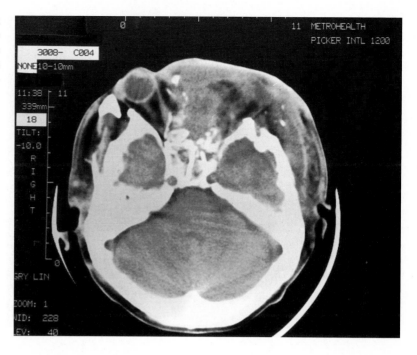

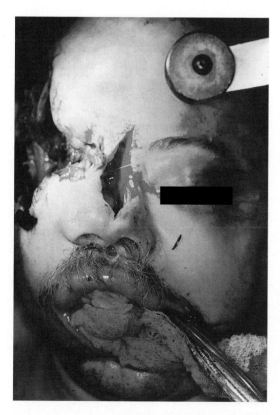

FIGURE 5.6 Note the soft tissue loss about the right midfacial region along with a total avulsion of the orbit (patient seen in Figure 5.5).

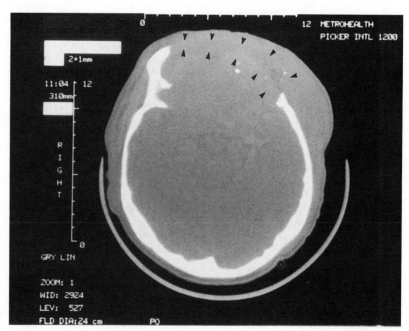

FIGURE 5.7 Note the large avulsed region of the frontal bone (arrows). The anterior frontal sinus table, posterior frontal sinus table, anterior cranial fossa, and portions of the left temporal bone are missing.

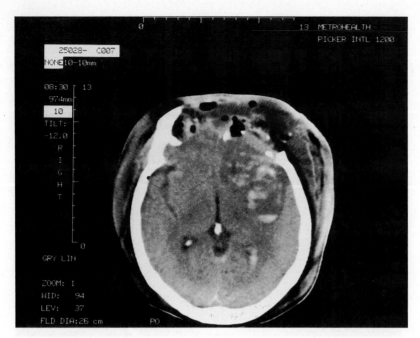

FIGURE 5.8 Note the gross neurologic damage that has been produced by this self-inflicted gunshot wound. A portion of the frontal bone has been avulsed. Numerous bullet fragments are noted within the brain and craniomaxillofacial soft tissues. Intracranial hemorrhage and pneumocephalus are also present.

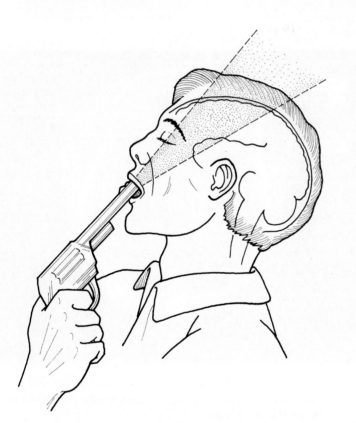

FIGURE 5.9 Handguns at close range yield high-energy injuries, which tend to avulse both hard and soft tissues. When held in the mouth, as is common in suicides, the midface and cranium are invariably affected.

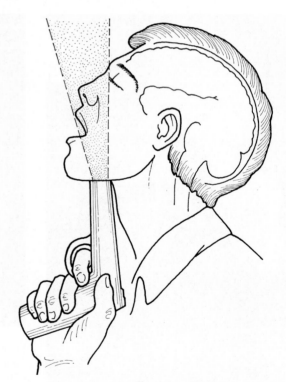

FIGURE 5.10 When the handgun is held at close range underneath the chin, the mandible is invariably affected.

Distribution

The actual loss of tissue associated with craniomaxillofacial wounds is fairly rare.[5] Although at first the facial tissues may appear absent, they tend to retract or roll under the wound margins. While statistics regarding the incidence of avulsion injuries are virtually nonexistent in the surgical literature, Osborn suggests in a survey of 9430 patients with maxillofacial injuries in the Vietnam conflict, that 9.4% exhibited avulsion of a significant portion of the mandible.[6] The trauma registry of the MetroHealth Medical Center (Cleveland, Ohio) for 1993 indicated that approximately 150 patients were admitted for the treatment of facial fractures. Of these, 66% were mandibular fractures and 33% midfacial. In this group, 1 patient sustained an avulsion injury of the mandible (1%), and 2 patients sustained avulsion injuries of the midface (4%). All were white males between 15 and 30 years of age, injured by firearms. It seems rational to assume that the patient profile of traumatic avulsion injuries would be similar to that of the general facial fracture population. Thus we can assume that this group would be mostly male (greater than 70%) and between the ages of 18 and 35 (mean age 30 years).[7,8]

Etiology

Handgun Injuries

Handguns propel low caliber projectiles at low velocities. Within 1 to 2 milliseconds after impact, a pressure wave from air in front of the missile distends the soft tissues up to four times the diameter of the projectile. Along with the temporary cavity is a permanent one that contains skin, clothing, necrotic tissue, and secondary projectiles. The projectile itself and the pressure wave of the temporary cavity cause damage to the muscle, bone, blood vessels, and nerves.[9] The muscles become contused, necrotic, and colonized with bacteria.[9] The blood vessels are crushed, ripped, displaced, or stretched.[9] This can result in arterial spasm, pseudoaneurysm, exudate production, thrombosis, and hemorrhage.[9] Nerves tend to become twisted with separation of nerve fibers[9] and become edematous. Gross comminution of the mandibular bone and drill-hole defects in the maxilla are common.[9] When a handgun is held beneath the chin or within the mouth, as is the case with many suicide attempts (Figures 5.9 and 5.10), all of the energy from the handgun is transferred to the patient. In this situation, the wound profile resembles that of a rifle injury with the associated avulsion of the soft and hard tissues. Those soft tissues which remain behind are compromised by edema, congestion, and contamination.

Rifle Injuries

Rifles project either low or high caliber projectiles at high velocity and are capable of causing injuries with a high amount of energy. The entrance wounds of these injuries tend to be stellate, with torn and irregular margins.[10] Exit wounds with rifles tend to be avulsive with defects that are more than two or three times larger than the entrance and which are stellate, saw tooth, or triangular in shape.[11] The temporary cavity in rifle wounds may be as high as eight times the diameter of the projectile.[11,12] Large amounts of muscle may be avulsed.

Large-diameter nerves are found to become grossly distended with rifle injuries. The myelin sheaths become protruded and deformed with axonal degeneration. Blood vessels damaged with rifles possess all of the characteristics outlined for handgun injuries but are also found to be more congested and thrombosed.[11] Veins reveal diapedesis of red blood cells as well as margination and pavementing of neutrophils.[11,12] Gross fragmentation and avulsion of the craniomaxillofacial bones are the rule with rifle injuries rather than the exception.[13] The remaining soft tissues are compromised by contusion, edema, congestion, and contamination with secondary projectiles and microorganisms.

Shotgun Injuries

Shotguns propel multiple low caliber spherical projectiles at low velocities. These hundreds of projectiles act collectively to injure the victim. Each individual pellet creates an entrance, temporary cavity, and permanent cavity characteristic of a handgun injury. A single pellet is relatively innocuous, multiple pellets more serious, but hundreds of pellets increase the mass of energy to create a devastating injury.[10,14] Because shotguns propel at low velocity, the energy dissipates greatly as the distance of the victim from the firearm increases.[14] Type III shotgun injuries (those within 3 yards or those with less than 10 cm of scatter) produce lethal avulsive injuries of both the soft and hard tissues.[15,16]

Explosions

Blast injuries are infrequently encountered. When they are, the victims are injured by multiple modalities. These patients initially sustain first degree burns from ignited explosives.[10] A blast wave of compressed air will then throw the patient through the air, which will create secondary injuries due to the fall.[10] Finally, the patient will be injured by the direct contact of exploded fragments.[10] These projectiles tend to be propelled at high or ultra-high velocities and injure with high or ultra-high energy. Victims close to the source of the explosion seldom survive. Those who do must be treated for burns, blunt, and penetrating injury.[17-19] The wounding profile will include both soft and hard tissue avulsion, compromised by the remaining soft tissues that are burned, contused, congested, and contaminated.

Occupational and Farm Injuries

Occupational and farm accidents have the potential for producing gross avulsive wounds or severe crush injuries.

Whether moving at low or high velocity, because of the magnitude of the mass of industrial machinery, the wheels or blades of tractors or combines, or the weight of steel I-beams and concrete walls, the injuries produced are either that of a high-energy impact or of a devastating crush. If the injury is that of a high-energy impact, large portions of soft and hard tissue will be avulsed.[20] If that of a crush injury, the vascular supply of the soft and hard tissues will be so compressed that large areas of bone and soft tissue will be rendered necrotic.[20]

Tearing Injuries

Bite injuries inflicted by the teeth of animals, tearing injuries caused by the blades of industrial machines, and ragged shearing wounds induced by machinery blades or saws can cause both avulsive injuries and contaminated crush injuries.[20–23] Animals such as dogs can bite with a force of 450 lbs/in^2. Their mouths are contaminated with a plethora of microorganisms.[21] Thus, grossly contaminated crush injuries can cause regions of soft tissue necrosis compromised with infection. In addition, the fangs of the teeth can avulse large areas of lip, cheek, scalp, the ears, or nose. Similarly, the blades of machinery or saws contaminated with airborne or earthen microorganisms can produce contaminated crush or soft tissue avulsive injuries just as the bites of animals can. On occasion, the underlying osseous structures may be penetrated, fractured, fragmented, or avulsed.

Abrasion Injuries

The last mechanism in the production of avulsion injuries is that caused by abrasion. It is extremely rare that a victim will be dragged by a moving object. Even if a victim falls off a moving motorcycle and slides, frequently the maxillofacial region is protected by a helmet or face mask. Under these circumstances the characteristic "road rash" explains the damage to the overlying soft tissues. Infrequently, the osseous tissues will also be avulsed.

Summary

From the limited resources available, it appears that the traumatic defect patient population is composed mostly of young males. These individuals routinely have been injured by high-energy wounding mechanisms. While the amount of energy should be a guide to the patient's evaluation and assessment, it should be understood that the clinician must treat the wound and not the etiology.[24]

References

1. Nordlicht S. Facial disfigurements and psychiatric sequelae. *NYS J Med.* 1979;79(9):1382–1384.

2. Ivy RH, Curtis L. Fractures of the mandible: an analysis of 100 cases. *Dent Cosmos* 1926;68:439–446.

3. Graham TW, Williams PC, Harrington T, et al. Civilian gunshot wounds to the head: A prospective study. *Neurosurgery* 1990;27:696–700.

4. Suddaby L, Weir B, Forsyth C. The management of 22 calibre gunshot wounds of the brain: a review of 49 cases. *Can J Neurol Sci.* 1987;14:268–272.

5. Powers MP, Bertz J, Fonseca RJ. Management of soft tissue injuries. In: Fonseca RJ, Walker RV, eds. *Oral and Maxillofacial Trauma.* Philadelphia: W.B. Saunders; 1991: ch 23.

6. Osborn D. Reconstructive surgery for maxillofacial injuries. In: Fonseca RJ, Davis WH, eds. *Reconstructive Preprosthetic Oral and Maxillofacial Surgery.* Philadelphia: W.B. Saunders; 1986: ch 10.

7. Haug RH, Prather J, Indresano AT. An epidemiologic survey of facial fractures and concomitant injury. *J Oral Maxillofac Surg.* 1990;48:926–932.

8. Vetter JD, Topazian RG, Goldberg MH, et al. Facial fractures occurring in a medium sized metropolitan area: recent trends. *Int J Oral Maxillofac Surg.* 1991;20:214–216.

9. Haug RH. Management of low-caliber, low-velocity gunshot wounds of the maxillofacial region. *J Oral Maxillofac Surg.* 1989;47:1192–1196.

10. Haug RH. Gunshot wounds to the head and neck. Topic 10. In: Kelly JP, ed. *OMS Knowledge Update, Part II.* Chicago: AAOMS Publishing; 1995:TRA 65–82.

11. Wang ZG, Fang SX, Liu YQ. Pathomorphological observations of gunshot wounds. *Acta Clin Scand Suppl.* 1986;508:185–195.

12. Wang Z, Tang C, Chen X, et al. Early pathomorphologic characteristics of the wound tract caused by fragments. *J Trauma.* 1988;28:S89–S95.

13. Suneson A, Hansson HA, Seeman T. Central and peripheral nervous damage following high energy missile wounds in the thigh. *J Trauma.* 1988;28:S197–S203.

14. Ordog GJ, Wasserberg J, Balasubramanian S. Shotgun wound ballistics. *J Trauma.* 1988;28:624–631.

15. Walker MC, Poindexter JM. Principles of management of shotgun wounds. *Surg Gynecol Obstet.* 1990;170:97–105.

16. Glezer JA, Minard G, Croce MA, et al. Shotgun wound of the abdomen. *Am Surgeon.* 1993;59:129–131.

17. Fackler ML, Bellamy RF, Malinowski JA. A reconsideration of the wounding mechanism of very high velocity projectiles—importance of projectile shape. *J Trauma.* 1988;28:S63–S67.

18. Ellis S. Maxillofacial surgery and the trouble in Northern Ireland. *Br Dent J.* 1990;168:411–412.

19. Phillips YY. Primary blast injuries. *Ann Emerg Med.* 1986; 15:1446–1450.

20. Cameron D, Bishop C, Sibert JR. Farm accidents in children. *Br Med J.* 1992;305:23–25.

21. Morgan JP, Haug RH, Murphy MT. Management of facial dog bite injuries. *J Oral Maxillofac Surg.* 1995;53:435–441.

22. Fukuta K, Jackson IT, Topf JS. Facial lawn mower injury treated by a vascular costochondral graft. *J Oral Maxillofac Surg.* 1992;40:194–198.

23. Marks RB, Fort F. Chain saw injury of the maxillofacial region. *J Oral Maxillofac Surg.* 1986;44:240–243.

24. Fackler ML. Wound ballistics: a review of common misconceptions. *JAMA* 1988;259:2730–2736.

6
Etiology, Distribution, and Classification of Craniomaxillofacial Deformities: Review of Nasal Deformities

John G. Hunter

The nose is the central feature of the human face, both anatomically and aesthetically. The normal, natural nose is made up of thin mucosal lining, sculptured alar cartilages, bone and cartilage struts that buttress the dorsum and side walls, and a conforming canopy of thin skin which compliments the face in color and texture.[1]

The nose is a pyramidal structure; its apex projects anteriorly, and its base attaches to the facial skeleton. The nasal pyramid consists of four parts: the *bony pyramid*, consisting of the paired nasal bones and projecting frontal processes of the maxillae; the *cartilaginous vault*, consisting of the paired upper lateral cartilages, which are attached to the deep surface of the more cephalic nasal bones; the *lobule*, consisting of the nasal tip, paired lower lateral alar cartilages, alae, vestibular regions, and columella; and the *nasal septum*. The alar cartilages articulate with the caudal edge of the upper lateral cartilages and the supporting septum. The nasal septum consists of the quadrilateral cartilage, perpendicular plate of the ethmoid, and the vomer, with minor contributions from the maxilla and palatine bone.[2]

In addition to its obvious aesthetic significance, the functional importance of the nose cannot be overemphasized. The nose plays major roles in humidification, warming and filtration of inspired air, immune function, and olfaction. Disruption of these nasal functions adversely affects an individual's sense of well-being and quality of life, as well as having significant health implications.[3]

Deformities of nasal structures are legion, ranging from subtle contour irregularities to devastating malformations or complete absence. Nasal deformities have been described as resulting from the following, among others: intrauterine and maternal (extrauterine) exposures; as components of hereditary conditions and craniofacial clefts; congenital cysts and encephaloceles; trauma in the prenatal, natal, and postnatal periods; tumors and tumor ablation; infections; and iatrogenic causes.

Regardless of etiology, significant nasal deformities can have lifelong consequences for those afflicted. They represent a formidable challenge for the surgeon seeking to restore nasal form, function, or both. In this chapter, the more common congenital, developmental, and acquired nasal deformities, particularly those involving the nasal bones, will be reviewed.

Congenital Nasal Deformities

Embryology

Congenital malformations of the nose are rare, with posterior choanal atresia probably occurring most frequently.[4] Although teratogenic influences may occur anytime up to birth, the sixth to eighth weeks and the fourth month of gestation are critical. Nasal anomalies arise as primary embryologic defects or as secondary to defects in other facial units, such as cleft lip and palate.[5]

An understanding of the normal events in the embryologic development of the face and nose facilitates understanding congenital nasal deformities, especially cleft lip and palate nasal deformities and the rare craniofacial clefts. The embryologic development of the face takes place between the fourth and eighth weeks of gestation. The midportion of the face develops immediately anterior to the forebrain by differentiation of the frontonasal prominence. The ectodermal nasal placodes arise from either side of the frontonasal prominence cephalic to the stomodeum. Elevation of mesoderm at the placode margins produces a horseshoe-shaped ridge, which opens inferiorly. The median and lateral nasal processes are formed from the placode limbs.[6]

The paired median nasal processes merge with the frontonasal prominence to form the frontal process. As the structures enlarge, the frontonasal process is displaced in a cephalic direction. The median nasal processes coalesce in the midline in the sixth week, while their caudal segments, the globular processes, coalesce as they expand above the midportion of the stomodeum. The premaxilla, philtrum, columella, nasal tip, cartilaginous septum, and primary palate arise from the paired median elements. The more cephalic frontonasal processes narrow to form the nasal dorsum and radix, while the lateral nasal processes form the nasal alae.[6]

In Utero Exposures

Either intrauterine or extrauterine disease may cause nasal developmental deformities. Exposure to maternal medications and illnesses during the sixth, seventh, and eighth weeks of embryologic development may result in deformities of olfactory and nasal structures.[7]

Extrauterine diseases, such as measles, chicken pox, and syphilis, are known to cause defective nasal development. Maternal medications may also affect the developing fetus. Exposure to hydantoin in this critical period may result in fetal hydantoin syndrome. Its features include midface hypoplasia and depression of the nasal dorsum, as well as heart defects, growth and mental retardation, cleft lip or palate, and epicanthal folds. Between 5% and 10% of children of mothers with seizure disorders taking hydantoin during early pregnancy develop the full syndrome.[8]

Another maternal medication implicated in defective nasal development is warfarin, an oral anticoagulant. Although it is well known that warfarin use in late pregnancy may result in fetal or placental hemorrhage, potential teratogenic effects of the drug were unappreciated until 1966, when the congenital warfarin syndrome was first described. This syndrome includes nasal bone deformities, stippling of bone, optic atrophy and mental retardation. Hypoplasia of the nasal bones is the most common anomaly reported. The nose is flat, the nasal septum is short, and a deep groove between the ala and nasal tip is sometimes present. The nasal abnormality usually results in breathing and feeding difficulties. The exact mechanism of warfarin teratogensis is uncertain. As low-molecular-weight warfarin can cross the placenta, the bone deformities are believed to be due to microhemorrhage into fetal cartilages, which subsequently heal by calcification, giving the bones a stippled appearance on x-ray.[4]

Nasal obstruction has also been reported in newborn children of mothers taking reserpine during the first trimester. In these cases, the cartilaginous nasal capsule, beginning about the third month, gradually becomes replaced by bone.[7]

Intrauterine exposure to ethanol in the first trimester of pregnancy may also result in fetal alcohol syndrome, a mild form of holoprosencephaly. It is characterized by a narrow forehead, short palpebral fissures, a small short nose and midface, and a long upper lip with deficient philtrum.[9]

Chromosome Disorders: Nasal Manifestations

Chromosome disorders can result from abnormalities of chromosome number, sex chromosome type or number, or individual chromosome rearrangements such as inversions, translocations, and deletions. Nasal defects are seen in many chromosome disorders.

Trisomy 21 (Down syndrome) is a fairly common chromosome disorder with an increasing risk of occurrence with advancing maternal age (1 in 50 at age 45). Multiple craniofacial anomalies are present, including a small nose with flat dorsum. Nasal deformities are also seen in the following chromosome disorders: Trisomy 13 (broad, flat nasal dorsum); 9p trisomy (bulbous nose); 4p syndrome (broad nasal tip); XXXY syndrome (saddle nose deformity).[8]

Nasal Deformities in Hereditary Conditions

Cleft Lip Nasal Deformity

One of the most common congenital anomalies of the nose is that seen in association with cleft lip deformities. Some degree of nasal deformity is present in all cleft lip patients, even those with incomplete clefts (Figure 6.1). While the cleft lip nasal deformity is usually characteristic, its severity varies with each case and is directly related to the extent of the lip deformity. In bilateral clefts, a double-sided nasal deformity occurs, reflecting the degree of anomaly present on each side (Figure 6.2).[5,10]

Components of the nasal deformity include defects of the alar cartilage on the cleft side, the septum, columella, and nasal tip, and the entire nasal pyramid. Maxillary clefting and hypoplasia and malpositioning of maxillary segments contribute significantly to nasal asymmetry. Anatomic and functional deformities of the orbicularis oris muscle also contribute to the nasal deformity.[10]

The etiology of the cleft lip nasal deformity is debated. An intrinsic defect or deficiency of growth of the medial and lat-

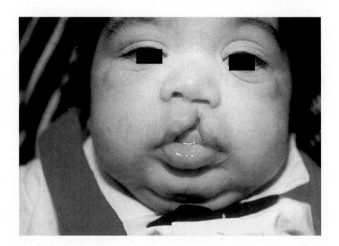

FIGURE 6.1 Unilateral incomplete cleft lip. Note characteristic nasal deformity.

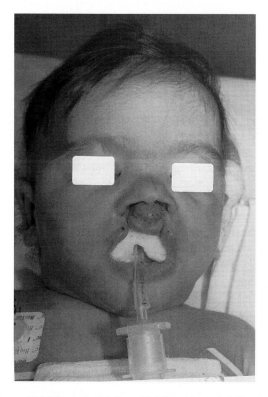

FIGURE 6.2 Bilateral cleft lip with bilateral nasal deformity.

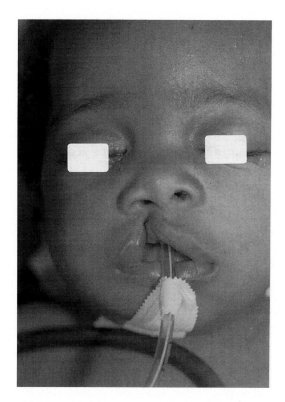

FIGURE 6.3 The nasal deformity associated with a unilateral cleft lip.

eral nasal processes, with an absence of mesodermal penetration of the soft tissues in the cleft region, has been postulated. Multifactorial inheritance and environmental influences have been demonstrated. The degree of severity of the deformity is related to the embryologic period in which the disturbance occurs.[10]

Cleft lip nasal deformities result from tissue deficiency of the cleft lip, a deficiency of the maxilla, or abnormal pull on the nasal structures. The role of tissue deficiencies extrinsic to the nose has been emphasized.[10]

The nasal deformity of a unilateral cleft lip is characterized by the following (Figure 6.3):

1. Deviation of the caudal septum and nasal spine to the cleft side by the unrestricted muscle pull of the normal side
2. Displacement of the alar base laterally and inferiorly by unopposed muscle forces, with retrodisplacement owing to maxillary hypoplasia on the cleft side
3. The nasal dome is lower on the cleft side and the ala flattened, with inward buckling. Increased nostril circumference results
4. The medial crus of the alar cartilage is displaced, and the columella shorter, on the cleft side. The columella is obliquely oriented, with its dorsal end slanted toward the noncleft side
5. The nasal floor is absent in complete clefts

6. The nasal bone on the cleft side is affected by growth and muscle pull. Unrestricted noncleft side pull deviates the cleft side nasal bone medially and vertically

The deformity of a bilateral cleft simply duplicates these deformities, adds the effects of an unstable premaxilla, and accentuates the lack of definitive columellar and philtral columns (Figure 6.2).[5]

Maxillonasal Dysplasia (Binder's Syndrome)

Maxillonasal dysplasia, or Binder's syndrome, is a distinct malformation characterized by a flattened nasal profile on a retruded base. The syndrome's etiology, although unknown, has been postulated to be either a congenital malformation or to occur secondary to midface trauma. A hereditary association has been reported but remains undefined. Prior to its description in 1962, the anomaly had not been clearly differentiated from other forms of midface hypoplasia, such as Crouzon and Apert syndromes, and posttraumatic nasomaxillary retrusion.[11,12]

The syndrome results in hypoplasia of the maxilla and nose, while sparing the malar region. The flattened nasal profile is characteristic. Associated with the nasomaxillary deformity is an excessively obtuse or absent nasofrontal angle, shortened columella, flattened alae, and class III malocclusion. The skeletal deformity causing the anomaly is typically a palpable depression in the anterior nasal floor and localized maxillary hypoplasia in the alar base region.[11,12]

Craniofacial Synostoses Syndromes

Craniosynostosis denotes premature fusion of one or more sutures in either the cranial vault or base. Most clinical observations are isolated suture synostoses that occur in a sporadic fashion. There are rare, inherited, distinct craniofacial synostosis syndromes that share common features, such as midface hypoplasia and facial and limb deformities, along with suture synostoses. Among the more common anomalies, such as Apert, Crouzon, and Pfeiffer syndromes, nasal deformities are commonly seen. Inheritance is usually autosomal dominant.[13]

The nasal deformities usually seen are hooked, flat nose (Crouzon, Apert) and flat nasal dorsum (Pfeiffer, Saethre-Chotzen syndromes). The nasal deformities are seen in association with, and probably secondary to, maxillary hypoplasia.[8]

Holoprosencephaly

Holoprosencephaly refers to a group of anomalies resulting from partial or complete failure of the anterior neural tube to form cerebral hemispheres with ventricles, so that there is only one forebrain cavity in severe cases.[9]

Holoprosencephaly is characterized by a wide range of facial anomalies, ranging from premaxillary agenesis through cebocephaly to cyclopia and ethmocephaly. The defects result from well-defined loss of midline tissues in the face, secondary to midline deficiency of the anterior neural plate, leading to small medial nasal prominences. Inheritance is mostly sporadic, but chromosome abnormalities should be excluded. Maternal exposure to ethanol has been demonstrated to be causative. Indeed, one of the mildest forms of holoprosencephaly is fetal alcohol syndrome.

Nasal deformities, as expected, run the gamut from complete absence (arrhinia), proboscis deformity, or cebocephaly (single nostril) in severe cases to the small, short nose seen in fetal alcohol syndrome.[8,9]

Frontonasal Dysplasia

Another rare anomaly with distinct nasal deformities is frontonasal dysplasia. Central features include hypertelorism, bifid nasal tip, or complete midline splitting of the nose. Other features seen include median cleft palate and anterior encephalocele. Inheritance is usually sporadic.[8]

Achondroplasia

Achondroplasia is a bone dysplasia characterized by short stature, large head with prominent forehead, midface hy-

poplasia, lumbar lordosis, and extremity deformities. A saddle nose deformity with short, flat nasal bones is present in most cases. Inheritance is autosomal dominant, but 70% to 80% of cases are new mutations.[8]

Miscellaneous

Numerous dysmorphic syndromes have nasal deformities as minor features. These conditions and the nasal anomaly present include the following: Rubinstein-Taybi syndrome (prominent hook nose with broad dorsum); multiple pterygium syndrome (saddle nose deformity); cerebro-ocular-facio-skeletal syndrome (COFS) (prominent nasal dorsum); Greig cephalopolysyndactyly syndrome (flat dorsum); tricho-rhino-phalangeal syndrome (bulbous dorsum); and Marden-Walker syndrome (flat dorsum).[8]

Rare Craniofacial Clefts

Craniofacial clefts exist in a multitude of patterns and degrees of severity. Although they often appear initially bizarre, most craniofacial clefts occur along predictable embryologic lines. Their exact incidence is unknown, and estimates of their occurrence vary widely. Bilateral involvement may occur. Among the rare craniofacial clefts, nasal involvement is relatively common.[6]

Two theories are most commonly postulated for facial cleft formation—failure of fusion of the facial processes or failure of mesodermal migration and penetration. Any mishap interfering with normal craniofacial embryologic development, occurring between the fourth and eighth week of gestation, may lead to cleft formation.[6]

Although a number of classification systems for craniofacial clefts exist, the Tessier classification[14] (Figure 6.4) is most widely employed today and will be used here. The following rare craniofacial clefts involve the nose:

No. 0 cleft (median craniofacial dysrhaphia). Midline cleft of the face. The cleft goes through the midline of the nose, with nasal septal thickening or duplication, and through the columella, maxilla, and upper lip. The nose is often bifid, with broad flattened nasal bones. Arrhinia or a proboscis deformity may occur. The No. 0 cleft includes most midline deformities described in other classification systems, including frontonasal dysplasia and holoprosencephaly. Cephalic continuation of the cleft, with cranial involvement, is the No. 14 cleft.

No. 1 cleft (paramedian craniofacial cleft). The No. 1 cleft passes through the dome of the alar cartilage with notching of the dome region of the nostril. The skeletal component of the cleft passes between the nasal bone and the frontal process of the maxilla. Although the septum is spared, the nasal bone on the involved side may be absent.

No. 2 cleft. The No. 2 cleft may be a transition between the No. 1 and No. 3 clefts. The cleft is slightly more lateral

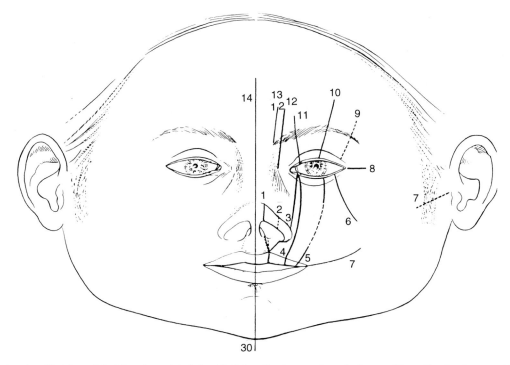

FIGURE 6.4 Tessier classification of facial and cranial clefts. Cleft localization on the soft tissues. (From Tessier, by permission of *J Maxillofac Surg.* 1976;4:69–92)

than the No. 1 cleft. The lateral aspect of the nose is flattened and the nasal bridge is broad.

No. 3 cleft (oculonasal cleft). The No. 3 cleft is a medial orbitomaxillary cleft extending through the lacrimal portion of the lower eyelid. The cleft undermines the base of the nasal ala. Hypoplasia of the lateral aspect of the nose is evident.[14]

Nasal Gliomas and Encephaloceles

Nasal gliomas and encephaloceles are rarely lesions with similar appearance and embryogenesis. Gliomas are deposits of cranial tissue in an extradural site, which have not maintained an attachment to the central nervous system. Approximately 15% of gliomas have a fibrous connection to the subarachnoid space. Encephaloceles maintain a connection to the central nervous system but are histologically identical to gliomas.[5]

An encephalocele is a protrusion of part of the cranial contents through a defect in the skull. The mass may contain meninges (meningocele), meninges and brain (meningoencephalocele), or meninges, brain and part of the ventricular system (meningoencephalocystocele).[15]

Nasal Encephalocele

The site of the defect in nasal encephalocele development is between the frontal and ethmoid bones, corresponding to the foramen cecum. It has been suggested that in the development of nasal encephaloceles the cranial content protrusion exits first, with subsequent bone formation around it.[15]

The bony defects associated with frontal and nasal encephaloceles have been included in many craniofacial classification systems. Frontonasal encephaloceles may be classified as Tessier No. 14 clefts.[14]

Nasal encephaloceles are classified into three groups according to the site of facial protrusion: nasofrontal, nasoethmoidal, or nasoorbital:

Nasofrontal type. The protrusion passes through a defect in the frontoethmoidal junction and passes directly forward between the frontal and nasal bones.

Nasoethmoidal type. The protrusion is lower and passes through a defect in the frontoethmoidal junction, emerging between the nasal bones and the upper lateral cartilages. Variations of this defect include nasal gliomas and midline nasal cysts and sinuses.

Nasoorbital type. The protrusion passes from the frontoethmoidal junction down behind the nasal bones, then extending laterally through a defect between the lacrimal bone and the frontal process of the maxilla. The lesion presents as a protrusion in the soft tissue between the nose and the lower eyelid.[15,16]

Lower nasofrontal and nasoethmoidal encephaloceles increase the distance between the frontal and nasal bones or between the nasal bones and the nasal cartilages, giving rise to a long-appearing nose. Furthermore, by displacing the medial orbital wall laterally, telecanthus or true hypertelorism may occur. Other clinical features include either soft tissue swelling in response to the protrusion or a wrinkled area due to collapse of the encephalocele.[15]

The prognosis for patients with nasal encephaloceles is excellent. Any brain tissue involved is from the frontal lobe and its sacrifice is not associated with significant neurological deficits.[15,16]

Nasal Gliomas

Most nasal gliomas are noticed at birth or in early childhood. They may be extranasal (60%), intranasal (30%), or combined intranasal and extranasal (10%). Extranasal gliomas are smooth, firm compressible masses that usually occur along the nasomaxillary suture or glabella. They occasionally occur in the nasal midline. Unlike encephaloceles, extranasal gliomas rarely cause bony defects. Intranasal gliomas may result in nasal airway obstruction or septal deviation. They appear as firm, noncompressible polypoid masses within the nasal cavity. Widening of the nasal bony pyramid and hypertelorism are possible with large gliomas.[5]

Nasal Dermoids

Nasal dermoids are congenital ectodermal cysts seen at or shortly after birth. They comprise between 1% and 2.5% of all dermoids. Being uncommon, diagnosis is often delayed. The time lag to diagnosis allows growth and increases the probability of infection, thereby complicating definitive removal.[17]

Nasal dermoid cysts contain skin appendages—hair follicles, sweat glands, and sebaceous glands. They represent areas of embryonal epithelium that survive along nasal bone fusion lines. A true dermoid cyst may occur subcutaneously on the nasal dorsum superficial to the nasal bones without a cutaneous opening. They therefore appear as slowly enlarging masses that may gradually deform the underlying nasal skeleton. However, a dermoid sinus, with or without a cyst, is an extensive lesion extending into nasal cartilage and bone. The dermoid cyst with sinus is usually visible at birth, and its punctum is usually located at the nasal osteocartilaginous junction. Discharge of casseous material and the presence of a hair tuft are diagnostic. Deep extension of the sinus tract occurs in 45% of cases. It may be predicted when nasal bone splaying or hypertelorism are present.[5,7]

Although very uncommon, intracranial extension of nasal dermoids through the cribiform plate may occur. Nasal dermoids may result in significant deformities, including dorsal saddling, open-roof deformity, and extensive scarring.[17]

Nasal Injuries

Nasal Trauma in the Prenatal and Natal Periods

Injuries to the nose, secondary to pressure effects, occur more often than is commonly appreciated during pregnancy and parturition.[7,18] Dislocation of the nasal septum may influence both the quantitative and qualitative development of maxillary, premaxillary, and nasal structures. Facial asymmetries and dental malocclusions may result.[7]

Persistent in utero pressure may result in fetal compression effects. Fetal compression may cause a number of deformities, including nasal-tip depression, saddle-nose deformity, micrognathia, craniostenosis, cleft deformities, and positional deformities of the limbs. Maternal uterus malformations are a common association.[8]

Owing to its prominent location, the nose is at particular risk to injury during the birth process. Of vaginally delivered white babies, about 7% have marked nasal deformities and 30% to 50% have temporary nasal flattening at birth. The temporary flattening results from dislocation of the septum during parturition; the degree of compression and resulting flattening is a function of the relationship between fetal head size and maternal pelvis size.[7]

Two basic types of septal deformity are seen in the newborn: anterior nasal deformity and combined septal deformity. These deformities may occur independently or together. They are considered to be acquired from different types of pressure on the fetus during pregnancy or parturition[18]:

The anterior nasal deformity is due to direct trauma and occurs in approximately 4% of normal vaginal deliveries. It is rarely seen following cesarean section. It is usually associated with asymmetry of the external nares, bending of the anterior septal cartilage, and distortion of the bony nasal pyramid and the septal cartilage-nasal spine junction. Minor deformity and cartilage bending is usually self-reducing. If the deformity persists beyond three days, however, deformity of the nasal bones is also present.

The combined septal deformity is a true facial deformity, caused by compression of the maxilla. The result is malocclusion, elevation of the palatal arch, and compression of the septum against the base of the skull. The orientation of the distorting pressure forces determines the type and degree of deformity seen. Manipulation is required to expand the maxilla and straighten and realign the septum. Indications for manipulation are stuffy nose, respiratory problems and cyanotic attacks, feeding problems, and sticky, infected eyes.[18]

Nasal Injuries in Childhood

As the most exposed and prominent feature of the face, the nose naturally bears the brunt of many injuring forces. It is, in fact, the most frequently injured facial structure.[19] Nasal injuries in childhood are often so seemingly trivial that neither the mother nor the child remembers when they occurred. Apparently mild injuries may result in a poorly functioning nose, a major aesthetic deformity later in life, or both. Early injuries are frequently difficult to diagnose. They may influence developmental patterns that affect function as the child matures. External nasal deformities seen in adulthood may result from a combination of apparently minor childhood injuries and growth factors.[7] The adverse consequences of nasal injuries during childhood is also reflected by the observation in a large series reviewing septal deformities present at birth that the incidence of straight septa was 42%, while in adult surveys, only approximately 20% are straight.[18]

Nasal injuries in childhood, as noted earlier, frequently have a profound effect on subsequent nasomaxillary growth and development, even after accurate diagnosis and proper treatment. Any child presenting with a nasal injury must also be evaluated for the presence of a septal hematoma. A septal hematoma presents as a bulging collection between the septal cartilage and overlying mucoperichondrium, and it may obstruct the nasal airway. If it is not promptly evacuated, pressure necrosis of the septal cartilage, with possible subsequent collapse of the nasal dorsum, may occur, resulting in saddle nose deformity.[20]

Septal abscess is an uncommon but serious cause of nasal deformities in children. Septal abscesses are usually the result of untreated or inadequately treated septal hematomas, which subsequently become infected. Marked nasoseptal destruction involving both the cartilaginous septum and the upper lateral cartilages may result.[7]

When cartilage is destroyed by hematoma or abscess, it is replaced by fibrous tissue. Scar retraction and loss of support of the lower two-thirds of the nose results in saddling of the dorsum, retraction of the columella, and widening of the alar base. Traumatic loss of the cartilaginous septum in early childhood may also cause maxillary hypoplasia. Injuries to the septum may also lead to buckling and twisting or cartilaginous hypertrophy with resultant nasal airway obstruction.

Facial fractures in adults, especially those of the midface, tend to be fragmented, whereas incomplete fractures predominate in childhood. Only 1% of facial fractures occur before age six; 5% occur prior to age 12. The frequency, distribution, and pattern of facial bone fractures begin to mirror those observed in adulthood by early adolescence. In most large series, fractures of the nasal bones and mandible account for the majority of pediatric maxillofacial fractures.[20] Although bony injuries are frequently discussed, injuries to the cartilaginous portions of the nose occur much more frequently than fractures in children, and, as stated earlier, may have a profound effect on subsequent development.

Nasal dorsum hematomas occur less frequently than septal hematomas, but if inadequately treated, they may result in significant nasal deformity. They usually result from direct blunt trauma to the dorsum with avulsion of the upper lateral cartilages from the nasal bones. Subsequent dissecting bleeding occurs. Pressure necrosis of the underlying nasal bone and/or upper lateral cartilage can result in depression or saddling.[7]

Nasal Injuries in Adolescence and Adulthood

Nasal fractures are said to account for 39% of all facial fractures. One extensive survey demonstrated an annual incidence of 53.2 per 100,000 population.[21,22] Although considered a relatively unimportant injury, optimal treatment of nasal fractures is needed to prevent long-term cosmetic and functional deformities (Figure 6.5).[21]

Blunt trauma caused by assault or fighting, motor vehicle accidents, and sports injuries is the most common cause of nasal fractures in adults.[19] Lateral fractures (Figures 6.6a,b) (66%), linear fractures (20%), and frontal fractures (13%) are most commonly observed. Septal fractures occur approximately 14% of the time, always in association with a fracture of the external nose (Figure 6.7).[22]

Closed reduction of depressed or deviated nasal fractures is the norm, with no manipulation required for linear fractures. Long-term follow-up following fracture reduction, compared with a noninjured control group, revealed that secondary deformities—saddling or dorsal hump formation—occurred infrequently and that most deformities seen were of little consequence.[21]

Nasal Tumors

Primary tumors of the skin—basal cell carcinoma, squamous cell carcinoma, and malignant melanoma—are fairly frequent causes of nasal deformity, either as a result of direct invasion of underlying nasal structures or as a consequence of tumor

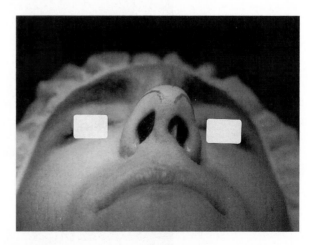

FIGURE 6.5 Cosmetic and functional deformity resulting from untreated nasal fracture. Note deviation of the nasal lobule to the left, with displacement of the caudal cartilaginous septum.

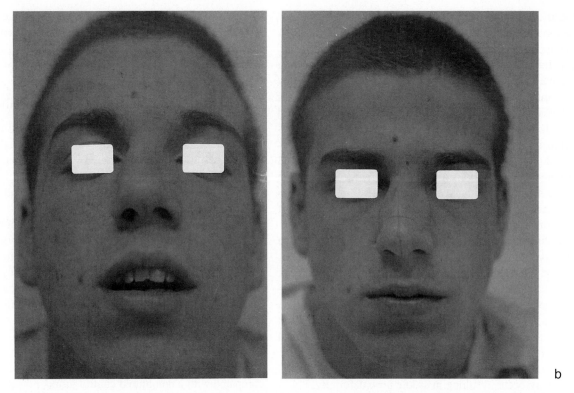

FIGURE 6.6 (a,b) Visible nasal deformity after lateral fracture. Note deviation of the nasal pyramid to the right following blunt trauma.

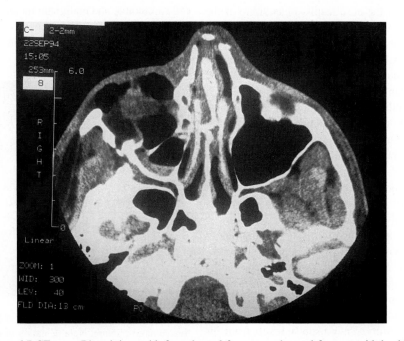

FIGURE 6.7 CT scan. Blunt injury with frontal nasal fracture and septal fracture with buckling.

ablation. Tumor invasion or surgical resection of the various nasal subunits up to total nasal amputation may be seen.[23]

Primary nasal tumors, however, are quite rare, with an annual incidence of less than 1 per 100,000 population in the United States. Squamous cell carcinoma is the most common primary malignant tumor of the nose. Squamous cell carcinoma can originate from the vestibule, lateral nasal wall, turbinates, meatus, or septum. Adenocarcinoma, chondrosarcoma, primary nasal malignant melanoma, and hemangiopericytoma are very rare nasal malignancies.[24] As with the more common overlying skin tumors, primary nasal malignancies and their ablation may result in significant nasoseptal deformity.

Benign tumors of the nose are even rarer than malignant lesions. In decreasing order of frequency, the more common benign nasal tumors are osteoma, hemangioma, papilloma, and angiofibroma.[24]

Nasal bone hemangiomas may be bony or mixed bony and soft tissue. They present as slowly enlarging masses at the nasal radix. Destruction of the involved nasal bone may occur, and ablation requires nasal bone resection.[25]

Nasal Deformities Resulting from Systemic Disease

Autoimmune disorders and infectious agents are often overlooked and poorly understood causes of nasal deformity and tissue destruction. Systemic diseases with nasal manifestations are often insidious in their early presentation, frequently resulting in delayed diagnosis and treatment. Systemic diseases with nasal manifestations are characterized as follows: autoimmune and connective tissue, lymphoma-like, granulomatous, and infectious.[26]

Systemic diseases with potentially deforming nasoseptal manifestations include:

Wegener's granulomatosis is a systemic vasculitis with preferential involvement of the respiratory tract. The disease usually beginning with limited organ involvement progressing to a disseminated vasculitis with upper airway, lung, and kidney manifestations. Wegener's granulomatosis may result in diffuse nasal mucosal ulceration, septal perforation, and nasal dorsal defects or collapse.

Relapsing polychondritis is an autoimmune connective tissue disorder characterized by intermittent cartilage inflammation, causing chondrolysis and atrophy. Cell-mediated immunity to cartilage has been demonstrated in vitro. Nasal cartilage involvement results in eventual collapse and saddle nose deformity.

Polymorphic reticulosis (T-cell lymphoma), formally known as *lethal midline granuloma*, and idiopathic midline destructive disease (IMDD) are lymphoma-like diseases that may manifest as destructive lesions or ulcerations causing nasal deformity. IMDD is a diagnosis of exclusion in patients who

manifest midline nasal necrosis with no specific etiology such as infection, tumor, or Wegener's granulomatosis. Fungal and atypical bacterial opportunistic infections may result in destructive lesions of the nose and septum. Potentially deforming infections include rhinoscleroma, tuberculosis, histoplasmosis, rhinosporidiosis, and mucormycosis.[26]

Nasal Deformities Resulting from Cocaine Abuse

The destructive effects of cocaine on the nasal cavity and septum are well known to otolaryngologists and plastic surgeons. Epistaxis and nasal congestion frequently occur in the occasional intranasal cocaine abuser. Other common findings include excessive "sniffing," sinusitis, diminished olfaction, and crusting. A severe form of rhinitis medicamentosa may accompany cocaine use, progressing to chronic injury of the nasal mucosa and perichondrium. Ultimately, ischemic necrosis of the septum and subsequent perforation may result.[27,28]

More serious nasal findings related to cocaine insufflation include osteocartilaginous necrosis, alar necrosis, and saddle deformity. The deleterious effects seen are due to both the profound vasoconstriction and local ischemia, leading to reperfusion injury, caused by topical cocaine, as well as chemical irritation by adulterants present in the drug itself.[27,28]

Recently, midline nasal destruction secondary to cocaine abuse, mimicking IMDD but less fulminant in its course, has been described.[27]

Iatrogenic Nasal Deformities

Aesthetic rhinoplasty and functional septorhinoplasty are undoubtedly the most common causes of significant iatrogenic nasal deformities. In the best of hands, secondary surgery of the nose is necessary in approximately 5% to 10% of rhinoplasty patients. Usually, the secondary procedure required is minor and involves further nasal reduction, such as rasping a small residual hump or correcting a persistent septal deviation.[29]

Overresection of the nasal osteochondrous skeleton during primary rhinoplasty results in more significant nasal deformities, including the supratip deformity, wide nasolabial angle, low radix, and inverted V deformity.[30] Saddle nose deformity may result from combining radical submucous resection (Killian) of the cartilaginous septum, along with either resection of a large dorsal hump or, more commonly, overzealous lowering of the dorsum.[29]

Orthognathic and craniofacial surgery may also result in iatrogenic nasal deformities. Standard hypertelorism operations have been demonstrated to interfere with subsequent anterior facial growth and have been complicated by gradual resorption of the reconstructed complex.[31]

References

1. Burget GC, Menick FJ. Nasal support and lining: the marriage of beauty and blood supply. *Plast Reconstr Surg.* 1989;84:189–203.

2. Graney DO, Baker SR. Anatomy. In: Cummings CW, Fredrickson JM, Harker LE, et al., eds. *Otolaryngology—Head and Neck Surgery.* 2nd ed. St. Louis, MO: Mosby Year Book; 1993:627–639.

3. Leopold DA. Physiology of olfaction. In: Cummings CW, Fredrickson JM, Harker LE, et al., eds. *Otolaryngology—Head and Neck Surgery.* 2nd ed. St. Louis, MO: Mosby Year Book; 1993:640–664.

4. Zakzouk MS. The congenital warfarin syndrome. *J Laryngol Otol.* 1986;100:215–219.

5. Pashley NRT. Congenital anomalies of the nose. In: Cummings CW, Fredrickson JM, Harker LE, et al., eds. *Otolaryngology—Head and Neck Surgery.* 2nd ed. St. Louis, MO: Mosby Year Book; 1993:702–712.

6. Kawamoto HK. Rare craniofacial clefts. In: McCarthy JG, ed. *Plastic Surgery.* Philadelphia: W.B. Saunders; 1990:2922–2973.

7. Hinderer KH. Nasal problems in children. *Pediatr Ann.* 1976;5:499–509.

8. Baraitser M, Winter R. *A Colour Atlas of Clinical Genetics.* London: Wolfe Medical Publications; 1983.

9. Johnston MC. Embryology of the head and neck. In: McCarthy JG, ed. *Plastic Surgery.* Philadelphia: W.B. Saunders; 1990:2451–2495.

10. Jackson IT, Fasching MC. Secondary deformities of cleft lip, nose and cleft palate. In: McCarthy JG, ed. *Plastic Surgery.* Philadelphia: W.B. Saunders; 1990:2771–2877.

11. Holmstrom H. Clinical and pathologic features of maxillonasal dysplasia (Binder's syndrome): significance of the prenasal fossa on etiology. *Plast Reconstr Surg.* 1986;87:559–567.

12. Demas PN, Braun TW. Simultaneous reconstruction of maxillary and nasal deformity in a patient with Binder's syndrome (maxillonasal dysplasia). *J Oral Maxillofac Surg.* 1992;50:83–86.

13. McCarthy JG, Epstein FJ, Wood-Smith D. Craniosynostosis. In: McCarthy JG, ed. *Plastic Surgery.* Philadelphia: W.B. Saunders; 1990:3013–3053.

14. Tessier P. Anatomical classification of facial, craniofacial and latero-facial clefts. *J Maxillofac Surg.* 1976;4:69–92.

15. Jackson IT, Tanner NSB, Hide TAH. Frontonasal encephalocele—"long nose hypertelorism." *Ann Plast Surg.* 1983;11:490–500.

16. David DJ, Sheffield L, Simpson D, et al. Frontoethmoidal meningoencephaloceles: morphology and treatment. *Br J Plast Surg.* 1984;37:271–284.

17. Kelly JH, Strome M, Hall B. Surgical update on nasal dermoids. *Arch Otolaryngol.* 1982;108:239–242.

18. Gray LP. Prevention and treatment of septal deformity in infancy and childhood. *Rhinology.* 1977;15:183–191.

19. Kern EB. Acute nasal trauma. In: Rees TD, Baker DC, Tabbal N, eds. *Rhinoplasty, Problems and Controversies.* St. Louis, MO: C.V. Mosby; 1988:392–396.

20. Hunter JG. Pediatric maxillofacial trauma. *Pediatr Clin North Am.* 1992;39:1127–1143.

21. Illum P. Long term results after treatment of nasal fractures. *J Laryngol Otol.* 1986;100:273–277.

22. Illum P, Kristensen S, Jorgensen K, et al. Role of fixation in the treatment of nasal fractures. *Clin Otolaryngol.* 1983;8:191–195.

23. Burget GC, Menick FJ. Nasal reconstruction: seeking a fourth dimension. *Plast Reconstr Surg.* 1986;78:145–157.

24. DeSanto LW. Neoplasms. In: Cummings CW, Fredrickson JM, Harker LE, eds. *Otolaryngology—Head and Neck Surgery.* 2nd ed. St. Louis, MO: Mosby Year Book; 1993:754–764.

25. Bise RN, Jackson IT, Smit R. Nasal bone hemangiomas: rare entities treatable by craniofacial approach. *Br J Plast Surg.* 1991;44:206–209.

26. McDonald TJ. Manifestations of systemic disease. In: Cummings CW, Fredrickson JM, Harker LE, et al., eds. *Otolaryngology—Head and Neck Surgery.* 2nd ed. St. Louis, MO: Mosby Year Book; 1993:713–722.

27. Sercarz JA, Strasnick B, Newman A, et al. Midline nasal destruction in cocaine abusers. *Otolaryngol Head Neck Surg.* 1991; 105:694–701.

28. Mattson-Gates G, Jabs AD, Hugo NE. Perforation of the hard palate associated with cocaine abuse. *Ann Plast Surg.* 1991;26: 466–468.

29. Rees T. Secondary rhinoplasty: basic considerations. In: Rees TD, Baker DC, Tabbal N, eds. *Rhinoplasty, Problems and Controversies.* St. Louis, MO: C.V. Mosby; 1988:292–298.

30. Labrakis G. The universal of early childhood: nature's aid in understanding the supratip deformity and its correction. *Ann Plast Surg.* 1992;29:55–57.

31. Mulliken JB, Kaban LB, Evans CA, et al. Facial skeletal changes following hypertelorism correction. *Plast Reconstr Surg.* 1986; 77:7–16.

7
Review of Benign Tumors of the Maxillofacial Region and Considerations for Bone Invasion

Joachim Prein

Tumors in the maxillofacial region are located in the soft and hard tissues. Those located in the facial skeleton are rare and can be of dental origin (odontogenic) or arise from bony tissues (osteogenic). No matter whether they are benign or malignant, clinically they often are symptomless for a long time. Only rarely do they cause pain. Even on x-ray films their appearance is very uniform. Most of them present as mono- or polycystic lesions. Even the distinction of whether these lesions are well delineated or not does not help to determine whether a tumor is benign or malignant.[1]

Although examinations with computed tomography (CT) or magnetic resonance imaging (MRI) give much more precise information about the contents and delineation of these lesions, in most of the cases it is not possible to establish a diagnosis. This can only be done through a biopsy and a histologic examination. These biopsies should always be open biopsies to receive sufficient material in quantity and quality. This is important because many benign or malignant tumors can present with histologically similar pictures.

This is true for odontogenic tumors (e.g., for the ameloblastoma and its variants, such as ameloblastic fibroma or ameloblastic fibroodontoma). Also, it may be difficult to differentiate between fibrous dysplasia and ossifying fibroma, osteoblastoma and osteosarcoma, or desmoplastic fibroma and fibrosarcoma.

A very close cooperation between the clinician, pathologist, and radiologist is mandatory to receive an exact diagnosis. The pathologist needs all clinical and radiologic information because tumors that are histologically similar may have different diagnoses according to their different anatomic locations. A correct treatment plan can, of course, only be established with a precise preoperative diagnosis.

Odontogenic Tumors and Tumorlike Lesions

Tumors and tumorlike lesions of dental origin are less common than those of osseous origin. Most reflect a state out of the development of a tooth. Because epithelial and mesenchymal tissues are involved in the formation of tooth bud, both components can be involved in the formation of an odontogenic tumor. Most odontogenic tumors are benign, and some are not even tumors, but rather tumorlike lesions or hamartomas, such as all odontomas. Therefore, most are clinically as well as radiologically and histologically well delineated and can be treated with curettage, enucleation, or sometimes fenestration. Their radiologic appearance is very uniform and often resembles a follicular cyst (Figure 7.1).

An infiltrative pattern of growth into the bony structures has histologically only been observed with ameloblastomas (Figure 7.2) and ameloblastic fibrosarcomas.

Because of size and location of some benign lesions, such as keratocysts, myxomas, or adenomatoid odontogenic tumors, it may be necessary to perform a complete resection of the involved bony area and a reconstruction thereafter. Characteristic of keratocysts is their high rate of recurrence (between 32% and 63%). In some instances, it has been reported that intraosseous carcinomas have developed out of keratocysts.

Table 7.1 mentions odontogenic lesions that necessitate a curettage or enucleation only, and according to size and location, a defect filling with cancelleous bone (Figures 7.3 and 7.4).

The ameloblastoma is a locally aggressive tumor that necessitates a complete resection with clear margins. Neither radiologic characteristics, such as mono- or polycystic appearances, nor resorption of tooth roots, nor the different histologic subgroups allow a differentiation between more or less aggressive tumors. Until a few years ago, resorption of tooth roots has been interpreted as pathognomonic for ameloblastomas. Meanwhile, this phenomenon has been observed in connection with several odontogenic and nonodontogenic tumors and tumorlike lesions. It was found, however, that it does not indicate a higher aggressivness of the lesion. Table 7.2 shows a list of lesions in which radiologically resorptions of tooth roots have been observed.

Although in rare instances true malignant ameloblastomas with lymph node or skeletal metastases have been described, a neck dissection together with the resection of the tumor is

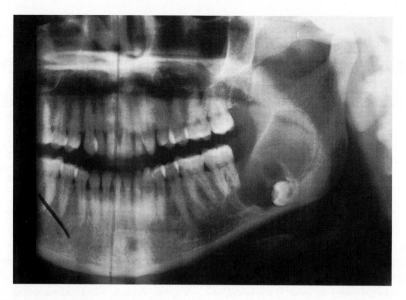

FIGURE 7.1 Cystic lesion in the left mandibular angle region with a retained molar. The x-ray appears similar to a follicular cyst. Within the cyst wall, an ameloblastoma was found.

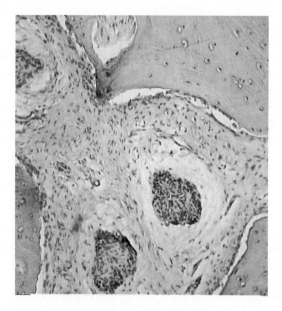

FIGURE 7.2 Epithelial islets pathognomonic for an ameloblastoma are found to infiltrate the bony structures.

TABLE 7.1 Benign odontogenic tumors and tumorlike lesions.

Adenomatoid odontogenic tumor
Ameloblastic fibroma and myxoma
Odontogenic myxoma and fibroma
Dentinoma
Cementoma
Cementifying fibroma
Odontoma
Calcifying epithelial odontogenic tumor
Calcifying odontogenic cyst
Odontogenic keratocyst
Follicular and radicular cysts

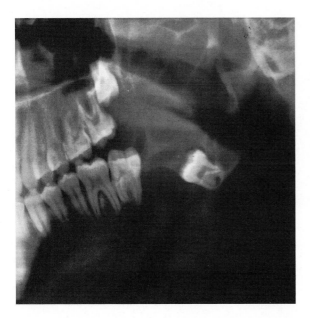

FIGURE 7.3 Extensive polycystic lesion in the left ramus and mandibular angle area in an 18-year-old man. The swelling was painless and the patient did not complain about loss of sensitivity in his left lower lip. Diagnosis: odontogenic keratocyst.

not indicated. As far as clinical behavior is concerned, the ameloblastoma can be compared with a basalioma. Infrequently, ameloblastic fibrosarcomas or ameloblastic odontosarcomas are observed. Regional metastasis have not been described with these.[2-4]

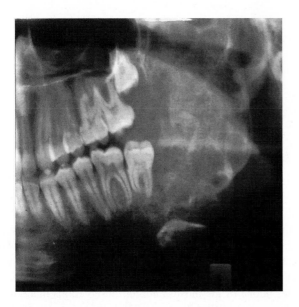

FIGURE 7.4 Although the lesion was very extensive and reached into the area of the joint, conservative treatment with curettage and filling of the cavity with autogenous cancellous bone was performed. The patient will remain in a follow-up control for many years.

Histomorphologically, several types of ameloblastomas are described. The attempt to assign different grading ranks to the various types has not proven to be clinically sound. Particularly in connection with the description of malignant ameloblastomas, the acanthous type ameloblastoma has been misinterpreted as squamous cell carcinoma or adenoid cystic carcinoma or adenocarcinoma.

Ameloblastomas are predominantly located in the mandible and rarely appear before the age of 18. This is an important criterion because it helps in some instances to differentiate between ameloblastoma and lesions such as ameloblastic fibromas and myxomas.

In most instances, after complete resection of the tumor with the bone, a primary reconstruction with a reconstruction plate and a free bone graft is performed. Only rarely and depending on size and location of the defect is a primary reconstruction with a microvascular graft indicated. The most important precondition for a successful primary reconstruction is a reliable stabilization with plates and screws together with a reliable closure of the soft tissues around the grafts. The following case clearly demonstrates this.

A 41-year-old patient presented with a symptomless moderate swelling of his left mandibular angle area. On x-ray, a polycystic lesion was found and, after an open biopsy, it was diagnosed as an ameloblastoma.

After resection of the tumor through a partial mandibulectomy the defect was bridged with a 2.7 reconstruction plate. A bone graft was taken from the iliac crest and the bony defect immediately reconstructed.

Two years after the removal of the tumor the plate was removed on the patient's request. As a rule we do not remove these plates because they are not responsible for any resorption of the bone graft through stress protection. At the occasion of the plate removal, dental implants were inserted into the bone graft (Figures 7.5–7.7).

TABLE 7.2 Lesions with possible tooth root resorption on x-rays.

Ameloblastoma
Ameloblastic fibroma
Odontogenic myxoma
Adenomatoid odontogenic tumor
Cementoma
Calcifying odontogenic cyst
Odontogenic keratocyst
Ossifying fibroma
Fibrous dysplasia
Desmoplastic fibroma
Eosinophilic granuloma
Giant-cell granuloma
Hemangioma
Osteosarcoma
Plasmocytoma

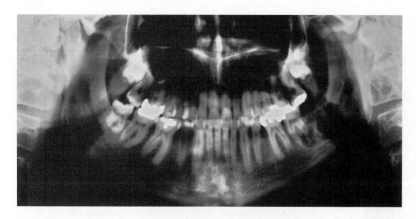

FIGURE 7.5 Polycystic lesion in the left mandibular retromolar and angle area. Diagnosis: ameloblastoma.

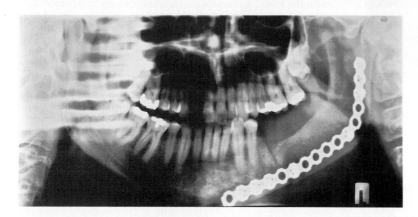

FIGURE 7.6 Reconstruction of the mandibular defect with a reconstruction plate and an autologous bone graft taken from the iliac crest.

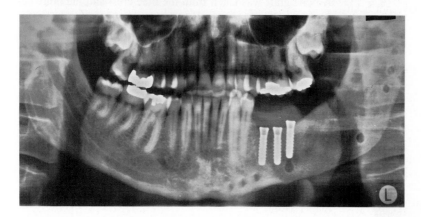

FIGURE 7.7 Two years after the reconstruction, the reconstruction plate was removed and dental implants inserted.

Nonodontogenic Tumors and Tumorlike Lesions Within the Facial Bones

Mesenchymal tumors in the jaw bone have other characteristics compared with those of the same name in the postcranial skeleton. They are less often benign than odontogenic tumors. Some appear almost exclusively in facial bones, such as the osteoma and the ossifying fibroma, and some, such as the giant-cell tumor, are not found in the facial bones. On the other hand, the giant cell granuloma, except as a brown tumor with hyperparathyroidism, is not observed outside the fa-

cial bones. For the pathologist, however, it may be difficult or impossible to differentiate between a giant cell tumor and a giant cell granuloma. Therefore, precise information about the clinical situation is mandatory for the pathologist. Recognizing that giant cell tumors do not appear in the facial bones is one of the most important observations made in recent years. Until the mid-1970s, many patients were overtreated with mutilating resections because giant-cell granulomas were misinterpreted as giant-cell tumors.

An important diagnostic sign is the vitality of the teeth. They often remain vital although their roots are located in the empty spaces of the cystic lesions (Figures 7.8 and 7.9).

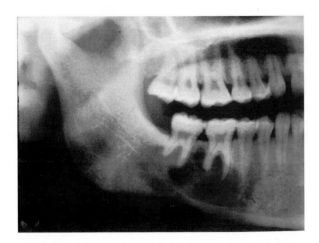

FIGURE 7.8 Extensive cystic lesion in the right horizontal part of the mandible surrounding the roots of the teeth 44, 45, 46, and 47. All teeth remained vital. Diagnosis: giant-cell granuloma.

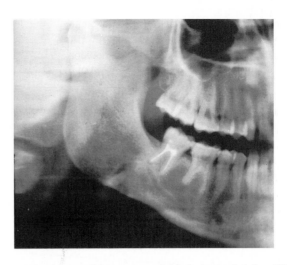

FIGURE 7.9 After careful curettage of this lesion and defect filling with autogenous cancellous bone, only tooth 47 lost its vitality.

The establishment of a special registry for tumors of the facial skeleton including odontogenic lesions in 1971 by the German-Austrian-Swiss Association for the Study of Tumors of the Face and Jaws (DÖSAK) and the analysis of all the giant-cell lesions in the registry has led to the recognition that malignant giant cell tumors do not appear in the facial skeleton.

It was in 1974 that the DÖSAK sponsored a symposium under the chairmanship of Professors Uehlinger and Remagen during which several reclassifications had to be done.

In benign tumors, one has in general to differentiate between cartilaginous, osteofibrous, cystlike lesions, and lesions that derive from the vessels. Most of the round-cell tumors and lymphatic tumors are malignant. On x-ray examinations it is rarely possible to establish a diagnosis, because very few pathognomonic signs exist. Lesions appearing in the mandible allow more often at least approximate conclusions than those in the maxilla, whereas on regular x-ray films a very monotonous appearance of the lesions is observed.

In the mandible, most appear to be cystlike, regardless of whether they are benign or malignant. Some allow at least approximate conclusions according to the degree of metaplastic bone formation, which is dependent on age and further activities within the tumor.

The following list mentions the main benign nonodontogenic lesions in the facial skeleton:

Chondroblastic:
    enchondroma
    chondroblastoma
    chondromyxoid fibroma
    osteochondroma

Osseous origin:
    osteoma
    osteoblastoma and osteoid-osteoma
    ossifying fibroma
    fibrous dysplasia

Histiocytosis x:
    Langerhans cell granuloma

Vascular origin:
    hemangioma

Probably semimalignant:
    desmoplastic fibroma

Unknown etiology:
    central giant-cell granuloma
    juvenile bone cyst
    aneurysmal bone cyst

Radical excision is necessary for all cartilaginous lesions because they have a strong tendency for recurrence. Resection or enucleation is sufficient for osteoma, osteoblastoma, ossifying fibroma, hemangioma, central giant-cell granulomas, and aneurysmal bone cysts.

A juvenile bone cyst is an empty hole without an epithelial lining. Apparently, the opening and the subsequent bleeding into the cavity initiates reossification of the area.

Surgical contouring, or in smaller lesions enucleation, is the treatment for fibrous dysplasia. Because of the tendency for recurrence or regrowth, clinical and radiologic follow-up for many years is indicated. The tendency toward malignant transformation is very low, although proven malignant transformation has been seen in connection with radiotherapy for a fibrous dysplasia.

The treatment of eosinophilic granuloma depends on its monostotic or multilocular appearance. Although desmoplastic fibroma may be considered as semimalignant and its growth pattern may be infiltrative into the cancellous areas of the bone, a first operative step can be enucleation for those well delineated on x-rays and more radical resection for those not well demarcated or in the case of recurrences.

Generally, radiotherapy is not indicated for any of the above-mentioned lesions. On the contrary, radiotherapy may be harmful since it may cause a transformation of some of these lesions into osteosarcomas. Radiotherapy may even cause secondary osteosarcomas without any lesions in this area.

References

1. Prein J, Remagen W, Spiessl B, Uehlinger E. *Atlas of Tumors of the Facial Skeleton. Odontogenic and Non-odontogenic Tumors.* New York: Springer Verlag; 1985.

2. Prein J, Remagen W, Spiessl B, Schafroth U. Ameloblastic fibroma and its sarcomatous transformation. *Pathol Res Pract.* 1979;11:123–130.

3. Pindborg JJ, Hjorting-Hansen E. *Atlas of Diseases of the Jaws.* Copenhagen: Munksgaard; 1974.

4. Takahashi K, Kitajima T, Lee M, Iwasaki N, Inoue SI, Matsue N, et al. Granular cell ameloblastoma of the mandible with metastasis to the third thoracic vertebra. *Clin Orthop.* 1985;197: 171–180.

8
Oral Malignancies: Etiology, Distribution, and Basic Treatment Considerations

Anna-Lisa Söderholm

Treatment Considerations

The most common oral malignancy (90% to 97%) is squamous cell carcinoma,[1,2] followed by adenocarcinomas of various types (2% to 3%).[1] Sarcomas, extranodal lymphomas[3–5] and metastases from distant cancers[6–8] are rare. Other malignant tumors, including melanomas and tumors of dental origin, occasionally occur in the oral and maxillofacial region.

Oral Squamous Cell Carcinoma

Epidemiology

Oral cancer is the fifth most common malignancy worldwide, with the incidence of new tumors per thousand estimated at 378.5 for all countries, with 272.3 in developing countries and 106.2 in developed countries.[9] Worldwide, however, a 3% to 4% relative frequency is usually encountered. For example, in Malaysia oral carcinomas ranks second among all histologically confirmed malignant tumors.[10–12] The approximate annual incidence rate in the United States is $1.2/10^5$ for squamous cell carcinoma (SCC) of the lip and $7/10^5$ (30.600 new cases) for oral SCC, which when combined constitutes approximately 3% of all reported malignancies in 1990.[2,13]

In the Scandinavian countries, the incidence of lip and oral cancer is fairly low.[14] The national cancer registries in the Scandinavian countries constitute ideal sources of material for epidemiological studies. The data in the Finnish Cancer Registry can be considered virtually complete in relation to coverage of cancers diagnosed in Finland.[15] In Finland, the mean age-adjusted incidence rates for 1991 were $3.1/10^5$ (lip), $2.3/10^5$ (oral) for males and $0.6/10^5$ (lip), $1.3/10^5$ (oral) for females.[16] The incidence of oral cancer decreased slowly but steadily from 1953 until 1976, especially in men,[17] but from 1977 on the figures have increased.[16]

Etiology

Tobacco use, especially smoking, is generally considered the main etiologic factor for mouth cancer. Other causes include alcohol abuse, some drugs, environmental factors, and viruses.[18–23] Analysis of the national Finnish Cancer Registry records of cancer of the lip, mouth, and pharynx for the occurrence of secondary primaries revealed 9092 cases diagnosed between 1953 and 1989. The observed numbers of patients were compared with the expected on the basis of the incidence rates in the Finnish population (Figure 8.1). There were 1130 patients (12%) with new tumors. The standardized incidence rate (SIR) of contracting a new cancer was 1.2 for lip cancer patients (95% CI 1.1–1.3) and 1.4 for patients with cancer of the oral cavity or pharynx 95% (CI 1.2–1.4) (Table 8.1). A concentration of the excess risk for tobacco-related new tumors in lip cancer patients, which, for example, is a significant excess risk of lung cancer (SIR 1.4), supports the role of smoking as a risk factor for lip cancer (Table 8.2). A variation of the relative risk by subsite and sex in oral cancer seemed more likely to support a multifactorial rather than a clearly tobacco-related etiology in these cancers[24] (Table 8.3). Analysis of the Finnish Cancer Registry material by occupation and social status pointed, on the other hand, in the case of oral cancer, more to an alcohol than smoking etiology. The role of occupational factors seemed to be minimal.[25] These figures from the Finnish Cancer Registry statistically are highly reliable since both the observed numbers of new tumors and the expected numbers relate to the same set of data.

Initial Symptoms

The symptoms of oral squamous cell carcinoma are often diffuse and nonspecific. For example, mucosal hyperplasia and different types of mucosal ulcers are common in elderly patients with dental prostheses, and malignant changes are often not recognized by the patients at an early stage. This creates an opportunity for dentists to detect early cancer when patients present with complaints concerning dental prostheses. The main presenting symptoms for cancer of the mandibular region are listed in Table 8.4.[26] The list also corresponds for other sites of the oral cavity. However, pain as the first complaint has been reported in 50% to 66% of intraoral carcinomas depending on the site,[2] an interesting and

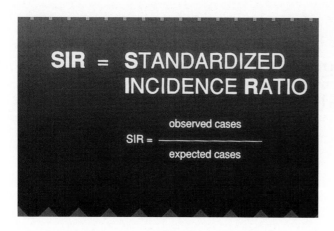

FIGURE 8.1 Standard incidence ratio (SIR).

TABLE 8.1 The excess risk of getting a new primary cancer among patients with lip cancer and cancer of the mouth and oropharynx respectively. The number of cases recorded in the national Finnish Cancer Registry 1953–1989 and SIR:s for a new primary cancer in these patients.[24]

Cancer type	Patients	Person-years at risk	New cancers	SIR
Lip	5633	51,951	901	1.2
Mouth and oropharynx	3454	15,764	229	1.4

TABLE 8.2 The excess risk (SIR:s) of getting a new primary cancer among patients with lip cancer in Finland 1953–1989 by site.[24]

New cancer	N	SIR
Lip	4	0.28
Mouth, pharynx	16	1.9
Larynx	23	2.0
Lung	269	1.4
Esophagus	18	1.2
Stomach	107	1.1
Colon	26	0.81

TABLE 8.3 The excess risk (SIR:s) of getting a new primary cancer among patients with cancer of the mouth and pharynx in Finland by site.[24]

New cancer	N	SIR
Lip	8	3.5
Mouth, pharynx	11	5.8
Larynx	1	0.54
Lung	52	1.8
Esophagus	5	1.4
Stomach	18	0.73
Colon	13	1.5
Thyroid gland	3	2.2
NHL*	4	1.5
Hodgkin's disease	2	2.7
Leukemia	9	2.3

* Non-Hodgkin's lymphoma

TABLE 8.4 Presenting symptoms and signs (one or several for each case) in 162 patients with oral carcinoma of the mandibular region.[26]

Symptom or sign	Number of patients	Percentage
Ulceration	103	64%
Palpable tumor alone	36	22%
Pain	28	17%
Soft tissue hyperplasia	19	12%
Symptoms of infection	6	4%
Paraesthesia	5	3%
Mobility of teeth	5	3%
Trismus	3	2%
Mandibular fracture	3	2%
Weight loss	2	1%
Delayed healing of extraction wound	1	1%

important symptom. Although a very early cancerous lesion may be painless, more advanced cancer lesions are not. In several studies, the interval between presenting symptoms and the tissue diagnosis of cancer has been reported to be approximately 4 months.[2,26,27]

Findings

At clinical examination, a nonhealing, indurated ulcer or firm lump is always suspicious for cancer. Premalignant lesions usually exist as leukoplakias or erythroplakias, while early frank invasive cancers may manifest as small, asymptomatic mucosal masses or ulcers. The role of the patient's own dentist, performing regular oral examinations including systematic inspection and palpation of the entire oral and oropharyngeal mucosa, is important. The examination always must be extended extraorally with bimanual palpation of the floor of the mouth, simultaneously with the submandibular and submental regions. Still, too few oral mucosal lesions are biopsied, and the follow-up of precancerous lesions is often neglected. Lesions classified as premalignant erythroplasia, leukoplakia, and lichen planus have to be thoroughly excised or regularly biopsied. If the histologic diagnosis is severe or moderate dysplasia, close follow-up is mandatory.[2]

Distribution by Site and Stage

Tongue cancer (ICD-7 140) represents 35% to 50% of the malignant tumors occurring in the oral area (Table 8.5).[2,13,24]

TABLE 8.5 Numbers of patients with cancer of the mouth and pharynx diagnosed between 1953 and 1989 in Finland by subsite.[24]

Site (ICD-7)	Number of patients	Person-years at risk
Tongue (141)	1,228	6,172
Oral cavity (143,4)	1,217	6,640
Pharynx (145,7,8)	1,014	2,952

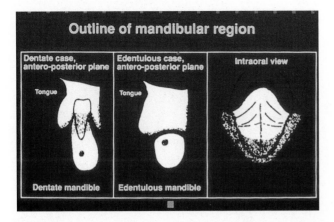

FIGURE 8.2 Outline of mandibular region.

TABLE 8.7 TNM classification of oral cancer.[28,29]

Primary tumor (T)

T_1 Tumor ≤ 2 cm in greatest dimension
T_2 Tumor >2 cm but ≤ 4 cm in greatest dimension
T_3 Tumor >4 cm in greatest dimension
T_4 Tumor invades adjacent structures

Regional lymph node (N)

N_0 No regional lymph node metastasis
N_1 Metastasis in a single ipsilateral lymph node, ≤ 3 cm in greatest dimension
N_2 Metastasis in a single ipsilateral lymph node, >3 cm but <6 cm in greatest dimension; in multiple ipsilateral lymph nodes, none >6 cm in greatest dimension; or in bilateral or contralateral lymph nodes, none >6 cm in greatest dimension
N_3 Metastasis in a lymph node >6 cm in greatest dimension

TNM stage groups:

I T_1N_0
II T_2N_0
III $T_{1-3}N_1$, T_3N_0
IV T_4, any of N_2, N_3, or distant metastatic disease

About one third of the oral cavity cancers (ICD-7 143–144) occur in the mandibular region (Figure 8.2).[26] This region represents an important, distinct entity associated with special problems related to the diagnosis, evaluation of bone extension, treatment planning, surgical techniques, reconstructive procedures, treatment results, and prognosis. The distribution of 162 cases of mandibular cancer is shown in Table 8.6.[26]

The TNM classification (UICC)[28,29] (Table 8.7) and staging system followed is generally that of the American Joint Committee for Cancer (AJCC) Staging and End Results Reporting (1988),[30] although several modifications and amplifications have been suggested for getting better prognostic reliability.[31,32] A large number of the tumors are, despite efforts toward earlier tumor detection, still advanced at diagnosis.[2,13,31,33,34] Involvement of the underlying bone (T_4) is common, both in the maxillary and mandibular areas (52%) (Figure 8.3).[26,34]

Clinical Examination and Diagnosis

Oral squamous cell carcinoma can usually be easily diagnosed by inspection of the oral mucosa and palpation by an experienced clinician (Figure 8.4a). However, initial carcinoma in connection with a leukoplakia or lichen planus might be neglected (Figure 8.4b). Histologic examination of a biopsy specimen gives the final diagnosis. No tumor should be treated without confirmation of the histologic examination. The biopsy should be adequate, and it should be obtained from a

representative portion of the tumor so that the pathologist can examine the tissue properly. In general, the most satisfactory biopsy of an intraoral lesion is the incisional biopsy (i.e., removal of a small portion). If, however, cancer is suspected in a very small lesion whose gross appearance would be altered by the biopsy, immediate referral would be preferred. It is of the utmost importance that the clinician who will apply the definitive treatment should see the extent of the lesion before the biopsy is taken in order to judge the extent of the resection or irradiation to be instituted.[2] For tumors in areas where biopsies are difficult to obtain (e.g., base of tongue or na-

TABLE 8.6 Location of 162 tumors in the mandibular region on diagnosis.[26]

Location	Males		Females		Total	
	N	%	N	%	N	%
Lower alveolar ridge	49	59%	50	63%	99	61%
Sublingual sulcus	27	33%	17	22%	44	27%
Lower buccal sulcus	3	3%	9	11%	12	8%
Retromolar area	4	5%	3	4%	7	4%
Totals	83	100%	79	100%	162	100%

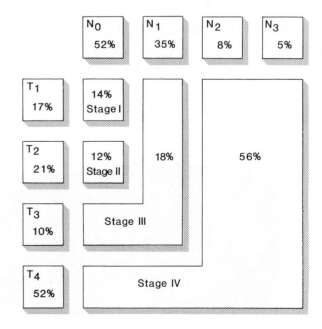

FIGURE 8.3 TNM classification and stage of 162 squamous cell carcinomas of the mandibular region diagnosed between 1973 and 1985 in Finland.[34]

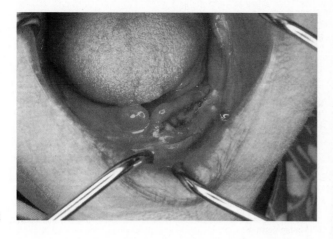

a

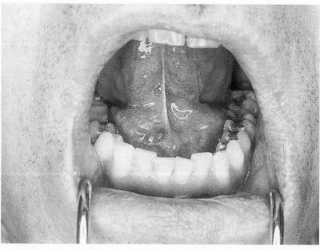

b

FIGURE 8.4 (a) A clinically obvious carcinoma of the left mandibular edentulous ridge in a 67-year-old female. The diagnosis was confirmed by biopsy. (b) A 0.5-cm area of erythroplasia in a 51-year-old man was excised. At histologic examination carcinoma in situ was found. Resection with 1.5-cm margins and reconstruction with local flaps from the tongue was performed. Histologic examination of the surgical specimen revealed infiltrative carcinoma.

sopharynx) it is necessary to perform the biopsy on the patient by fiberoscopy under general anesthesia. Lymph node biopsy is carried out only when a primary lesion cannot be identified, and in such instances, it is preferable for the entire lymph node to be excised. In clinically obvious cancer lesions, radiologic examination should be performed prior to the confirmatory biopsy for evaluating tumor extension and possible bone involvement. A thorough medical history, general health examination (including laboratory tests), and presurgical clearance, is, of course, mandatory.

Evaluation or Determination of Tumor Extension

For the evaluation of tumor extension in the middle and upper face, surrounding soft tissues in the mandibular region

and neck, computerized tomography (CT) and especially magnetic resonance imaging (MRI) are invaluable. For the detection of cervical lymph node metastasis according to several studies, ultrascan provides the most reliable information,[35] which can be combined with fine-needle aspiration biopsy. Preoperative assessment of possible lymph node spread is extremely important in treatment planning. Lymph node involvement at diagnosis is associated with poorer prognosis, which will influence the choice of reconstruction at the local tumor site.

Preoperative assessment of bone infiltration is one of the main problems in treatment planning in patients with cancer of the mandibular region. How large a resection is necessary? Mandibular bone involvement can occur at an early stage through small defects in the bony cortex and that type of in-

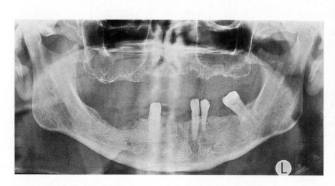

a

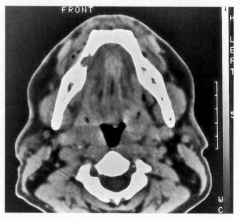

b

FIGURE 8.5 (a) Orthopantomogram of a 55-year-old male with a T_2 gingival squamous cell carcinoma of the right mandibular body region, showing diffuse local destruction at the upper margin. (b) Computerized tomogram of the same patient showing bone destruction of the right mandibular body, which is predominantly lingual.

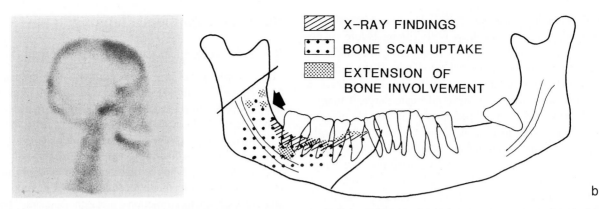

FIGURE 8.6 (a) Bone scan of a 40-year-old woman with squamous cell carcinoma of the right mandibular body area, presenting as gingival swelling around the third molar, which had recently been removed by her dentist. (b) Outline of x-ray findings, histologically determined bone involvement, and mandibular resection lines in the same patient. Histologic examination of the resected mandibular bone revealed deep bone infiltration along the periodontal pockets of the first and second molars into the spongiosa. Additionally, a few separate carcinoma islets were found in the ramus area.

filtration can vary.[29,36–38] Differences in spread pattern has been observed between radiated and nonradiated bone, indicating a more unpredictable spread into radiated bone.[39] In cases of squamous cell carcinoma of the mandibular region, plain radiographs are neither sensitive nor specific enough, except in advanced cases (Figure 8.5a). Computerized tomography (Figure 8.5b) has proven to be a good method for evaluating tumor invasion into bone.[40,41] However, it has clear limitations, and its sensitivity has been questioned by other authors.[42,43] Magnetic resonance imaging has many advantages over CT in assessing oral neoplasms, including increased spatial resolution, the absence of radiation exposure, and decreased dental artifacts. However, these different considerations concerning this more expensive modality in assessing bone involvement need further study.[43,44] Bone scanning (Figure 8.6a) provides valuable information regarding bone involvement in patients with tumors adjacent to bone.[45,46] The claims that bone scans give false positive results, usually owing to benign dental pathology, was not supported in a study comparing preoperative radiographs and bone scans with bone involvement observed through the careful analysis of histological sections of jaw specimens (Figure 8.6b).[47]

Prognosis

The prognosis of oral cancer is still poor, 32% to 44% (5-year survival, all cases; see Figure 8.7), despite new techniques developed in surgery, radiotherapy, and chemotherapy.[1,33,34,48] Limited lesions with a diameter of less than 2 cm have a much higher survival rate (67%) than advanced tumors (30%). However, at diagnosis most tumors are advanced (59% to 74%).[2,31,34] Despite efforts made for earlier detection of cancerous lesions, the observed tumor size at diagnosis has actually increased, not decreased as would be expected.[33] From a prognostic point of view, important factors influencing survival are tumor diameter and thickness, lymph node involve-

ment, distant metastasis at diagnosis, and age of the patient. However, still more important for prognosis is the type of treatment performed and therapeutic effect of treatment.[48]

Treatment Planning

The treatment for oral cancer is surgery, radiotherapy, or a combination therapy of the two. Chemotherapy has been widely used in combination therapy, but no actual influence on long-term survival (5 years) has been confirmed.[2] Small lesions may be treated by either radiotherapy or surgery alone, while the basis for adequate therapy in advanced cases

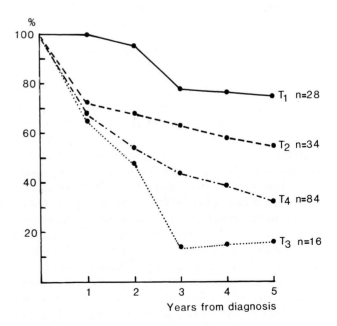

FIGURE 8.7 Relative survival for squamous cell carcinoma of the mandibular region by T classification.[26]

(T_3–T_4) is radical surgery.[31,34,49–51] The actual benefit of radiotherapy is controversial, as is its timing before or after surgery.[52] Many studies stress the central role of adequate surgical margins for prognosis.[48,49] However, if the tumor extension, histologic grade, or patient's general condition restricts the possibility to achieve adequate surgical margins, radiotherapy may permit a period of remission for many patients. On the other hand, radiotherapy increases postsurgical complication rates, can induce osteoradionecrosis, permanently decrease salivary flow and increase mucosal atrophy and caries incidence, and thereby adds to the patient's morbidity, disability, and inhibits rehabilitation to normal life. To avoid unnecessary osteoradionecrosis, preoperative dental care and timing of dental extractions are important. According to Silverman, the incidence is significantly higher if dental extractions are performed in the postoperative period.[2]

Sarcomas

Compared to squamous cell carcinoma in the oral region, other malignancies are rare. The estimated annual incidence of sarcomas, the second most common tumor of the jaws, is $0.05/10^5$. The treatment of choice is radical resection. Local recurrence is frequently a consequence of inadequate tumor excision. With large enough resections higher survival rates are achieved.[53–56] The assessment of the extent of bone involvement of sarcoma is more predictable to assess than in the case of carcinoma. Radiologic examination performed with plain radiographs (in several projections), tomograms, bone scans, and CT or MRI (for soft tissue involvement), preferably analyzed by one or more maxillofacial radiologists, is essential to ensure an informed opinion of bone involvement. This information will lead to large enough resections and higher survival rates.[34,56]

Other Malignant Tumors Involving the Mandible

Lymphomas of extranodal origin constitute about 25% of all lymphomas. Oral manifestations are seen in 3%–5% of these, with intraosseous origin in several cases.[3–5,57] The treatment of lymphomas generally consists of chemotherapy and radiotherapy, except in select cases in which resection of an isolated plasmacytoma prior to other treatment may be advisable.[57]

For the rare cases of melanoma of the oral cavity, a combination therapy including radical surgery and radiotherapy is usually indicated. Metastatic tumors with a predilection for bone metastases, such as carcinomas of the kidney, prostate, and breast,[6–8,58] are the most common in the oral cavity. The treatment is highly dependent on the type, metastatic pattern, and prognosis of the primary tumor. Salvage surgery owing to pathologic fracture of the mandible to restore oral function may be an indication for mandibular reconstruction in, for example, metastatic breast and kidney cancer.

Surgical Treatment Planning

Radical Excision at the Expense of Disability?

The principles governing cancer extirpation are the same in all oral regions. The tumor should be excised with large enough margins, preferably 2 cm, to ensure radicality. In cancer of the maxilla and midface, extension to the orbit or to the cranial base creates major problems for treatment planning. Is it possible to achieve radicality by extensive surgery, and in that case, is the patient ready to do without, for example, the other eye or the nose? Prosthetic reconstruction of the maxilla usually gives satisfactory functional and esthetic results. The same is true for reconstruction by epithesis of the eye and even the nose with respect to esthetics, but function is impossible to restore. Large resections of soft tissues, that is, the base of the tongue, greater than half of the tongue (subtotal glossectomy), or the entire anterior floor of the mouth, all represent difficult reconstruction problems that need to be taken into account in treatment planning. Can the patient accept severe difficulties with or complete inability to speak and eat normally? Is it appropriate to perform major surgery with extensive margins and sophisticated reconstructions in a patient over 85 years of age, if it would be understood that the risk of treatment complications and morbidity is actually higher than the risk for a recurrence during the patient's expected remaining lifetime? The studies done to create reliable prognostic parameters are very important to ensure that patients have a good quality of life for as long as possible.

Extent of Mandibular Resection

The treatment for cancers adjacent to or involving the mandible varies from radical symphysectomy or hemimandibulectomy with or without exarticulation to more conservative resections with preservation of continuity, depending on the stage, location, and signs of bone involvement observed.[37–39,43]

For the patient, conservative resection, such as resection of the lingual cortex adjacent to the tumor, is considerably less incapacitating than hemimandibulectomy (Figure 8.8a,b). Reconstructive surgery involves preprosthetic surgery with or without dental implants (Figure 8.8c). The results are often functionally good as well as esthetically pleasing (Figure 8.8d,e). However, owing to the preoperative radiologically determined extent of bone involvement, tumor extension, or atrophy of the mandible, such a resection is in many cases not possible, if our goal is radical surgery with large enough margins (1 to 2 cm), and a stable mandible with continuity left. Although several techniques have been described to preserve continuity, they may contribute to recurrences or pathologic fracture of the basal or buccal part of the mandible (Figure 8.9a,b). Therefore, adequate cancer surgery often results in a continuity defect of the mandible, which requires appropriate reconstruction.

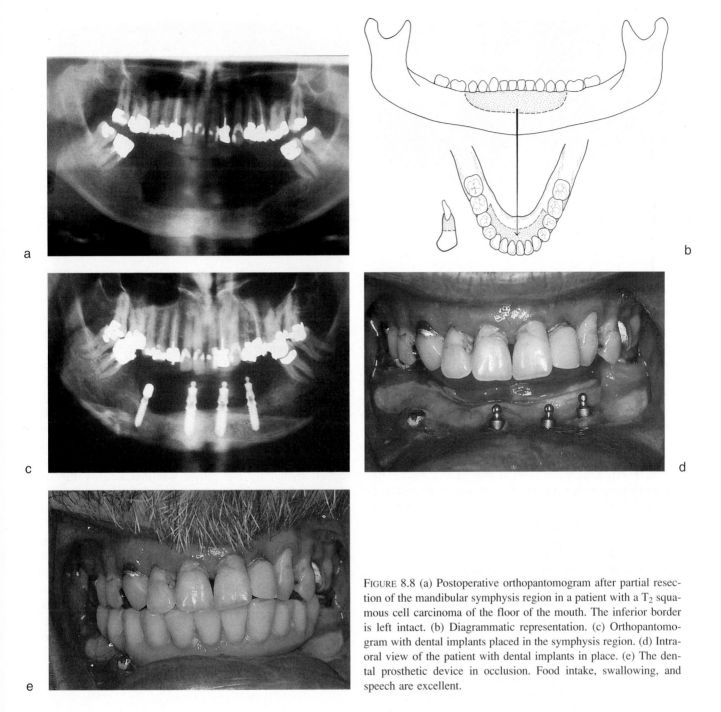

FIGURE 8.8 (a) Postoperative orthopantomogram after partial resection of the mandibular symphysis region in a patient with a T_2 squamous cell carcinoma of the floor of the mouth. The inferior border is left intact. (b) Diagrammatic representation. (c) Orthopantomogram with dental implants placed in the symphysis region. (d) Intraoral view of the patient with dental implants in place. (e) The dental prosthetic device in occlusion. Food intake, swallowing, and speech are excellent.

Considerations for Mandibular Reconstruction and Rehabilitation

Primary reconstruction of the mandible in patients with continuity loss owing to tumor surgery is important for functional as well as esthetic and psychosocial reasons.[59–63] The mandible is involved in important basic functions such as food intake, mastication, deglutition, and speech. It constitutes an essential part of the inferior framework of the face, a major part of an individual's appearance, and a modality for ex-

pression of one's personality. As part of the oral region, the lower jaw also has a basic psychosocial function. Therefore, even slight mandibular disability often causes extensive morbidity and psychological stress. Problems with food intake or speech make the patient a cripple in her own eyes more readily than if she has a stiff knee and requires a cane.

The basic goals for the primary reconstruction of mandibular defects are to restore function and esthetics as rapidly as possible. Owing to modern reconstruction techniques, the extent of mandibular resection can be determined by oncologic

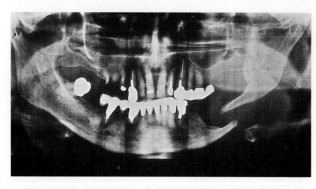 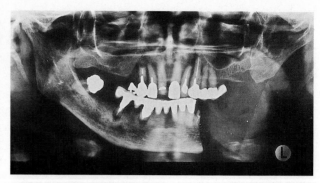

a   b

FIGURE 8.9 (a) Fracture of the mandible after partial resection for mandibular squamous cell carcinoma. (b) Orthopantomogram 15 years later at the time of a new squamous cell carcinoma in the buccal region on the same side.

considerations and not because of insurmountable difficulties with reconstruction. With the types of microvascular flaps presently used in cancer surgery, the necessary extent of the soft tissue ablation should be considered to ensure adequate anastomoses for the transplant. This must be considered in preoperative assessment and treatment planning.

The patient's age and general condition, diagnosis, and the size and location of the defect will correlate with the frequency of postoperative complications and problems. Cancer surgery combined with reconstructive procedures is time-consuming and places a great physical stress upon the patient, who is usually elderly and often in poor general health. Radiation therapy causes damage to host tissues as well as to bone and transplanted soft tissues. There are markedly elevated risks for all kinds of local and systematic complications. If pedicled flaps or microvascular transplants are needed to restore soft tissues,[64–70] problems may occur at the donor sites. Then, for example, there may be interference with walking for several weeks. We must always take into account the general health of the patient, the prognosis and the patient's overall well being, and the patient's quality of life.

Review of Continuous Long-Term Follow-Up

The importance of long-term follow-up for patients with reconstruction performed in the oral region has to be emphasized. The aim should be not only to diagnose but, if necessary, to treat possible recurrences or complications of surgery performed at an earlier stage.[71] The functional and psychosocial problems that patients experience are not always obvious during the initial months, when cure from the malignancy is the patient's major concern. By seeing patients according to a cancer follow-up protocol (Table 8.8)[72] for 5 years and thereafter on a yearly basis and through experimental studies on sheep, we have gained extensive insights about adequate requirements for reconstruction and rehabilitation.[71,73,74] We focus on what is of actual importance for each patient and on which disability is their greatest concern.

If the form and stability of the mandible is restored postoperatively, problems with food intake, mastication, deglutition, and speech can be minimized in patients with oral cancer. With primary reconstruction the patient can return to nearly normal life after 2 to 3 weeks. In elderly patients and patients with a poor prognosis, primary alloplastic reconstruction of the mandible is advantageous. The same can be true in patients with a low stress threshold. In our experience approximately 50% of postablation patients have such good oral function and facial appearance that major secondary reconstructive procedures after 2 to 3 years of follow-up were neither desired by the patient nor indicated by the surgeon.[62,75] Our treatment protocol has become more restrictive since we have noted that in many cases major secondary reconstructive procedures that include bone transplantation and sophisticated dental implant prosthetic rehabilitation are not always an agreeable patient experience. Morbidity during and after surgical procedures, repeated hospital stays, donor site complications, and frequent checkups disturb some patients more than a minimal permanent disability that the patient has already accepted. Therefore, especially in elderly patients with advanced cancer who require mandibular resection, primary alloplastic reconstruction can be considered a permanent reconstruction.[62]

TABLE 8.8 Oral cancer monitoring—follow-up protocol.

Clinical examination
Laboratory screening at every appointment, S-5-nucleotidase
Radiological examination:
    Chest x-rays 1 × per year for smokers
    Local x-rays only after consideration*
    CT, MRI, ultra scan if clinically indicated
Schedule:
    Every 1.5 months for up to 6 months after surgery
    Every 3 months for up to 36 months after surgery
    Every 6 months for up to 60 months after surgery
    Every 12 months continuously thereafter

*Special protocol for patients with reconstructions of the bony structures.

Reconstruction plates provide a simple solution with maximum benefit by permitting oral conditions that are easily maintained by the patient. With minimal interference of residual soft tissue function, reconstruction plates are an ideal solution, especially when the prognosis or general condition is questionable. It also must be kept in mind that although the hard tissue framework and the soft tissue bulk can be restored, diminished muscle and nerve function remains. Therefore, all remaining function should be preserved as undisturbed as possible in the course of surgical management.

Psychosocial Considerations

The patient's general health, possible drug or alcohol abuse, and psychosocial conditions may interfere with treatment planning. Major reconstructions demand cooperation and patience on the part of the patient. The patient's expectations of the end result may differ greatly from the surgeon's, which can sometimes have a negative impact on postoperative rehabilitation. Among cultures, the attitude toward disability and disfigurement varies considerably, and we have to realize that the concept of adequate treatment can vary considerably in different parts of our own country, among cultural subgroups in the same community, and worldwide.

Summary of Goals in Oral Cancer Treatment and Principles for Rehabilitation

Rice and Spiro[13] summarized the management goals in malignant tumor surgery and rehabilitation as follows.

To achieve increased survival and improved quality of survival by:

Emphasis on early detection.

Sound management of precancerous lesions.

Effective therapeutic measures that are the least disabling and disfiguring.

Early application of measures to achieve maximally feasible rehabilitation.

Effective palliation for those who cannot be cured.

The technique used in reconstruction should neither interfere with nor limit the extirpative operation and should not increase morbidity or mortality.

Intermediate restoration of form and function is desirable, especially when cure is doubtful.

Secondary cosmetic deformities should not be produced unless other treatment modalities are unavailable in the situation.

Extensive reconstructive surgery is seldom indicated when a prosthetic appliance can provide satisfactory rehabilitation.

Treat every patient individually and with respect for his or her dignity. The treatment performed always needs to be done for the patient's comfort and never for the surgeon's pride.[13]

References

1. Shklar G. *Oral Cancer*. Philadelphia: W.B. Saunders; 1984.
2. Silverman S Jr, ed. *Oral Cancer*. Washington, DC: American Cancer Society; 1990.
3. Fukuda Y, Ishida T, Fujimoto M, et al. Malignant lymphoma of the oral cavity: clinicopathologic analysis of 20 cases. *J Oral Pathol*. 1987;16:8–12.
4. Hashimoto N, Kurihara K. Pathological characteristics of oral lymphomas. *J Oral Pathol*. 1982;11:214–227.
5. Hotz G, Ho AD, Möller P. Zur Klinik, Immunohistochemie und Therapie maligner Non-Hodgkin-Lymphome im Kiefer-Gesichtsbereich. *Forschr Kiefer Gesichts Chir*. 1988;33:64–67.
6. Grätz KW, Sailer HF, Makek M. Ossäre Metastasen im Oberund Unterkiefer. *Dtsch Z Mund Kiefer Gesichts Chir*. 1990;14:122–131.
7. Löwicke G, Teuber S. Fernmetastasen im Unterkiefer. *Dtsch Z Mund Kiefer Gesichts Chir*. 1987;11:315–318.
8. Schwartz ML, Baredes S, Mignogna FV. Metastatic disease to the mandible. *Laryngoscope*. 1988;98:270–273.
9. Parkin DM, Laara E, Muir CS. Estimates of the wordwide frequency of sixteen major cancers in 1980. *Int J Cancer*. 1988; 41:184–187.
10. Krutchkoff DJ, Chen J, Eisenberg E, et al. Oral cancer: a survey of 566 cases from the University of Connecticut Oral Pathology Biopsy Service, 1975–1986. *Oral Surg Oral Med Oral Pathol*. 1990;70:192–198.
11. Muir C, Waterhouse J, Mack T, Powell J, Whelan S, eds. *Cancer Incidence in Five Continents*. Lyon: IARC Scientific Publications; 1987:88.
12. Waterhouse J, Muir C, Correa P, Powell J, eds. *Cancer Incidence in Five Continents III*. Lyon: International Agency for Research on Cancer; 1976.
13. Rice DH, Spiro RH, eds. *Current Concepts in Head and Neck Cancer*. Washington, DC: American Cancer Society; 1989.
14. Pindborg JJ. *Oral Cancer and Precancer*. Bristol, UK: John Wright & Sons Ltd.; 1980.
15. Teppo L, Pukkala E, Saxen E. Multiple cancer—an epidemiologic exercise in Finland. *J Natl Cancer Inst*. 1985;75:207–217.
16. Finnish Cancer Registry. *Cancer Incidence in Finland 1991. Cancer Statistics of the National Research and Development Centre for Welfare and Health*. Helsinki: The Institute for Statistical and Epidemiological Cancer Research; 1993.
17. Lindqvist C, Teppo L. Oral Cancer in Finland in 1953–1978. *Proc Finn Dent Soc*. 1982;78:232–237.
18. Blomqvist G, Hirsch J-M, Alberius P. Association between development of lower lip cancer and tobacco habits. *J Oral Maxillofac Surg*. 1991;49:1044–1049.
19. Boyle P, MacFarlane GJ, McGinn R, et al. International epidemiology of head and neck cancer. In: de Vries N, Gluckman JL, eds. *Multiple Primary Tumours of the Head and Neck*. New York: Thieme; 1990:80–138.
20. Jensen OM. *Cancer Morbidity and Causes of Death Among Danish Brewery Workers*. Lyons: International Agency for Research on Cancer; 1980.
21. Lindqvist C, Pukkala E, Teppo L. Second primary cancers in patients with carcinoma of the lip. *Community Dent Oral Epidemiol*. 1979;7:233–238.
22. Lindqvist C, Teppo L. Epidemiological evaluation of sunlight as a risk factor of lip cancer. *Br J Cancer*. 1978;37:983–989.

23. Snijders PJF, Cromme FV, van der Brule AJC, et al. Prevalence and expression of human papillomavirus in tonsillar carcinomas indicating a possible viral etiology. *Int J Cancer.* 1992;51:845–850.

24. Söderholm A-L, Pukkala E, Lindqvist C, et al. Risk of new primary cancer in patients with oropharyngeal cancer. *Br J Cancer.* 1994;69:784–788.

25. Pukkala E, Söderholm A-L, Lindqvist C. Cancers of the lip and oropharynx in different social and occupational groups in Finland. *Oral Oncol Eur J Cancer.* 1994;30B:209–215.

26. Söderholm A-L. Carcinoma of the mandibular region. *Br J Oral Maxillofac Surg.* 1990;28:383–389.

27. Rindum J, Pindborg JJ. Intraoral Cancer. *Ugeskrift Laeger.* 1986;149:8–9.

28. Spiessl B. Die TNM-Klassification (1987 neu aufgelegt). *Dtsch Z Mund Kiefer Gesichts Chir.* 1988;12:83–85.

29. UICC, International Union Against Cancer. *TNM Classification of Malignant Tumours,* 4th ed. Herbamanek P, Sobin LH, eds., Berlin: Springer-Verlag; 1987.

30. American Joint Committe for Cancer (AJCC). *Staging and End Results Reporting.* 1988.

31. Howalt H-P, Frenz M, Pitz H. Proposal for modified T-classification for oral cancer. *J Craniomaxillofac Surg.* 1992;21:96–101.

32. Jones GW, Browman G, Goodyear M, et al. Comparison of the addition of T and N integer scores with TNM stage groups in head and neck cancer. *Head Neck.* 1993;15:497–503.

33. Platz H, Fries R, Hudec M. Einführung in die "Prospektive DÖSAK-Studie über Plattenepithel-karzinome der Lippen, der Mundhöhle und der Oropharynx." *Dtsch Z Mund Kiefer Gesichts Chir.* 1988;12:293–302.

34. Söderholm A-L. Bone resection in the treatment of cancer of the mandibular region. Helsinki: 1991. Thesis.

35. Siegert R. Die nicht-invasive sonographische Diagnostik und ultraschallgeführte Punktion malignitätsverdächtiger Raumforderungen im Gesicht- und Halsbereich. *Dtsch Z Mund Kiefer Gesichts Chir.* 1989;13:186–191.

36. Lukinmaa P-L, Hietanen J, Söderholm A-L, et al. The histologic pattern of bone invasion by squamous cell carcinoma of the mandibular region. *Br J Oral Maxillofac Surg.* 1992;30:2–7.

37. McGregor AD, MacDonald DG. Routes of entry of squamous cell carcinoma into the mandible. *Head Neck.* 1988;10:294–301.

38. McGregor IA, MacDonald DG. Spread of squamous cell carcinoma to the nonirradiated edentulous mandible—a preliminary report. *Head Neck Surg.* 1987;9:157–161.

39. McGregor AD, MacDonald DG. Patterns of spread of squamous cell carcinoma to the ramus of the mandible. *Head Neck.* 1993;15:440–444.

40. Bahadur S. Mandibular involvement in oral cancer. *J Laryngol Otol.* 1990;104:968–971.

41. Close LG, Burns DK, Merkel M, et al. Computed tomography in the assessment of mandibular invasion by intraoral carcinoma. *Ann Otol Rhinol Laryngol.* 1986;95:383–388.

42. Schratter M, Mailath G, Imhof H, et al. Der Stellerwert bildgebender Verfahren bei primären Tumoren des Gesichtschädels. *Dtsch Z Mund Kiefer Gesichts Chir.* 1988;12:161–169.

43. Tsue T, McCulloch M, Girod DA, et al. Predictors of carcinomatous invasion of the mandible. *Head Neck.* 1994;16:116–126.

44. Ator GA, Abemayor E, Lufkin RB, et al. Evaluation of mandibular tumor invasion with magnetic resonance imaging. *Arch Otolaryngol Head Neck Surg.* 1990;116:454–459.

45. Bailey BJ. Surgical management of malignant tumors: considerations of mandibular invasion. In: Bailey BJ, Holt GR, eds. *Surgery of the Mandible.* New York: Thieme; 1987:45–59.

46. Baker HL, Woodbury DH, Krause CJ, et al. Evaluation of bone scan by scintigraphy to detect subclinical invasion of the mandible by squamous cell carcinoma of the oral cavity. *Otolaryngol Head Neck Surg.* 1982;90:327–336.

47. Söderholm A-L, Lindqvist C, Hietanen J, et al. Bone scanning for evaluating mandibular bone extension of oral squamous cell carcinoma. *J Oral Maxillofac Surg.* 1990;48:252–257.

48. Platz H, Fries R, Hudec M. Retrospective DÖSAK study on carcinomas of the oral cavity: results and consequences. *J Maxillofac Surg.* 1985;13:147–153.

49. Foote RL, Olsen KD, Davis DL, et al. Base of tongue carcinoma patterns of failure and predictors of recurrence after surgery alone. *Head Neck.* 1993;15:300–307.

50. Isaacs JH, Schnidtman JR. Outcome of treatment of 160 patients with squamous cell carcinoma of the neck staged N3a. *Head Neck.* 1990;12:483–487.

51. McQuarrie DG. Oral cancer. In: McQuarrie DG, Adams GL, Shons AR, Brown GA, eds. *Head and Neck Cancer: Clinical Decisions and Management Principles.* Chicago: Year Book Medical Publishers; 1996:219–243.

52. Söderholm A-L, Lindqvist L, Sankila R, et al. Evaluation of various treatments for carcinoma of the mandibular region. *Br J Oral Maxillofacial Surg.* 1991;29:223–229.

53. Clarc JL, Unni KK, Dahlin DC, et al. Osteosarcoma of the jaw. *Cancer.* 1983;51:2311–2316.

54. Delegado R, Maafs E, Alfeiran A, et al. Osteosarcoma of the jaw. *Head Neck.* 1994;16:246–252.

55. Russ JE, Jesse RH. Management of sarcoma of the maxilla and mandible. *Am J Surg.* 1980;140:572–576.

56. Söderholm A-L, Lindqvist C, Teppo L, et al. Bone resection in patients with mandibular sarcoma. *J Craniomaxillofac Surg.* 1988;16:224–230.

57. Söderholm A-L, Lindqvist C, Heikinheimo K, et al. Non-Hodgkin's lymphomas presenting through oral symptoms. *Int J Oral Maxillofac Surg.* 1990;19:131–134.

58. Meyer I, Shklar G. Malignant tumors metastatic to mouth and jaws. *Oral Surg Oral Med Oral Pathol.* 1965;20:350–362.

59. Gullane PJ. Mandibular reconstruction. New concepts. *Arch Otolaryngol Head Neck Surg.* 1986;112:714–719.

60. Gullane PJ, Havas TE. Mandibular reconstruction after cancer surgery. *Facial Plast Surg.* 1987;4:221–232.

61. Hellem S, Olofsson J. Titanium-coated hollow screw and reconstruction plate system (THORP) in mandibular reconstruction. *J Craniomaxillofac Surg.* 1988;16:173–183.

62. Lindqvist C, Söderholm A-L, Laine P, et al. Rigid reconstruction plates for immediate reconstruction following mandibular resection for malignant tumors. *J Oral Maxillofac Surg.* 1992;50:1158–1163.

63. Saunders JR Jr, Hirata RM, Jaques DA. Definitive mandibular replacement using reconstruction plates. *Am J Surg.* 1990;160:387–389.

64. Aviv JE, Urken ML, Vickery C, et al. The combined latissimus dorsi-scapular free flap in head and neck reconstruction. *Arch Otolaryngol Head Neck Surg.* 1991;117:1242–1250.

65. Buchbinder D, Urken ML, Vickery C, et al. Bone contouring and fixation in functional, primary microvascular mandibular reconstruction. *Head Neck.* 1991;13:191–199.

66. Codeiro PG, Hidalgo DA. Soft tissue coverage of mandibular reconstruction plates. *Head Neck.* 1994;16:112–115.

67. Mirante JP, Urken ML, Aviv JE, et al. Resistence to osteoradionecrosis in neovascularized bone. *Laryngoscope.* 1993;103:1168–1173.

68. Moscoso JF, Keller J, Genden E, et al. Vascularized bone flaps in oromandibular reconstruction. A comparative anatomic study of bone stock from various donor sites to assess suitability for enosseous dental implants. *Arch Otolaryngol Head Neck Surg.* 1994;120:36–43.

69. Urken ML, Buchbinder D, Weinberg H, et al. Functional evaluation following microvascular oromandibular reconstruction of the oral cancer patient: A comparative study of reconstructed and nonreconstructed patients. *Laryngoscope.* 1991;101:935–950.

70. Urken ML, Weinberg H, Vickery C, et al. The combined sensate radial forearm and iliac crest free flaps for reconstruction of significant glossectomy-mandibulectomy defects. *Laryngoscope.* 1992;102:543–558.

71. Söderholm A-L, Hallikainen D, Lindqvist C. Long-term stability of two different mandibular bridging systems. *Arch Otolaryngol Head Neck Surg.* 1993;119:1031–1036.

72. Söderholm A-L, Lindqvist C, Haglund C. Tumor markers and radiological examinations in the follow-up of patients with oral cancer. *J Craniomaxillofac Surg.* 1992;20:211–215.

73. Söderholm A-L, Lindqvist C, Skutnabb K, et al. Bridging of mandibular defects with two different reconstruction systems. *J Oral Maxillofac Surg.* 1991;49:1098–1105.

74. Söderholm A-L, Rahn BA, Suutnabb U, Lindquist C. Fixation with reconstruction plates under critical conditions: The role of screw characteristics. *Int J Oral Maxillofac Surg.* 1996;25:469–473.

75. Söderholm A-L, Lindqvist C, Laine P, et al. Primary reconstruction of the mandible in cancer surgery. A report of thirteen reconstructions according to the principles of rigid internal fixation. *Int J Oral Maxillofacial Surg.* 1988;17:194–197.

9
Craniomaxillofacial Bone Infections: Etiologies, Distributions, and Associated Defects

Darin L. Wright and Robert M. Kellman

Osteomyelitis is probably as old as mankind itself. The 500,000-year-old femur of the Java man (*Pithecanthropus erectus*) shows disease alterations that are consistent with a fracture complicated by osteomyelitis.[1] Descriptions of "purulent bones" with various methods of treatment including splinting, application of bandages and compresses, and burning are contained in the Smith Papyri (5000–3000 B.C.) and ancient Hindu and Chinese writings.[1]

Hippocrates, Galen, and Celsus all wrote of differing methods of treatment for osteomyelitis. Physicians following Celsus offered differing and often conflicting treatments. By the 16th century, amputation remained the mainstay of treating infected bone injuries.[1]

Prior to the discovery of bacteria by Pasteur in 1869, mechanical procedures (incision and drainage, removal of sequestra, and debridement) and immobilization of the affected extremity were the mainstays of treatment. The discovery of bacteria opened a new era in treatment. Lord Lister made use of phenol-soaked compresses; later, the German surgeon Franz Konig used local antiseptics and closed irrigation drainage. Ultimately, antibiotics were discovered, and they added a new dimension to the elimination of bacteria, which helped in the management of osteomyelitis.[1]

Since that time, the treatment of osteomyelitis has continued to evolve. Concomitant with this discovery, a decline in the incidence of osteomyelitis occurred.[2–5] This decline was in part due to early, aggressive, and sometimes inappropriate use of antibiotics at the first sign of infection; however, improvements in nutrition, better dental care, and better health education have also contributed.[2,6]

The goal of this chapter is to describe osteomyelitis in the craniomaxillofacial region. Etiology-specific treatments will be discussed in other chapters.

Terminology

The strict definition of *osteomyelitis* is an inflammation of the medullary portion of the bone. Inflammation of cortical bone is termed *osteitis*. In practice, this distinction is probably not important, as infection of the medullary cavity of the bone easily enters the Haversian systems and Volksman canals to involve the cortical bone with its periosteum.

Bones without a medullary cavity, such as the posterior wall of the maxillary sinus and posterior table of the frontal sinus, cannot be involved with osteomyelitis, but osteitis can and does occur in these areas. The treatment of bone infection varies little regardless of whether osteitis or osteomyelitis exists, so this distinction will not be emphasized.

Etiology

Osteomyelitis can be initiated from a contiguous focus of infection or from a hematogenous source.[2,4] The hematogenous route is a more common source for osteomyelitis in the long bones of children; however, in the maxillofacial region, spread from a contiguous source is the more typical etiology.[2,7] Thus patients with craniomaxillofacial osteomyelitis often give history or present with clinical findings indicating periodontal infection, sinusitis, and/or trauma.

Osteomyelitis is uncommon in the immunocompetent host. Considering the high incidence of local infections in the craniomaxillofacial region (e.g., sinusitis, pharyngitis, periodontitis) and the potentially pathogenic bacteria present in the upper aerodigestive tract, it is surprising that bone infection is not seen more frequently. One explanation for this may be the excellent blood supply normally present in this region.[2,4,8,9] Another may be the inherent resistance of the host.

On the other hand, osteomyelitis is seen more frequently in patients with vascular and immune compromise. Osteomyelitis is encountered more frequently in patients with vascular insufficiency (e.g., diabetes mellitus, sickle cell anemia, atherosclerosis, fibrous dysplasia, bone malignancy, Paget's disease, osteopetrosis, and those patients who have a history of radiation therapy or exposure to the bone-necrosing chemicals mercury, bismuth, and arsenic).[2,6,9–11] Facial bone infection is also more common in immunocompromised patients (i.e., those on immunosuppressive drugs or who have leukemia or agranulocytosis).[2,6,8–10,12] Paget's disease and osteopetrosis are included in this group as these patients suffer from neutropenia secondary to the bone marrow obliteration that accompanies these diseases. Patients who are malnourished or who are alcoholics also fall into this category as both conditions are known to lead to impaired immune function.[9,10] The organisms isolated from patients with immunosuppressive disorders are often opportunists differing from the organisms seen in immunocompetent individuals.[4]

As the prevalence of HIV infection with its concomitant immunosuppressive effects increases, it can be expected that osteomyelitis will be seen with greater frequency.[9] There have been multiple case reports describing osteomyelitis in individuals or very small groups of patients with HIV/AIDS, but a review of craniomaxillofacial bone infections in this group of patients has not been published. As expected in these patients, unusual organisms have been isolated (*Mycobacterium hemophilum* and *avium-intracellulare*, *Actinomyces naeslundii*, *Cytomegalovirus*, *Torulopsis glabrata*, *Salmonella*, and *Nocardia asteroides*).[13–18]

While many patients with osteomyelitis will have an identifiable illness predisposing them to infection, premorbid illness is not a prerequisite for infection to occur. In a recent study of osteomyelitis of the jaws, 17% of patients had no predisposing medical condition.[19] In treating patients with osteomyelitis, appropriate treatment of both the bone infection and of the underlying medical conditions must be instituted to optimize the outcome for the patient.

Pathogenesis

A common initiating feature in osteitis is the deposition of bacteria in bone. In true osteomyelitis, bacteria are deposited in the medullary cavity. The introduction of bacteria occurs infrequently by hematogenous spread or more commonly by direct spread. The bacteria may enter the medullary space after trauma in which natural barriers to infection, intact skin or mucosa, are violated either surgically or iatrogenically. Natural barriers to infection can also be violated when the abscess wall around periapical dental infections ruptures leading to seeding of the bone marrow.[20,21] In the frontal bone, infection spreads from an infected sinus via thrombophlebitic veins.[5]

Once infective material reaches the marrow cavity of the bone, an acute inflammatory reaction ensues with hyperemia, increased capillary permeability, and the influx of polymorphonuclear neutrophils.[2,21] As the inflammatory process develops, bacteria, dead inflammatory cells, and necrotic tissue accumulate, resulting in increasing intramedullary pressure.[2] As the pressure increases, venous stasis, which leads to more tissue edema, further impairs vascular flow to the involved bone. Ultimately, arterial blood flow is disrupted, and the pus within the medullary cavity is forced into the bone's nutrient vasculature, the Haversian and Volkmann's canals.[2]

Bacteria in the nutrient canals expose cortical bone to infection. In the final stages, pus enters the subperiosteal space, thereby elevating the periosteum. This further compromises the blood supply and makes it difficult for systemic antibiotics to reach the involved tissues.[2,6] Pus may break through overlying tissue, resulting in mucosal and/or cutaneous fistulae.

Using its natural defenses, the host will eventually attempt to wall-off the infection. Angiogenic factors in the inflamed area stimulate the formation of new blood vessels, which can cause bone lysis. Granulation tissue also forms and may completely surround fragments of necrotic bone (sequestra), and the body may attempt to further isolate the area of infection by forming a layer of new bone (involucrum) around the sequestrum (Figure 9.1a,b).[2,4,6,21] The formation of sequestra and involucra signify the conversion of the infection from an acute to a chronic process.

a 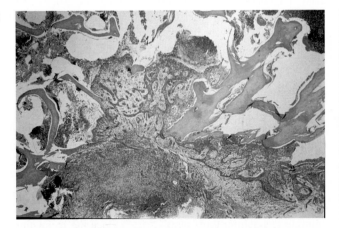 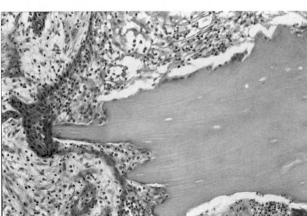 b

FIGURE 9.1 Chronic osteomyelitis with sequestrum in an acute phase in a human mandible under high magnification (a) and low magnification (b). (Courtesy of P.D. Dr. Med. G. Jundt, Institute of Pathology, Kantonspital Basel, Basel, Switzerland)

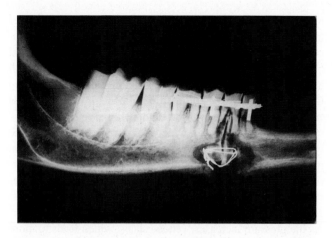

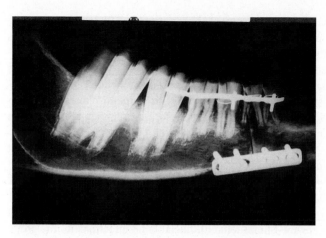

FIGURE 9.2 Radiograph of insufficient unstable fixation of an osteotomy in a sheep mandible. There is osteomyelitis with sequestrum formation. (Courtesy of Prof. Dr. Joachim Prein, Kantonsspital Basel, Basel Switzerland and Prof. Dr. Berton Rahn, Laboratory for Experimental Surgery, AO/ASIF Research Institute, Davos, Switzerland)

FIGURE 9.3 Insufficient stabilization of an osteotomy in a sheep mandible with a four-hole plate. There is osteomyelitis with sequestrum formation. (Courtesy of Prof. Dr. Joachim Prein, Kantonsspital Basel, Basel, Switzerland and Prof. Dr. Berton Rahn, Laboratory for Experimental Surgery, AO/ASIF Research Institute, Davos, Switzerland)

Radiographic Diagnosis of Craniomaxillofacial Bone Infections

Plain Radiographs

Plain radiographs are limited in their evaluation of osteomyelitis because 30% to 60% of the mineral content of the bone must be eliminated before it can be imaged radiographically (Figures 9.2 and 9.3).[2,6,22,23] Thus changes do not appear until at least ten days after the onset of infection. This disparity between the clinical situation and the radiographic findings is explained by two facts.[2,22] First, approximately 30% to 60% of the mineralized bone must be destroyed before significant radiographic changes occur. This degree of demineralization requires at least 4 to 8 days to occur, and the full extent of demineralization will not be apparent radiographically for up to 3 weeks. Second, the osteomyelitic process begins in the cancellous bone and progresses much more rapidly there than it does in the more resistant and dense cortical bone. The dense cortical bone is superimposed on the cancellous bone and, thus, obscures changes in the cancellous bone. Important radiographic findings that may eventually occur in osteomyelitis include periosteal reaction, osteoporosis, new bone formation, and sequestrum formation.[22]

As these radiographic findings can mimic those produced by malignant bone tumors, patients with unexplained osteomyelitis that is not responding as expected to treatment must be further evaluated for the possibility of malignancy.[2]

Computerized Tomography and Magnetic Resonance Imaging

Similar to plain radiographs, the bony changes on computerized tomography (CT) also lag behind the actual clinical situation. Magnetic resonance imaging (MRI) does not image bone but provides excellent resolution of surrounding soft tissues. Consequently, both CT and MRI are useful studies to evaluate complications of osteomyelitis (i.e., deep neck abscess formation, intracranial and intraorbital involvement, etc.). These studies may also be necessary in cases in which an underlying malignancy is suspected.

Radionuclide Imaging

Successful treatment of osteomyelitis depends on early diagnosis and rapid institution of therapy. Studies that are more sensitive to the early changes of osteomyelitis than plain radiographs are helpful. Radionuclide scans allow not only the early diagnosis of bone infection, showing changes as early as 24 hours after the onset of infection, but they also allow the determination of the proper timing for termination of therapy since scans return to normal after resolution of infection.[24]

Technetium Scan

Technetium accumulates at sites of osseous infection well before radiographic changes appear. Technetium phosphate compounds diffuse through the extracellular compartment to osseous tissue where the phosphate component binds to the hydration shell on the surface of hydroxyapatite crystals.[22] The greatest uptake occurs in less mature, less calcified bone. Areas of increased osteoblastic or osteoclastic activity concentrate technetium most avidly.[4,22–24] Once the technetium is incorporated in bone, its extracellular concentration decreases, promoting the diffusion of the radionuclide from the vascular to the extracellular space.[22] This diffusion reverses direction as the kidney excretes the technetium and the concentration in the extracellular space decreases. After approximately 4 hours, 30% to 40% of the injected activity will be excreted in the urine, while 55% to 60% is retained in bone.[22] Thus bone scanning at this time reflects the increase in activity of osteoblasts rather than increased vascular flow or extracellular concentration.

This principle forms the basis for the three-phase technetium bone scan.[6,22] The first phase is obtained after tracer injection and demonstrates the vascularity of the area of interest. In the second phase, which is obtained by scanning immediately after phase one, the extracellular uptake of tracer is imaged. Phase three is obtained 3 to 4 hours after tracer injection and reflects osteoblastic activity. The three-phase scan allows the differentiation of osteomyelitis from overlying soft tissue lesions.[6,22] In osteomyelitis, both the early (phases one and two) and late (phase three) scans will demonstrate increased technetium uptake. In soft tissue infection, the early scans will demonstrate increased uptake with decreasing uptake in the later phase-three scan.

Gallium Scan

Gallium-67-citrate is widely used to identify and localize inflammatory processes in the musculoskeletal system. Gallium binds to actively dividing cells, including white blood cells, tumor cells, and osteoblasts.[6] Its mechanism of localization is not known but is likely the result of several factors.[22,23] Gallium-67 binds to lactoferrin, which is found within leukocytes and transported to areas of inflammation. Lactoferrin is also released from leukocytes during bacterial phagocytosis. The free lactoferrin then binds to gallium, and the gallium-lactoferrin complex remains localized at the site of inflammation by binding to receptors on macrophages.

Gallium-67 and technetium scans are usually combined to identify sites of osteomyelitis.[6,22–24] While technetium-99m is very sensitive for evaluating sites of inflammation, it is not specific for infection.[22] Gallium-67 demonstrates only the site of infection without imaging the adjacent osteoblastic bone response of osteomyelitis. Thus when the two scans are combined, the diagnosis of active infection is more reliable.

The interpretation of sequential technetium-gallium scans can be difficult. At most centers, if both the gallium and technetium scan show increased uptake, especially if the gallium uptake exceeds that of technetium, the scan is interpreted as positive.[22] If the technetium scan is positive and the gallium scan is negative, the test is negative for infection.

The technetium scan remains positive long after the infection resolves as it reflects bone remodeling.[23] The gallium scan, however, is useful to follow the course of the disease and as a guide to termination of antibiotic therapy as the scan returns to normal after resolution of infection.

Indium White Blood Cell Scan

Both technetium and gallium scans have significant drawbacks as ideal agents to image bone infection. Technetium is sensitive but has poor specificity. Gallium uptake is increased at sites of noninfectious processes, including sites of tumors and new bone formation, leading to false positive results. Gallium uptake is often minimal at sites of low-grade infection leading to false negative results. Because of these drawbacks, radiolabeled leukocytes have been used to image sites of active infection.

The most ideally suited isotope for this application has been indium-111, which has a half-life of 67 hours allowing scanning to be performed over several days without exposing the patient to a large quantity of radiation or prolonged radiation.[22]

The indium-labeled leukocyte scan can be interpreted without a technetium bone scan.[22] If local accumulation of leukocytes occurs that is higher than surrounding bone activity, the scan is interpreted as positive. If no local accumulation occurs, the scan is negative. A technetium scan can be used as an overlay to better localize the infection.[22]

Experience with the indium-labeled-leukocyte scan is less than that of the technetium and gallium scans. The sensitivity of this scan is reported to be as high as 90% to 95% when imaged at 24 hours.[25] Despite this high sensitivity, a case of a false negative indium scan has recently been reported.[26]

Locations

Osteomyelitis may involve any bone in the craniomaxillofacial area; however, some bones are much more prone to involvement than others. For purposes of discussion in this chapter, craniofacial sites of involvement will be divided into lower third (mandible), middle third (maxilla, orbital bones, nasal bones, and zygoma), and upper third (frontal bone). In addition, a brief discussion of osteomyelitis of the cervical spine will also be presented as cervical osteomyelitis can be a complication not only of infections that occur in the head and neck, but also after commonly performed surgical procedures in the head and neck. Knowledge of the presentation and treatment of this potentially fatal complication is vital to surgeons who perform craniomaxillofacial surgery.

Osteomyelitis of the middle third of the face occurs much less frequently than osteomyelitis of the frontal bone or mandible.[2,6,20] The explanation for this lies in the very rich and diffuse blood supply to the maxilla. Additionally, the maxillary bone has a very small amount of medullary tissue and is composed of thin cortical plates.[2] Consequently, infection is less likely to become confined within the bone and more likely to dissipate into the paranasal sinuses and surrounding soft tissues.[2]

Osteomyelitis of the Mandible

Classification

Osteomyelitis can be classified as acute or chronic and suppurative or nonsuppurative.[2] The major focus of this chapter is the diagnosis and evaluation of patients with acute and chronic suppurative osteomyelitis. Brief descriptions of the nonsuppurative forms will be included for completeness.

Suppurative Osteomyelitis of the Mandible

Etiology

Osteomyelitis in the mandible can begin either hematogenously or spread from contiguous sites of infection. The hematogenous route is rarely seen. Most infections spread from contiguous sites, most commonly infected teeth, periodontal disease, and contaminated fractures.[2,4,6] Occasionally, spread from adjacent soft tissue infection is seen. Infection can also be introduced at the time of surgery on the mandible.

Many but not all patients with osteomyelitis of the mandible have conditions that predispose them to bone infection. These conditions include diseases that affect the peripheral vasculature as well as conditions that alter the host's ability to fight infection. These conditions must be identified and treated appropriately if the infection is to be treated adequately.

Posttraumatic Osteomyelitis of the Mandible (PTOM)

Posttraumatic osteomyelitis is characterized by infection and nonunion at a fracture site. This is probably one of the most frequent causes of osteomyelitis of the mandible. It can be considered a form of osteomyelitis associated with contiguous infection or direct trauma.[27] Mathog and Boies reviewed a series of 577 patients with mandible fractures and reported an incidence of osteomyelitis of 1.2%.[28] Treatment of PTOM will be discussed in detail in a later chapter.

Pathogenesis

By understanding the pathogenesis of osteomyelitis of the mandible, the clinical presentation of patients with this infection is easily understood. The infectious agent is introduced into the medullary cavity by periodontal infection, chronic movement of fracture fragments, or other mechanisms.[2] Once the agent has entered, an inflammatory response ensues with pus formation and accumulation. The intramedullary pressure increases sufficiently to cause venous stasis and ultimately arterial thrombosis.[2,4] Neural compression also develops, resulting in altered sensation (paresthesia, anesthesia, pain) in the distribution of the mental nerve. Ultimately, pus enters the subperiosteal space, culminating in devitalized bone and sequestration.[2] The pus can also penetrate the periosteum, leading to sub-periosteal abscesses with resultant cutaneous and mucosal fistulae.

Microbiology

In older reports on mandibular bone infection, *Staphylococcus aureus* and *Staphylococcus epidermidis* were cultured in approximately 90% of the cases in which organisms were isolated.[2] Many of these reports also had high rates of negative cultures, which was likely secondary to poor culturing techniques for anaerobic bacteria. It is probably unlikely that osteomyelitis is ever due solely to staphylococcal infection as studies using careful anaerobic culturing techniques are able to isolate anaerobes in nearly all cases.[29] Careful culturing techniques and prompt transportation to the laboratory are essential if anaerobic bacteria are to be consistently isolated. Most cases of mandibular osteomyelitis are mixed aerobic-anaerobic infections or strictly anaerobic.[2,10] Calhoun et al. in 1988 found polymicrobial infections in 93% of their 60 patients with an average of 3.9 organisms per patient.[10] *Streptococcus* species, *Bacteroides* species, *Lactobacillus* species, *Eubacterium* species, and *Klebsiella* species were seen most commonly in this study. Commonly isolated anaerobes include *Bacteroides* species, *Fusobacterium*, *Peptostreptococcus*, *Peptococcus*, and *Actinomyces*.[6] Aerobes isolated frequently include hemolytic streptococci, pneumococci, typhoid bacilli, acid-fast bacilli, and *E. coli*.

Actinomycotic Osteomyelitis

Actinomycotic osteomyelitis is an anaerobic infection that merits special attention. The jaw is the most common site of actinomycotic osteomyelitis.[30] *Actinomyces israelii* is the organism most frequently isolated in these cases.[31] The organism has been classified as a fungus in the past, but it is now known to be a slow-growing gram-positive filamentous anaerobic or microaerophilic bacteria. In addition, *A. israelii*, *A. naeslundii*, *A. viscosus*, and *A. odontolyticus* have also been reported as agents causing osteomyelitis.[31] Actinomyces are part of the normal oral flora and gain access to soft tissue and bone when there is a breakdown in host defense through associated disease (i.e., periodontal inflammation, direct spread from soft tissue infection) or direct trauma. The soft tissues are more commonly affected than the bone.[31] Actinomycotic infections are characterized by multiple abscesses, fistulae, and the presence of sulfur granules.

Clinical Findings

Acute Osteomyelitis

Patients presenting with osteomyelitis of the mandible should be questioned for a history of dental extraction, dental infection, trauma to the mandible, etc. In some cases, none of these historical factors will be elicited.

The clinical presentation of acute mandibular osteomyelitis will vary, depending on whether the infection is confined to the medullary cavity or has spread to accumulate subperiosteally.[6] Infection confined to the medullary cavity leads to altered sensation in the distribution of the mental nerve on the affected side secondary to neurovascular compression. There is usually indurated swelling over the affected area, and frequently teeth will be tender to percussion but do not loosen until later in the course of infection.[2,6] Tender regional adenopathy is almost always seen. As the infection spreads to involve the cortical bone and periosteum, severe, boring pain develops with a fluctuant intraoral and extraoral swelling over the affected area. The periosteum can be elevated to the temporomandibular joint, where a septic arthritis can occur. This is more common in children in whom the periosteum is less firmly attached than in adults.[2] Pathologic fracture, sequestration, and fistula formation occur later in the course of infection and bode the transition to chronic osteomyelitis.

In contrast to osteomyelitis of the long bones, osteomyelitis of the jaws is associated with relatively few systemic signs and symptoms.[2,4,6,8] The patient usually has a low-grade fever and may complain of malaise and fatigue. Laboratory findings reveal a mild leukocytosis (8,000–15,000 cells/mm^3) with a shift to the left. The erythrocyte sedimentation rate (ESR) may be elevated but does not reliably predict the severity or course of the disease. C-reactive protein (CRP) has been shown in some studies to be more useful than the ESR in reflecting the effectiveness of therapy and predicting recovery in bone infections.[32–35] Wannfors et al. studied CRP levels in chronic osteomyelitis of the jaws and found that a specific "mass of inflammation" was required before elevated CRP values could be detected.[36]

The body of the mandible is most frequently involved by osteomyelitis, followed by the anterior mandible, angle, ramus, and condyle.[10] The condyle is only rarely involved, and the coronoid process is involved even less frequently. The blood supply to the coronoid process and condyle is less dependent on flow through the inferior alveolar vessels than other areas of the mandible. The coronoid receives its blood supply from the temporalis muscle vessels, while the condyle is supplied by a branch of the arterial supply to the lateral pterygoid muscle in addition to branches from the inferior alveolar artery.[6]

Chronic Osteomyelitis

Chronic osteomyelitis is characterized by refractoriness to host defenses or to initial therapy.[2,6] Symptoms include localized pain and swelling. The patient may present with draining fistulae, pathologic fracture, or only localized pain and swelling. Trismus is a common complaint. Constitutional symptoms are rare.[37] In patients with osteomyelitis secondary to a fracture, mobility of the fracture will be present.

Imaging Studies

Plain Radiographs

Radiographic findings of suppurative osteomyelitis of the mandible are similar to those seen in other locations. The first radiographic changes will not be seen for at least 10 to 14 days after the onset of infection.[22] These will vary depending on the stage of the disease, but often scattered areas of bone destruction separated by normal areas of bone are seen.[2,4,6,8] Sequestra and involucra are seen once the infection is well established and indicate the transition to chronic disease. Subperiosteal deposition of bone or deposition of new bone on existing trabeculae may also be seen. When periosteal bone production is present, malignant bone-producing tumors must be included in the differential diagnosis.[2]

CT and MRI

Computed tomography and MRI are not particularly useful for the diagnosis of early osteomyelitis. Their use should be reserved for diagnosing complications or when malignancy is suspected. Similar to plain radiographs, bony changes also take 1 to 3 weeks to appear on CT.[6] Robinson et al. combined single-photon-emission CT with traditional x-ray CT to study anatomy and sequestrum activity.[38] They reported that the two examinations are complementary and aid in successful surgical and medical treatment of osteomyelitis. Further studies of this technique are required before its routine use can be advocated.

Radionuclide Studies

Radionuclide studies reveal changes in osteomyelitis as early as 24 hours after the onset of infection.[24] They provide confirmation of the diagnosis well before plain radiographs show significant change. As discussed earlier, the technetium scan is highly sensitive but poorly specific, and the gallium-67 scan also suffers from false positive and false negative images. The combination of the two scans, however, leads to a sensitivity of 98% with the gallium scan remaining positive for as long as infection is present. The conversion of the gallium scan to normal indicates the appropriate time to discontinue antibiotic therapy.

The indium-WBC scan has been less studied than the technetium and gallium scan, but it is purported to be highly sensitive and specific for osteomyelitis. Calhoun et al., however, found that the sensitivity of indium scans was 71% as opposed to the 95% sensitivity of the technetium scan.[10] Indium-WBC scan can be used to follow the course of the disease and similar to gallium indicates the appropriate time to terminate antibiotic therapy.

Nonsuppurative Osteomyelitis of the Mandible

Chronic Sclerosing Osteomyelitis

Chronic sclerosing osteomyelitis is also known as *sclerosing osteitis, multiple enostosis, local bone sclerosis, ossifying osteomyelitis, sclerosing cementoma, gigantiform cementoma,* and *sclerotic cemental masses of the jaws.*[2] It occurs either focally or diffusely. The focal form occurs most frequently in patients under the age of 20 years in association with low-grade dental infections.[2,4,8] Mild pain may be the patient's sole presenting complaint.[4] Radiographically, a circumscribed radiopaque mass of sclerotic bone associated with tooth roots is seen.[2] The sclerosis is thought to be the body's response to constant irritation.

True chronic diffuse sclerosing is difficult to diagnose and is often confused with fibro-osseous diseases such as fibrous dysplasia and florid osseous dysplasia.[9] It is seen mainly in patients in the mid-twenties to late forties and occurs more commonly in women (3:1 female to male predominance).[2,4,9] Blacks are affected more frequently than whites. Diagnosis in the early stages of the disease can be particularly difficult as early symptoms are vague and nonspecific.[2,9] Pain, swelling, and slight rises in temperature and/or ESR are seen. Later, patients develop unremitting, severe pain and frequently develop chemical narcotic analgesic dependencies. The ischemia, endosteal, and periosteal inflammation associated with the sclerosis produce the unremitting pain.[9] Characteristic radiographic changes include diffuse intramedullary sclerosis with ill-defined margins and focal areas of radiolucency within the sclerotic region.[2,4,9] This is also confirmed on histologic examination with findings of ischemia and irregular bony sclerotic changes (Figure 9.4). The disease may affect any region of the mandible, but the ramus and body are the most frequent sites of involvement.[9] The maxilla is rarely involved.

The etiology of chronic diffuse sclerosing osteomyelitis is obscure. While it has been most frequently attributed to an infectious process, negative cultures are frequently produced.[2,9] Studies using careful anaerobic culture techniques have shown this disease to be a form of actinomycotic osteomyelitis with *Eikenella corrodens* being cultured in approximately 50% of cases.[9]

Other studies have attempted to show immunologic aberrations in patients with diffuse sclerosing osteomyelitis, correlating the disease with specific HLA tissue types (HLA B13 and B27) and with hyperactive humoral immune response.[39] A recent report links diffuse sclerosing osteomyelitis with a systemic process that has characteristic skin and bone lesions and is known as *synovitis, acne, pustulosis, hyperostosis, osteitis* (SAPHO) *syndrome*.[40] The significance of the HLA, immunologic, and SAPHO associations remains to be proven.

Garre's Sclerosing Osteomyelitis

Garre's sclerosing osteomyelitis was first reported in 1893 by Carl Garre as an irritation induced focal thickening of the anterior tibia in young adults.[2] The first case of Garre's osteomyelitis in the mandible was reported by Pell et al. in 1955.[41] The etiology is thought to be secondary to low-grade infection or irritation that stimulates the periosteum to lay down new bone. It is seen most commonly in adolescents (mean age of 12) with a female-to-male predominance of 1.4 to 1. The most common inciting factor is an abscessed mandibular first molar.[41] As new bone is deposited, a localized, nontender bony enlargement is palpable, producing facial asymmetry. The asymmetric area is bony hard with normal overlying mucosa and skin; however, the gingivobuccal sulcus may be obliterated.[41] The periosteal proliferation does not cross the midline or involve only the lingual aspect of the mandible.[4] There are no systemic symptoms.

Radiographically, diffusely opaque reactive cortical bone is seen. It characteristically develops an "onion skin" pattern of successive layers of new bone deposition with the outermost layer appearing regular and well defined.[2,4,41] The radiographic appearance is not pathognomonic, and Ewing's sarcoma, osteosarcoma, and cortical hyperostosis must be ruled out. In the absence of dental pathology or with poor response to treatment, biopsy must be performed.

Neuralgia-Inducing Cavitational Osteonecrosis (NICO)

Low-grade osteomyelitis producing facial neuralgias is a controversial form of bone infection. Bouquot et al. named this entity neuralgia-inducing cavitational osteonecrosis (NICO) in 1992 after studying 135 patients with trigeminal neuralgia or atypical facial neuralgia.[42] Surgical specimens of every patient revealed intraosseous inflammation. Long-term pain reduction was achieved by Bouquot et al. in 91 of 103 neuralgia patients treated with curettage. Histologically, NICO has a distinct appearance from that of other forms of osteomyelitis. The etiology of NICO is obscure and widespread acceptance of it as a unique pathologic lesion capable of causing facial neuralgia is lacking.

Osteomyelitis of the Middle Third of the Face (Maxilla, Zygoma, Nose, and Orbit)

Osteomyelitis of the maxilla is a rare disease. It was first described by Rees in 1847 and scattered case reports have appeared in the literature since then.[43,44] It occurs much less fre-

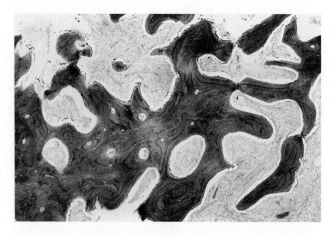

FIGURE 9.4 Chronic sclerosing osteomyelitis in a human mandible. (Courtesy of P.D. Dr. med. G. Jundt, Institute of Pathology, Kantonsspital Basel, Basel, Switzerland)

quently than osteomyelitis of the mandible with ratios of mandibular to maxillary osteomyelitis ranging from 3 to 1 to 19 to 1.[3,19,45] Maxillary involvement is seen much more frequently in younger patients and is the most common craniofacial location in newborn infants.[3]

The explanation for the paucity of cases of maxillary osteomyelitis is found by examining the bony anatomy of the maxilla and its blood supply. The maxilla is composed of thin cortical plates of bone with minimal amounts of medullary tissue.[45] Consequently, infection is less likely to be confined to the medullary space as it erupts early with subsequent dissipation of edema and pus into the soft tissues and paranasal sinuses. As the cause of maxillary osteomyelitis is most commonly dental infection, inflammation derived from maxillary infections often extends to the maxillary sinus and outer part of the cortex rather than spreading within the confines of the bone.[45] The maxillary blood supply is far more extensive than that of the mandible, which further reduces the incidence of osteomyelitis.[2]

Ischemia and aseptic necrosis of the soft and hard tissues of the maxilla is a rare complication of Le Fort I osteotomies.[3,46] While it is known that blood flow to the maxilla decreases in the operative and perioperative period after maxillary osteotomies, collateral blood flow likely maintains viability of the maxillary tissues. Necrosis and infection are therefore unlikely in an immunocompetent host with otherwise normal vasculature.

The most commonly affected area in the maxilla is the molar area because it is the region of the maxilla with the highest concentration of bone marrow.[45] In a study by Adekeye et al. of 141 patients with osteomyelitis of the middle and lower thirds of the face, localized involvement of the maxilla occurred in 24 (17%) patients, premaxillary involvement was seen in 6 (4%) patients, maxillary and malar involvement in 2 (1.5%) patients, and isolated nasal and malar involvement in 1 (0.7%) and 2 (1.5%) patients, respectively.[3]

The etiology and pathogenesis of osteomyelitis of the middle third of the face are similar to that described for osteomyelitis of the mandible.[2] Two forms of osteomyelitis of the middle third of the face deserve special attention: infantile osteomyelitis and osteoblastic osteitis.

Infantile Osteomyelitis

Infantile osteomyelitis usually occurs during the first 9 months of life and can be seen as early as 7 days postnatally.[43] The most common site of involvement is the maxilla. Early diagnosis and treatment are important as significant morbidity and mortality can result from delayed treatment. The etiology of this infection is thought to be secondary to contiguous spread through oral mucosal wounds incurred at the time of delivery or later from sucking on contaminated nipples.[2,43] Reports have been published of maxillary osteomyelitis occurring in infants suckling on a breast with an active mastitis. Spread from infected maxillary and ethmoid sinuses and from infected lacrimal sacs may also occur.[43,47] The hematogenous spread of pneumococci and streptococci to the maxilla has been reported.[43]

Once the maxilla is seeded and infection becomes established, the osteomyelitis runs a rapid course.[43,44,47,48] Infants with maxillary osteomyelitis present with hyperpyrexia, tachycardia, vomiting, and prostration. As the disease progresses, seizures may be seen. Local signs of infection include facial swelling with periorbital cellulitis and edema. Proptosis is common and purulent drainage from the ipsilateral nostril is seen almost universally. The intraoral examination reveals swelling of the maxilla. Subperiosteal abscesses can form as can fistulae through the palatal and alveolar mucosa.

Plain radiographs are of little help in diagnosing infantile osteomyelitis as they are invariably normal early in the disease and show only local bone sequestra in long-standing cases.[43] Computed tomographic (CT) scanning is useful to image orbital and intracranial complications of the disease. Radionuclide studies can be used in cases in which the diagnosis is in question.[43]

S. aureus, *S. pneumonia*, *S. pyogenes*, and *H. influenza* are the most common causes of infantile osteomyelitis.[2,43,47] *Citrobacter freundii* has also been reported as the causative agent.[47] *C. freundii* can cause severe meningitis and brain abscesses in neonates.

Complications of infantile osteomyelitis include blindness, meningitis, cerebral abscess, loss of tooth buds, necrosis of the zygoma, septicemia, and death.[2,43,44,47] The mortality rate has been reported as high as 4%.[49] Therefore, prompt diagnosis and institution of appropriate treatment are vital.

Osteoblastic Osteitis

Osteoblastic osteitis of the maxilla is a rare type of bone infection that usually occurs secondary to chronic maxillary sinusitis, recurrent episodes of acute sinusitis or as a postsurgical infection.[50] The posterior wall of the sinus is the most common site of involvement. The patient presents with vague, deep facial pain. The pain often goes undiagnosed until the infection spreads to the pterygomaxillary space or infratemporal space through anastomotic veins between these spaces and the maxillary sinus.[50] Once the infection spreads to these spaces, the patient develops trismus and temporal swelling. Involvement of the infraorbital nerve may cause a trigeminal neuralgia-like pain.[50]

Diagnosis of osteoblastic osteitis is radiologic. Bone thickening and sclerosis is seen in the involved bone often accompanied by sinus mucosal disease indicating the site of origin of the bone infection.[50] Scintigraphy is often useful for diagnosis of this entity.

Radiologic Diagnosis of Osteomyelitis of the Maxilla

Kaneda et al. studied eleven adult cases of maxillary osteomyelitis radiographically. The molar region was involved in seven cases.[45] The most common radiographic change was spotty osteolysis seen in seven cases. Osteolytic change is more commonly diffuse in the mandible. Osteosclerosis was seen in five cases, and sequestra in four.

The use of CT, MRI, and radionuclide studies in the diagnosis of osteomyelitis of the jaws is discussed in the section on osteomyelitis of the mandible.

Osteomyelitis of the Frontal Bone

Osteomyelitis of the cranial bones was discussed by the Roman physician Celsus in the first century A.D.[1] He recommended resection of the involved bone. It was not until the 17th century that osteomyelitis localized to the frontal bone was described by Fabricius Hildanus in his *Treatise of Surgery*.[5,51] In the following century, Percival Potts described the puffy tumor and was the first to associate this pericranial tumor with frontal extradural abscess.[5,51,52] Tilley in 1897 attributed frontal osteomyelitis to nasal sinus suppuration, suggesting that thrombophlebitis of the diploic vessels resulted in bacterial seeding of the bone.

Osteomyelitis of the frontal bone has become a relatively rare entity since the introduction of antibiotics. It is still seen more frequently than osteomyelitis of the middle third of the face.[51] The associated mortality has also decreased. Mortality rates for frontal osteomyelitis were reported as high as 60% in the preantibiotic era, but had dropped to 3.7% by the 1960s.[51] The disease continues to carry a high morbidity, including meningitis, brain abscesses, and severe forehead defects. Many of these complications can be averted if the disease is recognized early in its course and treated appropriately. Because of the decreasing incidence of frontal osteomyelitis, individual experience with the disease can be limited leading to delay in diagnosis and higher morbidity.

Etiology

Trauma and sinusitis can both lead to osteomyelitis of the frontal bone.[52–55] Fractures of the frontal sinus, especially when the nasofrontal duct is violated, can lead to osteomyelitis often months or even years after the fracture. Surgical trauma may also predispose the patient to osteomyelitis. Trauma to the frontal bone in patients with coexisting frontal sinus infection has culminated in osteomyelitis.[54] Osteomyelitis has also been reported in intranasal cocaine abusers and in patients who swim or dive with an acute bacterial sinusitis.[56] Osteomyelitis may also occur with the first episode of frontal sinusitis in the absence of trauma or as an acute infection su-perimposed on chronic sinus disease.[5,54] Many patients have a history of allergic rhinosinusitis.

Most cases of osteomyelitis are in the age range of 12 to 29, and most patients who have cerebral complications also fall into this age group.[5,51] This is explained by Woodward, who stated that the diploic system is proportionally larger and more active in adolescents and young adults.[57]

Predisposing medical illnesses are infrequently mentioned in the literature. There have been reports of osteomyelitis complicating fibrous dysplasia of the skull.[58] However, it appears that with frontal osteomyelitis, the most important etiologic factors are the presence of infection in the sinuses and/or injury to the frontal bone. Undoubtedly, host immunodeficiencies and vascular insufficiency may increase the likelihood of serious disease and lessen the effectiveness of treatment. These host deficiencies, if present, must be treated in conjunction with medical and surgical treatment of osteomyelitis.

Pathogenesis

Veins of the mucous membranes of the frontal sinuses communicate with the diploe of the inner and outer tables of the frontal sinus.[54] These diploic veins also drain the marrow cavity and frontal bone. There is direct communication between these veins and the intracranial venous sinus system.[51] The spread of infection in patients with frontal sinusitis occurs through these veins by causing thrombophlebitis and ultimately deposition of bacteria in the marrow cavity of the frontal bone. Once the Haversian systems of the inner and outer frontal tables become involved, there is rapid necrosis of bone with focal coalescence resulting in large areas of decalcified, decomposing bone.[5,51,54] As these veins cross suture lines, frontal osteomyelitis may appear in areas distant from the frontal sinus. Sequestra may form.

Infection may also spread to the frontal bone directly through congenital dehiscences in the intersinus septum or the posterior plate of the frontal sinus.

The usual spread of infection is upward into the frontal bone with eventual cortical breakthrough and the formation of a subperiosteal abscess, the Pott's puffy tumor.[51] Inferior extension can lead to orbital complications, including periorbital abscesses and draining sinocutaneous fistula. Cortical breakthrough in the posterior wall leads to the formation of epidural and subdural abscesses, meningitis, cavernous sinus thrombosis, and even brain abscess.

The pathogenesis of frontal osteomyelitis in fractures of the frontal sinus may result from direct implantation of bacteria into the marrow cavity through an open fracture or from extension of pyoceles along fracture lines.[51] Disruption of the nasofrontal duct can lead to the formation of a mucopyocele with subsequent osteomyelitis years after the injury.[59]

Microbiology

The bacteriology of frontal osteomyelitis is similar to that of chronic sinusitis.[60] *Staphylococcus* is the most common pathogen isolated from frontal osteomyelitis. Other aerobic pathogens include streptococci, *H. influenzae*, and *Neissera subflava*.[5,51,60,61] Gram-negative rods including *Escherichia coli*, *Proteus mirabilis*, and *Pseudomonas aeruginosa* have been isolated but seem to occur more frequently in diabetic and/or immunosuppressed patients. Anaerobic organisms are seen frequently, especially anaerobic streptococci. Mixed infections are common. Any organism can be isolated including fungi and mycobacteria.

Cultures are required to identify the causative agent. Cultures are obtained by early incision and drainage of abscesses or by frontal sinus trephination.

Clinical Findings

The presentation of osteomyelitis of the frontal bone depends on whether the process is acute or chronic and whether the anterior or posterior table is involved.[54] There is an acute fulminating form in which the patient presents with the sudden onset of high fever, leukocytosis, severe frontal pain, and advancing pitting edema and erythema of the forehead (Pott's puffy tumor), which frequently involved the upper eyelid on the affected side. These patients are extremely toxic, and if untreated, diplopia, proptosis, orbital abscess, cavernous sinus thrombosis, and cerebral complications may ensue, ultimately culminating in death within 24 hours to several days.[62] This form of frontal osteomyelitis appeared more frequently prior to the advent of antibiotics.[5]

A majority of the patients do not present with the fulminant form of infection but rather complain of some head pain and a low-grade fever.[54] Most will have frontal tenderness with pitting edema. Edema of the upper eyelid(s) is frequently present.

Patients with frontal bone osteomyelitis often give a history of trauma to the frontal area several days to several years prior to the onset of osteomyelitis.[51] A history of sinusitis or nasal/sinus surgery may also be elicited.[5]

In the chronic form of frontal osteomyelitis, there is no toxicity.[54,62] These patients may complain of intermittent or constant headache and low-grade fever. Swelling of the forehead and chronic draining fistula are often seen. Both sinocutaneous and sino-orbital fistulae can occur. Bony necrosis eventually occurs with severe forehead defects. A history of frontal trauma, sinusitis, or sinonasal surgery may be given.

Osteitis of the inner table is usually diagnosed only after a complication such as meningitis, epidural or subdural abscess, or a brain abscess has occurred.[54]

Laboratory studies are generally of no help in the diagnosis of frontal osteomyelitis. An equivocal white blood cell count and a normal erythrocyte sedimentation rate will be found in more than 50% of cases.[52]

Imaging Studies

Plain radiographs in evaluation of frontal osteomyelitis reveal no bony changes early in the course of the disease. While evidence of acute and/or chronic sinusitis, frontal bone or sinus fracture, pyocele, or soft tissue swelling may be seen early, bony changes lag 1 to 2 weeks behind the clinical progress of the disease.[54,63,64]

Radiographic changes begin with periosteal elevation.[5] Sclerosis and erosion of the sinus border occur later. "Motheaten" areas of bone destruction, resorption, and eventually sequestration will eventually occur. Thus plain radiographs are helpful in diagnosis but should never be relied upon to determine the extent of the disease.

Plain radiographs in the evaluation of suspected frontal osteomyelitis have largely been supplanted by CT scanning. The bony changes as imaged by CT lag behind the actual clinical situation but less so than plain radiographs. In addition, CT with enhancement is the best method of identifying areas of extracranial and intracranial infection as well as bony defects.[52,65] Serial CT scans are useful in the evaluation of new bony erosion or for following an intracranial process allowing earlier recognition and treatment of progressive or unresponsive disease.

Radionuclide Imaging

Technetium-99m MDP and gallium-67 bone scans are used to confirm the diagnosis of frontal osteomyelitis.[64] Uren et al. used gallium-67 scans to evaluate three patients with suspected frontal osteomyelitis.[66] In two of these patients the scans confirmed the diagnosis; however, the third patient had only a soft tissue abscess without osteomyelitis. Radionuclide studies are useful in delineating soft tissue and intracranial extensions of infection as well as following the infection to determine the appropriate time to terminate therapy.

Osteomyelitis of the Cervical Spine

Craniomaxillofacial surgeons must be aware of osteomyelitis of the cervical spine not only because patients may present with signs and symptoms localizing to the head and neck but because surgical procedures performed in the head and neck can lead to this complication. Although it occurs infrequently in otherwise healthy adults, cervical osteomyelitis must be diagnosed and treated early. Failure to do so can result in subluxation, dislocation, spinal cord compression, and death.[67–69] The cervical spine is less frequently affected by osteomyelitis than the lumbar or thoracic spine.[70]

Osteomyelitis of the cervical spine is more frequently the result of hematogenous seeding than direct extension.[70] The lower five cervical vertebrae and the body of the second vertebrae receive their blood supply from the vertebral or carotid arteries or their branches. Hematogenous dissemination can occur via the arterial or the venous systems.[70] Arterial spread likely occurs via nutrient posterior arterioles to the metaphyseal portion of the vertebral body.[69] Venous spread is facilitated by Batson's plexus, a valveless system of veins that travels the entire length of the vertebral column.[67,69] Bacteria can travel retrograde through this system of veins. Most commonly the causative bacteria arise from the pelvis following manipulation of the urinary tract or in association with a urinary tract infection.[67]

Of more interest to the maxillofacial surgeon are cases of cervical osteomyelitis that follow surgery in the head and neck. Cervical osteomyelitis has been reported after laryngectomy, tracheoesophageal puncture, cricopharyngeal myotomy, penetrating neck wounds, dental extractions, delayed repair of mandibular fracture, and other maxillofacial procedures.[71–77] The spread of infection in these cases is thought to occur via a system of pharyngovertebral veins that connect the pharyngeal venous system and upper cervical epidural sinuses.[67] Spread may also occur via lymphatics. As lymphatic drainage from the maxilla and oropharynx includes retropharyngeal nodes, a suppurative adenitis of these nodes could result in prevertebral fascia dehiscence and subsequent osteomyelitis.[67]

Adults are more commonly affected by cervical osteomyelitis than are children.[70] This is in part due to the hyperemia associated with osteoporosis but is more likely related to the change in vascular anatomy that occurs with age.[69,70] In children and young adults, vascular channels perforate the vertebral end-plates allowing bacteria access to the disc space. The adjacent vertebral bodies are affected secondarily. In the adult, there is no direct vascular communication between the vertebral body and the intervertebral disk. Consequently, hematogenously disseminated bacteria lodge in avascular areas adjacent to the subchondral bone.

As with other forms of osteomyelitis, certain medical illnesses increase the likelihood of infection.[69] Patients with diabetes mellitus, who are immunosuppressed, or who use illicit drugs intravenously appear to be particularly susceptible to cervical osteomyelitis.

Depending on bacterial virulence and host resistance, bacteria that are seeded into the vertebrae are either contained by the host with subsequent healing via fibrous or bony union, or complete destruction of the vertebral body can occur.[70] Destruction can result in paralysis and even death. Involvement of the odontoid process and craniovertebral regions can be particularly devastating and may result in meningitis, abscess of the medulla oblongata, and lateral atlantoaxial subluxation (Grisel's syndrome).[67,70]

Osteomyelitis of the cervical spine can result from infection by bacteria, fungi and parasites.[69,78] *Mycobacterium tuberculosis* may be the most common agent with the most common nontuberculous agent being *S. aureus*.[70,79,80] *Pseudomonas* is seen with greater frequency in intravenous drug users.[69]

Patients with cervical osteomyelitis may present with few complaints and a paucity of specific physical examination findings. Most commonly, patients complain of neck pain, anorexia, chills, night sweats, and malaise.[68–70] Cervical pain may be referred to the shoulders or scapular areas. Only when the process has progressed to nerve root compression are radiculopathy or paresis notable.[69,70] If the osteomyelitis is secondary to a retropharyngeal abscess or if an abscess has resulted from the osteomyelitis, the patient may present with more classic symptoms of a retropharyngeal abscess: dyspnea, dysphagia, odynophagia, or drooling.[81,82] Tenderness of the cervical spine and limited motion of the neck are seen on physical examination.

Diagnosis is established by history and physical examination, supplemented by needle biopsy of the affected area.[70] Important to the workup of these patients is a careful history of recent urinary tract infection or manipulation, surgery or trauma to the neck or face, etc. A high index of suspicion is required. Radiographic findings lag well behind the actual clinical situation and may not be helpful in the acute stages of the infection.[67,69,70,79] Findings will eventually include rarefaction of bone, disc space destruction, soft tissue swelling, and a sclerotic reaction. Early findings will include loss of prevertebral soft-tissue planes, and swelling can present with few bony x-ray changes evident.[70,79] Bone scanning may be necessary to confirm the diagnosis but can be problematic secondary to the presence of false positive scans in patients with degenerative disease of the spine.[79] Magnetic resonance imaging is more sensitive than CT or plain radiographs in diagnosing osteomyelitis, and it provides much better visualization of associated soft-tissue changes than radionuclide scans.[79]

Treatment requires long-term organism-specific antibiotic therapy (6 to 8 weeks).[67] Surgical drainage and debridement is often required, and cervical stabilization is vital. Many patients will eventually require bone grafting and spiral fusion.

Osteoradionecrosis (ORN)

Radiation therapy produces hypovascular, hypocellular, and hypoxic tissue.[83] Osteoradionecrosis (ORN) is primarily a problem of poor wound healing secondary to these changes rather than bacterial infection. Bacterial infection of the radiated bone can and does occur but is not the inciting event. Although ORN is fundamentally an avascular necrosis of bone rather than a primary bone infection, its inclusion and brief discussion here is warranted as secondary infection in irradiated bone is not uncommon.

The mandible is the most commonly involved site of osteoradionecrosis in the head and neck area.[84] The maxilla and skull are much less frequently involved. Osteoradionecrosis has also been reported in the hyoid and clavicular heads. The exact incidence of ORN after head and neck irradiation is unknown and ranges from 0.8% to 37%.[85] The incidence is higher when the primary tumor is located near bone.[85] The most likely time to develop ORN is within the first 12 months after the completion of radiation therapy, but it may occur many years after the completion of radiotherapy.[84,86]

The likelihood of developing ORN increases as the radiation dose increases; however, ORN has been reported even after doses as low as 2000 cGy.[84] Other authors have disputed the claim that the incidence of ORN correlates with the radiation dose. Bedwinek et al. and Carlson state that a threshold dose of 6000 cGy is required for spontaneous ORN to occur.[87,88]

There is an association of poor oral hygiene with the likelihood of developing ORN.[89] This likely relates to the increased incidence of periodontal infection in these patients.[85] Edentulous patients are less likely to develop ORN, and patients who require no dental extractions or who undergo extractions prior to radiation therapy have roughly equal incidences of ORN.[85] Patients who undergo extractions after radiation therapy, however, have a much higher incidence of ORN.

Patients with ORN can present in a number of ways, varying from painless intraoral areas of exposed mandible to painful pathologic fractures of the mandible with large orocutaneous fistulae and significant soft tissue loss.[84,85] The presence of exposed bone is an important but not absolute feature of ORN. In the early period after radiation therapy, exposed bone may be present secondary to mucosal lesions rather than actual bone damage.[85] If the bone remains exposed for 3 to 6 months, the bone is likely involved and cortical breakdown with sequestration may occur.

Diagnosis of ORN is based on history and physical examination supplemented by radiographic studies. Plain radiographs lag behind the actual course of the disease, but osteopenia is frequently seen. Radionuclide scans may be useful but can often be difficult to interpret in the postirradiated patient.[85]

References

1. Burri C. Historical review. In: *Post-Traumatic Osteomyelitis.* Bern, Switzerland: Hans Huber Publishers; 1975:11–17.
2. Topazian, RG. Osteomyelitis of the jaws. In: Topazian RG, Goldberg MH, eds. *Oral and Maxillofacial Infections.* Philadelphia: W.B. Saunders; 1994:251–288.
3. Adekeye EO, Cornah J. Osteomyelitis of the jaws: a review of 141 cases. *Br J Oral Maxillofac Surg.* 1985;23:24–35.
4. Nelson LW, Lydiatt DD. Osteomyelitis of the head and neck. *Nebraska Med J.* May 1987:154–163.
5. Harner SG, Newell RC. Treatment of frontal osteomyelitis. *Laryngoscope.* 1969;79(7):1281–1294.
6. Mercuri LG. Acute osteomyelitis of the jaws. *Oral Maxillofac Surg Clin North Am.* 1991;3(2):355–365.
7. Waldvogel FA, Medoff G, Swartz MN. Clinical types of osteomyelitis. *Osteomyelitis: Clinical Features, Therapeutic Considerations and Unusual Aspects.* Springfield: Charles C. Thomas; 1971:13–62.
8. Bieluch VM, Garner JG. Osteomyelitis of the skull, mandible and sternum. In: Jauregui LE, ed. *Diagnosis and Management of Bone Infections.* New York: Marcel Dekker. 1995:109–133.
9. Marx, RE. Chronic osteomyelitis of the jaws. *Oral Maxillofac Surg Clin North Am.* 1991;3(2):367–381.
10. Calhoun KH, Shapiro RD, Sternberg CM, Calhoun JH, Mader JT. Osteomyelitis of the mandible. *Arch Otolaryngol Head Neck Surg.* 1988;114:1157–1162.
11. Shaff MI, Mathis JM. Osteomyelitis of the mandible: an initial feature in late-onset osteopetrosis. *Arch Otolaryngol.* 1982;108:120–121.
12. Barasch A, Mosier KM, D'Ambrosio JA, Giniger MS. Postextraction osteomyelitis in a bone marrow transplant recipient. *Oral Surg Oral Med Oral Pathol.* 1993;75(3):391–396.
13. Yarrish RL, Shay W, LaBombardi VJ, Meyerson M, Miller DK, Larone D. Osteomyelitis caused by mycobacterium haemophilum: successful therapy in two patients with AIDS. *AIDS.* 1992;6(6):557–561.
14. Watkins KV, Richmond AS, Langstein IM. Nonhealing extraction site due to actinomyces naeslunii in patient with AIDS. *Oral Surg Med Pathol.* 1991;71(6):675–677.
15. Berman S, Jensen J. Cytomegalovirus-induced osteomyelitis in a patient with the acquired immunodeficiency syndrome. *South Med J.* 1990;83(10):1231–1232.
16. Rubin MM, Sanfilippo RJ. Osteomyelitis of the hyoid caused by torulpsis glabrata in a patient with acquired immunodeficiency syndrome. *J Oral Maxillofac Surg.* 1990;48(11):1217–1219.
17. Klein E, Trautmann M, Hoffman HG. Ciprofloxacin in salmonella infection and abdominal typhoid. *Dtsch Med Wochenschrift.* 1986;111(42):1599–1602.
18. Masters DL, Lentino JR. Cervical osteomyelitis related to nocardia asteroides. *J Infect Dis.* 1984;149(5):824–825.
19. Koorbusch GF, Fotos P, Goll KT. Retrospective assessment of osteomyelitis: etiology, demographics, risk factors and management in 35 cases. *Oral Surg Med Pathol.* 1992;74:149–154.
20. Moose SM, Marshall KJ. Acute infections of the oral cavity. In: Kruger GO, ed. *Textbook of Oral and Maxillofacial Surgery.* St. Louis, MO: C.V. Mosby; 1984:195–216.
21. Balm AJM, Tiwari RM, de Rucke BM. Osteomyelitis in the head and neck. *J Laryngol Otol.* 1985;99:1059–1065.
22. Prossor IM, Merkel KD, Fitzgerald RH, Brown ML. Roentgenographic and radionuclide detection of musculoskeletal sepsis. In: Hughes SPF, Fitzgerald RH, eds. *Musculoskeletal Infections.* Chicago: Year Book Medical Publishers, Inc.; 1986:80–111.
23. Strauss M, Baum S, Kaufman RA. Osteomyelitis of the head and neck: sequential radionuclide scanning in diagnosis and therapy. *Laryngoscope.* 1985;95:81–84.
24. Blahd WH, Rose JG. Nuclear medicine in diagnosis and treatment of diseases of the head and neck: II. *Head Neck Surg.* 1982;4:213–223.
25. Datz FL. Indium 111-labeled leukocytes for detection of infection: current status. *Semin Nucl Med.* 1994;24(2):92–109.
26. Redleaf MI, Angeli SI, McCabe BF. Indium 111-labeled white blood cell scintigraphy as an unreliable indicator of malignant external otitis resolution. *Ann Otol Rhinol Laryngol.* 1994;103(6):444–448.
27. Giordano AM, Foster CA, Boies LR, Maisel RH. Chronic osteomyelitis following mandibular fractures and its treatment. *Arch Otolaryngol.* 1982;108:30–33.
28. Mathog RH, Boies LR. Nonunion of the mandible. *Laryngoscope.* 1976;86:908–920.
29. Peterson LJ. Microbiology of head and neck infections. *Oral Maxillofac Clin North Am.* 1991;3(2):247–257.

30. Lewis RP, Sutter VL, Finegold SM. Bone infections involving anaerobic bacteria. *Medicine.* 1978;57:279–305.

31. Gupta DS, Gupta MK, Naidu NG. Mandibular osteomyelitis causes by actinomyces israelii. *J Maxillofac Surg.* 1986;14:291–293.

32. Roine I, Faingezicht I, Arguedas A, Herrera JF. Serial serum C-reactive protein to monitor recovery from acute hematogenous osteomyelitis in children. *Pediatr Infect Dis J.* 1995;14(1):40–4.

33. Unkila-Kallio L, Kallio MJ, Eskola J, Peltola H. Serum C-reactive protein, erythrocyte sedimentation rate, and white blood cell count in acute hematogenous osteomyelitis in children. *Pediatrics.* 1994;93(1):59–62.

34. Shih LY, Wu JJ, Yang DJ. Erythrocyte sedimentation rate and C-reactive protein values in patients with total hip arthroplasty. *Clin Orthop Relat Res.* 1987;(225):238–246.

35. Hedstrom SA. Immunoassay of acute phase reactants and latex-CRP as activity tests in chronic staphylococcal osteomyelitis. *Scand J Infect Dis.* 1983;15(2):161–165.

36. Wannfors K, Hansson LO. Plasma protein changes in chronic osteomyelitis of the jaws. *J Oral Pathol Med.* 1991;20(2):81–85.

37. Harris, LF. Chronic mandibular osteomyelitis. *South Med J.* 1986;79(6):696–697.

38. Robinson CB, Higginbotham-Ford EA. Determination of sequestrum activity by SPECT with CT correlation in chronic osteomyelitis of the head and neck. *J Otolaryngol.* 15(5):279–281.

39. Malmstrom M, Fryhrquist F, Kosunen TU, Tasanen A. Immunological features of patients with chronic sclerosing osteomyelitis of the mandible. *Int J Oral Surg.* 1983;12:6–13.

40. Kahn MF, Hayem F, Grossin M. Is diffuse sclerosing osteomyelitis of the mandible part of the synovitis, acne, pustulosis, hyperostosis, osteitis (SAPHO) syndrome? Analysis of seven cases. *Oral Surg Med Pathol.* 1994;75:594–598.

41. Lichty G, Langlais RP, Aufdemorte T. Garre's osteomyelitis: literature review and case report. *Oral Surg.* 1980;50(4):309–313.

42. Bouquot JE, Roberts AM, Person P, Christian J. Neuralgia-inducing cavitational osteonecrosis (NICO). Osteomyelitis in 224 jawbone samples from patients with facial neuralgia. *Oral Surg Oral Med Oral Pathol.* 1992;73(3):307–319.

43. Skouteris CA, Velegrakis G, Christodoulou, Helidonis E. Infantile osteomyelitis of the maxilla with concomitant subperiosteal orbital abscess: a case report. *J Oral Maxillofac Surg.* 1995;53:67–70.

44. Chohan BS, Parkash OM, Parmar IPS. Unusual complications of acute maxillary osteomyelitis in an infant. *Br J Ophthamol.* 1969;53:498–500.

45. Kaneda T, Yamamoto H, Suzuki H, Ozawa M. A clinicoradiological study of maxillary osteomyelitis. *J Nihon Univ School Dent.* 1989;31:464–469.

46. Dodson TB, Neuenschwander MC, Bays RA. Intraoperative assessment of maxillary perfusion during Le Fort I osteotomy. *J Oral Maxillofac Surg.* 1994;52(8):827–831.

47. Wong SK, Wilhelmus KR. Infantile maxillary osteomyelitis with cerebral abscess. *J Pediatr Ophthamol Strabis.* 1986;23(3):153–154.

48. Kapoor S, Kapoor MS, Sood GC. Osteomyelitis of the orbital bones. *J Pediatr Ophthamol.* 14(3):171–175.

49. Cavanaugh F. Osteomyelitis of superior maxilla in infants. *Br Med J.* 1960;1:468.

50. Tovi E, Benharroch D, Gatot A, Hertzanu Y. Osteoblastic osteitis of the maxillary sinus. *Laryngoscope.* 1992;102(4):426–430.

51. Bordley JE, Bischofberger W. Osteomyelitis of the frontal bone. *Laryngoscope.* 1967;77(8):1234–1244.

52. Blackshaw G, Thomson N. Pott's puffy tumor reviewed. *J Laryngol Otol.* 1990;104:574–577.

53. Tudor RB, Carson JP, Pulliam MW, Hill A. Pott's puffy tumor, frontal sinusitis, frontal bone osteomyelitis, and epidural abscess secondary to a wrestling injury. *Am J Sports Med.* 1981;9(6):390–391.

54. Montgomery WM, Cheney ML, Jacobs EE. Osteomyelitis of the frontal bone. *Ann Otol Rhinol Laryngol.* 1989;98:848–853.

55. Bordley JE, Bosley WR. Mucoceles of the frontal sinus: causes and treatment. *Ann Otol Rhinol Laryngol.* 1973;82(5):696–702.

56. Noskin GA, Kalish SB. Pott's puffy tumor: a complication of intranasal cocaine abuse. *Rev Infect Dis.* 1991;13:606–608.

57. Woodward FD. Osteomyelitis of the skull. *JAMA.* 1930;95:927.

58. Williams GT, Anderson W, Bryce DP. Osteomyelitis complicating fibrous dysplasia of the skull. *Arch Otolaryngol.* 1972;96:278–281.

59. Schramm VL, Maroon JC. Sinus complications of frontal craniotomy. *Laryngoscope.* 1979;89:1436–1445.

60. Baker AS. Role of anaerobic bacteria in sinusitis and its complications. *Ann Otol Rhinol Laryngol.* 1991;154(suppl):17–22.

61. Milo R, Schiffer J, Karpuch J, Sarfaty S, Shikar S. Frontal bone osteomyelitis complicating frontal sinusitis caused by haemophilus influenzae type a. *Rhinology.* 1991;29:151–153.

62. Hudson HK, Holcomb JL. Acute fulminating osteomyelitis of the frontal bone. *South Med J.* 1971;64(11):1313–1316.

63. Parker GS, Tami TA, Wilson JF, Fetter TW. Intracranial complications of sinusitis. *South Med J.* 1989;82(5):563–568.

64. Gardiner LJ. Complicated frontal sinusitis: evaluation and management. *Otolayngol Head Neck Surg.* 1986;95:333–343.

65. Belli AM, Dow CJ, Monro P. Radiographic appearance of frontal osteomyelitis in two patients with extradural abscess. *Br J Radiol.* 1987;60:1026–1028.

66. Uren RF, Howman-Giles R. Pott's puffy tumor: scintigraphic findings. *Clin Nucl Med.* 1992;17(9):724–727.

67. Tami TA, Burkus JK, Strom CG. Cervical osteomyelitis: an unusual complication of tonsillectomy. *Arch Otolaryngol Head Neck Surg.* 1987;113:992–994.

68. Battista RA, Baredes S, Krieger A, Fieldman R. Prevertebral space infections associated with cervical osteomyelitis. *Otolaryngol Head Neck Surg.* 1993;108(2):160–166.

69. Osenbach RK, Hitchon PW, Menezes AH. Diagnosis and management of pyogenic vertebral osteomyelitis in adults. *Surg Neurol.* 1990;33:266–275.

70. Forsythe M, Rothman RH. New concepts in the diagnosis and treatment of infections of the cervical spine. *Orthop Clin North Am.* 1978;9(4):1039–1051.

71. Ruth H, Davis WE, Renner G. Deep neck abscess after tracheoesophageal puncture and insertion of a voice button prosthesis. *Otolaryngol Head Neck Surg.* 1985;93(6):809–811.

72. Hosni AA, Rhys-Evans P. Cervical osteomyelitis and cord compression complicating pharyngeal myotomy. *J Laryngol Otol.* 1994;108:511–513.

73. Ell SR, Parker AJ, Limb D, Clegg RT. Osteomyelitis of the cervical spine following laryngectomy. *J Laryngol Otol.* 1992;106:1096–1097.

74. Cullen JR, Primrose WJ, Vaughn CW. Osteomyelitis as a complication of a tracheo-oesophageal puncture. *J Laryngol Otol.* 1993;107:242–244.

75. Diver JP, Murty GE, Bradley PJ. Cervical cord compression complicating tracheo-oesophageal puncture. *J Laryngol Otol.* 1991;105:1082–1083.

76. Hagadorn B, Smith HW, Rosnagle RS. Cervical spine osteomyelitis—secondary to a foreign body in the hypopharynx. *Arch Otolaryngol.* 1972;95:578–580.

77. Fein SJ, Torg JS, Mohnac AM, Magsamen BF. Infection of the cervical spine associated with a fracture of the mandible. *J Oral Surg.* 1969;27:145–149.

78. Rosendale DE, Myers C, Boyko EJ, Jafek B. Nocardia asteroides cervical osteomyelitis in an immunocompetent host. *Otolaryngol Head Neck Surg.* 1988;99(3):334–337.

79. Heary RF, Hunt CD, Wolansky LJ. Rapid bony destruction with pyogenic vertebral osteomyelitis. *Surg Neurol.* 1994;41:34–39.

80. Carpenter JL, Artenstein MS. Use of diagnostic microbiologic facilities in the diagnosis of head and neck infections. *Otolaryngol Clin North Am.* 1976;9(3):611–629.

81. Bartels JW, Brammer RE. Cervical osteomyelitis with prevertebral abscess formation. *Otolaryngol Head Neck Surg.* 1990; 102(2):180–182.

82. Faidas A, Ferguson JV, Nelson JE, Baddour LM. Cervical vertebral osteomyelitis presenting as a retropharyngeal abscess. *Clin Infect Dis.* 1994;18:992–994.

83. Marx RE. Osteoradionecrosis: a new concept of its pathophysiology. *J Oral Maxillofac Surg.* 1983;41:283–288.

84. Echavez M, Tami TA, Kelly K, Swift PS. Two unusual locations of osteoradionecrosis. *Otolaryngol Head Neck Surg.* 1992;106(2):209–213.

85. Sanger JR, Matloub HS, Yousif NJ, Larson DL. Management of osteoradionecrosis of the mandible. *Clin Plast Surg.* 1993; 20(3):517–530.

86. Som PM. Radiation osteitis of the facial bones. *Am J Otolaryngol.* 1992;13(5):310–311.

87. Bedwinek JM, Sjukovsky LJ, Fletcher GH, Daley TE. Osteonecrosis in patients treated with definitive radiotherapy for squamous cell carcinomas of the oral cavity and naso and oropharynx. *Radiology.* 1976;119:665–667.

88. Carlson ER. The radiobiology, treatment, and prevention of osteoradionecrosis of the mandible. *Recent Results Cancer Res.* 1994;134:191–199.

89. Mounsey RA, Brown DH, O'Dwyer TP, Gullane PJ, Koch GH. Role of hyperbaric oxygen therapy in the management of mandibular osteomyelitis. *Laryngoscope.* 1993;103:605–608.

10
A New Classification System for Craniomaxillofacial Deformities

Richard H. Haug and Alex M. Greenberg

The preceeding chapters have provided an excellent review of the various classification systems used to characterize congenital craniofacial deformities, cleft lip and palate deformities, posttraumatic deformities, postinfection deformities, and deformities acquired in the management of oncologic disease. While each of the previous classification schemes possess certain advantages in describing the individual defect or directing the surgical management for their particular anatomic region, neither is universal or all-inclusive when assessing the craniomaxillofacial deformity patient. An ideal system would account for each of the particular osseous structures that are absent (or about to be removed), the quantity and quality of the overlying soft tissues (i.e., skin and/or mucosa), the vascular supply available for microvascular reanastomosis, the presence of nerve tissue that could restore sensation and function, and the suitability of the tissues to allow prosthetic restoration of specialized structures (i.e., teeth, eyes, auricles, or the nose).

Grätz in 1986 developed a classification scheme for mandibular fractures based upon a review of 207 questionnaires from surgical centers in Basel, Frieburg, Innsbruck, Wels (Austria), and Zwolle (Netherlands) as part of his doctoral thesis.[1] Spiessl refined this system and presented it in a more complete form in 1989 as the AO/ASIF classification of mandibular fractures.[2] Haug and Greenberg extrapolated this refined system of mandibular fracture classification to include all craniomaxillofacial fractures in 1993.[3] Using this universal classification system for craniomaxillofacial fractures as an infrastructure, we have added information germane to the reconstruction of soft and hard tissue defects, extended the data pertaining to the quality and quantity of the soft tissues, and refined the system for universal application to all forms of craniomaxillofacial deformities requiring reconstruction.

General Description of the Scheme

The first consideration in the description of the craniomaxillofacial deformity patient is the particular anatomic region involved, based upon the underlying osseous structures (Table 10.1). The areas germane to this system are the mandible, maxilla, zygoma, cranial bones, nose, and nasoethmoidal region. The terminology for the particular site of the defect will be different for each anatomic region (Tables 10.2–10.7) and will be described in each of the individual sections to follow.

A major focus of this scheme is the type and quality of the soft tissue coverage that is available for reconstruction. The first consideration in the evaluation of the soft tissues is skin coverage (Table 10.1). Whether the skin is normal, is traversed by scars from previous surgery or lacerations, has been irradiated, is completely bound down by massive scarring, has been avulsed, or will be removed, all must be considered during the evaluation and prior to reconstruction. Similarly, the quality and quantity of the mucosal coverage for the mandible, maxilla, and nose must be assessed. The subclassifications will include normal mucosa, that which has been scarred by laceration or incision, that which has been irradiated or completely bound down, and that which is now absent or will be removed during resection. The next consideration of the soft tissues in the anticipation for reconstruction is the availability of a vascular supply for microvascular reanastomosis. The subclassifications include a vascular supply that is favorable, unfavorable, absent, or about to be removed. Finally, the availability of nerve tissue (trigeminal or facial) for repair, reanastomosis, or grafting in order to reestablish motor function and sensation must be assessed. This subclassification will include a nerve supply that is favorable, unfavorable, absent, avulsed, or about to be removed.

The restoration of specialized structures by the fabrication of prosthetic dentures, eyes, ears, and noses must be considered in the overall assessment and management of the reconstruction patient. The suitability of the tissue supporting these implant-borne prostheses will be subclassified as either favorable or unfavorable. Favorable conditions include the presence of healthy skin or mucosal tissue as well as a minimum of 8 to 10 cm of bone.

The classification system should be approached from inferior to superior, medial to lateral, and right to left. A / mark denotes left-sided deformity. The system is friendly to current data storage and retrieval systems.

TABLE 10.1 Classification of craniomaxillofacial deformities.

Bone		Location	Skin coverage		Mucosal coverage (for Mn, Mx, Na, Fr)		Vascular supply (for microvascular grafting)		Nerve supply (for anastomosis)		Prosthetic replacement (for specialized structures)	
Mn	Mandible	Varies with bone	S_1	Normal	M_1	Normal	V_1	Favorable	N_1	Favorable	Teeth	
Mx	Maxilla		S_2	Scarred	M_2	Scarred	V_2	Unfavorable	N_2	Unfavorable	PT_1	Favorable
Na	Nasal		S_3	Previously irradiated or completely bound down	M_3	Previously irradiated or completely bound down	V_3	Absent, avulsed, or to be removed	N_3	Absent, avulsed, or to be removed	PT_2	Unfavorable
Zy	Zygoma										Eye	
Fr	Frontal										PE_1	Favorable
Cr	Other cranial		S_4	Avulsed, absent, or to be removed	M_4	Absent, avulsed, or to be removed					PE_2	Unfavorable
											Auricle	
											PA_1	Favorable
											PA_2	Unfavorable
											Nose	
											PN_1	Favorable
											PN_2	Unfavorable

TABLE 10.2 Mandible deformities (Mn).

Location		Skin coverage		Mucosal coverage		Vascular supply		Nerve supply		Prosthetic replacement (of teeth)	
L_1	Precanine	S_1	Normal	M_1	Normal	V_1	Favorable	N_1	Favorable	PT_1	Favorable
L_2	Canine	S_2	Scarred	M_2	Scarred	V_2	Unfavorable	N_2	Unfavorable	PT_2	Unfavorable
L_3	Postcanine (body)	S_3	Previously irradiated or completely bound down	M_3	Previously irradiated or completely bound down	V_3	Absent, avulsed, or to be removed	N_3	Absent, avulsed or to be removed		
L_4	Angular										
L_5	Supra-angular (ramus)	S_4	Absent, avulsed, or to be removed	M_4	Absent, avulsed, or to be removed						
L_6	Condyle										
L_7	Coronoid										
L_8	Alveolus										

Mandibular Deformities

Mandibular deformities will be classified according to the following scheme (Tables 10.1 and 10.2, Figure 10.1). The precanine region includes the area between the canine teeth (symphysis of the mandible). The canine region includes deformities immediately adjacent to this area. The body region extends from the canine area to the region of the third molar. The supraangular region is ramus superior to the angle excluding the condyle and coronoid. Although unimportant in reconstruction, the coronoid has been included for the sake of completeness. The condyle region is of paramount importance in treating tumors to this area as well as such congenital deformities as Treacher Collins and hemifacial microsomia. The alveolar process has been included as a separate component in consideration of prosthetic reconstruction and for the repair of the cleft lip and palate.

The quality and quantity of the overlying skin and mucosa are considered according to the general scheme (Table 10.1). The condition of the inferior alveolar nerve should be assessed as favorable (normal), unfavorable (atrophic), or absent prior to treatment in order to consider the possibility of nerve graft-

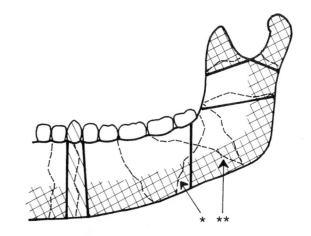

FIGURE 10.1 Location of mandibular deformities (Mn). (From Spiessl[2])

L_1	Precanine
L_2	Canine
L_3	Postcanine (body)
L_4	Angular
L_5	Supra-angular (ramus)
L_6	Condyle
L_7	Coronoid
L_8	Alveolar process

TABLE 10.3 Maxillary deformities (Mx).

Location		Skin coverage		Mucosal coverage		Vascular supply		Nerve supply		Prosthetic replacement (of teeth)	
L_1	Defects that involve the maxillae, palatine bones, and floor of the nose	S_1 S_2 S_3	Normal Scarred Previously irradiated or completely bound down	M_1 M_2 M_3	Normal Scarred Previously irradiated or completely bound down	V_1 V_2 V_3	Favorable Unfavorable Absent, avulsed, or to be removed	N_1 N_2 N_3	Favorable Unfavorable Absent, avulsed, or to be removed	PT_1 PT_2	Favorable Unfavorable
L_2	Defects that involve the antra										
L_3	Defects that involve the antra and nasal aperture	S_4	Absent, avulsed, or to be removed	M_4	Absent, avulsed, or to be removed						
L_4	Defects that involve the alveolus										

ing. The condition of the facial artery and vein must be assessed to determine the possibility of microvascular grafting. Favorable is a normal supply, while severe peripheral vascular disease is unfavorable. Finally, the quality and quantity of mucosa and alveolar bone for implant borne dental prostheses must be assessed.

Maxillary Deformities

The classification scheme of maxillary deformities takes into consideration only the maxillae and palatine bones (Tables 10.2 and 10.3, Figure 10.2). The types of deformity are as follows: those that involve the maxillae, palatine bones and the

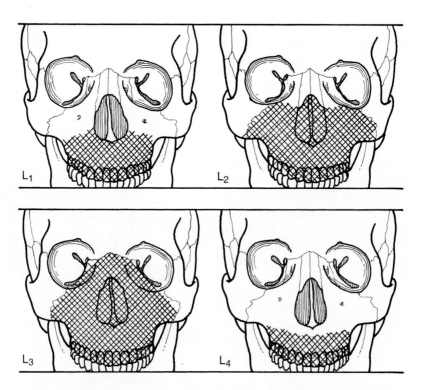

FIGURE 10.2 Location of maxillary deformities (Mx). (From Greenberg[3])

    L_1 Maxillae, palatine bones and floor of nose
    L_2 Those which involve the antra
    L_3 Those which involve the antra and nasal aperture
    L_4 Alveolar process

TABLE 10.4 Zygoma deformities (Zy).

Location		Skin coverage		Vascular supply		Nerve supply		Prosthetic replacement (of eyes)	
L₁	Arch	S₁	Normal	V₁	Favorable	N₁	Favorable	PE₁	Favorable
L₂	Supraarch (lateral	S₂	Scarred	V₂	Unfavorable	N₂	Unfavorable	PE₂	Unfavorable
	orbital rim)	S₃	Previously irradiated	V₃	Absent, avulsed,	N₃	Absent, avulsed,		
L₃	Body		or completely		or to be removed		or to be removed		
L₄	Orbital floor		bound down						
		S₄	Absent, avulsed, or						
			to be removed						

floor of the nose; those which include the antra; those that involve the antra and nasopharynx; and those that involve the alveolus. The quantity and quality of the skin must be assessed as described in the previous section. Next, the oral, nasal, and antral mucosa should be assessed for its quantity and quality. The condition of the facial artery for microvascular reanastomosis or temporal artery for rotational flaps are then assessed. The condition of the infraorbital nerve may be addressed if a repair is to be anticipated. Last, the condition of the alveolar structures as recipient sites for implant-borne dental prostheses are assessed.

Zygoma Deformities

The description of zygomatic defects are particularly important in the treatment of congenital deformities (Tables 10.1 and 10.4, Figure 10.3). These osseous subclassifications include the arch, supraarch region (lateral orbital rim), body, and orbital floor. The quality and quantity of the skin should be assessed. The quality and quantity of the antral mucosa in this situation is not important. The assessment of the facial nerve for reconstruction becomes important in the treatment of zygomatic deformities such as those in Treacher

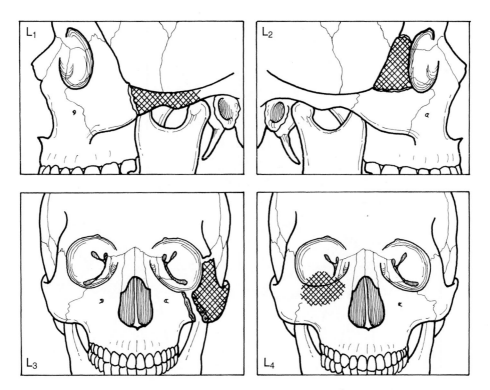

FIGURE 10.3 Location of zygoma deformities (Zy). (From Greenberg[3])

L₁   Arch
L₂   Supraarch (lateral orbital rim)
L₃   Body
L₄   Floor of orbit

TABLE 10.5 Nasal naso-orbital-ethmoid deformities (Na).

Location		Skin coverage		Mucosal coverage		Prosthetic replacement (of eyes or nose)	
L_1	Entire nasal bones	S_1	Normal	M_1	Normal	Eye	
L_2	Nasal bones and frontal	S_2	Scarred	M_2	Scarred	PE_1	Favorable
	process of maxilla	S_3	Previously irradiated	M_3	Previously irradiated	PE_2	Unfavorable
L_3	Nasal, ethmoid, frontal		or completely		or completely	Nose	
	process of maxilla, and nasal		bound down		bound down	PN_1	Favorable
	spine of frontal bone	S_4	Absent, avulsed,	M_4	Absent, avulsed	PN_2	Unfavorable
			or to be removed		or to be removed		

Collins syndrome. The capability of nerve preservation, reconstruction, or grafting should be considered. The quality of the facial artery for microvascular composite grafts or the temporal artery for rotation flaps should be assessed next. Lastly, the condition of the orbital floor and lateral orbital rim for an implant-supported prosthetic eye should be considered.

Nasal and Naso-Orbital-Ethmoid Deformities

The classification of the nasal deformity is as much soft tissue as osseous, but it begins with the assessment of the osseous structures (Tables 10.1 and 10.5, Figure 10.4). The location of the deformity includes the entire nasal bones; the nasal bones along with the frontal process of the maxilla, including the nasolacrimal duct; and finally, the nasal bones, ethmoid bone, frontal process of the maxilla and nasal spine of the frontal bone. The assessment of the quality and quantity of the skin and mucosa are of paramount importance. The vascular and nerve structures are ignored in the classification of this anatomic region. Last, the quality of tissues for a nasal prosthesis should be assessed. Favorability includes an evaluation of how many osseous walls are present. Is there enough bone to support osseointegrated implants? Is the quality of the soft tissue coverage favorable for the prosthesis?

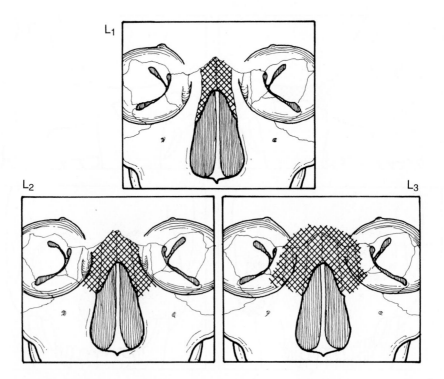

FIGURE 10.4 Location of nasal/naso-orbital-ethmoidal deformities (Na). (From Greenberg[3])
  L_1 Entire nasal bones
  L_2 Nasal bones and frontal process of maxilla
  L_3 Nasal, ethmoid, frontal process of maxilla, and nasal spine of frontal bone

TABLE 10.6 Frontal bone deformities (Fr).

Location		Skin coverage		Prosthetic replacement (of eyes)	
L_1	Supraorbital rim	S_1	Normal	PE_1	Favorable
L_2	Anterior table of the frontal sinus	S_2	Scarred	PE_2	Unfavorable
L_3	Posterior table of the frontal sinus	S_3	Previously irradiated or completely bound down		
L_4	Frontal sinus floor	S_4	Absent, avulsed, or to be removed		
L_5	Linear or other fractures of the frontal bone				

Frontal Bone Deformities

The frontal bone in this scheme is divided into five regions: the supraorbital rim, the anterior sinus wall, the posterior sinus wall, the floor of the sinus, and linear or other frontal bone fractures (Tables 10.1 and 10.6, Figures 10.5 and 10.6). The evaluation of the last three areas in reconstruction are particularly important to protect the cranial contents, assure isolation of the neurocranium from the nasopharynx, and provide cosmesis. The assessment of the overlying cutaneous structures is important. Last, an evaluation of the suitability of the supraorbital region for an implant borne ocular prosthesis must be addressed.

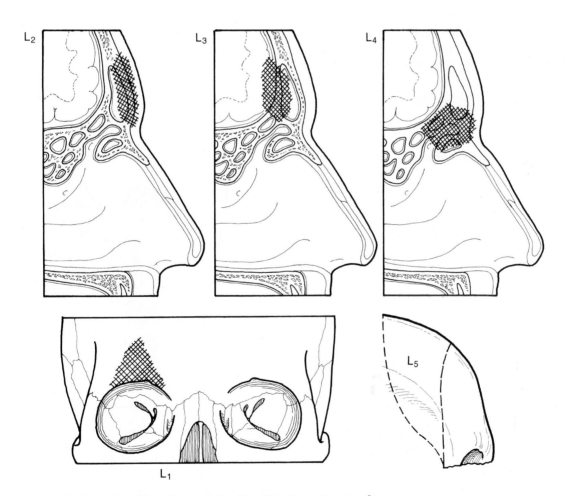

FIGURE 10.5 Location of frontal bone deformities (Fr). (From Greenberg[3])

    L_1 Supraorbital rim
    L_2 Anterior table of the frontal sinus
    L_3 Posterior table of the frontal sinus
    L_4 Sinus floor
    L_5 Linear or other fractures of the frontal bone

TABLE 10.7 Other cranial bone deformities (Cr).

Location		Skin coverage		Vascular supply		Nerve supply		Prosthetic replacement (of the auricle)	
L_1	Temporal	S_1	Normal	V_1	Favorable	N_1	Favorable	Auricle	
L_2	Parietal	S_2	Scarred	V_2	Unfavorable	N_2	Unfavorable	PA_1	Favorable
L_3	Occipital	S_3	Previously irradiated or completely bound down	V_3	Absent, avulsed, or to be removed	N_3	Absent, avulsed, or to be removed	PA_2	Unfavorable
L_4	Base of skull	S_4	Absent, avulsed, or to be removed						

Other Cranial Bone Deformities

The classification scheme for the other cranial bones includes the temporal, parietal, and occipital bones along with the base of the skull (Tables 10.1 and 10.7, Figure 10.6). The cutaneous structures should be assessed as in the previous sections. The facial and temporal arteries should be assessed to determine their suitability for microvascular grafting or rotational flaps. Lastly, the suitability of the temporal bone and mastoid process for an implant borne auricular prosthesis must be assessed.

Practical Application of the Classification System

This classification system is well ordered and should be approached from inferior to superior and medial to lateral. Right- and left-sided deformity is denoted by a / mark. As illustrated in Figure 10.7, a 40-year-old otherwise healthy man has sustained a traumatic avulsion from a high-energy rifle injury. He is devoid of the osseous structures of the right body of the mandible, right maxilla, right zygoma, right orbital floor, right supraorbital rim, and right medial nasal bones. The skin and mucosa of these areas are absent along with the globe. Thus this complex craniomaxillofa-

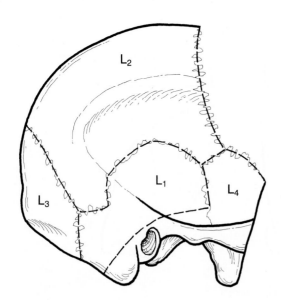

FIGURE 10.6 Location of other cranial bone deformities (Cr).

L_1 Temporal
L_2 Parietal
L_3 Occipital
L_4 Base of skull

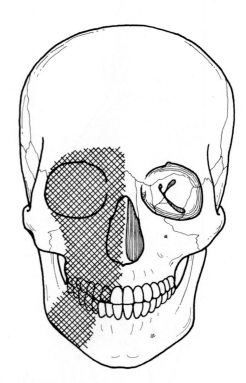

FIGURE 10.7 Illustrative case No. 1.
  A 40-year-old otherwise healthy male who has had a traumatic avulsive injury from a gunshot. He is devoid of the mandibular body, right maxilla, right zygomatic body, orbital floor, supraorbital rim, and medial nasal bones. The associated skin and mucosa as well as the orbit has been avulsed.
Mn $L_3L_8S_4M_4V_1N_3PT_2$
Mx $L_3L_4S_4M_4V_1N_3PT_2$
Zy $L_3L_4S_4M_4V_1N_3PE_2$
Na $L_4S_4M_4PE_2PN_1$
Fr $L_1S_4PE_2$

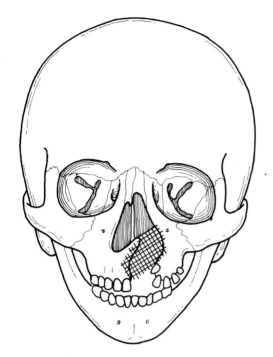

FIGURE 10.8 Illustrative case No. 2.

A four-year-old male with a complete cleft of the left lip, palate, and alveolus.

/ Mx $L_4S_4M_4V_1N_1PT_2$

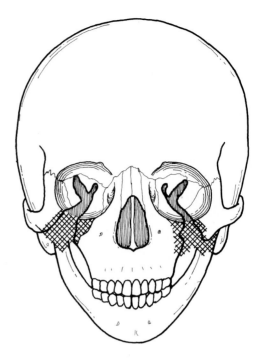

FIGURE 10.9 Illustrative case No. 3.

An 18-year-old male with incomplete penetrance of Treacher Collins syndrome. Bilateral clefts of the infraorbital rims and orbital floors are present. The right zygomatic body and mandibular condyles bilaterally are absent. All soft tissue coverage is satisfactory.

Mn $L_6S_1M_1V_1N_1PT_1$ / Mn $L_6S_1M_1V_1N_1PT_1$
Zy $L_3L_4S_1V_1N_1PE_1$ / Zy $L_4S_1V_1N_1PE_1$

cial defect can be considered Mn $L_3L_8S_4M_4V_1N_3PT_2$, Mx $L_3L_4S_4M_4V_1N_3PT_2$, Zy $L_3L_4S_4M_4V_1N_3PE_2$, Na $L_4S_4M_4PE_2PN_1$, Fr $L_1S_4PE_2$.

The case illustrated in Figure 10.8 is that of a 4-year-old with a complete cleft of the lip, alveolus, and palate on the left side. This craniomaxillofacial defect is classified as /Mx $L_4S_4M_4V_1N_1PT_2$. Note that the / mark denotes the left side.

The case illustrated in Figure 10.9 is that of an 18-year-old with Treacher Collins syndrome. The individual has bilateral clefts of the infraorbital rims and orbital floors. The right zygomatic body is absent. The mandibular condyles are absent bilaterally. All soft tissue coverage is satisfactory. This defect is classified as Mn $L_6S_1M_1V_1N_1PT_1$ / Mn $L_6S_1M_1V_1N_1PT_1$, Zy $L_3L_4S_1V_1N_1PE_1$ / Zy $L_4S_1V_1N_1PE_1$. Note that the classification progresses from inferior to superior and the medial to lateral.

While initially appearing lengthy, the description of deformities with this scheme is actually shorter than a conglomeration of other schemes. This new classification system focuses upon the anatomic region affected, the quality and quantity of the hard and soft tissues available, as well as the suitability for reconstruction of specialized structures. It is

universal in nature and thus can be used for congenital deformities, those acquired through trauma or infection, or those resulting from ablative tumor surgery. It is hoped with this new classification system that retrieval from data storage systems can provide information regarding patterns of deformity not previously attainable by prior classification systems.

References

1. Grätz K. Eine neue klassifikation zur Eintelung von Unterkiefer-frakturen. Dissertation. Universität Basel; 1986.
2. Spiessl B. Classification of fracures. In: Spiessl B, *Internal Fixation of the Mandible*. New York: Springer-Verlag; 1989: part 2, sect 2.
3. Haug RH, Greenberg AM. Etiology, distribution and classification of fractures. In: Greenberg AM, ed. *Craniomaxillofacial Fractures: Principles of Internal Fixation Using the AO/ASIF Technique.* New York: Springer-Verlag; 1993: ch 2.

Section II
Biomechanics of Internal Fixation and Dental Osseointegration Implantology

11
Craniomaxillofacial Bone Healing, Biomechanics, and Rigid Internal Fixation

Frederick J. Kummer

The basic orthopedic principles of bone healing and fixation biomechanics are applicable to craniomaxillofacial reconstructive surgery. In general, however, the emphasis is less on providing mechanical stability to resist high levels of applied physiological forces than on establishing rigid immobilization both to obtain proper, stable anatomic configuration and to promote rapid healing.[1] For each particular surgical application, there exists a variety of fixation techniques to achieve these goals. This chapter discusses fixation methods in general, as well as their biomechanical aspects as they influence bone healing, and relates these principles to several bone-specific clinical applications.

Principles of Bone Healing

The basic AO/ASIF principle of craniomaxillofacial surgery is rigid internal fixation achieved by functionally stable fixation of bone surfaces through the use of an appropriate device and its correct surgical application.[2–5] At present, related to the hardware system in current use in the craniomaxillofacial region, the process of stress shielding seems to be of little or no concern. The frequently observed process of bone resorption in the management of fractures in the human skeleton is now more often believed to be the result of interference with the vascular supply than the mechanical influences attributed to stress shielding.

Currently there exists controversy over whether completely rigid fixation is the optimal condition for bone healing. Although gross motion between two or more bone fragments usually leads to nonunion and fibrocartilage tissue formation, a low level of displacement (micromotion) appears to aid healing by providing a mechanical signal that stimulates the biological repair process.[6] The optimal frequency, waveform, and total number of cycles of this signal have yet to be determined.

Bone healing in the presence of a gap with minimal movement passes through several stages of repair with concurrent increases in mechanical strength: hematoma and inflammation, callus formation, replacement by woven bone, and finally remodeling into lamellar or trabecular bone (Figures 11.1 and 11.2). When there is direct bone apposition and compression of a rigidly fixed small gap, healing occurs more rapidly because the initial repair stages are minimized or eliminated. Perren has related this phenomenon to the concept of interfragmentary strain, where the local strain in the healing region (change in gap size divided by original gap size) influences the nature of the tissues formed.[7]

Healing also requires an adequate blood supply. In terms of operative technique, this means preserving the vascular supply of the bone and providing conditions for early revascularization (soft tissue preservation). Numerous studies have demonstrated a direct relationship between the quantity and quality of microvascular structures in the healing region and the rate of formation and mechanical properties of new bone.[5]

Fixation Methods and Devices

Wires, staples, pins, plates, and screws are the devices commonly used to achieve fixation. All are typically made of stainless steel (316L), titanium (or Ti-6A1-4V), or less commonly, cobalt-chromium alloy.[8] A renewed interest in biodegradable polymers such as polylactic acid, first proposed for these applications more than 20 years ago,[9] has recently led to their clinical use.[10] Research also continues into the use of various glues and adhesives for bone fixation.[11,12] The advantages and disadvantages of these materials and their relative strength, modulus (stiffness), corrosion resistance, and ease of imaging (MRI, CT) are discussed in a following chapter.

Wire

Wire fixation used as cerclage or a bone suture is less common in maxillofacial reconstruction. In either case, multiple wires are required to provide more rigid positional fixation. This necessitates achieving equal tension during tightening,

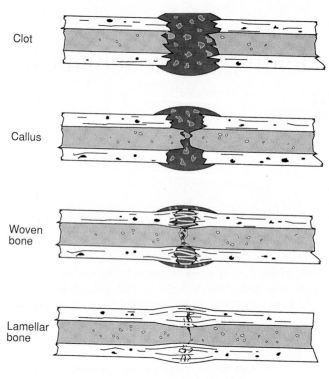

Clot

Callus

Woven
bone

Lamellar
bone

FIGURE 11.1 Stages of bone healing.

as loosening at one or more sites can provide a locus for motion and possible nonunion or malpositioning can result. Problems with wire fixation include the necessity and surgical complexity of making a hole in the bone and passing the wire through it, breakage during tightening or afterward due to fatigue (cyclic loading), and cut-through of the bone. In cerclage applications, there is some concern about compromise of the periosteal blood supply and resulting increased healing time required for revascularization.

Recent developments include wire tensioning/twisting instruments and the use of crimping systems to avoid the prob-

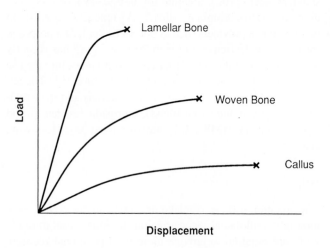

FIGURE 11.2 Mechanical behavior of healing bone.

lems with twisting or knot tying. Oriented polymers (e.g., Spectra) that do not stretch as do traditional suture materials can be used with a suture anchor system to eliminate the difficulty of looping a suture through bone. Wire fixation alone, however, does not provide functionally stable fixation.

Staples

Staples usually do not provide sufficient mechanical stability for permanent fixation, and their use often requires predrilling holes for the staple legs. Pneumatically driven staples can be used to rapidly tack fragments prior to a more rigid fixation, but insertion driving force must be carefully controlled to prevent untoward damage to the bone. Some staple designs can effect compression during insertion, such as prebent staple legs or fabrication from nitinol (an alloy that changes shape when heated to body temperature).

Pins

Kirschner wires, normally used to hold fragments prior to rigid fixation and for percutaneous pinning, in general lack sufficient mechanical stability for use as primary fixation. At least two should be used for each bone fragment, and they should not be inserted in a parallel manner to prevent "pistoning" of the fragment (Figure 11.3). Threaded pins provide additional stability because they minimize sliding of bone fragments; their removal, however, is more difficult. Occasionally, pinning is used in combination with a suture looped around the pin ends. This "tension band" technique provides significantly increased mechanical stability.

Screws

The major intrinsic factors that influence screw-holding power are the screw's outer thread diameter, configuration, and length; the extrinsic factors are bone quality, bone type, and screw insertion orientation and driving torque.[7,13] The two basic types of screw are cortical and cancellous, distinguished by thread design. Cancellous screws exhibit a greater distance between adjacent threads (pitch) and a higher ratio of outer thread diameter to body diameter (Figure 11.4). A screw's inherent holding power is a function of outer thread diameter multiplied by the length of threads within the bone. When used to hold two bone fragments together, screws are commonly used in a lag modality in which the proximal portion of the screw remains free within one fragment; this is accomplished either by using a screw design that has no proximal threads or by enlarging the hole in the proximal fragment, preferably with a washer under the screw head for adequate support. Insertion torque determines the force with which bone fragments are held together and creates the friction that inhibits their motion. Control of torque by use of a torque-limiting screwdriver is important to prevent stripping of the bone and screw-head failure.

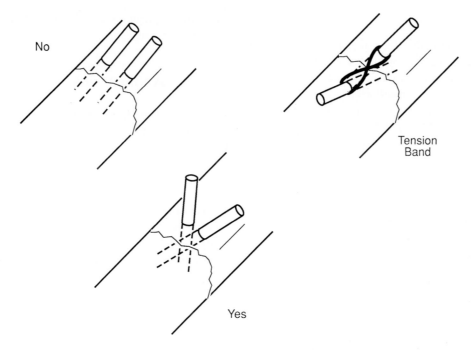

FIGURE 11.3 Pinning techniques for optimal fixation stability.

Because of anatomic constraints or surgical exposure, screws cannot always be inserted perpendicular to the bone axis, or the orientation of the ends of the bone fragments may not be perpendicular to the screw axis. In such cases, the screw's holding power is decreased, and a shear component of the holding force is created that acts to destabilize alignment (Figure 11.5). With the size of screws usually used in craniomaxillofacial surgery, self-tapping screws are in the range of 1.0 to 2.4 mm and pretapping is unnecessary. However, for screws 2.7 mm or longer, pretapping is still recommended. Pretapping of screws is usually not necessary and has been shown to have minimal effect on their holding ability; many screws are self-tapping by virtue of a modified design of the leading threads. Usually, two or more screws are required for proper function, although one screw has been suggested for some applications if sufficient interfragment ap-proximation can be achieved to create mechanical stability between the bone surfaces.[14,15]

Bone type and quality greatly influence screw-holding ability. Cortical bone is approximately 10 times stronger than cancellous bone.[16] The thickness of the cortex and degree of osteopenia (bone density) are thus critical for fixation strength and dictate the number of screws required for adequate stability.[17] Using screws in a bicortical manner appreciably increases the strength of fixation, although this is not possible for some maxillofacial reconstructions.[18]

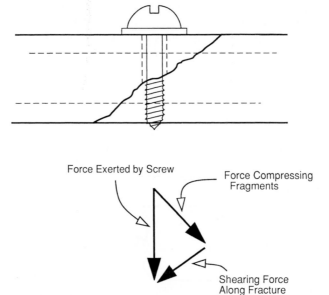

FIGURE 11.5 Forces created by lag screw fixation.

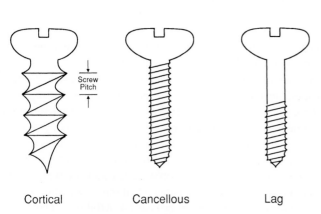

FIGURE 11.4 Types of bone screws.

Plates

Because anatomic constraints limit the number of screws that can be applied in a given region, screws are often combined with plates to achieve adequate stability and increased strength of fixation. Plates for maxillofacial reconstruction are often four holed. Unlike their counterparts in orthopedic applications, they are usually applied to only one side of the bone. Because of anatomic constraints such as soft tissue thickness, the plates are relatively thin, just thick enough to possess stiffness—a function of width multiplied by the height squared—sufficient to prevent motion due to flexion.

Plate screws should be inserted with a torque driver and their tightness double-checked after insertion of all screws. Some plates incorporate a countersunk screw hole slot to accommodate the screw head; the slot is eccentrically situated so that interfragmentary compression is achieved as the screw is tightened (Figure 11.6). An alternative strategy is to prebend the plate so that when the screws are tightened, the bone fragments are approximated. Some plates have threaded holes to engage the screws; in these designs, bicortical screw insertion is not essential for maximum stability.

Plates can also be used to span gaps created by severe fractures or tumor surgery, frequently with the help of bone grafts.[19] Unless the graft is an exact fit between the bone ends, the plate will bear the entire load across the defect. The bending moment on the plate, screw, and bone at the point of fixation linearly increases with defect size, requiring additional stabilization, particularly at the proximal end of the plate. Thus, as a general rule, at least three screws are needed at each end of the plate for this application. Using multiple-holed plates in this application allows one to select the best osseous sites for screw purchase and permits anchoring of the graft by additional screws.

Potential drawbacks to plate fixation are that it requires a larger exposure during surgery and that plate application may compromise periosteal blood supply. Some plate designs incorporate inferior feet or ridges to minimize the risk of the latter possibility. More flexible polymeric plates, currently in use, permit a greater degree of micromotion that may accelerate bone healing.

Surgical Applications

Among the several factors that must be weighed to determine the optimal fixation method for a specific application, two are fundamental. *Mechanical considerations* include the types (tension, bending, and/or torsion) and magnitude of forces to which the fixation will be subjected and whether these forces will be cyclic (e.g., chewing), in which case additional strength of fixation is required to compensate for possible fatigue of the supporting bone. *Bone quality* determines the strength available to support the fixation device. Other factors include surgical and anatomic considerations. For example, the exposure (possible scarring, vascular compromise), whether the device will fit adequately within the soft tissues, and whether neurovascular structures are at risk.

Evaluation of fixation strength can be accomplished by laboratory testing of implants in cadaver bone. One difficulty of such testing is to adequately simulate in the test model the complex forces to which the device or fixation technique would be subjected in vivo as well as the biological repair processes that would act to stabilize the fixation. Cadaver studies can also be used to determine those anatomic structures that would be at risk.

The alternative method of evaluating the efficacy of a particular fixation method is by means of a prospective study using clinical trials. In this case, proper study design must be observed, including specifying an appropriate number of patients, ensuring adequate follow-up, and selecting suitable techniques of data quantification so that the several parameters of interest can be statistically analyzed in a proper manner.

Mandibular Osteotomies

Osteotomies and fixation of the mandible represent the most highly mechanically loaded situation for maxillofacial reconstruction. Bending loads during mastication, created by the action of several muscles, are significant. By modeling these muscle forces and analyzing them mathematically, a resultant force (vector sum of separate forces) can be calculated and used for the design of experiments to test fixation stability in the laboratory.[20] Similar mathematical analyses can be used to ascertain optimal location and type of osteotomy. The location, in turn, determines the magnitude and direction of force to be applied to the fixation, while the type determines the degree of approximation of bone surfaces acting to augment the stability achieved by the fixation device itself.

Mandibular osteotomies are fixed by a variety of techniques: wiring, single or multiple screws, and miniplates. Laboratory studies have demonstrated that screw orientation, size, and insertion technique are critical for stability.[21] Three 2.7-mm-diameter screws along the superior border and two plates

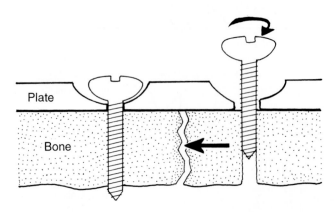

FIGURE 11.6 Screw hole mechanism of the self-compressing plate.

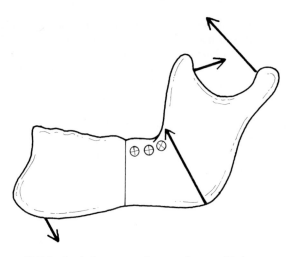

FIGURE 11.7 Optimal placement of screws for mandibular osteotomy showing muscle and reaction forces acting on the fixation (arrows not to scale).

have been shown to provide maximum fixation stability (Figure 11.7).

Orbitozygomatic Reconstruction

The principal aim of orbitozygomatic repair or reconstruction is to restore the anatomic configuration of the orbit. Loss of fixation stability can lead to nonunion or osseous displacement with severe sequelae (e.g., optic nerve damage).[22,23] Biomechanically, several muscles, particularly the masseter, will act upon the fixation, resulting in a tendency toward inferior bone fragment displacement. The original type of fixation used transcutaneous Kirschner wires. Clinical failure us-

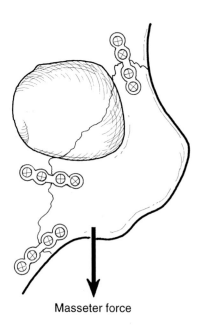

Masseter force

FIGURE 11.8 Optimal placements of plates for orbitozygomatic fracture fixation (adapted from Rohrich and Watumull[25]).

ing this method led to the use of two-point interosseous wiring and, later, three- and four-point wiring for increased stability. A more recent innovation has been the use of miniplates and screws for fixation (Figure 11.8). Laboratory cadaver studies comparing the stability achieved by these techniques demonstrated that the plating systems provide the most rigid fixation.[24,25] The major problem with plate fixation is the larger surgical exposure required and greater profile (thickness) of the plate beneath the soft tissue.

References

1. Rudderman RH, Mullen RL. Biomechanics of the facial skeleton. *Clin Plast Surg.* 1992;19:11–29.
2. Gruss JS, Phillips JH. Complex facial trauma: the evolving role of rigid fixation and immediate bone graft reconstruction. *Clin Plast Surg.* 1989;16:93.
3. Hobar PC. Methods of rigid fixation. *Clin Plast Surg.* 1992; 19(1):31–39.
4. LaTrenta GS, McCarthy JG, Breitbard AS, et al. The role of rigid skeletal fixation in bone-graft augmentation of the craniofacial skeleton. *Plast Reconstr Surg.* 1989;84:578.
5. Phillips JH, Forrest CR, Gruss JS. Current concepts in the use of bone grafts in facial fractures. Basic science considerations. *Clin Plast Surg.* 1992;19(1):41–58.
6. Lin KY, Bartlett SP, Yaremchuk MJ, et al. An experimental study on the effect of rigid fixation on the developing craniofacial skeleton. *Plast Reconstr Surg.* 1991;87:229.
7. Perren SM, Cordey J, Baumgart F, Rahn BA, Schatzker J. Technical and biomechanical aspects of screws used for bone surgery. *Int J Orthop Trauma.* 1992;2:31–48.
8. Lemons JE, Bidez MW. Endosteal implant biomaterials and biomechanics. In: McKinney RV Jr., ed. *Endosteal Dental Implants.* St. Louis, MO: C.V. Mosby; 1991.
9. Cutright DE, Hunsuck EE. The repair of fractures of the orbital floor using biodegradable polylactic acid. *Oral Surg.* 1972;33: 28–34.
10. Leenslag JW, Pennings AJ, Bos RRM, Rozema FR, Boering G. Resorbable materials of poly (L-lactide). VI. Plates and screws for internal fracture fixation. *Biomaterials.* 1987;8:70–73.
11. Sierra DH, Nissen AJ, Welch J. The use of fibrin glue in intracranial procedures: preliminary results. *Laryngoscope.* 1990;100(4):360–363.
12. Weber SC, Chapman MW. Adhesives in orthopedic surgery. A review of the literature and in vitro bonding strengths of bone-bonding agents. *Clin Orthop.* 1984;191:249–261.
13. Schatzker J, Sanderson R, Murnaghan JP. The holding power of orthopedic screws in vivo. *Clin Orthop.* 1975;108:115–126.
14. Foley WL, Frost DE, Paulin WB, et al. Internal screw fixation: comparison of placement pattern and rigidity. *J Oral Maxillofac Surg.* 1989;47:720.
15. Shetty V, Caputo A. Biomechanical validation of the solitary lag screw technique for reducing mandibular angle fractures. *J Oral Maxillofac Surg.* 1992;50(6):603–607.
16. Bidez MW, Misch CE. Issues in bone mechanics related to oral implants. *Implant Dent.* 1992;1(4):289–294.
17. Misch CE. Density of bone: effect on treatment plans, surgical approach, healing, and progressive bone loading. *Int J Oral Implantol.* 1990;6:23–31.

18. Ellis JA Jr., Laskin DM. Analysis of seating and fracturing torque of bicortical screws. *J Oral Maxillofac Surg.* 1994;52(5): 483–486 (disc 487–488).

19. Raveh J, Sutter F. Titanium coated hollow screw reconstruction plate system for bridging lower jaw defects: biomechanical aspects. *Int J Oral Maxillofac Surg.* 1988;17:267–274.

20. van Eijden TMGJ. Three-dimensional analyses of human bite-force magnitude and moment. *Arch Oral Biol.* 1991;36(7): 535–539.

21. Foley WL, Beckman TW. In vitro comparison of screw versus plate fixation in the sagittal split osteotomy. *Int J Adult Orthod Orthognath Surg.* 1992;7(3):147–151.

22. Jackson IT. Classification and treatment of orbitozygomatic and orbitoethmoid fractures—the place of bone grafting and plate fixation. *Clin Plast Surg.* 1989;16:77.

23. Rohrich RJ, Hollier LH, Watumull D. Optimizing the management of orbitozygomatic fractures. *Clin Plast Surg.* 1992; 19(1):149–165.

24. Davidson J, Nickerson D, Nickerson B. Zygomatic fractures: comparison of methods on internal fixation. *Plast Reconstr Surg.* 1990:25–32.

25. Rohrich RJ, Watumull D. The superiority of rigid plate fixation in the management of zygoma fractures and a long-term follow-up clinical study. *Plast Reconstr Surg.* 1991;18:58–61.

12
Metal for Craniomaxillofacial Internal Fixation Implants and Its Physiological Implications

Samuel G. Steinemann

Implants function as a temporary splint. In the form of a screw, a plate, or a pin, the implant stabilizes the fracture and supports forces in addition to those of functional load. Yet the implant is a foreign body. Is this foreign body an insult of the chemical, physiological, or mechanical kind for the living tissue?

Simpson et al.[1] made a comprehensive study of fracture-treatment implants of stainless steel, cobalt-base alloy, and titanium. Clinical symptoms of pain, swelling, and inflammation are observed with the first two metals but none with titanium. Local findings show sequestration for stainless steel and cobalt-base alloy implants, and inertness (i.e., absence of infection and a loose, vascularized tissue in contact with titanium implants (Figure 12.1). Such observations certainly distinguish the "2nd generation metal" titanium from the classical materials stainless steel and cobalt-chromium-molybdenum alloy.

Corrosion and Tissue Reaction

In the chemist's view, corrosion is the visible destruction of a metal. It may cause rupture of a structure or loss of function (e.g., by breakage of an implant). That was before the 1960s. This aspect is not important for modern metals in surgery because an attack is so small that a material loss is neither visible nor can it be weighed. More sensitive electrochemical methods are needed to measure corrosion, but experiments that reproduce the real conditions for a surgical implant in tissue are not simple.[2,3]

The polarization resistance method has been used for in vivo experiments,[2] with results shown in Figure 12.2. The method requires minimally invasive procedures and is characterized by reduction and oxidation reactions on the metal that are not forced and run freely.

The noble metals silver (Ag) and gold (Au) have a resistance to corrosion, lying about in the middle of the scale of the corrosion resistance. In the logarithmic scale of the polarization resistance, the number is 5 to 6, thus about 2 units or

a factor of 100 lower than high-grade stainless steel and titanium. Gold and silver do resist oxidation in air, but are much less resistant to corrosion in sea water and biological fluids. It is common experience that they lose polish after some time.

Metals having lower corrosion resistance than silver and gold (e.g., aluminum, molybdenum, and iron) show visible attack or oxidation in living tissue, and they are always surrounded by a pseudomembrane (i.e., such metals are sequestrated; however, without manifest pathological changes). This tissue reaction equals to a chemical insult. In fact, the group of metals iron (Fe) through silver corrodes so rapidly that supply and migration of oxygen cannot follow the consumption of the oxidant, so that the tissue starves of oxygen. This direct effect of corrosion is not specific for the metal of the implant. However, metals are released with the corrosion process and some of them are cell-toxic. Gerber et al.[4,5] and Rae[6] measured the toxicity by adding metal salts to embryonic bone rudiments and fibroblast cultures and observing inhibition reactions. Among the four elements shown in Figure 12.2, vanadium (V) is the most toxic and copper (Cu) the least toxic. This reaction equals to a major physiological insult.

The polarization resistance of stainless steel, cobalt-base alloy, and titanium is about the same for all three metals, but tissue reactions differ (see Figure 12.1). High corrosion resistance is apparently not sufficient to suppress a minor rejection reaction observed for the two classical alloys, which include cell-toxic nickel (Ni) and cobalt (Co) as essential components.

Fate of the Unwanted Reaction Product of Corrosion—Physiological Insult

The species of metal compounds ingested with nutrition and making the passage in the bloodstream (i.e., being metabolized) as well as those finally stored in organs and tissue are rather incompletely known.[7] However, most metals (other than alkali) in body fluids and tissue are bound to organic matter and exist in a stable, electrically uncharged form.

107

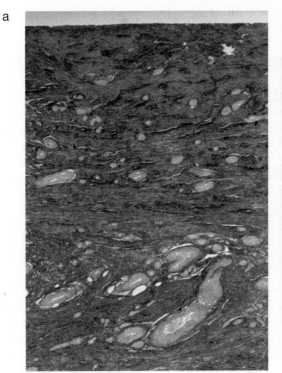 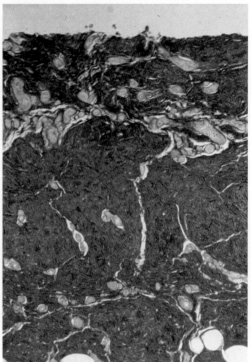

a   b

FIGURE 12.1 Optical micrographs of tissue in contact with a stain-less steel (a) and a commercially pure titanium implant (b). Biopsies are taken at metal retrieval about 1.5 years after operation. Blood and lymphatic vessels are seen throughout the contact zone for titanium but not in the case of stainless steel.

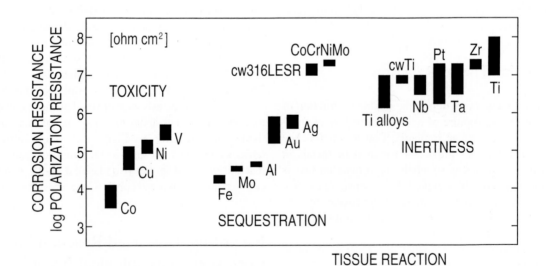

FIGURE 12.2 Data from in vivo corrosion experiments for various metallic elements and for practical alloys. The diagram has the following two coordinates: tissue reaction as abscissa, and polarization/corrosion resistance as the ordinate. Tissue reaction is grouped according to the three distinct forms of toxicity, sequestration, and inertness. Corrosion resistance is roughly proportional to the measured polarization resistance. It is noted that the useful scale in chemistry and biology is always the logarithmic one; thus differences over the series, for example, from cobalt (Co) to silver (Ag) to titanium (Ti), amount to factors of 1 to 100 to 10,000 in corrosion resistance. CoCrNiMo is wrought cobalt-base alloy, cw316LESR is cold-worked, remelted stainless steel, Ti alloys are Ti4Al4Mo, Ti6Al4V, and Ti15Mo.

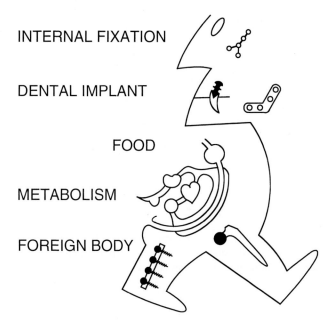

INTERNAL FIXATION

DENTAL IMPLANT

FOOD

METABOLISM

FOREIGN BODY

FIGURE 12.3 A sketch intended to illustrate that metals released from implants follow another reaction path than metals entering metabolism with nutrition.

Figure 12.3 suggests that metal release from implants involves a different path. It can be associated with the entry of the metal through a wound, which then undergoes corrosion. The unwanted reaction products of this corrosion are hydroxides, hydrous oxides, and oxides (i.e., sparingly soluble salts and occasionally complexes such as halides). These salts can be soluble or not in the tissue fluids (which are aqueous electrolytes), and they can be toxic or not.[8] To know the effects of this corrosion burden, the identity and stability of the hydrolysis products must be considered.

The word *hydrolysis* is applied to chemical reactions in which a substance is split or decomposed by water. What are the conversions of the metal salt, and does hydrolysis involve electrically neutral and ionic species, either the positively charged cation, the negatively charged anion, or both? These questions are addressed for two metallic biomaterials, stainless steel, with nickel as the main component, and titanium.

It is common to find that salts and oxides dissolve easily in strong acids and in strong bases and that the solubility of oxides is low around neutral pH values. Further, oxides dissociate and cations, either as bare ions or an ion comprising the hydroxide as ligand, dominate at low pH, while anions (always comprising the hydroxide ligand) exist at high pH. In between, uncharged aqueous species exist but must not dominate. Measurements of the kind are best represented as the solubility, or distribution curves of the various hydrolysis products. Diagrams have the two coordinates, acidity (i.e., pH of the solution) as abscissa and molar concentration of dissolved and precipitated species as the ordinate. Both are in logarithmic scale, which gives the straight lines.

The 2+ oxidation state of nickel is the important one, and in an aqueous environment the hydroxide is the first-formed corrosion product. Its dominant hydrolysis product under physiological conditions is the unhydrolyzed nickel cation with a concentration of about 1 mmol at the limit of hydroxide precipitation (Figure 12.4). The unwanted reaction product of corrosion is an ion.

In serum, the nickel concentration is about 10 nM, and in human skeletal muscle it is about 3 μM and less than the solubility limit. The metal concentration in the contact tissue around implants is still 100 times higher than that of normal muscle tissue and of the order of the toxicity threshold for nickel. The sequestration reaction for stainless steel implants is the consequence.

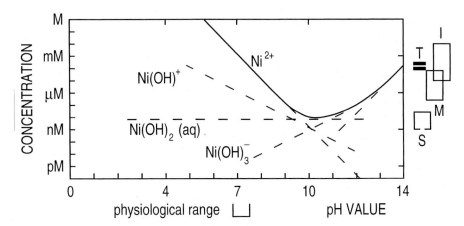

FIGURE 12.4 Distribution of hydrolysis products in solutions saturated with respect to nickel hydroxide [Ni(OH)$_2$]. The full line is the solubility limit expressed as the total concentration of two-valent Ni. Data for the concentration of nickel in serum (S), in muscle (M), in contact tissue around stainless steel implants (I), and toxicity levels (T) are added at right margin. Hydrolysis results are from Baes and Mesmer,[9] tissue concentrations of Ni are collected from many sources in Steinemann,[10] and toxicity levels are from Gerber et al.[4,6] and Rae.[6]

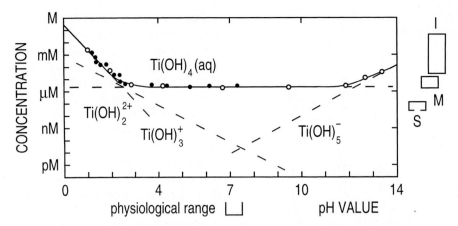

FIGURE 12.5 Solubility behavior of hydrous titanium-dioxide measured in sodium chloride and chlorate electrolytes.[9,10] The full line is the solubility limit and dashed lines are partial concentrations for the named species. Data for the concentration of titanium in serum (S), in muscle (M), and in contact tissue around implants (I) are added at right margin (numerous sources[10]).

Titanium is a reactive metal. In air and electrolytes, it forms spontaneously a dense and electrically insulating oxide film at its surface. The unwanted reaction product becomes a potent barrier against dissolution of the metal.

The constant solubility of titanium dioxide above a pH of around 3 and up to a pH of around 12 suggests that an electroneutral species dominates in solution (Figure 12.5). At physiological pH values, the first charged species is the cation $Ti(OH)_3^+$ with a concentration of not more than 0.1 nM, which is by orders of magnitude lower than the concentration of the always-present hydrogen ion in solution. The unwanted reaction product of corrosion is not an ion. This is an important finding because uncharged hydrolysis products have no affinity for reaction with organic molecules. Corrosion of titanium becomes, in fact, no chemical burden and its inert reaction in tissue is a sign of the basically different chemistry in solution.

In serum, the titanium concentration is about 0.1 μM, and in human skeletal muscle, it is about 5 μM. The muscle concentration of titanium equals the upper limit of solubility for the aqueous hydroxide, which is also the lower limit for precipitation of the solid oxide (about 3 μM). Solution chemistry thus provides a stringent, even simple homeostatic mechanism for the regulation of titanium in tissue: titanium is at saturation in tissue. The concentration of titanium in the contact tissue around implants is about 300 times higher than that of muscle tissue. These high concentrations seem representative for larger and loaded implants and include fretting and wear debris and residues from insufficient surface treatment. These metal and oxide particles beyond the solubility limit are deposited in tissue. Retrieval studies give no indication of any adverse reaction.

The in vivo corrosion experiments led us to distinguish for three forms of local tissue reaction (see Figure 12.2). The unwanted reaction product of corrosion is the cause. Tissue impregnation by corrosion products equals to a chemical insult, but it is crucial to ask whether it is an ion or an uncharged inorganic compound. With this distinction, toxicity is a major

physiological insult, and sequestration is a minor physiological insult, while inertness equals to no physiological insult.

The distinction between ions and uncharged inorganic compounds has a prolongation for immunologic reactions. Metals can act as haptens, that is, the ion can unite with a protein to form an antigen.[7,11] Such complex formation is known to occur with ions of nickel, cobalt, and chromium, but it is absent for titanium and a few other metals whose hydrolysis products in tissue fluids are not ions.

Note that no case of local or systemic reaction for titanium is documented.

Titanium has the surprising property that it can bind to living tissue and to bone. Dental surgeons use this quality for dental implants and call it *osseointegration*. The binding between the metal and bone resists forces along the interface (shear) and the perpendicular to the interface (tear off) and the adhesion is quite strong.[12] What is the glue? It is a true bonding interaction between hydroxyls in the ever-present surface titanium dioxide and the various ligands of organic matter.[13] These basic processes occur in atomic dimensions, and Listgarten[14] notes in his high-resolution transmission electron microscopic pictures that "there is no evidence of any space between the metallic surface and the bone." The affinity between bone and titanium may be termed *pseudobiological activity*.

Metal and Implants—Mechanical Properties and Manufacture

Titanium is not a rare metal, but its reduction from ore (ilmenite, an iron-titanium-oxygen compound, and rutile, an oxide of titanium) is not easy and in industrial scale succeeded only in the 1940s. The metal is used for aircraft, in chemical industry, and since the 1960s for surgical implants. Specifications for the application exist today.

AO/ASIF implants for craniomaxillofacial bone surgery are made from commercially pure (cp) titanium, with the excep-

TABLE 12.1 Mechanical properties of stainless steel, titanium, and bone.

Material	Yield strength, MPa	Ductility, %	Young's modulus, GPa
Cold-worked stainless steel	730	21%	190
cp titanium (grade 2)	280	(30%)	105
Cold-worked Ti (grade 4)	690	18%	105
Cortical bone	140		18

tion of a mandibular reconstruction set in stainless steel. Oxygen is added in small amounts, which increases the mechanical strength (Table 12.1). Grade 2 metal is used when malleability is more important than strength (thin bone, midface), while screws and loaded implants (mandible region) are made from the stronger, cold-worked metal. Shapes are obtained by machining (cutting, milling, drilling) operations.

Implants for head surgery must cause the smallest mechanical insult; a minimum volume and a smooth form is required (Figure 12.6). Titanium is the indicated material. It has good strength and high admissible strain to avoid overload of the implant. This admissible strain, equal to the ratio yield strength divided by Young's modulus, is 7% for cold-worked titanium, higher than that of stainless steel (4%), and about equal to that of bone (8%).

The last steps in fabrication are mechanical and chemical surface treatments. These processes augment the inertness of the implant. The matte yellow surface results from pickling in acid and the anodic oxidation that makes an implant inconspicuous in tissue and near the skin. This surface treatment further stabilizes an osteosynthesis. Experiments show that the release torque of small bone screws exceeds the in-sertion torque after 3 months.[15] Stainless steel screws, on the the contrary, always loosen with time.

Clinical Implications

Titanium implants are fully inert in tissue, and screws made of titanium integrate for a "solid mounting" of the osteosynthesis. Such behavior could suggest that we should "fit and forget" the fracture implant. The proposition is restricted to titanium and does not apply for stainless steel implants.

Head trauma, reconstructive, and corrective surgery can require large implants or a great number of small implants, sometimes in conjunction with dental implants to achieve functional rehabilitation. Some questions may emerge:

Is there a limit to the number or the surface area of implants that can be placed? Experience indicates no restrictions, based on the absence of foreign body reactions and the fact that living tissue is saturated with titanium. A larger size or greater number of implants is not a burden.

Is there an interaction among several implants? The answer is no. Mutual interaction between two plates or with a dental implant would at least require electrical contact.

Can another kind of insult occur? A bad mechanical situation may exist if solid mounting (i.e., stability of the osteosynthesis) is not achieved. Displacement by too much metal is a mechanical insult. Displacement can also limit indications for operations on children and adolescents.

Indications for removal of the implants do exist. Because of their favorable chemical and biochemical properties, titanium integrates easily and rapidly, especially for children. Thus removal should be done early.

a
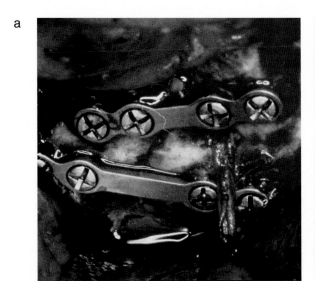

b
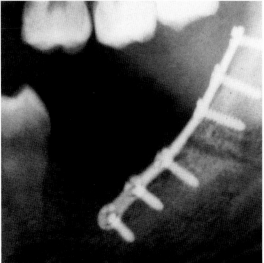

FIGURE 12.6 Smooth and malleable shapes with minimum volume are important for internal fixation implants in maxillofacial surgery. Fixation of a fractured mandible by two miniplates (a). Postopera-tive view of fracture fixation by a miniplate on the superior border of the mandibular angle (b). (Courtesy STRATEC Medical, Oberdorf, Switzerland)

References

1. Simpson JP, Geret V, Brown SA, Merritt K. Retrieved fracture plates—implant and tissue analysis. In: Weinstein A, Gibbons D, Brown S, Ruoff S, eds. *Implant Retrieval—Material and Biological Analysis.* NBS Spec. Publ. 601, 1981:395–422.
2. Steinemann SG. Corrosion of titanium and titanium alloys for surgical implants. In: Lütjering G, Zwicker V, Bunk W, eds. *Titanium, Science and Technology; Proc 5th Intl Conf Titanium.* Oberursel: Deutsche Gesellschaft Metallkunde. 1985:1373–1379.
3. Steinemann SG. Corrosion of implant alloys. In: Buchhorn GH, Willert HG, eds. *Technical Principles, Design and Safety of Joint Implants.* Seattle: Hogrefe & Huber Publishers; 1994: 168–179.
4. Gerber H, Perren SM. Evaluation of tissue compatibility of in vitro cultures of embryonic bone. In: Winter GD, Leray JL, de Groot K, eds. *Evaluation of Biomaterials.* Chichester: John Wiley & Sons, 1980:307–314.
5. Gerber HW, Moosmann A, Steinemann S. Bioactivity of metals—tissue tolerance of soluble or solid metal, tested on organ cultured embryonic bone rudiments. In: Buchhorn GH, Willert HG, eds. *Technical Principles, Design and Safety of Joint Implants.* Seattle: Hogreve & Huber Publishers; 1994:248–254.
6. Rae T. The toxicity of metals used in orthopaedic prostheses. *J Bone Joint Surg.* 1981;63-B:435–440.
7. Luckey TD, Venugopal B. *Metal Toxicity in Mammals, Vol. 1, Physiological and Chemical Basis.* New York: Plenum Press, 1977:39–91, 103–128.
8. Steinemann SG, Mäusli P-A. Titanium alloys for surgical implants—biocompatibility from physicochemical principles. In: Lacombe P, Tricot R, Béranger G, eds. *6th World Conf Titanium, France 1988.* Les Ulis: Les éditions de physique. 1988; 535–540.
9. Baes CF, Mesmer RE. *The Hydrolysis of Cations.* New York: John Wiley & Sons; 1976.
10. Steinemann SG. Tissue compatibility of metals from physicochemical principles. In: Kovacs P, Istephanous NS, eds. *Proc Symp Compatibility of Biomedical Implants*, vol. 94-15. Pennington, NJ: The Electrochemical Society, 1994:1–13.
11. Black J. *Biological Performance of Materials.* New York: Marcel Dekker; 1992:184–199.
12. Steinemann SG, Eulenberger J, Mäusli P-A, Schroeder A. Adhesion of bone to titanium. In: Christel P, Meunier A, Lee AJC, eds. *Biological and Biomechanical Performance of Biomaterials.* Amsterdam: Elsevier Science Publishers. 1986:409–414.
13. Gold JM, Schmidt M, Steinemann SG. XPS study of amino acid adsorption to titanium surfaces. *Helv Phys Acta.* 1989:62: 246–249. Idem. XPS study of retrieved titanium and Ti alloy implants. In: Heimke G, Soltész V, Lee AJC, eds. *Clinical Implant Materials—Advances in Biomaterials, vol. 9.* Amsterdam: Elsevier Science; 1990:69–74.
14. Listgarten MA, Buser D, Steinemann SG, Donath K, Lang NP, Weber H-P. Light and transmission electron microscopy of the intact interfaces between non-submerged titanium-coated epoxy resin implants and bone or gingiva. *J Dental Res.* 1992; 71: 364–371.
15. Eulenberger J, Steinemann SG. Lösemomente an Kleinschrauben aus Stahl und Titan mit unterschiedlichen Oberflächen. *Unfallchirurg.* 1990;93:96–99.

13

Bioresorbable Materials for Bone Fixation: Review of Biological Concepts and Mechanical Aspects

Riitta Suuronen and Christian Lindqvist

The development of biodegradable devices for fracture fixation and guided bone regeneration has been intense for three decades. An optimal device should not cause any local or systemic disorders and should degrade slowly, transferring the stress to the healing bone. Hence, it need not be removed after the fracture or defect has healed.

The first material to be used as biodegradable suture was catgut (collagen), which degrades proteolytically and disappears from tissue via phagocytosis, thus causing a local inflammation in the tissue. Modern suture materials are made of polyhydroxy acids (polyesters). Most widely used are polylactide (PLA), polyglycolide (PGA), and polydioxanone (PDS). In fracture fixation, PGA was the first material to be used by Schmitt and Polistina,[1] but their results were never reported in a scientific journal. The first reports on the use of PLA in the fixation of fractures or osteotomies were published by Cutright et al.[2] and Kulkarni et al.[3] Later, devices made of PGA and PDS were used successfully for fracture fixation in maxillofacial surgery.[4,5]

The development of PLA devices for maxillofacial surgery started in the 1970s, when Cutright et al.[2] used PLA sutures and Kulkarni[3] used PLA rods in the repair of experimental mandibular fractures. The following year, sheets of PLA were used in experimental blow-out fractures.[6] Better knowledge in material management has led to a wide use of biodegradable materials, and today PLA screws are routinely used in our department in the fixation of sagittal split osteotomies.[7]

Materials

The synthetic biodegradable materials most widely used in fracture fixation are high molecular weight alpha hydroxy acid polymers: polydioxanone (Figure 13.1), polyglycolide (Figure 13.2), and polylactide (Figure 13.3). Of these, PGA and PLA have received the most interest, partly because they can be self-reinforced to gain better strength properties.

Sterilization also contributes to the degradation rate. Ethylene oxide does not alter the polymer or cause degradation,[8] but it can introduce residues to the polymer.[9,10] By con-

trast, gamma radiation causes both chain-scissioring and cross-linking in the polymer[11] and can change its mechanical properties.[12,13] It also reduces the molecular weight of the polymer.[14]

Polydioxanone

Polydioxanone (Figure 13.1) is a colorless crystalline polymer. At room temperature it is rubberlike, its melting point being 110°C and glass transition temperature −16°C. It is degraded by hydrolysis, and the end products are excreted mainly in urine, some in feces, and some exhaled as CO_2.[15] It is completely resorbed in 6 months, and only a minimal foreign body tissue reaction in the vicinity of the implant can be seen.[15–17] Implants made of PDS can be sterilized by ethylene oxide.

These properties make it well suited for sutures. Because of its flexibility, it has been used in soft tissue, tendon, and ligament surgery,[18] and in orthopedic surgery (cords, pins, and screws).[19–25] Only a few studies have been published of its use in maxillofacial surgery.[5,26,27]

Polyglycolic Acid (Polyglycolide, PGA)

PGA is a hard, brownish crystalline polymer, which is insoluble in most solvents (Figure 13.2). It has a melting point of 224–226°C and glass transition temperature of 36°C.[28] It is degraded in hydrolysis, and it is also broken down by nonspecific esterases and carboxy peptidases. Monomeric units of glycolic acid can be excreted in urine or enzymatically converted to end products H_2O and CO_2 (Figure 13.4).[29] Depending on its molecular weight, purity, and crystallinity as well as the size and shape of the implant, it loses its mechanical strength in 6 weeks and is totally resorbed in a few months.[18,30] Degradation is faster in vivo than in vitro, supposedly because of cellular enzymes.[31] PGA is usually sterilized by using ethylene oxide.

Because it loses its mechanical strength rather quickly, it has been used mainly in sutures (e.g., Dexon, Davis and Geck, UK) and in rods and screws in fracture fixation of cancellous bone.[32–35]

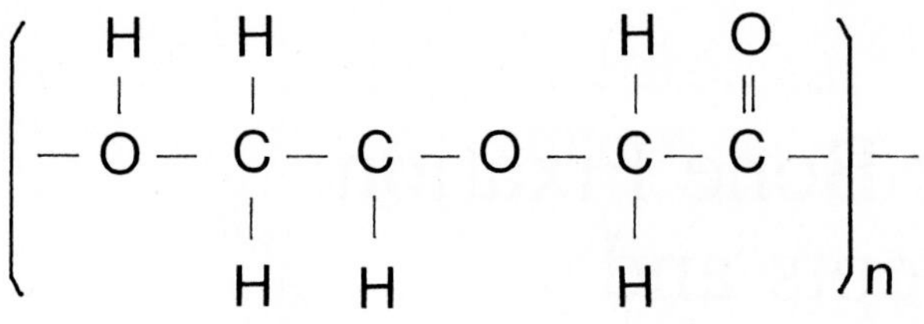

FIGURE 13.1 Polydioxanone (PDS).

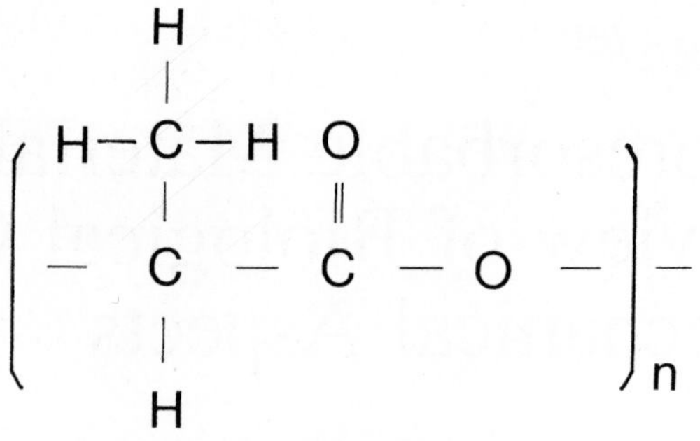

FIGURE 13.3 Polylactide (PLA).

Polylactic Acid (Polylactide, PLA)

Polylactic acid (Figure 13.3) is a pale, semicrystalline polymer with a melting point of 174°C and glass transition temperature of 57°C.[8] It can exist in four forms, depending on the L and D configuration.[36] It also is degraded in hydrolysis, its end products being H_2O and CO_2 (Figure 13.5). The strength retention time of PLA varies depending on the sterilization method and the properties of the material and implant, but it is considerably longer than PDS or PGA. The total resorption time of poly-L-lactide is several years.[37,38] A copolymer of D- and L-lactide, poly-DL-lactide (PDLLA), seems to degrade somewhat faster.[39] Cellular enzymes are supposed to enhance this reaction, too.[31]

PLA can be sterilized with ethylene oxide or steam[40] and high-strength self-reinforced implants can be sterilized with gamma radiation.[18] Gamma sterilization decreases significantly the molecular weight of PLA, and, hence, might enhance the degradation, resulting in shorter resorption time.[18]

Copolymers

PGA and PLA can be combined to form a copolymer. Its properties can be changed by varying the ratios of its components. By increasing the amount of PGA, the copolymer will degrade faster and vice versa. Today, a PLA/PGA copolymer suture material, polyglactin 910, is widely used (Vicryl®, Ethicon, Sollentuna, Sweden). Also, a copolymer of poly-L-lactide (PLLA) and poly-D-lactide (PDLA) can be manufactured, and by varying their ratio, the properties of this PDLLA can be changed.

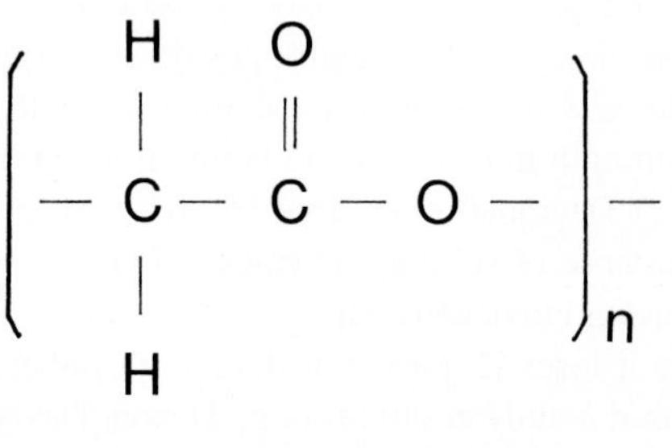

Self-Reinforcing Technique

The self-reinforcing (SR) technique developed by Törmälä et al.[41] has enabled the manufacture of polylactide and polyglycolide implants strong enough for fracture fixation. In this technique, polymeric fibers are bound together with a matrix of the same polymer without any adhesion promoters (Figure 13.6). These implants have high initial strength values and, therefore, are suitable for fracture fixation.[42]

Biocompatibility and Tissue Reactions

In general, all these materials have been well tolerated in living tissue. Local tissue responses depend on the rate of degradation and the biocompatibility of the components and degradation products of the polymer.[29] Cutright and Hunsuck[43] found that resorption of PLA was accomplished by a peculiar phagocytic process that started at 4 weeks and was still

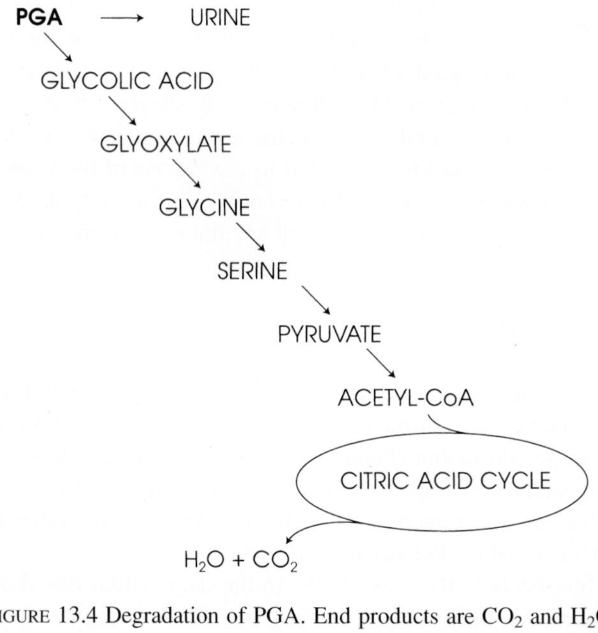

FIGURE 13.2 Polyglycolide (PGA).

FIGURE 13.4 Degradation of PGA. End products are CO_2 and H_2O.

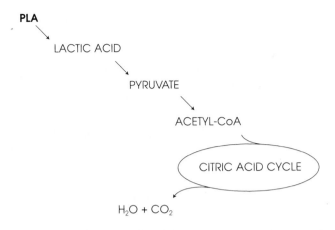

FIGURE 13.5 Degradation of PLA. Final products are CO_2 and H_2O.

continuing at 38 weeks. Phagocytic cells, giant cells, and villous projections were involved in this process. PLA tissue compatibility was found to be very good. Majola et al.[44] used SR-PLLA and SR-PDLLA/PLLA (40/60) rods on femoral osteotomies in rats and rabbits with follow-up times up to 2 years. Resorption of the implants started in the periphery and continued toward the center of the implant. Histologically, no evidence of inflammation or foreign body reaction could be seen. However, mild inflammatory reactions have been encountered surrounding the implant throughout the resorption period. Hatton et al.[45] evaluated SR-PGA membranes in rat bone cell cultures. In 2 weeks, cells had colonized the surface of the membrane, and after 3 weeks, bone cells penetrated the weave of the membrane, forming calcified collagenous bonelike tissue. At the same time, evidence of

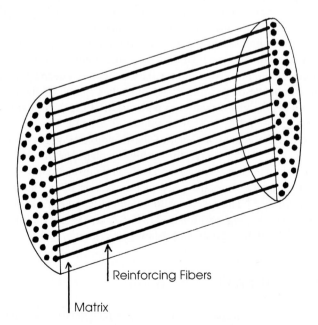

Reinforcing Fibers

Matrix

FIGURE 13.6 The self-reinforcing technique, in which fibers and binding matrix are of the same chemical composition.

resorption of PGA could be noticed. The authors conclude that this study supports previous reports on the osteoconductive activity of this material.

PDS elicited minimal or slight foreign body reactions when implanted in subcutaneous tissue in rats.[15] At 5 days, the reaction consisted primarily of macrophages and proliferating fibroblasts. At 91 days and later, no neutrophils were seen, and only macrophages and fibroblasts remained consistently present until the material was completely absorbed. After absorption, reactions were either absent or identified by the presence of a few enlarged macrophages or fibroblasts localized between otherwise normal muscle cells.

In humans, inflammatory foreign body reactions, which include a discharging sinus without infection, have been encountered in several clinical studies when PGA or PGA/PLA copolymer has been used.[33,35,46–48] This is demonstrated by an uncomfortable swelling in the operation area after a follow-up period of approximately 12 weeks. In these cases, implants have been placed directly under the skin, in areas where there is very little subcutaneous tissue. After drainage, the swelling disappeared in 3 weeks.[35] When the aspirate from the swelling was cytologically analyzed, mainly lymphocytes and some monocytes were found. The authors concluded that PGA is immunologically inert but induces mononuclear cell migration.[49]

Eitenmüller et al.[50] reported a clinically manifest foreign body reaction to nonreinforced PLLA plates and screws after fixation of an ankle fracture. In 4 of 25 patients, small fragments of degraded plate were pushed through the overlying skin 6 to 9 months postoperatively. No signs of infection could be noticed. Bergsma et al.[51] reported on a late tissue response on nonreinforced PLLA 3 years after fracture fixation in 6 of 10 patients. The plates and screws were placed directly under the skin at the frontozygomatic suture, with minimal subcutaneous tissue. The patients had clinically manifest intermittent swelling at the operation site. At reoperation, fragments of the polymer were removed and histological samples taken. In histological and electron microscopic evaluation, crystalline PLLA particles were found extracellularly and intracellularly together with numerous fibrocytes, macrophages, and giant cells. SR-PLLA pins have been used in the treatment of small-fragment fractures and osteotomies in 32 patients without signs of foreign body reaction 8 to 32 months postoperatively.[52]

Experimental Fracture Fixation

Orbital Blowout

Cutright and Hunsuck[6] used 1.5-mm-thick PLA sheets to repair experimental blowout fractures in 12 monkeys (*Macaca mulatta*). Bone was deposited immediately adjacent to the capsule surrounding the resorbing PLA. Healing was reported normal, but residual PLA could still be detected after 38 weeks.

Rozema et al.[53] studied the use of as-polymerized PLLA implants for the repair of blow-out fractures in 15 goats. The implants were concave, 0.4 mm thick and 30 mm in diameter, and they had perforations of 2 mm in diameter to allow tissue ingrowth. The artificial defects created in the bone and maxillary sinus epithelium were approximately 15 mm in diameter. Excess areas of each implant were trimmed using scissors. The implants were fixed to the infraorbital rim using one PGA suture. Follow-up times were up to 78 weeks, after which histological examinations were performed. After 3 weeks, the implants were totally covered by loose connective tissue. By 12 weeks, some growth into the perforations was evident. The epithelium at the roof of the maxillary sinus was normal. A thin layer of new bone was observable. After 19 weeks, a bony plate in apposition to the outer side of the connective tissue capsule was observed. By 78 weeks, new bone totally covered the antral and orbital sides of the implant and filled the perforations in the implant. No inflammatory reactions were seen. The authors concluded that the implant gave sufficient stability to the fracture for it to heal, but that a shorter absorption time (now estimated to be as long as 3.5 years) would be preferable.

Mandible

Sutures

In the beginning of the development of biodegradable materials, PLA sutures were used in the fixation of experimental mandibular midline fractures in *Macaca mulatta*.[2] The suture consisted of three strands, twisted together to form a 0.35-mm strand. Each 0.2-mm strand consisted of fibers of 28 mm in diameter. The healing was uneventful with a follow-up time up to 12 weeks.

Rods

Kulkarni et al.[3] used 1/8-in. (3.2-mm) PDLLA extruded rods in the fixation of mandibular fractures in dogs. The healing rate was the same as in a control group, in which similar stainless steel pins were used. The rods changed color to a whitish shade after 2 weeks. At 6 weeks they were "worm-eaten."

Plates and Screws

Getter et al.[54] reported on having used four-hole plates and non–self-tapping screws in the fixation of mandibular fractures in 6 dogs. During surgery, the plates and screws were fused into a one-piece system with a warm soldering iron, which ensured the stability of the fixation and inhibited movement between the screws and the plate. The fractures healed with secondary callus formation in 4 to 6 weeks. By 32 to 40 weeks, the plates and screws were completely degraded.

Gerlach et al.[55] used high-molecular-weight (800, 000) PLLA plates and screws to fix mandibular fractures in 12 adult beagle dogs. The plates were of the Sherman type with a cross section of $4 \times 9 \times 15$ mm and length of 45 mm. The thread diameter of the screw was 3 mm and that of the core 1.9 mm. Fracture healing was uncomplicated in all dogs, and the fractures consolidated after 4 weeks, although some screws broke. After 12 weeks, callus had disappeared.

Bos[56] has published a PhD thesis on the use of high-molecular-weight PLLA plates and screws in mandibular fractures in sheep and dogs. In pilot studies in two sheep and six dogs, a special clamp was used to produce a "natural" fracture, that is, one with serrated edges of the alveolar process, buccal cortex, and inferior border of the mandibular body area. The plates were bent to match the underlying bone using a heat gun. The follow-up time was from 3 to 11 weeks. Bos used a Champy-like 4-hole plate with monocortical screws. The plate was, however, 2.0 mm thick, 37 mm long, and 8 mm wide. The screws used had a thread diameter of 2.7 mm. Bos fixed fractures on one side of the mandible and placed unloaded plates on the other side of the mandible. After the follow-up, the plates were removed, but it was impossible to remove the screws after 3 weeks because they broke in the area between the screw head and thread. The results indicated that the plates subjected to loading had lost more of their tensile strength (about 90%) in 11 weeks than those not under stress (about 80%). The fractures healed uneventfully. No callus formation was seen. The authors concluded that use of their PLLA plates and screws resulted in good stability over a sufficiently long period of time for normal bone healing to occur.

In their early studies, Törmälä et al.[41,42,57] focused on developing SR-technique mainly for rod-shaped implants. The first clinical report on the use of biodegradable implants in weight-bearing fractures was that by Rokkanen et al.[32] From the late 1980s biodegradable screws and plates have been used successfully for the fixation of experimental mandibular osteotomies in 87 sheep. They have been used in three different osteotomies: condylar and body osteotomies and sagittal split osteotomies. No intermaxillary fixation has been applied in any of these cases.[7,58–64] These studies started by the fixation of condylar osteotomies with one SR-PLLA screw (Figures 13.7–13.9).[58,63] Then a multilayer SR-PLLA plate was used in the edentulous area of the mandible (Figures 13.10 and 13.11).[60,61] Finally, this multilayer plate was used with polylactide screws (Suuronen et al., unpublished data). SR-PLLA screws were also used in the fixation of sagittal osteotomies.[7,59] The results of these animal experiments were very encouraging, and today, SR-PLLA screws are routinely used in certain sagittal split osteotomies (Figure 13.12a–c).[7]

Clinical Fracture Fixation

The first clinical studies on the use of biodegradable materials in fracture surgery were carried out 20 years ago. In the beginning, the results were not very satisfying. Reports of repair of small numbers of zygomatic, mandibular, and orbital blow-

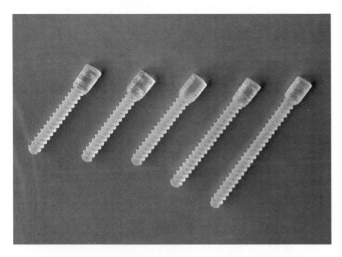

FIGURE 13.7 SR-PLLA screws, core diameter 2.7 mm.

out fractures were published in the international literature. Intermaxillary immobilization was necessary in most cases.

Orbital Floor/Wall Fractures

Cantaloube et al.[26] and Iizuka et al.[27] have reported the use of PDS plates for reconstruction of orbital floor defects greater than 10 mm in size. The dimensions of the bowl-shaped plates were 28 × 28 × 1 mm. The plates were easy to cut to suitable sizes. They were placed over the defect subperiosteally. They were fixed to the orbital rim with one or two 0.35-mm steel wires or sutures. The PDS was well tolerated by the body and did not give rise to clinically detectable inflammatory reactions. New bone formation, even hypertrophic bone, was seen. The authors concluded that the material retained its structural integrity long enough for a sufficiently rigid scar to be formed,

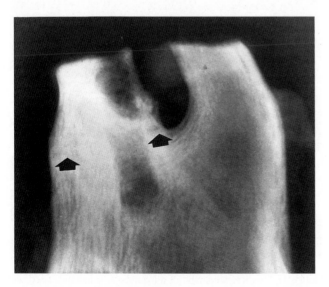

FIGURE 13.8 Mandibular condylar osteotomy fixed with SR-PLLA screw in sheep. The osteotomy line is barely visible (arrows). The screw is not radiopositive. Twelve weeks after the operation.

preventing delayed herniation of the orbital contents. Because of the thickness of the plate, overcorrection is necessary. As the plate biodegrades, the globe attains a correct position.

Sasserath et al.[65] reported the use of 0.15-mm-thick SR-PGA membranes in 20 blowout fractures. The sizes of the bony defects were not reported. The results were promising. Two patients complained of continuous infraorbital edema, which, according to the authors, was caused by poor residual drainage. The problem was solved by regular massage of the region.

Vert et al.[66] reported the use of small (2-mm-thick) PLLA/PGA composite plates reinforced with two-ply PGA fabric for repair of mandibular and skull fractures in 25 patients over a period of 2 years. The plates were warmed using an electric hair dryer and shaped to fit the bone. The plates were fixed using stainless steel screws. The first clinical results were good. There were no acute or chronic tissue reactions.

Zygoma

Gerlach[67] used poly-L-lactide screws and plates in 15 patients with zygomatic fractures. The plates were 2 mm thick, 8 mm wide, and 26 mm long. The plates were fixed using four screws. The outer diameter of each screw was 2.7 mm and the core diameter 1.9 mm. The implants were sterilized using ethylene oxide. Stabilization was good, and no side effects were noted during a follow-up period of 20 months.

Bos et al.[68] treated 10 patients with zygomatic fractures, using PLLA plates and screws. The plates had four holes, and they were slightly curved, 30 mm long, 6.7 mm wide, and 2 mm thick. The screws had a thread diameter of 2.7 mm. Shaping to the bone was achieved by heating the plate with a heat gun. Postoperative healing was good in all cases. However, after several years a foreign body reaction was observed in some patients.[51]

Mandible

Roed-Petersen[4] treated two young patients (a 15-year-old girl and a 23-year-old man) with unfavorable, severely dislocated fractures of the angle using PGA (Dexon®) sutures. The need for intermaxillary fixation was evident, and it was undertaken for 6 weeks. Healing was uneventful. One year after operation, radiography showed that the bur holes at the sites of the sutures had filled in.

Niederdellmann and Bührmann[5] used a PDS lag screw to fix a fracture of the mandibular angle. The screw core diameter was 3.2 mm and its thread diameter 4.5 mm. It is not stated whether or not MMF was applied.

Defect Repair and Membrane Technique

Biodegradable sheets and membranes can be used to prohibit faster-growing tissue (i.e., soft tissue) from intruding into bony defects, allowing the defect to be filled with new bone.

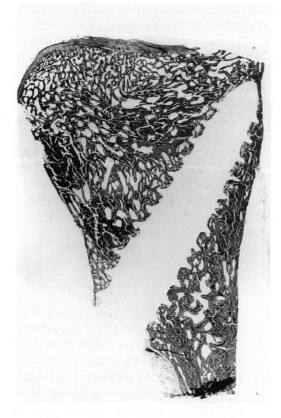

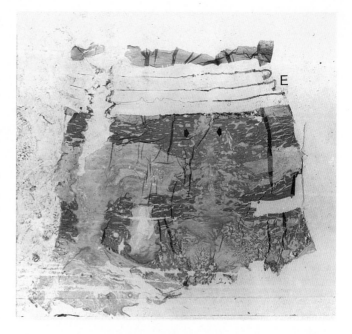

FIGURE 13.10 Histological section of a mandibular osteotomy fixed with SR-PLLA multilayer plate 6 weeks postoperatively. The 4-layer plate can be clearly seen (E). The osteotomy is still visible (arrows).

FIGURE 13.9 Histological section of mandibular condylar osteotomy 24 weeks postoperatively in sheep. The osteotomy cannot be detected. Degradation of the screw has not yet started.

For this purpose, PLA sheets have been used in the repair of oroantral fistulas.[69] Also, PGA membranes have been used in implant surgery, when implants have been placed into fresh experimental sockets.[70]

PLA matrix has been successfully used as a wound stabilizing implant in reconstructive periodontal surgery. Supra-alveolar circumferential periodontal defects were surgically created around mandibular premolars in beagle dogs. After 4 weeks of wound healing the use of PLA matrix significantly enhanced connective tissue repair. The authors conclude that the development of a biodegradable implant system aimed at stabilizing and supporting the healing wound seems a desirable direction for future research in regenerative periodontal procedures.

Use of Materials Today

Guided Bone Growth

Both PLA/PGA (Vicryl®, Ethicon, Sollentuna, Sweden) and SR-PGA (Biofix®, Bioscience, Tampere, Finland) membranes (Figures 13.13 and 13.14) are currently used in periodontal reconstructive and oral surgery,[71] as well as in orthognathic surgery (Le Fort I osteotomies). The biodegradable

membranes prevent the ingrowth of soft tissue to bone defects, allowing new bone ingrowth. In implant surgery, the use of resorbable membrane simultaneously with the implant insertion immediately after extraction, other interventions, except for the abutment placement procedure, are avoided. These SR-PGA membranes have also been used in places where

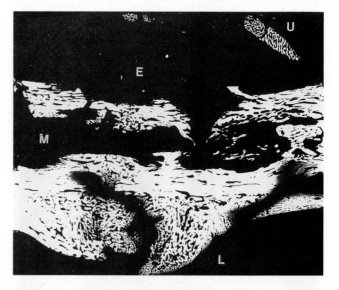

FIGURE 13.11 Microradiograph of a mandibular osteotomy fixed with SR-PLLA multilayer plate 12 weeks postoperatively. A prominent callus can be seen on the lingual side (L) and inside the mandibular canal (M), as well as on top of the plate (U). The plate itself is not visible (E).

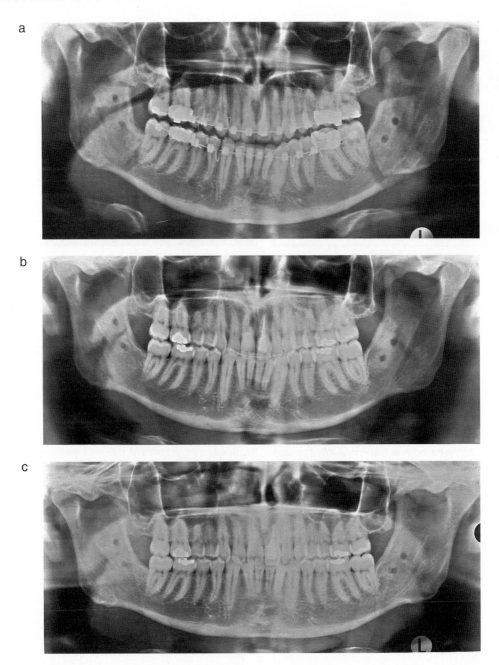

FIGURE 13.12 Sagittal osteotomy fixed with biodegradable SR-PLLA screws. (a) Postoperative ortopanthomogram; (b) 9 months postoperatively; (c) 15 months postoperatively.

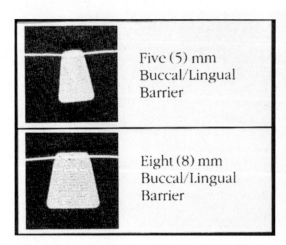

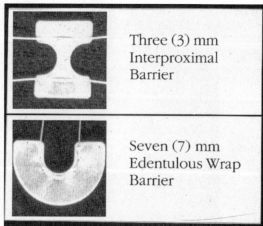

FIGURE 13.13 PLA/PGA membrane (Vicryl®).

bone is lost due to periodontitis, and in rescue procedures in infected bone resorption around implants.[71]

Fracture Fixation

The use of self-reinforced poly-L-lactide (SR-PLLA) implants in fracture fixation started in orthopedic surgery. It has been gradually extended to the field of oral and maxillofacial surgery. The implants used have to be strong enough to allow free movement of the jaws postoperatively. Only this can be considered the aim of research work, because the side effects caused by wiring the jaws together with intermaxillary fixation after open reduction of the fracture or osteotomy must be avoided whenever possible.

Orbital Floor/Wall Fractures

Today in clinical use are concave PDS plates and PGA sheets (Figures 13.14 and 13.15).[27] The disadvantage of using these

plates is the thickness of the plate. When placed in the orbit, double vision is almost always a consequence for a couple of weeks. This situation is corrected when the plate degrades. Today, a thinner sheet is also available (PDS® Ethicon). In some patients the material has extruded through the skin when resorption starts. The reason for this phenomenon is still unknown.

SR-PGA membranes (Biofix®) have been used in blow-out fractures in a multicenter study in Europe. It was found that the membranes conformed well to the topography of the orbital floor and provided adequate initial support. The authors conclude that SR-PGA membrane appears to be a suitable alternative to traditional nonresorbable materials for orbital floor repair and may reduce the incidence of long-term complications associated with currently used alloplastic materials.[65,72]

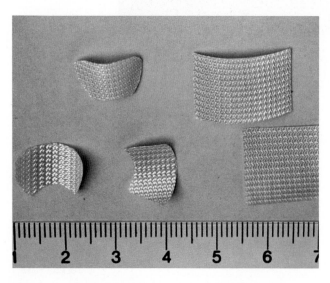

FIGURE 13.14 PGA membrane (Biofix).

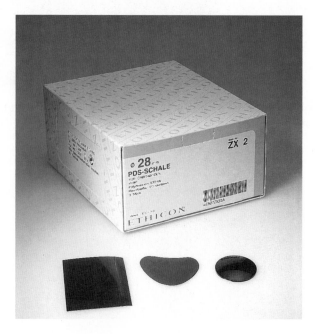

FIGURE 13.15 PDS concave disc and sheet.

Sagittal Split Osteotomies

In our department, those sagittal osteotomies that do not have a bony gap between the buccal and lingual bone fragments are today fixed with SR-PLLA screws (Biofix®, Figure 13.12a–c). The screws are available in two sizes, with a core diameter of 2.7 or 2.0. With the longest follow-up in sagittal osteotomies now being more than 6 years, we believe that we probably can widen the range of use to other fractures and osteotomies of the facial skeleton, too.

Costochondral Arthroplasty

Biofix®-screws have been used to fix the rib transplant lateral to the mandibular ramus in costochondral arthroplasty (see Chapter 30).

Future Prospects

New Materials

New biodegradable materials for maxillofacial and orthopaedic surgery are constantly being studied. A copolymer of polylactide/poly-E-caprolactone seems to be a promising material for bone filling. Also an experimental polyorthoester (POE) has shown very good properties in tissue tolerance. However, these materials require extensive investigation before they can be used clinically.

New Applications: Bioactive Composites

Adding drugs to these biodegradable polymers has been studied for several years.[73] However, these studies have dealt with controlled drug release only, without a simultaneous fracture fixation or tissue growth guidance. In the future, it might be possible to add, for example, antibiotics to these screws and membranes to inhibit bacterial ingrowth or growth factors to accelerate healing and bone ingrowth into the defect area.

References

1. Schmitt E, Polistina R. Polyglycolic acid prosthetic devices. US Patent 3 463 158: Aug. 26, 1969.
2. Cutright DE, Hunsuck E, Beasley JD. Fracture reduction using a biodegradable material, polylactic acid. *J Oral Surg.* 1971;29: 393–397.
3. Kulkarni RK, Moore EG, Hegyeli AF, Leonard F. Biodegradable poly(lactic acid) polymers. *J Biomed Mater Res.* 1971;5: 169–181.
4. Roed-Petersen B. Absorbable synthetic suture material for internal fixation of fractures of the mandible. *Int J Oral Surg.* 1974;3:133–136.
5. Niederdellmann H, Bührmann K. Resorbierbare Osteosyntheseschrauben aus Polydioxanon (PDS). Dtsch Z Mund Kiefer Gesichtschir 1983;7:399–400.
6. Cutright DE, Hunsuck E. The repair of fractures of the orbital floor using biodegradable polylactic acid. *Oral Surg.* 1972;33:28–34.
7. Suuronen R, Laine P, Pohjonen T, Lindqvist C. Sagittal ramus osteotomies fixed with biodegradable screws: A preliminary report. *J Oral Maxillofac Surg.* 1994;52:715–720.
8. Vert M, Christel P, Chabot F, Leray J. Bioresorbable plastic materials for bone surgery. In: Hastings GW, Ducheyne P, eds. *Macromolecular Biomaterials.* Boca Raton, FL: CRC Press; 1984:119–142.
9. Handlos V. The hazards of ethylene oxide sterilization. *Arch Pharm Chem Sci.* 1979;7:147–157.
10. Handlos V. Kinetics of the aeration of ethylene oxide sterilized plastics. *Biomaterials.* 1980;1:149–157.
11. Gupta MC, Deshmukh VG. Radiation effects on poly(lactic acid). *Polymer.* 1983;24:827–830.
12. Gilding DK, Reed AM. Biodegradable polymers for use in surgery—polyglycolic/poly(lactic acid) homo- and copolymers: 1. *Polymer.* 1979;20:1459–1465.
13. Lähde H, Pohjonen T, Heponen V-P, Vainionpää S, Rokkanen P, Törmälä P. In vitro degradation of poly-L-lactide fibres. In: *Abstract book of the IVth International Conference on Polymers in Medicine and Surgery.* Leeuwenhorst, Holland; 1989:7/1–7/4.
14. Spenlehauer G, Vert M, Benoit JP, Boddaert A. In vivo and in vitro degradation of poly(D,L lactide/glycolide) type microspheres made by solvent evaporation method. *Biomaterials.* 1989;10:557–563.
15. Ray JA, Doddi N, Regula D, Williams JA, Melveger A. Polydioxanone (PDA), a novel monofilament synthetic absorbable suture. *Surg Gynecol Obstet.* 1981;153:497–507.
16. Craig PH, Williams JA, Davis KW, Magoun AD, Levy AJ, Bogdansky S, et al. A biologic comparison of polyglactin 910 and polyglycolic acid synthetic absorbable sutures. *Surg Gynecol Obstet.* 1975;141:1–10.
17. Ala-Kulju K, Verkkala K, Ketonen P, Heikkinen L, Harjola PT. Polydioxanone in coronary vascular surgery. *J Cardiovasc Surg.* 1989;30:754–756.
18. Vainionpää S, Rokkanen P, Törmälä P. Surgical applications of biodegradable polymers in human tissues. *Prog Polym Sci.* 1989;14:679–716.
19. Blatter G, Meier G. Augmentation der korakoklavikulären Bandnaht. Vergleich zwischen Drahtcerclage, Vicrylband und PDS-Kordel. *Unfallchirurg.* 1990;93:578–583.
20. Claes L, Burri C, Kiefer H, Mutschler W. Resorbierbare Implantate zur Refixierung von osteochondralen Fragmenten in Gelenkflächen. *Akt Traumatol.* 1986;16:74–77.
21. Gay B, Bucher H. Tierexperimentelle Untersuchungen zur Anwendung von absorbierbaren Osteosyntheseschrauben aus Polydioxanon (PDS). *Unfallchirurg.* 1985;88:126–133.
22. Greve H, Holste J. Refixation osteochondraler Fragmente durch resorbierbare Kunststoffstifte. *Akt Traumatol.* 1985;15:145–149.
23. Mäkelä EA. Healing of epiphyseal fracture fixed with a biodegradable polydioxanone implant or metallic pins. An experimental study on growing rabbits. *Clin Mater.* 1988;3:61–71.
24. Ochsner PE, Ilchmann TH. Zuggurtungsosteosynthesen mit resorbierbaren Kordeln bei proximalen Humerusmehrfragmentbrüchen. *Unfallchirurg.* 1991;94:508–510.
25. Plaga BR, Royster RM, Donigian AM, Wright GB, Caskey PM. Fixation of osteochondral fractures in rabbit knees. A comparison of Kirschner wires, fibrin sealant, and polydioxanone pins. *J Bone Joint Surg.* 1992;74-B:292–296.
26. Cantaloube D, Rives JM, Bauby F, Andreani JF, Dumas B. Utilisation de la cupule en PDS dans les fractures orbito-malares. *Rev Stomatol Chir Maxillofac.* 1989;90:48–51.

27. Iizuka T, Mikkonen P, Paukku P, Lindqvist C. Reconstruction of orbital floor with polydioxanone plate. *Int J Oral Maxillofac Surg.* 1991;20:83–87.

28. Frazza EJ, Schmitt E. A new absorbable suture. *J Biomed Mater Res Symp.* 1971;1:43–58.

29. Hollinger JO, Battistone GC. Biodegradable bone repair materials. Synthetic polymers and ceramics. *Clin Orthop.* 1986;207:290–305.

30. Gerlach KL, Eitenmüller J. In vivo evaluation of 8 different polymers for use as osteosynthesis material in maxillo-facial surgery, In: Pizzoferrato A, Marchetti PG, Ravaglioni A, Lee ACJ, eds. *Biomaterials and Clinical Applications.* Amsterdam: Elsevier Science Publisher B.V., 1987:439–445.

31. Williams DF. Some observations on the role of cellular enzymes in the in-vivo degradation of polymers. In: Syrett BC, Acharya DA, eds. *ASTM Special Technical Publications: Corrosion and Degradation of Implant Materials.* Philadelphia: American Society for Testing and Materials; 1979:61–75.

32. Rokkanen P, Böstman O, Vainionpää S, Vihtonen K, Törmälä P, Laiho J, et al. Biodegradable implants in fracture fixation: Early results of treatment of fractures of the ankle. Lancet 1985; 1:1422–1424.

33. Hirvensalo E. Fracture fixation with biodegradable rods: forty-one cases of severe ankle fractures. *Acta Orthop Scand.* 1989; 60:601–606.

34. Partio EK, Böstman O, Hirvensalo E, Vainionpää S, Vihtonen K, Pätiälä H, et al. Self-reinforced absorbable screws in fixation of displaced ankle fractures: A prospective clinical study of 152 patients. *J Orthop Trauma.* 1992;6:209–215.

35. Böstman O, Hirvensalo E, Mäkinen J, Rokkanen P. Foreign body reactions to fracture fixation implants of biodegradable synthetic polymers. *J Bone Joint Surg (Br).* 1990;72-B: 592–596.

36. Holten CH. Lactic acid. In: *Verlag Chemie.* Weinheim; 1971: pp 221–231.

37. Suuronen R, Pohjonen T, Hietanen J. Long-term degradation of self-reinforced poly-L-lactide (SR-PLLA) plates in vivo and in vitro, in press.

38. Rozema FR, Bos RRM, Pennings AJ, Jansen HWB. Poly(L-lactide) implants in repair of defects of the orbital floor: An animal study. *J Oral Maxillofac Surg.* 1990;48:1305–1309.

39. Majola A, Vainionpää S, Mikkola HM, Törmälä P, Rokkanen P. Absorbable self-reinforced polylactide (SR-PLA) composite rods for fracture fixation: Strength and strength retention in the bone and subcutaneous tissue of rabbits. *J Mater Sci Mater Med.* 1992;3:43–47.

40. Rozema FR. Resorbable poly(L-lactide) bone plates and screws. Tests and applications. PhD Thesis, University of Groningen, The Netherlands, 1991, 107 p.

41. Törmälä P, Rokkanen P, Laiho J, Tamminmäki M, Vainionpää S. US Patent 4, 743, 257. May 10, 1988.

42. Törmälä P. Biodegradable self-reinforced composite materials; manufacturing structure and mechanical properties. *Clin Mater.* 1992;10:29–34.

43. Cutright DE, Hunsuck E. Tissue reaction to the biodegradable polylactic acid suture. *Oral Surg.* 1971;31:134–139.

44. Majola A, Vainionpää S, Vihtonen K, Mero M, Vasenius J, Törmälä P, et al. Absorption, biocompatibility and fixation properties of polylactic acid in bone tissue: an experimental study in rats. *Clin Orthop.* 1991;268:260–269.

45. Hatton PV, Walsh J, Brook IM. The response of cultured bone cells to bioresorbable polyglycolic acid and teflon reinforced silicone membranes for use in orbital floor fracture repair. *Clin Mater.* 1994;17:71–80.

46. Hoffmann R, Krettek C, Haas N, Tscherne H. Die distal radiusfraktur. Frakturstabilisierung mit biodegradablen Osteosynthese-stiften (Biofix). Experimentelle Untersuchungen under erste klinische Erfahrungen. *Unfallchirurg.* 1989;92:430–434.

47. Böstman OM. Osteolytic changes accompanying degradation of absorbable fracture fixation implants. *J Bone Joint Surg (Br).* 1991;73-B:679–682.

48. Böstman OM. Intense granulomatous inflammatory lesions associated with absorbable internal fixation devices made of polyglycolide in ankle fractures. *Clin Orthop.* 1992;278:193–199.

49. Santavirta S, Konttinen YT, Saito T, Grönblad M, Partio E, Kemppinen P, et al. Immune response to polyglycolic acid implants. *J Bone Joint Surg (Br).* 1990;72-B:597–600.

50. Eitenmüller J, David A, Muhr G. Treatment of ankle fractures with complete biodegradable plate and screws of high molecular weight polylactide. In: Proceedings of 92 Congrés Francais de Chirurgie. 1990; Paris.

51. Bergsma EJ, Rozema FR, Bos RRM, de Bruijn WC. Foreign body reactions to resorbable poly(L-lactide) bone plates and screws used for the fixation of unstable zygomatic fractures. *J Oral Maxillofac Surg.* 1993;51:666–670.

52. Pihlajamäki H, Böstman O, Hirvensalo E, Rokkanen P, Törmälä P. Absorbable pins of self-reinforced poly-L-lactic acid for fixation of fractures and osteotomies. *J Bone Joint Surg.* 1992;74-B:853–857.

53. Rozema FR, Bos RRM, Pennings AJ, Jansen HWB. Poly(L-lactide) implants in repair of defects of the orbital floor: an animal study. *J Oral Maxillofac Surg.* 1990;48:1305–1309.

54. Getter L, Cutright DE, Bhaskar SN, Augsburg JK. A biodegradable intraosseus appliance in the treatment of mandibular fractures. *J Oral Surg.* 1972;30:344–348.

55. Gerlach KL, Krause HR, Eitenmüller J. Use of absorbable osteosynthesis material for mandibular fracture treatment of dogs. In: Pizzoferrato A, Marchetti PG, Ravagliori A, Lee ACJ, eds. *Biomaterials and Clinical Applications.* Amsterdam: Elsevier Science Publisher B.V.; 1987:459–464.

56. Bos RRM. Poly(L-lactide) osteosynthesis. Development of bioresorbable bone plates and screws. Groningen, The Netherlands: University of Groningen; 1989. Thesis.

57. Törmälä P, Vainionpää S, Kilpikari J, Rokkanen P. The effects of fibre reinforcement and gold plating on the flexural strength of PGA/PLA copolymer materials in vitro. *Biomaterials.* 1987;8:42–45.

58. Suuronen R. Comparison of absorbable self-reinforced poly-L-lactide screws and metallic screws in the fixation of mandibular condyle osteotomies. Experimental study in sheep. *J Oral Maxillofac Surg.* 1991;49:989–995.

59. Suuronen R, Laine P, Sarkiala E, Pohjonen T, Lindqvist C. Sagittal split osteotomy fixed with biodegradable, self-reinforced poly-L-lactide screws. *Int J Oral Maxillofac Surg.* 1992; 21:303–308.

60. Suuronen R, Pohjonen T, Vasenius J, Vainionpää S. Comparison of absorbable self-reinforced multilayer poly-L-lactide and metallic plates in the fixation of mandibular body osteotomies: An experimental study in sheep. *J Oral Maxillofac Surg.* 1992; 50:255–262.

61. Suuronen R, Pohjonen T, Wessman L, Törmälä P, Vainionpää S. New generation biodegradable plate for fracture fixation. Comparison of bending strengths of mandibular osteotomies fixed with absorbable self-reinforced multi-layer poly-L-lactide plates and metallic plates. An experimental study in sheep. *Clin Mater*. 1992;9:77–84.

62. Suuronen R. Biodegradable self-reinforced polylactide plates and screws in the fixation of osteotomies in the mandible. PhD Thesis. University of Helsinki, Finland, 1992.

63. Suuronen R, Törmälä P, Vasenius J, Wessman L, Mero M, Partio E, et al. Comparison of shear strength of osteotomies fixed with absorbable self-reinforced poly-L-lactide and metallic screws. *J Mater Sci Mater Med*. 1992;3:288–292.

64. Suuronen R, Manninen M, Pohjonen T, Laitinen O, Lindqvist C. Mandibular osteotomy fixed with biodegradable plates and screws: an animal study. *Br J Oral Maxillofac Surg*. 1997;35:341–348.

65. Sasserath C, Van Reck J, Gitani J. Utilisation d'une membrane d'acide polyglycolique dans les reconstructions de plancher orbitaire et dans les pertes de substances osseuses de la sphère maxillo-faciale. *Acta Stomatol Belg*. 1991;88:5–11.

66. Vert M, Christel P, Chabot F, Leray J. Bioresorbable plastic materials for bone surgery. In: Hastings GW, Ducheyne P, eds. *Advances in Biomaterials*. Amsterdam: Elsevier Science Publishers; 1990;9:573–578.

67. Gerlach KL. Treatment of zygomatic fractures with biodegradable poly(L-lactide) plates and screws. Clinical implant materials. In: Heimke G, Soltész U, Lee ACJ, eds. *Advances in Biomaterials*. Amsterdam: Elsevier Science Publishers; 1990;9:573–578.

68. Bos RRM, Boering G, Rozema FR, Leenslag JW. Resorbable poly(L-lactide) plates and screws for the fixation of zygomatic fractures. *J Oral Maxillofac Surg*. 1987;45:751–753.

69. Gerlach KL. Absorbierbare Polymere in der Mund- und Kieferchirurgie. *Zahnärtzliche Mitteilungen*. 1988;78:1020–1024.

70. Muhonen J, Suuronen R, Sarkiala E, Oikarinen VJ, Happonen RP. Effect of polyglycolic acid membrane on bone regeneration around titanium fixtures implanted in bone sockets. *J Mater Sci Mater Med*. 1994;5:40–42.

71. Pajarola GF, Sailer HF. SR-PGA membranes in dental surgery. In: Rokkanen P, Törmälä P, eds. *Self-Reinforced Biodegradable Polymeric Composites in Surgery*. Boca Raton: CRC Press, in press.

72. McVicar I, Hatton PV, Brook IM. Self-reinforced polyglycolic acid membrane: a bioresorbable material for orbital floor repair. *Br J Oral Maxillofac Surg*. 1995;33:220–223.

73. Heller J. Biodegradable polymers in controlled drug delivery. *CRC Crit Rev Ther Drug Carrier Syst* 1985;1:39–90.

14
Advanced Bone Healing Concepts in Craniomaxillofacial Reconstructive and Corrective Bone Surgery

Tomas Albrektsson, Lars Sennerby, and Anders Tjellström

When working with experimental oral implants at our biomaterials unit in Gothenburg during the 1960s, Brånemark et al.[1] observed that there seemed to be a direct bone anchorage of the metallic devices. At that time proper methods were not available to verify the presence of direct bone anchorage, which is why the osseointegration of metal implants was not generally recognized until well into the 1980s.[2] In Brånemark's early concept, osseointegration was a feature of c.p. titanium alone and characterized by an almost complete cortical bone encapsulation of the foreign material. This is in contrast to our present knowledge when, in fact, many look upon bone anchorage of metallic implants to be a primitive foreign body reaction that is observed to occur with numerous metals of varying biocompatibility.[3] Furthermore, it is now understood that in reality the osseointegrated interface consists of a mixture of bone and soft tissue.[4] The reason osseointegration (which at present is best defined as a stability concept)[5] has survived as a relevant important contemporary term is related to the clinical superiority of osseointegrated craniofacial implants compared to soft tissue anchored devices that have a high failure rate. There is substantial evidence that a biocompatible metal such as c.p. titanium shows a stronger bony interface response than other metals, which lends support to the early concept.[6] The osseointegrated, clinical implant, which is similar to the experimental version, does not have complete encapsulation in bone. With retrieved c.p. titanium oral implants, an average bony interface of about 80% has been reported.[7]

However, osseointegration is not dependent only on the type of biomaterial. Albrektsson et al. summarized[8] the then-current knowledge of six different factors important for osseointegration: biocompatibility, design, and surface condition of the implant, the state of the host bed, the surgical technique at insertion, and the loading conditions. With control of these factors Brånemark et al.[9] were able to demonstrate a high percentage of clinical success with osseointegrated oral implants, as well as with skin-penetrating extraoral ones. To some investigators,[10] the reason for the good clinical results (despite penetration of oral or skin soft tissues that theoretically would seem likely to result in infections and sub-sequent implant loss) relates to the implant stability. According to this theory, implant failure owing to infection and soft tissue problems is unlikely if fixture stability is maintained, a notion with some clinical support at least with Brånemark-type implants.[11,12] Implant failure would then occur mainly because of overload that would result in gradual bone saucerization. Whether the osseointegration of an oral implant is mainly threatened by so-called peri-implantitis[13] or over-load[14] remains a controversial issue, and presently it seems as though the predominantly quoted failure mode is mainly related to the background of the investigator (i.e., periodontics versus prosthodontics).

This chapter will first discuss oral implants with an emphasis on grafting techniques to augment the severely resorbed maxilla. Our aim is to present the background to and current results of various ways of augmenting maxillary bone. The chapter will end with an overview of extraoral, osseointegrated implants in the auricular, nasal, and orbital bone bed. In this part of the chapter we will briefly discuss the clinical outcome in radiated bone and the use of hyperbaric oxygen.

Bone Grafting and Endosseous Implants

Reconstruction of the craniomaxillofacial region may require a combination of bone grafting and placement of endosseous implants for anchorage of extraoral as well as intraoral prostheses. The incorporation of the graft and the integration process of the implants individually are complex healing situations that must be successful for an acceptable clinical outcome. Owing to the extent of tissue loss, various types of grafts and different strategies for placement of the implants may be used. The implants can be inserted in conjunction with grafting or after primary healing of the graft. A third option is preformed osseointegration surgery, in which implants are placed at the donor site in the planned graft prior to its transfer to the recipient bed.

By definition, a bone-grafting procedure is either a transplantation or an implantation. The former involves surgical transfer of living tissue, with or without vascular supply, from a donor site to a recipient bed. The latter comprises the surgical insertion of a nonliving biocompatible material. The use of free autologous bone grafts clearly dominates in the scientific literature, although allogeneic and alloplastic grafts and implants have been used as well. To minimize necrosis of autologous grafts and thereby improve the healing and incorporation process, grafts with an internal blood supply may be considered (i.e., free-vascularized or pedicled grafts).

Basic Principles of the Integration of Grafts and Implants

Bone healing occurs as a two-step process, with woven bone initially formed rapidly by osteoblasts in a random manner, for instance, to bridge a defect. This immature bone has poor biomechanical properties, owing to its lack of organization and its low mineral content. In the next step, the immature bone will be replaced by lamellar bone via a coupled osteoclastic/osteoblastic activity, known as *creeping substitution*, which originally was described based on histologic sections by Axhausen[15] and for the first time was observed in vivo by Albrektsson.[16] Bone-metabolizing units (BMUs; i.e., cutting and filling cones in cortical bone) will result in the formation of secondary osteons or haversian systems in cortical bone and bone-structural units in trabecular bone. Any surgical intervention in bone will provoke such a well-programmed and complex tissue response, which aims at regeneration of the traumatized tissues. In the ultimate healing situation, the repair will proceed until the tissues are completely restored (i.e., all voids are filled with lamellar bone). Frequently however, bone defects heal incompletely and/or with an admixture of bone and fibrous scar tissue, depending on the influence of several factors such as nutrition, pressure, instability, competition from adjacent tissues, etc. If stability, adequate blood supply, and the prevention of soft tissue collapse and ingrowth in a bone defect can be provided, the bone defect will undergo complete healing. In essence, if the conditions are favorable, bone will fill in and be condensed and remodeled in any space and toward any surface. In introducing a graft/implant in a bone defect, the healing process may be influenced by the graft or implant itself: passively, by its action as a mechanical barrier and by its mobility, and actively, by interaction between the graft/implant surface or molecules released from it and the biological environment. For example, an autologous graft may enhance the healing process owing to the presence of viable cells and bone inductive agents in the graft, while a fresh allograft will have a negative influence, since an immunological reaction will be elicited due to the lack of histocompatibility. In conclusion, the outcome of a grafting/implantation procedure depends on the extent to which the present circumstances allow the newly formed bone from the recipient bed to fill voids and undergo remodeling (Figure 14.1).

Healing of Free Autologous Bone Grafts

The healing of a free autologous bone graft is determined by the vascular supply at the recipient bed and to some still unknown extent by the survival of the cells in the graft. The graft is incorporated by the enveloping of a complex of necrotic old bone with viable new bone. Since sufficient nutrition is a prerequisite for any cellular activity, the ability of newly formed vessels to penetrate the graft is crucial to the repair process. This process differs when comparing the healing of cortical bone grafts with that of cancellous bone grafts, due to their three-dimensional structures. Morphologically, cortical bone is built up by densely packed circular, parallel, and interstitial bone lamellae around haversian and Volkmann's canals. Cancellous bone is porous and appears as a lattice of rods, plates, and arches, generally described as trabeculae, in between which marrow tissue is present. A larger surface of the cancellous bone graft is consequently within reach of cells and vessels from the recipient site as compared to the cortical bone graft. Vascular ingrowth has been demonstrated, in vivo, to occur 30% more rapidly into cancellous, as compared to cortical, bone grafts.[16] Furthermore, owing to the large surface area, more bone marrow cells and cells lining the bone surfaces (which possibly can survive and take part in the repair) are present in cancellous bone grafts as compared to cortical bone grafts.

Cancellous Grafts

After the surgical trauma, a hemorrhage is formed around and in the graft. A number of mediators are released from the tissue, as well as from the fluid and cellular components of the blood, which stimulate migration of inflammatory cells, phagocytes, and mesenchymal pluripotential cells by chemotaxis. Depending on the kind of stimuli, the mesenchymal cells proliferate and differentiate into endothelial cells, fibroblasts, and osteoblasts, resulting in the formation of vessels and new connective tissue. The revascularization may occur as a result of end-to-end anastomoses of the host vessels with those of the graft within a few hours after grafting.[17] Revascularization of a cancellous bone graft may be completed after a few weeks. Bone formation can occur without the preceding resorption by osteoclasts, which is in contrast to cortical bone grafts. Osteoblasts line the surfaces of the old trabeculae and start to produce osteoid, which sequentially becomes mineralized to immature bone. On radiographs, this can be seen as an increase in radiolucency. Cores of necrotic bone will consequently be entrapped in the newly formed bone. In the final remodeling stage, the immature newly formed bone and the necrotic bone will be resorbed by osteoclasts and replaced with mature lamellar bone by BMUs, and with time, the cancellous bone graft will be totally replaced.

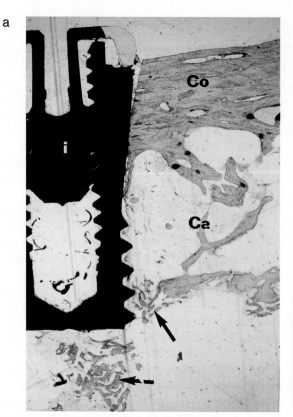

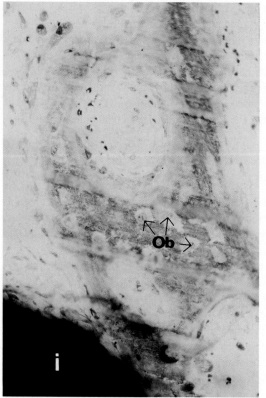

FIGURE 14.1 (a) Ground section of a conical Brånemark System implant (i) removed 4 weeks after insertion in an onlay iliac crest bone graft in the maxilla of a patient. There are no signs of bone formation or resorption in the cortical bone (Co) of the graft. However, bone formation (arrows) is evident around the apex of the implant in the cancellous and the marrow part of the graft (Ca) near the recipient side. (b) Close-up showing solitary bone formation in the vicinity of the implant (i). Osteoblasts (Ob) are being trapped in a mineralized matrix.

Cortical Bone

The initial healing phase of cortical bone grafts is identical to that of cancellous bone grafts. The most apparent difference is in the rate of revascularization, since this takes at least twice as long for cortical bone grafts as for cancellous ones. Complete revascularization usually occurs within 2 months. As stated earlier, it is this difference that is most likely attributed to the structural differences. In cortical bone grafts, vascular penetration is primarily the result of osteoclastic resorption and vascular ingrowth into previously existing Volkmann's and haversian canals. The resorption of the internal cortical bone proceeds by enlargement of haversian canals followed by the apposition of new bone by osteoclasts (i.e., as creeping substitution). In this way, the repair of cortical grafts results in an admixture of viable and necrotic bone.

Healing of Vascularized Autologous Bone Grafts

If the graft has an internal vascular supply (i.e., free vascularized and pedicled grafts), it does not necessarily become necrotic or require a lengthy process of incorporation. The graft will heal with the recipient bone at either end by a process that is analogous to fracture healing.

Healing of Allogeneic and Alloplastic Grafts

Allogeneic grafts are widely used in orthopedic reconstructive surgery. However, fresh allografts are treated to avoid an immunological reaction and rejection of the graft. Such treatments include deep freezing, freeze drying, chemical processing with chloroform-methanol, paracetic acid, hydrogen peroxide, etc. Most of the allogeneic grafts used in oral surgery today are demineralized or mineralized freeze-dried grafts. These materials have, however, poor biomechanical properties and are suitable to fill defects and cavities. The healing process of allogeneic and alloplastic materials follows the same principles as for the incorporation of an autologous graft (i.e., penetration of vessels and bone condensation) provided that an immunological reaction toward the graft can be prevented. However, the bone-forming process is delayed as compared to autologous grafts, which is attributed to the absence of living cells in the graft. Overall, allografts appear to undergo decreased incorporation as compared to autologous grafts.

Factors of Importance for Successful Incorporation and Maintenance of a Graft

Vascular Supply

A free graft placed in a defect within the skeletal envelope is surrounded by highly vascularized bone surfaces, which provides the optimal conditions for revascularization of the graft. This is in contrast to the situation in which the graft extends beyond the skeletal borders so that there is a reduced surface of the host bone, which can provide contact for the graft with vessels and osteogenic cells. Moreover, the situation with such defects is that the degree of spontaneous healing is high, while bone is not likely to form spontaneously beyond the skeletal borders. In the former situation, probably any type of graft can be successfully incorporated. In the latter case, however, greater demands are at hand, and large differences might be found when comparing different types of grafts and surgical procedures. When vascularized grafts are used, the incorporation does not depend entirely on contributions from the local tissue of the recipient bed.

Stability

It is well known that stability of the bone-bone, bone-graft, or bone-implant interface is crucial for bone formation to occur. Mesenchymal cells are sensitive to strain and may differentiate into fibroblasts or chondroblasts if micromovements are present in the healing area. The graft may be stabilized with screws or wires, but it is also the biomechanical properties of the graft itself that can be of importance for its stability.

Biocompatibility

The implantation of any biological or inorganic material in the human body elicits a tissue reaction in response to the surgery and to the material itself. The tissue response to the transplant/implant can either be the result of a specific immunological reaction, as in the case of nonself biological transplants or implants (e.g., allografts, xenografts), or be of a nonspecific character. The specific reaction correlates to the degree of matching of major histocompatibility antigens (transplantation antigens) between donor and recipient. Specifically, an activation of B- and T-lymphocytes results in the production of antibodies and direct actions between T-lymphocytes and the foreign cells, leading to rejection of the transplant. The nonspecific reaction is related to factors other than the antigenic properties of the implanted material. The nonspecific reaction is induced by the interaction between biomolecules, cells, and the surface of the implant, and it is related to the chemical and physical properties of the implant surface. Moreover, it is well known that the macroscopic de-

sign, such as the pore size of alloplasts, or the thread design of an implant, as well as the topography of the implant surface can modify the tissue response. From a host-acceptance point of view, it is likely that autologous bone is the preferred grafting material.

Prevention of Soft Tissue Ingrowth

Complete healing of large bone defects cannot be expected, since soft tissue will occupy the defect by ingrowth, collapse, or both. The bone healing can be enhanced in such a situation by using a physical barrier for guided tissue regeneration (GTR). The barrier will hinder ingrowth of soft tissues and seclude the defect so that only bone cells will have access to the defect. It is reasonable to consider that there is some degree of competition between soft tissue and bone tissue formation during the incorporation of a graft. In that respect, it is possible that a porous graft (i.e., a cancellous bone graft) is more prone to soft tissue ingrowth than a nonporous graft (i.e., cortical bone graft). Theoretically, a corticocancellous graft may be better incorporated, when the cancellous layer is oriented toward the defect since the cortical layer will act as a barrier to prevent soft tissue ingrowth into the cancellous part of the graft. Moreover, it may also be important to pack voids between the graft and the recipient bone surfaces with particulate bone grafts. In the literature, some authors have suggested that barrier membranes should be used to enhance the incorporation of bone grafts. However, to date it is not clear if any of the various types of alloplastic membranes are superior to an intact periosteum.

Loading

It is well known that unloaded grafts are usually completely resorbed with time. However, several studies indicate that the graft will maintain its dimensions when implants are inserted and loaded (Figure 14.2).

Experimental Studies of Grafts and Implants

Albrektsson[16] used a rabbit tibial model in which he had inserted a specially constructed c.p. titanium implant that would enable in vivo visualization of the pending bone graft (Figure 14.3). Following transplantation, repeated inspections were performed at varying times for follow up of the remodelling of the graft structures (Figure 14.4). In this manner it was possible to compare the vascular activity before and after grafting and to monitor the ingrowth of new vessels. In cancellous bone, this was observed to occur at a maximal rate of some 1.2 to 0.4 mm a day, while cutting cones invaded cortical bone at a maximal rate of 30 to 40 μm a day.

Donath et al.[18] compared the healing of Tübingen implants in vascularized and free iliac crest grafts in a sheep model. Bone segments of identical size were osteotomized in both left and right iliac crests of eight animals. The blood supply to the graft was kept intact on one side, while the vessels were

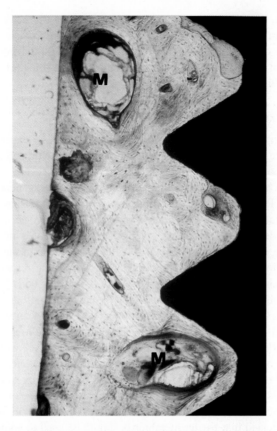

FIGURE 14.2 Ground section showing the bone implant interface of a Brånemark System implant removed 3 years after insertion in an iliac crest onlay graft in the maxilla. Normal lamellar bone with marrow cavities (M) and an apparently direct contact between bone and implant is seen.

cut on the contralateral site. The segments were repositioned and fixed with ostheosynthesis plates and screws, after which one or two Tübingen implants were placed in the grafts. The animals received fluorochromes during a 1- to 12-week healing period. After sacrifice, the histological analysis showed that the implants became osseointegrated in the vascularized graft and that soft tissue encapsulated the free graft. It was concluded that the immediate placement of implants in free bone grafts cannot be recommended, which is in contradistinction to the results presented by other researchers.[19,20] Neukam et al.[19] demonstrated the integration of Brånemark System implants in onlay grafts inserted into the mandibles of 10 minipigs. In that study, mandibular defects were created 3 months following the removal of the premolars in the minipigs, and free grafts were transplanted from the iliac crest and stabilized with two implants into the defects. The authors observed osteoneogenesis with direct contact between the recipient bone and the implants and between the bone graft and the implants at 3 and 5 months. These authors concluded that their experimental and clinical experiences provided the basis for expecting good long-term results when using onlay osteoplasties and simultaneous insertion of implants. Similar results were presented by Lew et al.,[20] who performed a

comparison of the integration of Brånemark implants in free corticocancellous block grafts and particulate corticocancellous grafts. The iliac crests in 17 dogs were used as experimental sites. On one side, a block of corticocancellous bone was osteotomized and the cortical bone at one end of the bone block was removed. The same procedure was performed on the other side, but the graft was additionally sectioned into 2- to 3-mm segments. The corticocancellous block graft was placed in the contralateral defect and stabilized with a 20-mm-long implant. An implant was inserted on the other side and the nonburied portion of the implant was covered with bone particles. Light microscopy and microradiography were performed on the specimens, including the implant and the surrounding bone, taken at 1, 2, and 3 months after surgery. Both types of grafts were determined to be viable through the evaluation of fluorescent labels. The bone density appeared to be greater with a higher degree of bone/implant contact calculated by morphometry in the block grafts, as compared to the particulate ones. The authors concluded that the osseointegration of titanium implants developed more rapidly in corticocancellous bone blocks, as compared to the particulate bone grafts.

In a rabbit model, Lundgren et al.[21] studied the integration of Brånemark System implants in particulate autologous grafts. One implant was inserted in the tibias of eight rabbits in such a way that five threads were not covered with bone on one side. On the test side, particulate cortical bone grafts from the calvarium were packed over the exposed implant surfaces, and covered with a bioresorbable polylactide barrier. At the control side, only particulate bone grafts were applied over the implant threads. Histology from 12-week-old specimens showed significantly thicker bone at the test side, with osseointegration occurring to the same degree on both the test and control sides. It was concluded that the barrier probably stabilized the grafts and prevented the ingrowth of soft tissue and resorption of the bone particles during the healing period.

The integration of titanium implants in dog alveolar ridges augmented by allogeneic material was evaluated by Pinholt et al.[22] Six weeks after the removal of two premolars in all quadrants via block resections, the ridges were augmented with allogeneic demineralized and lyophylized dentin or bone. A total of 32 titanium implants were inserted in the augmented regions of 10 dogs 5.5 months later and followed for another 3.5 months, at which time the animals were killed and specimens retrieved. All implants were encapsulated by a fibrous tissue containing a few multinuclear giant cells and some other inflammatory cells. The graft material was without signs of remineralization, except when there was contact with the recipient bone surfaces.

Clinical Histology of Implants in Bone Grafts

In 1989, Riediger et al.[23] presented histology from a patient treated with a vascularized iliac crest graft and Tübingen implants. The patient had been reconstructed following the re-

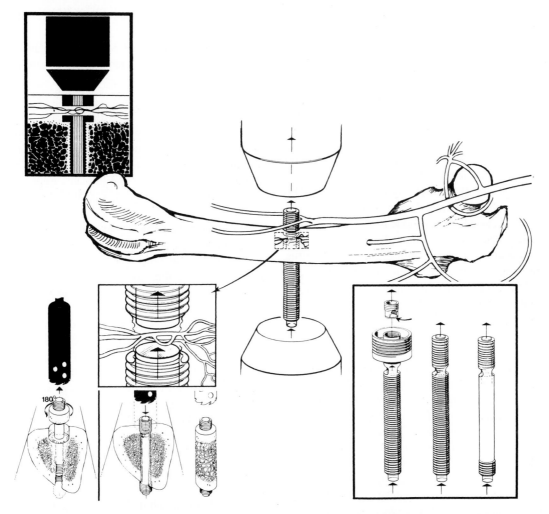

FIGURE 14.3 Albrektsson-constructed titanium implants permitting direct visualization of bone graft remodelling and revascularization. The implants, existing in slightly different designs (bottom right), were inserted through long bones in various animals. Bone and vascular tissue invaded a space that went straight through the body of the titanium chamber. Grafting was performed when the ingrown bone and vessels were found to be in a steady-state situation (bottom left). In this manner, it became possible to inspect bone tissue before the graft-bone complex was transplanted in an autologous or allologous manner.

a

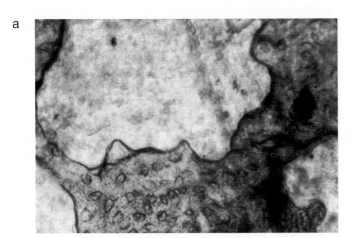

b

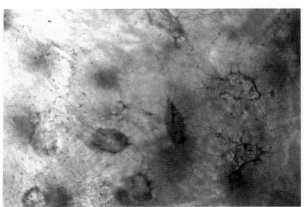

FIGURE 14.4 (a) Low-power view from bone chamber at 4 weeks after autologous transplantation with bone tissue (darker with numerous rounded bodies representing osteocyte lacunae) undergoing resorption. The depicted bone was completely resorbed and replaced with invading soft tissue (light), when inspected a couple of weeks later. (b) Osteocyte lacunae with visible canaliculae in living bone after autologous transplantation.

section of a mandibular segment because of a tumor. Three years later the patient had a recurrence, and the graft and implants were removed. The implants were clinically stable at the time of removal, with direct bone contact observed at the apical portion of the implants, while soft tissue and epithelium contact were observed at the coronal portion of the implant.

Nyström et al.[24] presented histology of one patient who died 4 months after an onlay grafting procedure and immediate placement of six Brånemark System implants. The grafted bone from the iliac crest demonstrated signs of resorption, but also areas where new bone formation was seen on old trabeculae. There was only a patchy contact between the grafted bone and the implants, with the major part of the interface consisting of soft tissues. Bone condensation into the implant threads was evident in some areas, both in the graft and in the recipient bone.

Histology from a patient who died 8 months after a sinus elevation procedure was reported by GaRey et al.[25] Freeze-dried cortical allografts and resorbable hydroxyapatite had been used in conjunction with immediate placement of "root-formed" implants. One of the two implants studied was totally submerged in bone, and the microscopical examination revealed a bone interface, while the other implant had a minimal amount of bone in the interface. The authors concluded that "eight months would not have been enough healing time prior to loading for this patient."

Jensen and Sennerby[26] used small test implants of c.p. titanium to study osseointegration in patients that had undergone sinus augmentation with radiated mineralized cancellous allografts (RMCA) or autografts and immediate placement of Brånemark System implants. The test implants were inserted through the buccal bone into the grafts and were removed at abutment connection 6 to 14 months later. The histological examination of the specimens revealed a minor degree of bone formation and osseointegration when using allografts. Most of the specimens contained nonviable particles of the allograft. Bone formation was evident only in the cortical passage. However, in one specimen of the particulate cancellous autograft/titanium interface, mature lamellar bone in direct contact with the implant was observed. The study indicated that autologous bone grafts are preferable to allografts.

Clinical Use of Grafts and Implants

Cortical Bone Grafts and Implants

In 1994, Donovan et al.[27] reported on the clinical outcome of two techniques using calvarial bone grafts and Brånemark System implants. With the first technique, the grafts were placed as horizontal onlays and inlays for immediate insertion of the implants. After an average follow-up time of 18 months, 98% of the initially inserted 43 implants were still clinically stable. The second technique involved the fixation of calvarian strips as vertical onlay grafts and the de-

layed insertion of implants 6 to 8 months later. Using this approach, 86% of the 50 implants inserted were considered to be successful.

Cancellous Bone Grafts and Implants

Breine and Brånemark[28] used tibial cancellous bone chips and bone marrow packed around titanium implants inserted in the atrophied maxilla or mandible of 18 patients. The result was not satisfactory as 75% of the implants were lost and a dramatic resorption of the graft was observed during the first years.

Cancellous bone particles have been used for maxillary sinus augmentation and were first described by Boyne and James in 1980.[29] In 3 of 14 cases treated, blade implants were inserted 12 weeks after the augmentation procedure. No signs of resorption were evident during the 1 to 4 years the implants were followed.

Jensen[30] described the clinical outcome of using cancellous autografts for sinus augmentation and the immediate ($n =$ 179) and delayed ($n = 43$) insertion of Brånemark System implants. The lateral wall of the sinus was covered with an e-PTFE barrier to prevent the ingrowth of soft tissue into the augmented sinus cavity. Delayed implant placement improved the overall implant survival rate, 93% versus 81%. More implant failures occurred when less alveolar bone was available inferior to the sinus cavity.

Corticocancellous Bone Grafts and Implants

Preformed Endochondral Grafts and Implants

Brånemark introduced the technique of bone graft preformation on theoretical grounds. The idea was to insert, as a guide, a mold together with fixation screws at the donor site several months before the actual grafting. As the mold was shaped in accordance with the estimated needs at the recipient site, the advantage of the preformed bone graft would be that it had already remodeled before grafting. The grafting procedure would be less traumatic since the separation surgery had been partially performed during the initial surgical procedure. Experimental studies in rabbits confirmed that the preformation procedure indeed produced a highly viable graft.[31] One variety of the preformed bone graft was applied clinically by Tjellström et al.[32,33] The authors inserted titanium molds into the tibias of humans. The mold had a canal that was preformed as an ossicular bone graft. Bone tissue invaded the canal and 6 months later the molds were removed with a trephine, which upon opening ossicular "self-cast" grafts were found inside. In a total of 11 cases, such preformed ossicular bone was grafted to the middle ear, and when evaluated 5 years later,[34] the grafts continued to demonstrate very adequate function.

Breine and Brånemark[28] placed implants in a preformed tibial graft 3 to 6 months prior to harvesting the graft and transplanting it to the maxilla. During the follow-up period of 1 to 8 years, more than 50% of the implants had failed. Lindström et al.[35] used the preformation technique to obtain large bone grafts to treat defects resulting from the ablation of major mandibular tumors. In addition to molds, fixation screws and "oral implants to be" were inserted at the donor site and allowed to be incorporated in the intended bone graft before disruption of the vascular connections. The actual grafting was performed 4 to 5 months after the first surgical procedure when adequate remodelling of the grafts had occurred. Of the five patients, two died from metastatic disease within a year after surgery, and three others had experienced good graft and implant function for follow-up periods ranging from 5 to 10 years.

Although theoretically advantageous, the preformation principle is time-consuming and troublesome for patients in that it involves a two-stage surgical procedure. Furthermore, it is questionable as to whether the technique really results in an improved outcome compared to routine procedures. Therefore, at the Göteborg University clinic, the procedure was abandoned many years ago.

Other Types of Endochondral Bone Grafts and Implants

In a study by Keller et al. in 1987,[36] 9 patients were treated with iliac corticocancellous grafts and immediate placement (5 patients) or delayed placement (4 patients) of titanium implants. Of 28 immediately placed implants 4 (14.3%) were removed owing to clinical mobility, and 5 (23%) of 21 delayed implants failed.

In a Swedish and an international multicenter study, Albrektsson et al.[37] reported on 42 implants inserted in grafted mandibles with only one failure over a follow-up period of 1 to 5 years. In the maxilla, 183 implants were inserted in grafted bone and 50 of those failed over a follow-up of 1 to 5 years.

The use of iliac onlay-grafts and immediate insertion of titanium implants in patients with severely resorbed maxillae and mandibles was reported by Neukam et al. in 1989.[19] Of 110 implants inserted in 21 patients, 13 failed (11.8%) during an observation period of up to 4 years. The overall survival rate was higher in the upper jaws (95.95%) as compared to the lower jaws (82.0%).

Adell et al.[38] reported on the outcome of 124 implants inserted together with iliac onlay grafts in 23 patients who were followed from 1 to 10 years. Seventeen of the patients had stable fixed prostheses, 5 had overdentures, and 1 patient returned to using a complete denture. Of the originally placed fixtures, 8.1% were lost during the healing period until the abutment connection and 73.8% of the implants were still in function after 5 years of loading. The mean marginal bone resorption during the first year in function was 1.49 mm and 0.1 mm/year thereafter. Similar results were presented by Gunne et al.[39] using the same technique. In that study, 30 patients divided into a development group (10 patients) and a routine group (20 patients) were followed for 3 years. Of the total 177 implants inserted, 43 failed during the observation period (24.3%). However, the implant survival rate was higher in the routine group (87.5%). The remodeling of the residual ridge was also studied, and it was concluded that a reduction of height and faciopalatal width of the grafted area was observed during the first year.

This technique was applied to the partially edentulous patient by Schliephake et al.[40] Fifty-five Brånemark System implants were inserted in 16 patients. Two implants (3.6%) failed because of wound dehiscence and subsequent infection, and another 2 implants were left as "sleepers." No further implants failed during the 2- to 80-month period of loading.

In 1989, Sailer[41] described a new method for augmentation of the atrophied maxilla in conjunction with installation of titanium implants. He would perform a Le Fort-1 osteotomy, placed iliac corticocancellous bone blocks to obturate the floor of the nose and maxillary sinus, and simultaneously inserted titanium implants as a single-step surgical procedure. The maxilla/graft complex was held in position with the use of osteosynthesis screws and plates. None of the 35 implants in 5 patients failed during the follow-up period of 0 to 13 months. Using the same technique, Isaksson reported a survival rate of only 68% of the first 10 cases with 57 implants placed. However, Isaksson[42] had a considerably longer follow-up time, 33 to 95 months, as compared to Sailer in which the implants in 2 of the 5 patients had not yet been uncovered.

Intramembranous Grafts and Implants

In a series of publications, Jensen et al.[43–45] have described the use of autologous intramembranous corticocancellous bone grafts taken from the chin and immediate insertion of implants for augmentation of the severely resorbed maxilla. The grafts were taken from the chin by the use of specially made instruments that permitted preparation of the implant sites through the tapping stage at the donor site prior to harvesting and transfer to the recipient site. The grafts were used as onlays or sinus grafts or as a combination of the two. In a preliminary report in 1990, they presented the results of 107 implants inserted in 26 patients. The overall implant survival rate was 93.5% after a follow-up of 6 to 26 months. All 7 implants lost had been inserted in a combination of onlay and sinus grafts. Four of the lost implants were removed due to wound dehiscence and exposure of the grafts. An average marginal bone resorption of 1 to 2 mm was observed in this study. The authors suggested that this minor bone resorption was attributed to the intramembranous origin of the graft bone. In 1994, Jensen et al.[45] reported the outcome of different procedures when inserting implants in the maxilla. In one group, chin transplants were used as onlays and sinus grafts for immediate placement of implants. Of 152 implants, 17 (11.2%) failed to integrate or lost the integration during the 13- to 58-month follow-up period.

A two-stage technique of using intramembraneous retromolar or chin grafts and ITI implants was presented by

Krekeler et al.[46] The grafts used as buccal onlays and fixated by osteosynthesis screws were allowed to heal for 4 to 6 months prior to installation of the implants. None of the 47 implants installed in 30 patients failed during the 1-year follow-up period. The marginal bone loss was reported to be less than 1 mm.

Allogeneic Grafts and Implants

Allogeneic allografts have mostly been used for sinus lift procedures. Jensen and Greer[47] reported on the use of radiated mineralized cancellous allograft and immediate insertion of implants in the augmented maxillary sinus. Of 38 implants, 8 (21.1%) failed during the 2.5-year follow-up. They also used demineralized cancellous allografts for sinus augmentation and immediate placement of implants, and lost 10 (45.5%) of 22 implants.

In 1993, Small et al.[48] reported on the use of demineralized freeze-dried cortical bone mixed with 50% hydroxyapatite for maxillary sinus augmentation and immediate placement of cylindrical implants. Of 111 implants placed in 45 sinus grafts in 27 patients, 76 were used for anchorage of dental prostheses. None of the 76 implants failed during a 1- to 5-year period of loading.

Vascularized Grafts and Implants

In a study by Riediger et al.[23] a microsurgical technique using vascularized iliac crest grafts and immediate insertion of implants for the replacement of mandibular and maxillary segments, owing to tumor surgery, trauma, or infection, was described. The graft was taken in such a way that the deep circumflex iliac artery and vein could be used for anastomosis with the facial artery and vein. In the 1989 study, 46 Tübingen implants and 15 IMZ implants where placed in 22 iliac crest grafts. Two of the Tübingen implants were lost during the healing period. In 1991, Riediger and Ehrenfeld[49] reported on the use of the same technique for augmentation of the atrophied mandible. Three of 12 Tübingen implants, 2 of 12 IMZ, and none of 8 Brånemark implants failed during the up to 34-month follow-up period.

Craniomaxillofacial Prostheses

There are two major indications for inserting skin-penetrating, craniofacial implants. One is related to the stable fixation of a bone-anchored hearing aid, which is useful for patients with certain types of hearing disorders. The other indication is related to craniofacial reconstruction with the stable anchorage of a facial prostheses. Patients in the latter category may represent congenital malformations, cancer-surgery deformities, or facial trauma injuries with ear loss (Figure 14.5).

Skin-Penetrating Implants for External Hearing Aids

The indication for treatment may not represent the most appropriate example of craniomaxillofacial reconstructive bone surgery, as the primary indication for surgery is a hearing disorder. Nevertheless, the first patients to be treated with skin-penetrating implants received those for the indication related to hearing impairment,[50] and we have gained invaluable experience on skin-penetrating implants from treating such patients. In a review of the first 100 patients who were treated with skin-penetrating implants and external hearing aids, Tjellström and Granström[51] came to the conclusion that 90%

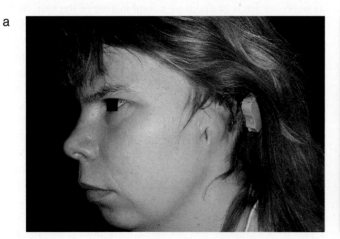

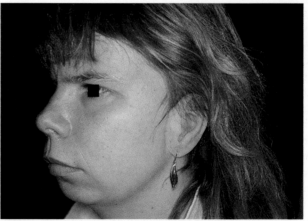

FIGURE 14.5 (a) Patient with a thalidomide embryopathy who had a conventional bone-conducting hearing aid until 1979. She received a bone-anchored hearing aid (BAHA) the same year and showed a clear speech improvement after surgery. Her ability to hear particularly high-frequency sounds was greatly improved. (b) The same patient had bilateral ear atresia. She was operated on both sides in 1992 and received bone-anchored silicone ear replacements (b).

of the implants were still stable after a follow-up of between 8 and 16 years. Five percent of the implants had been removed due to trauma, whereas another 5% had lost their integration for other reasons. About 80% of the patients were without or experienced only a single episode of adverse soft tissue reactions, with the majority of those complaints treated without any associated problems with the bone-anchored implants. In a more detailed analysis of soft tissue reactions around skin-penetrating implants, Tjellström[52] divided the problems into five categories in which 0 implied no irritation and 4 meant infection leading to removal of percutaneous implant. Of all 1739 observations made in 1989, 92.5% of those were of grade 0, 4.1% of grade 1 (redness), 1.8% of observations were of grade 2 (moist), 1.5% of observations were of grade 3 (granulation), and only 0.1% of all observations were of grade 4. There were similar results for skin-penetrating auricular prostheses and no tendency for increased problems over time. The average score of all observations was found to be 0.14. The author concluded that adverse skin reactions were not a major problem with the type of permanent skin penetrating implants used in the study.

Skin-Penetrating Implants for Stable Anchorage of Facial Prostheses

The great advantages with skin-penetrating implants in conjunction with facial prostheses are the stability of the devices and the improved aesthetics (Figure 14.6). Psychologically, the patients often regard the implant and prosthesis to be "self" rather than "nonself." The first patient with skin-penetrating fixtures for the anchorage of an auricular prosthesis was treated at the University of Göteborg in 1979.[53]

When evaluating the outcome of skin-penetrating fixtures, Jacobsson et al.[54] came to the conclusion that implant survival in the auricular area was 95.6%, and in the orbital region it was only 67.2%. These statistics were based on 234 auricular and 81 orbital consecutively inserted fixtures followed up from 6 months to more than 5 years. The comparatively poor result in the orbit region is partly explained by previous irradiation in that 16 of 19 mobile orbital implants had been inserted in previously irradiated bone beds. Excluding irradiated cases, the implant survival in the orbit region was much improved in that only 3 of 38 placed implants were lost, for a survival of 92%. The interesting question is whether hyperbaric oxygen treatment will improve the long-term survival of orbital implants inserted into previously irradiated bone beds. Jacobsson et al.[54] were the first to suggest criteria for success with respect to skin-penetrating maxillofacial implants. Their criteria were based on the guidelines for oral implants suggested by Albrektsson et al.[55] and included implant immobility, soft tissue reactions of 0 and 1 in a minimum of 95% of all observations, and the absence of persistent pain, infections, or paresthesia. Wolfaardt et al.[56] compared the Swedish (Göteborg University), Canadian (University of Alberta), and U.S. (University of San Antonio) experiences with skin-penetrating fixtures. In regions other than those quoted earlier, altogether 53 implants were placed in the nonirradiated nasal region for an average success rate of 83%. Only 10 implants were placed in the irradiated, nasal region for a success rate of 80%. One difference from the Swedish experience was the much better outcome of 28 Canadian implants inserted in the irradiated orbit, where there was a 96.4% success rate. Of a total of 1365 implants inserted at all 20 participating centers (13 in the United States, 6 in Canada, and 1 in Sweden), 1290 or 94.5% had integrated in the bone.[56]

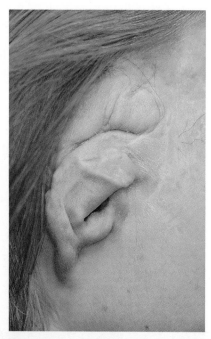

a

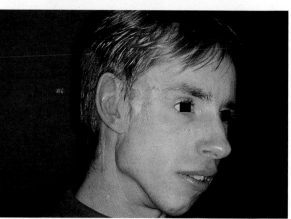

b

FIGURE 14.6 Patient with hemofacial microtia initially treated by conventional plastic surgery. The figure shows the plastic-surgically created ear after some 40 surgical interventions. This patient was initially operated with implants in 1983 but had then decided that he wanted to keep his surgically made ear as depicted in (a). The resultant prosthesis had therefore quite bulky proportions (b). In 1993, the patient decided that his ear fragments from plastic surgery could be removed and it was then easier to provide him a better-fitting artificial silicone ear on skin-penetrating implants.

One central issue with respect to craniofacial, skin-penetrating implants is trying to increase survival rates in previously irradiated bone. Granström et al.[57] concluded that even heavily irradiated bones could integrate the implants and bear the load from the prosthesis. There were no major complications such as wound infection, fistulation, or osteoradionecrosis reported after surgery. Nevertheless, there was an increased loss of implants with time after irradiation, particularly in the orbital region. The authors reported that hyperbaric oxygen treatment (HBO) reduced the number of implant losses. In another study,[58] the problem of postimplantation irradiation was addressed, in which 32 implants were placed before irradiation. Two of those were removed from the temporal bone in a secondary surgical intervention, and 2 others were lost from the frontal bone region during chemotherapy. Osteoradionecrosis developed in 3 of 11 patients. The authors recommended the subsequent removal of all prostheses, frameworks, and abutments before irradiation, whereas the fixtures should be allowed to remain in the bone but should be covered with skin or mucosa.

Craniomaxillofacial Implants in Children

The youngest child, to the knowledge of the authors, ever operated with an implant aimed for permanent skin penetration was 6 months old and suffering from Mb Apert. However, the implant was later removed on request of the parents before any second-stage surgery was performed. Histology demonstrated some 47% bone-to-implant contact, and the threaded region was filled out by bone to some 79% (Figure 14.7).

One problem with operating on children is, of course, that their cortex is thin compared to adults, but children have, on the other hand, a better bone-forming capability. The outcome

a

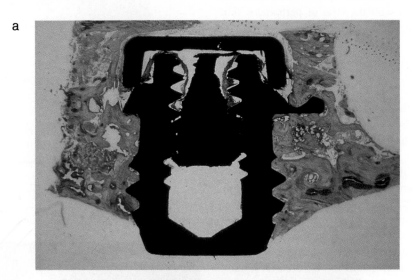

b

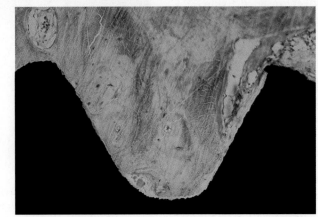

FIGURE 14.7 (a) We have experience with about 100 implants inserted in children. In children with hearing disorders, we have sometimes operated on patients as young as 3 years, whereas craniofacial disorders are often not operated until the child reaches puberty. The youngest child to receive a bone-anchored implant that we know of was operated on in a European clinic at the age of 6 months. Indication for surgery was Morbus Apert. However, the implant was later removed on request from the parents. (b) The implant of (a) that was never loaded showed some 47% bone-to-implant direct contact.

of 59 consecutively inserted skin-penetrating implants in 30 children was reported by Jacobsson et al.[54] Of those implants, 16 were inserted in an equal number of patients with the indication of impaired hearing. In this group we operated on the youngest patients, down to an age of 3 years, as we hoped to establish an improved feedback situation with a bone conduction hearing aid, in turn leading to better social development. The average age of this patient group was 9.3 years compared to 10.6 years for the 14 patients with 43 implants inserted with the indication to anchor a facial prosthesis. The follow-up time of all patients ranged between 1 and 144 months. The skin reactions and the clinical results did not differ significantly from the situation in adults, and there was an average fixture survival rate of 96.6%

Tjellström[59] has pointed out that in selecting young patients for auricular prostheses, the most important factor is for the child to be clearly motivated for this type of surgery. Sometimes there is a parental guilt complex in the background instead of a true problem for the patient. It is extremely important that the child understand that the skin has to be carefully cleaned to avoid soft tissue reactions and that the prosthesis will have to be remade every 2 to 3 years.

Stability of Maxillofacial Implants and Histological Examinations

In an investigation approved by the Göteborg University ethical committee, two implants were inserted in the temporal bone of patients, although only one was necessary to attach the hearing aid. One of these screws was later removed with a torque-gauge analyzer revealing an average removal torque of 42.7 Ncm over an average follow-up of 107 months.[60] Yamanaka et al.[61] inserted 31 similar implants in the temporal bone. The implants were divided into three groups depending on the time of implantation. Group 1 ($n = 10$), with an average follow-up of 3.4 months, demonstrated an average removal torque of 39.3 Ncm; group 2 ($n = 7$), with an average follow-up of 15.6 months, demonstrated an average removal torque of 67.9 Ncm; and group 3 ($n = 14$), with an average follow-up of 69 months, demonstrated an average removal torque of 96.4 Ncm. Thus there was a clear tendency of an increasing removal torque with increasing time.

Retrieval analyses have confirmed a good bone-interfacial response as the reason for the torque needed for implant removal.[62] One implant removed for psychological reasons at 9 months after insertion demonstrated a bone mineral contact percentage of 54 and a mean bone area of 84%. In a case in which the reason for implant removal was "insufficient hygiene," inflammatory cells, macrophages, and osteoclasts were observed, but there was nevertheless an average bone-to-metal contact of 78% and a mean bone area of 90% at 18 months after implant insertion. Another patient who had been irradiated with 90 Gy and had four implants inserted some 5 months later was available for re-

trieval analyses post mortem another 2 years later. Bone remodelling was then still active. Mean percentage of bone-to-metal contact was about 40 and mean bone area in the implant threads was 75%. Another patient received irradiation of 50 Gy and cytostatics for the treatment of a partial maxillectomy for squamous cell carcinoma. Two years later, three fixtures were placed in the orbital region. When these implants were removed because of pain and other discomfort 3 years later, it was demonstrated that they had penetrated into the frontal sinus and were covered by a mucous membrane. The bone structure did not appear very normal, and there were numerous empty osteocyte lacunae without any bone to implant direct contact.

Conclusion

An essential aspect of every new clinical procedure is the careful documentation of short- and long-term results so that techniques that truly represent new, advanced modes of treatment can be properly differentiated from questionable procedures that at best are theoretically advantageous. An example of the latter category is the preformed bone graft. New grafting techniques, such as sinus lift procedures, which are now presented as more or less routine at numerous meetings, are still difficult to properly evaluate owing to differences in graft selection and implant types. Therefore, they should be used with some caution at the present time. By contrast, several good papers have been published on the outcome of onlay bone grafts, which at the current level of knowledge are much better documented than other more novel types of grafting procedures. In craniomaxillofacial surgery, a thorough clinical documentation has at all times accompanied the advancement of threaded titanium implants, which is why we now have substantial documentation of the excellent outcome of such implants inserted in the temporal bone, in contrast to the less reliable outcome of the same implant inserted in previously irradiated orbit bone. This has resulted in our trying new techniques, such as hyperbaric oxygen treatment, to improve results of orbital implants. The authors are convinced that when introducing new implant techniques, a meticulous mode of clinical documentation joined with the supervision of university ethical committees should replace what is commonly seen today; specifically, a series of relatively poorly controlled human experiments supervised by numerous clinical entrepreneurs.

References

1. Brånemark P-I, Breine U, Lindström J, et al. Intra-osseous anchorage of dental prostheses I. Experimental studies. *Scand J Plast Reconstr Surg.* 1969;3:81–93.

2. Albrektsson T. The response of bone to titanium implants. *CRC Critical Reviews in Biocompatibility.* 1985;1:53–84.

3. Donath K, Laass M, Günzl HJ. The histopathology of different foreign-body reactions in oral soft tissue and bone tissue. *Virchows Arch A Pathol Anat.* 1992;420:131–137.

4. Johansson C, Albrektsson T. Integration of screw implants in the rabbit. A 1-year follow-up of removal of titanium implants. *Int J Oral Maxillofac Implants.* 1987;2:69–75.

5. Zarb G, Albrektsson T. Osseointegration—A requiem for the periodontal ligament?—An editorial. *Int J Periodont Res Dent.* 1991;11:88–91.

6. Johansson C. On tissue reactions to metal implants. Göteborg, Sweden: University of Göteborg; 1991. PhD Thesis.

7. Albrektsson T, Eriksson A, Friberg B, et al. Histologic investigations on 33 retrieved Nobelpharma implants. *Clin Mater.* 1993;12:1–9.

8. Albrektsson T, Brånemark P-I, Hansson HA, Lindström J. Osseointegrated titanium implants. Requirements for ensuring a long-lasting, direct bone anchorage in man. *Acta Orthop Scand.* 1981;52:155–170.

9. Brånemark P-I, Zarb G, Albrektsson T, eds. *Osseointegration in Clinical Dentistry.* Berlin/Chicago: Quintessence; 1985.

10. Ten Cate R. The gingival junction. In: Brånemark PI, Zarb G, Albrektsson T, eds. *Tissue Integrated Prostheses.* Chicago/Berlin: Quintessence; 1985:145–153.

11. Apse P. Clinical and microbiological aspects of the periodontal and periimplant sulcus: a cross-sectional study. Toronto, Canada: University of Toronto; 1987. MSc Thesis.

12. Carmichael R, Apse P, Zarb G, McCulloch C. Biological, microbiological, and clinical aspects of the peri-implant mucosa. In Albrektsson T, Zarb G, eds. *The Brånemark Osseointegrated Implant.* Chicago/Berlin: Quintessence; 1989:39–78.

13. Marinello C. Resolution of experimentally induced periimplantitis. Göteborg, Sweden: Göteborg University; 1995. MSc Thesis.

14. Hoshaw S. Investigation of bone modeling and remodeling at a loaded bone-implant interface. Troy, NY: Rensselaer Polytechnic Institute; 1992. PhD Thesis.

15. Axhausen, G. Die patologisch-anatomischen Grundlagen der Lehre von freien Knochentransplantation beim Menschen und beim Tier. *Med Klin.* 2 1908; Beiheft 23.

16. Albrektsson, T. Repair of bone grafts. A vital microscopic and histological investigation. *Scand J Plast Reconstr Surg.* 1980;14:1–12.

17. Albrektsson, T. In vivo studies of bone grafts. The possibility of vascular anastomoses in healing bone. *Acta Orthop Scand.* 1980;51:9–17.

18. Donath K, Hillman G, Ehrenfeld M, Riediger D. Enossale Einheilung Tübinger Implantate in frei und gefäßgestielt replantierte Beckenkammsegmente. Eine tierexperimentelle Studie. *Z Zahnärztl Implantol.* 1991;VII:58–61.

19. Neukam FW, Scheller H, Günay H. Experimentelle und klinische Untersuchungen zur Auflagerungsosteoplastik in Kombination mit enossalen Implantaten. *Z Zahnärztl Implantol.* 1989;V:235–241.

20. Lew D, Marino AA, Startzell JM, Keller JC. A comparative study of osseointegration of titanium implants in corticocancellous block and corticocancellous chip grafts in canine ileum. *J Oral Maxillofac Surg.* 1994;52:952–958.

21. Lundgren AK, Sennerby L, Lundgren D, Taylor Å, Nyman S. Bone augmentation at titanium implants using autologous bone grafts and a bioresorbable barrier. An experimental study in the rabbit tibia. *Clin Oral Implant Res.* 1996;8:82–89.

22. Pinholt EM, Haanaes HR, Donath K, Bang G. Titanium implant insertion into dog alveolar ridges augmented by allogeneic material. *Clin Oral Implant Res.* 1994;5:213–219.

23. Riediger D, Ehrenfeld M, Donath K. Tübinger Implantate im vaskularisierten Beckenkammtransplantat. Klinische Ergebnisse und morphologische Befunde. *Z Zahnärztl Implantol.* 1989;V: 137–141.

24. Nyström E, Kahnberg KE, Albrektsson T. Treatment of the severely resorbed maxillae with bone graft and titanium implants. Histologic review of autopsy specimens. *Int J Oral Maxillofac Implants.* 1993;8:167–172.

25. GaRey DJ, Whittaker JM, James RA, Lozada JL. The histologic evaluation of the implant interface with heterograft and allograft materials. An eight month autopsy report. Part II. *J Oral Implant.* 1991;XVII:404–408.

26. Jensen OT, Sennerby L. Histological analysis of titanium microimplants placed in conjunction with maxillary sinus floor augmentation. *Int J Oral Maxillofac Implants,* 1997.

27. Donovan MG, Dickerson NC, Hanson LJ, Gustafson RB. Maxillary and mandibular reconstruction using calvarial bone grafts and Brånemark implants. A preliminary report. *J Oral Maxillofac Surg.* 1994;52:588–594.

28. Breine U, Brånemark P-I. Reconstruction of alveolar jaw bone. *Scand J Plast Reconstr Surg.* 1980;14:23–48.

29. Boyne PJ, James RA. Grafting of the maxillary sinus floor with autogenous marrow and bone. *J Oral Surg.* 1980;38:613–619.

30. Jensen OT. Guided bone graft augmentation. In: Buser, Dahlin, Schenk, eds. *Guided Bone Regeneration in Implant Dentistry.* Chicago: Quintessence; 1994:235–264.

31. Albrektsson T, Brånemark P-I, Eriksson A, Lindström J. The preformed autologous bone graft. An experimental study in rabbits. *Scand J Plast Reconstr Surg.* 1978;12:215–223.

32. Tjellström A, Lindström J, Albrektsson T, Brånemark P-I, Hallén O. A clinical pilot study on preformed, autologous ossicles I. *Acta Otolaryngol (Stockh).* 1978;85:33–39.

33. Tjellström A, Lindström J, Albrektsson T, Brånemark P-I, Hallén O. A clinical pilot study on preformed, autologous ossicles II. *Acta Otolaryngol (Stockh).* 1978;85:232–242.

34. Tjellström A, Albrektsson T. Five-year follow-up of preformed, autologus ossicles in tympanoplasty. *J Laryngol Otol.* 1985;99: 729–733.

35. Lindström J, Brånemark P-I, Albrektsson T. Mandibular reconstruction using the preformed autologus bone graft. *Scand J Plast Reconstr Surg.* 1981;15:29–38.

36. Keller EE, Van Roekel NB, Desjardins RP, Tolman D. Prosthetic-surgical reconstruction of the severely resorbed maxilla with iliac bone grafting and tissue-integrated prostheses. *Int J Oral Maxillofac Implants.* 1987;2:155–164.

37. Albrektsson T, Dahl E, Enbom L, Engevall S, et al. Osseointegrated oral implants. A Swedish multicenter study of 8139 consecutively inserted Nobelpharma implants. *J Periodontol.* 1988; 59:287–296.

38. Adell R, Lekholm U, Gröndal K, et al. Reconstruction of severely resorbed edentulous maxillae using osseointegrated fixtures in immediate autogenous bone grafts. *Int J Oral Maxillofac Implants.* 1990;5:233–246.

39. Gunne J, Nyström E, Kahnberg KE. Bone grafts and implants in the treatment of the severely resorbed maxillae: A 3-year follow-up of the prosthetic restoration. *Int J Prosth.* 1995;8:38–45.

40. Schliephake H, Neukam FW, Scheller H, Bothe KJ. Local ridge augmentation using bone grafts and osseintegrated implants in the rehabilitation of partial edentulism. Preliminary results. *Int Oral Maxillofac Implants.* 1994;9:557–564.

41. Sailer HF. A new method of inserting endosseous implants in totally atrophic maxillae. *J Craniomaxillofac Surg.* 1989;17: 299–305.

42. Isaksson S. Evaluation of three bone grafting techniques for severely resorbed maxillae in conjunction with immediate endosseous implants. *Int Oral Maxillofac Implants.* 1994;9:679–688.

43. Jensen J, Krantz-Simonsen E, Sindet-Petersen S. Reconstruction of the severely resorbed maxilla with bone grafting and osseointegrated implants. A preliminary report. *J Oral Maxillofac Surg.* 1990;48:27–32.

44. Jensen J, Sindet-Petersen S. Autogenous mandibular bone grafts and osseointegrated implants for reconstruction of the severely atrophied maxilla: a preliminary report. *J Oral Maxillofac Surg.* 1991;49:1277–1287.

45. Jensen J, Sindet-Pedersen S, Oliver AJ. Varying treatment strategies for reconstruction of maxillary atrophy with implants. Results in 98 patients. *J Oral Maxillofac Surg.* 1994;52:210–216.

46. Krekeler G, ten Bruggenkate C, Osoterbeek HS. Verbesserung des Implantatbettes durch Augmentation mit autologem Knochen. *Z Zahnärztl Implantol.* 1993;IX:231–236.

47. Jensen OT, Greer R. Immediate placement of osseointegrated implant into maxillary sinus augmented with mineralized cancellous allograft and Gore-Tex. Second stage surgical and histological findings. In: Laney W, Tolman D, eds. *Tissue Integration in Oral, Orthopedic and Maxillofacial Reconstruction.* Chicago: Quintessence; 1992:321–333.

48. Small SA, Zinner ID, Panno FV, Shapiro HJ, Stein JI. Augmenting the maxillary sinus for implants. Report of 27 patients. *Int J Oral Maxillofac Implants.* 1993;8:523–528.

49. Riediger D, Ehrenfeld M. Mikrochurigische Beckenkammtransplantate in Kombination mit enossalen Implantaten. Ein neues Verfahren zur Rehabilitation extrem atrophier Kiefer. *Z Zahnärztl Implantol.* 1991;VII:178–183.

50. Tjellström A, Lindström J, Albrektsson T, et al. The bone-anchored auricular episthesis. *Laryngoscope.* 1981;91:811–815.

51. Tjellström A, Granström G. Long-term follow-up with the bone-anchored hearing aid: A review of the 100 patients between 1977 and 1985. *ENT J.* 1994;73:21–23.

52. Tjellström A. An analysis of soft tissue reactions around skin-penetrating implants. In: Yanagihara N, Suzuki J, eds. Transplants and Implants in Otology. II. Amsterdam/New York: Kugler; 1992:2–3.

53. Tjellström A, Lindström J, Albrektsson T, et al. Osseointegrated titanium implants in the temporal bone. A clinical study on bone-anchored hearing aids. *Am J Otol.* 1981;2:303–310.

54. Jacobsson M, Tjellström A, Fine L, Andersson H. A retrospective study of osseointegrated skin-penetrating titanium fixtures used for retaining facial prostheses. *Int J Oral Maxillofac Implants.* 1992;7:523–528.

55. Albrektsson T, Zarb G, Worthington P, Eriksson RA. The long-term efficacy of currently used dental implants: A review and proposed criteria of success. *Int J Oral Maxillofac Implants.* 1986;1:11–25.

56. Wolfaardt J, Wilkes G, Parel S, Tjellström A. Craniofacial osseointegration: the Canadian experience. *Int J Oral Maxillofac Implants.* 1993;8:197–204.

57. Granström G, Tjellström A, Brånemark PI, Fornander J. Bone-anchored reconstruction of the irradiated head and neck cancer patient. *Otolaryngol Head Neck Surg.* 1993;108:334–343.

58. Granström G, Tjellström A, Albrektsson T. Postimplantation irradiation for head and neck cancer treatment. *Int J Oral Maxillofac Implants.* 1993;8:495–500.

59. Tjellström A. The relevance for a child of the BAHA and auricular prosthesis. In: Fior R, Pestalozza G, eds. *The Child and the Environment: Present and Future Trends.* Amsterdam: Elsevier Science Publishers BV; 1993:251–255.

60. Tjellström A, Jacobsson M, Albrektsson T. Removal torque of osseointegrated craniofacial implants. A clinical study. *Int J Oral Maxillofac Implants.* 1988;3:287–289.

61. Yamanaka E, Tjellström A, Jacobsson M, Albrektsson T. Long-term observations on removal torque of directly bone-anchored implants in man. In: Yanagihara N, Suzuki J, eds. *Transplants and Implants in Otology II.* Amsterdam/New York: Kugler; 1992:112–117.

62. Johansson C, Tjellström A, Albrektsson T, Sennerby L. Retrieved extraoral implants. Biomaterials Club 3rd Winter meeting, Val Gardena, Italy. 1993.

15
The ITI Dental Implant System

Hans-Peter Weber, Daniel A. Buser, and Dieter Weingart

The current ITI Dental Implant System (Institut Straumann AG Waldenburg, Switzerland) was developed in 1985–1986 on the scientific basis and clinical experience of more than 10 years with earlier ITI implants (F-type Hollow Cylinder,[1] TPS, or Swiss screw[2]). The initial development of these implants was the result of a collaboration between the University of Berne, Switzerland, with Dr. André Schroeder and the Institut Straumann, Waldenburg, Switzerland. Today, the system consists of three different basic shapes: the full-body screw, the hollow screw, and the hollow-cylinder implant (Figure 15.1).[3,4] All implants are titanium plasma sprayed (TPS) in their bone-anchoring section, which comes in various lengths. The transmucosal portion is smoothly machined. Although it has been used in Europe and Japan since the mid-1980s, the ITI Dental Implant System was only introduced to the North American market in 1990 (Straumann USA, Cambridge, MA). The descriptions found in the following represent the system with implants and components as they are available in the United States at the time of preparation of this chapter.

Implant Designs and Surgical Instrumentation

Full-Body-Screw (S) Implant

The S implant is the successor of the TPS, or Swiss, screw.[2] The S implant is available in diameters of 4.1 mm (standard) and 3.3 mm (diameter reduced). Both types come in lengths (bone-sink depths) of 8 to 16 mm. Thread profile and head geometry are the same for both and are also identical to the HS implants later described.[3–5] The screw threads improve the primary stability of the implant in its bony bed. Thus sufficient primary stability can also be achieved in implant sites with a spongy bone structure. Today, the full-body screw is the most important ITI implant, and it is universally indicated in recipient sites with a vertical bone height of 10 mm or more. The S implant is also the implant of choice for maxillofacial surgical applications such as

ridge augmentations involving bone grafts as described in detail in Chapter 17. From a mechanical view point, the standard diameter S implant is the strongest of the ITI family. To our knowledge, not one implant fracture has been reported worldwide to date.

The implant bed is prepared with three different spiral drills of increasing diameter (Figure 15.2).[5] Confirmation of the sink depth, tapping of the screw thread, and placement of the implant are performed with the same instruments as are used for the HS implant. For the diameter-reduced screw, only the first two spiral drills, a diameter-reduced depth gauge, and a diameter-reduced tap are used.

Furthermore, a ratchet and a guidance key are necessary to screw thread the bone walls of the recipient site and to insert the implant. In implant sites with a normal or high bone density, the thread is cut in the entire length of the bone cavity prior to the insertion of the implant to avoid primary pressure peaks after placement of the implant. In implant sites with more spongy bone, the thread is cut only in the coronal portion of the cavity, and the implant is inserted in a self-tapping mode to achieve sufficient primary stability.[7]

Above the bone crest, the diameter of the smoothly machined implant neck flutes out to 4.8 mm to better match the diameter of a natural tooth. This allows for an emergence profile for aesthetic and functionally designed restorations. If necessary, the bone-sink depth of the implant can be varied by the surgeon during implant placement to enhance the aesthetic aspect.

Hollow-Screw (HS) Implant

The HS implant has a hollow design in its apical (bone-anchoring) portion, which also has systematically arranged perforations in the sides of the implant that allow for bone ingrowth and, therefore, an increased anchoring surface.[3–8] Like the full-body screw, the HS implant is threaded in its bone-anchoring portion allowing for improved primary stability. With these characteristics (i.e., threaded hollow perforated body design) this implant is preferably used for implant sites with reduced vertical bone heights of 8 to 10 mm.

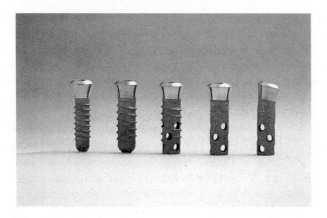

FIGURE 15.1 The ITI dental implants from right to left: diameter reduced solid screw, standard diameter solid screw, hollow screw, hollow cylinder straight and angled.

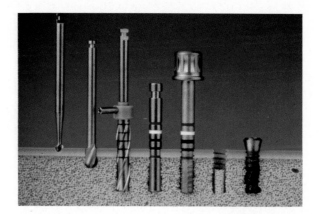

FIGURE 15.3 Instruments for hollow screw site preparation.

The HS implant is available in sink depth of 8, 10, and 12 mm. The preparation of the bone cavity is carried out with the following instruments: three round burs of increasing diameters, a predrill, and a trephine mill (Figure 15.3).[3–7] An internal irrigation system is available for the trephine mill to reduce the risk of bone-damaging temperatures. Extended experimental tests[6] demonstrated that this cooling system allows the reduction of the temperature in the peri-implant bone structure during preparation, which is important for the avoidance of postoperative bone necrosis. In addition, the same instruments (tap, ratchet, guidance key) as for the standard-diameter full-body screw are used to cut the screw thread into the bone wall of the recipient site and to insert the implant. Regarding tapping implant sites of different bone quality and sink depth of the implant, the same principle is applied as for S implants.[7]

Hollow-Cylinder (HC) Implant

In its basic outline, the HC implant is the successor of the ITI type-F implant,[1] which was first used clinically in 1979, generally for the treatment of edentulous mandibles and occasionally for single-tooth replacements or other indications.[9,10] The modified HC implant was specifically developed for single-tooth replacements in the anterior maxilla.[3,4] The HC implant is available both in a straight and an angled version (15° angulation in the neck portion). Both types are identical in their bone-anchoring section with an outer diameter of 3.5 mm. The angled HC implant is mainly used in indications with a maxillary anterior alveolar protrusion, a frequently found condition in that jaw region (Figure 15.4). HC implants are available in three different lengths of 8-, 10-, and 12-mm

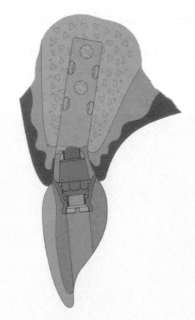

FIGURE 15.4 Use of angled hollow cylinder to correct the angulation between implant axis and crown, i.e., in sites with anterior alveolar protrusion.

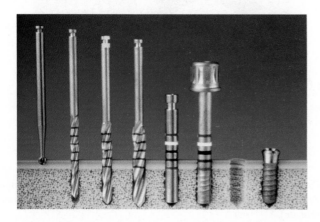

FIGURE 15.2 Instruments for solid screw site preparation.

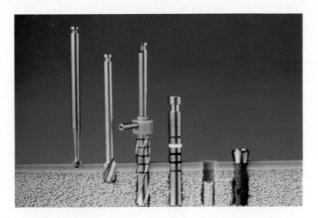

FIGURE 15.5 Instruments for hollow cylinder site preparation.

sink depth. They are press-fit implants, which achieve the required primary stability with the preparation of a precise, congruent implant bed. The instruments necessary for bone preparation are in part the same as for the HS implant (Figure 15.5): three round burs of increasing diameters, predrill, trephine mill, and a color-coded depth gauge. However, tap, ratchet, and guidance key are not necessary. To insert the implant, the insertion device is attached to the implant top in the sterile ampoule. The implant is then removed from the ampoule and placed into the bone cavity until a slight resistance is detectable. Subsequently, the inserting device is removed, and the implant is tapped to its final position using a special tapping instrument and a mallet. The gentle press-fit after insertion allows for good primary stability in recipient sites with a firm bone structure.

ITI Implant Material and Tissue Reactions

ITI implants are endosseous implants that are anchored in the bone and penetrate the soft tissue cover. Therefore, the implant surface is not only in contact with the bone but also with the mucosa.

Since their inception 20 years ago, ITI implants have been made of commercially pure titanium with a TPS surface in the bone-anchoring section. This coating procedure, first described by Hahn and Palich,[11] was introduced in implant dentistry for the first time with ITI implants in 1974. It creates a rough and microporous implant surface, with a porosity between 30 and 50 μm (Figure 15.6). The oxide film responsible for the biocompatibility of titanium forms on this sprayed layer. Therefore, the biocompatibility of the TPS surface is equivalent to a solid titanium body. Technical details of this procedure and the TPS surface were described by Steinemann.[12]

Bone

Direct bone apposition onto TPS surfaces was clearly shown at the beginning of the research project in animal experiments, and results were reported by Schroeder and coworkers in 1976 and 1978 using a new histologic technique with nondecalcified sections.[13,14] This phenomenon of direct bone-implant contact is often termed *osseointegration*,[15] or *functional ankylosis*.[16] Light-microscopic images demonstrate the anchorage of titanium implants with osseointegration (Figure 15.7). The

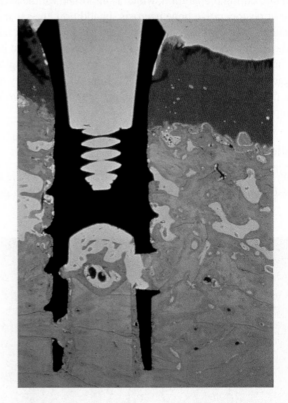

FIGURE 15.7 Micrograph demonstrating direct bone-to-implant contact (osseointegration) to TPS surface (experimental sample from primate).

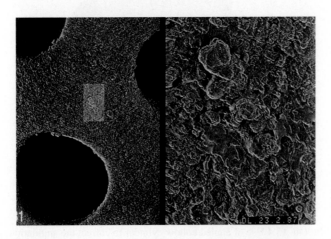

FIGURE 15.6 Titanium-plasma-sprayed surface (TPS) in a close-up view.

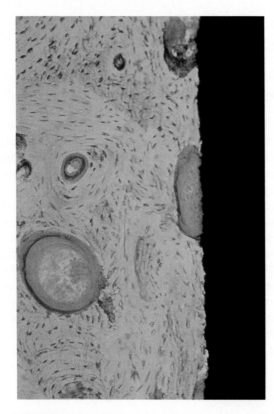

FIGURE 15.8 Direct bone-implant contact without interpositioning of soft tissue. Blood vessels in contact with implant surface (experimental sample from canine model).

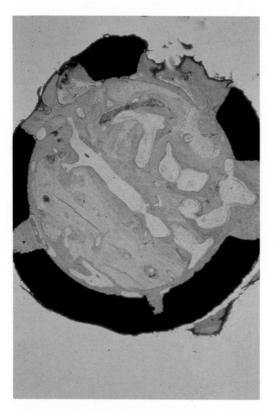

FIGURE 15.9 Osseointegration in apical section of hollow-cylinder implant, cross-sectional view (human explant).

higher magnification reveals the direct apposition of newly formed bone onto the surface of titanium implants with a TPS surface without an intervening layer of connective tissue. The vitality of the bone is demonstrated by the presence of osteocytes and blood vessels close to the implant surface (Figure 15.8). Osseointegration was also confirmed on a few human implants, which had to be removed (e.g., due to recurrent peri-implant infections in the crestal area; see Figure 15.9). Furthermore, direct bone-implant contact was also demonstrated in scanning electron-microscopic analyses, as well as in a transmission electron-microscopic study by Listgarten et al.[17] using titanium evaporated epoxy resin implants (Figure 15.10). Osseointegration is generally not observed to have 100% bone contact along a given implant surface. The extent of bone-implant interface depends mainly on three factors: (1) the implant and surface material used; (2) the roughness of the implant surface; and (3) the density of the surrounding bone.

As mentioned earlier, ITI implants have been coated with a TPS surface since their inception in 1974 as this porous titanium surface offers several advantages from a clinical point of view. An animal study in rats demonstrates that the TPS surface accelerates bone apposition during early wound heal-

ing.[18] TPS implants revealed the first visible bone-implant contact after 7 days of healing, whereas smooth titanium implants demonstrated the first contacts after 21 days. In a study of miniature pigs, titanium implants with TPS coatings demon-

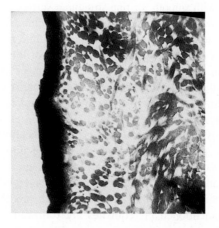

FIGURE 15.10 Direct bone apposition to TPS surface in electron microscopic view (magnification 16,000, sample from canine experiment with TPS coated epoxy implants).

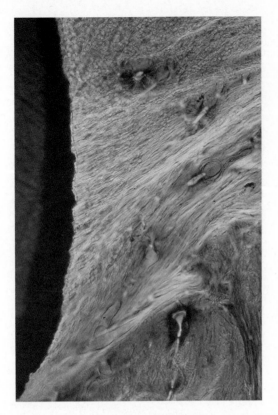

FIGURE 15.11 Supracrestal connective tissue fibers in perpendicular orientation to TPS coated implant surface (cross-sectional view).

Supracrestal Connective Tissue and Epithelium

Dental implants are not covered by a closed integument. The fact that they penetrate the mucosa and are consequently exposed to the environment of the oral cavity with all its possible contaminants creates a delicate problem. Thus the components of the soft tissue cover (i.e., the supracrestal connective tissue as well as the epithelium) have to act as an important barrier between the internal and external environment if long-term function is to be expected.[26]

As demonstrated above, bone as mineralized connective tissue adheres to the rough TPS surface. Therefore, it could be expected that a similar reaction would occur when the nonmineralized supracrestal connective tissue directly contacted the TPS surface, and when the implant post is located in keratinized attached mucosa. Light-microscopic experiments on TPS-coated implants placed in monkeys[16] or beagle dogs[28] demonstrated a fiber orientation perpendicular to the implant surface (Figure 15.11). However, studies in beagle dogs evaluating titanium implants with smooth or sandblasted surfaces[17,29] revealed no evidence of perpendicular fiber attach-

strated a significantly higher percentage of direct bone-implant contact in cancellous bone when compared to smooth- or fine-structured titanium surfaces.[19] And finally, a study in sheep revealed significantly higher removal torques for TPS implants when compared with smooth- or fine-structured titanium implants.[20] Summarizing these studies, it can be concluded that titanium implants with TPS surfaces achieve significantly faster and better bone anchorage when compared with titanium implants with smooth- or fine-structured surfaces.

To achieve osseointegration of ITI implants, four prerequisites need to be fulfilled: (1) biocompatible material; (2) atraumatic surgical technique using a slow drilling technique to prevent overheating of the bone; (3) primary implant stability; and (4) a healing period of 3 to 4 months without direct loading.[7] As already mentioned, ITI implants were designed as nonsubmerged implants. If placed as such, they are not covered by the oral mucosa during healing and penetrate the crestal mucosa from the time of implant placement. In contrast to the frequently stated requirement for a submerged implant placement,[15] nonsubmerged ITI implants achieve osseointegration with high predictability if the aforementioned prerequisites are followed.[7,21–25] This clinical fact observed over more than 20 years has been confirmed in the recent past by several experimental studies.[13,14,16,17,19,26–30]

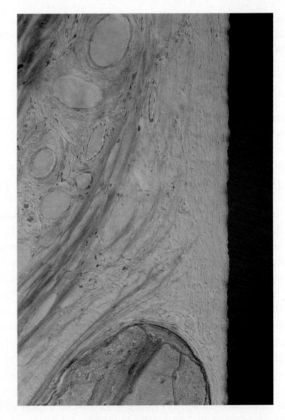

FIGURE 15.12 Absence of perpendicular fibers close to the implant surface. Collagen fibers with a parallel orientation distant from the implant surface. Blood vessel and cell-free zone in contact with implant surface.

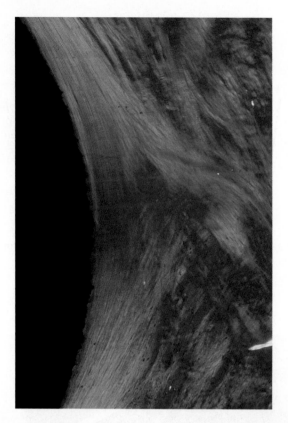

FIGURE 15.13 Circular fibers around implant post in cross-sectional view (canine experiment).

ment to the tested nonporous titanium surfaces. The connective tissue in direct contact with the implant post was mainly dominated by circularly oriented collagen fibers. This inner zone of connective tissue was free of blood vessels and resembled most likely an inflammation-free scar-tissue formation (Figure 15.12). The obvious difference to the aforementioned studies with perpendicular fiber attachment can probably be explained by the difference in the surface characteristics.

Based on biological considerations for successful maintenance of healthy peri-implant soft tissues, ITI implants have a smoothly machined titanium surface in the transmucosal section to reduce the risk of plaque accumulation. Thus it has to be expected that a similar arrangement of circularly oriented connective tissue fibers is predominantly present around ITI implants in patients due to the smooth surface in the supracrestal area (Figure 15.13).

Different light-microscopic studies using nonsubmerged titanium implants in different animal models[16,28–30] demonstrated no evidence of an epithelial downgrowth to the bone-crest level. The micrographs revealed the formation of a peri-implant sulcus, with the most apical epithelial cells being located approximately 1 mm above the bone-crest level (Figure 15.14). The epithelial structures around titanium implants are similar to those found around teeth (i.e., sulcular

epithelium-like and, more apically, junctional epithelium-like cell layers along the implant surface; see Figure 15.15).

Prosthodontic Concept

Abutments

Various abutments are available for the two-part ITI implants. They consist of a number of conical abutments for screw-retained and/or cemented restorations including an angled abutment (Figure 15.16), an octagonal abutment for screw-retained restorations only, and the retentive anchor used for implant treatments with overdentures. The abutments all have the same apical portion fitting to the inner top portion of the implant with an M2 (2-mm) screw and an 8° cone (Figure 15.17). This cone-to-screw interface serves as a nonrotational friction fit or mechanical lock on the basis of the Morse taper principle. It has shown to be three to four times as strong as a conventional, flat-coupling screw connection.[31] To secure the abutments into this nonrotational fit, they are inserted with a torque of 35 Ncm using a special torque instrument (Figure 15.18).

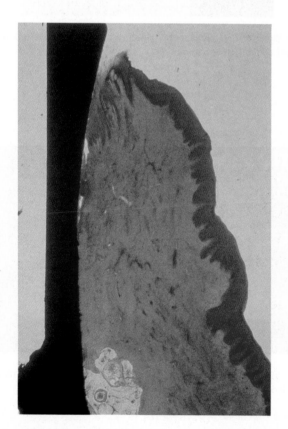

FIGURE 15.14 Microradiograph demonstrating peri-implant soft tissue morphology. At the top apical extension of peri-implant epithelium. At the bottom is the crestal bone height. Connective tissue contact height extends from the crestal bone height to the epithelium.

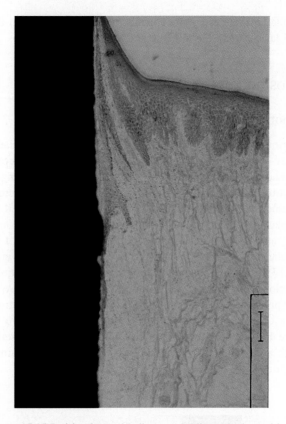

FIGURE 15.15 Peri-implant epithelium resembling sulcular and junctional epithelium at natural teeth.

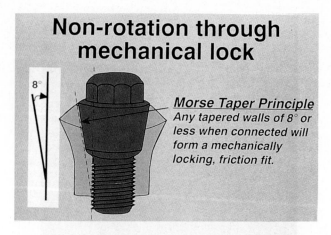

FIGURE 15.17 Cone-to-screw design (Morse taper principle) for rotation safe anchorage of abutment in implant.

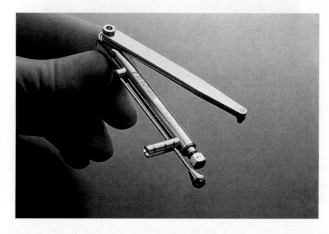

FIGURE 15.18 Torque instrument for abutment insertion (35 Ncm) and tightening of occlusal screws (20 Ncm).

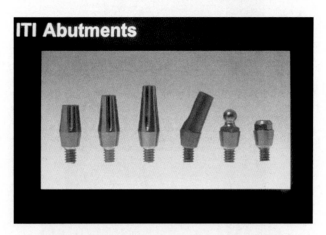

FIGURE 15.16 ITI abutments. From left to right: Solid abutments, angled abutment retentive anchor, and octa-abutment.

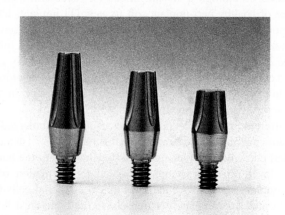

FIGURE 15.19 Solid conical abutments (4-mm, 5.5-mm, and 7-mm height) for cemented restorations.

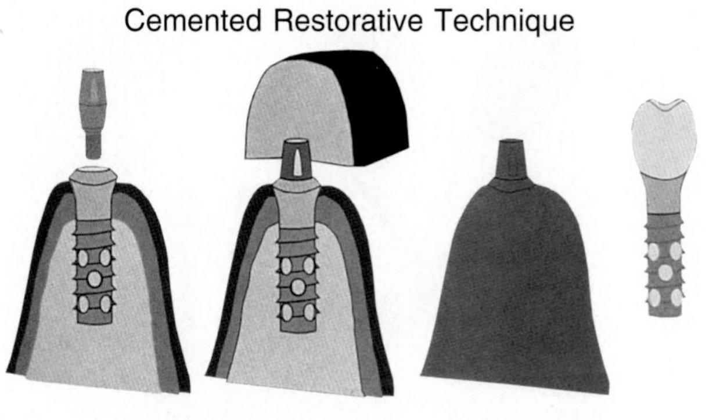

Cemented Restorative Technique

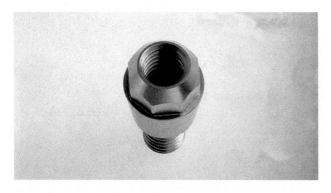

FIGURE 15.20 Schematic overview of restorative steps for cemented restorations.

Non-Repositionable Transfer Technique

a

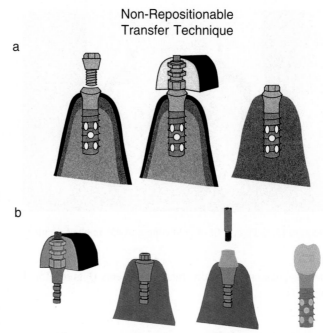

b

FIGURE 15.22 (a,b) Schematic overview of procedural steps for screw-retained restorations with the octa-abutment concept and its prefabricated components.

Conical Abutments

The conical abutments come as solid abutments without internal screw threads in heights of 4, 5.5, and 7 mm, for cementation of restorations (Figure 15.19). They are especially easy to use and, therefore, save time and reduce costs. After placement of the conical abutment, an impression is made, a stone cast is poured, and the crowns or fixed partial dentures are waxed directly to the stone model and then completed as conventional crown-bridge work (Figure 15.20).

Octa-abutment for Screw-Retained Restorations

For screw-retained prostheses, the Octa-system with different prefabricated parts for accurate transfer and laboratory procedures has been added to the ITI armamentarium in the more recent past.[31] The top of the Octa-abutment has eight sides and is 1.5 mm high (Figure 15.21), with an M2 screw hole in its top to retain the restoration. This 2-mm occlusal screw limits the occurrences of screw loosening or fractures commonly reported for implant restorations. The Octa-abutment is anchored in the implant with the same cone-to-screw interface as the con-

ical abutments described earlier, and they provide a nonrotational friction fit. Transfer copings are used for impressions. Once an impression is made, one-piece analogs are secured into the transfer copings and die stone poured. After the stone has set, the transfer copings are removed. Prefabricated gold copings made from nonoxidizing, high gold-content alloys with a high melting range are placed on the analogs. Long wax-up or guide screws are used to secure the copings on the analogs and to create the space for the future occlusal screw access canal. The frame of the future restoration is then waxed and cast to the copings. In case of porcelain-fused-to-gold restorations, the porcelain is added thereafter. It is important that for such restorations, a layer of gold compatible with the ceramic material to be used is cast onto the copings. Gold copings with an octagonal inside are chosen for single-tooth cases, whereas gold copings with rounded insides are used for fixed partial dentures. The step-by-step procedure for screw-retained restorations is summarized in Figure 15.22a,b. The prefabricated gold copings have an outstanding precision, which can be documented in SEM images (Figure 15.23). The resistance of the implant-abutment-superstructure complex to lateral forces is superior due to the precise component fit and even enhanced by the 45° inclination of the implant shoulder. Angled abutments and a transversal screw retention concept have been added to the prosthodontic concept more recently. For instructions on their use, the reader is referred to the respective, detailed system literature. They assist the restorative dentist in overcoming im-

FIGURE 15.21 Octa-abutment for screw-retained restoration in close-up view.

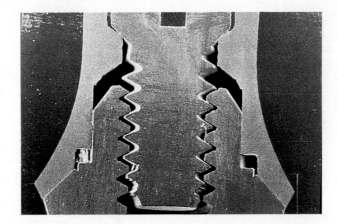

FIGURE 15.23 Precise fit of gold coping to 45° implant shoulder.

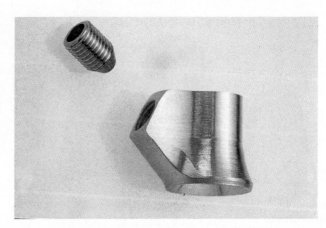

FIGURE 15.25 Transverse screw coping for single-tooth restorations.

plant angulation and/or divergence problems (Figures 15.24 and 15.25).

Overdentures on Bars

In cases in which support for dentures is needed, two to four implants can be placed and restored with a gold bar and an overdenture after completion of implant healing.[9,10] Prefabricated gold copings, gold bars with round or oval profile, and gold clips or bar sleeves are the available components. Note that these gold copings are different from the ones used for

cast restorations. The bar-retaining copings are only to be used to affix prefabricated bar segments via soldering procedure, in that they are fit tightly onto the bars and fitted into the denture as retentive elements (Figures 15.26–15.28).

Overdenture on Retentive Anchors

When moderate additional retention is required for a mandibular or maxillary denture, two implants can be placed, and round (retentive) anchors are inserted in the implants after the 3- to 4-month healing period.[32] Because no reopening surgery is necessary, the restorative phase begins at the end of this healing period. Female matrices are processed into the denture to fit tightly to the retentive anchors with a simple impression and pick-up method (Figures 15.29–15.31).

Case Reports

Figures 15.32 to 15.37 show illustrative examples from case reports.

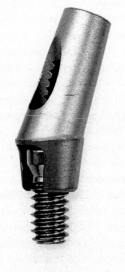

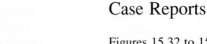

FIGURE 15.24 Angled abutments to correct angulation problems in fixed partial denture cases.

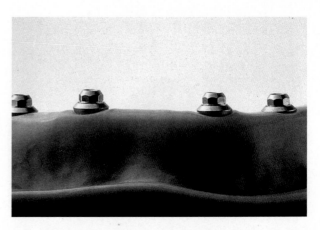

FIGURE 15.26 Octa-abutments on four implants for bar-retained overdenture.

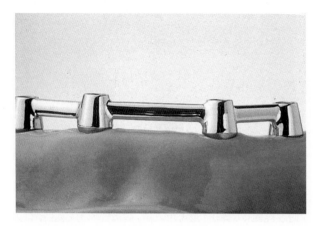

FIGURE 15.27 Gold bar in place. Bar segments are soldered to gold copings different from the ones used for cast restorations.

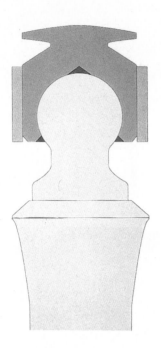

FIGURE 15.30 Schematic illustration of function of gold matrix on retentive anchor. The presence of the polyethylene sleeve around the matrix is important for proper retentive function of the matrix.

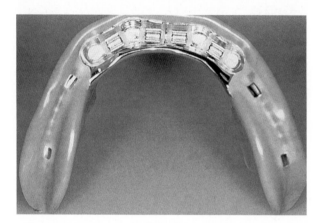

FIGURE 15.28 Finished overdenture demonstrating bar clips in situ. A metal lingual plate for strength and minimizing interference with tongue function is recommended as shown.

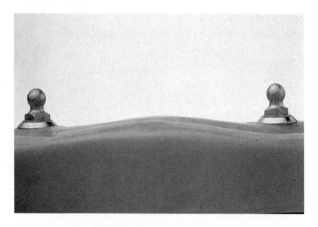

FIGURE 15.29 Retentive anchor in close-up view.

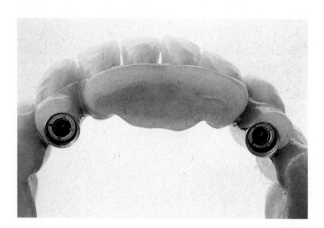

FIGURE 15.31 Tissue side of overdenture with retentive matrices in place.

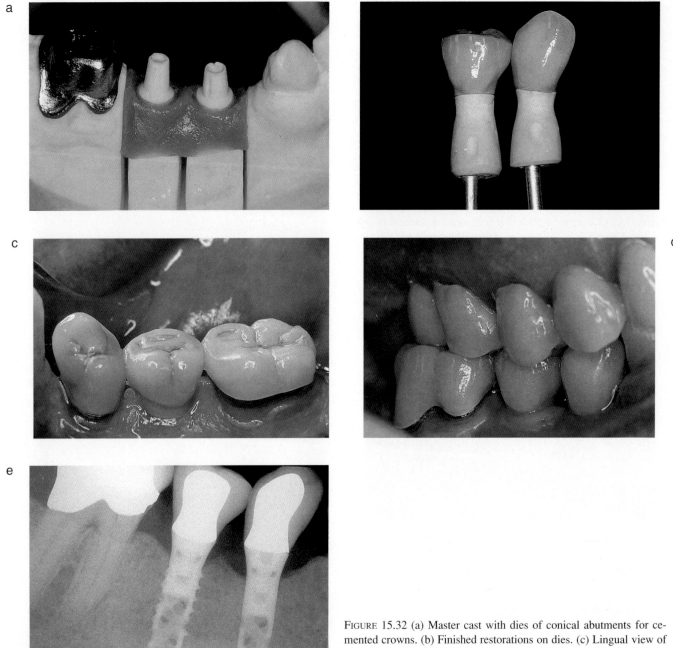

FIGURE 15.32 (a) Master cast with dies of conical abutments for cemented crowns. (b) Finished restorations on dies. (c) Lingual view of cemented restorations. (d) Buccal view of cemented resotrations. (e) Radiographic control 3 years after implant placement.

a

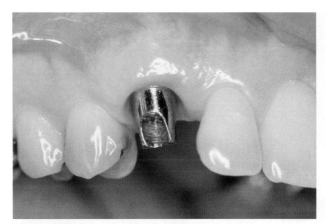

b

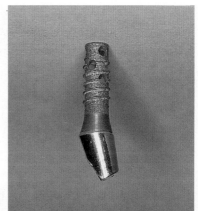

c

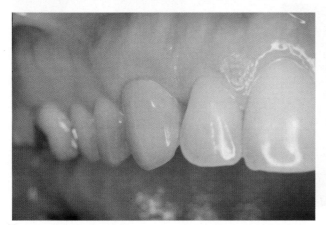

d

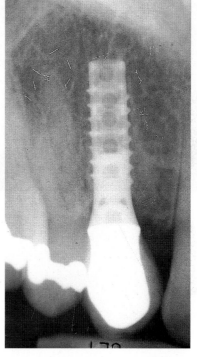

FIGURE 15.33 (a) Custom-angled abutment in case with maxillary alveolar protrusion in right canine area. Note the placement of the implant below tissue level for aesthetic crown emergence. (b) View of custom angled abutment on an HS implant. The custom angled abutment was waxed and cast on an octogonal gold coping and then custom milled. (c) Procelain-fused-to-metal crown in place. (d) Radiographic control at 3 years after crown insertion.

a

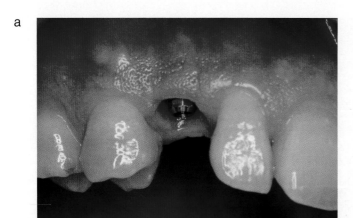

b

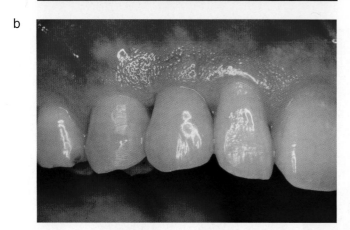

c

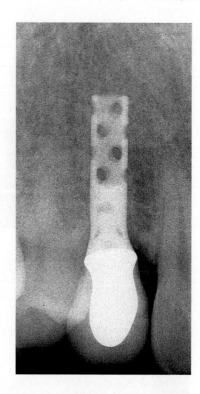

FIGURE 15.34 (a) Octa-abutment placed for screw-retained restoration in area of the right canine. Note again the deeper implant placement for aesthetic purposes. (b) Final restoration in place. (c) Radiographic control 2 years after insertion.

a

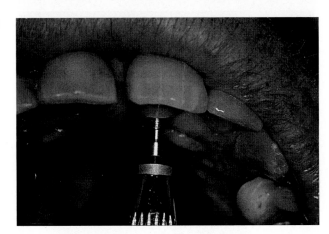

b

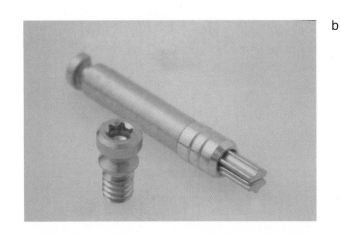

c

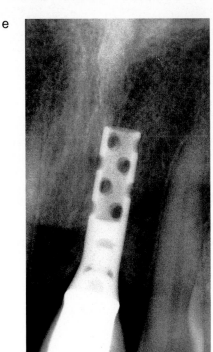

d

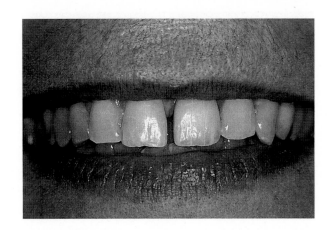

e

FIGURE 15.35 (a) Crown post inserted in octa-abutment for fixation of crown via transversal screw in area of missing upper left central incisor. (b) Close-up view of crown post and SCS screwdriver. (c) Fixation of crown with transversal screw. (d) Aesthetic appearance of completed tooth replacement. (e) Radiographic control 2 years after crown insertion.

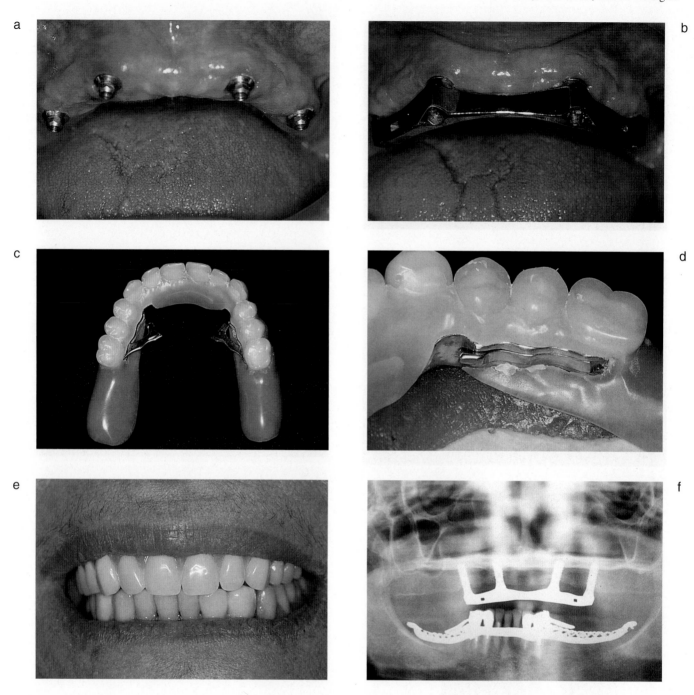

FIGURE 15.36 (a) Octa-abutments on four implants placed in maxillary edentulous patient. (b) High-profile milled bar in situ. (c) Palate-free overdenture with bilateral custom fabricated locks which can be easily opened and closed by the patient. (d) Close-up view of one of the locks. (e) Frontal view of final prosthesis. (f) Radiographic control at 1 year.

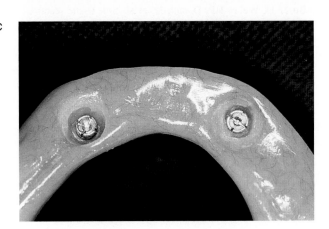
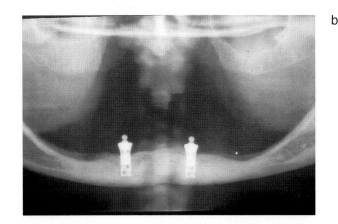
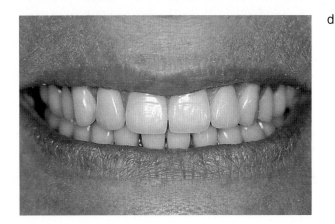

a b c d

FIGURE 15.37 (a) Retentive anchors in place. (b) Radiographic control at 4 years. (c) Retentive anchor matrices processed in lower overdenture. (d) Frontal view of final prostheses (i.e., lower overdenture, upper complete denture).

References

1. Sutter F, Schroeder A, Straumann F. ITI Hohlzylinder Systeme. *Prinzipien Methodik Swiss Dent.* 1983;4:21.
2. Babbush CA, Kent JN, Misiek DJ. Titanium plasma-sprayed (TPS) screw implants for the reconstruction of the edentulous mandible. *J Oral Maxillofac Surg.* 1986;44:274.
3. Sutter F, Schroeder A, Buser D. The new concept of ITI hollow cylinder and hollow screw implants. Part I: Engineering and design. *Int J Oral Maxillofac Implants.* 1988;3:161.
4. Buser D, Schroeder A, Sutter F, Lang NP. The new concept of ITI hollow-cylinder and hollow-screw implants: Part 2, Clinical aspects, indications, and early clinical results. *Int J Oral Maxillofac Implants.* 1988;3:173.
5. Sutter F, Schroeder A, Buser D. Das neue ITI-Implantatkonzept. Technische Aspekte und Methodik. *Quintessenz.* 1988;39: (Teil 1)1875–XX; (Teil 2)2057.
6. Sutter F, Krekeler G, Schwammberger AE, Sutter FJ. Das ITI-Bonefitimplantatsystem: Implantatbettgestaltung. *Quintessenz.* 1991;42:541.
7. Buser D, Weber HP, Brägger U. The treatment of partially endentulous patients with ITI hollow-screw implants: Pre-surgical evaluation and surgical procedures. *Int J Oral Maxillofac Implants.* 1990;5:165.

8. Sutter F. Raveh J. Titanium-coated hollow screw and reconstruction plate system for bridging of lower jaw defects: Biomechanical aspects. *Int J Oral Maxillofac Surg.* 1988;17:267.
9. Schroeder A, Maeglin B, Sutter F. Das ITI-Hohlzylinderimplantat Typ-F zur Prothesenretention beim zahnlosen Kiefer. *Scheiz Monatsschr Zahnheilk.* 1983;93:720.
10. ten Bruggenkate CM, Muller K, Oosterbeek HS. Clinical evaluation of the ITI (F-type) hollow cylinder implant. *Oral Surg Oral Med Oral Pathol.* 1990;70:693.
11. Hahn H, Palich W. Preliminary evaluation of porous metal surfaced titanium for orthopedic implants. *J Biomed Mater Res.* 1970;4:571.
12. Steinemann S. The properties of titanium. In: Schroeder A, Sutter F, Krekeler G, eds. *Oral Implantology: Basics-ITI Hollow Cylinder.* New York: Thieme Medical Publishers; 1991:37–58.
13. Schroeder A, Pohler O, Sutter F. Gewebsreaktion auf ein Titan-Hohlzylinderimplantat mit Titan-Spritzschichtoberfläche. *Schweiz Monatsschr Zahnheilk.* 1976;86:713.
14. Schroeder A, Stich H, Straumann F, Sutter F. Über die Anlagerung von Osteozement an einen belasteten Implantatkörper. *Schweiz Monatsschr Zahnheilk.* 1978;88:1051.
15. Brånemark PI, Hansson BO, Adell R, et al. Osseointegrated implants in the treatment of the edentulous jaw. Experience from a 10-year period. *Scand J Plast Reconstruct Surg II.* (suppl 16), 1977.

16. Schroeder A, van der Zypen E, Stich H, Sutter F. The reactions of bone, connective tissue and epithelium to endosteal implants with titanium-sprayed surfaces. *J Maxillofac Surg.* 1981;9:15.

17. Listgarten MA, Buser D, Steinemann S, Donath K, Lang NP, Weber HP. Light and transmission electron microscopy of the intact interface between bone, gingiva and non-submerged titanium-coated epoxy resin implants. *J. Dent Res.* 1992;71:364–371.

18. Kirsch A, Donath K. Tierexperimentelle Untersuchungen zur Bedeutung der Mikromorphologie von Titanimplantatoberflächen. *Fortschr Zahnärztl Implantol.* 1984;1:35.

19. Buser D, Schenk RK, Steinemann S, Fiorellini JP, Fox C, Stich H. Influence of surface characteristics on bone reactions to titanium implants: a histomorphometric study in miniature pigs. *J Biomed Mater Res.* 1991;25:889.

20. Wilke HJ, Claes L, Steinemann S. The influence of various titanium surfaces on the interface shear strength between implants and bone. *Adv Biomater.* 1990;9:309.

21. Buser D, Weber HP, Lang NP. Tissue integration of non-submerged implants. *Clin Oral Implants Res.* 1990;1:33.

22. Buser D, Weber HP, Brägger U, Balsiger C. Tissue integration of one-stage ITI implants: 3-year results of a longitudinal study with hollow-cylinder and hollow-screw implants. *Int J Oral Maxillofac Implants.* 1991;6:405.

23. Buser D, Sutter F, Weber HP, Belser U, Schroeder A. The ITI Dental Implant System: basics, indications, clinical procedures and results. *Clark's Clin Dentistry.* 1992;5:1–22.

24. Mericske-Stern R. Clinical evaluation of overdenture restorations supported by osseointegrated implants: a retrospective study. *Int J Oral Maxillofac Implants.* 1990;5:375.

25. Mericske-Stern R, Steinlin-Schaffner T, Marti P, Geering AH. Peri-implant mucosal aspects of ITI implants supporting overdentures. A five-year longitudinal study. *Clin Oral Implants Res.* 1994;5:9–18.

26. McKinney R, Steflik DE, Koth DL. Per, peri, or trans? A concept from improved dental terminology. *J Prosthet Dent.* 1984; 52:267.

27. Gotfredsen K, Rostrup E, Hjøerting-Hansen E, Stoltze K, Budtz-Jørgensen E. Histological and histomorphometrical evaluation of tissue reactions to endosteal implants in monkeys. *Clin Oral Implants Res.* 1991;2:30.

28. Buser D, Stich H, Krekeler G, Schroeder A. Faserstrukturen der periimplantären Mukosa bei Titan-Implantaten. Eine tierexperimentelle Studie am Beagle-Hund *Z Zahnärztl Implantol.* 1989; 5:15.

29, Buser D, Weber HP, Donath K, et al. Soft tissue reactions to non-submerged unloaded titanium implants in beagle dogs. *J Periodontol.* 1992;63:225.

30. Weber HP, Buser D, Donath K, Fiorellini JP, Doppalapudi V, Paquette DW, et al. Comparison of healed tissues adjacent to submerged and non-submerged unloaded titanium dental implants. A histologic and histometric study in beagle dogs. *Clin Oral Implants Res.* 1996;7:11.

31. Sutter F, Weber HP, Sorensen J, Belser U. The new restorative concept of the ITI Dental Implant System: engineering and design. *Int J Periodont Rest Dent.* 1993;13:408.

32. Mericske-Stern R, Geering AH. Implantate in der Totalprothetik: Die Verankerung der Totalprothese im zahnlosen Unterkiefer durch zwei Implantate mit Einzelattachment. *Schweiz Monatsschr Zahnmed.* 1988;98:871.

16
Localized Ridge Augmentation Using Guided Bone Regeneration in Deficient Implant Sites

Daniel A. Buser, Dieter Weingart, and Hans-Peter Weber

The use of osseointegrated implants anchored in the jawbone with direct bone-implant contact has become an increasingly important treatment modality for the replacement of missing teeth.[1,2] To expect a predictable long-term prognosis for osseointegrated implants, a sufficient volume of healthy bone should be available at possible recipient sites. Thus a careful presurgical evaluation is essential to obtain the necessary information about the quality of the bone, the vertical bone height, and the orofacial bone width. When this analysis reveals that the width of the alveolar ridge is insufficient at desired implant locations, reconstructive surgery is needed if endosseous implants are to be used. One augmentation technique is based on the principle of guided tissue regeneration using barrier membranes, which was initially developed for periodontal regeneration.[3,4] A comprehensive text on guided bone regeneration in implant dentistry has been published by Buser et al.[5]

This principle has been tested for the regeneration of bone tissue in different types of bone defects as well as around dental implants.[4–23] These studies have in common that barrier membranes were placed over bone defects and closely adapted to the surrounding bone surface, creating a secluded space between the bone and the membrane. With the placement of a barrier membrane, preference is given to bone-forming cells that originate from adjacent bone to populate and regenerate these defects with bone, since competing soft tissue cells from the mucosa are excluded from these defects. Control sites without membranes demonstrate incomplete bone regeneration and the presence of soft tissue within the defects. For the regeneration of bone defects using barrier membranes, the term guided bone regeneration (GBR) is preferable since this term describes the purpose of the membrane application more precisely than does the term guided tissue regeneration (GTR).

In combination with the placement of endosseous implants, two different applications of GBR are possible: (1) the simultaneous approach using membranes to regenerate bone defects around an inserted implant; and (2) the staged approach using membranes for localized ridge augmentation and placement of implants 6 months later into the newly regenerated alveolar ridge in a separate surgical procedure.

The clinical testing of GBR in patients for implant indications started at the University of Bern in 1988, and the potential of both treatment options was demonstrated.[11,12] From these early experiences it could be concluded that the biological principle of GBR for ridge enlargement is predictable. However, factors such as soft tissue management, placement of membranes with the provision of sufficient space for bone regeneration, primary flap closure, and postsurgical infection control influence the prognosis to a great degree and must be optimized.

Consequently, the surgical procedures were refined and technical modifications developed to improve the predictability of the GBR technique.[21–23]

In implant patients with an insufficient bone volume, the surgical approach to be chosen depends on three selection criteria. If the intrasurgical status demonstrates: (1) an implant cannot be inserted with primary stability; (2) an implant cannot be inserted in an appropriate position from a prosthetic point of view; or (3) the peri-implant bone defect would be relatively extended, the simultaneous application of a barrier membrane, and an implant would have certain risks. Therefore, the staged approach is preferred in these situations since it reduces the risk for compromise or failure of the result.

The goal of the staged approach is a localized ridge augmentation and subsequent placement of endosseous implants into the newly formed alveolar ridge after a healing period of 6 months.

Based on current experimental and clinical knowledge, a healthy individual with normal healing capacity and an alveolar bone (defect) site rendering the opportunity for vascularization and colonization with bone-forming cells is a good candidate for GBR procedure. Additionally, the following clinical and/or technical prerequisites need to be fulfilled for predictable success with ridge augmentation procedures.

Appropriate Barrier Membrane

An appropriate membrane to serve as a barrier is necessary. The mostly used e-PTFE (Teflon) membrane (GTAM, W.L. Gore and Associates, Flagstaff, AZ) is a nondegradable membrane. The structure of this membrane does not allow the penetration of cells through the membrane, which is an important factor for its success as a physical barrier. Numerous experimental studies in animals have demonstrated that this membrane material is bioinert and allows complication-free tissue integration, provided that submerged healing without direct contact to the oral cavity can be achieved (for review, see Buser et al.[5]). Biodegradable membranes have also been tested in animals and humans with successful outcomes for periodontal indications.[24–28] In these indications, the use of biodegradable membranes gains from the advantage of avoiding a second surgical procedure for membrane removal. However, the advantage of using biodegradable membranes for implant indications is not considerable since most surgical sites have to be reopened anyway, either for abutment connection (simultaneous approach) or for implant placement (staged approach). Biodegradable membranes may have an advantage over nondegradable, bioinert membranes for implant indications, with further research needed for outcomes.

Primary Soft Tissue Healing

It has been clearly demonstrated in clinical applications and confirmed in experimental studies (for review, see Buser et al.[5]) that a closed healing of the regeneration site is a prerequisite for a predictable result. When a soft tissue dehiscence occurs, the exposure of the membrane leads to its contamination with bacteria from the oral cavity and frequently to an infection in the membrane site within 2 to 3 months, when the membrane remains in place. Since infected membranes cited have an increased risk for a compromised surgical result, early membrane removal is generally recommended in cases of soft tissue dehiscences.[23] Therefore, an appropriate flap design has to be chosen for predictable achievement of primary soft tissue healing. Placement of a barrier membrane changes the conditions for the healing of a soft tissue wound. In the presence of a barrier membrane, the soft tissue flap is separated from the bone. As a consequence, the primary soft tissue healing depends mainly on a sufficient vascular supply of the soft-tissue flaps, and the soft tissue wound cannot be supported by granulation tissue derived from the underlying bone. Clinical experience has demonstrated that crestal incisions do not allow the predictable achievement of primary soft-tissue healing. The modified incision technique using a lateral incision on the palatal aspect with a combined split-thickness and full-thickness flap design clearly reduced the frequency of postoperative soft tissue complications. Other important factors for primary soft tissue healing are careful handling of the soft tissue flap using fine surgical instruments and retraction sutures during surgery as well as

tension-free wound closure with appropriate mattress and interrupted sutures. Furthermore, a perioperative medication with nonsteroidal anti-inflammatory drugs and the local extraoral application of cold packs in the surgical area are useful to reduce postoperative swelling.

Membrane Adaptation and Fixation to Surrounding Bone

Close adaptation is necessary to achieve a sealing effect to prevent the ingrowth of soft tissue cells derived from the gingival connective tissue because these cells are able to compete with bone-forming cells in the created space underneath the membrane. In addition, stabilization of the membrane is useful for maintaining close adaptation of the membrane to the bone during wound closure. Clinical applications with the specially designed mini-screws (Memfix System, Institut Straumann AG, Waldenburg, Switzerland)[21–23] or pins[29,30] have documented their effectiveness for membrane adaptation and stabilization.

Creation and Maintenance of Secluded Space

A membrane-protected space allows the ingrowth of angiogenic and osteogenic cells so that bone regeneration is undisturbed by competing nonosteogenic soft tissue cells.[14] It is important to differentiate between space-making defects, such as an extraction socket with intact bone walls, and non–space-making defects. Non–space-making defects, including sites for localized ridge augmentation, are more demanding because the membrane is not supported by local bone walls. In these defects, standard e-PTFE membranes are susceptible to partial collapse caused by the soft tissue cover during healing.[14,23] Therefore, membrane support for space maintenance is important.

Attempts have been made to solve this clinical problem in recent years. One possible solution is the use of stiffer membranes (i.e., reinforced e-PTFE membranes with titanium mesh) as recommended for periodontal indications.[31] However, clinical testing must demonstrate if stiffer membranes also have value for ridge augmentation procedures. Membrane-supporting devices such as mini-screws[21–23] or pins[29,30] have been used. The surgical results were improved, but partial membrane collapse lateral to the support posts still posed a problem. It became obvious that an appropriate filling material was needed in non–space-making defects. Autogenous bone is still considered the material of first choice for bone defect grafting.[32,33] Consequently, autografts were used to further optimize the ridge augmentation procedure. It was expected that the combination of autogenous bone grafts and e-PTFE augmentation material would improve the outcome of ridge augmentation procedures because the autograft would not only serve as a membrane-supporting device to maintain the created space but also act as an osteoconductive scaffold to accelerate bone regeneration.

It is important to understand the biological behavior of autografts with respect to graft incorporation and repair and the differences between cortical and cancellous autografts. These details have been intensively studied in numerous experimental studies in orthopedic surgery (for review, see Burchardt[32,33]). Cancellous autografts are rapidly revascularized, and they are completely repaired by creeping substitution. In contrast, revascularization of cortical autografts is slow and occurs through existing haversian canals. Remodeling of cortical autografts is also slow and results in a mixture of necrotic and new viable bone.

Based on this biological knowledge of graft incorporation and graft repair, corticocancellous block grafts placed in the center of the augmentation area and combined with smaller bone particles surrounding the block graft were subsequently used. This surgical approach is based on two assumptions. First, the cortical portion of the graft facing to the buccal aspect of the crest is used to reestablish the missing buccal cortex. Although this new cortex will be a mixture of necrotic and new viable bone, it offers good mechanical stability and is less susceptible to resorption than cancellous bone. Second, the cancellous portion of the graft is placed in direct contact to the host bone in the area where the implant will be placed during second surgery. The host bone surface is perforated during the surgical procedure to activate bone formation and to open the marrow space, allowing fast ingrowth of blood vessels. It can be expected that this portion of the graft will undergo rapid revascularization and graft remodeling. In addition, the preparation of an implant bed during second surgery will further activate bone remodeling in this area. These assumptions, however, are based on orthopedic literature, and histologic details of graft incorporation and repair underneath barrier membranes are not yet documented. Experimental studies evaluating these aspects are currently in progress.

Corticocancellous block grafts can be harvested either in the retromolar area of the mandible or in the chin, where the cortical layer normally has an appropriate thickness of 2 to 3 mm. The harvesting is uncomplicated and feasible within the extension of the same surgical flap. The block graft should be appropriately applied to the recipient site. First, rigid fixation of the graft is important. A bone-graft fixation screw should be used because it allows precise positioning of the graft and prevents micromovements of the graft underneath the membrane during healing. Second, the block graft must be placed with its cortical layer facing buccally and the can-

cellous portion of the graft in direct contact of the host bone, as discussed previously. Based on more than 6 years of experience with the combination of 3-PTFE membranes and autografts, treatment outcome can clearly be optimized in both maxillary and mandibular sites,[21–23] as demonstrated in the clinical examples presented at the end of this section. When autografts and the GBR technique are combined, the membrane has a double function. First, it serves as a physical barrier to protect the created space against nonosteogenic cells derived from the mucosa. Second, the membrane serves as a graft preservation device, protecting the autograft from postoperative resorption. It has been documented that autogenous bone graft applied in ridge augmentation procedures without membranes show resorption of up to 50% after 6 months of healing.[34] Resorption in ridge augmentation cases has not been observed when bone grafts were protected by a membrane. This clinical observation has been confirmed in patients undergoing vertical alveolar ridge augmentation utilizing autografts from the iliac crest.[35] As an alternative to autografts, mineralized and demineralized freeze-dried bone allografts have been used as a membrane-supporting device in ridge augmentation procedures as well,[15, 36–40] and some of these publications have presented encouraging clinical results.[37,39,40] Allografts have the advantage that no harvesting procedure is necessary. However, histologic details of allograft incorporation and their substitution underneath barrier membranes and adjacent to implants are not sufficiently known for each material at present and need further investigation to provide information concerning their predictability for clinical outcomes.

Healing Time

A last factor important for achieving predictable results is a sufficiently long healing period. It has been demonstrated that sites of early membrane removal attain less gain in bone height.[41–43] However, the exact healing period for ridge augmentation procedures with the GBR technique is not known at present. A histologic study involving extended defects in the alveolar ridge in foxhounds revealed almost complete cortical and cancellous bone repair and an onset of bone remodeling after 4 months of healing in membrane-covered defects.[14] These defects are surgically created and no osteoconductive filler was used. The study confirmed that bone regeneration and bone maturation is a time-dependent process, even in an animal known for its rapid healing. Based on this fact, a healing period of 9 months has been used during the development of this technique for ridge augmentation procedures in large bone defects. Clinical experience has proven this length of time to be efficacious.[12, 21–23] However, it can be speculated that the healing period may be shortened when membranes combined

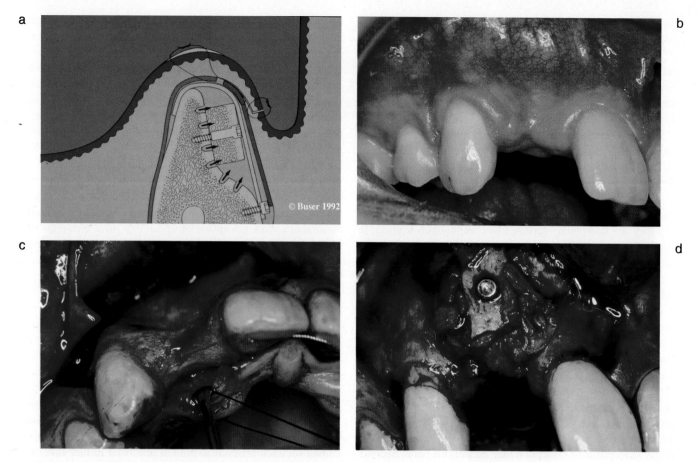

FIGURE 16.1 Staged approach of guided bone regeneration. (a) Schematic overview of staged approach to augment a deficient alveolar ridge. Note lateral split-thickness/full-thickness incision and wound-closing technique. (b) Patient with missing right lateral incisor. Compromised width of alveolar site. (c) Mucoperiosteal flap elevated; deficient alveolar bone site does not allow placement of implant. (d) Corticocancellous bone block graft secured with bone fixation screw. Small autologous bone chips are arranged around block graft.

with autogenous bone grafts are used because of the excellent osteoconductive properties of autografts. This expectation has been confirmed in more than 30 cases with a healing period of 6 months.

Summary

Over the past several years, the ridge augmentation procedure using e-PTFE membranes and autografts has proven to be an efficient and predictable surgical technique.[21–23] This technique uses a staged approach, which has numerous advantages over a simultaneous approach in large bone defects in the alveolar process. First, it provides a larger bone surface available to contribute to new bone formation, because no implant is inserted in the defect area. With a simultaneous approach, the inserted implant reduces the exposed bone surface and its marrow space as a source of angiogenic and osteogenic cells. Second, the implant positioning can be optimized from a prosthetic point of view because the implant is placed when the new crest is already reestablished. Following confirmation of the treatment outcome, this allows a much easier preparation of the recipient site and a better initial stability for the implant. Third, the staged approach offers advantages with respect to

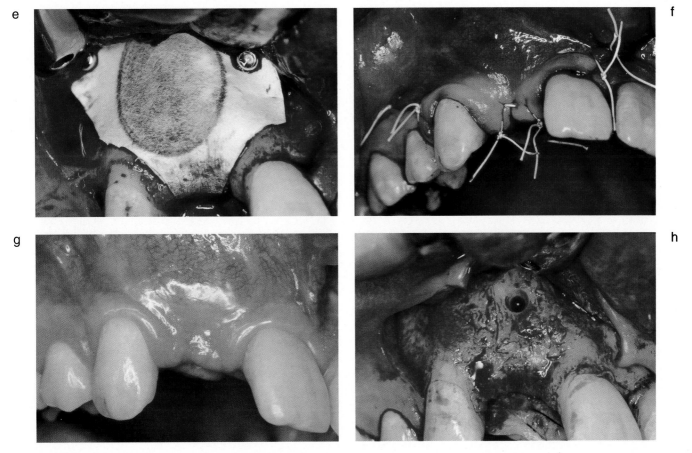

FIGURE 16.1 *Continued.* (e) GTAM membrane adapted and secured with miniature fixation screws (Memfix System, Institut Straumann AG, Waldenburg, Switzerland). (f) Primary flap closure with Gore-Tex sutures. (g) Postoperative follow-up at 7 months. (h) Reopening surgery, Memfix screws and membrane removed.

Continued.

bone maturation because new bone formation is activated twice by the local release of growth factor.[44] The first activation occurs during membrane surgery, when the cortical layer is perforated prior to graft placement. The second activation occurs during implant placement, when the implant recipient site is prepared in the newly formed alveolar crest. Finally, it can be assumed that better bone apposition to the titanium surface can be achieved with a staged approach because the "travel distance" for osteogenic elements to the implant surface is much shorter. Thus the staged approach should be the treatment of choice for large bone defects in the alveolar process, whereas the simultaneous approach can be used in smaller defects. The question of whether bone regenerated using the barrier technique is "for real" has recently been answered in two dog experiments.[14, 45] These studies have shown that the newly regenerated bone closely resembled the structure of preexisting alveolar bone,[14,45] and osseointegration of unloaded and loaded implants in these regenerated bone sites occurred identically as for preexisting bone.[45]

Case Reports

Figures 16.1 and 16.2 show illustrative examples from case reports.

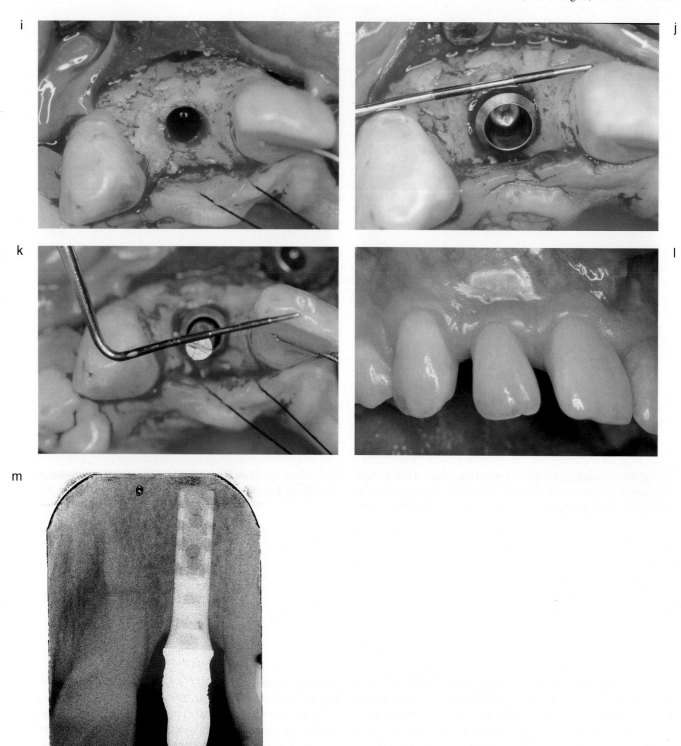

FIGURE 16.1 *Continued*. (i) Result of alveolar augmentation in an occlusal view. Site prepared for ITI Hollow-Cylinder (HC) implant in ideal position. (j) Implant placed to correct vertical level (i.e., shoulder apical to cementoenamel junction of neighbor teeth). (k) HC implant in proper axis direction for screw-retained restoration with screw access in the cingulum area of the future crown. (l) Final restoration (porcelain-fused-to-metal) in place. (m) Radiographic control.

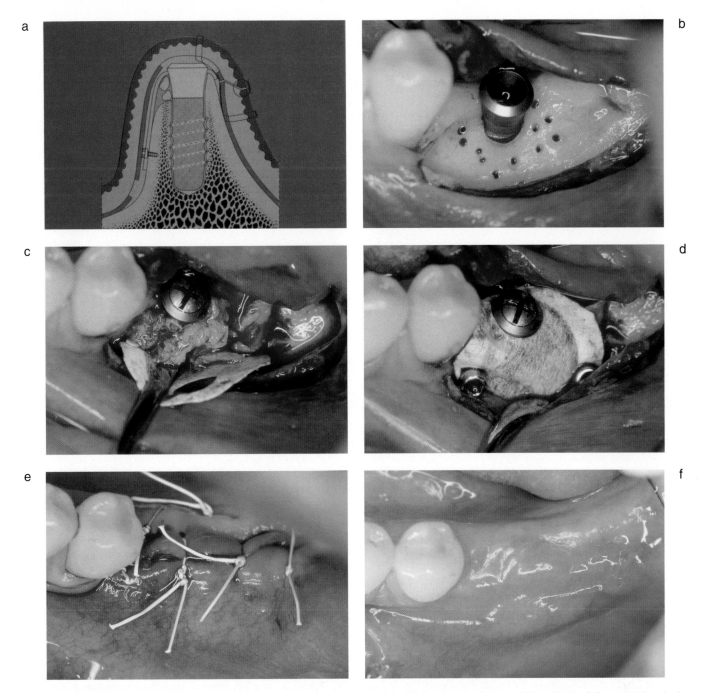

FIGURE 16.2 Simultaneous approach of guided bone regeneration. (a) Schematic overview on simultaneous approach for alveolar ridge augmentation. Note incision technique as in staged approach. (b) Implant placed in area of lower left first molar. Note buccal alveolar dehiscence. Surrounding bone is perforated with a small round bur to promote bleeding and a source for cells with bone-forming po- tential. (c) Autologous bone particles obtained from implant bed preparation (bone core) placed in area of dehiscence. Small closure screw placed in implant. (d) GTAM membrane adapted as "poncho" over implant and secured with two Memfix screws. (e) Primary wound closure. (f) Postoperative follow-up at 1 month.

Continued.

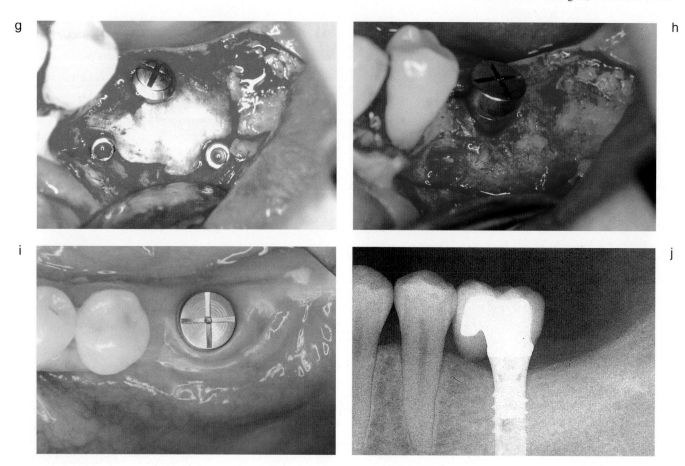

FIGURE 16.2 *Continued*. (g) Reopening surgery at 6 months. (h) Result of augmentation. Small implant closure screw replaced with transmucosal healing cap. (i) Postoperative follow-up 3 weeks after reopening surgery. (j) Radiographic control 1 year after crown insertion.

References

1. Brånemark P-I, Zarb GA, Albrektsson T, eds. *Tissue-Integrated Prostheses: Osseointegration in Clinical Dentistry*. Chicago: Quintessence; 1985.

2. Schroeder A, Sutter F, Krekeler G, eds. *Oral Implantology. General Basics and ITI-Hollow-Cylinder System*. New York: Thieme Medical; 1991.

3. Nyman S, Lindhe J, Karring T. Reattachment-new attachment. In: Lindhe J, ed. *Textbook of Clinical Periodontology*. 2nd ed. Copenhagen: Munksgard; 1989:450–476.

4. Dahlin C, Linde A, Gottlow J, et al. Healing of bone defects by guided tissue regeneration. *Plast Reconstr Surg*. 1988;81:672–676.

5. Buser D, Dahlin C, Schenk RK, eds. *Guided Bone Regeneration in Implant Dentistry*. Chicago: Quintessence; 1994.

6. Dahlin C, Sennerby L, Lekholm, et al. Generation of new bone around titanium implants using a membrane technique: An experimental study in rabbits. *Int J Oral Maxillofac Implants*. 1989;4:19–25.

7. Dahlin C, Gottlow J, Linde A, et al. Healing of maxillary and mandibular bone defects using a membrane technique. *Scand J Plast Reconstr Hand Surg*. 1990;24:13–19.

8. Seibert J, Nyman S. Localized ridge augmentation in dogs: a pilot study using membranes and hydroxylapatite. *J Periodontol*. 1990;61;157–165.

9. Becker W, Becker B, Handlesman M, et al. Bone formation at dehisced dental implant sites treated with implant augmentation material: a pilot study in dogs. *Int J Periodont Rest Dent*. 1990; 10:93–101.

10. Lazarra RJ Immediate implant placement into extraction sites: Surgical and restorative advantages. *Int J Periodont Rest Dent*. 1989;9:333–343.

11. Nyman S, Lang NP, Buser D, et al. Bone regeneration adjacent to titanium dental implants using guided tissue regeneration: a report of two cases. *Int J Oral Maxillofac Implants*. 1990;5: 9–14.

12. Buser D, Brägger U, Lang NP, et al. Regeneration and enlargement of jaw bone using guided tissue regeneration. *Clin Oral Implants Res*. 1990;1:22–32.

13. Jovanovic S, Spiekermann H, Richter EJ. Bone regeneration around titanium dental implants in dehisced defect sites: a clinical study. *Int J Oral Maxillofac Implants* 1992;7:233–241.

14. Schenk RK, Buser D, Hardwick WR, Dahlin C. Healing pattern of bone regeneration in membrane-protected defects. A histologic study in the canine mandible. *Int J Oral Maxillofac Implants*. 1994;9:13–29.

15. Gotfredsen K, Warrer K, Hjørting-Hansen E, et al. Effect of

membranes and hydroxyapatite on healing in bone defects around titanium implants. An experimental study in the monkey. *Clin Oral Implants Res.* 1991;2:172–178.

16. Warrer K, Gotfredsen K, Hjøerting-Hansen E, et al. Guided tissue regeneration allowing immediate implantation of dental implants into extraction sockets. An experimental study in the monkey. *Clin Oral Implants Res.* 1991;2:166–171.

17. Wachtel HC, Langford A, Bernimoulin JP, et al. Guided bone regeneration next to osseointegrated implants in humans. *Int J Oral Maxillofac Implants.* 1991;6:127–135.

18. Becker W, Becker B. Guided tissue regeneration for implants placed into extraction sockets and for implant dehiscences: surgical techniques and case reports. *Int J Periodont Rest Dent.* 1990;10:377–392.

19. Jovanovic SA, Giovannoli JL. New bone formation by the principle of guided tissue regeneration for peri-implant osseous lesions. *J Parodontol.* 1992;11:29–39.

20. Magnusson I, Batich C, Collins BR. New attachment formation following controlled tissue regeneration using biodegradable membranes. *J Periodontol.* 1988;59:1–12.

21. Buser D, Dula K, Belser U, Hirt HP, Berthold H. Localized ridge augmentation using guided bone regeneration. I. Surgical procedure in the maxilla. *Int J Periodont Rest Dent.* 1993;13:29–45.

22. Buser D, Dula K, Belser U, Hirt HP, Berthold H. Localized ridge augmentation using guided bone regeneration. II. Surgical procedure in the mandible. *Int J Periodont Rest Dent.* 1995;15:13–29.

23. Buser D, Dula K, Hirt HP, Schenk RK. Lateral ridge augmentation using autografts and barrier membranes. A clinical study in 40 partially edentulous patients. *J Oral Maxillofac Surg.* 1996;54:420–432.

24. Fleisher N, De Waal H, Bloom A. Regeneration of lost attachment in the dog using Vicryl absorbable mesh (polyglactin 910). *Int J Periodont Rest Dent.* 1988;8(2):45–54.

25. Chung KM, Lakin LM, Stein MD, et al. Clinical evaluation of a biodegradable collagen membrane in guided tissue regeneration. *J Periodontol.* 1990;61:732–741.

26. Schultz AJ, Gager AH. Guided tissue regeneration using absorbable membrane (polyglactin 910) and osseous grafting. *Int J Periodont Rest Dent.* 1990;10:8–15.

27. Zappa U. Resorbierbare Membranen. I. Parodontale Geweberegeneration unter Verwendung von resorbierbaren Membranen-klinische Aspekte. *Schweiz Monatsschr Zahnmed.* 1991;101:1147–1155.

28. Zappa U. Resorbierbare Membranen. II. Parodontale Geweberegeneration unter Verwendung von resorbierbaren Membranen—Histologische Aspekte. *Schweiz Monatsschr Zahnmed.* 1991;101:1321–1331.

29. Fugazzotto P. Ridge augmentation with titanium screws and guided tissue regeneration: Technique and report of a case. *Int J Periodont Rest Dent.* 1993;13:335–339.

30. Becker W, Becker BE, McGuire MK. Localized ridge augmentation using absorbable pins and e-PTFE barrier membranes: a new surgical technique. Case reports. *Int J Periodont Rest Dent.* 1994;14:49–61.

31. Tinti C, Vincenzi G, Cochetto R. Guided tissue regeneration in mucogingival surgery. *J Periodontol.* 1993;64:1184–1191.

32. Burchardt H. Biology of bone transplantation. *Orthodont Clin North Am.* 1987;18:187–196.

33. Burchardt H. Biology of bone graft repair. *Clin Orthop Relat Res.* 1983;174:28–42.

34. ten Bruggenkate CM, Kraajenhagen HA, van der Kwast WAM, et al. Autogenous maxillary bone grafts in conjunction with placement of ITI endosseous implants. A preliminary report. *Int J Oral Maxillofac Surg.* 1992;21:81–84.

35. Jensen O. Guided bone graft augmentation. In: Buser D, Dahlin C, Schenk RK, eds. *Guided Bone Regeneration in Implant Dentistry.* Chicago: Quintessence; 1994:235–264.

36. Buser D, Berthold H. Knochendefektfüllung im Kieferbereich mit Kollagenvlies. *Dtsch Z Mund Kiefer Gesichtschir.* 1986;10:191–198.

37. Nevins R, Mellonig JT. Enhancement of the damaged edentulous ridge to receive dental implants: A combination of allograft and the GoreTex membrane. *Int J Periodont Rest Dent.* 1992;12:97–111.

38. Becker B, Lynch S, Lekholm U, et al. A comparison of three methods for promoting bone formation around implants placed into immediate extraction sockets: e-PTFE membrane alone, or with either PDGF and IGF-I, or DFDB. *J Periodontol.* 1992;63:929–940.

39. Shanaman RH. The use of guided tissue regeneration to facilitate ideal prosthetic placement of implants. *Int J Periodont Rest Dent.* 1992;12:226–265.

40. Nevins R, Mellonig JT. The advantages of localized ridge augmentation prior to implant placement: a staged event. *Int J Periodont Rest Dent.* 1994;14:97–111.

41. Simion M, Baldoni M, Rossi P, Zaffe D. A comparative study of the effectiveness of e-PTFE membranes with and without early exposure during the healing period. *Int J Periodont Rest Dent.* 1994;14:167–180.

42. Becker W, Dahlin C, Becker BE, et al. The use of e-PTFE barrier membranes for bone promotion around titanium implants placed into extraction sockets: a prospective multicenter study. *Int J Maxillofac Implants.* 1994;9:31–40.

43. Lekholm U, Becker W, Dahlin C, et al. The role of early vs late removal of GTAM membranes on bone formation around oral implants placed in immediate extraction sockets: an experimental study in dogs. *Clin Oral Implants Res.* 1993;4:121–129.

44. Schenk RK. Bone regeneration: biologic basis. In: Buser D, Dahlin C, Schenk RK, eds. *Guided Bone Regeneration in Implant Dentistry.* Chicago: Quintessence; 1994:49–100.

45. Buser D, Ruskin J, Higginbottom F, Hardwick R, Dahlin C, Schenk RK. Osseointegration of titanium implants in bone regenerated in membrane-protected defects: a histologic study in the canine mandible. *Int J Oral Maxillofac Implants.* 1995;10:666–681.

17
The ITI Dental Implant System in Maxillofacial Applications

Dieter Weingart, Daniel A. Buser, and Hans-Peter Weber

In severe trauma cases, after jaw resection in tumor surgery, and especially in cases of severe atrophy of the maxillary or mandibular alveolar ridge, a direct implant placement using the one-stage approach with ITI implants as described in Chapter 15 is often not possible. Also, the technique of guided bone regeneration discussed in that chapter would not be an efficient method to restore areas of such extended and severe alveolar atrophy. Therefore, a vertical augmentation with bone grafts most frequently obtained from the iliac crest is the method of choice in patients presenting with such conditions (Figures 17.1–17.4). As with guided bone regeneration, two methods regarding timing of implant placement may be differentiated: (1) implant insertion simultaneously with the bone grafts in which instance the implants serve to stabilize the grafts to the basal bone; and (2) stage approach, that is, the bone grafts are stabilized by means of miniplates or screws, which are removed after graft healing at which time the implants are inserted (Figures 17.1 and 17.2).

As a prerequisite for the use of free bone grafts, a maximum wound closure during the healing phase is required. Accordingly, the implants in this indication need to be inserted to the bone level, and the mucoperiosteal flap must cover the implants after suturing. A modification of the standard ITI Dental Implant System was necessary to allow that at the time of second-stage surgery (i.e., after bone-graft healing and osseointegration of the implants) transmucosal extensions can be attached. For this purpose, the ITI Extender System was developed.[1–5] The available extensions allow the adaptation of the peri-implant mucosa to this transmucosal component (Figure 17.5d).

After completion of soft tissue healing following second-stage surgery, any of the prosthetic abutments of the regular ITI system may be placed on top of the extensions, and the superstructure is fabricated according to standard procedures.

Surgical Procedure

As outlined earlier, the implants used for the stabilization of bone grafts are to be inserted into the transplants in a submerged manner, mainly for reasons of infection prophylaxis

and prevention of graft resorption. The ITI full-body screws, available in lengths of 6 to 16 mm, are used for these indications. Owing to their flared neck, the ITI screw implants function as tension screws, building up an interfragmentary compression between the natural bone bed of the jaw bone and the bone transplant (Figure 17.6e).

The surgical augmentation procedure and the implantation with ITI screw implants as well as the use of the transgingival extension system is documented step by step in Figures 17.5 and 17.6. At first surgery, the implant (ITI FS) is inserted to its shoulder into the bone graft and covered with a small closure screw. The mucoperiosteal flap is then positioned over the bone graft and implants (Figure 17.6g). At second-stage surgery following a healing phase of 3 to 6 months, the implants are exposed, the healing caps removed, and the basal screws and the mucosa cylinders are inserted and covered with healing caps (Figures 17.5a–d). After completion of wound healing (3 to 4 weeks), the prosthetic phase is started with the insertion of the abutments after removal of the healing caps.

Mechanical Aspects

At second-stage surgery, it is important to consider that the basal screw and the mucosa cylinder are used in corresponding pairs and in accordance with the standard lengths (Figure 17.7). The microgaps between the implant and the extension parts are kept as small as technically possible.

This transgingival unit of the extender system has been mechanically tested under different loading conditions. As a result of preliminary tests with different designs, an integrated attachment (basal screw) was chosen. As usual for ITI secondary components, its apical portion comprises an 8° cone and a 2-mm screw for attachment to the implant. This cone-to-screw design provides a frictional fit, eliminating the risk of loosening of the basal screw. The design of the coronal portions of the basal screw consists of a threaded part to which the corresponding mucosa cylinder is attached (Figure 17.7). It is preferably tightened with a torque meter adjusted to approximately 35 Ncm.

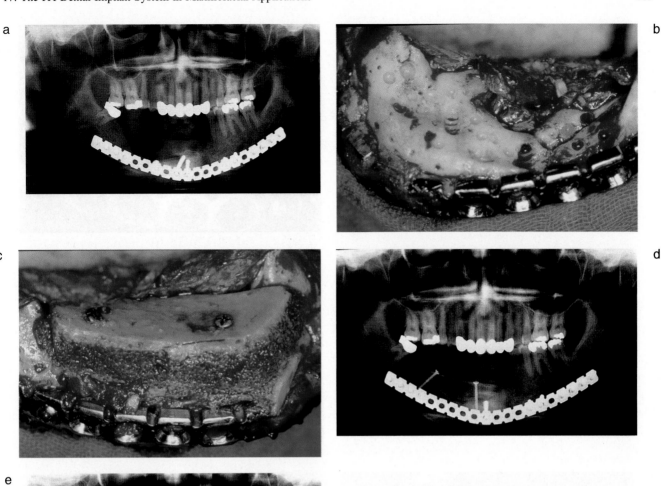

FIGURE 17.1 (a) Situation after a comminuted fracture of the mandible with a defect in the region of the right alveolar ridge stabilized with an AO 2.7 reconstruction plate. (b) The defect is exposed. The remaining vertical bone height in the premolar area is only 3 to 4 mm. (c) An autogenous corticocancellous iliac bone graft is adapted with two lag screws. (d) Radiological control 6 months after bone grafting before implant placement. (e) Situation after mandibular reconstruction and implant placement of ITI full-body screw. For transgingival elongation, the ITI Extender System is inserted.

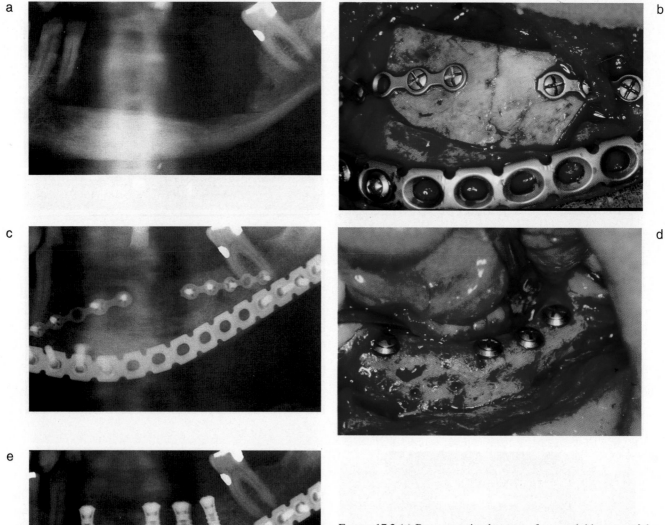

FIGURE 17.2 (a) Bone resection because of an ameloblastoma of the mandible. (b,c) After pathohistological evaluation of the resection border, reconstruction of the mandible with an autogenous cortico-cancellous iliac bone graft. Fixation of the graft with AO 2.0 mini-plates, and stabilization of the mandible with an AO 2.4 universal plate. The alveolar nerve was preserved and lateralized. (d,e) The ITI full-body screw implants are inserted 5 to 6 months after bone grafting.

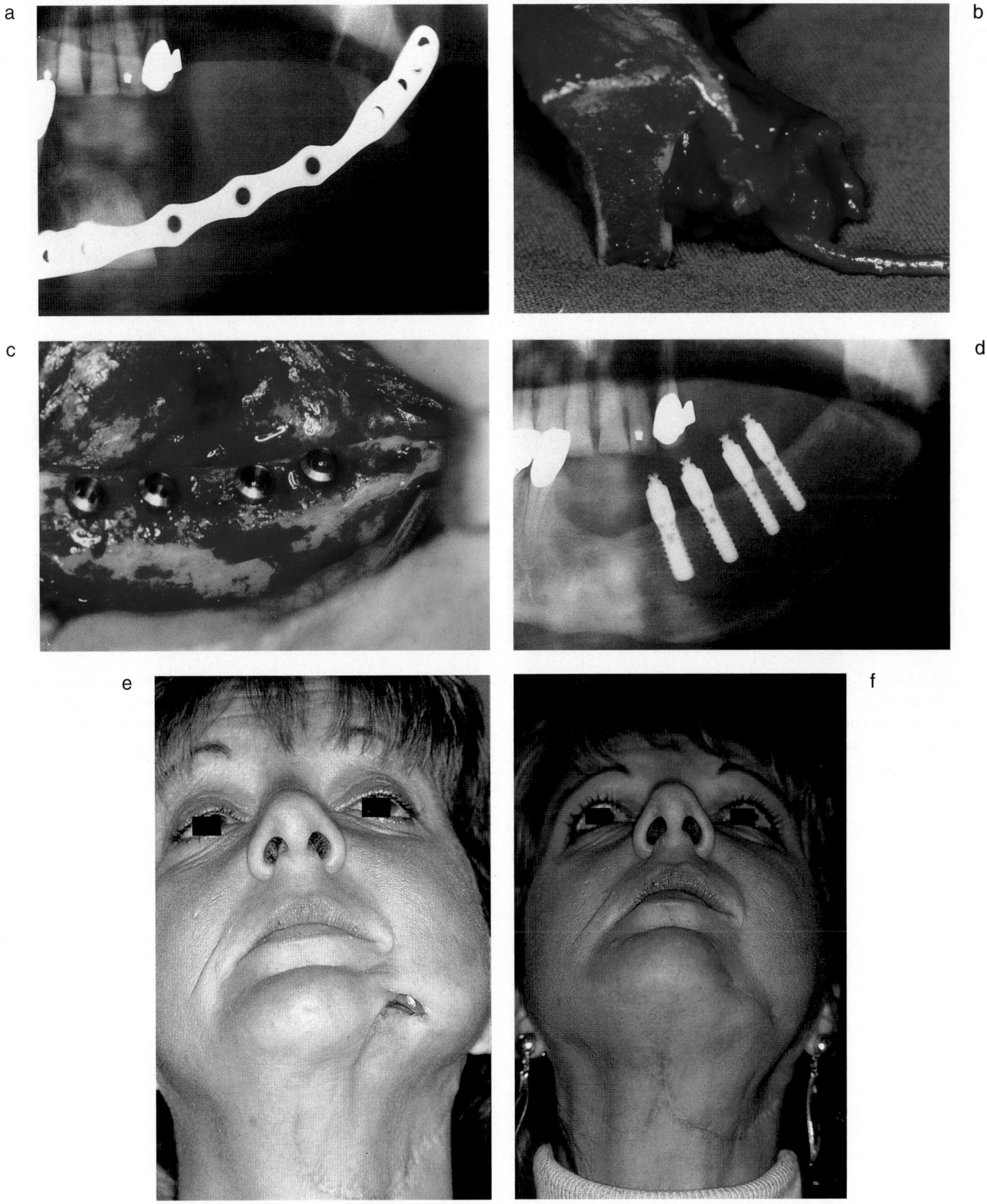

FIGURE 17.3 (a) Situation after resection in the left mandible because of a carcinoma of the floor of the mouth. (b) Restoration by microsurgically revascularized iliac crest bone graft. (c) The implants are inserted into the bone graft during a second-stage approach. (d) Good osseointegration of the implants in the grafted bone with only minimal vertical resorption. The ITI Extender System was inserted 3 months following implant placement. (e) Preoperative extraoral aspect of the patient, with perforation of the reconstruction plate through the skin. (f) Postoperative extraoral aspect of the patient following mandibular reconstruction with revascularized iliac bone graft and implant placement.

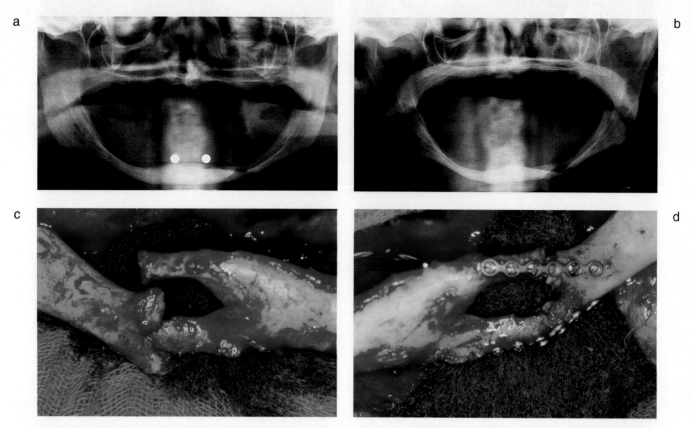

FIGURE 17.4 (a) Extreme atrophy of the mandibular alveolar ridge. Measurements for evaluating the vertical height were performed. Patient refused an augmentation procedure. (b) Situation 2 years later. Increase of alveolar ridge atrophy. Patient came back with a fracture of the extremely atrophied left mandible. (c) Intraoperative sit-uation after an extraoral approach: Fracture and dislocation occurred because there was no bone in the middle of the mandibular ridge. (d) Initial stabilization of fracture with miniplate fixation to allow anatomic segment positioning for reconstruction plate application in the same operation.

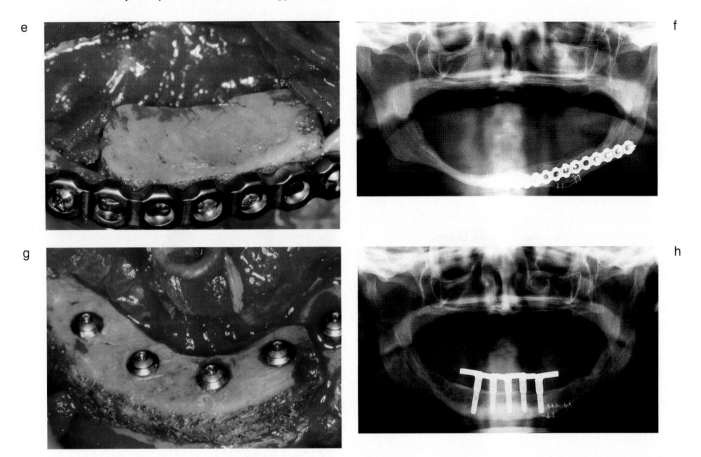

FIGURE 17.4 *Continued*. (e) Stabilization of the fracture with an AO 2.4 reconstruction plate and simultaneous bone grafting with autogenous iliac bone. (f) Radiological control 6 months after fracture treatment and augmentation on the left side of the mandible. (g) Augmentation on the anterior and right region of the mandible: the implants are inserted through the corticocancellous bone graft into the mandible (see Figure 17.6). Good interfragmentary compression between the natural bone bed of the jaw bone and the bone transplant due to implant configuration and a certain lag-screw effect. (h) Situation after posthodontic treatment with a bar suprastructure: the ITI Extender System in place. Compare the bony situation with (b). Increase in vertical bone height and titanium microplate for fracture adaption still in place.

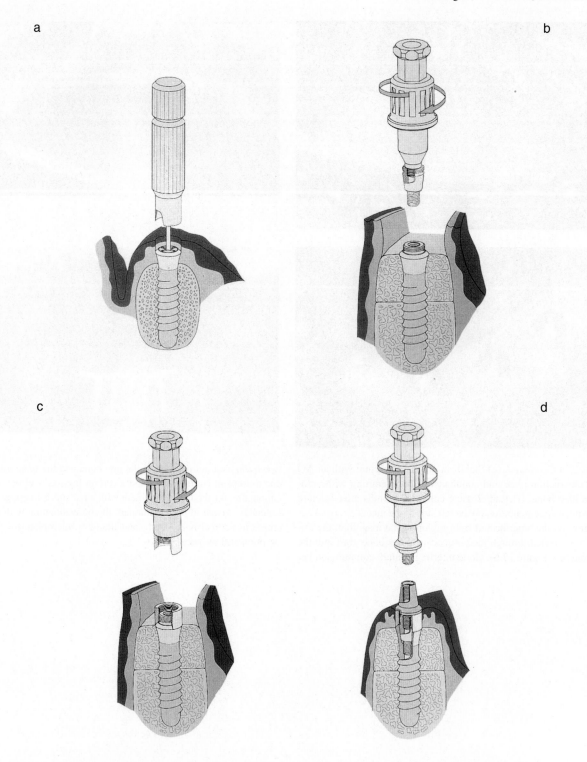

FIGURE 17.5 (a) After the healing phase, the implants are exposed either by incision or by punching. The basal screw (b) and the mucosa cylinder (c) are inserted with a special insertion instrument. (d) The assembled transgingival elongation system.

a

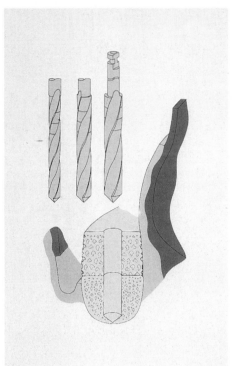

b

c

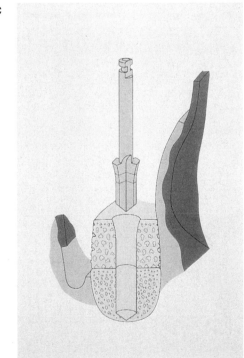

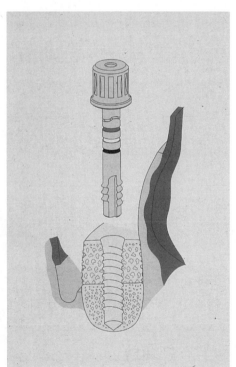

d

FIGURE 17.6 Step-by-step representation of the surgical sequence. After vestibular incision and adoption of the transplant, the implant bed is prepared in the usual way. (a) Marking with the round bur.

(b) Drilling to the desired depth with three spiral drills. (c) Profiling of the neck portion. (d) The next step is to pretap the thread in accordance with the depth.

Continued.

e

f

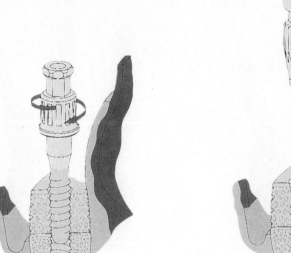

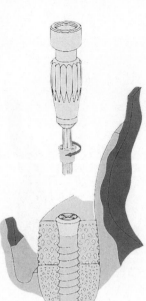

g

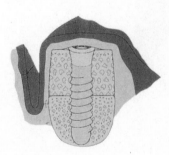

FIGURE 17.6 *Continued*. (e) The implant is introduced with a standard insertion instrument through the bone graft into the ridge. (f) Insertion of the closure screw into the subgingival positioned implant. (g) The situation after suturing the periosteum and the mucosa.

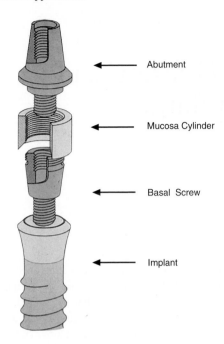

FIGURE 17.7 Parts of the ITI Extender System.

With regard to their coronal configuration, the prosthetic components of the extender system correspond to those of the standard ITI Dental Implant System (conical abutment, retentive anchor, and octa-abutment) and are also manufactured from pure titanium. Any of these abutments can be attached to the mucosa cylinder.

Maximum tightening moments of more than 400 Ncm could be achieved with the new transgingival unit compared with 125 Ncm observed with a conventional 2-mm flat coupling screw. Additional dynamic loading tests proved that the loosening moment remained approximately 10% above the tightening moment after 2,000,000 cycles.[4]

Summary

Positive experience and results with endosteal implants in the field of standard oral implantology led to an extension of the indication to implantations into transplants. In these cases, the simultaneous use of screw implants facilitated optimal graft adaptation and fixation. Originally, ITI implants were designed for a transmucosal (one-stage) implant placement. Using bone-graft procedures, it is necessary to cover the bone graft with a soft tissue flap to get satisfactory incorporation of the bone. These cases need second-stage surgery and a special abutment device.

The extender system presented here provides a simple method of restoring ITI implants placed in combination with autogenous bone transplants with various prosthetic superstructures.

References

1. Asikainen P, Sutter F. The new distance system for the submergible use of the ITI-Bonefit Implants. *J Oral Implantol.* 1990;4:48–54.
2. Sutter F, Weingart D, Mundwiler U, Sutter F, Asikainen P. ITI implants in combination with bone grafts: design and biomechanical aspects. *Clin Oral Implants Res.* 1990;5:164–172.
3. Weingart D, Strub JR, Schilli W. Kieferchirurgisch-prothetisches Konzept zur implantologischen Versorgung bei unterschiedlichem Atrophiegrad des zahnlosen Patienten. *Z Stomatol.* 1992;3:137–145.
4. Sutter F, Weber HP, Sorensen J, Belser U. The new restorative concept of the ITI Dental Implant System: design and engineering. *Int J Periodont Rest Dent.* 1993;13:409–431.
5. Weingart D, Strub JR, Schilli W, Schenk R, Kleinheinz J, Hürzeler B. Mandibular ridge augmentation combining onlay iliac bone graft with endosseous implant placement in dogs. *J Dent Res.* 1993;72:204–205.

18

Maxillary Sinus Grafting and Osseointegration Surgery

Jeffrey I. Stein and Alex M. Greenberg

Posterior maxillary dental implant reconstruction for advanced alveolar ridge atrophy has become possible through bone grafting procedures involving the maxillary sinus. This procedure involves augmentation of either the internal or the external aspects of the sinus, or both. Bone grafting of the external aspect is usually performed with guided bone regeneration using allogeneic, autogenous cortical, or corticocancellous grafts as onlays with immediate or delayed implant placement.[1] Sandwich techniques of bone grafting both the external ridge and the internal sinus with simultaneous dental implant placement has also been reported.[2] Sailer and Keller et al. have reported the use of iliac crest bone grafts with the immediate placement of dental implants with Le Fort I osteotomies.[3,4] However, this is a more extensive technique with increased possibilities for morbidity in this older patient population.

What has become the most common procedure for this region of reconstruction, however, is the sinus lift graft procedure, which was first reported in 1976 at the Alabama Implant Congress by Tatum et al.[5] This procedure is further supported by Jensen et al., who prefer sinus grafting as opposed to onlay grafts, which tend to have greater resorption.[6] In this technique, a bony window in the lateral sinus wall is infractured, and the sinus membrane is preserved intact and elevated superiorly. Initially, Tatum's technique involved the use of autologous bone. A bone graft of various reported compositions is placed, and immediate or delayed dental implant placement is performed. A review of the literature reveals that this new procedure has various reports and that several methods of bone grafts have been proposed. The reports of sinus lifting technique are basically the same with regard to the type of incisions, lateral sinus wall osteotomy, sinus membrane elevation, and use of root form implants. It is with regard to various types of bone grafts that numerous authors report differences in their methods.

Tatum et al. reported more than 1500 cases using either 100% autogenous bone of iliac crest origin, demineralized freeze-dried bone, or irradiated bone and some experience with mixtures of these types with various forms of hydroxyapatite.[5] Jensen et al. reported only the use of 100% autoge-

nous iliac crest cancellous bone grafts.[6] Raghoebar et al. reported 25 patients who had various autogenous bone grafts of iliac crest (22), symphysis (2), and maxillary tuberosity (1) origin.[7] Block and Kent advocate the use of a 1:1 mixture of autogenous bone with demineralized bone.[8]

Vlassis et al. reported using a mixture of demineralized allogeneic bone gel (Grafton; Musculoskeletal Transplant Foundation, Little Silver, NJ, USA) and resorbable hydroxyapatite (Osteogen; Stryker, Kalamazoo, MI, USA).[9] Fugazzotto reported the use of a 1:1 mixture of demineralized bone and resorbable tricalcium phosphate (Augmen; Miter and Co.).[10] Moy et al. have performed a comprehensive histomorphometric investigation regarding four different maxillary sinus grafting materials, which consisted of autogenous symphysis bone (44.4% bone), hydroxyapatite (20.3% bone), hydroxyapatite and demineralized bone, 7:1 (4.6% bone), and hydroxyapatite and autogenous symphysis bone, 1:1 (59.4% bone).[11]

Treatment Planning

A multitude of prosthetic and surgical alternatives exist for treatment of the partially or completely edentulous posterior maxilla. It must first be determined if conventional nonimplant dentistry is a viable alternative. Numerous questions need to be addressed. In the partially edentulous patients, are the remaining teeth in sufficient number, periodontally fit, and strategically located to serve as abutments for a traditional fixed bridge or removable partial denture? In complete edentulism, a determination must be made whether a denture can be fabricated with satisfactory retention. If not, would an implant supported overdenture be acceptable to the patient? In the presence of advanced atrophy with altered ridge relationships, will esthetic and occlusal demands be reasonably met without skeletal correction?

If implant treatment is to be considered, initial factors to be evaluated are the patient's age, medical history, and psychologic status. The patient's tolerance for surgery and a prolonged treatment time with the possibility of an extended pe-

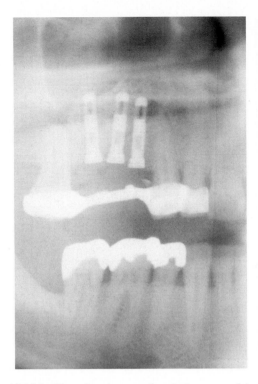

FIGURE 18.1 Maxillary sinus bone graft and placement of three dental implants to prevent fracture of a long span fixed bridge and failure of natural tooth abutments.

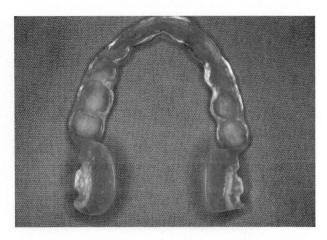

FIGURE 18.2 Surgical guide stent for bilateral maxillary sinus bone graft and dental implant placement.

riod without a prosthesis needs to be assessed. The surgical-restorative team must have a clear comprehension of the patient's complaints and desires and of each other's vision of the final restoration. Many individuals may not wish to further compromise remaining teeth to serve as abutments (Figure 18.1). Frequently, the only desire stated may be for a plan that would allow for a fixed rather than a removable prosthesis.

Load requirements must be delineated. Nonaxial loading from malaligned abutments/fixtures as well as long edentulous spans, more posterior locations, parafunctional habits, increase in crown/root (implant) ratio, and an opposing natural dentition all place a greater strain on the restoration. This problem is further compounded because the posterior maxillary bone density, especially in long-standing edentulism, is spongy with fewer trabeculae. Compromised stress-bearing capacity is inherent. Modification of the treatment plan needs to account for these biomechanical demands. If inadequate natural abutments are present, the use of fixture(s) generally restored as a free-standing unit should be considered (Figure 18.1). Fixture load tolerances are elevated by positioning implants along the long axis of force vectors as well as by increasing fixture number, length, diameter, and available surface area for osseointegration. This plan may be accomplished by altering the implant surface coating via plasma spraying.

These and future determinations are made on the basis of the initial patient discussion, examination, mounted cast evaluation, and diagnositc setup. These casts can later be utilized

for fabrication of a surgical guide stent (Figure 18.2). Radiographic assessment is an essential element of the workup. Minimally, a panoramic radiograph supplemented by periapical films is necessary. The magnification factors must be known either by comparison to a standard measure placed in the region under examination or by use of a film with a measured grid. From these radiographs, the periodontal-endodontic status of the remaining teeth are first considerations. Short- and long-term prognostic determinations as to the viability of teeth individually and whether they may serve as abutments needs to be judged. Edentulous areas as well as the tuberosity-pterygoid plate region should be surveyed for pathology and quantitatively assessed for vertical bone heights. A qualitative assessment of bone type may also be approximated. If no panoramic machine is available, the maxillary sinus may be screened with a Waters' view (Figure 18.3).

Should further radiographic data be necessary, or to delineate sinus pathology or septae detected on plain films, a

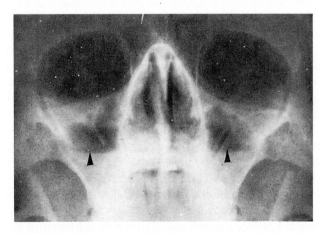

FIGURE 18.3 Waters' view demonstrating bilateral air/fluid levels indicating sinus infection (black arrows).

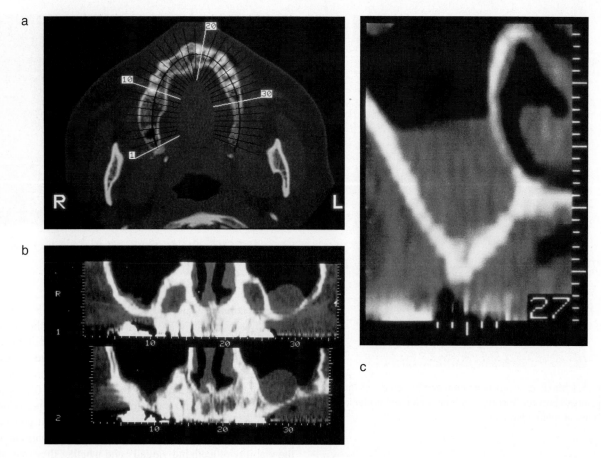

FIGURE 18.4 Computerized tomography scan reformatted with dental software. (a) Axial plane with numerically identified 3-mm sectional cuts correlated to each cross-sectional view. (b) Chronic left maxillary sinus membrane thickening and subantral bone atrophy. (c) Cross-sectional view also demonstrating left maxillary sinus membrane thickening and advanced subantral alveolar bone atrophy.

computed tomographic (CT) study should be ordered.[12,13] Patients with a significant history of sinus disease or smoking considering a sinus lift procedure also are required to obtain CT scanning. Reformatted CT utilizing specialized dental software will clearly demonstrate the residual bone length, width, and angulation. Qualitative bone assessment is also enhanced. Stents with radiopaque markers may be used to delineate prosthetically desirable implant locations in all views. Study and cross-referencing of the various dimensions will demystify and facilitate treatment planning (Figures 18.4a–c). Availability, cost, and additional radiation exposure dictate the need for CT scanning are made on an individual case-by-case basis.

Once it is evident that the residual dentition cannot serve as abutments and a fixed or removable restoration is desired, an implant treatment plan must be developed. Assessment of bone density and volume of individualized implant sites in light of biomechanical demands is critical. Generally, bone rising vertically 10 mm or more with adequate width to encase the fixture circumferentially permits utilization of the standard surgical approach. Minor vertical deficiencies may

be compensated for by placing the fixture apex slightly beyond the sinus floor and allowing for secondary bony doming. This can also be accomplished by localized apical sinus lifts which enhance length by imploding the fixture site sinus floor via an osteotome technique described later.[14,15] Localized width deficiencies may be augmented via a guided tissue regeneration procedure with simultaneous fixture placement or as a staged procedure. Fixture sites approximating 7 mm of height, particularly if poor bone quality is evident, require alternative planning. In this intermediary range, if biomechanical forces are not excessive, bony ridge inadequacies may be compensated by increasing the number or the diameter of fixtures utilized.

Unfortunately, minimum bony thresholds are frequently not met. Posterior maxillary atrophy inferiorly (crestally) and laterally results from periodontal disease and postextraction disuse resorption. Pneumatization of the maxillary sinus further compromises the residual alveolus. This expansion of the maxillary antrum results from a slight increase in intrasinus pressure during expiration, inducing osteoclastic activity in the periosteal layer of the Schneiderian membrane. The resid-

a

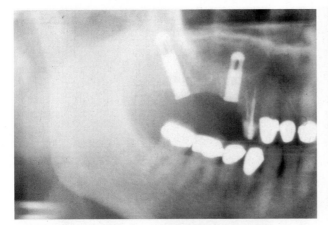

b

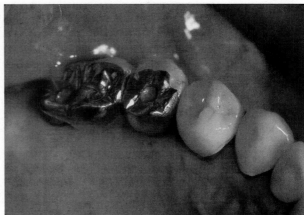

c

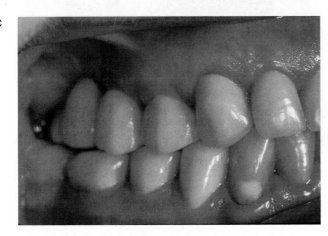

FIGURE 18.5 Posterior maxillary implant reconstruction without sinus grafting. (a) Panoramic radiograph with dental implants placed in the maxillary tuberosity and second premolar site in order to avoid sinus bone grafting. (b) Occlusal clinical view of fixed implant prosthesis. (c) Right buccal clinical view.

ual ridge may be narrow with a medial inclination and of minimal osseous volume.

If inadequate bone is present for traditional fixture placement, an alternative to subantral grafting to be considered is to bypass this region and place a fixture within the maxillary tuberosity, possibly extending into the pterygoid plates[16–18] (Figures 18.5a–c and 18.6a–c). This will provide a distal abutment for bridge fabrication. This option is only viable for short spans and if mesial and distal fixtures are of sufficient length and diameter. Excessive angulation of the distal fixture as well as other unfavorable biomechanical factors will commonly preclude implementation of this procedure.

The use of a distal cantilevered pontic is often entertained at this junction. Commonly, this is at the misguided prodding of the patient in their desire "to keep it simple" and avoid a graft procedure. The strain placed on the distal fixture in a cantilevered situation, especially if it is short or in poor quality bone, may lead to fixture failure or fracture (Figures 18.7a,b), or possible frequent abutment–prosthetic screw loosening or fracture. Similar considerations contraindicate the use of excess anterior lever arms when only posterior fixtures are available in the totally edentulous situation.

Restoration of the severely atrophic posterior maxilla re-

quires graft augmentation by either Le Fort I osteotomy with an autogenous interpositional corticocancellous graft,[3,4,19] an onlay corticocancellous graft, or a maxillary antrostomy with membrane elevation and a subantral graft, commonly referred to as a sinus lift or sinus inlay graft procedure. Limited indication exists for the Le Fort I approach. Because of the procedure's complexity and its lowest success rate of osseointegration at 68%,[20] the Le Fort I approach should be reserved for those patients who require a major correction of a class III ridge relationship. The maxillary onlay graft is a procedure of potentially greater complexity and postoperative complications, with a lower osseointegration success rate than the sinus inlay graft. Inital onlay results reported range from 50% to 90% but appear to approach 80% to 90% with experience.[2,19–24] An onlay graft procedure is indicated in lieu of the sinus inlay approach in the following circumstances: when severe buccal alveolar resorption would necessitate palatal implant placement or angulation, excessive interocclusal space would result in an unfavorable prosthesis/implant ratio, maxillary anterior augmentation is required, or when the patient has significant sinus disease or smoking addiction. It should be noted that anterior atrophy or posterior buccal atrophy may be alternatively addressed with adjunctive graft-

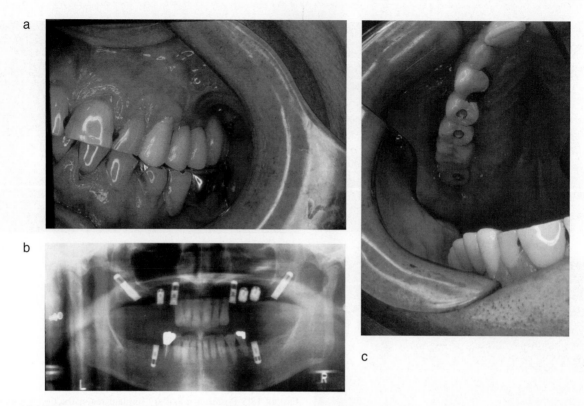

FIGURE 18.6 Bilateral posterior maxillary implant prosthesis supported with tuberosity and Subantral implants. (a) Left buccal clinical view. (b) Panoramic radiograph. (c) Left occlusal clinical view.

ing procedures (i.e., nasal inlay graft, localized guided tissue regeneration) in combination with the sinus lift technique.

The sinus lift procedure has, comparatively, the highest success rate and may be of less complexity and morbidity. Contraindications to sinus elevation and augmentation include sinusitis, presence of a cyst, tumor, or displaced root tip. These conditions may interfere with normal sinus drainage through the ostium, leading to a mucopurulent accumulation within the antrum. Sinus pathology must be resolved before grafting

to permit a well-ventilated, draining, aseptic antrum. Sinus inlay grafting alone will not address excess intermaxillary space or correct major skeletal discrepancies in the transverse or anteroposterior dimension. Alternative or adjunctive procedures should be considered. Smoking may be a relative to absolute contraindication depending on severity. Bain and Moy[25] reported smokers have more than twice the failure rate, 11.3% versus 4.8%, compared to nonsmokers in standard implant cases. Impaired polymorphonuclear neutrophil (PMN) func-

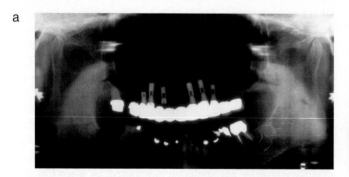

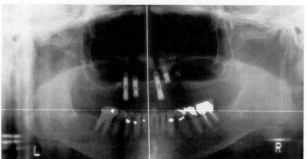

FIGURE 18.7 Failure of bilateral cantilevered prosthesis with resultant implant fractures. (a) Panoramic radiograph demonstrates right single cantilever and left double cantilever. (b) Panoramic radiograph following removal of fixed bridge. Right distal implant removed with retained implant apex, and left two distal implants with retained implant apices.

tion as well as local and systemic vasoconstrictive effects are believed responsible. Increased complications and failure have been evident in heavy smokers undergoing the sinus elevation procedure.[26–28] It is recommended that smoking be discontinued 2 months preoperatively and throughout the healing period.[29] Clinical data have yet to clearly define necessary time parameters. Patient compliance with such requirements is frequently difficult to monitor and achieve, despite new spoking cessation treatments.

Anatomy

The maxillary sinus is a paired, pyramidally shaped, pneumatic cavity occupying the body of the maxilla. The base of the pyramid lies medially, serving as the lateral nasal wall. This medial sinus wall–lateral nasal wall merges with the anterior wall to form the tallest vertical strut of the maxilla. Posteriorly, the maxillary antrum abuts the pterygoid plates. The lateral sinus wall is contiguous with the buccal plate of the alveolar bone. Superiorly, the sinus roof helps form the orbital floor. Inferiorly, the floor of the maxillary sinus extends below the level of the nasal cavity. Bony septae (buttress) frequently join the medial or the lateral walls to reinforce the sinus cavity. These septae may divide the sinus into two or more cavities that may or may not communicate.

The dimensions and capacity of the sinus demonstrate marked variability, dependent on sinus expansion. It is the largest of the four paranasal sinuses, with an approximate height at the base of 35 mm. The mediolateral base width is 35 mm, which tapers to 25 mm in the first molar regions. Its anteroposterior depth is generally in excess of 30 mm. The maxillary antrum has an average volume capacity of 15 ml.

The sinus is lined with a thin delicate pseudostratified ciliated cuboidal to columnar epithelium tightly bound to and indistinguishable from the underlying periosteum. The periosteum has few elastic fibers and is loosely bound to bone, facilitating surgical elevation. In the lining there are three glandular cell types—goblet, mucous, and serous—with the latter two concentrated near the ostium. Approximately 2 liters of fluid is produced per day. The fluid layer is divided into an outer gel-like mucous layer for transport that overlies a less viscous serous fluid layer surrounding the cilia. The cilia beat in a coordinated undulating manner, propelling a blanket of mucus and intrasinus debris toward the ostium for drainage into the nose.

The ostium is located along the superior aspect of the medial wall, 25 to 35 mm above the antral floor, and drains through the anterior aspect of the middle meatus. The ostium is a ductlike orifice 3.5 × 6 mm in cross section, extending superomedially 3.5 to 10 mm in length. The ostium position, high on the medial wall, is further hindered by the ductlike configuration, making passive (gravitational) drainage ineffective.

The sinus functions to lighten the weight of the skull and to warm and debride inhaled air, as well as acting as a resonance chamber for voice modulation. Normal sinus function requires the patency of the ostium, a functioning ciliary apparatus, and secretions qualitatively and quantitatively appropriate.

The arterial vasculature to the maxillary antrum derives from branches of the internal maxillary artery (ethmoidal, infraorbital, facial, and palatine). Venous drainage medially is into the sphenopalatine vein while the remaining walls drain through the pterygomaxillary plexus. Innervation is provided by branches of the trigeminal nerve, second division (lateral posterior superior nasal, superior alveolar, and infraorbital nerves).

Sinus inlay grafting in reports discussed previously has demonstrated success rates generally well in excess of 90%. In managing the severely atrophic posterior maxilla, this procedure most frequently fulfills a cardinal goal of surgery, which is to obtain a successful if not optimal long-term outcome with the least amount of intervention, complications, and risks. This statement is particularly valid if the procedure morbidity can be further decreased by performing it in one stage (simultaneous graft and implant insertion) and if the graft material utilized does not necessitate an iliac crest or mandibular symphyseal donor site. Various graft materials that have been successfully used independently or in combination are autogenous, allogeneic, alloplastic, and xenogeneic.

Selection of Graft Material

The graft material selected must be able to provide long-term support for an implant-borne prosthesis. Present materials utilized alone or in combination include autologous, allogeneic (demineralized freeze-dried bone), alloplastic (synthetic hydroxyapatite), and xenogeneic grafts. A potential additional class of bone substitutes likely to be available in the near future are genetically engineered osteoinductive bone morphogenic proteins. The characteristics of the ideal subantral graft material are that it be nontoxic, nonantigenic, nonmigratory, infection resistant, readily available, easily fabricated, inexpensive, strong, resilient, capable of functional remodeling, provide ease of manipulation, minimize surgical time, eliminate donor morbidity, eliminate need for general anesthesia, enhance early stability of implants, and permit long-term osseointegration.

Bone Healing

Autologous bone grafts may be cortical, cancellous, or corticocancellous in composition. These type of grafts contain many live cells capable of osteogenesis. Success of any graft is dependent on a variety of host and surgical factors. In selecting which graft material to utilize, whether autologous in nature or a substitute, the healing process of autogenous bone grafts must be clearly comprehended.[30]

Axhausen[28] delineated a two-phase healing model of bone grafts. During phase 1, cortical and cancellous grafts heal similarly, with blood coagulated around transplanted bone and an acute inflammatory reaction evident. Initial grafted cell survival is through nutrient diffusion followed by angiogensis from the graft bed. Transplanted cells proliferate and differentiate to form osteoid surrounding avascular grafted trabeculae. With progressive osteoid deposition, the graft becomes joined with new bone. The quantity of bone regenerated is directly proportional to the amount of cellular density of transplanted bone cells that survived. By the end of week two, inflammation has decreased, and fibrous granulation tissue around the graft and increased osteoclastic activity are present. Osteocytes die, as evidenced by vacant lacunae. Necrotic tissue in the Haversian system is removed by macrophages.

Cancellous grafts are rapidly revascularized by host ingrowth and end-to-end anastomosis by the end of week two. Primitive mesenchymal cells differentiate into osteogenic cells. These cells together with transplanted osteogenic cells differentiate into osteoblasts that envelop cores of necrotic bone with osteoid, which is then replaced completely by new bone strengthening the graft.

Cortical grafts behave differently and are revascularized slowly, taking approximately 1 to 2 months. Remodeling differs in that repair is driven by osteoclastic, not osteoblastic, resorption. Neovascularization is facilitated by osteoclastic bone resorption through and following along preexisting Haversian and Volkmann's canals. This initial resorptive component, which begins within the first 4 weeks, is followed by appositional bone deposition sealing off bone from further osteoclastic activity. This process is termed creeping substitution. Areas of necrotic bone may persist and are histologically unique to cortical bone healing. New bone continues to form via creeping substitution until the graft is remodeled. The early osteoclastic component with delayed osteoblastic activity leads to early mechanical weakness, which may last 6 weeks to 6 months. Maturation to normal bone strength may require 1 to 2 years.

These differing processes between cortical and cancellous graft behavior occur predominately during Axhausen's phase 2. This phase begins during week two and becomes critical in weeks four and five. Fibroblasts and other mesenchymal cells from the host bed differentiate into osteoblasts and begin to produce new matrix. This programming of cells is termed osteoinduction and is believed to be regulated by bone matrix proteins. BMP (bone morphogenic protein), the best known, is an acid-insoluble, oligosaccharide glycoprotein of low molecular weight (15,000–18,000). Additionally, passive ingrowth of osteogenic cells occurs from the surrounding bone with the grafted bone acting as a scaffold or new bone formation, a process designated as osteoconduction. Neovascularization, osteogenesis, osteoinduction, and osteoconduction combined with osteoclastic activity derived from circulating monocytes allow for continued resorption, remodeling, and replacement, eventually leading to an incorporated bone graft.

Autogenous Grafts

Autologous bone is the gold standard by which other graft materials are judged. Sinus inlay grafting utilizing an iliac crest particulate cancellous graft was first performed by Tatum[5,29] in the 1970s and later published by Boyne and James.[30] Jensen et al.[6] similarly described the use of a particulate cancellous graft into which implants were placed 4 to 5 months later. Simultaneous one-stage implant and graft insertion was reported by Tatum[5,29] and by Block and Kent[8,26] utilizing cancellous chips, and by Keller et al.[4,19,31] and others[7,32–34] using a corticocancellous block.

Autogenous bone has been a reliable source of immunocompatible viable bone cells to allow for osteogenesis. Via transplanted osteoprogenitor cells and their osteoconductive and osteoinductive properties, bone is produced and maintained to stabilize fixtures. Graft healing is generally accelerated in comparison to other material, allowing for implant insertion at 4 to 6 months in a staged procedure, or facilitates earlier fixture uncovering at 6 to 8 months for single-stage implant graft procedures. The major disadvantages of autogenous bone grafts relates to the donor site morbidity, additional surgical time, anesthesia, and cost. The potential for graft resorption in cases of delayed implant placement may also exist.

A cancellous graft contains particulate medullary bone and hematopoietic marrow with the highest concentration of osteogenic cells. This graft type allows for rapid revascularization and bone production. Available intraoral sources of cancellous bone may be within the surgical field from fixture preparation sites or the maxillary tuberosity. Additional volume can be obtained from the mandibular symphysis, extraction sites, or the retromolar pad–ramus region. Should large quantities be necessary, the iliac crest is an abundant source. Autologous grafts should be stored in saline, not hypotonic or hypertonic solutions, which may cause osteogenic cell death before transplant. Unlike intraoral sources, which are membranous in nature, the iliac crest provides endochondral bone and may be more prone to resorption. This seems to be of minimal if any clinical significance in terms of fixture integration and long-term stability. Particulate cancellous bone is readily combined and osteogenically enhances allogeneic, alloplastic, and xenogeneic material that may serve as a volume expander or the bulk of the graft. The major drawbacks of a cancellous graft to those previously stated for autogenous bone in general are associated with excess resorption and an inability, as all particulate grafts, to rigidly stabilize and maintain implant position and angulation where minimal alveolar bone exists.

The corticocancellous block graft is indicated in such situations to allow for rigid fixture stabilization. Immediate fixture placement, particularly of threaded types, allows for precise implant positioning as well as rigid primary stabilization of the graft, thereby minimizing mobility and resultant resorption. Corticocancellous grafts provide greater initial strength and possibly less postremodeling resorption than cancellous grafts. However, because of slow revascularization block grafts are more prone to infection and weakness during early remodeling. When the graft is subjected to force transmission by direct loading through the implants, it is not known whether a corticocancellous or a particulate cancellous graft will behave differently. Shaping, placement, and stabilization of a corticocancellous block is more technically demanding. Sinus septae must be removed to optimize the interface between the donor block and its bed. Residual voids between the block and the sinus walls are packed with particulate bone. In cases in which the sinus membrane has been perforated, there is less risk of fragment migration and dissemination than when only a particulate cancellous graft is utilized.

Corticocancellous blocks may be harvested from the symphysis. The iliac crest is used if a large graft is necessary and commonly when a bilateral augmentation is planned. Iliac crest bone harvesting increases the relative magnitude of the overall procedure in comparison to utilizing other graft materials to be discussed. Faltering patient motivation and acceptance, if not frank objection, may be encountered. Graft procurement from the iliac crest usually entails hospitalization, general anesthesia, increased blood loss, surgical time, cost, convalescence, and possibly the need for a second surgeon. Donor site morbidity may include gait disturbances (related to disruption of the tensor fascia latae and psoas major muscles), neurosensory deficits (lateral femoral cutaneous nerve), scarring, and abdominal and urologic complications (hernia, meralgia parathetica, adynamic ileus, hematoma, seroma, pain, and infections). Tibial plateau bone grafts may also be a consideration, especially for outpatient or in office ambulatory procedures.

Intraoral graft procurement from the symphysis, ramus, extraction sites, tuberosity, or sinus retromolar pad eliminates many of these disadvantages. Problems of donor site morbidity, neurosensory complication (inferior alveolar, mental, and lingual nerves), increased surgical time, inadequate graft volume, and cost, however, still persist and dictate consideration of alternative graft materials for sinus lift procedures. Particular care is needed in harvesting bone from the tuberosity. One must avoid invasion into the sinus. Utilizing the tuberosity may compromise the primary procedure, eliminate a potential implant recipient site, and make retention of a transitional prosthesis during the healing period difficult. However, harvesting bone from regions other than the surgical field once again may raise patient objections.

Allogeneic Grafts

Allogeneic grafts have been quite successful as a volume expander in combination with autologous grafts or for providing osteoconductive properties with hydroxyapatite of various forms. Allografts are materials taken from another individual within the same species. Mineralized allografts possess osteoconductive properties, but are unacceptable because of slower revascularization and resorption with increased infection liability. Demineralized allografts are capable of more predictable repair. Minerals may be removed by means of an acid treatment, then washed and freeze-dried (lyophilized). This demineralized freeze-dried bone (DFDB) retains bone morphogenic protein (BMP) and thus osteoinductive activity.[35] DFDB is available as cancellous or cortical chips (1–5 mm) or powder (250–1000 μm). Demineralized freeze-dried cortical powder of 250–500 μm particle size provides enhanced osteoinductivity and surface area compared to the other forms. A 20-min saline reconstitution period is minimally necessary.

DFDB should be obtained from a reputable, accredited bank that adheres to the guidelines and standards of the American Association of Tissue Banks (AATB). The AATB criteria delineate protocols for donor selection and screening, recovery techniques, testing, processing, storage, distribution, and record keeping. All donors are screened and tested to exclude transmissible diseases, infections, malignancy, toxic exposures, parenteral drug use, immunosuppression, and other disease states, Donor tissue undergoes extensive serologic assays with aerobic-anaerobic microbiologic monitoring from recovery throughout processing, including sampling at final packaging.[36,37] Buck et al.[38] in 1989 estimated the risk of HIV transmission as 1 in 1.2 million allograft procedures. Introduction in 1991 of the polymerase chain reaction test has proven to be an extremely sensitive screen for HIV and further diminishes the risk. Patient education is critical in minimizing anxiety and objection to allografts. Clinicians should utilize only those tissue banks that abide by AATB guidelines and employ advanced tissue testing and processing technique.

Urist,[35] Reddi and Hascall,[39] Glowacki et al.,[40] and many others[27,41,42] over the past 30 years have delineated the osteoinductive healing process of DFDB. DFDB has no osteoprogenitor cells and serves to enhance phase 2 bone healing. The graft is initially bound by fibrin and fibronectin, followed by mesenchymal cell proliferation and chemotaxis to the graft. These pluripotential cells differentiate into chrondroblasts, hematopoietic cells, and osteoblasts, eventually producing bone. Adequate oxygenation as determined by local vascularity is critical to this process.

DFDB as a lone subantral graft material has been somewhat unpredictable.[8,43–45] Extended healing periods of 12 to 16 months, prolonged rubbery consistency, and comparatively sparser bone formation contraindicate its routine use alone as an independent subantral graft material. However, success is evident in the high 90th percentile since the mid- to late 1980s with DFDB as part of a composite graft with autologous bone or hydroxyapatite porous[46] or resorbable.[10,43,47–49] In a 2.5-year period, Smiler et al.[43] reported 95% success using DFDB with a xenogeneic material, Bio-Oss (Osteohealth, Shirley, NY, USA) in a 1:3 proportion in 21 graft sites with 56 implants.

DFDB composite grafts may enhance bone formation compared to either component used independently.[50] This allograft does not demonstrate antigenicity and provides predictable results. As an autograft expander, it may be synergistic for bone formation while diminishing donor site morbidity and other unfavorable consequences when larger autologous grafts would be otherwise necessary. If autogenous bone is not utilized, the osteoinductive features of DFDB appear to complement the osteoconductive properties of alloplastic materials. This provides an excellent subantral graft option with a healing period of 9 to 12 months.

Alloplastic Grafts

The use of synthetic hydroxyapatite as the sole graft material or in combination with autografts or allografts has been expanding during the past 10 years. Hydroxyapatite (HA) is a natural mineral component of hard tissue composing 97% of enamel, 70% to 80% of dentin, 50% to 60% of cementum, and 60% to 70% of bone. HA is biocompatible, nontoxic, nonantigenic, readily available, inexpensive, and a time-efficient material. Synthetic HA is derived from calcium phosphate crystals compacted under high pressure (10,000–20,000) and temperature (1100°–1300°C). This fusion process is termed sintering. Porosity size approximating 100 μm is necessary for effective bony ingrowth. Somewhat larger porosity size allows for more rapid bone infiltration.[51]

A frequently utilized form of HA is derived by a hydrothermal chemical exchange reaction from coral (family Portidae) commercially available as Interpore 200 (Interpore, Irvine, CA, USA). This HA is a highly organized material with a pore average of 230 μm and a labyrinth of continuous uniform interconnected porosities averaging 190 μm.[50] The pore percentage is uniform with a solid-to-void ratio of 1. Porous forms of HA provide a passive scaffold for bony infiltration. It is an osteophilic and osteoconductive material encouraging bony ingrowth from the surrounding graft bed into areas where bone would not otherwise form. It does not possess any intrinsic osteogenic potential and lacks the bone matrix proteins required for osteoinduction. Bony infiltration is enhanced by increasing the exposed surface area of surrounding bone. Bone formation is slower and less predictable in regions further distant from the recipient bone bed. Creation of a three-wall defect by adequately reflecting the medial sinus wall mucoperiosteum is critical for graft maturation with this material as well as others discussed. The contribution to bone formation from the imploded lateral cortical sinus wall is somewhat speculative.

Natural occurring porous HA structure mimics the macrostructure of bone, optimizing fibrovascular invasion and new bone incorporation. Following osteogenic cell ingrowth, osteoblasts organize on the HA surface with apposition of lamellar bone until the final regeneration of cortical bone in the form of osteons. Normal bone healing is evident on the surface of both porous and nonporous HA. The bond between HA and bone consists of an amorphous zone rich in mucopolysaccharides with calcification evident. Cells directly attach to the HA by collagen fibers.

Dense, sintered HA has low microporosity. Resorbability of HA is dependent on density, crystal size, and porosity. High-density HA of relatively large particle size as well as HA derived from coral are slowly resorbable or essentially nonresorbable in vivo.[50] A nonsintered (nonceramic) graft material composed of small crystal clusters is a nonporous resorbable form of HA marketed as Osteogen (Stryker, Kalamazoo, MI, USA). As osteoclasts resorb this form of HA, new bone formation is facilitated through osteoconduction with HA acting as a mineral reservoir.

Tatum,[29] Misch,[47,48] Smiler et al.,[43] and Smiler and Holmes,[52] followed by numerous clinicians,[46,49,53,54] began reporting the use of HA as an independent or combination subantral graft material in the mid- to late 1980s. Predictable successful outcomes generally approaching 100% were evident with HA or HA in combination with autologous grafts or allogeneic grafts. Smiler et al.[43] in 1992 published a 100% success rate on the use of Interpore in 66 sinus lifts on 36 patients with 198 implants supporting a prosthesis. Histomorphometric examination confirmed bony ingrowth into the porous HA granules. Core biopsies on specimens demonstrated bone present in as much as 10 mm of the 12-mm core length, with a mean amount of HA covered by bone ingrowth of 40.9% and a mean bony ingrowth of 23.10%. Small and Zinner[46] reported on a 6-year experience using Interpore 200 in a 1:1 ratio with demineralized freeze-dried cortical bone. To date (in yet unpublished data) in 68 sinus lifts only 4 of 211 implants have failed, for a success rate of 98%. Limited histomorphometric and volume fraction studies were consistent with Smiler's results (Figures 18.8a–d) (Ralph E. Holmes, Department of Plastic Surgery, University of California, San Diego, CA). Approximately equal thirds of HA, bone, and soft tissue were noted in the consolidated subantral augmentation. Resorbable HA has also demonstrated predictable successful outcomes as an independent or as a composite graft in multiple reports.[9,43,53,55]

A multitude of varying proportions in composite grafts have been suggested. Many clinicians have utilized an alloplast as a minor component serving as an autograft extender when less than optimal autologous bone was available. Others, wishing to limit donor site morbidity, used only readily available autogenous bone in whatever limited quantities from intraoral sites, generally harvested from the tuberosity or fixture osteotomies as a supplement to the predominant HA component. Autologous bone serves to enhance the osteogenic, osteoinductive, and osteoconductive potential of the graft. Similarly, DFDB providing osteoinductive properties is added by some with this mix or with HA only. On the basis of core biopsies studying bone volume and clinical consistency, it appears that DFDB should be limited maximally to 50% or less of the composite graft.[43–46] Further bone volume fraction studies considering healing time variabilities appear necessary to determine the optimal graft material or combination proportions.

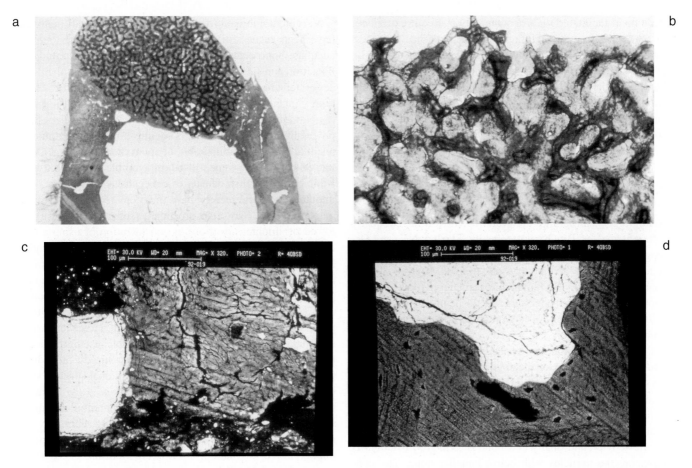

FIGURE 18.8 Histomorphometic and volume fraction studies of core biopsies from human sinus bone grafts with Interpore 200 hydroxyapatite and demineralized freeze dried bone in a 1:1 ratio (courtesy of Ralph Holmes, MD, Department of Plastic Surgery, University of California San Diego, San Diego, California). (a) Routine stain low power reveals mixture of bone regeneration and ingrowth into Interpore 200 pores. (b) High power light photomicrograph. (c) Scanning electon micrograph of mature new bone growth with fibrous tissue. (d) Scanning electron micrograph of bone growth in relation to hydroxyapatite Interpore 200 granules.

Predominantly anecdotal evidence suggests the minimal healing period for autogenous grafts is 4 to 6 months for fixture placement in a two-stage procedure, and 6 to 9 months for a one-stage protocol. DFDB alone, which is not recommended, takes approximately 12 to 16 months to mature. HA alone necessitates a wait of 9 to 12 months until abutment surgery in simultaneous graft/implant insertion or 6 months until fixture placement if staged with an additional 9 months to allow for osseointegration. HA-DFDB combinations require 9 months minimally in a one-stage procedure or fixture placement no earlier than 6 months post grafting in a two-stage procedure.

Autologous grafts or autologous-dominated combinations demonstrate the fastest healing and the highest bone volume fractions. Despite these results, similar high levels of clinical success in the development and maintenance of osseointegration is apparent with HA as a solitary graft or in combination as an equal or dominant component mixed with allogeneic grafts. It must be kept in mind that the ultimate goal of the sinus lift procedure is stable long-term osseointegration. Pragmatically, porous nonresorbable HA combined with readily available autologous bone or possibly DFDB ($\leq 50\%$) would seem a prudent choice.

HA grafts or combinations, owing to their particular nature, may not provide adequate fixture positional stability. Cases of extreme osseous atrophy leaving an eggshell residual ridge may dictate a staged procedure or use of a corticocancellous graft to allow for reliable implant positioning. Additional disadvantages of HA to consider are increased healing time and an increase in difficulty in implant site preparation because of the HA hardness compared to autogenous grafts. Although HA independently or as part of a composite graft does not satisfy all the criteria for an ideal graft material, it has demonstrated clinical success equal if not superior to other graft options. It does so with the advantage of eliminating or limiting donor site morbidity, hospitalization, general anesthesia, cost, operative time, and potential disease transmission. HA lacks toxicity and antigenicity and permits a direct bone bond facilitated via osteoconduction. In our experience of 68 sinus lifts with 211 implants, we have had a success rate of 98% utilizing a composite graft consisting of 50% Interpore 200 with 50% DFDB, and locally available intraoral bone from the tuberosity or implant preparation sites is substituted on a volume basis for the DFDB when available. The autologous bone fraction constituted 0% to 25% of the final composite graft.

Xenogeneic Grafts

Xenografts (heterografts) are grafts taken from a genetically different species. BioOss (Osteohealth, Shirley, NY) and Osteograf/N (Ceramed, Lakewood, CO, USA) are calcium-deficient carbonate apatite crystals derived from a bovine source. Osteograf/N (Ceramed) has a smaller particle size than BioOss. This natural bone mineral is chemically and physically identical to bone. It is deorganified and deproteinated to render it nonantigenic. As a result of deproteination it does not possess osteoinductive capacity. Because of its natural structure and network of macropores, micropores, and small crystal formations, it provides considerably greater surface area than synthetic HA.[27] This natural porous HA undergoes a three-phase healing process. Initially particles are surrounded by host bone, then particles are resorbed by osteoclastic activity, and finally new bone is formed by osteoblasts replacing the particles with dense lamellar bone. The conversion rate is dependent on cellularity and other local and systemic factors.

Initial short-term reports of less than 3 years of these materials combined with autogenous bone in varying proportions are encouraging.[43,56] Utilization in composite grafts with either autogenous bone or DFDB seems promising but optimal fractions need to be defined. Further long-term evaluation of these xenografts as an independent antral graft material or as a composite graft is necessary.

Selection of Endosseous Implant

Endosseous fixtures approximately 15 mm in length and 4 mm in diameter are generally utilized to optimize the bone–implant surface area interface. Narrower diameter implants may be necessary when only a thin crestal ridge remains. Use of a wider diameter fixture in such circumstances may lead to residual ridge fracture. Shorter fixtures are indicated for patients with skeletal vertical deficiency with decreased sinus height or when the level of the superior horizontal osteotomy is inappropriately placed. The maximal number of implants allowing 2 mm of spacing between fixtures should be placed. At 2 to 3 months preoperatively, any tooth with a poor long-term prognosis is extracted to permit bone healing for fixture placement and sufficient time for soft tissue closure.

Varying combinations of implant types and graft materials have been successful. Uncoated screw-type fixtures require adequate bone quantitatively and qualitatively for initial stabilization and success. It is well documented that implant success rates are lower in type IV bone, particularly for screw-type implants.[57–59] This most likely results from an inability to obtain initial (bi)cortical stabilization. In subantral grafting procedures, threaded implants require a minimal amount of residual bone for stabilization, of approximately 5 mm. Qualitatively, the bone may still be unfavorable, presenting with a thin cortex and low density of trabeculae. Use of screw-type implants more frequently may therefore require the implementation of a two-stage procedure (subantral grafting followed by implant insertion) or consideration of using a corticocancellous block to enhance stabilization. Threaded fixtures and corticocancellous blocks stabilize each other reciprocally. Screw-type fixtures are very successful when employed for subantral grafting when a sufficient residual alveolus is present. These are most commonly used with a predominantly autogenous graft material. However, when minimal bone volume or density is available, use of threaded-type implants would mandate a more complex procedure. Complexity may be in the form of an additional surgical step, increased treatment time, or the necessity of using an autogenous corticocancellous block from the mandibular symphysis or iliac crest. This increase in complexity seemingly derives from some clinicians' interest in utilizing one type of implant universally and procedures are modified as necessary around the "chosen" implant. As there are well-documented simplified alternatives for extremely deficient bone status that use coated cylinders, frequently with nonautogenous graft material, and are equally or more successful, logic would dictate reassessment of such planning.

Plasma-sprayed cylinders do not require as rigid initial stability as screw-type implants and possess a significally higher surface area for integration. HA-coated fixtures, owing to their osteoconductive surface, stabilize earlier than non-HA-coated implants. In subantral grafting procedures, unlike those in other regions, problems relating to HA coating dissolution, bacterial colonization of the roughened surface with resultant bone loss, and fixture failure have not been encountered. This may be because the basilar bone of the sinus floor does not resorb as easily, and therefore the HA surface is not exposed to the oral environment. A fixture with a polished titanium collar should be used. Coating variabilities among manufacturers must also be considered in selecting fixtures. HA coatings with higher crystallinity percentages have lower dissolution rates and are therefore desirable. Inadequate data are currently available for the use of coated screw-type implants. HA-coated implants have been successfully implemented in one-stage simutaneous graftng and insertion procedures in extremely poor residual bone situations.[46] Cylinders do not provide as satisfactory rigid stabilization as threaded fixtures when a corticocancellous graft is used.

In summary, titanium threaded fixtures, HA, or titanium plasma-sprayed cylinders have all been successfully utilized in the sinus lift procedure. However, in situations of diminished bone volume and density, the plasma-sprayed fixtures, particularly those that are HA coated, appear useful if a one-stage procedure is desired.

One-Stage Versus Two-Stage Procedure

The advantages of simultaneous subantral grafting and implant insertion are the avoidance of the trauma of a second surgery, reduction in total treatment time, and the possibility of providing a stimulus to the graft for consolidation around the fixtures. For press-fit implants, 3 mm or possibly even less of residual bone may be adequate for proper immediate positioning and stabilization.[8,46] Fixture displacement may be further avoided by minimal countersinking of the preparation site. This will necessitate corresponding relief to a removable prosthesis or use of a fixed temporary prosthesis to avoid premature loading. Utilizing HA-coated implants will facilitate early stabilization because bonding with bone may begin to occur as early as 4 weeks. Care in packing the particulate graft so as to avoid deflection of the implant body is necessary. Corticocancellous blocks if utilized are best stabilized rigidly by screw-type fixtures. Healing periods required are 6 to 8 months for autogenous grafts, 9 to 12 months for HA grafts, and 9 months for HA combined with autogenous bone or DFDB.

The advantages of a two-stage approach are possibly better control of implant alignment as well as less risk of fixture displacement and better tolerance to iatrogenic premature loading. Aside from the obvious disadvantage of additional surgery and treatment time, there are concerns about autogenous graft disuse resorption or pneumatization should significant delays in implant insertion occur. Fixtures may be placed 4 to 6 months following autogenous grafts and uncovered 5

to 6 months later. For HA grafts and combinations with autologous or DFDB, the waiting period is 6 to 9 months, depending on proportions. A longer bone maturation phase is necessary to account for a graft subjected to osteoconductive revitalization.

Surgical Technique

Preoperatively, the patient rinses with chlorhexidine gluconate, and ingests an appropriate antibiotic (discussed later), glucocorticoid, and NSAID are administered. The procedure may be performed in the office or hospital under local anesthesia, with sedation or general anesthesia. The patient is prepped, draped, and then infiltrated with a local anesthetic containing a vasoconstrictor. The sinus boundaries are indentified by radiographic evaluation and fiberoptic transillumination.

Incision and Reflection

In the totally edentulous posterior maxilla, a horizontal anteroposterior incision is made slightly palatal to the crest from the region of the hamular notch to the canine region (Figures 18.9a,b and 18.10). Anteriorly and posteriorly, vertical releasing incisions are placed approximately 1 cm beyond the vertical walls of the antrum. The relief incisions are brought from the palate horizontal and laterally over the crest and extended superiorly toward the vestibule anteriorly. The posterior vertical release should remain conservative so as to contain the buccal fat pad. A full-thickness mucoperiosteal flap is reflected superiorly to 5 mm beyond the proposed superior horizontal osteotomy or the malar buttress if encountered first. Once adequate exposure to the residual alveolar crest and the lateral wall of the maxilla has been attained, multiple 3-0 silk sutures are used to suture the flap laterally to the cheek in a self-retentive fashion.

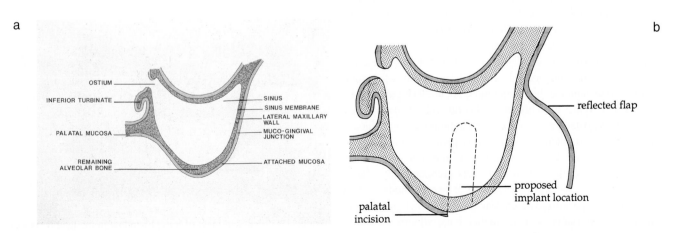

FIGURE 18.9 Design of incision for sinus bone grafting. (a) Incision at crest of alveolar ridge. (b) Reflected flap and planned position of implant.

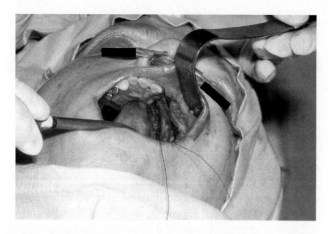

FIGURE 18.10 Clinical view of incision at alveolar ridge with buccally retracted flap.

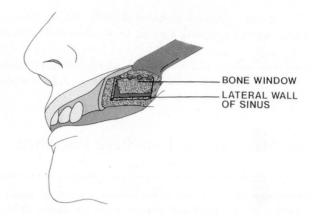

FIGURE 18.11 Diagram of buccally retracted flap and creation of bone window in the lateral wall of the maxillary sinus.

Osteotomy

Once again, on the basis of radiographs and fiberoptic illumination, the sinus boundaries are defined. A surgical marking pencil may be used to delineate the location and extent of the antrostomy. Using a high-speed drill with a small round diamond bur under saline irrigation, a rectangular box with rounded corners or an ovoid osteotomy is scored just within the anterior, posterior, and inferior extent of the sinus. The inferior horizonal cut is minimally 2 mm above the alveolar crest to facilitate Schneiderian membrane reflection. This cut may need to be placed slightly superiorly to leave sufficient buccal bone to place fixtures simultaneously while avoiding a ridge fracture. It is also important to make the inferior horizontal osteotomy within the antrum and above the thicker alveolar bone. The further superior the cut is made, however, the more difficulty is encountered in raising the membrane inferiorly. This horizontal osteotomy extends approximately 25 mm from the anterior sinus border to the molar region posteriorly as necessary. Full anterior extension is necessary to avoid blind spots during sinus membrane elevation and grafting. The superior horizontal osteotomy parallels the inferior at a level to permit placement of 15-mm-long implants. The horizontal osteotomies are then connected with parallel rounded vertical cuts. Once the bony window is accurately scored, the osteotomies are completed using the diamond bur in a delicate paintbrush stroke until the bluish hue of the membrane is apparent (Figures 18.11 and 18.12). When mobility of the lateral wall of the window is noted, the osteotomy is complete circumferentially. Should these cuts be complete and immobility persist, a sinus septum may be suspected. Radiographic review and transillumination will likely reveal the presence of septa preoperatively. These sinus septa may be negotiated in one of two methods. A thin osteotome or specialized curette can be used to section the septa inferiorly. Alternatively, two smaller bone windows may be created on either side of the septae partition.

Membrane Reflection

A curved side of a dull surgical curette displaces the bony window slightly inward. The concave portion is positioned between the membrane and the inferior margin of the residual alveolus. The inferolateral membrane is reflected with a sliding motion anteroposteriorly. The Schneiderian membrane has few elastic fibers and is easily separated from its underlying bone. Maintaining contact with bone throughout, the mucoperiosteal lining is released circumferentially around the outer window margin. With increasing medial and superior mobility of the bony window, the membrane can next be raised to the medial sinus wall. Vertically, the mucoperiosteal lining is reflected anteriorly, posteriorly, and medially to accomodate placement of 15-mm fixtures. The attainment of adequate height should be measured. The bony window has simultaneously been infractured and hinged superiorly (Figure 18.13). Membrane reflection without perforation is facilitated by utilizing specialized sinus membrane elevators of appro-

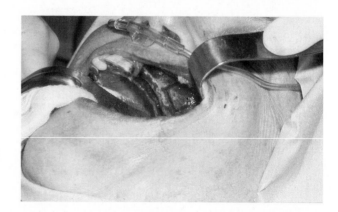

FIGURE 18.12 Clinical view of buccal window in the lateral wall of the maxillary sinus.

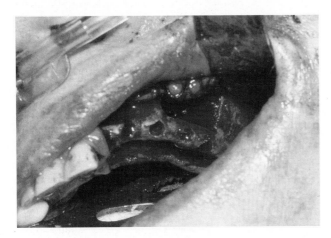

FIGURE 18.13 Clinical view of infractured buccal window of lateral wall of the maxillary sinus with osteotomy sites prepared for dental implants.

priate curvature and size. These curettes should always lie subperiosteally against bone. Under direct visualization the rounded back is used to elevate the soft tissue. With an intact sinus membrane, a bellows effect will be observed during breathing, with the hinged lateral sinus wall rising and falling.

Graft and Fixture Insertion

In a two-stage procedure, the antral void is obturated with a graft material. For one-stage procedures, after completion of the sinus membrane elevation a surgical guide stent is placed and stabilized (Figure 18.14). Receptor sites for implants are prepared. Minimal if any countersinking may assist in stabilizing fixtures, if necessary. Placement of a particulate graft is facilitated by loading the graft into a small-diameter glass syringe, which will allow for easier manipulation, control, and access to the medial aspects of the recipient bed (Figure

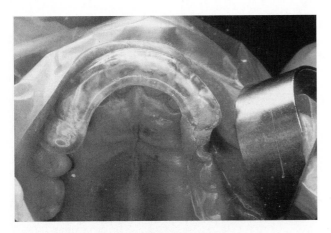

FIGURE 18.14 Example of surgical guide stent for exact placement of osteotomies for dental implants.

18.15). Alternatively, a 3-cc plastic syringe with the tip cut off may be used. The graft material is compacted initially in the medial half and extreme anterior and posterior aspects of the antral void (Figures 18.16 and 18.17). Press-fit fixtures are subsequently inserted, and the residual lateral aspect and the regions between implants are condensed with graft material (Figures 18.18 and 18.19). Observation and care in placement of the lateral graft is necessary to prevent any deflection of the fixtures in cases of severe atrophy. A plastic or titanium instrument can be used to reorient the displaced implant if necessary.

If the screw-type fixtures are utilized with a particulate graft, the fixtures may need to be placed before graft insertion. This will prevent washout of the graft material from the cooling irrigant but complicates medial graft placement. If an autogenous corticocancellous block is chosen as the graft material, it must be custom shaped to the bed. With the cortical surface lying superiorly, the graft is rigidly stabilized with fixtures. Residual voids should be packed with particulate graft material.

The lateral wall of the maxilla is restored to normal contour with particulate graft material. A resorbable membrane such as a collagen sheet or laminar bone is custom fitted to prevent extravasation of material and to delay fibrous tissue invasion. The flap is repositioned and sutured closed with 3-0 slowly resorbable sutures (Figure 18.20). Rarely, a periosteal releasing incision will be necessary to attain a tensionless closure.

Postoperative Management

Glucocorticoids and analgesics are prescribed in anticipation of mild to moderate edema and pain. Antibiotics are administered for a 7- to 10-day period. Amoxicillin clavulanate is commonly prescribed. This antibiotic will provide coverage against the typical oral organisms (anaerobic gram-negative rods, aerobic and anerobic streptococci) as well as common sinus pathogens (*Streptococcus pneumoniae, Haemophilus influenzae, Staphylococcus aureus, Branhamella catarrhalis,* and numerous anaerobes).[60] Alternative antibiotics are either clindamycin or cefaclor, which have no or low cross-sensitivity, respectively. Chlorhexidine gluconate 0.12%, as an antiseptic rinse twice daily is additionally recommended. Sinus mucosa inflammation and edema may obstruct the ostium and lead to an infection. Short-term use of a systemic or topical decongestant, particularly if membrane perforation has occurred, may be prophylactically efficacious. These oral and nasal preparations containing sympathomimetric amines vasoconstrict the vascular bed and relieve congestion. Antihistamines are not routinely indicated.

Instructions are similar to other oral surgical procedures with sinus involvement. Temporization with an appropriately adjusted fixed toothborne prosthesis may be immediate. Retaining a nonrestorable, noninfected tooth may be worthy to act as

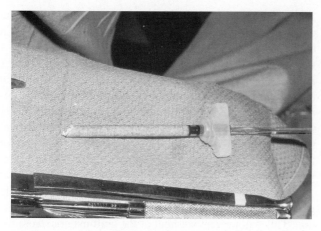

FIGURE 18.15 Glass syringe filled with particulate bone graft.

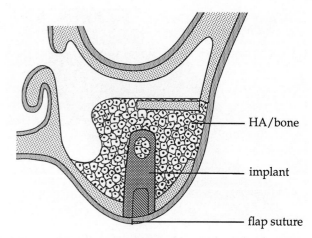

FIGURE 18.18 Cross-sectional diagram demonstrating placement of dental implants and complete bone grafting beneath sinus membrane.

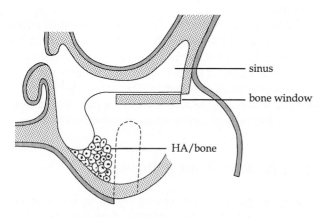

FIGURE 18.16 Cross-sectional diagram before insertion of dental implants; bone graft is placed along medial sinus wall.

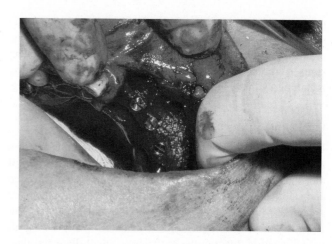

FIGURE 18.19 Clinical view of placement of dental implants and completion of bone grafting with complete filling of buccal window.

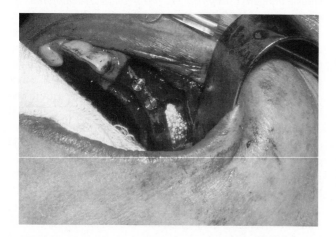

FIGURE 18.17 Clinical view before insertion of dental implants; bone graft is placed along medial sinus wall for medial placement of bone graft.

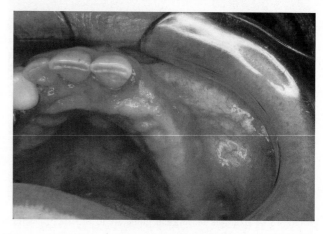

FIGURE 18.20 Clinical view of healed incision with closure of mucosa overlying bone graft and implants.

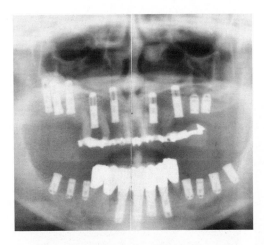

FIGURE 18.21 Panoramic radiograph of bilateral posterior maxillary partial edentulism with right maxillary sinus bone graft and implants, left subantral implant placement, retention of teeth for interim prosthesis, and total mandibular dental implant prosthesis reconstruction.

an interim abutment (Figure 18.21). More commonly, a removable prosthesis may be inserted after 2 or preferably 4 weeks (Figure 18.22a,b). The soft tissue-bearing prosthesis must then be appropriately relieved to avoid encroachment on the implants, particularly if not fully countersunk. Premature loading may cause micromovement and implant failure to osseointegrate.

Abutment Surgery and Progressive Bone Loading

Patients are followed clinically and when necessary radiographically during the healing period. At the appropriate time, depending on the residual bone and the graft material utilized, abutment placement surgery is performed (Figure

23a,b). The incision should be midcrestal or slightly palatal to allow transposition of keratinized tissue buccally. Tissue height in excess of 3 mm will impair maintenance and should be trimmed.

Implants are most at risk during the first year of function as the result of stresses exceeding physiologic limits. The degree of bone contact and the density of the supporting bone will determine whether a load placed upon an implant is tolerable.[48] The fabrication and insertion of an occlusally adjusted acrylic temporary with a metal substructure for 12 months allows additional time for bone maturation as well as incremental loading of the bone (Figures 18.24, 18.25, and 18.26). Progressive implant loading will enhance the amount of desirable mature lamellar bone to develop at the interface. The increase in trabeculae in contact with the implant and in the immediate surrounding bone will improve implant survival. Additionally, early temporization provides for immediate patient gratification (Figure 18.27a,b). It allows the restorative dentist time to perfect the final prosthesis while ameliorating the patient's desire to "finish up" after a prolonged surgical period. Temporization can also permit the use of sinus bone grafted implants for use as posterior anchorage for fixed orthodontic treatment until idealized tooth positions allow final prosthesis fabrication or additonal implant placement (Figure 18.28a–d).

Complications

Sinus Membrane Perforation

Tearing of the Schneiderian membrane is the most common complication of the sinus lift procedure. These defects usually result from excess depth penetration during the initial osteotomy, right-angle bone window corners, and presence of sinus septa,

a
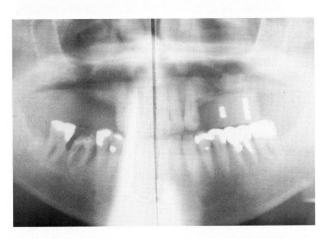

b
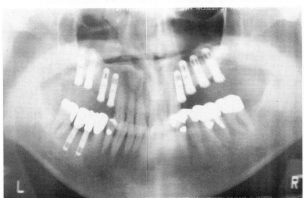

FIGURE 18.22 Bilateral posterior maxillary partial edentulism reconstructed with maxillary sinus bone grafts and placement of dental implants, with removable partial denture temporization possible ow-

ing to the presence of anterior dentition. (a) Preoperative panoramic radiograph. (b) Postoperative panoramic radiograph.

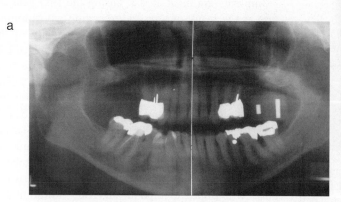

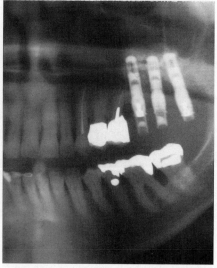

FIGURE 18.23 Unilateral posterior maxillary partial edentulism reconstructed with maxillary sinus bone grafts and placement of dental implants and fixed prosthesis. Placement of cementable post type abutments after exposure of implants allows acrylic temporization and early loading prior to final prosthesis fabrication and insertion. (a) Preoperative panoramic radiograph. (b) Postoperative panoramic radiograph.

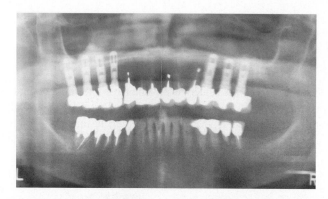

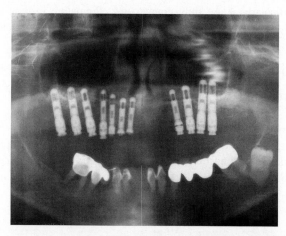

FIGURE 18.24 Postoperative panoramic radiograph with staged bilateral maxillary sinus bone grafts and placement of dental implants with fixed prosthesis. Left maxillary sinus bone graft and placement of dental implants with permanent fixed bridge, right maxillary sinus bone graft with cast metal temporary prosthesis for early loading.

FIGURE 18.25 Postoperative panoramic radiograph with total maxillary dental implant reconstruction with bilateral maxillary sinus bone grafts and placement of dental implants. Placement of temporary abutments and fabrication of temporary acrylic prosthesis following exposure of bilateral sinus bone grafts and dental implants and removal of remaining anterior maxillary teeth and placement of dental implants. Temporary fixed bridge allows early loading and transitional period until remaining maxillary implants can be utilized in the fabrication of a permanent fixed prosthesis.

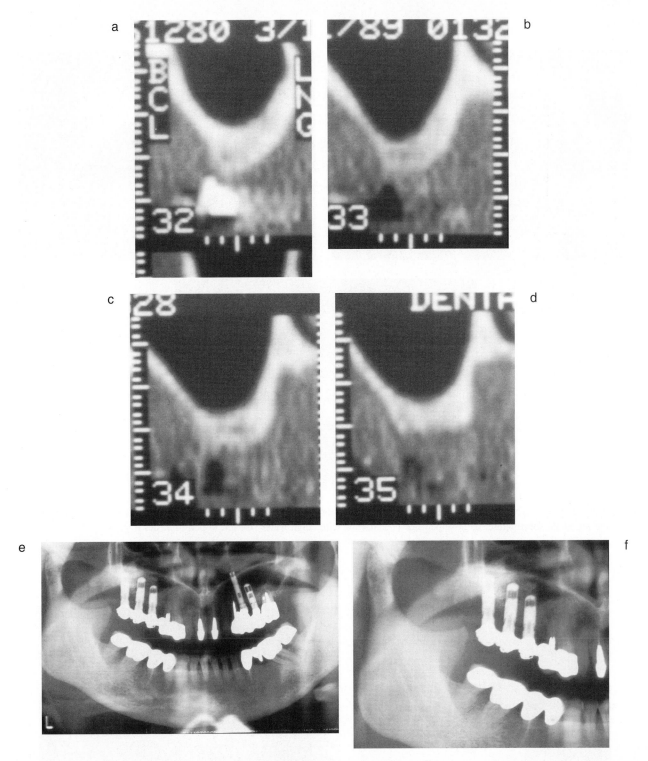

FIGURE 18.26 Right posterior maxillary sinus bone graft with dental implant reconstruction demonstrating adequate subantral bone to stabilize immediate placement of implants and bone graft. Early progressive loading is permitted with a temporary fixed bridge reinforced with a metal substructure. Preoperative CT scan reveals adequate subantral bone to stabilize immediate placement of dental implants with sinus bone graft: (a) tooth #4 site, (b) tooth #3 site, (c) tooth #2 site, (d) tooth #1/tuberosity site. (e) Postoperative panoramic radiograph of postoperative view with temporary cast metal reinforced prosthesis for early loading. (f) Postoperative panoramic radiograph close-up view.

Continued.

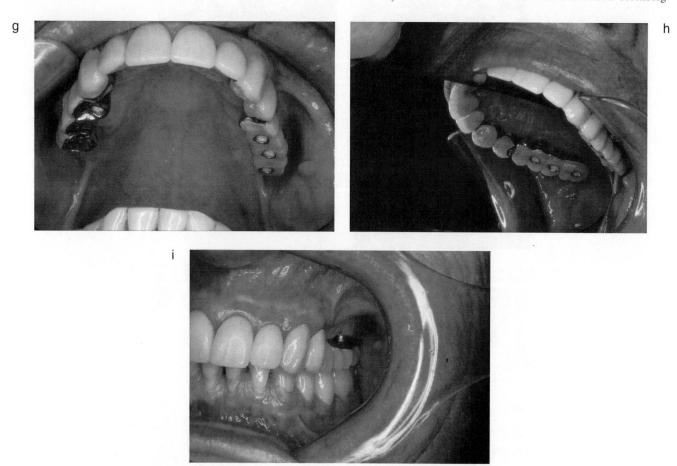

FIGURE 18.26 *Continued.* (g) Postoperative occlusal view with temporary prosthesis. (h) Postoperative lingual view with temporary prosthesis. Note the metal substructure. (i) Postoperative buccal view with "high water" design to permit easier hygiene.

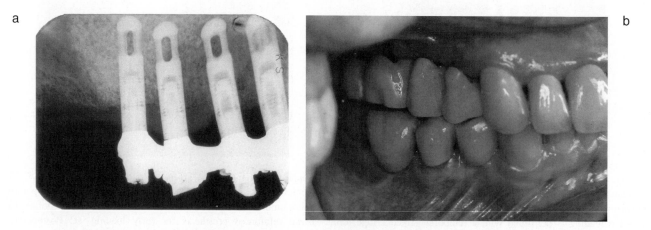

FIGURE 18.27 Right posterior maxillary sinus bone graft and implant placement with temporary metal substructure temporary prosthesis with natural crown emergence for better soft tissue site development and esthetics, and early loading. (a) Postoperative panoramic radiograph. (b) Postoperative buccal view.

a
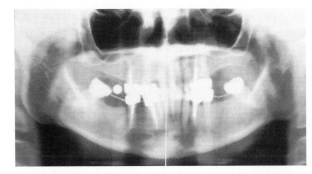

b
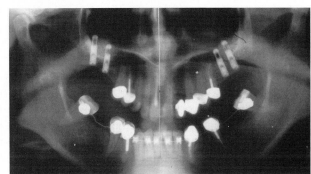

c
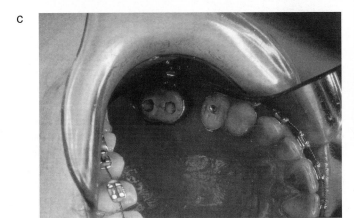

d
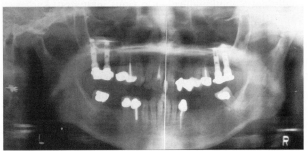

FIGURE 18.28 Bilateral posterior maxillary edentulous ridges with decreased vertical dimension and placement of bilateral maxillary sinus bone grafts and placement of dental implants. Sinus bone grafted dental implants with temporary bridges placed for early loading and use as posterior anchorage for fixed orthodontic treatment. (a) Preoperative panoramic radiograph with fixed orthodontic me-chanics for mandibular molar uprighting. (b) Postoperative panoramic radiograph. (c) Clinical occlusal view with temporary fixed prosthesis and fixed orthodontic appliances. (d) Post completion of fixed orthodontic treatment preparation for additional mandibular dental implant placement.

and most commonly occur inferiorly during the initiation of si-nus membrane elevation and anteriorly if the osteotomy was in-adequately extended and the reflection is being performed blindly. Earlier in the development of the procedure develop-ment, the osteotomy was designed so as to be incomplete su-periorly. Subsequently, the superiorly hinged bony window was greenstick fractured inwardly. The modified osteotomy design and membrane reflection technique as described earlier will pre-vent and decrease perforation frequency. Membrane defects in-crease early and late complications. Tears in the membrane in-crease bacterial and mucus ingress into the graft, increasing the risk of infection and decreasing graft density, respectively. Egress of graft material through the defect into the residual si-nus proper will decrease the graft volume as well as potentially block the ostium and impair drainage (Figure 18.29).

Appropriately managed sinus perforations are generally of minimal consequence. When a defect is noted, further mem-brane elevation should be performed distally, working toward the perforation circumferentially; this will prevent further en-largement of the tear. With enhanced membrane elevation, particularly along the medial wall, the membrane frequently

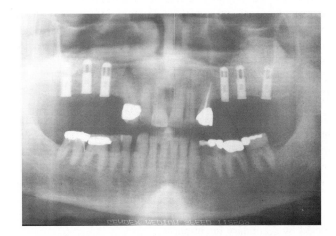

FIGURE 18.29 Postoperative panoramic radiograph with bilateral maxillary sinus bone grafts and dental implant placement. Left max-illary sinus extravasation of bone graft into the space above the si-nus membrane perforation causing decreased bone graft volume, blockage of ostium, and impaired sinus drainage.

folds upon itself, sealing the opening. If small residual defects persist they are best occluded with a customized resorbable collagen sheet. Alternatively, laminar bone may be utilized as a patch for larger defects. The graft material, which normally should be compacted in all directions, is passively condensed toward this region. Extensive large defects may necessitate aborting the procedure. All internal septa should then be removed in anticipation of reentry months later.[29] Ironically, patients with a history of sinus disease have a thicker membrane that is more resistant to perforation. Sinus membrane thickening in the absence of active sinus disease is usually not a contraindication to sinus inlay graft surgery.

Residual Ridge Fracture

In the presence of minimal crestal bone or an excessively inferior horizontal osteotomy, a ridge fracture may occur. This is an uncommon event and will occur during either fixture site preparation or insertion in eggshell ridges. A one-stage procedure must then be aborted and a two-stage procedure instituted. The antral void is grafted inclusive of the fractured region. Fixture insertion is performed following the period required for graft maturation.

Hemmorhage

Significant hemorrhage is rarely a problem. If the initial horizontal incision is placed too far palatal, the greater palatine artery may be lacerated. Increased bleeding from the lateral flap may occur if the periosteum is violated. Sinus membrane perforation may result in low-grade hemorrhage as well as postoperative epistaxis. If bleeding is not self-limiting, hemostasis is attained by conventional methods.

Parathesia

Temporary neurosensory deficits of the infraorbital nerve may occur with excess superior flap reflection or improper retractor positioning. Greater palatine nerve distribution paresthesia may occur with an incision placed to medially or excessive medial flap reflection or traction.

Delayed Soft Tissue Healing

Superficial wound dehiscence and necrosis may occur if the horizontal incision is placed excessively palatal. This results in ischemia to the distal edges of the lateral flap as it crosses over the ridge. Prolonged elevated pain, infection, implant exposure, or loss of graft material may occur. Local wound care is supplemented with use of analgesics, chlorhexidine gluconate rinses, and possibly antibiotics until healing is completed by secondary intention.

Infection

Wound infection and acute sinusitis are infrequent and generally transient in nature. Initial care is predominately pharmacologic with an antibiotic protocol based on culture and sensitivity tests. Prolonged infections will significantly impair bone volume and maturation. Surgical management is with incision and drainage, and if refractory, open debridement and antrostomy or middle meatus widening may be necessary. Regrafting may be considered after a prolonged healing period. Chronic sinusitis is not evident and, anecdotally, patients have reported improvement over preoperative sinus states. It is conjectured that the subantral augmentation enhances drainage by elevation of the floor superiorly in closer proximity to the ostium.

Displaced or Malposed Implant

In one-stage procedures, inadequate crestal bone may lead to displaced or malposed fixtures. The crest will be thin and medial, resulting in bodily palatal implant placement or buccal emergence angulation. This will result in unfavorable biomechanics or prosthetic compromise requiring the burying of a fixture (Figure 18.30) or the use of an angled abutment (Figure 18.31) or an overdenture in lieu of a fixed restoration. Fixtures inadequately stabilized by crestal bone may be deflected during graft placement. Similarly, fixtures may be totally displaced into the subantral graft by a poorly adjusted prosthesis during the initial healing period. These complications may be avoided by having bone adequate for prosthetically desirable implant positioning and to provide sufficient stabilization. A two-stage procedure deferring fixture insertion is necessary if these criteria are not met.

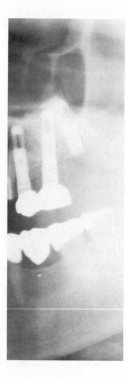

FIGURE 18.30 Postoperative panoramic radiograph close-up view reveals left maxillary sinus bone graft with implant placement. Malposed most posterior implant that could not be utilized in the final prosthesis owing to poor position.

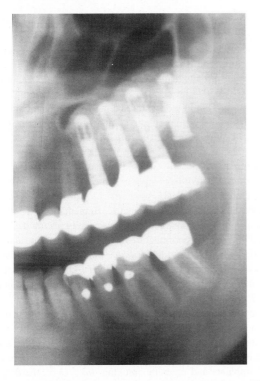

FIGURE 18.31 Postoperative panoramic radiograph left maxillary sinus bone graft with placement of dental implants. Poorly angled middle position fixtures requiring use of angulated abutments. The distal most implant could not be utilized in the final prosthesis.

Deficient Graft

Insufficient new bone volume or density will result in failure or loss of osseointegration. Supplementation with alternative materials should be considered. This regrafting may be performed with minimal morbidity in that the osteotomy, lateral access, and sinus elevation are preexisting.

Osteotome Sinus Floor Elevation

Summers[14,15] has described a simpler, less invasive method of immediate implant insertion utilizing specialized serial osteotomes (Figure 18.32; Implant Innovations, West Palm Beach, FL, USA) in patients with a minimum of 5–6 mm of residual crestal bone. In this technique, bone of the implant recipient site is conserved and serially impacted upward. Bone graft material may be then added to the osteotomy site apically. Further malleting pressure from the osteotome and the graft causes infracturing of the sinus floor and elevation of the membrane. Additional graft material may then be incrementally added to gain additional height. With this technique, the sinus floor may be elevated and grafted, allowing for placement of a 10-mm-long fixture (Figure 18.33). Further multicenter studies are still necessary to determine the efficacy of this procedure. Extensive malleting necessary in the preparation of multiple sites may be disconcerting to the unsedated patient.

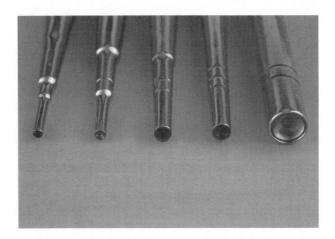

FIGURE 18.32 Summers Osteotomes of various sizes (Implant Innovations, Inc., Palm Beach Gardens, FL).

Conclusion

Osseous deficiencies quantitatively and qualitatively have made the posterior maxilla the least predictable region of endosseous implant placement. Sinus membrane elevation with subantral augmentation utilizing a variety of graft materials, including many that are nonautogenous in nature, has produced bone capable of responding to biomechanical demands. Endosseous implants may be placed simultaneously or as a staged procedure, which achieves and maintains long-standing osseointegration. This provides a suitable foundation for an appropriately designed prosthesis following bone maturation. Techniques described here provide for low morbidity, few risks, and minimal and manageable complications, and may be performed in an office setting under local anesthesia. Introduced by Tatum in the 1970s and more widely performed for more than 15 years, sinus lift grafting has been highly successful in providing implant predictability equivalent to any intraoral region.

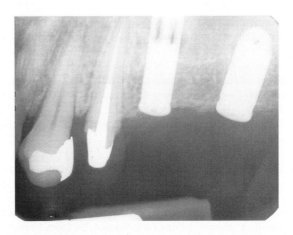

FIGURE 18.33 Summers technique for maxillary sinus bone grafting and placement of two dental implants.

References

1. Jensen J. Reconstruction of the atrophic alveolar ridge with mandibular bone grafts and implants (abstract). *J Oral Maxillofac Surg.* (special issue) 1990:125.
2. Brein V, Bránemark P-I. Reconstruction of the alveolar jaw bone. An experimental and clinical study of immediate and preformed autologous bone grafts in combination with osseointegrated implants. *Scand J Plast Reconstr Surg.* 1980;14:23–48.
3. Sailer HF. A new method of inserting endosseous implants in totally atrophic maxilla. *J Craniomaxillofac Surg.* 1989;17:299–305.
4. Keller EE, VanReokel NB, Desjardins RP, Tolman DE. Prosthetic-surgical reconstruction of the severely resorbed maxilla with iliac bone grafting and tissue integrated prosthesis. *Int J Oral Maxillofac Implants.* 1987;2:155–165.
5. Tatum OH, Leibowitz MS, Tatum CA, Borgner RA. Sinus augmentation rationale development, long-term results. *NY State Dent J.* 1993;5:43–48.
6. Jensen J, Simonson EK, Sindet-Pederson S. Reconstruction of the severely resorbed maxilla with bone grafting and osseointegrated implants: a preliminary report. *J Oral Maxillofac Surg.* 1990;48:27–34.
7. Raghoebar GM, Brouwer TJ, Reintsoma H, VanDort RP. Augmentation of the maxillary sinus floor with autogenous bone for the placement of endosseous implants: a preliminary report. *J Oral Maxillofac Surg.* 1993;51:1198–1203.
8. Block MS, Kent JN. Maxillary sinus grafting for totally and partially edentulous patients. *J Am Dent Assoc.* 1993;124:139–143.
9. Vlassis JM, Húrzeler MB, Quinones CR. Sinus lift augmentation to facilitate placement of nonsubmerged implants: a clinical and histologic report. *Pract Periodontol Restor Dent.* 1993;2:15–23.
10. Fugazzotto PA. Maxillary sinus grafting with and without simultaneous implant placement: technical considerations and case reports. *Int Periodontics Restor Dent.* 1994;14:544–551.
11. Moy PK, Lundgren S, Holmes RE. Maxillary sinus augmentation: histomorphometric analysis of graft materials for maxillary sinus floor augmentation. *J Oral Maxillofac Surg.* 1993;51:857–862.
12. Williams MY, Mealey BL, Hallman WW. The role of computerized tomography in dental implantology. *Int J Oral Maxillofac Implants.* 1992;7:373–380.
13. Kraut R. Radiologic planning for dental implants. In: Block MS, Kent JN, eds. *Endosseous Implants for Maxillofacial Reconstruction.* Philadelphia: WB Saunders; 1995:113–133.
14. Summers RB. A new concept in maxillary implant surgery: the osteotome technique. *Compend Contin Educ Dent.* 1994;2:152–160.
15. Summers RB. The osteotome technique: Part 3. Less invasive methods of elevating the sinus floor. *Compend Contin Educ Dent.* 1994;8:698–708.
16. Bahat O. Osseointegrated implants in the maxillary tuberosity: report on 45 consecutive patients. *Int J Oral Maxillofac Implants.* 1992;7:459–467.
17. Khayat P, Nader N. The use of osseointegrated implants in the maxillary tuberosity. *Pract Periodontol Aesth Dent.* 1994;4:53–61.
18. Graves SL. The pterygoid plate implant: a solution for restoring the posterior maxilla. *Int J Periodontol Restor Dent.* 1994;14:513–523.
19. Keller EE. Composite graft reconstruction of advanced maxillary resorption. In: Block MS, Kent JN, eds. *Endosseous Implants for Maxillofacial Reconstruction.* Philadelphia: WB Saunders; 1995:504–536.
20. Isaksson S. Evaluation of three bone grafting techniques for severely resorbed maxilla in conjunction with immediate endosseous implants. *Int J Oral Maxillofac Implants.* 1994;9:679–688.
21. Bránemark PI, Zarb GA, Albrekitsson T. *Tissue-Integrated Prosthesis Osseointegration in Clinical Dentistry.* Carol Stream, IL: Quintessence; 1985.
22. Adell R, Lekholm V, Grondahl K, Bránemark PI, Lindstrom J, Jacobson M. Reconstruction of the severely resorbed edentulous maxillae using osseointegrated fixtures in immediate autogenous bone grafts. *Int J Oral Maxillofac Implants.* 1990;5:233–246.
23. Jensen J, Sindet-Pederson S, Oliver AJ. Varying treatment strategies for reconstruction of maxillary atrophy with implants. *J Oral Maxillofac Surg.* 1994;52:210–216.
24. Kahnberg KE, Nystrom E, Bartholdsson L. Combined use of bone grafts and Bránemark fixtures in the treatment of severely resorbed maxillae. *Int J Maxillofac Implants.* 1989;4:297–304.
25. Bain CA, Moy PK. The association between the failure of dental implants and cigarette smoking. *Int J Oral Maxillofac Implants.* 1993;8:609–615.
26. Block MS, Kent JN. *Endosseous Implants for Maxillofacial Reconstruction.* Philadelphia: WB Saunders; 1995.
27. Buckley MS. Bone substitutes. *Sel Read Oral Maxillofac Surg.* 1995;4:2.
28. Axhausen W. The osteogenetic phases of regeneration of bone, a historical and experimental study. *J Bone Joint Surg.* 1956;38A:593–601.
29. Tatum OH. Maxillary and sinus implant reconstruction. *Dent Clin North Am.* 1986;30:207–229.
30. Boyne PJ, James RA. Grafting of the maxillary sinus floor with autogenous marrow bone. *J Oral Surg.* 1980;38:613–616.
31. Keller EE, Eckert SE, Tolman DE. Maxillary antral and nasal one stage inlay composite graft: preliminary report on 30 recipient sites. *J Oral Maxillofac Surg.* 1994;52:438–447.
32. Loukota RA, Isaksson SG, Linner ELJ, Blomquist JE. A technique for inserting endosseous implants in the atropic maxilla in a single stage procedure. *Br J Oral Maxillofac Surg.* 1992;30:46–49.
33. Hall DH, McKenna SJ. Bone graft of the maxillary sinus floor for Branemark implants: a preliminary report. *Oral Maxillofac Surg Clin North Am.* 1991;3:869–875.
34. Hirsch JM, Erickson I. Maxillary sinus augmentations using mandibular bone grafts and simultaneous installation of implants. *Clin Oral Implant Res.* 1991;2:91–96.
35. Urist MR. Bone formation by autoinduction. *Science* 1965;150:893.
36. Marx RE, Carlson ER. Tissue banking safety: caveats and precaution for the oral and maxillofacial surgeon. *J Oral Maxillofac Surg.* 1993;51:1372–1379.
37. Buck BE, Malinin TI. Human bone and tissue allografts: preparation and safety. *Clin Orthop Relat Res.* 1994;303:8–17.
38. Buck BE, Malinin TI, Brown MD. Bone transplantation and human immunodeficiency virus: an estimated risk of AIDS. *Clin Orthop Relat Res.* 1989;240:129–136.

39. Reddi AH, Hascall VC. Changes in proteoglycan types during matrix reduced cartilage bone and marrow formation. *Proc Natl Acad Sci USA.* 1977;55:89.

40. Glowacki J, Altobelli D, Mulliken JB. Fate of mineralized and demineralized osseous implants in cranial defects. *Calcif Tissue Int.* 1981;33:71.

41. Lindholm TS, Nilsson OS, Lindholm TC. Extraskeletal and intraskeletal new bone formation induced by demineralized bone matrix combined with marrow cells. *Clin Orthop Relat Res.* 1982;171:251–255.

42. Wittbjer J, Palmer B, Robbin M, Thorngren KG. Osteogenetic activity in composite grafts of demineralized compact bone and marrow. *Clin Orthop Relat Res.* 1983;173:229–238.

43. Smiler DG, Johnson PW, Lozada JL, Misch C, Rosenlicht JL, Tatum OH, Wagner J. Sinus lift grafts and endosseous implants: treatment of the atropic posterior maxilla. *Dent Clin North Am.* 1992;36:151–188.

44. Collins T, Small S, Shepherd N, Buser D, Parel SM. Sinus floor elevations and the status of membranes. Panel discussion. *Int J Oral Maxillofac Implants.* 1994;9(suppl):85–96.

45. Becker W, Becker BE, Caffesse R. A comparison of demineralized freeze-dried bone and autologous bone to induce bone formation in human extraction sockets. *J Periodontol.* 1994;65:1128–1133.

46. Small SA, Zinner ID, Panno FV, Shapiro HJ, Stein JI. Augmenting the maxillary sinus for implants: report of 27 patients. *Int J Oral Maxillofac Implants.* 1993;8:523–528.

47. Misch CE. Maxillary sinus augmentaion for endosteal implants: organized alternative treatment plans. *Int J Oral Implantol.* 1987;4:49–58.

48. Misch CE. *Contemporary Implant Dentistry.* St. Louis: CV Mosby; 1993.

49. Whitaker JM, James RA, Lozada J, Cordova C, GaRey DJ. Histological response and clinical evaluation of autograft and allograft material in the elevation of maxillary sinus for the preparation of endosteal dental implant sites. Simultaneous sinus elevation and root form implantation: an eight month autopsy report. *J Oral Implantol.* 1989;15:141–144.

50. Wittfbjer J, Palmer B. Osteogenetic activity in composite grafts of demineralized compact bone and marrow. *Clin Orthop.* 1988;173:209.

51. Klinge B, Alberius P, Isaksson S, Jonsen J. Osseous response to implanted natural bone mineral and synthetic hydroxylapatite ceramic in the repair of experimental skull bone defects. *J Oral Maxillofac Surg.* 1992;50:241–249.

52. Smiler DG, Holmes RE. Sinus lift procedure using porous hydroxyapatite: a preliminary report. *J Oral Implantol.* 1987;13:239–253.

53. Wagner J. A $3^1/_2$ year clinical evaluation of resorbable hydroxyapatite Osteogen (HA resorb) used for sinus lift augmentation in conjunction with the insertion of endosseous implants. *J Oral Implantol.* 1991;17:152–164.

54. Tidwell JK, Blijdorp PA, Stoelinga PJW, Brouns JB, Hinderks F. Composite grafting of the maxillary sinus for placement of endosteal implants. A preliminary report of 48 patients. *Int J Oral Maxillofac Surg.* 1992;21:204–209.

55. Vassos DM, Petrick DK. The sinus lift procedure: an alternative to the maxillary subperiosteal implant. *Pract Periodontal Dent.* 1992;9:14–19

56. Dario LJ, English R. Chin bone harvesting for autogenous grafting in the maxillary sinus: a clinical report. *Pract Periodontol Restor Dent.* 1994;9:87–91.

57. Jaffin RA, Berman CL. The excessive loss of Branemark fixtures in type IV bone: a 5-year analysis. *J Periodontol.* 1991;62:2–4.

58. Bahat O. Treatment planning and placement of implants in the posterior maxillae: report of 732 consecutive Nobelpharma implants. *Int J Oral Maxillofac Implants.* 1993;8:151–161.

59. Fugazzotto PA, Wheeler SL, Lindsay JA. Success and failure rates of cylinder implants in type IV bone. *J Periodontol.* 1993;64:1085–1087.

60. Schow SR. Infections of the maxillary sinus. *Oral Maxillofac Surg Clin North Am.* 1991;32:343–353.

19
Computerized Tomography and Its Use for Craniomaxillofacial Dental Implantology

Morton Jacobs

Recently, permanent dental implantation has gained wide acceptance because of the well-documented long-term surgical successes.[1] In the past, preoperative x-ray evaluation has included lateral views of the skull, intraoral dental, and panoramic films. More recently, the use of coronal computed tomography (CT) has added another dimension to this evaluation.[2–3] The use of coronal CT has several important limitations. In older patients, it may not be possible because of cervical osteoarthritis. Even under the best of circumstances, it may not be entirely possible to obtain scans exactly perpendicular to the long axis of the mandible or maxilla. Perhaps the most serious drawback, however, are the beam-hardening artifacts generated by dental restorations already in the patient's mouth (Figure 19.1).

The latest improvement in preoperative x-ray evaluation is the availability of sophisticated computer programs, such as the Dentascan (GE Medical Systems, Milwaukee, WI), which reformats standard axial CT images into a series of cross-sectional oblique images that are oriented perpendicular to the curvature of the jaw.[4–6] Additional panoramic CT images and 3D surface renderings are also available with the computer program. From a practical standpoint, the patient is positioned comfortably in a supine position with the head restrained to avoid motion artifacts between images, which would ultimately affect image quality. The lowest possible technical factors are used in combination with a bone algorithm, which enhances spatial resolution. Scanning is performed in the dynamic mode with contiguous or overlapping 1.0-mm-thick sections to again enhance spatial resolution. The images are oriented as nearly parallel to the mandible or maxilla as possible. If both the upper and lower jaw are to be scanned in one sitting, the head has to be repositioned to obtain the correct angulation (Figure 19.2). This serves two purposes: (1) It ensures the fewest number of slices, thereby reducing the x-ray exposure to the patient; and (2) it minimizes geometric distortion.

The computer program relies on the technique of reformatting. In a very simple way, the digital information inherent in the actual CT images are placed in the computer memory. The software program then rearranges this information to obtain the desired series of images.

An axial CT image is selected from the series that corresponds to the roots of any remaining teeth. The physician or technologist then draws in a line corresponding to the curvature of the jaw (Figure 19.3). A series of lines is then prescribed perpendicular to this reference line (Figure 19.4). An oblique cross-sectional image is then obtained corresponding to each cut line, which represents a true cross section that corresponds to the curvature of the jaw (Figure 19.5). In addition, five panoramic tomographic sections are generated by the software program. The central image corresponds to the original prescribed cut line (Figure 19.6) with two on either side, buccally and lingually. Easy cross-referencing is possible among the axial, oblique, and panoramic images. The axial and panoramic images are used for orientation purposes to identify the edentulous areas in the jaw. Once these are localized, measurements of width and thickness of the bone are made from the oblique images. Frontal and lateral 3D surface renderings are shown in Figure 19.7.

These sophisticated computer programs can be used to determine the suitability and appropriate site of implant placement and the possible need for augmentation ridge surgery. Postoperatively, these imaging studies can show failure of an implant to osseointegrate to bone, improper placement of an implant, and violation of important structures.

Let us now determine how the program can be helpful to the surgeon in preoperative evaluation. In the mandible, the surgeon needs to know thickness of alveolar bone, the contour of the alveolar ridge, and the position of the inferior alveolar nerve. In Figure 19.8, we can see the most common appearance of the inferior alveolar nerve, which images as a small dark hole surrounded by a faint cortical line. This is seen in approximately 50% of cases. The next most common appearance is a lucent area without a distinct cortical line and rounded, as seen in Figure 19.9. In this situation, visualization of the nerve depends on a normal amount of trabecular bone remaining in the body of the mandible. Figure 19.10 demonstrates the situation occurring when there is an osteopenic mandible with marked resorption of bony trabecula. Despite the excellent quality of images, the nerve cannot be easily recognized consistently on all the films. In this case, a

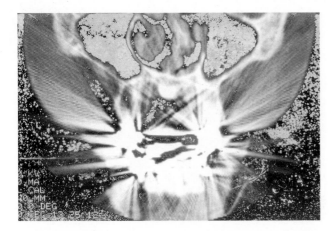

FIGURE 19.1 Direct coronal CT demonstrates severe degradation of image quality secondary to dental restoration in the patient's mouth.

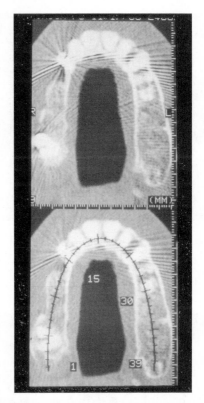

FIGURE 19.3 Prescription of reference line used for generation of oblique cross-sectional images.

a

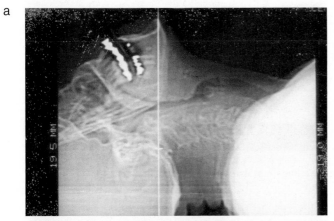

b

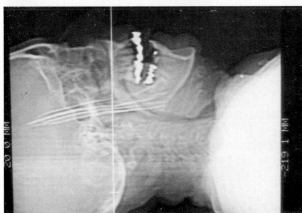

FIGURE 19.2 Sagittal digital radiograph demonstrates patient positioning required for (a) mandibular and (b) maxillary studies. For the mandibular examination, the inferior border of the mandible is perpendicular to the table top, whereas for the maxillary study the hard palate is perpendicular to the table top.

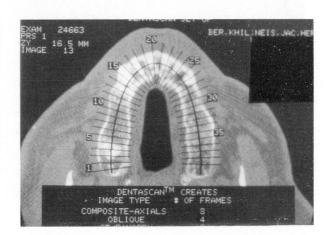

FIGURE 19.4 Oblique cross-sectional images oriented perpendicular to the jaw along the reference line.

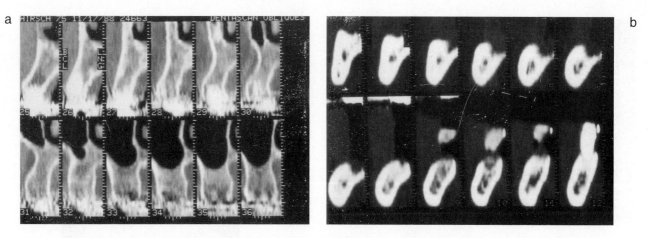

FIGURE 19.5 Series of computer-generated cross-sectional images in (a) maxillary and (b) mandibular examinations.

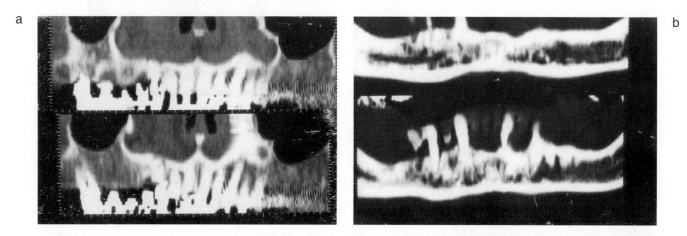

FIGURE 19.6 Computer-generated panoramic images along reference line in (a) maxillary and (b) mandibular examinations.

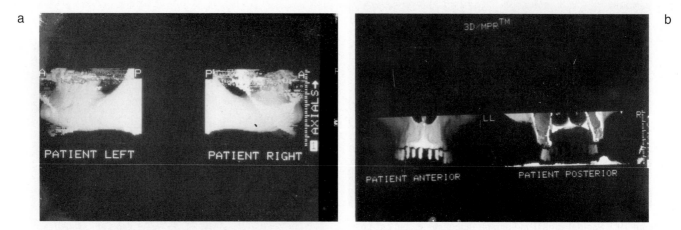

FIGURE 19.7 3D computer-generated surface renderings in (a) mandibular and (b) maxillary studies.

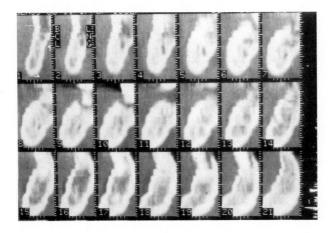

FIGURE 19.8 Oblique cross-sectional images demonstrating inferior alveolar nerve. Typical appearance of nerve surrounded by thick cortical line.

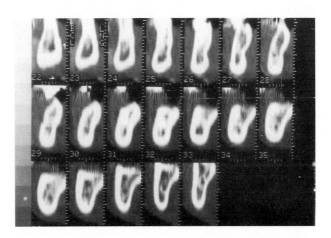

FIGURE 19.9 Oblique cross-sectional images of inferior alveolar nerve appearing as a rounded lucency in body of mandible without distinct cortical line.

precise determination of the position of the nerve is not possible radiographically. Fortunately, this occurs in only 10% to 15% of cases. The position of the nerve relative to the buccolingual cortices is readily determined as is the amount of remaining bone between the nerve and the crest of the ridge. The contour of the ridge is also well demonstrated. Any significant downward sloping is easily recognized.

Several clinical cases are now presented that highlight the usefulness of the Dentascan program. Figure 19.11 demonstrates a severely resorbed mandible in an elderly patient. Under normal circumstances, the mental foramen exists approximately one third of the way from the crest of the alveolar ridge. In this case, the mental foramen and nerve lie at the ridge with no cortical bone covering the nerve. Resorptive changes are present both anteriorly and posteriorly in the mandible, precluding successful intraosseous implantation.

Figure 19.12 demonstrates another patient with a severely resorbed mandible posteriorly with only a small amount of bone covering the inferior alveolar nerve. There is, however, a small area of exposure of the nerve posteriorly in the body of the mandible. The central position of the nerve within the body of the mandible precluded successful positioning of implants either buccally or lingually in the mandible. There is, however, adequate bone anteriorly for fixture placement.

The next two cases highlight the value of the technique in marginal situations. Panoramic view in the first case suggested lack of sufficient bone for implantation. The oblique images (Figure 19.13) show a severely resorbed alveolar ridge with little bone remaining between the nerve and the crest of the ridge. The position of the nerve, however, which can be seen hugging the lingual cortex, allowed successful fixture placement buccally in the body of the mandible. In the next case, preliminary radiographic examination suggested adequate bone for implantation as suggested by the panoramic image (Figure 19.14a). The oblique view (Figure 19.14b), however, demonstrates significant buccolingual atrophy with

a

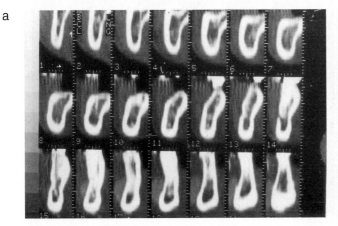

b

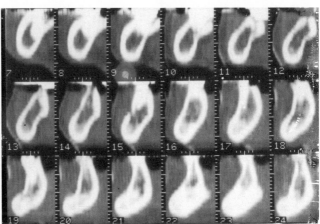

FIGURE 19.10 Osteopenic mandible with resorption of bony trabecula. The inferior alveolar nerve cannot be discerned.

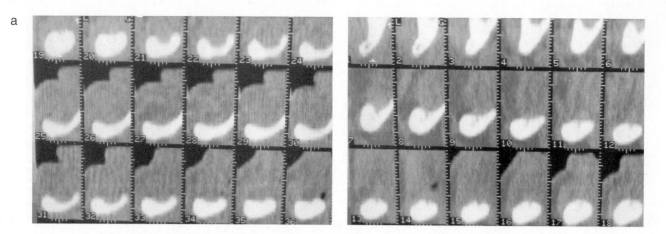

FIGURE 19.11(a+b) Examples of marked bony resorption of the alveolar ridge in the mandible. Inferior alveolar nerve is visualized at the crest of the ridge with little or no bony covering.

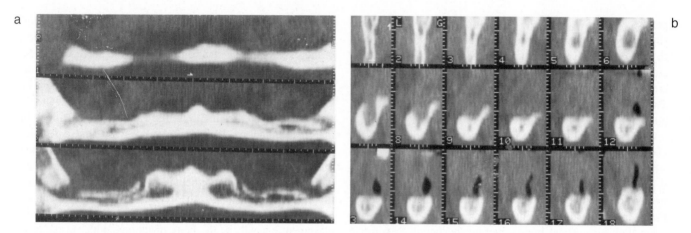

Figure 19.12 Severely resorbed mandible with localized area of exposure of the nerve seen on both (a) panoramic and (b) axial images.

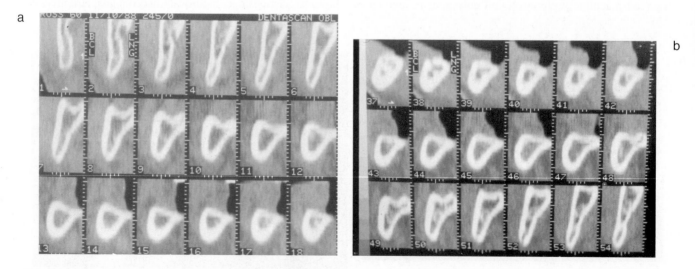

FIGURE 19.13 (a,b) This demonstrates a marginal case with marked resorption of alveolar ridge initially precluding fixture placement. Position of nerve adjacent to the lingual cortex allowed fixture placement buccal to the nerve.

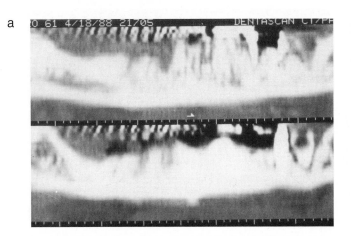

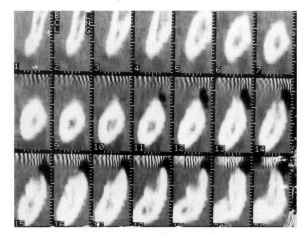

FIGURE 19.14 Appearance of adequate bone on plain film taken before the examination and panoramic images (a) suggest adequate bone. Oblique cross-sectional images (b), however, demonstrate buccolingual atrophy requiring alveolectomy or bone graft augmentation. Considerably less bone is available for final fixture placement.

sharp, tapered pointing of the ridge. The patient required alveolectomy and considerably less bone was therefore available for fixture placement. In both cases Dentascan imaging aided presurgical planning and influenced final decision-making.

Postoperatively, these imaging techniques are useful in assessing adequacy of osseointegration. Normally successful osseointegration demonstrates a tight metal-to-bone contact. Failure of osseointegration is evident by absent metal-to-bone contact with a lucent zone around the fixture representing fibrous tissue. Axial and oblique cross-sectional images in this case demonstrate fibrous osseointegration of the left incisor and premolar fixtures (Figure 19.15).

Violation of the mandibular canal by either improper drilling, fixture placement, or secondary infection can result in permanent injury to the inferior alveolar nerve. Usually, however, once it is recognized and adequate measures undertaken, this can be avoided.

In the following case (Figure 19.16), an implant placed in

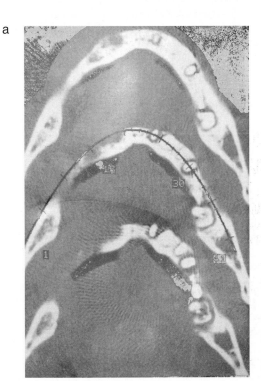

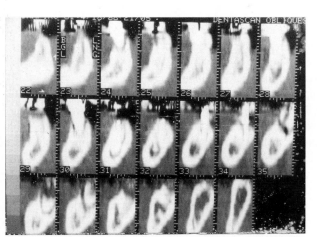

FIGURE 19.15(a) Axial view and (b) oblique cross sectional images demonstrating fibrous osseointegration involving left incisor and premolar fixtures demonstrating faint lucent zone on original axial and oblique cross-sectional images.

a

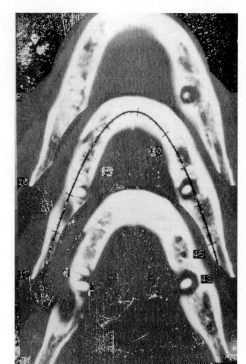

b

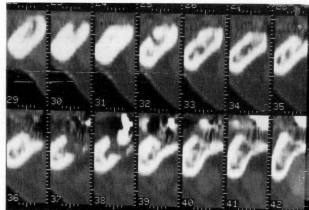

d

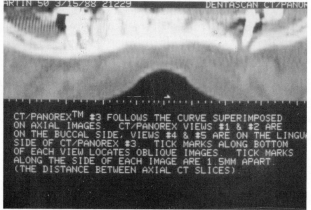

c

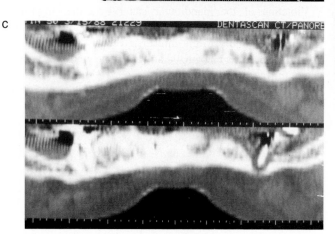

CT/PANOREX™ #3 FOLLOWS THE CURVE SUPERIMPOSED
ON AXIAL IMAGES. CT/PANOREX VIEWS #1 & #2 ARE
ON THE BUCCAL SIDE. VIEWS #4 & #5 ARE ON THE LINGU
SIDE OF CT/PANOREX #3. TICK MARKS ALONG BOTTOM
OF EACH VIEW LOCATES OBLIQUE IMAGES. TICK MARKS
ALONG THE SIDE OF EACH IMAGE ARE 1.5MM APART
(THE DISTANCE BETWEEN AXIAL CT SLICES).

FIGURE 19.16 Postoperative infection demonstrated on (a) axial, (b) oblique cross sectional, and (c,d) panoramic images as localized area of bony resorption around the fixture. Exposure of the inferior alveolar nerve and adjacent lingual cortex.

the immediate extraction site in the left molar region developed a localized infection within the tooth socket. There is extensive erosion of bone with exposure of the inferior alveolar nerve and the adjacent lingual cortex.

Improper implant placement is illustrated in the next case (Figure 19.17). The patient experienced paresthesia of the right lower left lip and chin after improper implant placement in the molar region. The implant is seen on the same axial image as the inferior alveolar nerve. Oblique cross-sectional images confirm violation of the canal by the fixture. Once removed, the paresthesia quickly resolved. In the maxilla, the surgeon again needs to know the height of alveolar bone, the contour of the ridge, and sinus pathology.

In our first case, a commonly encountered problem is recognized—the large incisive canal. The axial image (Figure 19.18a) shows generalized resorption of the alveolar ridges.

A large incisive canal is demonstrated which often accompanies the generalized resorptive change. This often limits fixture placement in the anterior premaxillary region. This change is again confirmed on oblique and panoramic images (Figures 19.18a,b). The next case highlights an interesting problem and an instructive case. In Figure 19.19a we see edentulous areas in the posterior alveolar regions. Adequate bone is present for fixture placement and no significant buccolingual atrophy is seen on oblique images (Figure 19.19b). Interestingly, the surgeon encountered great difficulty at operation owing to the softness of the bone. Perhaps the only limiting factor at the present time with many of these computer programs is the assessment of textural abnormalities of bone.

The problem of buccolingual atrophy, particularly in the premaxilla, is illustrated in Figure 19.20. Despite adequate height

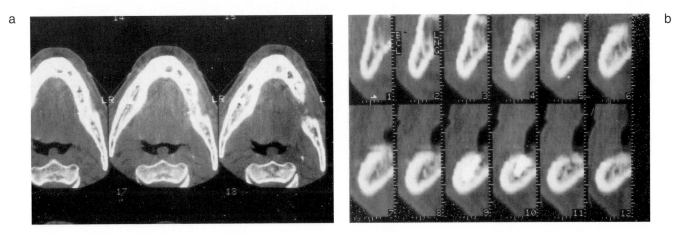

FIGURE 19.17 Improper fixture placement demonstrated on (a) axial and (b) oblique cross-sectional images. Involvement of the inferior alveolar nerve by the fixture is seen to excellent advantage.

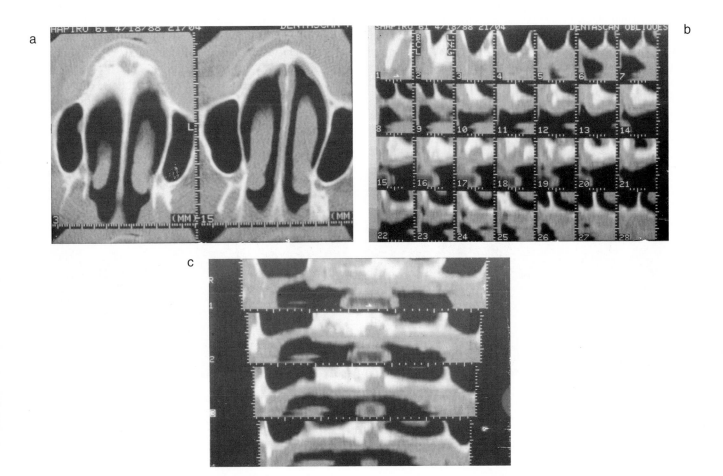

FIGURE 19.18 Severe resorptive changes within the maxillary ridge. Associated enlargement of the incisive canal is seen on (a) original axial, (b) oblique cross-sectional, and (c) panoramic images.

a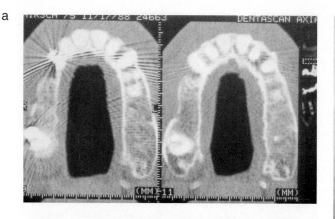

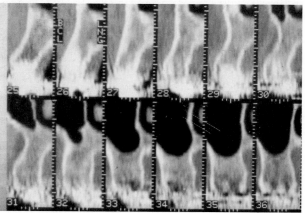 b

FIGURE 19.19 Edentulous area in posterior maxilla on the left with adequate bone for fixture placement (a). Softness of bone encountered at surgery was not recognized on preoperative imaging (b).

of the ridge, the severe buccolingual atrophy recognized on both axial and oblique views precludes fixture placement at the desired positions without further bone graft augmentation. In the next case, we see a situation of asymmetrical buccolingual atrophy. Adequate bone is seen on the right, but the severe buccolingual atrophy and tapering of the premaxilla on the left dictates an alveolectomy prior to fixture placement (Figure 19.21).

An interesting technique is illustrated in the following case.

The patient is scanned with a plastic stent with gutta percha markers placed at the sites where the surgeon wants to place fixtures. The radiologist can comment about the adequacy of bone at each site, permitting a direct correlation with the surgeon (Figure 19.22)

The final series of cases demonstrates the use of the Dentascan program in assessing maxillary sinus pathology with regard to posterior fixture placement. Figure 19.23 illustrates a

a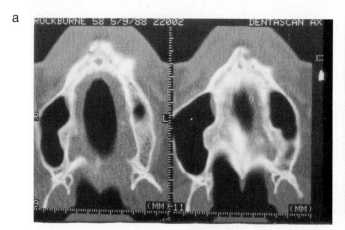

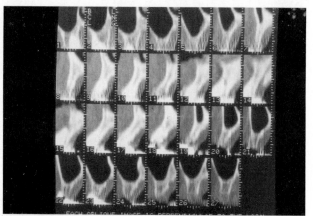 b

FIGURE 19.20 Severe buccolingual atrophy demonstrated on (a) axial and (b) oblique cross-sectional images.

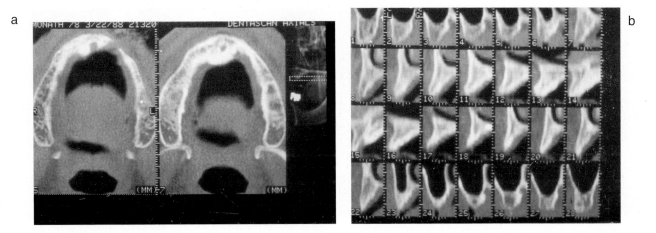

FIGURE 19.21(a) Axial and (b) oblique cross sectional images of asymmetrical buccolingual atrophy on the left required alveolectomy prior to fixture placement.

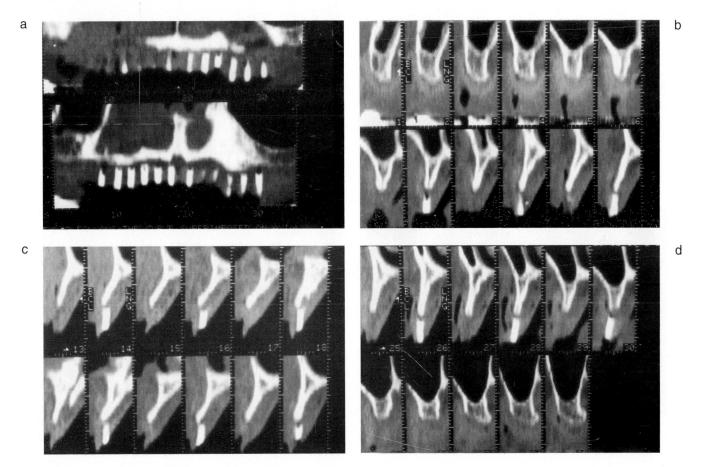

FIGURE 19.22 Patient scanned with radiopaque markers where surgeon desires to place fixtures. Direct correlation is available between (a) panoramic and (b–d) oblique cross-sectional images.

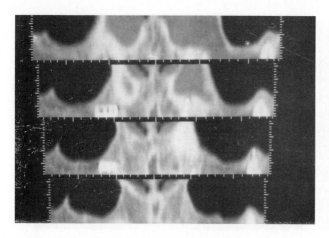

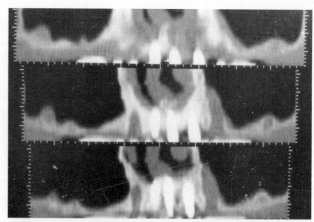

a

FIGURE 19.23 Normal panoramic image demonstrating clear maxillary sinuses with no inflammatory disease.

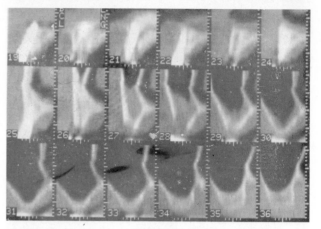

b

normal case without evidence of sinus pathology. The normally aerated sinuses are seen without abnormal tissue adjacent to the bone. Figure 19.24 shows inflammatory disease within the inferior recess of the right maxillary sinus imaging as polypoid soft tissue interposed between the alveolar ridge and aerated sinuses. Violation of the maxillary sinus by an implant is seen as possibly accounting for the infection. Although very accurate in defining soft tissue disease, the exact nature is uncertain. It may represent either submucosal edema, retained se-

FIGURE 19.25 Failed implants filled with granulation tissue is seen extending into the alveolar recess of the left maxillary incisor on both (a) panoramic and (b) oblique cross-sectional images.

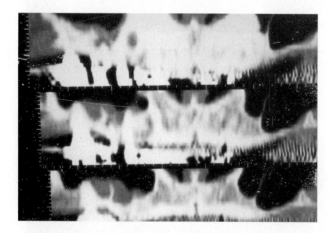

FIGURE 19.24 Polypoid mucosal thickening within the alveolar recess right maxillary sinus.

cretions, or inflammatory tissue. Figure 19.25 again demonstrates inflammatory disease in the left maxillary sinus on both oblique and panoramic images. Three normal implants are seen within the anterior maxilla. Two failed implant sites are seen filled with granulation tissue. Infection extends into the alveolar recess of the left maxillary antrum.

The use of multiplanar reconstruction programs combined with CT scanning has greatly enhanced the success of intraosseous dental implantation. Although not necessary in every case, its use in difficult or marginal cases can often aid the surgeon in preoperative evaluation and surgical planning. Imaging of the maxillary sinus and posterior mandibular nerve-bearing regions, however, is often essential.

References

1. Albrektsson T, Lekholm U. Osseointegration: current state of the art. *Dent Clin North Am.* 1989;33:537–544.
2. DelBalso AM, Hall RE. Advances in maxillofacial imaging. *Curr Probl Diagn Radiol.* 1993;22:96–103.
3. Rothman SLG, Chafetz N, Rhodes ML, Schwartz MS. CT in the preoperative assessment of the mandible and maxilla for endosseous implant surgery. *Radiology.* 1988;168: 171–175.
4. Schwartz MS, Rothman SLG, Rhodes ML, Chafetz N. Computed tomography. I. Preoperative assessment of the mandible for endosseous implant surgery. *Int J Oral Maxillofac Implants.* 1987;2:137–141.
5. Schwartz MS, Rothman SLG, Rhodes ML, Chafetz N. Computed tomography. II. Preoperative assessment of the maxilla for endosseous implant surgery. *Int J Oral Maxillofac Implants.* 1987;2:143–148.
6. Abrahams JJ. Anatomy of the jaw revisited with dental CT software program. *AJNR.* 1993;14:979–990.

20A
Radiographic Evaluation of the Craniomaxillofacial Region

Dorrit Hallikainen, Christian Lindqvist, and Anna-Lisa Söderholm

Panoramic and Plain Film Radiography and Conventional Tomography

Preoperative radiographic evaluation of patients undergoing corrective or reconstructive bone surgery aims to evaluate the nature and extent of the lesion or deformity and to provide the surgeon with anatomic mapping of structures that are important in treatment planning. Follow-up examinations are performed to confirm healing and to discover complications at an early stage.

The selection of the most appropriate imaging method in each case has to take into account the diagnostic capability and cost-effectiveness of the investigation. Plain films are still used frequently, as for example in graft evaluation.[1,2] Plain films, panoramic radiography, and conventional tomography can be performed at low cost and a low radiation dose, as compared to computed tomography (CT) examination, which exposes the imaged area to a substantially higher radiation dose.[3]

Good image quality is essential, and special attention must be paid to quality assurance. The entire chain of image acquisition, from selection of equipment to patient positioning, exposure, and dark-room processing has to be carefully controlled.

Imaging Methods

Panoramic Radiography

The panoramic view is the basis of imaging the dentition and mandible.[4] It corresponds to plain film in other parts of the skeleton because the entire mandible is within the image layer of a single exposure. The form of the image layer and the direction of the beam (i.e., the projection) varies from one machine to the next, and several image layer profiles may be programmed into a single panoramic unit. In purely dental imaging, an orthoradial projection is usually the goal because it minimizes crown overlapping. An orthoradial projection, however, causes more ghost shadows of the opposite ramus than an oblique projection and may give origin to very dis-

torted shadows in patients with metal fixation devices in the ramus or angular area. When the opportunity exists to select the projection in panoramic radiography, the lowest orthoradial beam direction is recommended for patients with bone plates (Figure 20A.1).

The use of panoramic radiography is well established in imaging the dentition and the entire mandible, but its use in other parts of the facial skeleton and in coned-down views has, until now, been limited. The panoramic technique of using rotating narrow-beam radiography is useful in imaging various parts of the facial skeleton, when image layer forms different from the conventional techniques are applied.[5,6] Panoramic radiography of the middle face is usually carried out using a cylindrical image layer. It gives a good overall view of the midface. It can be complementary to plain films, or it can replace Waters' and Caldwell projections (Figure 20A.2).[5,7]

Detailed narrow-beam radiography is a term used for coned-down views of various parts of the jaws.[6] With this method, an area of 3×3 cm is imaged using the panoramic technique and a magnification of 1.7. The diagnostic capability of this technique has proven to be in dental radiology of the same quality as in periapical radiography.[8,9] These findings may be partly owing to the understanding that detailed narrow-beam radiography includes four projections of the same area, and the images are stereoscopic pairs (Figure 20A.3). Detailed narrow-beam radiography is in our experience suitable for bone structure evaluation of the mandible and the alveolar process of the maxilla.[10]

Plain Films

Basic plain film series for the upper jaw include Waters', Caldwell, and lateral projections, often supplemented with a submentovertex view.[11] For the mandible, Towne's and submentovertex projections are usually considered the standard series.

The plain films provide an overview of the lesion or deformity, and at follow-up examinations, they are used to evaluate the location of fixation plates and screws. Usually plain films do not permit early detection of subtle bone changes, such as those seen with infection or bone-graft failure.

a 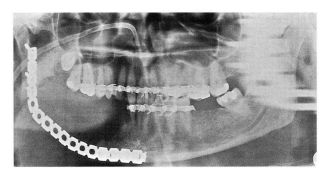 b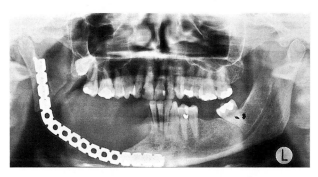

FIGURE 20A.1 (a) A panoramic image taken with orthoradial projection. Ghost shadows originating from the plate are present on the contralateral side. (b) A panoramic image of the same patient with a more oblique projection. There are no ghost shadows from the metal plate. There is no overlapping of teeth crowns and a part of the atlas overlaps the ramus.

Multidirectional Tomography

Multidirectional, cross-sectional tomography is valuable both in preoperative mapping of the jaws and for the postoperative follow-up of bone grafts, fracture fixation, and reconstruction plate and screw fixation.

Linear tomography is not recommended because the technique uses linear blurring motion, which causes spurious con-

a

b

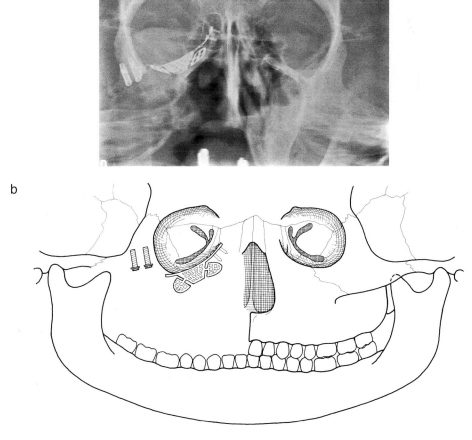

FIGURE 20A.2 (a) A panoramic image of the middle face demonstrates a large defect of the right maxilla and zygoma, metal devices of the orbital floor, and implants inserted to the frontal process of the right zygoma. (b) A diagrammatic representation of (a).

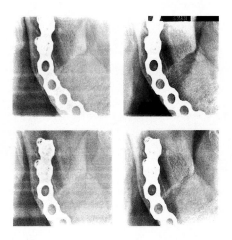

FIGURE 20A.3 An example of detailed narrow-beam radiography. The examination includes four different projections, which is helpful in the evaluation of bone structure details. This example shows the proximal part of a bone graft the day following surgery.

tours. As a result the blurring artifacts cannot be separated from the real image, with subsequent misinterpretation.[12]

Mandibular height and form, and location of the mandibular canal can be assessed by using cross-sectional tomography.[13] The alveolar ridge of the upper jaw can be evaluated in a similar manner.[14,15] Cross-sectional tomography is also useful in the diagnosis of cortical resorption under reconstruction plates, screw loosening, and bone healing.[10,16]

Imaging Sequence and Interpretation

The Upper Jaw

Before surgery, a Waters' view may be complementary to the anthropomorphic measurement evaluations. Waters' view provides an overview of the deformity. Preoperative management of complex cases require CT, and 3-D reconstruction is very valuable.[4] A postoperative Waters' view is often sufficient for the assessment of osteosynthesis plate location (Figure 20A.4), although in general plain films are of limited use in follow-up of the upper jaw.

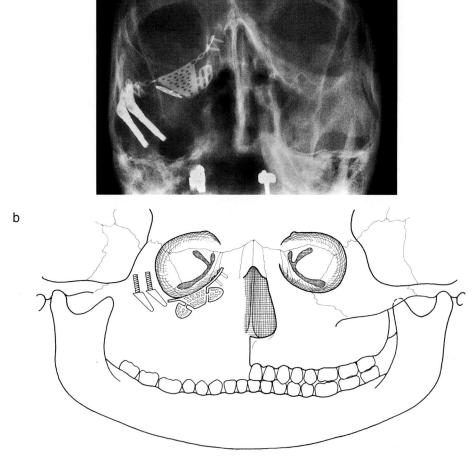

FIGURE 20A.4 Waters' view after surgery is sufficient to show the implant abutments in place. (Same patient as in Figure 20A.2). (b) A diagrammatic representation of (a).

The Lower Jaw, Corrective Surgery

Prior to operation, the anthropomorphic measurements are co-ordinated with a panoramic radiograph, Towne's projection, and axial view to determine the status of the dentition and the shape of the mandible.

Cross-sectional multidirectional tomography of the planned osteotomy site is recommended to assess location of the mandibular canal and the form, height, and thickness of the mandible (Figure 20A.5).

The first follow-up examination is performed the day after surgery, and it should include a panoramic and a Towne's projection. Positioning the patient for a submentovertex view causes considerable pain and discomfort and should be avoided in the early postoperative period. The osteotomy sites are then evaluated: amount of correction, location of fixation material, and any indications of unfavorable correction, including the temporomandibular joints.

To evaluate the healing process, a follow-up schedule of examinations at 1, 3, and 6 months is suitable, as long as the clin-

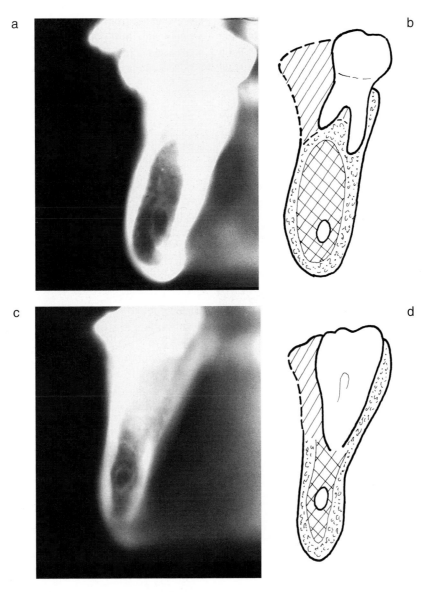

FIGURE 20A.5 (a) Cross-sectional tomography of the right lower jaw at the level of the distal molar area. The mandibular canal is clearly visible lingually. The patient was a 46-year-old woman with retrognathia. (b) A diagrammatic representation of (a). (c) Preoperative examination of a 26-year-old woman with prognathia. Cross-sectional tomography of the right molar area shows the mandibular canal, which is located centrally. The thickness of the lower jaw at the level of the canal is only 8 mm. (d) A diagrammatic representation of (c).

ical course is uneventful. If the first follow-up examination reveals inadequate correction or any indications of complication, the examination schedule is adjusted. In these situations, the examination can include detailed narrow-beam images as well as multidirectional tomography, with particular attention directed toward signs of infection and delayed union.

The Lower Jaw, Reconstructive Surgery

The preoperative examination should include at least a panoramic radiograph, Towne's projection, and an axial view. Depending on the underlying lesion other examinations, such as detailed narrow-beam images, conventional tomography, or CT, may be obtained.[10] The first follow-up examination is performed on the first postoperative day, and it should include a panoramic and Towne's radiographs. The height of the bone graft is measured from the panoramic image, which will be used as reference for further measurements. This is an exception to the general rule that measurements should not be taken from panoramic images.[10,17]

The magnification on a panoramic image is not constant, but varies in different parts of the image. This is remarkable, especially in the horizontal direction, where even a slight change in patient positioning has considerable influence on the horizontal dimensions.[17] This variability is not as considerable in the vertical direction, so measurements from successive images of the same patient's region of interest are sufficiently accurate to permit, for example, graft-height assessment (Figures 20A.6 and 20A.7).

The overall location of the reconstruction plate and screws are evaluated from the panoramic and Towne's images. The second and third follow-up examinations are scheduled 2 weeks and 1 month after the operation. It is possible to recognize evidence of infection 2 weeks after surgery.[18] Early

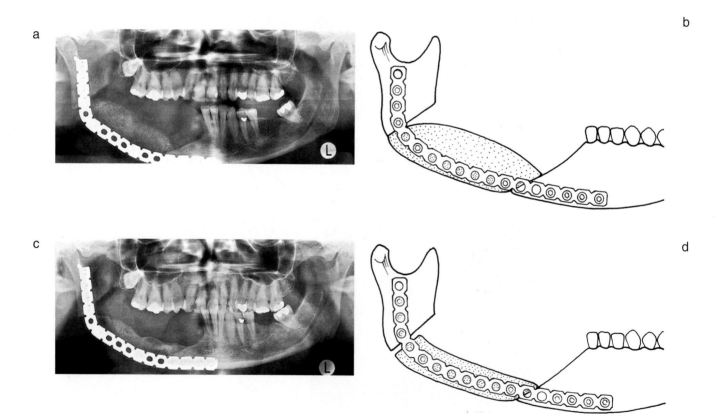

FIGURE 20A.6 (a) A panoramic image taken 2 days after graft surgery. The height of the graft can be measured in the vertical direction. (b) A diagrammatic representation of (a). (c) A panoramic image of the same patient 8 months after insertion of the graft. There is moderate resorption of the graft, which has diminished in height. Good healing is seen at the medial end, but there is still a gap between graft and mandible in the angular area, indicating delayed healing. (d) A diagrammatic representation of (c).

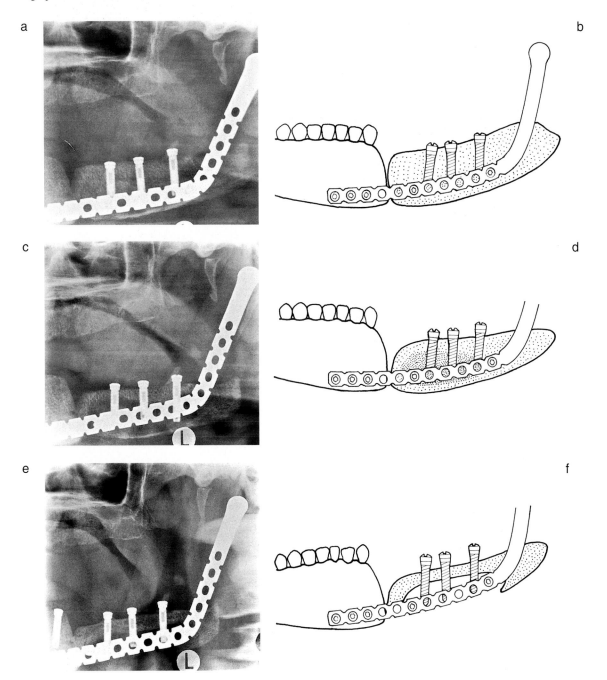

FIGURE 20A.7 (a) A panoramic image taken 3 days after graft surgery. Note height and density of the graft. (b) A diagrammatic representation of (a). (c) A panoramic image of the same patient 2 months later. The graft has diminished in height, and there is a marked radiolucent defect, indicating resorption within the graft. (d) A diagrammatic representation of (c). (e) A panoramic image 8 months after graft surgery. The height of the graft is approximately one third of the original height, indicating ongoing and marked resorption, but no signs of infection. (f) A diagrammatic representation of (e).

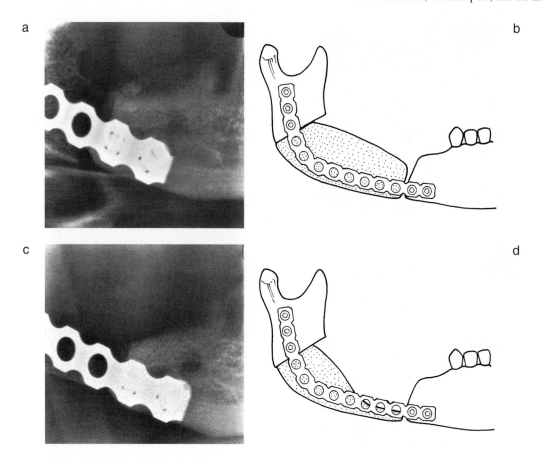

FIGURE 20A.8 (a) Example of massive graft resorption. A detailed image of the medial end of a bone graft on the day following surgery. The graft height corresponds to the mandible. (b) A diagrammatic representation of (a). (c) The same patient 4 months later. The graft has dimished in height; the upper border is visible through the holes in the plate. The resorption exceeds 30% and indicates graft failure. (d) A diagrammatic representation of (c).

graft failure can be diagnosed 1 month postoperatively.[10] In these examinations, a panoramic and Towne's projection are complemented with detailed narrow-beam images (Figure 20A.8). Cross-sectional tomography is undertaken if the detailed images show excessive graft resorption or signs of infection (Figure 20A.9).

The schedule for further follow-up examinations depends on the findings at 1 month after surgery, with any signs of infection, significant graft resorption, or slow healing requiring closer follow-up. In nonvascularized grafts, some degree of bone resorption regularly appears, in which slight resorption (where the height of the graft diminishes 0% to 15% within the first 3 months) is a reliable sign of good healing.[10]

On the other hand, resorption exceeding 30% always indicates graft failure, and if this condition is recognized early, it can influence patient care and the timing of further treatment. Moderate graft resorption of 15% to 30% may appear for several reasons, but it always indicates the need for thorough and regular follow-up, and leads to more efficient treatment of these complications.

Infection appears as patchy bone loss, with blurring of the trabecular pattern and increased sclerosis, and detailed images are suitable for the interpretation of the signs of infection.[18]

Cross-sectional tomography is useful in discovering cortical resorption under the fixation plate, where some degree of resorption is often seen, although massive resorption usually indicates diminished stability. Screw loosening is easy to evaluate on cross-sectional images (Figure 20A.10).[16]

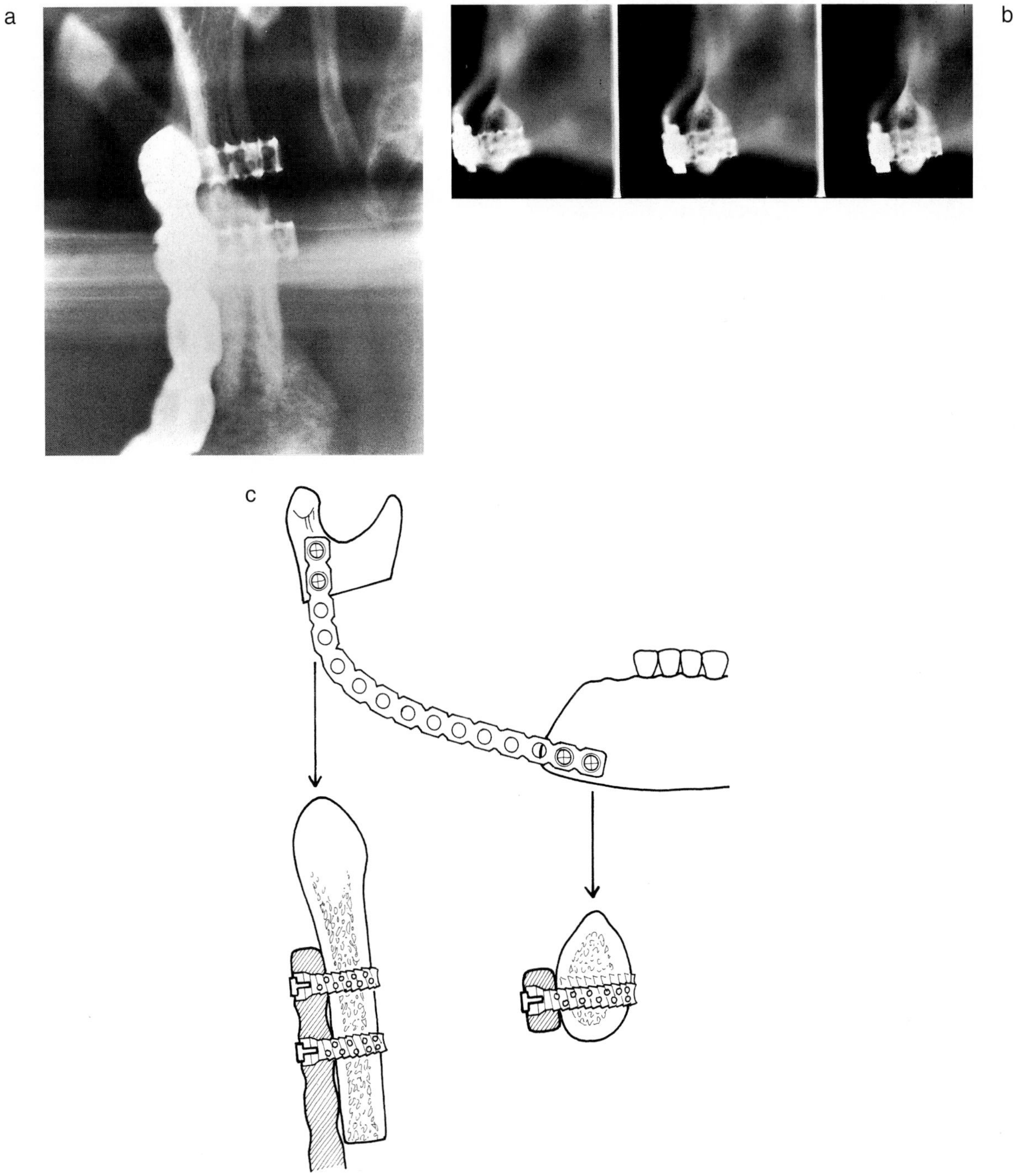

a

b

c

FIGURE 20A.9 (a) A detailed image in the posteroanterior direction of the condylar fragment shows two screws in good position. No signs of bone resorption. (b) A cross-sectional tomography of the mandibular body area (same patient). Three consecutive cuts show the body screws in good position. (c) A diagrammatic representation of (a) and (b).

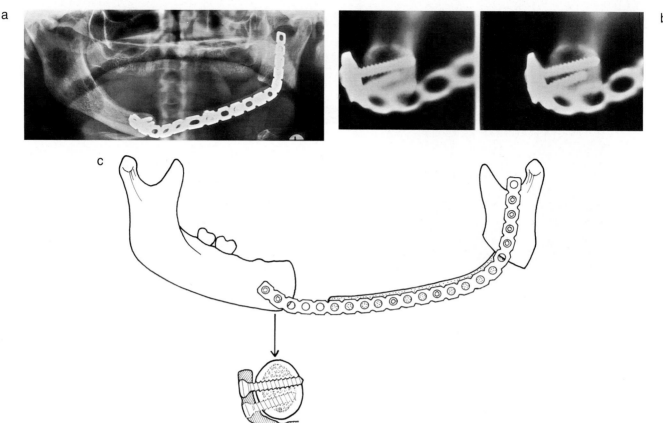

FIGURE 20A.10 (a) A panoramic image of a 59-year-old patient shows a reconstruction plate and a vascular, fibular graft. There is a gap between the mandibular symphysis and the medial end of the graft. (b) Cross-sectional tomography of the symphyseal area demon-strates a gap between the plate and mandible. Only one screw is bi-cortical. These findings indicate loosening of the screws. (c) A dia-grammatic representation of (a) and (b).

Conclusion

Panoramic radiography, plain films, and multidirectional tomography are still valuable tools in examinations for reconstructive bone surgery of the mandible. The imaging procedure must be selected according to the specified diagnostic task, and good image quality is a necessity. Close collaboration between clinician and radiologist is essential for an optimal result.

References

1. Bowerman J, Huges L. Radiology of bone grafts. *Radiol Clin North Am.* 1975;13:67–77.
2. Murphey M. Imaging aspects of new techniques in orthopedic surgery. *Radiol Clin North Am.* 1994;32:201–225.
3. Ekestubbe A, Thilander A, Gröndahl K, et al. Absorbed doses from computed tomography for dental implant surgery: comparison with conventional tomography. *Dentomaxillofac Radiol.* 1993;22:13–17.
4. Wolford L, Henry C. Preoperative and postoperative imaging evaluation of patients with maxillofacial deformities. *Radiol Clin North Am.* 1993;31:221–231.
5. Hallikainen D, Paukku P. Panoramic zonography. In: DelBalso A, ed. *Maxillofacial Imaging.* Philadelphia: WB Saunders; 1990:1–33.
6. Tammisalo E, Hallikainen D, Kanerva H, et al. Comprehensive oral x-ray diagnosis: scanora (R) multimodal radiography. A preliminary description. *Dentomaxillofac Radiol.* 1992;21:9–15.
7. Paukku P, Tötterman S, Hallikainen D, et al. Comparison of the visibility of the anatomical structures of the facial skeleton in panoramic zonography and linear tomography. *Eur J Radiol.* 1983;3:177–179.
8. Tammisalo T, Luostarinen T, Vähätalo K, et al. Comparison of periapical and detailed narrow-beam radiography for diagnosis

of periapical bone lesions. *Dentomaxillofac Radiol.* 1993;22: 183–187.

9. Tammisalo T, Vähätalo K, Luostarinen T, et al. Comparison of periapical and narrow-beam radiography for diagnosis of periodontal pathology. *Dentomaxillofac Radiol.* 1994;23:97–101.

10. Söderholm A, Hallikainen D, Lindqvist C. Radiologic follow-up of bone transplants to bridge mandibular continuity defects. *Oral Surg Oral Med Oral Pathol.* 1992;73:253–261.

11. Hall R, DelBalso A, Carter L. Radiography of the sinonasal tract. In: DelBalso A, ed. *Maxillofacial Imaging.* Philadelphia: WB Saunders; 1990:139–207.

12. Littleton J. *Tomography: Physical Principles and Clinical Applications.* Baltimore: Williams & Wilkins; 1976:33–75.

13. Hallikainen D, Iizuka T, Lindqvist C. Cross-sectional tomography in evaluation of patients undergoing sagittal split osteotomy. *J Oral Maxillofac Surg.* 1992;50:1269–1273.

14. Ekestubbe A, Gröndahl H. Reliability of spiral tomography with the Scanora (R) technique for implant planning. *Clin Oral Implants Res.* 1993;4:195–202.

15. Gröndahl K, Ekestubbe A, Gröndahl G. A multimodal unit for comprehensive dento-maxillofacial radiography. *Dental Update.* 1993;20:436–440.

16. Söderholm A, Hallikainen D, Lindqvist C. Long-term stability of two different mandibular bridging systems. *Arch Otolaryngol Head Neck Surg.* 1993;119:1031–1036.

17. Welander U, McDavid W, Tronje G. Theory of rotational panoramic radiography. In: Langland O, Langlais R, Morris C, eds. *Principles and Practice of Panoramic Radiology.* Philadelphia: WB Saunders; 1982:37–63.

18. Iizuka T, Lindqvist C, Hallikainen D, et al. Infection after internal fixation of mandibular fractures. A clinical and radiological study. *J Oral Maxillofac Surg.* 1991;49:585–593.

20B
Atlas of Cases

Christian Lindqvist, Dorrit Hallikainen, and Anna-Lisa Söderholm

Regular radiologic examinations are essential in follow-up of bone grafts. Radiologic examination contributes to the evaluation of bone healing and complications such as infection or graft failure. It is possible to recognize signs of infection 2 weeks after surgery.[1] Early graft failure can be diagnosed 1 month postoperatively.[2] In nonvascular grafts, some degree of bone resorption regularly appears. Slight resorption, where the height of the graft diminishes 0% to 15% within the first 3 months, is a reliable sign of good healing. Massive resorption exceeding 30% always indicates graft failure. Moderate graft resorption of 15% to 30% may appear for several reasons, but it always indicates the need for thorough and frequent follow-up and should lead to an active treatment of the problems.[2]

Radiologic follow-up examinations are scheduled on the first postoperative day, and 2 weeks and 1 month after the operation. The schedule for further follow-up depends on the findings 1 month after surgery.

The examination should include a panoramic image and a Towne's radiograph and detailed narrow-beam images complemented with cross-sectional tomography when necessary.

The use of other imaging modalities (e.g., CT, MRI) in follow-up depends on the possibilities to overcome interpretation problems caused by metal artifacts.[3]

All the cases presented here illustrate clinical problems. The first case (Figure 20B.1) shows good bony healing between graft and mandible but resorption within the graft, ongoing for more than 3 years.

The second case (Figure 20B.2) illustrates a good final result in spite of delayed union and plate fracture.

The third case (Figure 20B.3) shows moderate graft resorption, which was due to infection. Intensive therapy resulted in a good final result.

The fourth case (Figure 20B.4) shows delayed but otherwise uneventful healing.

The fifth case (Figure 20B.5) illustrates delayed union, which was caused by hyperparathyroidism. After parathyroidectomy bony healing was achieved, and the final result is good.

The sixth case (Figure 20B.6) shows delayed healing in a spontaneous fracture of an irradiated, edentulous mandible. Bone grafting and insertion of implants achieved a good final result.

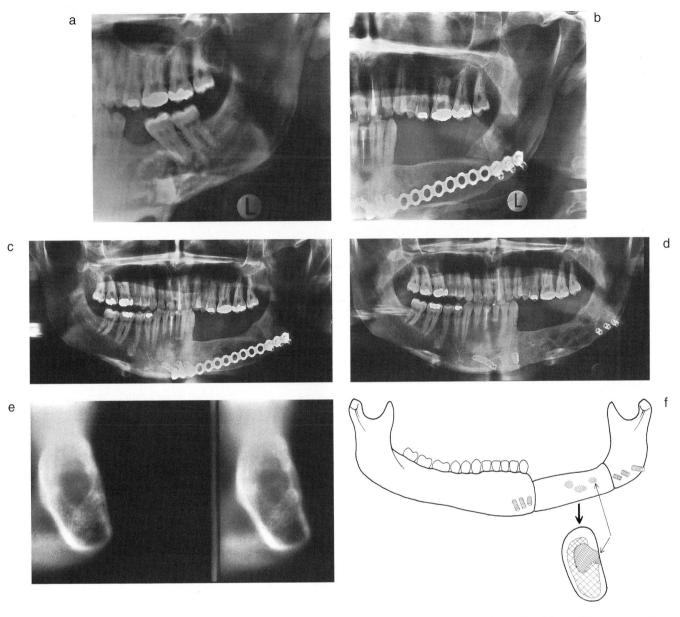

FIGURE 20B.1 (a) Panoramic image of a 32-year-old male with Pindborg's tumor (CEOT) to the left. (b) Panoramic image 6 months after the operation. The border between graft and the angular area is still sharp, and the bony union is not complete. (c) Situation 14 months after the operation. There is complete bony union between graft and mandible. However, areas of bone resorption are seen within the graft. (d) Situation 27 months after the operation. The plate has been removed, and the height of the graft is preserved, but bone resorption within the graft seems to continue. (e) Cross-sectional tomography 27 months after operation. Two consecutive cuts. There is good cortical lining of the graft, but it has a central area of radiolucency (bone resorption). (f) A diagrammatic representation of (e).

a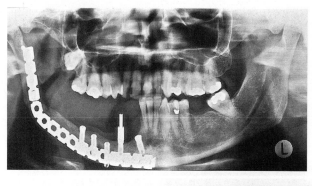

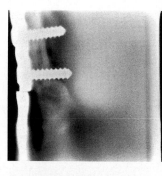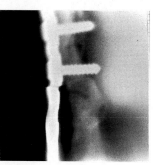b

c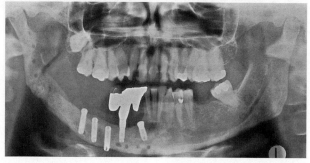

FIGURE 20B.2 (a) Panoramic image of a 40-year-old female 4 years after primary operation for SCC of mandibular gingiva of the molar area and 20 months after transplantation of an iliac bone graft. The plate has fractured. There is good bony union medially between graft and mandible, but a defect at the angular border. (b) Cross-sectional tomography also shows the plate fracture. A thin bony bridge is seen lingually. (c) Panoramic image 5 months later. There is complete union between graft and mandible; the plate has been removed.

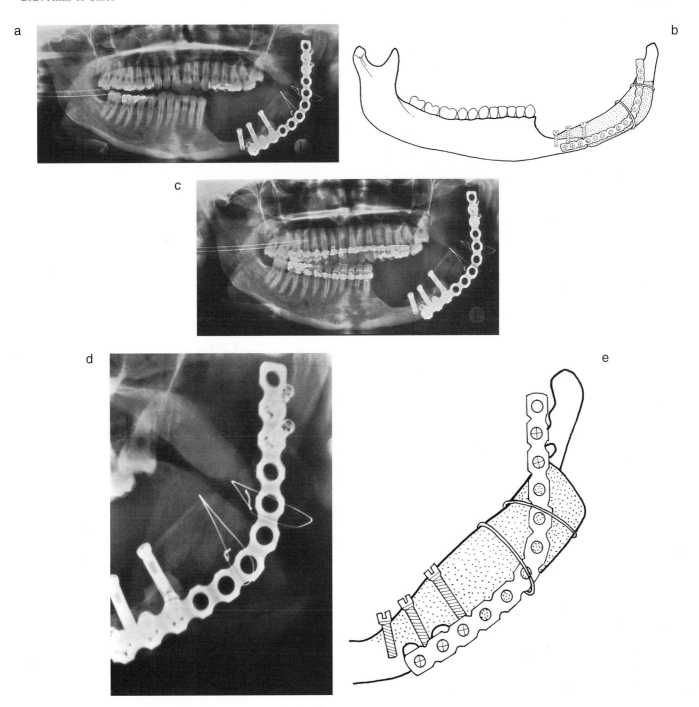

FIGURE 20B.3 (a) Panoramic image of a 23-year-old female 1 month after surgery for recurrent ameloblastoma. There is moderate resorption of the graft, especially in the mesial part, due to infection. (b) A diagrammatic representation of (a). (c) Panoramic image 2 months later. The resorption has increased. (d) Detailed image of the ramus area shows the contours of the graft. (e) A diagrammatic representation of (d).

Continued.

f

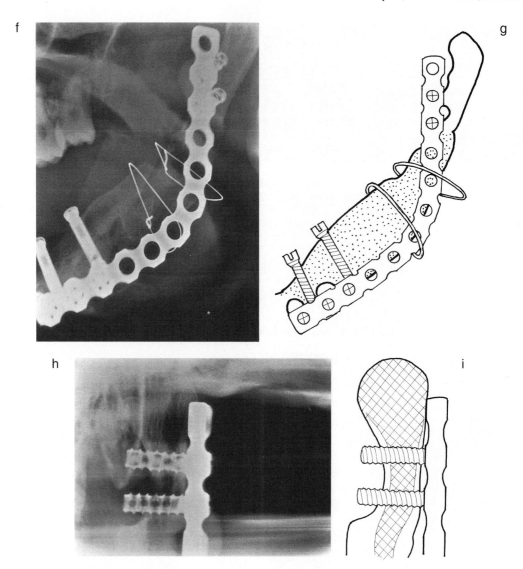

g

h

i

j

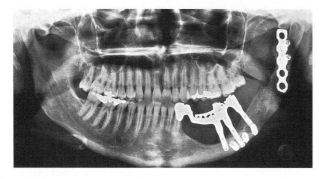

FIGURE 20B.3 *Continued*. (f) Detailed image of the ramus 13 months after the operation shows good healing. (g) A diagrammatic representation of (f). (h) Detailed posteroanterior image of the condylar area. The buccal cortex is preserved, and there is complete union between graft and mandible. (i) A diagrammatic representation of (h). (j) Panoramic image 4 years later. A part of the plate was removed, and dental implants with suprastructure are in use. The patient is symptom free.

a

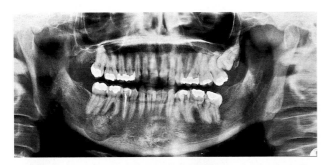

b

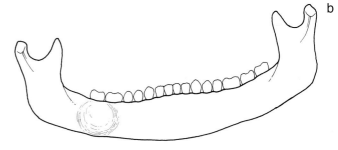

c

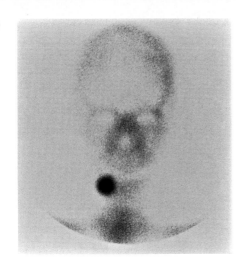

d

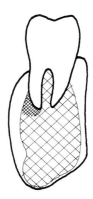

e

FIGURE 20B.4 (a) Panoramic image of a 31-year-old female shows an atypical ossifying fibroma in the mandible. (b) A diagrammatic representation of (a). (c) Cross-sectional tomography shows expansion and bulging of the lingual cortex and a radiolucent area at the lower border revealing that the tumor has growth potential. (Courtesy Pertti Paukku, M.D. Helsinki University Central Hospital, Department of Diagnostic Radiology.) (d) A diagrammatic representation of (c). (e) Nuclear scan shows strongly increased uptake in the right mandibular body.

Continued.

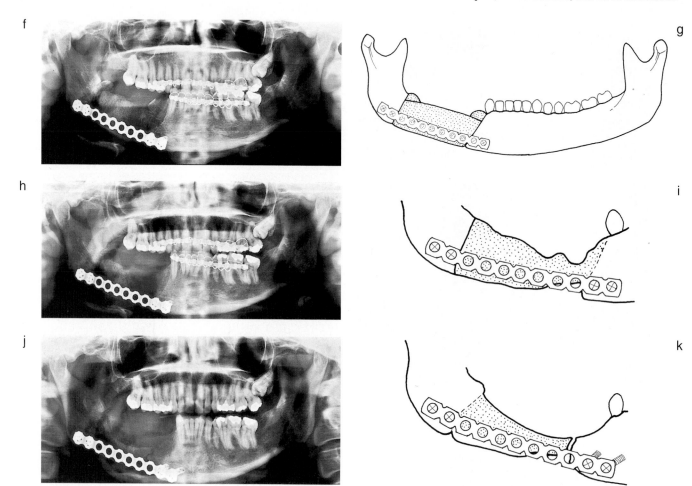

FIGURE 20B.4 *Continued.* (f) Immediate postoperative panoramic image. (g) A diagrammatic representation of (f). (h) Panoramic image 3 months after surgery. There is moderate resorption of the graft but no signs of infection or loosening. (i) A diagrammatic representa-

tion of (h). (j) Panoramic image 6 months after surgery. There is still a radiolucent border between graft and mandible indicating delayed union. No signs of complications. (k) A diagrammatic representation of (j).

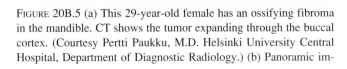

FIGURE 20B.5 (a) This 29-year-old female has an ossifying fibroma in the mandible. CT shows the tumor expanding through the buccal cortex. (Courtesy Pertti Paukku, M.D. Helsinki University Central Hospital, Department of Diagnostic Radiology.) (b) Panoramic im- age 1 day after resection of the mandibular left body. (c) A dia- grammatic representation of (b). (d) Panoramic image 3 months af- ter transplantation of bone graft. The border between mandibular an- gle and graft is still sharp. (e) A diagrammatic representation of (d).

Continued.

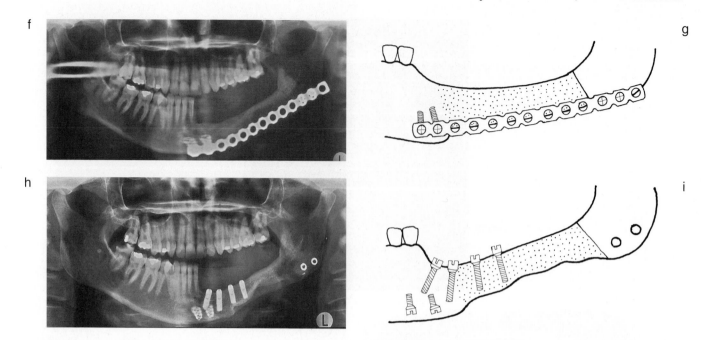

FIGURE 20B.5 *Continued.* (f) Panoramic image 10 months after bone transplantation. There is good bony union mesially, but the distal border between graft and angle is still visible, indicating delayed union. (g) A diagrammatic representation of (f). (h) Situation 42 months after primary operation. The plate has been removed and dental implants inserted into the graft. (i) A diagrammatic representation of (h).

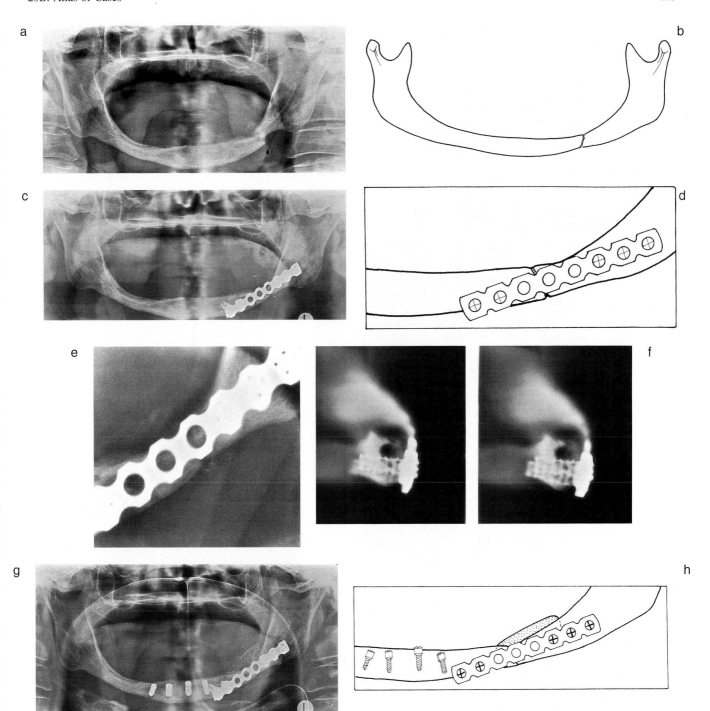

FIGURE 20B.6 (a) Spontaneous fracture of irradiated edentulous mandible in a 66-year-old female. (b) A diagrammatic representation of (a.) (c) Fracture stabilized with THORP. (d) A diagrammatic representation of (c). (e) Detailed image 8 months after fixation. The fracture is still visible, and there is delayed union. (f) Cross-sectional tomography of the parasymphyseal area reveals good screw fixation. There is some fragmentation of the atrophied alveolar crest. The mandibular canal is clearly visible above the screws. (g) Panoramic image taken the day after transplantation of bone graft and insertion of dental implants. (h) A diagrammatic representation of (g).

Continued.

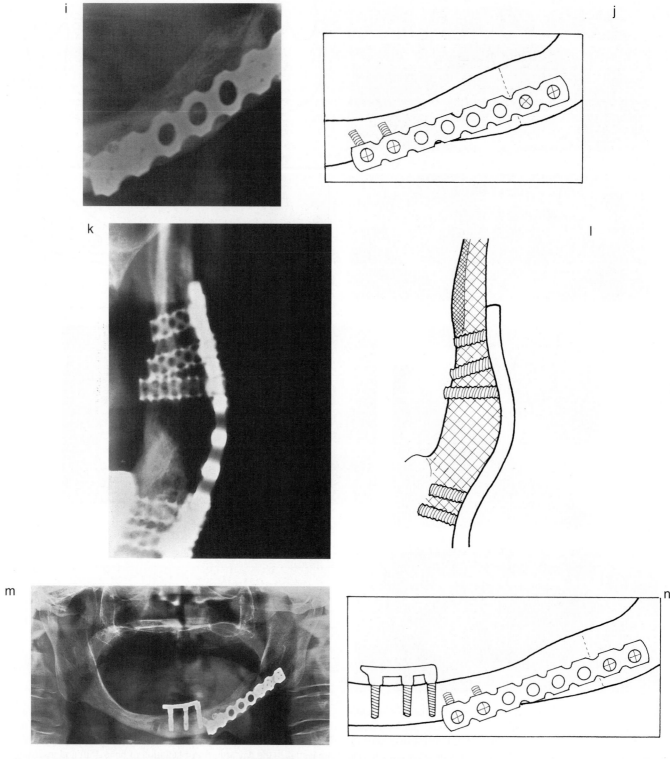

FIGURE 20B.6 *Continued.* (i) Detailed image 1 year after graft surgery shows good bony healing. (j) A diagrammatic representation of (i). (k) Detailed image in posteroanterior direction confirms good bony union. (l) A diagrammatic representation of (k). (m) Panoramic im- age 13 months after surgery. The plate is still in place. The dental implants have been connected with a bar. (n) A diagrammatic representation of (m).

References

1. Iizuka T, et al. Infection after internal fixation of mandibular fractures. A clinical and radiological study. *J Oral Maxillofac Surg.* 1991;49:585–593.

2. Söderholm A, Hallikainen D, Lindqvist C. Radiologic follow-up of bone transplants to bridge mandibular continuity defects. *Oral Surg Oral Med Oral Pathol.* 1992;73:253–261.

3. Tartaglino L, Flanders A, Vinitski S, Friedman D. Metallic artifacts on MR images of the postoperative spine: reduction with fast spin-echo techniques. *Radiology.* 1994;190:565–569.

21A
Prosthodontic Considerations in Dental Implant Restoration

James H. Abjanich and Ira H. Orenstein

Osseointegrated implant dentistry was originally developed to address the special needs of the edentulous lower jaw.[1–3] Many patients who were unable to manage a complete lower denture had four to six implants placed in the anterior mandible upon which a rigid prosthesis was fabricated. From this early success, there emerged an effort to expand the uses of endosseous implants to restore a variety of edentate conditions.

As with any developing technology, dental implantology has become a highly complex and sophisticated treatment modality rooted in fundamental principles. Surgeons are opening texts from earlier school days to reacquaint themselves with the dynamics of bone biology. Similarly, restorative dentists are relearning basic biomechanical concepts. There has been a resurgence in research addressing bone healing, biomaterials, and implant biology.

The need for a strong interdisciplinary relationship between the surgeon and restorative dentist cannot be overstated. Dental implantology should be prosthetically driven. It is the patient's intention to have dental function restored, often emphasizing a highly aesthetic result. The final prosthetic tooth position governs all phases of implant therapy. Fixture placement, possibly incorporating plastic procedures, must be executed with coordinated precision. Treatment planning and delivery is now fraught with nuances and subtleties that mandate accurate communication among the members of the interdisciplinary team. Toward that end, it is the goal of the authors of this chapter to expand the surgeon's scope of understanding of restorative implant dentistry. It is through this sharing of knowledge that the implant team can be most effective.

Basic Principles

Surgical Stent

The surgical phase of implant placement requires a vision of the final prosthesis. The stent provides the surgeon with a three-dimensional prescription for implant placement. It will convey the proper position, angulation, and number of fixtures to be placed. Implant diameter, length, and the relationship to anatomic structures can also be evaluated.

Radiographic markers (e.g., gutta percha, ball bearings, metal wires, barium sulfate) can be incorporated into the stent and worn by the patient during CT scanning and conventional radiographic procedures.

For the edentulous arch, a trial setup or existing ideal denture can be replicated into clear acrylic with a denture duplicating flask (e.g., Lang Denture Duplicator Flask, Lang Dental Mfg. Co., Inc., Wheeling, IL, USA). A window is cut in the stent, which defines the perimetric limits of implant placement. A perspective of the relationship between the proposed implant location and the desired tooth position is maintained. This design allows flexibility in alternate site selection. The stent should take into account flap design and be relieved to accommodate tissue retraction. It should be stable and provide good visual access to the surgical site[4,5] (Figure 21A.1) while in position.

The same principles can be applied to the partially edentulous patient. A diagnostic wax-up is made on a stone model and replicated in clear acrylic as previously described. Acrylic resin is then added to the incisal and occlusal surfaces of adjacent teeth to orient and stabilize the stent. A window is made through the occlusal surfaces demarcating the potential implant sites.

The CT scan[6] can be reformatted from conventional transaxial scan images into cross-sectional views that are perpendicular to the long axis of the jaw. These reformatted images help the clinician to visualize bony topography and vital structures. Technology with computed tomographic (CT) radiology is rapidly progressing. Software (Simplant, Columbia Scientific Inc., Columbia, MD, USA) that allows the operator to superimpose implant facsimiles of different lengths and widths on reformatted images is available (Figure 21A.2). Scans taken with stents that incorporate radiopaque markers permit visualization of the labial and incisal tooth contours in relation to the bony topography and proposed implant orientation.

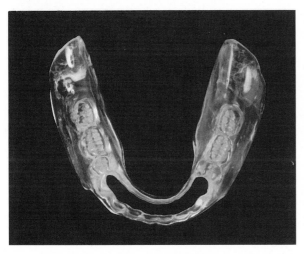
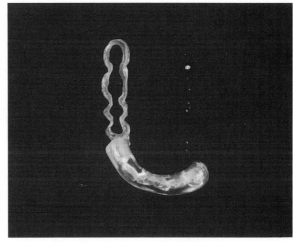

FIGURE 21A.1 Surgical templates for the (a) completely and (b) partially edentulous mandible.

Bone

Bone quality and volume are of paramount importance to the surgeon placing implants. Lekholm and Zarb[7] developed a system for classifying bone quality and volume that has become widely accepted (Figure 21A.3). Misch and Judy,[8] and Jensen[9] developed similar site-specific systems of bone classification. Initial rigid fixation is desirable for osseointegration to occur. This is best achieved by engaging cortical bone. Misch[10] described three criteria for rigid fixation: (1) atraumatic bone preparation; (2) close adaptation of living bone to a biocompatible implant surface; and (3) absence of movement at the interface between the bone and implant during healing. He also suggested that bone quality may influence such factors as the drilling rate, sequence, countersinking, length and number of implants placed, healing time, occlusal scheme, and the need for progressive loading.

Jaffin and Berman[11] reported an overall implant failure rate of 35% in quality-four (Q-4) bone using threaded titanium fixtures. Implant design and surface characteristics may influence success in various bone qualities. Manufacturers seek to develop implant designs that lend themselves for use in poor quality bone (i.e., self-tapping implants, hydroxyapatite coatings, plasma-sprayed surfaces). It is important for the restorative dentist to consider bone quality from a biomechanical standpoint. Generally, the anterior mandible has the densest bone followed by the posterior mandible, anterior maxilla, and posterior maxilla.[12] Low-density bone requires a longer healing period to maximize bony adaptation to the implant surfaces.

Forces

Implants best tolerate compressive forces.[13] Compression is an apically directed force along the long axis of the implant. Tensile forces (coronally directed along the implant axis) are not as well tolerated. Shear forces (off-axis loads) have the potential to be the most destructive to the integrity of the implant–bone complex.

It is not always possible to position fixtures ideally to achieve optimal force distribution. The surgeon may have to

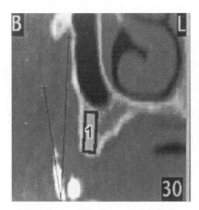
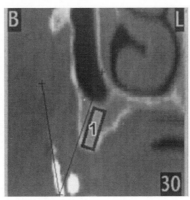
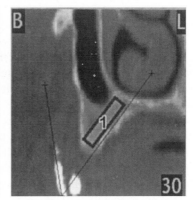

FIGURE 21A.2 Reformatted CT scan. Superimposed implant analog can be oriented to determine optimum placement. (Courtesy of Simplant, Columbia Scientific Inc., Columbia, MD, USA)

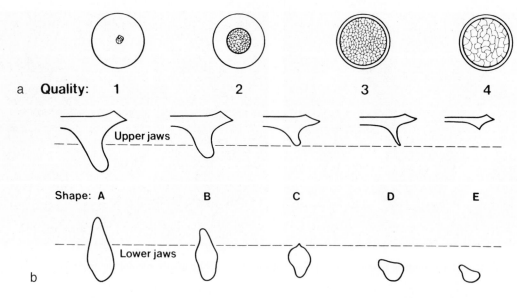

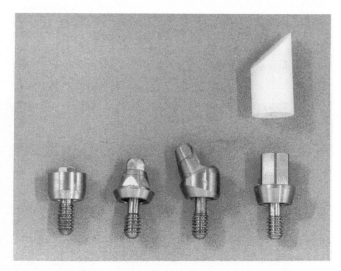

FIGURE 21A.3 Lekholm and Zarb's classification of bone (a) quality and (b) quantity. (From Lekholm and Zarb,[7] by permission of Quintessence Publishing Co.)

angle an implant from the ideal position when bone volume is limited or in an attempt to engage cortical bone. The restorative dentist may need to modify the treatment accordingly.

It is well documented that bone density increases in relation to physiologic stress.[14] The concept of progressive prosthetic loading was developed in an effort to optimize maturation of bone around implants.[15,16] The restorative dentist gradually increases the forces applied to the implant–bone interface over time. This can be achieved in a variety of ways specific to the type of prosthesis. The interval between appointments may be increased to allow more time for bone remodeling to occur. Temporary removable prostheses should be frequently relined with tissue conditioner and selectively relieved. Fixed acrylic temporary restorations should initially have a narrow occlusal table, no occlusion on pontics, and no cantilever occlusion. Loads should be concentrated onto the most favorable implants. Over time, the provisional prosthesis can be modified to mimic the final result.

Abutment Selection

In most situations the surgeon should defer the final abutment selection to the restorative dentist. A healing abutment should be placed at the time of uncovering, which emerges slightly coronal to the soft-tissue level.

The restorative dentist addresses many factors when choosing a final abutment. The proposed tooth position and contour as it relates to implant orientation will contribute to the determination of abutment length, width, and angulation. The single-tooth restoration must be antirotational. The abutment-prosthesis complex should be cleansable.[17]

Premachined abutments are available in a variety of de-

signs (Figure 21A.4). Standard cylindrical abutments are used where they do not compromise aesthetics (i.e., mandibular hybrid prosthesis, bar-retained overdenture). Aesthetic abutments allow the final prosthesis to end at or below the gingival margin. Angled abutments redirect the orientation of misaligned implants. The clinician can choose between abutments that employ screw or cement retention of the final prosthesis.

The use of custom abutments is becoming the procedure of choice for many practitioners (Figure 21A.5). These abutments can be waxed and cast to develop proper emergence profiles and maximize aesthetic potential. Implant alignment

FIGURE 21A.4 Nobel Biocare abutments. (Nobel Biocare, USA, Inc., Yorba Linda, CA.) From left to right: Standard, EsthetiCone, Pre-Angled, CeraOne®.

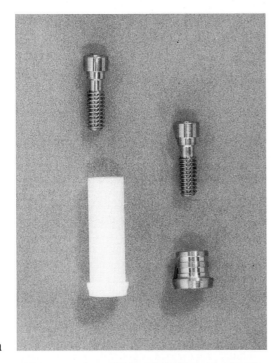

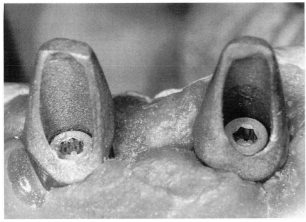

FIGURE 21A.5 (a) Implant Innovations Inc., Palm Beach Gardens, FL custom abutment components; plastic (left) and gold alloy (right). (b) Custom abutments (viewed on soft tissue cast) fabricated from plastic UCLA-type patterns.

can be corrected to control the path of insertion of the prosthesis. Short abutments can often be milled with minimal taper and grooves to increase prosthesis retention. Abutment inventory is vastly reduced.

The recently developed high-strength all-ceramic abutments (Ceradapt™, Nobel Biocare, USA, Inc., Yorba Linda, CA) by Prestipino and Ingber in conjunction with Nobel Biocare, USA, Inc. (Yorba Linda, CA) is currently being investigated for clinical usefulness.[18–20] They are said to be safe to prepare intraorally without generating heat to the implant

body and are more resistant to scratching than titanium during maintenance procedures. The aesthetic potential of these abutments is excellent.

At times, it may be difficult or impossible for the restorative dentist to choose the proper abutment intraorally. Repositioning the surgical stent may provide the necessary spatial relationship between the proposed abutment and tooth position. When selection remains difficult, it becomes necessary to directly impression the implants.[21] A stone master model with implant analogs is generated and articulated at the correct vertical dimension. A diagnostic wax-up is made and a buccal putty matrix is fabricated to establish a tooth-abutment perspective. This procedure is particularly helpful when fabricating custom abutments.

Screw Versus Cement Retention of Prosthesis

Implant prostheses can be either screw- or cement-retained. Many instances require this decision to be made prior to surgery as it may influence the desired implant position as detailed in the "Single Tooth Restorations" section of this chapter. When the patient has been treatment-planned to receive an anterior screw-retained prosthesis, it is generally advisable to direct implants for the access hole to exit the cingulum area. This will often necessitate placing a labial ridge-lap to meet aesthetic demands. The screw-retained prosthesis access channel can interfere with aesthetics if an implant is angled too far labially and can compromise the tongue space when oriented lingually. Angled abutments can redirect the access opening. When using UCLA-type abutments that screw-retain the prosthesis directly to the implant body (i.e., because of limited intermaxillary space or for better control of emergence profile) redirection of the access opening is impossible. Lingually positioned fixtures are often best restored with a one-piece screw-retained prosthesis to reduce bulk, which could otherwise affect phonetics and comfort (Figure 21A.6). Difficult cases that require screw-retention with fine control of exit holes can sometimes be restored with prostheses that incorporate mesostructures (see the "Complications" section in this chapter). These restorations are often very complex, costly, and bulky, reinforcing the need for accurate implant placement.

Cemented prostheses eliminate the aesthetic and surgical limitations associated with the screw access opening. Custom abutments often employ cement retention of the overlying prosthesis and offer the greatest control of emergence profile and aesthetics.

The restorative dentist may not wish to place a cement-retained prosthesis where intermaxillary space is limited. Alveoloplasty and/or countersinking of implants below the crest of bone might otherwise be necessary to achieve the height requirement for cement retention. The decision to do this is not without potential consequences as the surgeon may be sacrificing precious crestal cortical bone and reducing the

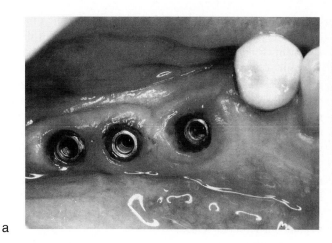
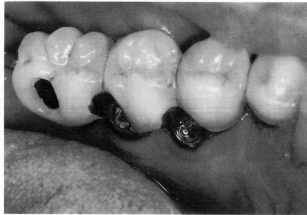

a   b

FIGURE 21A.6 (a) Severe lingual placement of implants. (b) One-piece screw-retained restoration minimizes lingual bulk.

potential implant length. In such situations, a screw-retained prosthesis may be the better choice as the vertical height requirement is less.

The cemented prosthesis is more likely to fit passively than its screw-retained counterpart. This factor is important to the surgeon and restorative dentist troubleshooting the ailing implant. A screw-retained prosthesis that does not fit passively may induce implant overload with potential failure if not corrected.

The restorative procedures associated with cemented prostheses closely parallel those of the conventional crown and bridge.[22]

Completely Edentulous

Many edentulous patients are unable to function with conventional complete dentures. Patients with advanced bone resorption and thin overlying mucosa have ridges that provide minimal stability and resistance to motion. This causes continual irritation and limits mastication and speech. Other patients cannot tolerate a palatal section due to severe gagging. A small group is psychologically unable to confront their edentulous state and completely rejects the concept of complete dentures.[23] These concerns have made dental implantology useful for the restoration of many edentulous arches.

Immediately following the extraction of all teeth in an arch, bone is rapidly resorbed.[24] During the first year of edentulism there is an average decrease in bone height of 4 to 5 mm in the mandible and 2 to 3 mm in the maxilla.[25] A ratio of 3 or 4:1 has been demonstrated for long-term bone loss of the mandible and maxilla, respectively. Carlsson found the mean mandibular height reduction 5 years after tooth extraction to be 12.5 mm (ranging from 2 to 14.5 mm).[26] Patients who have initial rapid bone loss tend to continue to demonstrate greater long-term ridge resorption. There is a poor correlation between ridge size and time of edentulism as significant individual variation exists.

The maxillary edentulous arch will resorb in a superior and lingual direction. The outer cortical plate is thinner, and as a result, resorption from the facial aspect tends to be more rapid. As the maxilla resorbs, it becomes smaller in all dimensions. The mandibular outer cortex is generally thicker than the lingual except in the molar region. The mandibular width is greatest at its inferior border and therefore appears to widen in the posterior region as resorption progresses in an inferior and lateral direction.

The horizontal and vertical bony resorptive patterns produce narrowing of the maxilla and expansion of the mandible.[27] The resulting unfavorable ridge relationships can have many effects. The decrease in maxillary anterior arch circumference necessitates unfavorable lingual implant placement, a poor crown-to-implant ratio, and reverse occlusion (crossbite)[28] (Figure 21A.7).

Although the mandible suffers a greater magnitude of resorption, restoration of the edentulous maxilla remains more challenging. The anterior mandible widens toward the inferior border. The absence of a mandibular residual ridge does not influence the use of implants since the width and depth of basal bone below the floor of the mouth is usually substantial with a prominent inferior cortex.[29] It is usually possible to place fixtures here in the presence of advanced resorption. On the contrary, the maxillary ridge may resorb yielding bone that is too narrow and of insufficient height. The nasal fossa and maxillary sinus may limit implant length.

The aesthetic considerations are very different for both jaws. Aesthetic restoration of the mandible is usually straightforward because the interface between the implant abutments and prosthesis is well hidden by the lower lip. Conversely, the upper arch carries with it a host of aesthetic and functional concerns. The implant-prosthesis interface will sometimes be visible, thereby necessitating meticulous fixture placement within the confines of the body of the prosthetic tooth. The restoration will often employ aesthetic abutments. The maxillary prosthesis may require a prosthetic flange to replace hard and soft tissue for facial support. A major concern with any maxillary pros-

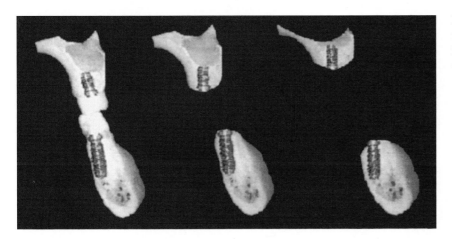

FIGURE 21A.7 Progression of bone resorption in the maxilla and mandible as it relates to implant position. (From Bahat,[28] by permission of *Int J Oral Maxillofac Implants*)

thesis is speech-related to air flow and tooth position. Air that escapes between the superior aspect of the prosthesis and the ridge can most profoundly affect fricative sounds (*f, v, th, s, z, sh, j, ch*). Lingual implant placement and a concurrent palatally placed prosthesis may disrupt lingual alveolar sounds (*t, d, n, l*). In many situations, therefore, restoration of the edentulous maxilla is best accomplished using an overdenture.

Full-arch implant-supported restorations can be fixed (screw- or cement-retained) or patient-removable (overdenture). The fixed restoration can be porcelain fused to metal or a hybrid prosthesis using acrylic resin to affix stock denture teeth to a custom frame. Overdentures can incorporate varying degrees of tissue support and can be retained by bars and retention clips, stud attachments, or magnets.

The spark erosion restoration has the rigidity of a fixed prosthesis coupled with the advantages of a conventional implant-retained overdenture as will be discussed in the "Edentulous Maxilla" section of this chapter.

Several factors should be considered when choosing between a fixed or removable restoration.[30] Fixed prostheses are usually preferred by the patient whenever possible. They require sufficient fixture support and distribution. The cantilever length will depend upon the amount of implant support, bone quality, crown-to-implant ratio, anteroposterior (A-P) spread (to be discussed in the "Fixed Mandibular Reconstructions" section of this chapter) and opposing occlusal forces. When facial support from hard and soft tissues is correct a fixed option is often preferred. Trial setups with and without a flange can determine whether additional support is necessary. Fixed reconstructions may be preferred when knife-edged ridges with minimal denture-bearing area provide poor support for tissue-borne overdentures. Fixed restorations generally require less interarch space. The removable overdenture may require less complicated treatment planning and decreased expense. It is indicated when confronted with less bone for fewer implants. Overdentures allow greater ease for achieving aesthetics. They should be used when a flange is necessary to support facial structure that has been lost from resorption or trauma. Removable

flanges can be fabricated for fixed reconstructions, but they are usually not durable and attract plaque. Overdentures may be indicated when increased functional capacity of a fixed prosthesis may exceed the load-bearing limit of a weaker opposing jaw.[31] A fixed restoration should never be promised to a patient. The treatment plan should always be flexible, and the overdenture restoration should not be viewed as a second-rate service (Figure 21A.8).

Edentulous Mandible

Fixed Mandibular Prosthesis

The high level of implant and prosthesis stability associated with mandibular osseointegrated restorations is well documented.[32,33] Adell[32] reported that 99% of mandibular prostheses remained continuously stable through a 15-year follow-up period; 100% fixture survival is not required for continuous prosthesis stability when adequate fixture redundancy has been incorporated into the treatment plan. The high success rate is reflective of the good bone quality generally found in the anterior mandible. Brånemark's original protocol called for the placement of four to six fixtures between the mental foramena. The prosthesis was connected to an abutment cylinder via a gold screw. This gold screw is the weak link and will protect the implant from potential overload. It is preferable for the prosthesis or abutment retaining screw to break prior to loss of integration or implant fracture. The classic mandibular prosthesis is a hybrid design, which uses acrylic resin to process stock denture teeth to a screw-retained precisely fitting framework.

The success of implant-retained prosthodontic restorations depends largely on the ability to achieve a precise, passive fit. The healthy natural tooth will typically flex 100 μm vertically and horizontally. The fixture will hardly flex (10 μm vertically and horizontally).[33] Carlsson demonstrated that an angular prosthesis gap of 50 μm requires a 200-μm correction of the fixture apex to alleviate the resultant forces.[34] Any stress produced by the prosthodontic restoration will remain

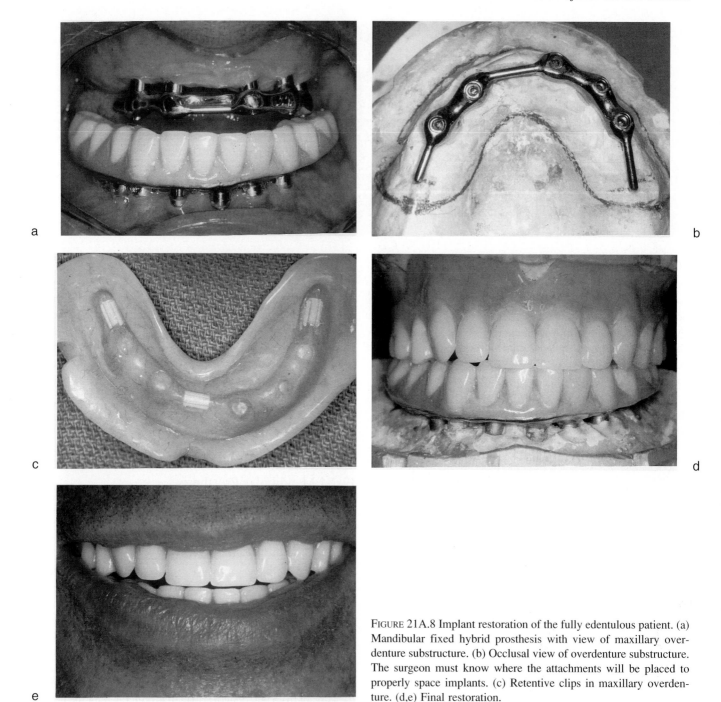

Figure 21A.8 Implant restoration of the fully edentulous patient. (a) Mandibular fixed hybrid prosthesis with view of maxillary overdenture substructure. (b) Occlusal view of overdenture substructure. The surgeon must know where the attachments will be placed to properly space implants. (c) Retentive clips in maxillary overdenture. (d,e) Final restoration.

there since the rigid implant has limited adaptability.[35] It is therefore critical to minimize static misfit forces. Even when the prosthesis appears to clinically have an acceptable fit, a significant force may be introduced when the framework is screwed into position (Figure 21A.9).[36]

Transfer Copings for Master Cast Fabrication

Precise reproduction of implant position with the master cast is imperative especially for screw-retained prostheses. Con-

troversy surrounds the issue of master-cast accuracy derived from open-tray square transfer copings (direct technique) versus smooth unsplinted copings (indirect technique). Assif[37] and Carr[38] concluded that splinted square copings retained in the impression were better than tapered unsplinted transfer copings that were reseated. Zarb[39] suggested affixing floss along square abutments to form a matrix for resin splinting. Self-cure acrylic shrinks upon polymerization. Ivanhoe[40] advocates splinting copings on a preliminary cast with light-cured resin, while Lechner[41] uses autopolymerized acrylic. The resin

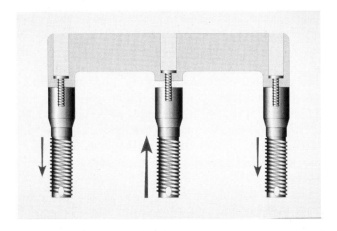

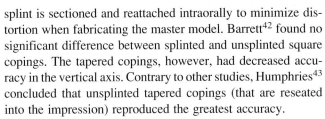

FIGURE 21A.9 A screw-retained prosthesis with a misfit will generate destructive tensile forces.

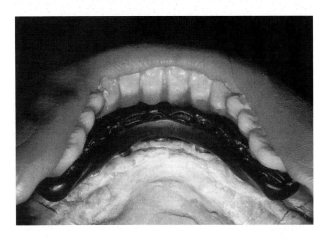

FIGURE 21A.10 Facial putty matrix with denture teeth guides the technician with substructure wax-up.

splint is sectioned and reattached intraorally to minimize distortion when fabricating the master model. Barrett[42] found no significant difference between splinted and unsplinted square copings. The tapered copings, however, had decreased accuracy in the vertical axis. Contrary to other studies, Humphries[43] concluded that unsplinted tapered copings (that are reseated into the impression) reproduced the greatest accuracy.

Transfer copings that can be retained in impression material do not have to be reseated, thereby eliminating a potential source of error. Copings splinted with acrylic should be sectioned and reannealed with minimal material to reduce distortion. Tapered copings that are reseated may need to be used in limited access regions as they require less vertical height.

Verification of the Master Cut

Prior to fabricating the wax pattern, verification of the master cast accuracy[41,44] will minimize sectioning and resoldering of frameworks. Gold cylinders can be placed on the abutment replicas and connected with acrylic resin. The joints are sectioned and reconnected with minimal material to reduce polymerization shrinkage. The assembly is checked in the mouth to verify acceptable clinical fit, which is usually agreed to be within 30 μm. If the index is inaccurate, it is sectioned and reannealed in the mouth, and a corrected stone master model is generated. Each subsequent step (i.e., porcelain application) can be checked for distortion by replacement of the prosthesis on the verified master model. All cylinders must simultaneously seat without tightening multiple screws. One terminal screw is placed, and the fit of the prosthesis checked. If this is acceptable the other terminal screw is inserted and the original one removed. Intermediate screws can then be placed and fit reassessed. For cement-retained prostheses, master-cast verification may be less critical.

Substructure Fabrication

Prior to substructure fabrication, a diagnostic setup should be verified in the patient's mouth to establish aesthetics, pho-

netics, vertical dimension, and occlusion. A putty matrix is constructed to relate the final tooth position to the master cast (Figure 21A.10). The substructure is correctly waxed to be strong and rigid and to adequately support the veneering material (denture teeth or porcelain). Porcelain is particularly vulnerable to fracture if it is not properly supported. Substructure thickness when using porcelain veneering with implants compared to natural teeth can result in a much thicker metal frame. This has the distinct advantages of reducing flexure and decreasing the possibility of tensile fracture of porcelain. The increased rigidity permits distribution of static loading more evenly thereby decreasing the potential for sudden impact loading with better distribution to the implants.[45]

Gold and silver-palladium are the most popular materials employed to fabricate substructures. Recently, Nobel Biocare, USA, Inc. (Yorba Linda, CA) introduced Brånemark System Custom Solutions' Procera method to fabricate accurate titanium frameworks.[46,47] The process begins with the creation of a light-cured resin substructure, which is sectioned into several pieces. Prefabricated titanium rod stock elements that include the abutment (standard or Estheticone) are placed in a copy milling machine (similar to a key cutter) with the resin pieces to replicate their shape. The resulting individual titanium elements are welded with a stereo laser that minimizes framework warpage. This technology produces the most accurate fitting frameworks to date (less than 30-μm gap on master model analogs).

Biomechanical Considerations for Mandibular Fixed Reconstructions

The final prosthetic treatment decision is based upon several biomechanical factors. They include the number, length, and angulation of fixtures, bone quality, crown height to implant ratio, opposing occlusion, and the A-P (anteroposterior) spread[48] of implants.

The classic lower fixed implant reconstruction has five to six fixtures placed between the mental foramena. Four have been used when opposing a complete denture with all other factors favorable. However, the prosthesis is at a greater risk of failure in the absence of fixture redundancy. When fixtures are not placed distal to the mental foramina, cantilever extensions are necessary.

There is considerable variation in the literature regarding proper cantilever extension. Mandibular cantilever lengths have been suggested not to exceed 20 mm[49,50] (while not exceeding 10 mm in the maxilla). Shackleton[51] reported significantly better prosthesis survival when cantilevers do not exceed 15 mm. The A-P spread will have a profound effect on this decision.

The A-P spread is the distance between the fulcrum and a line through the most anterior implant (Figure 21A.11). A curved implant distribution is more capable of resisting the bending moments generated on cantilever sections. Calculations reveal that posterior cantilever extensions should be less than two times the A-P spread.[52] A horizontal arrangement of four to six fixtures would therefore not adequately support a customary cantilever length. Other factors that decrease potential cantilever length include opposing natural dentition, poor bone quality, short or poorly angled implants, poor crown-to-implant ratio, parafunction, and fewer than six implants.

Severely resorbed mandibles can sometimes have an extremely unfavorable crown-to-implant ratio of 3:1. When this is coupled with a poor A-P spread the potential for overload exists, and a fixed prosthesis may be contraindicated.

Lindqvist et al.[53] found that biting force on a cantilever results in compression (better accepted by fixtures) on the distal fixture and tension (potentially destructive) on the anterior fixture. As a result, medial fixtures show more bone loss when compared to the distal fixtures (fulcrum). Sullivan[54] demonstrated that an additional 5-mm separation of the distal fixtures decreases the tensile forces by 2.5 times. White et al.[55] used a photoelastic model to demonstrate that the highest stresses from forces exerted on distal cantilevers are concentrated on the ridge crest of the distal surface of the distal implant.

Situations arise in which more posterior occlusion is necessary than can be cantilevered from fixtures between the mental foramina. The lower anterior teeth are often the last to be lost. Patients who have worn an upper complete denture over a removable partial prosthesis with natural anterior teeth may have severe maxillary anterior ridge resorption with flabby redundant tissue. A fixed lower implant-supported bridge with only bicuspid occlusion may yield a tipping and unstabilizing effect, whereas a complete denture or overdenture can provide a full complement of posterior teeth. Alternatively, additional fixtures can be placed posterior to the mental foramina to fabricate a fixed prosthesis. Bruxers may also benefit from additional posterior implant placement. Zarb[56] reported fractures of abutment screws and gold screws despite accurate framework fit and proper occlusion.

Patients with a full complement of maxillary molars (concerns for supereruption) and those who desire more posterior occlusion may require additional posterior fixtures.

Anterior and posterior fixtures splinted in one piece around the lower arch may subject the bone–implant interface to stress-induced microdamage due to the flexure inherent in the mandible on opening.[57] With sufficient posterior fixtures, the fabrication of three independent sections should be considered. When only one terminal fixture can be placed on both sides, the concept of cantilever rests[58] can be incorporated. These distal fixtures are not rigidly connected to the framework. They function as vertical stops that reduce torque on anterior fixtures, thereby negating the harmful effects of long cantilevers.

Veneering Materials

Biomechanical concerns have been raised addressing the need to dampen impact forces on osseointegrated implants.[59] Various ways to reduce impact load have been suggested. The intramobile element used in the IMZ system is said to simulate the periodontium. Brånemark suggested the use of acrylic resin occlusal surfaces to decrease impact stresses. A study by Gracis et al.[60] showed resin to decrease impact force 50% over metal and porcelain occlusal surfaces. Davis suggested that porcelain is more appropriate than resin for patients who brux.[61] Porcelain will stiffen the framework and provide more even stress distribution to implants. Naert[62] has clinically shown that when compared to resin, porcelain as an occlusal

A-P Spread

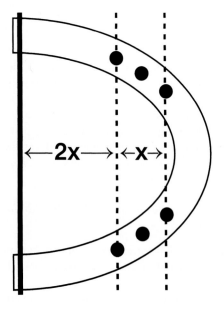

FIGURE 21A.11 A-P spread. Cantilever extensions (2×) should never exceed two times the distance between the anterior fixture(s) and posterior fulcrum (×).

material did not influence the marginal bone height around implants. To date, the clinical significance of impact loading of implants and its relationship to occlusal materials remains unanswered.

Resin and porcelain each have specific indications. Both have a long record of success with conventional dental restorations. Resin is usually indicated when the opposing occlusion is of the same material. Porcelain is more color stable. When porcelain is used, one should consider the potential for framework distortion during firing. For longer spans, postsoldering of shorter sections will minimize this effect. Acrylic wears more rapidly than porcelain and therefore can create iatrogenic occlusal changes over time.

Occlusal Considerations

When considering an occlusal scheme, the weakest component concept should be employed. When a lower fixed osseointegrated reconstruction opposes a maxillary complete denture, the bone of the premaxilla must be protected. There should be no anterior contacts in centric, and a balanced occlusion is developed in excursions. The masticatory forces generated with a fixture-assisted lower fixed prosthesis approach that of the natural dentition. This increased biting force may result in fracture of a previously stable maxillary denture. It is therefore advisable to incorporate cast metal reinforcement in the opposing prosthesis.

When a lower fixed fixture-assisted bridge opposes another implant bridge or natural dentition, a mutually protected occlusion is developed. Protrusive and lateral excursions on the anterior teeth will disclude the posterior dentition, thereby protecting distal cantilever extensions and implants placed in soft bone from lateral forces.

When full-arch implant reconstructions oppose each other, emphasis is placed on protecting the upper cantilevers. If the upper arch has an anterior cantilever and the lower has posterior cantilevers, protection of the upper prosthesis will usually still take precedence.

Removable Mandibular Prosthesis

Brånemark's original prosthodontic protocol called for a screw-retained fixed prosthesis that could not be removed by the patient. The use of overdentures retained by two or more fixtures has since been proven to be successful. Multicenter studies demonstrate mandibular overdenture success rates similar to those observed for fixed prostheses.[63,64] Feine et al.[65] found long-bar mandibular overdentures to provide similar chewing efficiency when compared to mandibular fixed full-arch prostheses. Overdentures have several advantages over complete dentures. Prosthesis retention, stability, tissue sensitivity, oral hygiene, chewing efficiency, and speech are improved. Bone atrophy is reduced. After the extraction of mandibular anterior teeth, there is an average of 4 mm of vertical bone loss in the first year. The mandible will have a four-fold greater loss of height when compared to the maxilla during the next 25 years.[66] With the placement of overdenture fixtures long-term bone loss may stabilize at 0.1 mm per year around implants. A reduced extension of the lingual denture flange may improve patient comfort and tongue mobility without necessarily sacrificing function.[67] Overdentures may be indicated for maxillofacial patients who have undergone resective surgical procedures.

Overdentures present several advantages over fixed appliances. Fabrication time and cost may be reduced. Hygiene access is improved. Overdentures can replace lost facial support. Sometimes fixture support is insufficient to place a fixed prosthesis. Overdentures provide more posterior teeth to function against the opposing arch (when compared to a fixed prosthesis with distal cantilevers).

Several design considerations should be addressed depending on the number and distribution of implants. Bars with retentive clips as well as ball attachments have been used successfully.

Corrosion and tarnish of intraoral magnets have raised questions as to their acceptability for intraoral use.[68]

Bar-Retained Overdentures

Two implants supporting a bar can effectively stabilize a lower denture (Figure 21A.12). Rotation of the prosthesis around the bar permits the soft tissue to share the occlusal load and minimizes torsional forces on the implants. To achieve this the bar and clip must be perpendicular to the sagittal plane[69] (Figure 21A.13). These same principles apply when restoring tooth-supported bar-retained overdentures.[70]

The shape of the bar will influence rotation. A round bar (e.g., Hader bar, APM Sterngold, Attleboro, MA, USA) allows free rotation. The pear-shaped Dolder bar (APM Sterngold, Attleboro, MA, USA) permits less rotation, and finally the parallel-sided Dolder bar allows the least amount of movement. The two fixtures should be placed in the canine regions. If additional implantation for a future fixed prosthesis is anticipated, a site between the implant and mental foramen should be preserved. A distal bar extension should never be used with two implants.

Three-splinted implants will greatly negate the ability of the denture to rotate if there is no straight bar section perpendicular to the sagittal plane. The third implant is sometimes placed for security to maintain the viability of the overdenture prosthesis in the event of implant failure. It is sometimes possible to cantilever a small section with retentive elements distal to the last fixtures when opposing a stress-broken prosthesis.[71] The addition of these cantilever extensions must be weighed against the potential introduction of implant overload.

Four implants can sometimes support a fixed prosthesis but will also act as well-positioned overdenture abutments. Two fixtures are placed in the cuspid sites and two just anterior to the mental foramina. A clip will be placed anteriorly, and re-

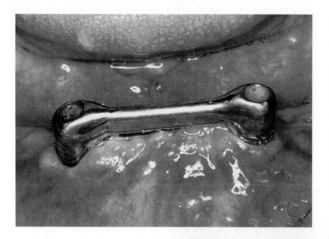
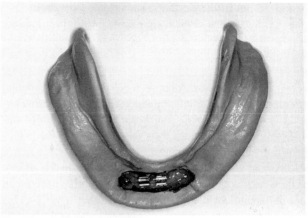
a   b

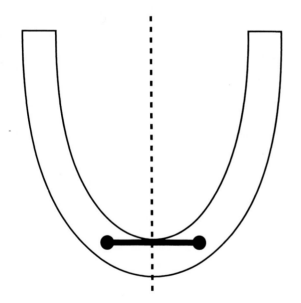
c

FIGURE 21A.12 (a) Mandibular implant-supported overdenture bar, (b) denture with retentive clips, and (c) stud attachments. Bar and stud attachments can significantly stabilize a mandibular denture.

silent extracoronal attachments are situated immediately distal to the posterior fixtures. Rotation of the denture and posterior lifting are significantly reduced (Figure 21A.14a,b).

Tissue-supported mandibular overdentures generally function better in the presence of adequately attached gingiva as the tissue borders are more stable.

Overdentures can be totally implant-supported in some situations when five or more implants are present.

Stud-Retained Overdentures

Naert et al.[72] found no difference in implant success or clinical performance of prosthetic treatment in the mandible for two nonsplinted versus splinted implants. A variety of stud attachments are available to retain mandibular overdentures. The ball attachment has been widely used with great success.[73] This prefabricated mechanism is less expensive and quicker to fabricate than a cast or soldered bar. The appropriate height (1 to 2 mm above the gingiva) is selected, and the attachment is screwed directly into the implant. The female retaining cap is inserted into the denture with autopolymerizing acrylic (Figure 21A.12c).

FIGURE 21A.13 A mandibular overdenture bar when supported by two implants should be oriented perpendicular to the midsagittal plane.

a

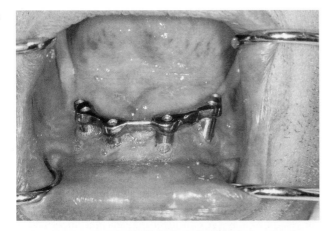

b

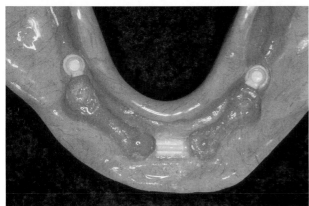

FIGURE 21A.14 (a) For implant design with splinted bar. "Passive" rotation from anterior clip and posterior resilient attachments. (b) Denture with anterior clip and posterior ERA attachments.

Occlusal Considerations

The mandibular overdenture should have a balanced scheme of occlusion. There are no anterior contacts in centric. In protrusive and lateral excursions, both anterior and posterior teeth will touch.

Edentulous Maxilla

The edentulous maxilla presents the greatest challenge to implant reconstruction. Aesthetic demands, anatomic limitations, resorption patterns, and phonetic considerations are just a few of the many restorative concerns that must be addressed. The variability of implant placement will also require flexibility in the design of the final prosthesis. The patient should never be promised a maxillary fixed restoration. The need to replace lost facial support will require most maxillary arches to be restored with overdentures or spark erosion prosthesis.

It is more difficult to achieve and maintain osseointegration in the maxilla. The fixture survival rate decreases approximately 10% from that found in the mandible.[1] It is wise to employ the concept of fixture redundancy. Ideally, the max-

illary treatment plan should be overengineered, calling for the placement of as many properly positioned implants as is possible.

Significance of Maxillary Resorption Patterns

As the maxilla resorbs, the ridge moves superior and medial. The bone available for implant placement is therefore often palatal to the original tooth position. This may result in crowding of the tongue and compromised speech. A posterior crossbite or labial cantilever may be necessary to regain former tooth relationships. Anterior teeth positioned for esthetics and phonetics may be far removed from the implants. Labial resorption can result in lost facial support, which can be restored with a labial flange. An overdenture or spark erosion prosthesis will permit optimal hygiene maintenance when a flange is required.

The extent of ridge resorption has been classified by Desjardins as minimal, moderate, or severe.[74] This greatly influences prosthesis design.

Minimal resorption usually permits fabrication of a fixed restoration. This is generally found in newly edentulous patients or patients who will be rendered edentulous. The fixtures can therefore be placed in an appropriate buccolingual, mesiodistal, and coronogingival position to support aesthetic, phonetic, and emergence profile requirements. This situation lends itself to the use of ceramometal restorations (Figure 21A.15a,b). Implants can be placed where the teeth previously existed. Ideal biomechanical distribution of six or more fixtures is often possible.

Moderate resorption will usually require a labial flange to restore facial support and esthetics. Overdenture therapy is often indicated. If sufficient fixture support and distribution is possible, a spark erosion prosthesis can be used. Diagnostic setups with and without a labial flange should be used to determine whether additional facial support is necessary.

Severe resorption may require bone grafting procedures. There is insufficient bone height, and what is present is in a palatal position. Whenever possible, implant placement with simultaneous bone grafting will save considerable time. These patients should almost exclusively be treated with overdentures as precise fixture positioning is hard to achieve.

Maxillary Implant Positioning and Distribution

The maxilla can be divided into three regions when discussing implant location.

The **cuspid** area generally provides the most predictable location with good bone height, width, and arch position.[75] It should be viewed as the primary site for implant placement.

The **posterior** areas vary as potential regions for implant placement. It is not uncommon to find Q-4 bone here, reinforcing the need for as much fixture support as possible. The maxillary sinus may limit bone height and width. There is a higher failure rate with 7-mm fixtures.[76] Where less than

a

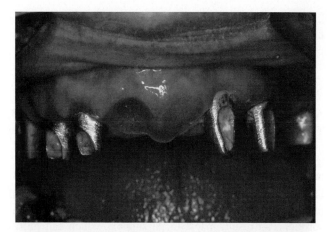

b

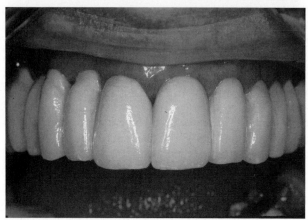

FIGURE 21A.15 (a) Full arch implants restored with custom abutments. (b) Porcelain fused to metal cemented prosthesis.

10 mm of bone is available in the sinus region a graft should be considered. Wide-diameter implants may sometimes be used under the sinus. They have increased surface area requiring less fixture length, and may also engage buccal and lingual cortical bone.

The **anterior** areas provide the third region for implant placement. If sufficient bone exists to place fixtures in the canine and posterior regions, it may be possible to fabricate a fixed prosthesis without involving the premaxilla[77] if doing so would compromise aesthetics or create excessive bulk in an overdenture. Where possible, two fixtures can be placed in the central incisor sites. Fixtures should not be placed lingual to the incisive papilla as this can affect speech and restrict tongue movements.

As a general rule, prudence dictates the placement of as many implants as is possible when restoring the edentulous maxilla.

Maxillary Fixed Prosthesis

Jemt[78] reported a 5-year cumulative fixture and prosthesis survival rate of 92.1% and 95.9%, respectively, for fixed prostheses supported by osseointegrated implants in the edentulous maxilla. During the first year of function, speech problems were the most common patient complaint. The most frequent adjustments to the prosthesis were related to resin fracture.

The maxillary fixed prosthesis can be fabricated with porcelain fused to metal or as a hybrid case. When a porcelain-to-metal restoration is considered, ideal implant placement is imperative to optimize aesthetics, phonetics, and effective hygiene. The fixtures must be positioned mesiodistally within the tooth confines. Interproximal or lingual fixtures will compromise aesthetics. A flange may be necessary to hide the implant(s), complicating hygiene access. The fixture head should be positioned 2 to 4 mm apical to the marginal tissue and exit just palatal to the proposed labial gingival interface. Local bone anatomy may prevent ideal implant placement and require the use of angled or custom abutments.

The maxillary hybrid design must be very different than its mandibular counterpart. The mandible classically shows 2 mm of abutment to facilitate hygiene. The maxilla has stringent requirements. Air and salivary flow between the top of the prosthesis and the ridge may compromise speech. The prosthesis should be initially abutted to the ridge crest. The borders can be later adjusted as needed for hygiene access.

Maxillary Removable Prosthesis

The maxillary overdenture is indicated when lost facial support necessitates the use of a prosthetic labial flange. Hygiene will be greatly facilitated with this design. Flanges incorporated into fixed restorations compromise hygiene access. Fixture number and distribution may biomechanically rule out the possibility of a fixed restoration. Overdentures usually permit tissue support to assist the implants with force dissipation. Treatment cost and time are often less than for fixed prostheses.

The implant failure rate associated with maxillary overdentures is higher than reported for fixed implant prostheses.[79] This fact supports the recommendation that the maximum number of implants be placed when fabricating an upper overdenture. Rotation and torquing associated with overdentures may contribute to their increased failure rate. Langer[80] suggests rigidly splinting maxillary fixtures to compensate for the less-favorable bone quality. Unsplinted stud attachments in the maxilla have been associated with a higher failure rate than splinted maxillary implants supporting overdentures. In the presence of adequate fixture and facial support the potential for overload may be better controlled with a fixed restoration. Overdenture maintenance is greater than for fixed prostheses supported by implants.[81] Fatigue fractures of the resin and clips along with mucosal problems surrounding implants have been observed. Fewer phonetic disturbances have been documented.

It is imperative that the surgeon knows where the restorative dentist plans to place attachments so that the implants can be spaced to accommodate them. Attachment mechanisms near the incisive papilla should be used judiciously as over-bulking of the prosthesis in this region can annoy the tongue and interfere with phonetics.

Maxillary Spark Erosion Prosthesis

The spark erosion prosthesis combines the best aspects of both the fixed and removable design.[82] A primary 2° tapered milled bar is fabricated on the master cast. The secondary casting is made to fit over the primary bar with great intimacy via the spark erosion process. Retention comes from the minimal taper, parallel pins, and direct swivel latch attachment. The swivel latch is placed on the lingual of the upper (and labial of lower) prosthesis.

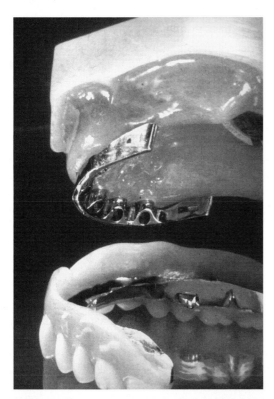

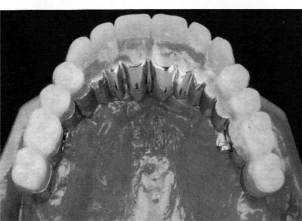

FIGURE 21A.16 Maxillary spark erosion prosthesis. (a) Milled bar with mating prosthesis. (b) Prosthesis has the stability of a fixed restoration.

This prosthesis is totally implant-supported and will have the retention and function of a fixed restoration while maintaining the advantages of a removable design. A labial flange can be incorporated, and correct tooth position achieved. The patient can easily remove the prosthesis by unlocking the lingual swivel latch, facilitating hygiene access (Figure 21A.16a,b).

Partially Edentulous

Clinicians have expanded the use of endosseous implantology to treat the partially edentulous patient. Naert et al.[83] demonstrated a cumulative implant success rate of 96.1% and 95.9% for the maxilla and mandible, respectively, during a 6-year prosthodontic study. Jemt et al.[84] found 98.6% implant success with free-standing fixed partial prostheses after 1 year. Zarb and Schmitt[85,86] experienced 94.3% fixture survival during 2.6 to 7.4 years of loading for the posterior partially edentulous and a 91.5% implant success rate for anterior restorations during loading periods ranging from 2 to 8 years. These studies support the consideration of endosseous implantology as an adjunct to restoring the partially edentulous arch.

Sullivan[87] notes that approximately 17 to 20 million Americans are partially edentulous. Implant-supported prostheses can be considered for those patients who experience difficulty wearing a removable partial denture. This is a common finding in patients with unilateral edentulism. Implant-supported prostheses may also provide an acceptable alternative to extensive crown and bridge procedures on natural teeth.

Bone density and volume often present problems when considering implant-borne restorations. Knife-edged ridges often necessitate extensive alveoloplasty. The mandibular canal, maxillary sinus, and nasal fossa may limit implant length.

Posterior Considerations

The mandibular canal often limits implant length. When the posterior mandible has a broad bony base, a wide-diameter implant may be considered, which can engage the buccal and lingual cortical plates for greater stability. Wide implants increase the bone–implant interface when vertical height is limited. They also provide a better emergence profile for molar teeth and improved axial loading (Figure 21A.17a,b). Bone augmentation may sometimes be considered. Reformatted CT scanning may permit good visualization of the relationship of the mandibular canal to the proposed implant orientation. It is sometimes possible to use a longer fixture by placing it buccal or lingual to the canal. The mandibular nerve has been surgically repositioned to permit longer implant placement.[88]

The posterior maxilla often presents several obstacles to achieving predictable implant rehabilitation. Kopp[89] stated that the replacement of bilateral posterior edentulous areas in the maxilla with osseointegrated implants is difficult if not impossible. Bone density in this region tends to be the

a

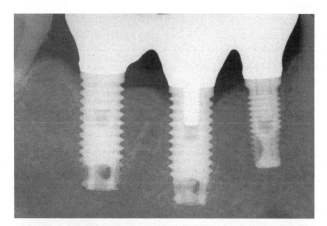

b

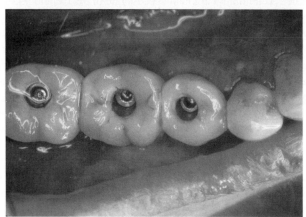

FIGURE 21A.17 (a) Radiograph: the combination of wide platform molars and standard premolar allows for more natural emergence profile. (b) Screw access chambers in final prosthesis.

poorest with Q-3 and Q-4 bone being a common finding. The surgeon may prefer to use self-tapping implants in softer bone to avoid stripping bone threads, which can occur during standard tapping procedures. Alternatively, press-fit implants that are easier to install may be considered. Maxillary bone resorbs from buccal to lingual, often necessitating that restorations be cantilevered buccally for proper cheek support and occlusion. The maxillary sinus tends to pneumatize with age, reducing the amount of vertical bone height available for implant placement. A reformatted CT scan may be indicated to relate proposed implant placement to the orientation of the maxillary sinus. Wide implants, maxillary sinus bone augmentation, or both may be considered when bone height is limited.[90] It is generally recommended that the surgeon wait 9 months to 1 year before uncovering implants that have been placed in the posterior maxilla that was treated with sinus augmentation (a great variation in healing times has been reported for various graft materials[91]). Carefully planned onlay grafts that do not encroach excessively on intermaxillary space can improve the crown-to-implant ratio.

Clinicians may encounter difficulty working in the posterior regions of patients with limited intermaxillary opening. When this occurs, it may be advantageous to employ press-

fit implants as the osteotomy site is easier to prepare and placement does not require mounting tools. Tilting the implants slightly mesially may permit easier access for the surgeon and restorative dentist. Impressioning of implants or abutments using the indirect coping technique described earlier requires less vertical space.

Supereruption of teeth opposing an edentulous area may limit intermaxillary space. Occlusal equilibration with possible tooth devitalization and periodontal crown lengthening may be necessary (Figure 21A.18). Segmental osteotomy may be considered when supereruption is severe. Alveoloplasty of the edentulous ridge may also be performed when sufficient bone will remain for fixture placement.

Biomechanically, implants tolerate forces better when they turn the arch to create a curved support system.[92] Posterior partially edentulous restorations often have the implants oriented in a straight line in response to jaw anatomy, creating a distinct mechanical disadvantage. Furthermore, molar biting forces can be four times greater than in the incisor region.[13] These factors, coupled with the lower bone density, decreased available bone height, and maxillary buccal cantilevering often encountered in the posterior region, suggest the need for careful treatment planning for posterior partially edentulous restorations. Implant support should be maximized, and progressive loading as described earlier should be considered. A mutually protected occlusion that disarticulates the posterior prosthetic teeth in lateral excursions is recommended (lateral forces generate shear stresses on fixtures).

Anterior Considerations

Anterior restorations often present several challenges. Implants must be positioned to permit natural tooth emergence angles, particularly for the patient with a high smile line. Fixtures placed too lingually compromise the tongue space and interfere with phonetics. Lingual or interproximal positioning may require ridge-lapping of the final prosthesis, which can complicate oral hygiene procedures. The nature of bone resorption in the anterior maxilla often necessitates that implants be directed labially. The restorative dentist must compensate by using angled machined abutments or custom abutments or mesostructures to redirect the implants. In severely resorbed, defective, and injured ridges bone grafting may be required to idealize implant positions on placement.

Final tooth position for anterior restorations commonly creates a mutually protected occlusion that disoccludes posterior teeth in excursions. Anterior implants may therefore be exposed to lateral forces. The consequences of this are not known to date. Fortunately in the maxilla, the cuspid region usually provides a good site for implant placement as it lies anterior to the maxillary sinus and posterior to the nasal fossa.

The hard- and soft tissue housing of the final prosthesis may need to be evaluated from a cosmetic perspective. The surgical stent relates these tissues to the final tooth position

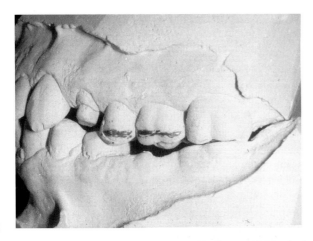

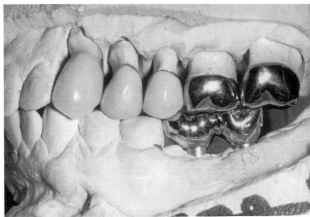

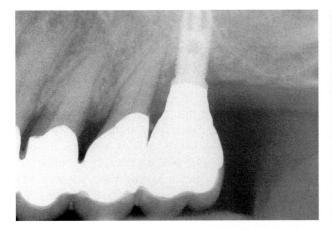

FIGURE 21A.18 (a) Supereruption of maxillary posterior segment. (b,c) Correction of occlusal plane coupled with mandibular alveoloplasty allowed for restoration with two mandibular fixtures.

and may help determine whether augmentation procedures would enhance the result.

Connecting Implants to Natural Teeth

Controversy surrounds the issue of whether and how to connect implant-supported restorations to natural teeth (Figure 21A.19a,b). Weinberg[93] states that implants have less than 10 μm of movement under horizontal loads, while well-supported teeth display movements of 100 μm to 500 μm under similar conditions. He warns that differential mobility would concentrate excess horizontal forces around the implants' crestal bone. Skalak[94] and Sullivan[95] suggest that rigid splinting of implants to teeth can create biomechanical complications due

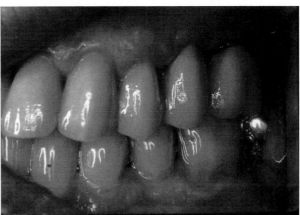

FIGURE 21A.19 (a) Radiograph: direct implant to natural tooth connection. (b) Final prothesis (part of a full arch reconstruction).

to uneven force distribution, resulting in implant overload. Increasing the distance between implant and tooth abutments potentiates greater tortional force on the fixture(s). Ericsson et al.[96] reported favorable clinical results over 6 to 30 months in six cases in which Brånemark implants were rigidly splinted to natural teeth. Åstrand et al.[97] studied 23 patients with Kennedy Class I mandibles. For each patient, on one side a Brånemark implant was joined to a natural tooth with a rigid prosthesis while a two-implant-supported prosthesis was placed on the contralateral side. After 2 years of function the results revealed no statistical difference between the two prosthetic groups. It should be noted that these prostheses opposed a maxillary complete denture. These studies were of relatively short duration, and no long-term data exist to date.

Rangert et al.[98] rigidly joined a Brånemark implant to a tooth using an in vitro model to perform mechanical tests. He found that the screw joints that attach the gold cylinder and abutment to the implant form a flexible system that matches the vertical mobility of natural teeth. The study also revealed that transverse mobility of the tooth should be limited to prevent screw loosening.

The IMZ implant system (Nobel Biocare, USA, Inc., Yorba Linda, CA) attempts to resolve the discrepancy between implant and tooth mobility by incorporating a resilient intramo-

bile element (IME) that is said to simulate a tooth's periodontium. Kirsch[99] adds that joining implants to natural teeth may increase proprioception through the prosthesis.

The Periotest (Siemens AG, Bensheim, Germany) is a mechanical device designed to objectively measure tooth mobility and has since been adopted for use with dental implants.[100,101] Measuring the relative mobility of the fixture and tooth abutments used to support a prosthesis may help determine the type of connection to use. Multiple abutting of natural teeth can be employed to reduce their relative mobility. Periotest can also be employed to verify osseointegration at implant uncovering.

Implants can be joined to natural teeth with a variety of nonrigid connectors (i.e., semiprecision attachments). This arrangement minimizes the transfer of force from the movement of natural teeth in function to the implant component of the prosthesis. The female portion of the attachment is placed in the tooth section, and the male in the implant section. This allows depression of the natural teeth during functional loading without direct force transfer to the implants. Nonrigid attachments also permit retrievability of implant-borne segments (Figure 21A.20). This technique sometimes has complications with natural tooth intrusion.

Implants can be rigidly joined to natural teeth while maintaining retrievability. Teeth can be prepared to receive telescopic copings, which are permanently cemented. The final prosthesis is seated over the copings and implant abutments. Retention to the implant portion can be accomplished with screws or temporary cement, while the tooth component is retained with temporary cement (Figure 21A.21). Implants can also be joined to natural tooth in a nonretrievable format. When there are many more teeth than implants, it may not justify overcopings and a retrievable case. A direct cementation to the natural teeth and implants can be performed.

Nonrigid attachment and telescopic cases can become complex and expensive, and they require additional reduction of tooth structure.

There is no clear concensus regarding the proper management of the tooth–implant connection. It is generally felt that implant-supported prostheses should be freestanding whenever possible (Figure 21A.22a,b).

Abutment Intrusion

Ericsson et al.[96] observed tooth abutment intrusion when nonrigidly connected to an implant. Reider and Parel[102] and others have also reported this finding. English[103] proposes several possible etiologies for this phenomenon (Figure 21A.23a,b). To date, the cause remains a mystery. Intrusion can be prevented by placing a U-shaped pin between the male and female portions of semiprecision attachments while preserving some resiliency. When implants are rigidly connected to natural teeth that have telescopic copings, placement of horizontal screws through the bridge into the overcopings will help prevent root intrusion while maintaining retrievability.

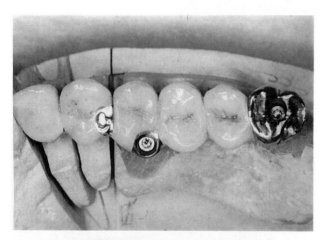
a

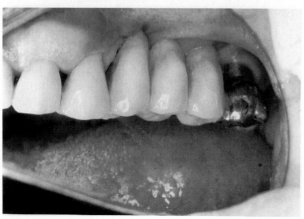
b

FIGURE 21A.20 (a,b) Nonrigid attachment of implants to natural teeth.

a 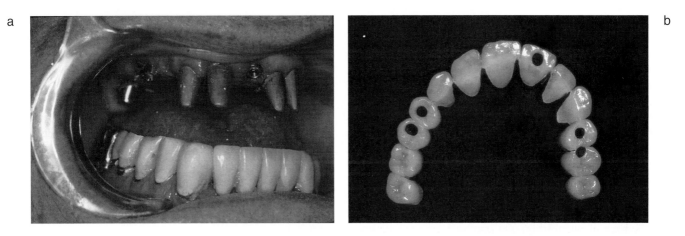 b

FIGURE 21A.21 (a) Maxillary implants and natural teeth with copings. Telescopic copings on natural teeth allow retrievability while minimizing potential for decay. (b) Prosthesis with screw access channels.

a 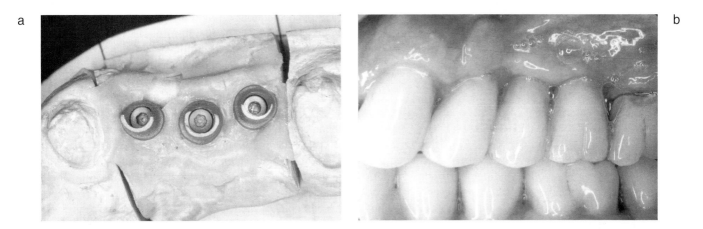 b

FIGURE 21A.22 (a) Custom abutments on implant lab analogs with triad effect. (b) Splinted implants are freestanding and not connected to adjacent reconstruction of the natural teeth.

a 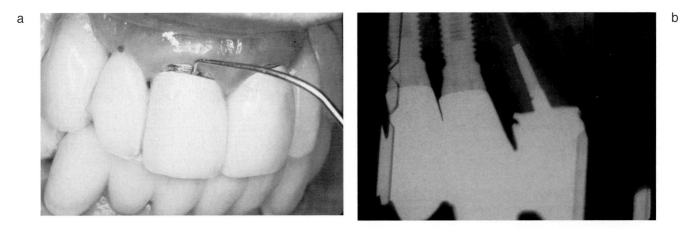 b

FIGURE 21A.23 (a) Intrusion of natural tooth with overcoping (part of full arch implants/natural tooth reconstruction). (b) Radiograph: misfit of coping and bridge due to intrusion.

From the time of implant placement, the restorative dentist plays a critical role in assisting with the osseointegration process. The patient is provided with a temporary restoration that was made prior to surgery. If the prosthesis is removable, there should be maximum soft tissue coverage and vertical stops on teeth to prevent it from settling onto the implant sites. The undersurface of the prosthesis should be relieved and in some cases relined with tissue conditioner in the areas of fixture placement to prevent micromovement. Sometimes extraction of hopeless teeth adjacent to the implant sites can be delayed, and they can be used to support the temporary restoration.

Impressions of the implant bodies (or abutments if placed at the time of uncovering) and opposing arch can be taken and poured at or soon after uncovering. A bite registration is performed. These models can be useful in a variety of ways. A fixed or removable temporary prosthesis as previously described can be made at this early stage. These "study models" can aid in abutment selection. A custom tray can be made for the final impression to be taken when the tissues have healed. If a temporary prosthesis will not be worn, the surgeon and restorative dentist must confirm that the healing abutment or permanent abutment is not contacting the opposing dentition as this could induce implant overload and failure.

Single Tooth Restorations

Osseointegrated implants have been successfully used to replace a single missing tooth. Jemt and Pettersson[104] reported a 98.5% cumulative implant success rate over a 3-year follow-up period. Similar findings have been cited by Schmitt and Zarb[105] and Laney et al.[106]

A single implant-supported tooth may be indicated to address a variety of situations.[107–109] Patients are often reluctant to have adjacent intact dentition or existing bridgework disturbed for conventional crown and bridge procedures. Young individuals with large pulp horns on adjacent teeth are at an increased risk of pulp exposure. A single tooth implant supported restoration may be used to fill a pontic space that is larger than the tooth being replaced. It may provide a simple solution in the presence of short teeth with a close bite. One posterior implant-supported tooth may be all that is necessary when a posterior cantilever or conventional partial denture will not suffice.

Single tooth replacement requires precise treatment planning and execution. A stent with opaque markers can be worn during CT scanning to accurately relate the remaining bone to the contours of the proposed restoration. The template also relates final tooth position to the remaining soft tissues and can aid in determining when hard and/or soft tissue augmentation should be performed. Hard- and soft tissue augmentation procedures often coupled with barrier membrane techniques often permit more optimal implant placement (Figure

21A.24). The surgeon should select the longest implant that the site will allow. The implant must have an antirotational mechanism. The surgical stent will help the surgeon properly direct the fixture.

Faciolingual orientation of the implant is largely dependent on the mode of prosthetic connection to be used in the final restoration. Optimal esthetics and tissue emergence is often achieved with a screw- or cement-retained prosthesis on a custom abutment.

When screw retention is chosen, the fixture should be directed for the access opening to coincide with the cingulum region or central fossa. Labial ridge-lapping may be necessary to achieve proper contours of anterior teeth (Figure 21A.25).

Cemented prostheses eliminate the cosmetic and surgical restrictions created by the screw access chamber. Often in the anterior region, the surgeon can position the implant slightly labially to more closely coincide with the long axis of a tooth root and potentiate a natural emergence angle. (N.B.: Excessive labial implant positioning can result in irreversible aesthetic and functional compromise. When in doubt, it is best to err on the side of lingual implant placement.)

When there is collapse of the facial plate, soft and/or hard tissue augmentation should be considered.

Apicocoronal implant positioning will affect the emergence profile of the tooth being replaced. As a general rule, the crest of the fixture should be located 2 to 4 mm apical to the cementoenamel junction of the adjacent dentition[110] (Figure 21A.26), thereby permitting the replacement to emerge from under the gingiva at a width that corresponds to that of a natural tooth. When recession is present, the fixture should be placed 2 to 4 mm apical to the marginal gingiva unless the lip will conceal the neck of the restoration and the result will be consistent with the patient's expectations. Emergence angle is also affected by implant width. Narrow implants exist that may be employed to replace narrow teeth (i.e., lower incisors). They may also be used in ridges that are knife-edged as a result of bone resorption (when bone augmentation will not be performed). Wider teeth require more apical positioning of narrow fixtures. Wide bony beds that will support larger teeth may lend themselves to the use of wide-diameter implants.

Mesiodistal orientation of the implant is again dependent on the prosthetic tooth position and will impact on proximal contours and recreation of natural papillae. Placement should generally coincide with the mesiodistal midline of the replacement tooth.

Access for implant uncovering can impact on final gingival contours. Vertical incisions that bisect interproximal papillae are less likely to produce papillary blunting with unsightly open triangular spaces. "Cookie-cutter-type" tissue punches sacrifice keratinized tissue and should not be used. Stage-two surgery provides an opportunity to perform plastic procedures that augment keratinized tissue and reshape gingival architecture as needed to optimize aesthetics.

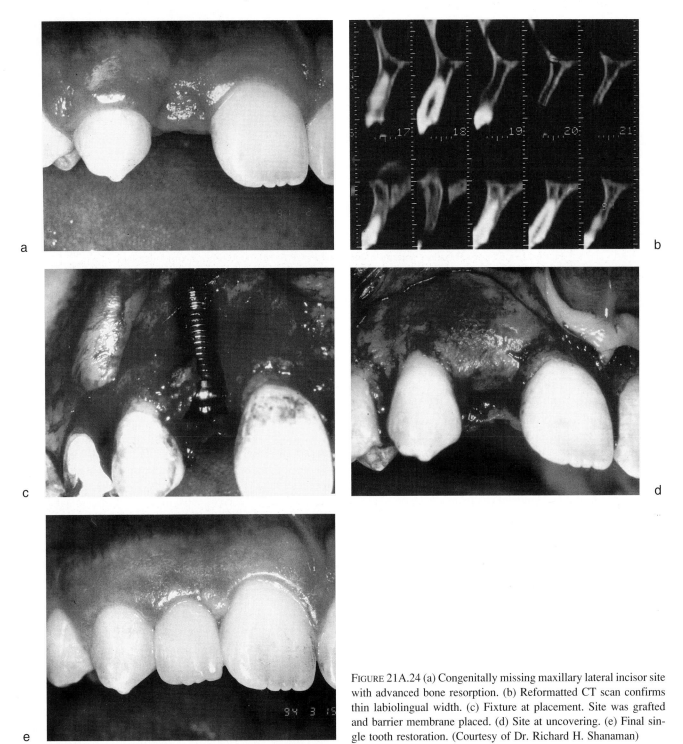

FIGURE 21A.24 (a) Congenitally missing maxillary lateral incisor site with advanced bone resorption. (b) Reformatted CT scan confirms thin labiolingual width. (c) Fixture at placement. Site was grafted and barrier membrane placed. (d) Site at uncovering. (e) Final single tooth restoration. (Courtesy of Dr. Richard H. Shanaman)

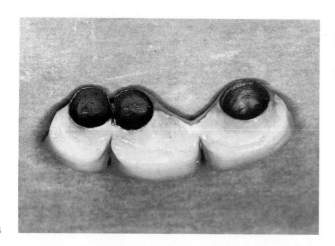

a

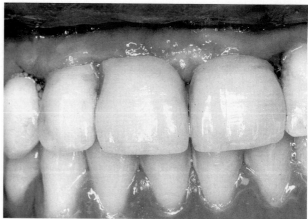

b

FIGURE 21A.25 (a,b) Maxillary anterior implant supported fixed bridge necessitating ridge lap.

Abutment selection was discussed earlier. The single tooth abutment must be antirotational. Lazarra[111] introduced the Emergence Profile System (Implant Innovations, Inc., Palm Beach Garden, FL, USA) that permits selection of a healing abutment that gradually widens from the implant coronally (Figure 21A.27). The permanent Emergence Profile abutment is selected and placed after tissue healing is complete and the final impression is taken using copings that conform to the gingival taper. Good access to the implant and abutment is maintained with less tissue impingement during prosthodontic procedures.

When aesthetic control of gingival contours must be maximized (i.e., anterior single tooth replacement with a high lip line), a custom healing abutment can be made. Upon implant insertion at stage-one surgery, a fixture impression coping is placed and an impression made. The impression and coping are removed, the cover-screw secured, and the surgery completed. An implant analog is attached to the impression coping and a model is fabricated that relates the implant to the

remaining dentition. A temporary crown that closely resembles the final restoration is produced which is inserted at the time of implant uncovering.

The implant team will often have to decide whether to place an implant immediately after tooth extraction or to allow time for healing to take place. Immediate fixture placement following extraction was first advocated by Barzilay and colleagues.[112] Facial bone resorption is kept to a minimum, and the extraction socket may help with mesiodistal implant orientation (avoiding adjacent roots). The patient's waiting period for the final prosthesis is reduced. Immediate treatment presents several potential problems. Implants should not be placed in the presence of acute infection. Primary stability of the implant is desirable and is sometimes difficult to achieve when the socket is wider than the implant. Primary soft tissue closure can be difficult to achieve and may necessitate coronal flap mobilization with resultant reduction of keratinized tissue. Bone augmentation coupled with barrier mem-

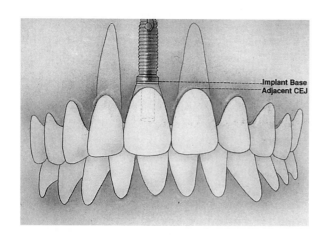

FIGURE 21A.26 Generally the implant base should be placed 2 to 4 mm apical to the adjacent gingival margin. (From Parel and Sullivan,[47] by permission of Taylor Publishing Co., Dallas, TX, USA)

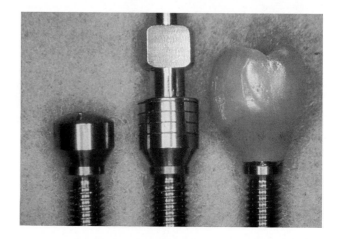

FIGURE 21A.27 Implant Innovations Inc. Emergence Profile System. From left to right: healing abutment, impression coping, final restoration. (Courtesy of Implant Innovations Inc., Palm Beach Gardens, FL, USA)

brane techniques may be indicated. Tarnow and Fletcher[113] suggest allowing the extraction socket to heal for 8 to 10 weeks prior to fixture placement. This facilitates primary soft tissue closure without sacrificing keratinized tissue. The only disadvantage is the potential for osseous resorption during the 8- to 10-week waiting period. Langer[114] has suggested cutting a hopeless tooth to the osseous crest and allowing tissue overgrowth for 3 to 4 weeks. The hopeless root is then extracted. The additional soft tissue will provide better closure during implant placement. Mensdorff-Pouilly[115] and colleagues compared immediate and primary immediate (placed 6 to 8 weeks postextraction) implants. The immediate implants showed a tendency toward deeper pocket formation and an increased frequency of membrane dehiscence. This may reflect the poorer quality of soft tissue coverage. Nevins and Mellonig[116] advocate a staged approach when immediate and primary immediate implant placement is not possible. When indicated, the alveolar bone is initially reconstructed with guided tissue regeneration in combination with bone grafts. After a 10-month waiting period the fixtures are placed.

The implant team must pay particular attention to biomechanics when replacing single teeth. Contacts should be light in centric and absent in lateral excursions. Fixtures should be directed to receive axial loads whenever possible and particularly in the posterior region where occlusal forces are greater. Single tooth restorations are particularly subject to rotational forces around the long axis of the implant. It is sometimes possible to replace a single missing molar with two implants[117] to minimize these rotational forces and provide additional support for the replacement tooth. When bone volume permits, a wide-diameter implant should be used. This will allow occlusal forces between the cusp tips to be directed over the implant body.

Several potential noteworthy complications are associated with the single tooth replacement. The most common problem reported by Jemt and Pettersson[104] and others is loosening and fatigue of the abutment screw, which sometimes leads to fistulae and gingival hyperplasia. Possible causes include rotational forces and inaccurate fit of custom cast abutments at the interface with the implant head. Screw loosening decreases over time. Nobel Biocare's CeraOne® (Nobel Biocare, USA, Inc., Yorba Linda, CA) system incorporates a new gold-palladium screw that is tightened with a torque-controller to 32 Ncm and is reported by Boudrias[118] to show no clinical signs of loosening. Other complications include devitalization of adjacent roots, implant failure, bone loss, or both; loss of gingival height and papillae; and poor aesthetics resulting from improperly directed implants.

Complications

Implant Failure

Long-term osseointegration has been documented to be 93% for individual implants in the anterior mandible and 84% in the maxilla.[3] The causes for decreased maxillary implant success are probably multifactorial. Maxillary bone quality is often poorer than its mandibular counterpart. Anatomic obstacles (i.e., maxillary sinus, nasal fossa) coupled with decreased bone volume secondary to resorption often call for the use of short implants, which Jemt[76] has shown to have a higher rate of failure than longer implants in the maxilla. Short implants are usually placed in regions of significant resorption, which results in a high crown-to-implant ratio. Aesthetics, phonetics, occlusion, and lip and cheek support often necessitate significant facial positioning of maxillary fixed prostheses. The resulting cantilever can produce off-axis forces and difficulty with hygiene due to excessive ridge-lapping. The overall effect is a lower rate of implant success observed in the maxilla. It therefore becomes prudent to always inform the patient that it may be necessary to employ a secondary treatment plan in the event of implant failure. A patient should never be promised a fixed prosthesis. This is particularly important when bone grafting procedures are performed, which make it difficult to accurately predict final fixture location.

Several prosthetic factors can contribute to implant bone loss and failure. Achieving and maintaining osseointegration begins at the treatment-planning stage. Anticipated prosthesis design must take into consideration adequate implant support and distribution. A surgical template helps assure proper fixture orientation. The temporary prosthesis should be adequately relieved to prevent micromovement of fixtures during the integration phase. Upon uncovering, healing or permanent abutments should not contact opposing dentition and temporization that promotes progressive loading as previously discussed should be considered. The final prosthesis should fit passively and the occlusion refined. The design should permit full hygiene access to all implant abutment and prosthesis surfaces.

The impact of parafunctional habits should be minimized by providing additional implant support where possible. The prosthesis should be durable, and a night guard should be considered.

Fixture failure is most obviously evidenced by mobility. This may not be apparent if a splinted prosthesis is not routinely removed at recall visits. Radiographic evidence of a mobile fixture often reveals a lucent area between the implant and surrounding bone. The gingival collar may be inflamed and hyperplastic. No attempt should be made to save mobile implants. They should be removed as soon as possible and the remaining prosthesis evaluated for adequate support and possible modification or removal.

The potential for implant failure may be evidenced in more subtle ways. Maximal crestal bone loss should be 1.5 mm within the first year after surgery and 0.1 mm every year thereafter.[119] When bone loss appears to be excessive, it behooves the implant team to attempt to identify the problem and intervene expeditiously.

The gingival tissues may often provide the earliest evidence of an ailing implant in the forms of inflammation, hyperplasia, pocketing, fistula formation, and recession. Implant overload may be manifest by pocket formation in the absence of gingival inflammation. Loosening of abutment screws may cause hyperplasia and fistula formation as observed by Jemt et al.[120] for single tooth restorations. Plaque retention may cause gingival inflammation, and the patient must be encouraged to actively participate in a comprehensive hygiene program. Despite the patient's best intentions, several obstacles may preclude optimal hygiene performance. The restoration may not permit full access to the prosthesis-abutment-implant interfaces. Titanium abutments may scratch easily and encourage plaque adherence. Exposed hydroxylapatite, fixture threads, or plasma-sprayed implant surfaces may similarly attract plaque.

Implant Fracture

Naert et al.[121] observed a 0.5% rate of fixture fracture when supporting a complete fixed prosthesis. Fracture of implants is directly attributable to biomechanical overload and can occur with any prosthesis type. The etiology should be sought to minimize recurrence of this problem. The fractured fragment need not be removed if it is free of pathology and if the site is not needed for fixture replacement. If the implant fractures at the neck, it may still be usable by adapting a UCLA-type abutment to the fracture interface with Duralay resin (Reliance Dental Mfg. Co., Worth, IL, USA) and casting a custom abutment. Implant trephines can be employed to assist in removal of unwanted fractured segments.

Loose and Fractured Screws

Loosening of abutment and prosthetic retaining screws is a common observation. There are several possible etiologies for this finding, including inadequate tightening of screws, biomechanical overload, and poor fit of the prosthesis. Nobel Biocare, USA, Inc. (Yorba Linda, CA) developed a torque control device that can be used to tighten Brånemark-implant component screws with a precise amount of force. The gold retaining screw and abutment screw receive 10 Ncm and 20 Ncm of torque, respectively. Nobel Biocare acknowledges the increased likelihood of screw loosening encountered with single tooth restorations and has developed a gold-palladium screw for their CeraOne® single tooth abutment that is tightened to 32 Ncm. Paragon (Paragon Implant Company, Encino, CA, USA) developed an implant design with an internal hexagon that joins an abutment that has a 1° tapered external hexagon (Taper-Lock mating system). The resulting antirotational frictional fit is said to reduce the frequency of abutment screw loosening. Some implant systems utilize a Morse taper design to establish a secure implant abutment connection.

Fracture of abutment and prosthetic retaining screws can occur for any of the same reasons as screw loosening. Walton et al.[122] found replacement of fractured gold screws to be the most common repair for fixed implant-supported prostheses. Nobel Biocare designed the gold retaining screw to be the "weak link" to protect the implant body from overload

and/or fracture. A fractured screw indicates biomechanical breakdown, and its etiology must be determined to prevent greater adverse sequelae.

Removal of broken screws can at times present a challenge. If the gold screw fractures so that a portion remains inside the abutment screw and it cannot be readily retrieved, the easiest solution is to remove and replace the abutment screw with a new one. The greater problem arises when the abutment screw fractures within the screw channel of the implant body and cannot be reached with a narrow forceps. When the abutment screw fractures, it almost always loosens first. The section remaining in the implant can usually be teased out. An explorer tip can be placed near the edge of the screw and rotated counterclockwise. If this is not successful, another method of retrieval calls for placing a small eccentric notch into the superior portion of the screw fragment with a quarter-round bur being careful not to damage the internal threads of the screw channel. An explorer tip is then inserted into the notch, and the fragment is backed out. Implant Innovations, Inc. (Palm Beach Gardens, FL, USA) manufactures a screw-removing system for Brånemark and Brånemark-compatible implants that protects the internal threads of the fixture from damage during retrieval. Ultrasonic scalers are also useful in rotating fractured abutment screws out.

Stripped Threads

Clinicians should be careful to avoid stripping the internal fixture threads. This problem can occur when engaging the fixture mount during implant surgery or when connecting abutments or fixture impression copings. All connections should be smooth with no binding. Proper use of torque-control devices assures appropriate tightening of screws. Nonpassive seating of prostheses that are screw-retained directly to the implant heads may cause thread damage. Some prostheses are cemented to abutments that are screw-retained to the implant. If an abutment screw loosens, the prosthesis must often be removed to reaccess the loose screw. The internal implant threads are particularly vulnerable to damage when the prosthesis is being tapped off.

Implant Innovations, Inc. (Palm Beach Gardens, FL, USA) manufactures a tapping tool designed to rethread the damaged internal screw channel of Brånemark and Brånemark-compatible implants. It is easy to use and provides precise tapping within minutes.

Prosthodontic Solutions for Compromised Implant Placement

Poor implant position creates an all-too-common dilemma. Implant position should incorporate the biomechanical, functional, and aesthetic principles previously discussed. This is best achieved through proper planning and stent fabrication. The severely off-angled implant often requires complex management.

The need for coordinated planning of implant placement between the surgeon and restorative dentist cannot be overstated. Despite careful communication and proper stent use, several anatomic limitations will restrict ideal positioning. The nasal fossa, maxillary sinus, incisive canal, and inferior alveolar nerve will often prevent optimal placement. Bony undercuts can result in flared maxillary fixtures to avoid apical perforations without bone grafting. Mandibular posterior implants may require a lingual tilt to avoid the retromylohyoid fossa. Advanced ridge resorption in the maxilla may yield palatally positioned implants. The surgeon's attempt to engage cortical plates may yield a less favorable emergence position. Residual ridge height, width, shape, and relationship to the opposing arch can compromise fixture orientation. Bone grafting procedures that improve implant position, length, and distribution should be considered on a case by case basis. Only with optimal placement can the ultimate restorative result be achieved. The restorative dentist may employ several strategies when restoring fixtures with compromised orientation.

Prefabricated angled abutments are available with a variety of tilts. They are usually connected directly to the fixture. Depending upon the abutment type, the prosthesis can be either screw- or cement-retained.

Custom abutments allow the restorative dentist to optimize control of orientation, emergence profile, and retention. A plastic or gold UCLA-type pattern is custom waxed and cast, enabling one to control angulation of the implant post. All-plastic patterns should be machined with a lapping tool after casting to ensure precise fit to the implant. Patterns should be cast in an alloy with less than 9% silver. Metals with high silver content deform more easily, which can accelerate wear at the screw and implant interfaces.[123] Custom abutments are particularly useful in the maxillary anterior region where, due to ridge inclination, screw-access holes would often exit the labial of the tooth, severely compromising esthetics.

Mesostructures can be fabricated on some or all of a series of abutments. This substructure is usually screw-retained and houses the overlying suprastructure. The suprastructure will be veneered with the aesthetic tooth material (i.e., porcelain, denture teeth, or composite resin). Mesostructures offer an advantage when porcelain fused to metal restorations are used. After firing large sections of porcelain, distortion of the substructure can occur. Since the mesostructure is not veneered, its fit to the implants would not be altered and would not yield additional stress after ceramic firing. Mesostructures should be reserved for situations in which severely misaligned implants cannot be managed by more conventional means. These prostheses greatly increase cost and complexity, and they can be bulky. Suprastructures that are cement retained can still be retrievable when a provisional luting agent is used.

Tube and screw attachments are prefabricated with a gold alloy. The female portion can be incorporated into the mesostructure and the male into the suprastructure, yielding a retrievable screw-retained prosthesis. This can be utilized with severely off-angled implants (Figure 21A.28).

Lingual positioned implants are most ideally restored with a screw-retained prosthesis (refer to Figure 21A.6a,b). The framework must be designed to be flush with the ridge at the interface of the screw access chamber and the mucosal surface in order to avoid tongue impingement and altered phonetics. If sufficient countersinking has not been performed with implant heads close to the marginal gingiva, framework connection will likely be directly to the implants to further minimize bulk. These frameworks can be extended labially to support veneering materials. Angulated or custom abutments are less than ideal in these cases since the resulting prosthesis may be too bulky.

Interproximal positioning of implants can cause problems in visible areas where aesthetics is important. This is particularly relevant to cases with minimal resorption in conjunction with a high lip line. Fixtures that emerge between teeth can be masked with a flange where necessary (using pink porcelain or acrylic). If sufficient redundancy exists, the problematic fixture may be buried and not used. A flange is never a good substitute for proper mesiodistal implant positioning.

Interproximal positioning of fixtures often occurs in the posterior mandible. In an attempt to avoid the mental foramen on its distal side, the surgeon will often place the implant between the second premolar and first molar position. This problem may repeat itself as subsequent posterior implants are placed. In some instances it may be better to keep the first site distal to the mental foramen vacant to avoid this aesthetic problem.

Esthetic Complications

Implant prostheses can be host to a variety of esthetic complications. The complete maxillary fixed prosthesis as originally described by Brånemark[124] was designed to stand 1 to 2 mm from the gingiva to facilitate oral hygiene procedures. Unfortunately, many patients experienced difficulty with phonetics as air escaped under the prosthesis. For some patients, this problem abates over time as the upper lip adapts to limit excessive air flow by creating a seal against the prosthesis. For others the problem continues, and a removable labial flange can be fabricated from silicone or resin to help correct phonetic and aesthetic deficiencies. Unfortunately, the patient expecting a fixed prosthesis ends up with "removable gingiva." These veneers tear easily, attract plaque, and require frequent remakes.[125] For patients with a high smile line, minimal maxillary ridge resorption, or both, implants in the incisor region should precisely correspond to the final tooth positions. If this cannot be achieved, one might consider not placing implants in this area. Short maxillary posterior cantilevers may present aesthetic problems if the buccal corridor is not adequately supported. For patients with severe maxillary and/or mandibular ridge resorption, complete fixed prostheses may not be capable of adequately replacing missing hard and soft tissue, resulting in deficient facial support. This problem can be avoided by fabricating a diagnostic setup of teeth to help choose between a fixed prosthesis and an over-

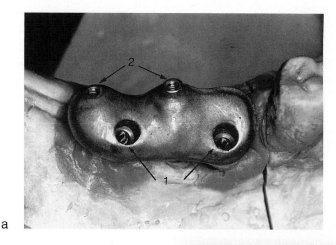

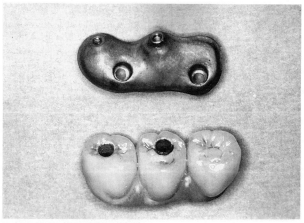

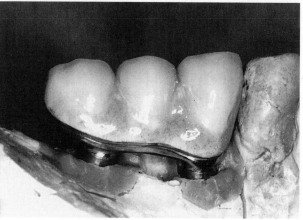

FIGURE 21A.28 Mesostructure prosthesis with tube and screw retention. (a) Substructure: retained to implant analogues (1); tube and screw attachments (2) Implant screws. (b) Substructure (top) and suprastructure retained by tube and screw attachments (bottom). (c) Final prosthesis.

denture design. If the tooth position does not approximate the ridge, a removable design may be appropriate. When fabricating a fixed prosthesis with acrylic resin and denture teeth, it is necessary to opaque the metal substructure when the acrylic is less than 2 mm thick.

Removable overdentures present with far fewer aesthetic complications. When vertical space is limited, retention clips may create bulking of acrylic in areas that are either visible or annoying to the tongue. This problem may be minimized by performing selective alveoplasty at the time of surgery and choosing a retentive mechanism with reduced vertical and/or horizontal dimensions. Alternatively, a fixed prosthesis may be the treatment of choice in jaws with minimal resorption and limited intermaxillary space.

The single tooth replacement is most vulnerable to aesthetic complications that have been detailed previously.

Patient Expectations

A potentially serious complication associated with implant therapy is the development of false expectations on the part of the patient. The fully edentulous patient may accept implant treatment to construct a fixed prosthesis only to realize that the treatment plan must be changed later on. The removable prosthesis should not be considered inferior. Each has its advantages and limitations as previously described.

Failure of Restorative Materials

Several potential complications exist concerning the choice of restorative materials. Johansson and Palmqvist[126] found fractures of acrylic suprastructure resin or artificial teeth in 22% of full-arch implant-supported fixed prostheses during an observation period of 3 to 8 years. Jemt[76] found this problem to be most prevalent in the maxillary arch. Acrylic artificial teeth can wear over time with resulting occlusal changes. Denture teeth also require more room for placement than porcelain and will fracture if made too thin. Porcelain, on the other hand, shrinks on firing and can deform the underlying metal with a resulting loss of passivity of fit.

Walton and MacEntee[127] noticed an increased rate of repairs of complete dentures opposing implant-supported prostheses. This potential problem can be minimized by reinforcing such dentures with a metal framework. These investigators also observed that removable implant prostheses require three times as many adjustments and two times as many repairs as fixed implant-supported prostheses. The most common repair needed for removable prostheses were associated with retention clips, whereas the most common repair for fixed prostheses involved fracture of gold screws.

Complete implant-supported fixed prostheses are vulnerable to framework fracture at the cantilever extension joints. These regions should be designed with adequate bulk to resist biomechanical forces.

Maintenance

As with conventional prosthodontic rehabilitation, long-term success with implant-supported restorations depends on patient compliance with maintenance procedures. The impact of plaque and calculus formation upon implant surfaces is currently under investigation. George et al.[128] found a correlation between implants with gingival inflammation and the presence of pathogens associated with periodontitis. Maintenance of a clean permucosal environment begins at stage-two uncovering. Upon suture removal or initial tissue healing the surgeon will instruct the patient to gently brush the healing or permanent abutments. Access for patient hygiene procedures is optimal at this point. Sulcular areas lacking keratinized mucosa tend to be more sensitive, and the dentist should confirm that these sites are not being avoided. Abutments should not be occluding against the opposing dentition and temporary prostheses should be appropriately relieved, relined with resilient material, or both to prevent implant overload. Temporary removable prostheses should be cleaned by the patient regularly. Temporary fixed restorations should be designed to mimic the final prosthesis, giving the patient an opportunity to develop oral hygiene skills at this early phase.

Upon delivery of the final prosthesis, recall intervals should be established appropriate to the patient's needs. The patient, hygienist, and dentist must all use instruments that will not scratch abutment surfaces. Plastic (Nobel Biocare, USA, Inc., Yorba Linda, CA), gold-plated (Hu-Freidy, Chicago, IL, USA), and graphite (Premier Dental Products Co., Norristown, PA, USA) scalers as well as plastic pressure-sensitive periodontal probes (e.g., Sensor Probe, Pro-Dentec, Batesville, AR, USA) have been developed specifically for implant maintenance procedures. SofScale Calculus Scaling Gel (Ash/Dentsply International, York, PA, USA) softens calculus, thereby facilitating the ease of its removal. At home, the patient can incorporate conventional tooth brushing and flossing as well as heavier flosses (e.g., Oral-B Super Floss, Oral B Laboratories, Redwood City, CA, USA) and Butler Implant Floss (John O. Butler Company, Chicago, IL, USA) and end-tufted brushes (e.g., Lactona Double-End Interdental Brush, Lactona Corporation, Montgomeryville, PA, USA) into the daily routine. (Figure 21A.29). Electric mechanical brushes may be recommended by some dentists and/or preferred by patients.

The use of chlorhexidine gluconate (Peridex, Procter and Gamble, Cincinnati, OH, USA) concurrent with various phases of implant therapy and maintenance is being investigated and has been shown to reduce the rate of infectious complications to stage two uncovering (Dental Implant Clinical Research Group, Ann Arbor, MI, USA). The dentist may elect to take advantage of the retrievable nature of most implant prostheses. Removing the restoration at appropriate intervals allows the dentist and hygienist to visualize areas of plaque and calculus accumulation. This is particularly appro-

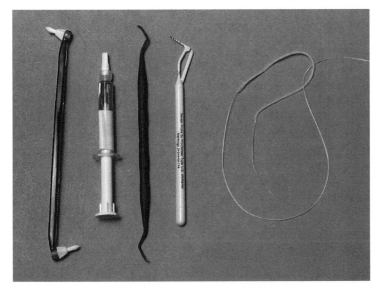

FIGURE 21A.29 Oral hygiene aids from left to right: Interdental brush (Lactona Corp. Montgomeryville, PA, USA); SofScale Calculus Scaling Gel (Ash/Dentsply International, York, PA, USA); graphite scaler (Premier Dental Products Co., Norristown, PA, USA); Sensor Probe (Pro-Dentec, Batesville, AR, USA); Oral-B Super Floss (Oral-B Laboratories, Redwood City, CA, USA).

priate for restorations that require ridge-lapping, where oral hygiene measures are more complex. Implants can be checked for mobility and the gingival areas readily examined and pockets probed. Secure abutment connections can be verified. Radiographs should be taken to monitor crestal bone levels and confirm the integrity of the implant-bone interface. Threads on Brånemark implants are machined at 0.5-mm intervals and can be used to gauge bone loss.[129]

The prosthesis should be regularly examined for evidence of bruxism and occlusal changes that can lead to biomechanical overload. Acrylic and porcelain fractures are more readily repaired when prostheses are retrievable. Overdenture retentive elements should be adjusted and replaced when necessary. Over time, hard and soft tissues resorb from beneath overdentures that are fixture- or tissue-supported, making the implant components increasingly vulnerable to biomechanical overload. Such prostheses should be relined as needed and the retentive elements carefully replaced incorporating techniques that maintain resiliency of the prosthesis when indicated.

Periotest was discussed earlier as a tool that may help assess osseointegration. The same instrument may be employed during maintenance visits to confirm integration and to observe changes in bone density surrounding implants. It is possible that the earliest signs of implant overload may be captured, thereby permitting immediate intervention. The usefulness of Periotest for implant therapy is currently being investigated (Dental Implant Clinical Research Group, Ann Arbor, MI).

References

1. Brånemark P-I, Zarb GA, Albrektsson T. *Tissue-Integrated Prostheses Osseointegration in Clinical Dentistry*. Chicago: Quintessence Publishing Co. Inc.; 1985.
2. Brånemark P-I, Hansson BO, Adell R, Breine U, Lindstrom J, Hallen O, Ohman A, et al. Osseointegrated implants in the treatment of the edentulous jaw. Experience from a 10-year period. *Scand J Plast Reconstr Surg*. Suppl 1977;16:1–132.
3. Adell R, Lekholm U, Rockler B, et al. A fifteen year study of osseointegrated implants in the treatment of the edentulous jaw. *Int J Oral Surg*. 1981;6:387–416.
4. Monson ML. Diagnostic and surgical guides for placement of dental implants. *J Oral Maxillofac Surg*. 1994;52:642–645.
5. Orenstein IH. The surgical template: a prescription for implant success. *Implant Dent*. 1992;1:182–184.
6. Weinberg LA. CT scan as a radiologic data base for optimum implant orientation. *J Prosthet Dent*. 1993;69:381–385.
7. Lekholm U, Zarb GA. Patient selection and preparation. In: Branemark P-I, Zarb GA, Albrektsson T, eds. *Tissue-Integrated Prostheses Osseointegration in Clinical Dentistry*. Chicago: Quintessence Publishing Co. Inc.; 1985:199–209.
8. Misch CE, Judy KW. Classification of partially edentulous arches for implant dentistry. *Int J Oral Implantol*. 1987;4:7–13.
9. Jensen O. Site classification for the osseointegrated implant. *J Prosthet Dent*. 1989;61:228–234.
10. Misch CE. Density of bone: effect on treatment planning, sur-
gical approach, and healing. In: Misch CE, ed. *Contemporary Implant Dentistry*. St Louis: Mosby Year Book, Inc.; 1993: 469–485.
11. Jaffin RA, Berman CL. The excessive loss of Brånemark fixtures in type IV bone: a 5-year analysis. *J Periodontol*. 1991;62:2–4.
12. Orenstein IH, Synan WJ, Truhlar RS, et al. Bone quality in patients receiving endosseous dental implants: DICRG interim report no. 1. *Implant Dent*. 1994;3:90–94.
13. Bidez MW, Misch CE. Force transfer in implant dentistry: basic concepts and principles. *J Oral Implantol*. 1992;18:264–274.
14. Aloia JF, Cohn SH, Ostuni Ja, et al. Prevention of involutional bone loss by exercise. *Ann Intern Med*. 1978;89:356–358.
15. Misch CE. Progressive bone loading. In: Misch CE, ed. *Contemporary Implant Dentistry*. St Louis: Mosby Year Book, Inc.; 1993:623–650.
16. Misch CE. Implant success or failure: clinical assessment. In: Misch CE, ed. *Contemporary Implant Dentistry*. St Louis: Mosby Year Book, Inc.; 1993:29–42.
17. Jaggers A, Simons AM, Badr SE. Abutment selection for anterior single tooth replacement: a clinical report. *J Prosthet Dent*. 1993;69:133–135.
18. Prestipino V, Ingber A. Esthetic high strength implant abutments. Part I. *J Esthetic Dent*. 1993;4:29–36.
19. Prestipino V, Ingber A. Esthetic high-strength implant abutments. Part II. *J Esthetic Dent*. 1993;5:63–68.
20. Kvarnstrom B. Personal communication. Nobelpharma Inc., Chicago, IL. April 1995.
21. Baumgarten HS, Salama H, Nelson A. Abutment head selection as a prosthetic discipline. *Compendium*. 1991;12:942–947.
22. Chiche GJ, Pinault A. Considerations for fabrication of implant-supported posterior restorations. *Int J Prosthodont*. 1991;4:37–44.
23. Friedman N, Landesman HM, Wexler M. The influence of fear, anxiety, and depression on the patient's adaptive responses to complete dentures. Part 1. *J Prosthet Dent*. 1987;58:687–689.
24. Davidoff SR, Steinberg MA, Halperin A. The implant-supported overdenture: a practical implant-prosthetic design. *Compendium*. 1993;14:722–730.
25. Carlsson G, Haraldson T. Fundamental aspects of mandibular atrophy. In: Worthington P, Brånemark P-I, eds. *Advanced Osseointegration Surgery: Applications in the Maxillofacial Region*. Chicago: Quintessence Publishing Co. Inc.; 1992;109–118.
26. Carlsson GE, Persson G. Morphologic changes of the mandible after extraction and wearing of dentures: a longitudinal, clinical and x-ray cephalometric study covering 5 years. *Odontol Rev*. 1967;18:27–54.
27. Hickey JC, Zarb GA. The edentulous state. In: Hickey JC, Zarb GA, eds. *Boucher's Prosthodontic Treatment for Edentulous Patients*. St. Louis: C.V. Mosby Co.; 1980:3–43.
28. Bahat O. Treatment planning and placement of implants in the posterior maxillae: report of 732 consecutive Nobelpharma implants. *Int J Oral Maxillofac Implants*. 1993;8:151–161.
29. Watson RM, Davis DM, Forman GH, et al. Considerations in design and fabrication of maxillary implant-supported prostheses. *Int J Prosthodont*. 1991;4:232–239.
30. DeBoer J. Edentulous implants: overdenture versus fixed. *J Prosthet Dent*. 1993;69:386–390.

31. Parel SM. Implants and overdentures; the osseointegrated approach with conventional and compromised applications. *Int J Oral Maxillofac Implants.* 1986;1:93–99.

32. Adell R, Eriksson B, Lekholm U, et al. A long-term follow-up study of osseointegrated implants in the treatment of totally edentulous jaws. *Int J Oral Maxillofac Implants.* 1990;5:347–359.

33. Weinberg LA, Kruger B. Biomechanical considerations when combining tooth-supported and implant-supported prostheses. *Oral Surg Oral Med Oral Pathol.* 1994;78:22–27.

34. Carlsson L. Built-in strain and untoward forces are the inevitable companions of prosthetic misfit. *Nobelpharma News.* 1994;8:5.

35. Gyllenram F. Optimal clinical fit is a multi-dimensional issue. *Nobelpharma News.* 1994;8:4.

36. Jemt T, Carlsson L, Boss A, et al. In vivo load measurements on osseointegrated implants supporting fixed or removable prostheses: a comparative pilot study. *Int J Oral Maxillofac Implants.* 1991;6:413–417.

37. Assif D, Fenton A, Zarb G, et al. Comparative accuracy of implant impression procedures. *Int J Periodont Restor Dent.* 1992;12:112–21.

38. Carr AB. Comparison of impression techniques for a five-implant mandibular model. *Int J Oral and Maxillofac Implants.* 1991;6:448–55.

39. Zarb GA, Jansson T. Prosthodontic procedures. In: Brånemark P-I, Zarb GA, Albrektsson T, eds. *Tissue-Integrated Prosthesis Osseointegration in Clinical Dentistry.* Chicago: Quintessence Publishing Co. Inc.; 1985.

40. Ivanhoe JR, Adrian ED, Krantz WA, et al. An impression technique for osseointegrated implants. *J Prosthet Dent.* 1991;66:410–411.

41. Lechner S, Duckmanton N, Klineberg I. Prosthodontic procedures for implant reconstruction. 2. Post-surgical procedures. *Aust Dent J.* 1992;37:427–432.

42. Barrett MG, de Rijk WG, Burgess JO. The accuracy of six impression techniques for osseointegrated implants. *J Prosthodont.* 1993;2:75–82.

43. Humphries RM, Yaman P, Bloem TJ. The accuracy of implant master casts constructed from transfer impressions. *Int J Oral Maxillofac Imp.* 1990;5:331–336.

44. Goll GE. Production of accurately fitting full-arch implant frameworks. Part 1. Clinical procedures. *J Prosthet Dent.* 1991;66:377–384.

45. Parel SM, Sullivan DY. *Esthetics and Osseointegration.* Dallas: Taylor Publishing Co.; 1989.

46. Jemt T, Linden B. Fixed implant-supported prostheses with welded titanium frameworks. *Int J Periodont Restor Dent.* 1992;12:177–184.

47. Nadeau P. Personal communication. Nobelpharma Inc. Chicago, IL. April 1995.

48. English CE. The critical a-p spread. *Implant Soc.* 1990;1:2–3.

49. Hobo S, Ichida E, Garcia LT. Fully bone anchored prostheses. In: Hobo S, Ichida E, Garcia LT, eds. *Osseointegration and Occlusal Rehabilitation.* Tokyo: Quintessence Publishing Co. Ltd., 1989:163–186.

50. Naert I, Quirynen M, van Steenberghe D, et al. A study of 589 consecutive implants supporting complete fixed prosthesis. Part 2. Prosthetic aspects. *J Prosthet Dent.* 1992;68:949–956.

51. Shackleton JL, Carr L, Slabbert JC, et al. Survival of fixed implant-supported prosthesis related to cantilever lengths. *J Prosthet Dent.* 1994;71:23–26.

52. Takayama H. Biomechanical considerations on osseointegrated implants. In: Hobo S, Ichida E, Garcia LT, eds. *Osseointegration and Occlusal Rehabilitation.* Tokyo: Quintessence Publishing Co. Ltd.; 1989:265–280.

53. Lindqvist L, Rockler B, Carlsson G. Bone resorption around fixtures in edentulous patients treated with mandibular fixed tissue-integrated prosthesis. *J Prosthet Dent.* 1988;59:59–63.

54. Sullivan DY. Implant restoration of the edentulous maxilla. Presented at the American College of Prosthodontists annual scientific session, New Orleans, Hyatt Regency Hotel, 3–5 November 1994.

55. White SN, Caputo AA, Anderkvist T. Effect of cantilever length on stress transfer by implant-supported prostheses. *J Prosthet Dent.* 1994;71:493–499.

56. Zarb GA, Schmitt A. The longitudinal clinical effectiveness of osseointegrated dental implants: the Toronto study. Part 3: Problems and complications encountered. *J Prosthet Dent.* 1990;64:185–194.

57. Fischman B. The rotational aspect of mandibular flexure. *J Prosthet Dent.* 1990;64:483–485.

58. McCartney JW. Cantilever rests: an alternative to the unsupported distal cantilever of osseointegrated implant-supported prostheses for the edentulous mandible. *J Prosthet Dent.* 1992;68:817–819.

59. Skalak R. Aspects of biomechanical considerations. In: Brånemark P-I, Zarb GA, Albrektsson T, eds. *Tissue-Integrated Prosthesis Osseointegration in Clinical Dentistry.* Chicago: Quintessence Publishing Co. Inc.; 1985:117–128.

60. Gracis SE, Nicholls JI, Chalupnik JD, et al. Shock-absorbing behavior of five restorative materials used on implants. *Int J Prosthodont.* 1991;4:282–291.

61. Davis DM, Rimrott R, Zarb GA. Studies on frameworks for osseointegrated prostheses. Part 2. The effect of adding acrylic resin or porcelain to form the occlusal superstructure. *Int J Oral Maxillofac Implants.* 1988;3:275–280.

62. Naert I, Quirynen M, van Steenberghe D, et al. A six-year prosthodontic study of 509 consecutively inserted implants for the treatment of partial edentulism. *J Prosthet Dent.* 1992;67:236–245.

63. Johns RB, Jemt T, Heath MR. A multicenter study of overdentures supported by Branemark implants. *Int J Oral Maxillofac Implants.* 1992;7:513–522.

64. Mericske-Stern R, Zarb GA. Overdentures: an alternative implant methodology for edentulous patients. *Int J Prosthodont.* 1993;6:203–208.

65. Feine JS, Maskawi K, de Grandmont P, et al. Within-subject comparisons of implant-supported mandibular prostheses: evaluation of masticatory function. *J Dent Res.* 1994;73:1646–1656.

66. Pietrokovski J. The bony residual ridge in man. *J Prosthet Dent.* 1975;34:456–462.

67. Arbree NS, Chapman RJ. A comparison of mandibular denture base extension in conventional and implant-retained dentures. *J Prosthet Dent.* 1991;65:108–111.

68. Drago CJ. Tarnish and corrosion with the use of intraoral magnets. *J Prosthet Dent.* 1991;66:536–540.

69. Lewis S. Implant-retained overdentures. *Compendium.* 1993;14:1270–1283.

70. Dolder EJ, Durer GT. *The Bar-Joint Denture*. Chicago: Quintessence Publishing Co. Inc.; 1978.

71. Davidoff SR, Steinberg MA, Halperin A. The implant-supported overdenture: a practical implant-prosthetic design. *Compendium*. 1993;14:722–730.

72. Naert I, Quirynen M, Hooghe M, et al. A comparative prospective study of splinted and unsplinted Brånemark implants in mandibular overdenture therapy: a preliminary report. *J Prosthet Dent*. 1994;71:486–492.

73. Donatsky O. Osseointegrated dental implants with ball attachments supporting overdentures in patients with mandibular alveolar ridge atrophy. *Int J Oral Maxillofac Implants*. 1993;8:162–166.

74. Desjardins RP. Prosthesis design for osseointegrated implants in the edentulous maxilla. *Int J Oral Maxillofac Implants*. 1992;7:311–320.

75. Friberg B, Jemt T, Lekholm U. Early failure in 4,641 consecutively placed Branemark dental implants. A study from stage 1 surgery to the connection of completed prostheses. *Int J Oral Maxillofac Implants*. 1991;6:142–146.

76. Jemt T. Failures and complications in 391 consecutively inserted fixed prostheses supported by Brånemark implants in edentulous jaws: a study of treatment from the time of prosthesis placement to the first annual checkup. *Int J Oral Maxillofac Implants*. 1991;6:270–276.

77. Taylor TD. Fixed implant rehabilitation for the edentulous maxilla. *Int J Oral Maxillofac Implants*. 1991;6:329–337.

78. Jemt T. Fixed implant-supported prostheses in the edentulous maxilla. A five-year follow-up report. *Clin Oral Implants Res*. 1994;5:142–147.

79. Johns RB, Jemt T, Heath MR, et al. A multicenter study of overdentures supported by Branemark implants. *Int J Oral Maxillofac Implants*. 1992;7:513–522.

80. Langer B. Personal communication. New York, NY. March 1995.

81. Jemt T, Book K, Linden B, et al. Failures and complications in 92 consecutively inserted overdentures supported by Branemark implants in severely resorbed edentulous maxillae: a study from prosthetic treatment to first annual check-up. *Int J Oral Maxillofac Implants*. 1992;7:162–167.

82. Van Roekel NB. Prosthesis fabrication using electrical discharge machining. *Int J Oral Maxillofac Implants*. 1992;7:56–61.

83. Naert I, Quirynen M, van Steenberghe D, et al. A six-year prosthodontic study of 509 consecutively inserted implants for the treatment of partial edentulism. *J Prosthet Dent*. 1992;67:236–245.

84. Jemt T, Lindén B, Lekholm U. Failures and complications in 127 consecutively placed fixed partial prostheses supported by Brånemark implants: from prosthetic treatment to first annual checkup. *Int J Oral Maxillofac Implants*. 1992;7:40–44.

85. Zarb GA, Schmitt A. The longitudinal clinical effectiveness of osseointegrated dental implants in posterior partially edentulous patients. *Int J Prosthodont*. 1993;6:189–196.

86. Zarb GA, Schmitt A. The longitudinal clinical effectiveness of osseointegrated dental implants in anterior partially edentulous patients. *Int J Prosthodont*. 1993;6:180–188.

87. Sullivan DY. Prosthetic considerations for the utilization of osseointegrated fixtures in the partially edentulous arch. *Int J Oral Maxillofac Implants*. 1986;1:39–45.

88. Smiler DG. Repositioning the inferior alveolar nerve for placement of endosseous implants: technical note. *Int J Oral Maxillofac Implants*. 1993;8(2):145–150.

89. Kopp CD. Brånemark osseointegration prognosis and treatment rationale. *Dent Clin North Am*. 1989;33:701–731.

90. Tatum OH Jr, Lebowitz MS, Tatum CA, et al. Sinus augmentation: rationale, development, long-term results. *NY State Dent J*. 1993;59:43–48.

91. Smiler DG, Johnson PW, Lozada JL, et al. Sinus lift grafts and endosseous implants. Treatment of the atrophic posterior maxilla. *Dent Clin North Am*. 1992;36(1):151–186.

92. English CE. The critical a-p spread. *Implant Soc*. 1990;1:2–3.

93. Weinberg LA, Kruger B. Biomechanical considerations when combining tooth-supported and implant-supported prostheses. *Oral Surg Oral Med Oral Pathol*. 1994;78:22–27.

94. Skalak R. Aspects of biomechanical considerations. In: Brånemark P-I, Zarb GA, Albrektsson T, eds. *Tissue-Integrated Prosthesis Osseointegration in Clinical Dentistry*. Chicago: Quintessence Publishing Co. Inc.; 1985:117–128.

95. Sullivan DY. Prosthetic considerations for the utilization of osseointegrated fixtures in the partially edentulous arch. *Int J Oral Maxillofac Implants*. 1986;1:39–45.

96. Ericsson I, Lekholm U, Brånemark P-I, et al. A clinical evaluation of fixed-bridge restorations supported by the combination of teeth and osseointegrated titanium implants. *J Clin Periodontol*. 1986;13:307–312.

97. Åstrand P, Borg K, Gunne J, et al. Combination of natural teeth and osseointegrated implants as prosthesis abutments: a 2-year longitudinal study. *Int J Oral Maxillofac Implants*. 1991;6:305–312.

98. Rangert B, Gunne J, Sullivan DY. Mechanical aspects of a Brånemark implant connected to a natural tooth: an in vitro study. *Int J Oral Maxillofac Implants*. 1991;6:177–186.

99. Kirsch A. The IMZ osseointegrated system. Presented at the Interpore IMZ seminar, Baylor University, Dallas, 3–4 May 1986.

100. Olivé J, Aparicio C. The Periotest method as a measure of osseointegrated oral implant stability. *Int J Oral Maxillofac Implants*. 1990;5:390–400.

101. Teerlinck J, Quirynen M, Darius P, et al. Periotest: an objective clinical diagnosis of bone apposition toward implants. *Int J Oral Maxillofac Implants*. 1991;6:55–61.

102. Reider CE, Parel SM. A survey of natural tooth abutment intrusion with implant-connected fixed partial dentures. *Int J Periodont Restor Dent*. 1993;13:334–347.

103. English CE. Root intrusion in tooth-implant combination cases. *Implant Dent*. 1993;2:79–85.

104. Jemt T, Pettersson P. A 3-year follow-up study on single implant treatment. *J Dent*. 1993;21:203–208.

105. Schmitt A, Zarb GA. The longitudinal clinical effectiveness of osseointegrated dental implants for single-tooth replacement. *Int J Prosthodont*. 1993;6:197–202.

106. Laney WR, Jemt T, Harris D, et al. Osseointegrated implants for single-tooth replacement: progress report from a multicenter prospective study after 3 years. *Int J Oral Maxillofac Implants*. 1994;9:49–54.

107. Orenstein IH, Petrazzuolo V. A new angle on restoring anterior teeth with root-form implants: clinical report. *Implant Soc*. 1993;3:10–16.

108. Scher EL. Use of an osseointegrated implant to replace a single anterior tooth. *Int J Oral Implantol*. 1990;6:11–12.

109. Saadoun AP, Sullivan DY, Krischek M, et al. Single tooth implant-management for success. *Pract Periodontics Aesthet Dent.* 1994;6:73–80.

110. Sullivan DY, Sherwood RL. Considerations for successful single tooth implant restorations. *J Esthet Dent.* 1993;5:118–24.

111. Lazzara RJ. Managing the soft tissue margin: the key to implant aesthetics. *Pract Periodontics Aesthet Dent.* 1993;5:81–88.

112. Barzilay I, Grazer GN, Canton J, et al. Immediate implantation of pure titanium implants into extraction sockets. *J Dent Res.* 1988;67:234.

113. Tarnow D, Fletcher P. The 2-3 month post-extraction placement of root form implants: a useful compromise. *Implants: Clin Rev Dent.* 1993;2(1):1–8.

114. Langer B. Spontaneous in situ gingival augmentation. *Int J Periodont Restor Dent.* 1994;14:525–35.

115. Mensdorff-Pouilly N, Haas R, Mailath G, et al. The immediate implant: a retrospective study comparing the different types of immediate implantation. *Int J Oral Maxillofac Implants.* 1994;9:571–578.

116. Nevins M, Mellonig JT. The advantages of localized ridge augmentation prior to implant placement: a staged event. *Int J Periodont Restor Dent.* 1994;14:97–111.

117. Balshi TJ. First molar replacement with an osseointegrated implant. *Quintessence Int.* 1990;21:61–65.

118. Boudrias P. The implant-supported single-tooth restoration. Preoperative evaluation and clinical procedure. *Dent Clin North Am.* 1993;37:497–511.

119. Hobo S, Ichida E, Garcia LT. Complications and maintenance. In: Hobo S, Ichida E, Garcia LT, eds. *Osseointegration and Occlusal Rehabilitation.* Tokyo: Quintessence Publishing Co., 1989:239–254.

120. Jemt T, Lekholm U, Gröndahl K. A 3-year follow-up study of early single implant restorations ad modum Brånemark. *Int J Periodontics Restorative Dent.* 1990;10:340–349.

121. Naert I, Quirynen M, van Steenberghe D, et al. A study of 589 consecutive implants supporting complete fixed prostheses. Part II: prosthetic aspects. *J Prosthet Dent.* 1992;68:949–956.

122. Walton JN, MacEntee MI. Problems with prostheses on implants: a retrospective study. *J Prosthet Dent.* 1994;71:283–288.

123. Zinner ID, Panno FV, Abrahamson BD, et al. Prosthodontic solutions for compromised implant placement. *Int J Prosthodont.* 1993;6:270–278.

124. Zarb GA, Jansson T. Prosthodontic procedures. In: Brånemark P-I, Zarb GA, Albrektsson T, eds. *Tissue-Integrated Prostheses Osseointegration in Clinical Dentistry.* Chicago: Quintessence Publishing Co. Inc.; 1985;241–282.

125. Parel SM, Balshi TJ, Sullivan DY, et al. Gingival augmentation for osseointegrated implant prostheses. *J Prosthet Dent.* 1986;56:208–211.

126. Johansson G, Palmqvist S. Complications, supplementary treatment and maintenance in edentulous arches with implant-supported fixed prostheses. *Int J Prosthodont.* 1990;3:89–92.

127. Walton JN, MacEntee MI. Problems with prostheses on implants: a retrospective study. *J Prosthet Dent.* 1994;71:283–288.

128. George K, Zafiropoulos GG, Murat Y, et al. Clinical and microbiological status of osseointegrated implants. *J Periodontol.* 1994;65:766–770.

129. Hobo S, Ichida E, Garcia LT. Complications and maintenance. In: Hobo S, Ichida E, Garcia LT, eds. *Osseointegration and Occlusal Rehabilitation.* Tokyo: Quintessence Publishing Co.; 1989:239–254.

21B
Overdenture Case Reports

Alex M. Greenberg

Overdentures have been an excellent solution for the management of the completely edentulous patient.[1–4] By using a minimum of two to three implant fixtures, stabilization attachments can be utilized for improved retention of the complete denture. Individual ball type, ERA, spark erosion, clip bar, and modified Dalbo attachments may be used as the retentive element(s). When sufficient implants are in place, overdentures can have retention that nearly replicates the stability of fixed prosthetics in function, while allowing superior cleansability and oral hygiene. Multiple maxillary dental implants[5–7] can allow the elimination of palatal coverage, which is poorly tolerated by many patients, and provide patients with better taste sensation and phonetics.

The following are cases that represent maxillary and mandibular overdenture treatment.

Case 1

Completely edentulous mandible reconstructed with 3-screw type dental implants and fabrication of a bar with three ball attachments and an overdenture (Figures 21B.1–21B.5). (Dental implant surgery: Alex M. Greenberg, DDS, Oral and Maxillofacial Surgeon, New York, NY. Implant prosthodontics: Ava Thaw, DDS, Prosthodontist, Private Practice, New York, NY.)

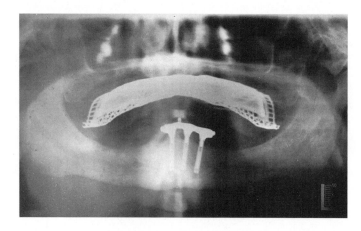

FIGURE 21B.1 Panoramic radiograph demonstrating 3-screw type dental implant fixtures of the anterior mandible with overdenture bar.

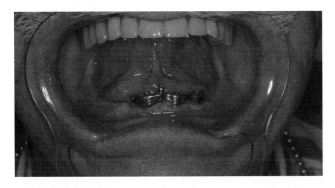

FIGURE 21B.2 Frontal view of edentulous mandible with overdenture bar. Note the unfavorable floor of mouth and tongue position relative to the edentulous ridge.

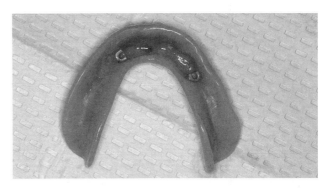

FIGURE 21B.4 View of overdenture base and three o-rings.

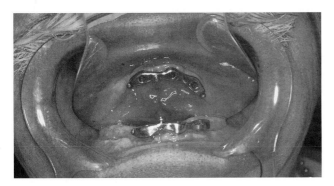

FIGURE 21B.3 Occlusal view of edentulous mandible with overdenture bar.

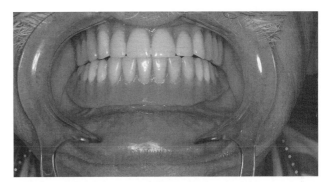

FIGURE 21B.5 Mandibular overdenture in occlusion with maxillary fixed bridge.

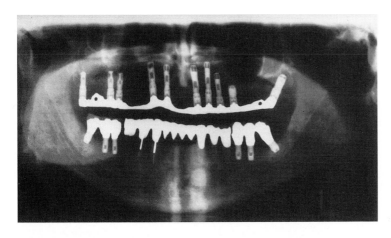

FIGURE 21B.6 Panoramic radiograph demonstrating 10 maxillary dental implant fixtures as well as the overdenture bar and bilateral posterior skirts for push–pull Lew attachments.

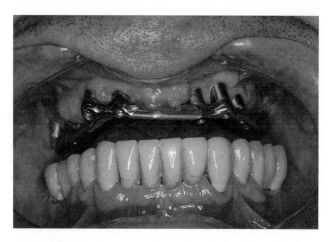

FIGURE 21B.7 Frontal view of maxillary overdenture bar and occlusal clearance.

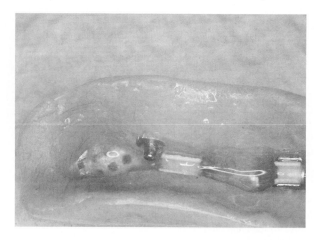

FIGURE 21B.10 Close-up view of overdenture base with Lew attachment pushed into position.

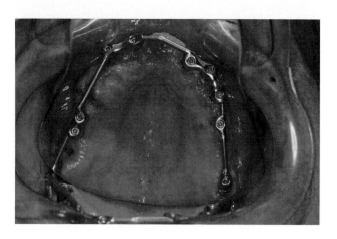

FIGURE 21B.8 Occlusal view of maxillary overdenture bar.

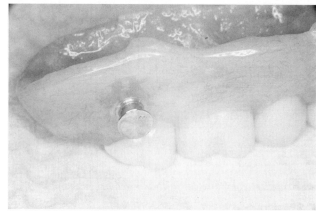

FIGURE 21B.11 Close-up buccal view of Lew attachment push–pull button.

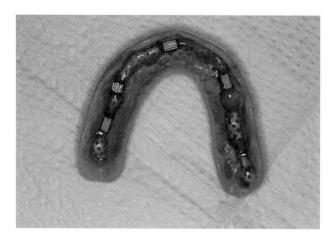

FIGURE 21B.9 View of overdenture base and 5 Hayder nylon clips. Note the absence of palatal coverage.

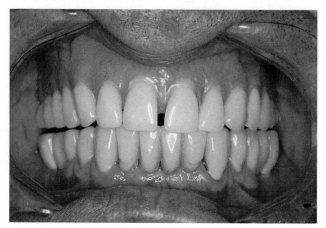

FIGURE 21B.12 Maxillary overdenture in opposing mandibular fixed bridge.

Case 2

Completely edentulous maxilla reconstructed with 10 dental implants, fabrication of continuous bar with posterior bilateral skirts for Lew attachments, 5 Hayder clips, and overdenture (Figures 21B.6–21B.12). (Dental implant surgery: Alex M. Greenberg, DDS, Oral and Maxillofacial Surgeon, New York, NY. Implant Prosthodontics, Joel Hirsch, DDS, Prosthodontist, Private Practice, New York, NY.)

References

1. Branemark P-I, Zarb GA, Albrektsson T. *Tissue Integrated Prostheses*. Quintessence: Chicago, 1987:283–287.
2. Worthington P, Branemark P-I. *Advanced Osseointegration Surgery: Applications in the Maxillofacial Region*. Chicago: Quintessence, 1992:233–247.
3. Misch CE. *Contemporary Implant Dentistry*. St. Louis: Mosby-Yearbook, 1993:223–240.
4. Jemt T, Chai J, Harnett J, Heath MR, et al. A 5-year prospective multicenter follow-up report on overdentures supported by osseointegrated implants. *Int J Oral Maxillofac Implants*. 1996; 11:291–298.
5. Misch LS, Misch CE. Denture satisfaction: a patient's perspective. *Int J Oral Implant*. 1991;7:43–48.
6. Floystrand F, Karlsenk, Saxegaard E, Orstavik JS. Effects on retention of reducing the palatal coverage of complete maxillary dentures. *Acta Odontol Scand*. 1986;44(2):77–83.
7. Lundqvist S. Speech and other oral functions. Clinical and experimental studies with special reference to maxillary rehabilitation on osseointegrated implants. *Swed Dent J*. (suppl) 1993;91:1–39.

Section III
Craniomaxillofacial Reconstructive and Corrective Bone Surgery

22
AO/ASIF Mandibular Hardware

Joachim Prein and Alex M. Greenberg

The AO/ASIF mandibular systems of instruments and titanium implants have been developed primarily for the correction of deformities, distraction osteogenesis, reconstruction of defects, and fixation of fractures of the mandible. The mandibular system consists of stronger and larger screws and plates than those utilized in the craniofacial modular system. These are necessary because of the dynamic functional forces acting on the mandible, as compared to the static forces associated with the maxilla. Stronger implants are also required because the mandible is a heavier, thicker, and articulated bone with varied mechanical loading. The mandibular modules are organized according to screw sizes—2.0 mm, 2.4 mm, 3.0 mm, and 4.0 mm. Implant systems with screws sizes less than 2.0 mm are rarely applied in mandibular surgery. These hardware systems based on screw size are uniform worldwide, as approved by the AO/ASIF Maxillofacial Technical Commission. There are some differences in tray or module configurations depending on the distributor (Synthes Maxillofacial in North America and STRATEC and Mathys for the rest of the world). The different mandibular systems, which range in size from 2.0 mm to 4.0 mm, are arranged in color-coded trays or modules. The Synthes Maxillofacial system for North America is called the Modular Fixation System (Figures 22.1 and 22.2a,b), while the Mathys and STRATEC system from Europe is the Compact MF System (Figures 22.3 and 22.4). Not only are these modules organized by screw size, but also by type of surgery performed—trauma, reconstruction, or orthognathic. For the latest surgical technique of bone distraction, a separate Mandible Distractor Module Set has been developed (Appendix A.1).

The instrumentation for mandibular corrective surgery is contained within the module of the craniofacial modular system. Both the North American and European systems have separate trays that contain the universal instruments. The North American system has two trays, of which the top tray contains the transbuccal instruments as follows: 2.0 mm/2.4 mm Trocar with obturator; 2.0-mm and 2.4-mm obturators; cheek retractor ring; cheek retractor blade 1.5-mm, 2.0-mm, 1.8-mm, and 2.4-mm drill guides; 1.5-mm/2.0-mm insert drill guide; 1.8-mm neutral drill guide; 1.8-mm compression drill guide; 2.4-mm depth gauge (measures up to 40 mm) in regular and extra large; wide screwdriver handle; narrow screwdriver handle; cruciform screwdriver (self-retaining) for 2.0-mm and 2.4-mm screws; cruciform screwdriver with holding sleeve for 2.0-mm and 2.4-mm screws; tap handle; counter/sink; and 1.8-mm DCU drill guide (neutral and load). The lift-out lid for the auxiliary bin of the top tray contains 1.8 and 2.4-mm pins for countersink; 2.0-mm and 2.4-mm taps; 1.8-mm × 125-mm drill bit; and 2.4-mm × 125-mm drill bit. The bottom universal instrument tray contains plate holding forceps; bone reduction forceps (short and long); bending pliers for 2.0-mm/2.4-mm plates locking; bending pliers for 2.0-mm/2.4-mm plates nonlocking; universal bending irons (2); bending pliers for 2.4-mm plates; 3-in-1 Bending Pliers for 2.0-mm plates (Figure 41.19); shortcut plate cutters (2); plate cutter for 2.0-mm/2.4-mm plates (double action), ratcheting screwdriver (Figure 22.27), and battery powered screwdriver (Figure 22.28). The STRATEC and Mathys systems include the same instruments, which may be placed in either one or two trays at the bottom of the graphic case (Figure 22.5a,b).

2.0 Mandible Locking Plate System (MLP) Module

Color: Blue (Synthes Maxillofacial for North America and Compact MF for Europe and Worldwide)
Indications: Trauma, simple to unstable fractures, microvascular reconstructive surgery, and orthognathic surgery

The 2.0-mm MLP system module (Figure 22.6) contains plates and screws for the management of simple to unstable fractures. The plates are available in 3 thicknesses (1.0 mm, 1.3 mm, 1.5 mm) to accommodate a wide range of indications. The module contains 2.0-mm self-tapping and self-drilling locking and nonlocking gold-colored star drive-headed screws available in 5, 6, 8, 10, 12, 14, 16, and 18 mm. 2.4-mm teal colored emergency screws are available in the same lengths.
Number embossed markers attach to the top of each modular

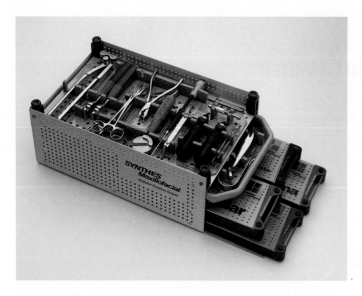

FIGURE 22.1 Mandibular Modular Fixation System Graphic Case. (Courtesy Synthes Maxillofacial, Paoli, PA)

a

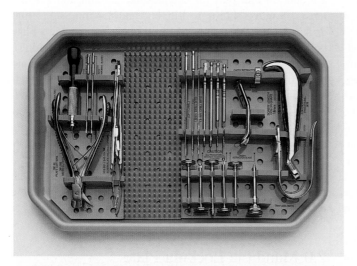

b

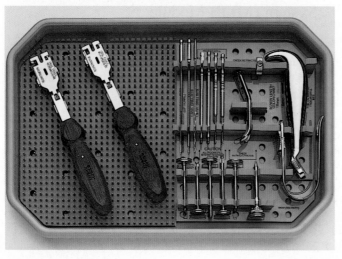

FIGURE 22.2 (a,b) Mandibular Modular Fixation System Universal Instrument Trays. (Courtesy Synthes Maxillofacial, Paoli, PA)

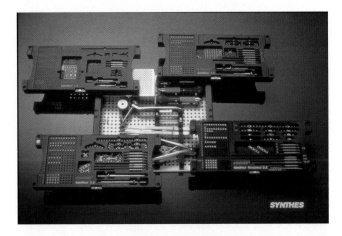

FIGURE 22.3 Compact MF System modules and instrument tray. (Courtesy of STRATEC Medical, Oberdorf, Switzerland and Mathys LTD Bettlach, Bettlach, Switzerland)

screw row indicate the screw length for the customized module in use. Self drilling screw markers have a white background and self tapping screw markers have a black background. Corresponding drill bits for plate fixation are 1.5 mm. Drill bits are available in J latch, Jacob's chuck, Universal, and mint quick coupling. A tap is available for pretapping holes before the placement of screws in dense cortical bone. Long and short star drive screw driver (self retaining) for both the regular and ratchet type screw drivers is included. There are 1.5 mm regular and threaded drill guides. The 2.0 MLP module includes mini thickness implants as follows (Figure 22.7): malleable straight 4 and 6 holes, mini straight narrow 4 and 6 hole, adaption 20 hole, tension band 4 hole, broad straight 4 hole, and broad curved 4 hole. Intermediate thickness implants as a straight 6 hole and straight 12 hole. Large thickness implants as straight 6 hole, straight 12 hole, and straight 20 hole. Angled implants as: crescent angled 3 × 3

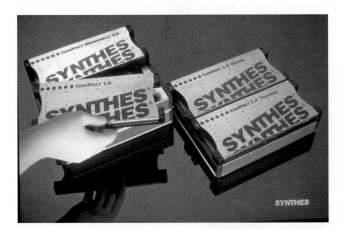

FIGURE 22.4 Compact MF System Graphic Case. (Courtesy of STRATEC Medical, Oberdorf, Switzerland and Mathys LTD Bettlach, Bettlach, Switzerland)

holes, angled 4 × 4 holes, angled left 6 × 21 holes, and angled right 6 × 21 holes.

2.0 Mandible Trauma

Module Color: Blue (Synthes Maxillofacial for North America and Compact MF for Europe and Worldwide)

The 2.0 Mandible Trauma module (Figures 22.8, 22.9, and 22.10) contains 2.0-mm fluted self tapping screws in 4-, 6-, 8-, 10-, 12-, 14-, 16-, and 18-mm lengths (up to 24 mm) and 2.4-mm emergency teal-colored screws in 6-, 8-, 10-, 12-, 14-, 16-, and 18-mm lengths (up to 24 mm). Number-embossed markers attach to the top of each modular screw row indicate the screw length for the customized module in use. The corresponding drill bits for plate fixation are 1.5 mm × 110 mm (3). For lag screw technique, the 2.0-mm × 110-mm (3) drill bit is for the gliding hole, and the 1.5-mm drill bit is for the threaded hole. The drill bits are available in Stryker J Latch, Jacob's Chuck, Universal, or Miniquick coupling. A tap is available for pretapping holes before the placement of extra-long screws in thick cortical bone. A cruciform screwdriver blade (self-retaining) for 1.5-mm/2.0-mm screws is included. The 2.0 mandible miniplates are thicker (1.0 mm) and stronger than the 2.0-mm miniplates for the midface. The Synthes Maxillofacial System (Figure 22.8b) includes limited contact implants as follows: straight plate; narrow (4, 6, and 8 holes); straight plates, broad (4, 6, and 8 holes); curved plate (narrow) (4 and 6 holes); and curved plate (broad) (4 and 6 holes). Other implants include adaption plate (20 holes), DCP (4, 5, 6, 7, and 8 holes), DCP (angled) 4 × 4 holes (8 holes); mandible strut plate 4 × 4 holes (8 holes), LC-EDCP (4 and 6 holes).

The Compact MF 2.0 Mandible System consists of a combination 2.0 midface/mandible module and a separate 2.0 unilock/locking plate system. The STRATEC and Mathys 2.0 Mandible system (Figure 22.8a) includes miniplates with center space (2, 4, and 6 holes); miniplates (2, 4, or 20 holes); miniplates twisted 70° with center space, left, and right (6 holes); mini DCP (20 holes); and LC miniplate with center space (4 and 6 holes). These plates are mainly used for simple mandibular fractures with good bony buttresses, either as single-plate fixation or a two-plate fixation system (one plate along the tension side, and the other on the pressure side of the fracture).

2.4 mm Mandible Trauma Module

Colors: Red (Compact MF for Europe and Worldwide)
Purple (Synthes Maxillofacial for North America)
Indications: Simple to complex mandibular fractures including comminution and avulsive defects.

The 2.4 Mandible Trauma system consists of one module in North America and two modules in Europe and Worldwide

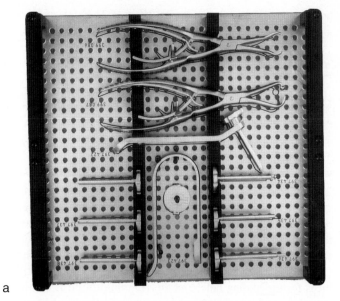

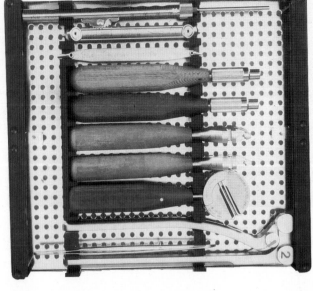

a

b

FIGURE 22.5 (a) Compact MF 2.4-mm universal instrument tray containing trocar system and bone-and-plate holding forceps. (b) Compact MF 2.4-mm universal instrument tray containing depth gauge, drill guides, screwdriver handles, plate cutters, and plate bender. (Courtesy of STRATEC Medical, Oberdorf, Switzerland and Mathys LTD Bettlach, Bettlach, Switzerland)

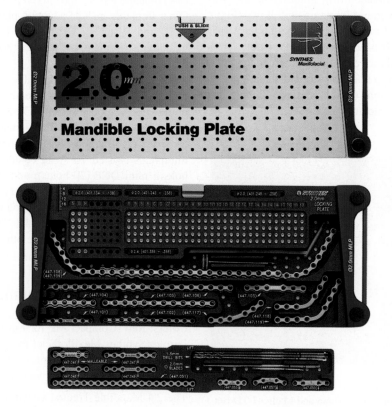

FIGURE 22.6 A 2.0 Mandible Locking Plate Module Set. (Courtesy of Synthes Maxillofacial, Paoli, PA)

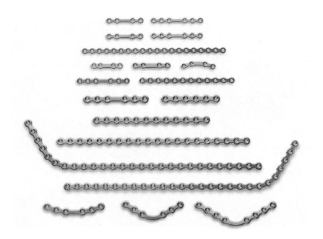

FIGURE 22.7 2.0 Mandible Locking Plate System selection of implants. (Courtesy of Synthes Maxillofacial, Paoli, PA)

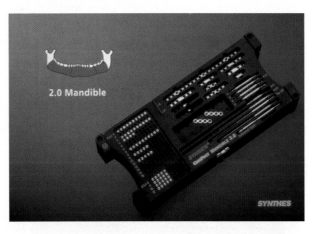

FIGURE 22.9 Compact MF 2.0 Mandible Trauma Module with lift-out tray for 2.0 Midface Plates. (Courtesy of STRATEC Medical, Oberdorf, Switzerland and Mathys LTD Bettlach, Bettlach, Switzerland)

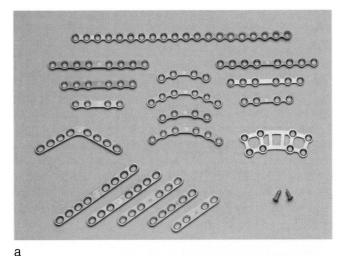

a

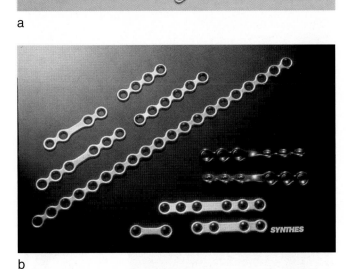

b

FIGURE 22.8 (a) 2.0-mm Mandible Trauma Module selection of implants for North America. (Courtesy of Synthes Maxillofacial, Paoli, PA) (b) Compact MF 2.0 Mandible Trauma Module selection of implants for Europe and worldwide. (Courtesy of STRATEC Medical, Oberdorf, Switzerland and Mathys LTD Bettlach, Bettlach, Switzerland)

(2.4-mm Trauma and 2.4-mm UniLock/Locking Reconstruction Plate systems) (Figures 22.11, 22.12, and 22.13). The 2.4-mm trauma module contains plates and screws for the management of more extensive, complex, fragmented, and avulsive fractures, as compared to the 2.0-mm trauma module. The plates are thicker for example, 1.65 mm for the straight LC-DCP and 2.0 mm for the crescent LC-DCP. The module contains 2.4-mm gold-colored self-tapping screws 6-, 8-, 10-, 12-, 14-, 16-, and 18-mm screws (20, 22, 24, 26, 28, and 30 are also available). The Synthes Maxillofacial Module includes an additional pop-up tray that contains 2.4-mm gold-colored self-tapping 32-, 34-, 36-, 38-, and 40-mm screws. Emergency 2.7-mm teal-colored screws in 6-, 8-, 10-, 12-, 14-, 16-, and 18-mm lengths (available up to 30 mm). Number-embossed markers attach to the top of each modular screw row indicate the screw length for the customized module in use. The corresponding drill bits for plate fixation are 1.8 mm × 100 mm (3 each). For lag-screw technique, the 2.4 mm × 100 mm (3 each) is used for the gliding hole and the 1.8 mm × 100 mm drill bit for the threaded hole. The drill bits are available as J-Latch, Jacob's chuck, or mini/quick coupling. Although the screws are self-tapping, a tap is included for those instances where pretapping is necessary, such as long lag screws in solid cortical bone of the symphysis. The implants include the limited contact LC-DCP (straight 4, 5, and 6 holes); LC-DCP crescent (4 and 6 holes); 2.4-mm tension band plates (4 and 6 holes); universal fracture plate (straight) (8, 10, and 24 holes), and angled 3 × 3 (6 holes) and 4 × 4 (8 holes) (Figure 22.11). The 3 × 3- and 4 × 4-angled universal fracture plates are indicated for mandibular angle fractures, and they are similar to reconstruction plates in that they are three dimensionally bendable. However, as the universal fracture plate thickness is 2.0 mm, compared to 2.5 mm for reconstruction plates, they are weaker and should not be used in higher load-bearing situations (i.e., avulsive defects).

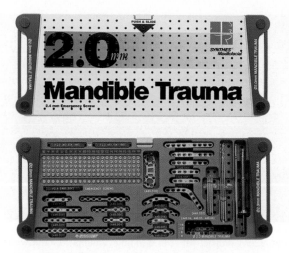

FIGURE 22.10 2.0-mm Mandible Trauma Module for North America. (Courtesy of Synthes Maxillofacial Maxillofacial, Paoli, PA)

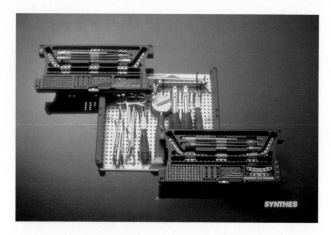

FIGURE 22.12 Compact MF 2.4-mm Mandible Trauma and 2.4 UniLock Reconstruction modules. (Courtesy of STRATEC Medical, Oberdorf, Switzerland and Mathys LTD Bettlach, Bettlach, Switzerland)

2.4-mm Microvascular Module

Color: Purple (Synthes Maxillofacial/North America availability only).

Indications: Mandibular continuity defect reconstruction with microvascular anastamosed bone grafts.

The 2.4-mm Microvascular Module (Figures 22.14 and 22.15) contains 2.4-mm self-tapping screws in 6-, 8-, 10-, 12-, 14-, 16-, and 18-mm lengths (available up to 40 mm), and emergency screws in 6-, 8-, 10-, 12-, 14-, 16-, and 18-mm lengths

(available up to 40 mm). The corresponding drill bits are 1.8 mm × 100 mm (3 each) for plate fixation and 2.4 mm × 100 mm for lag-screw technique. The implants come as microvascular plates (straight) (12, 14, 16, 18, 20, 22, and 24 holes), microvascular plate (angled) 4 × 8 (12 holes), right and left, 4 × 16 (20 holes), right and left, 5 × 17 (22 holes), right and left, microvascular plate, double angle 4 × 20 × 4 (28 holes), 5 × 22 × 5 (32 holes), and 6 × 24 × 6 (36 holes) (Figure 22.14). Corresponding templates are also available for these plates. These plates are similar to the universal fracture plates.

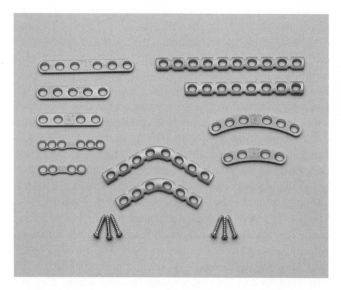

FIGURE 22.11 2.4-mm Mandible Trauma Module selection of implants. (Courtesy of Synthes Maxillofacial, Paoli, PA)

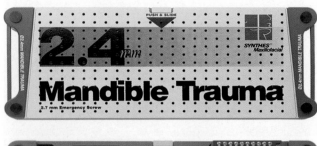

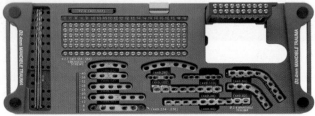

FIGURE 22.13 2.4 mm Mandible Trauma Module for North America. (Courtesy Synthes Maxillofacial, Paoli, PA)

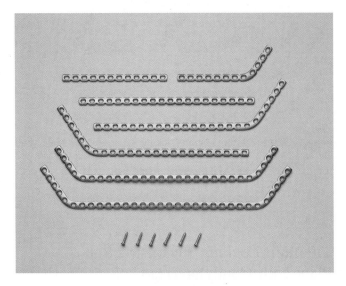

FIGURE 22.14 2.4-mm Microvascular Module selection of implants. (Courtesy of Synthes Maxillofacial, Paoli, PA)

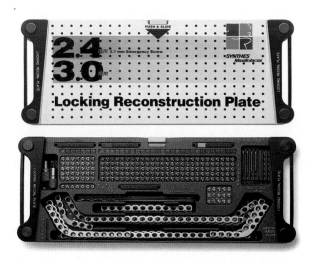

FIGURE 22.16 A 2.4 mm/3.0 mm Locking Reconstruction Plate Module. (Courtesy of Synthes Maxillofacial, Paoli, PA)

2.4/3.0 mm Locking Reconstruction Plate System Module

Colors: Purple (Compact MF for Europe and Worldwide) Black (Synthes Maxillofacial for North America) Indications: Mandibular continuity defect reconstruction with and without bone grafts, and complex mandibular fractures including comminution and avulsive defects.

The 2.4 mm/3.0 mm Locking Reconstruction Plate System module contains reconstruction plates with threaded plate holes and corresponding threaded head screws is indicated for posttraumatic and postablative defects (Figures 22.16 and 22.17).

The plate is the same thickness as the standard reconstruction plate. Plate fixation may also be performed with standard nonlocking 2.4-mm screws. The special locking screws only permit perpendicular screw angulation (Figure 22.18) and are placed using special color-coded threaded drill guides (Figure 22.19) while the regular 2.4-mm self-tapping screws allow a 40° angulation within the plate hole. It consists of 2.4-mm self-tapping gold-colored screws in 8-, 10-, 12-, 14-, 16-, and 18-mm lengths, with corresponding teal-colored 2.7-mm emergency screws in 8-, 10-, 12-, 14-, 16-, and 18-mm lengths. These screws allow a 40° angulation within the plate holes. The 2.4-mm locking screws are purple colored and come in 8-, 10-, 12-, 14-, 16-, and 18-mm lengths (up to 24 mm), and the 3.0-mm locking screws are colored aqua and

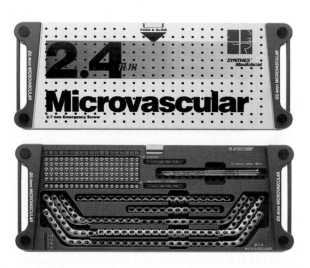

FIGURE 22.15 2.4-mm Microvascular Module. (Courtesy of Synthes Maxillofacial, Paoli, PA)

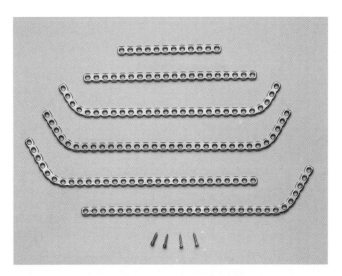

FIGURE 22.17 A 2.4 mm/3.0 Locking Reconstruction Plate Module selection of implants. (Courtesy of Synthes Maxillofacial, Paoli, PA)

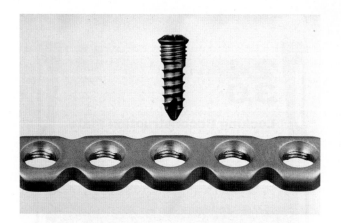

FIGURE 22.18 A 2.4 mm/3.0 mm Locking Reconstruction Plate with threaded hole and corresponding threaded locking screw. (Courtesy of Synthes Maxillofacial, Paoli, PA)

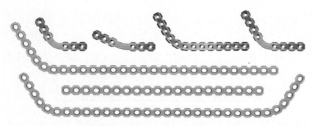

FIGURE 22.20 A 2.4 mm/3.0 mm Locking Reconstruction Plate Module selection of implants including Crescent and Angled types. (Courtesy of Synthes Maxillofacial, Paoli, PA)

Titanium Locking Reconstruction Plate with Condylar Head

Indications: For temporary reconstruction in patients undergoing ablative tumor surgery requiring the removal of the mandibular condyle.

The Titanium Locking Reconstruction Plate with Condylar Head is available as left and right implants in three sizes (3 × 16 holes, 4 × 18 holes, 5 × 20 holes (Figure 22.21). 2.4 mm self-tapping cortex screws are available in 6-40 mm in 2 mm increments; 2.4-mm locking screws in 8-24 mm in 2 mm increments; and 3.0 mm locking screws in 8-24 mm in 2 mm increments. 3-mm locking screws are recommended for osteoporotic bone. The implant size can be selected with the use of the Titanium Locking reconstruction Plate with Condylar Head Planning Template for measurement of the ramus height from a radiograph. Intraoperatively a template can be used to determine the shape and length of the desired implant, and should be aligned with the inferior border of the mandible. For Europe and worldwide use, a titanium locking plate with condylar head is available.

are available in 8-, 10-, 12-, 14-, 16-, and 18-mm lengths (up to 24 mm). The side bin contains 3.0-mm screws in 20-, 22-, and 24-mm lengths. The drill bits are color coded with 1.8-mm × 125-mm purple coded (3 each) and 2.4-mm × 125-mm aqua coded (3 each). The implants come as locking reconstruction plates (straight) (12 and 20 holes), the locking reconstruction plate (angled) 6 × 23 (29 holes), left and right, locking reconstruction plate (double-angled) 4 × 20 × 4 (28 holes), 5 × 22 × 5 (32 holes), and 6 × 24 × 6 (36 holes), crescent 3 × 3 holes, angled 3 × 3 holes and 4 × 4 holes, angled left and right 5 × 8 holes, with corresponding templates (Figure 22.20).

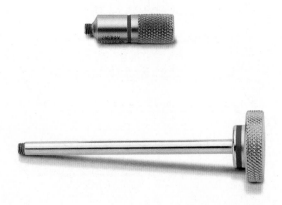

FIGURE 22.19 Threaded drill guide which when engaged into the holes of the 2.4 mm/3.0 mm Locking Reconstruction Plate, allow the preparation of perpendicular holes. (Courtesy of Synthes Maxillofacial, Paoli, PA)

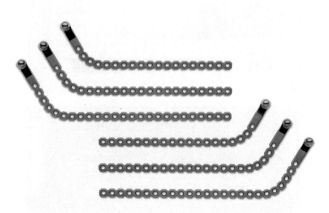

FIGURE 22.21 Left and right: Titanium Locking Reconstruction Plate with Condylar Head implants. (Courtesy of Synthes Maxillofacial, Paoli, PA)

4.0-mm Titanium Hollow Screw Reconstruction Plate (THORP) Set

North America:
4.0-mm Titanium Hollow Screw Reconstruction Plate (THORP) Set (Synthes Maxillofacial)
Europe, Asia, South America, Africa:
4.0-mm Titanium Hollow Screw Reconstruction Plate (THORP) Set (STRATEC and Mathys)

Indications: Rarely used except for large mandibular continuity defect reconstruction with and without bone grafts, and complex mandibular fractures. The 4.0-mm Titanium Hollow Screw Reconstruction Plate (THORP) Set (Figure 22.22a,b) was developed to permit noncompressive stabilization with the avoidance of bone resorption under the plate and its associated unstable fixation. These features have particular advantages for the fixation and healing of bone grafts. The titanium hollow THORP screws permit bone ingrowth and added stabilization. The THORP set contains 4.0 mm titanium THORP screws of 8-, 10-, 12-, 14-, 16-, 18-, and 20-mm lengths which are intended for removal, and 4.0 titanium hollow THORP

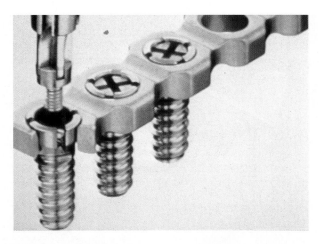

FIGURE 22.23 Locking screw insertion in THORP screw head case. (Courtesy of Synthes Maxillofacial, Paoli, PA)

screws 8-, 12-, 14-, 16-, 18-, and 20-mm lengths which are not generally intended for removal. 1.8 mm titanium locking screws 5 mm in length (Figure 22.23) are inserted into the head of the 4.0 mm titanium solid and hollow THORP screws in order to lock the plate to these bone penetrating screws. The corresponding drill bits to be used are 3.0 mm × 130 mm, which after the hole is prepared is then widened with a 4.0 mm tap. The implants come as 4.0 Titanium THORP Reconstruction Plates Straight (10, 12, 14, 16, 20, and 24 holes) (Figure 22.22b), 4.0-mm Titanium THORP Reconstruction Plates, Angled 5 × 15 (20 holes) Right and Left, and 4.0 Titanium THORP Reconstruction Plates, and Angled 6 × 24 (30 holes) Right and Left Corresponding bending templates are also available for these plates. Additional instruments include the 3.0-mm Drill Guide for 4.0-mm screws to ensure perpendicular screw placement (Figure 22.22a) 4.5-Bending Inserts are for use within the plate holes to prevent deformation during bending and are removed with a corresponding Bending Insert Removal Pliers. Other instruments include a Tap for 4.0 mm Screws, Cruciform Screwdriver Shaft, Self Retaining for 4.0 mm Titanium THORP Screws, Cruciform Screwdriver Shaft for 1.8-mm Titanium Locking Screw, Conical Extraction Screw, 4.5-mm Reamer for Titanium THORP plates (to redefine plate holes following bending), and Bending Irons (2), Depth Guide, handle with Quick Coupling (1), Drill Guide Handle (1), Torque Indicating Screwdriver Handle with Quick Coupling (1), and Transbuccal Instruments.

Mandible Fix Bridge

Indications: Mandibular tumor and resective surgery.

This fixation device allows the remaining mandibular segments to be maintained in their preoperative positions following the resection of an anterior mandibular segment in order to permit the application of a THORP, microvascular, or

a

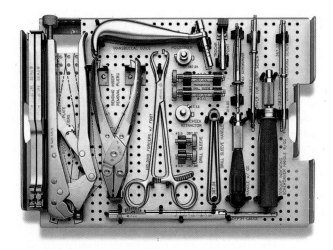

b

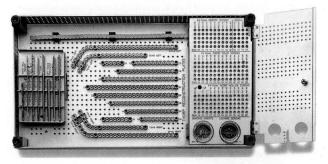

FIGURE 22.22 4.0-mm Titanium Hollow Screw Reconstruction Plate (THORP) Set within graphic case. (a) Lift out tray with instruments at top. (b) Implants, screws, drills, taps, reamer, and screwdriver shafts at bottom of graphic case. (Courtesy of Synthes Maxillofacial, Paoli, PA)

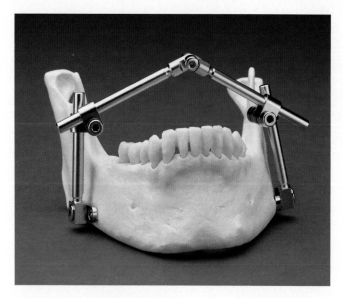

FIGURE 22.24 The Mandible FixBridge assembly in place prior to partial anterior resection of the mandible. (Courtesy of Synthes Maxillofacial, Paoli, PA)

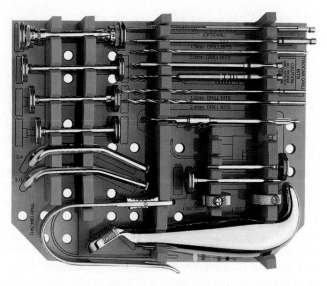

FIGURE 22.26 Universal Trocar System Insert B system tray. (Courtesy of Synthes Maxillofacial, Paoli, PA)

locking reconstruction plate with or without immediate bone grafting (Figure 22.24). The device is placed prior to resection and then the Mandible FixBridge assembly is removed to allow resection, after which the device is reapplied and an appropriate THORP, microvascular, or locking reconstruction plate is contoured and fixated.

The Universal Trocar System

This is a comprehensive system supporting all transbuccal surgical applications for the placement of 2.0-3.0 mm screws (Figure 22.25). It contains (Figure 22.26) 2.0-mm and 2.4-mm cannulas and obturators, handle size specific color coded drill guides for 2.4-mm cannula: 1.8-mm, 1.8-mm DCU Neutral, 1.8-mm DCU compression, 1.8-mm threaded, 2.4-mm threaded, 1.8-mm insert (lag screw), 2.4-mm and 2.0-mm cannula: 1.5-mm. Cheek retractors come as the malleable C-retractor cheek retractor rings and cheek retractor blades. The malleable C-retractor and cheek retractor blades can rotate.

Ratcheting Screwdriver

The ratcheting screwdriver is used for the manual placement of screws using a swivel mechanism that allows independent

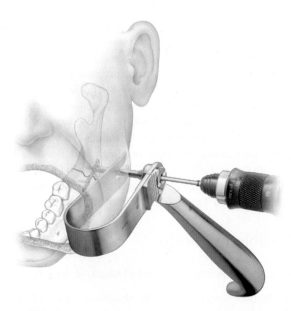

FIGURE 22.25 Universal transbuccal instrumentation with trocar system and ratcheting screwdriver. (Courtesy of Synthes Maxillofacial, Paoli, PA)

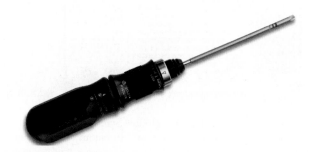

FIGURE 22.27 Ratcheting screwdriver. (Courtesy of Synthes Maxillofacial, Paoli, PA)

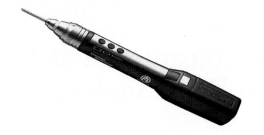

FIGURE 22.28 Battery powered screwdriver system. (Courtesy of Synthes Maxillofacial, Paoli, PA)

movement of the handle for forward and reverse ratchet, as well as for rigid use (Figure 22.27). The hex coupling allows quick connection to the screwdriver blades for 1.5-mm, 2.0-mm, 2.4-mm, and 3.0-mm screws.

Battery Powered Screwdriver

This battery powered cordless screwdriver (Figure 22.28) uses a rechargeable battery pack. A battery charger recharges 2 battery packs at a time. It is used for the 1.3-mm StarDrive and Cruciform Screwdriver blades and for short and long 1.5-mm/2.0-mm cruciform screwdriver blades.

23

Aesthetic Considerations in Reconstructive and Corrective Craniomaxillofacial Bone Surgery

R. Gregory Smith and Luc M. Cesteleyn

Although the bony architecture of the face is a major component in the perception of facial harmony, it must not be viewed as the most important. The truly aesthetic face is defined by the abstract interplay of symmetry, balance, projection, and animation created within the soft tissue envelope overlying its bony foundation.

Concepts of Facial Harmony

Many attempts have been made to quantify facial beauty dating back to early times. Da Vinci was a student of body proportion and symmetry. His studies furnished important data upon which many modern concepts of facial beauty are based.[1] In the study of facial harmony, symmetry is one of the most obvious yet most critical concepts to appreciate, especially when dealing with the facial bony base. The aesthetic face requires reasonable symmetry. Any disturbance of equality of the facial halves is usually quite obvious to even the most casual observer. When planning a surgical procedure (either reconstructive or cosmetic), the surgeon must have symmetry as a primary goal.[2] Even with the use of state-of-the-art rigid internal fixation to align bony fragments, this is not always possible, especially in the trauma patient. The following two examples will illustrate this concept. The patient in Figure 23.1a,b is shown preoperatively after multiple midface and mandible fractures and postoperatively after multiple reconstructive procedures. Final symmetry was achieved after realignment of bony segments using rigid internal fixation, and later insertion of a right malar implant to compensate for overlying soft tissue atrophy on the right and previous overprojection of the zygoma on the left. The patient in Figure 23.2a,b is shown preoperatively status post open reduction with rigid internal fixation of a displaced left zygomaticomaxillary complex fracture, operated elsewhere. The patient felt this fracture was still minimally displaced and requested reoperation. The postoperative view shows near-perfect reduction of this fracture with the use of microplates via a bicoronal approach. At a separate operation, the patient's preexisting congenital facial asymmetry of the lower half of

the face was corrected. Improved facial symmetry resulted with improvement in overall aesthetic balance.

Balance among the aesthetic units of the face plays a very important role in creating facial harmony. The facial units that should be systematically studied preoperatively include the forehead, nose, eyes, malar prominences, lips, chin, and mandibular angles.[3] No one feature should overpower the interrelationship between units. Features that are out of proportion should be considered for change during the planned cosmetic or reconstructive procedure. Once again, several examples will serve to illustrate the concept of balance. Figure 23.3a,b demonstrate a patient, preoperatively and postoperatively, who was treated for multiple complaints of facial imbalance in the areas of the malar prominences, chin, and mandibular angles. His facial balance was dramatically improved by placement of malar and mandibular angle implants and performance of a rigidly fixated bony genioplasty. The patient in Figure 23.4a,b shows preoperative and postoperative results after a rigidly fixated bony genioplasty and full face/neck liposuction. Again, remarkable improvement was achieved by reestablishing more favorable facial balance of the aesthetic units.

The projection of bony aesthetic units provides contours over which the facial soft tissue may drape. Lack of appropriate projection of the underlying facial skeleton leads to an amorphous facial appearance, which often appears more aged or plain.[4,5] The facial units appear to blend together and inelastic soft tissue may sag in the older patient, adversely impacting facial aesthetics as seen in Figure 23.5a,b.

Maintenance of jaw and bony landmark projection is imperative to accentuate the transitions between the aesthetic units of the face. This concept is especially important in craniomaxillofacial and orthognathic surgery.

Two patients who lack important areas of facial projection are illustrated by the following examples. Figure 23.6a,b show preoperative and postoperative views of a Treacher-Collins syndrome patient treated by cranial bone reconstruction of the zygomas, orthognathic surgical correction of malocclusion with rigid fixation, lower lid-switch blepharoplasties, malar implant insertion, and conservative rhinoplasty. In this case, both hard and soft tissues required

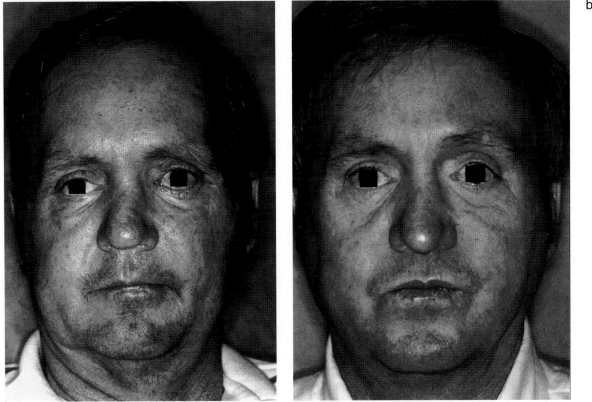

FIGURE 23.1 (a) Patient shown preoperatively status post multiple midface and mandibule fractures. (b) Patient shown postoperatively status post reduction of multiple midface and mandible fractures and placement of right malar implant.

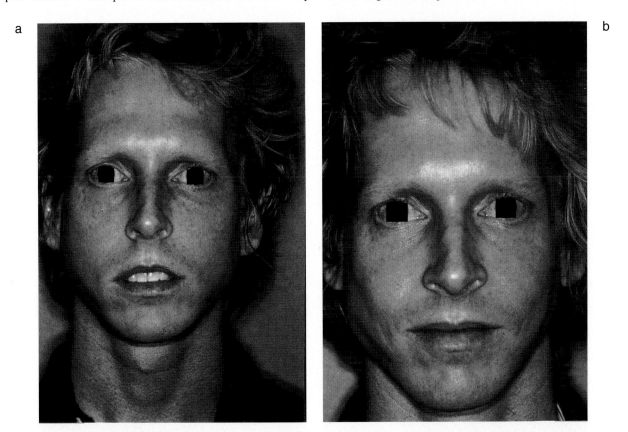

FIGURE 23.2 (a) The patient shown preoperatively status post open reduction of left zygomatic maxillary complex (ZMC) fracture operated elsewhere. (b) The patient shown postoperatively status post reoperation of left ZMC fracture and reduction via micro-miniplates and status post Le Fort I maxillary osteotomy and bilateral sagittal split mandibular osteotomies with rigid internal fixation. Greater facial balance has been achieved.

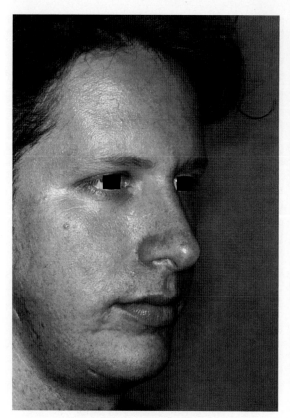 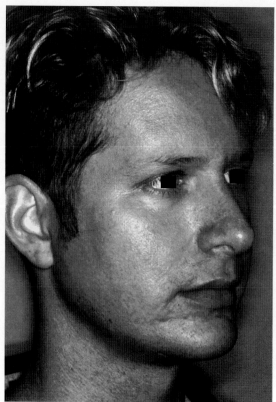

FIGURE 23.3 (a) The patient shown preoperatively with facial imbalance secondary to malar deficiency, mandibular angle deficiency, and genial deficiency. (b) The patient shown postoperatively after placement of bilateral malar implants, mandibular angle implants, and rigidly fixated advancement bony genioplasty.

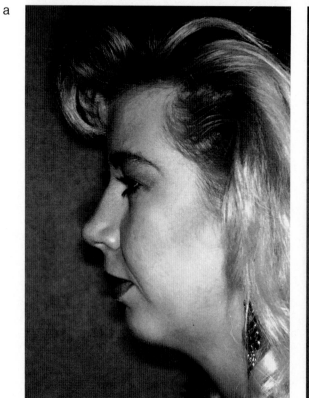 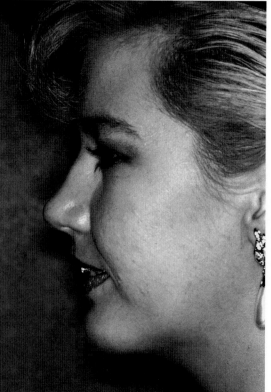

FIGURE 23.4 (a) Patient shown preoperatively with genial deficiency and increased facial liposity. (b) Patient shown postoperatively status post rigid fixated bony genioplasty and full face/neck liposuction.

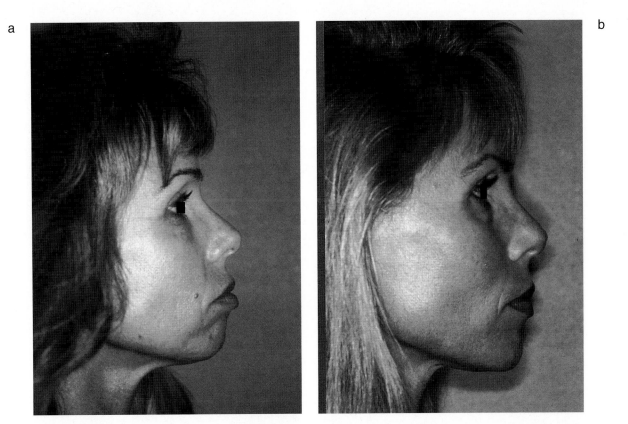

FIGURE 23.5 (a) Patient shown preoperatively with genial and malar deficiency. (b) Patient shown postoperatively status post placement of bilateral malar implants and rigidly fixated advancement bony genioplasty.

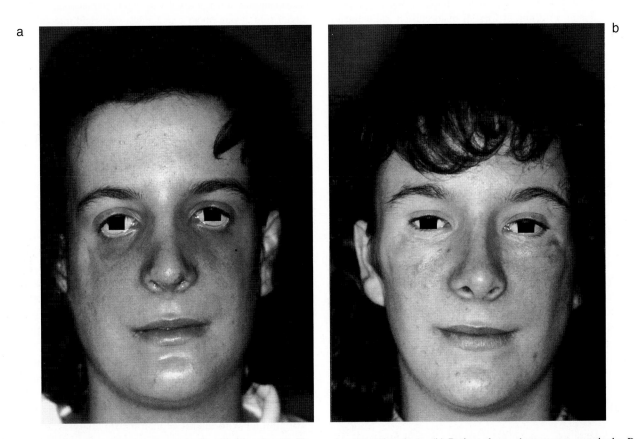

FIGURE 23.6 (a) Patient shown preoperatively with Treacher-Collins syndrome with absent zygomas. The patient is also status post-orthognathic surgical correction of her malocclusion and has had con-servative rhinoplasty. (b) Patient shown 1 year postoperatively. Pa-tient shown status post cranial bone graft reconstruction of zygomas, lower lid-switch blepharoplasties, and placement of malar implants.

a

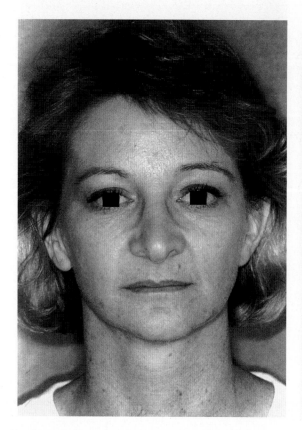

b

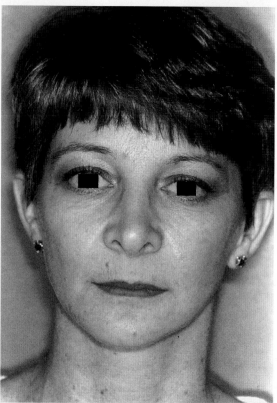

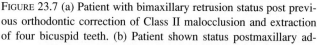

FIGURE 23.7 (a) Patient with bimaxillary retrusion status post previous orthodontic correction of Class II malocclusion and extraction of four bicuspid teeth. (b) Patient shown status postmaxillary advancement and down grafting with rigid internal fixation, bilateral sagittal split advancement osteotomies, with rigid internal fixation, and conservative rhinoplasty.

augmentation to achieve the appearance of adequate projection. The patient in Figure 23.7a,b had undergone four previous bicuspid extractions and orthodontic treatment of a class II malocclusion, which left her with a sunken-in appearance secondary to maxillomandibular deprojection. The postoperative views show the correction achieved with application of internal rigid fixation to allow downgraft advancement of the maxilla and advancement of the mandible, which was combined with simultaneous conservative rhinoplasty. Reestablishment of proper facial projection has achieved dramatic improvement.

Finally, facial animation plays a paramount role in the aesthetic appearance of the face. In short, if the soft tissues do not move, no alteration of the amount of symmetry, balance, and projection will make it aesthetic. Often, major soft tissue injuries to muscle, skin, and nerves leave little chance of normal animation, even if the bony framework is restored to a normal position. Knowledge and skill in soft tissue repair is mandatory for the surgeon. However, coverage of these areas is beyond the scope and mission of this text.

Quantifying Facial Harmony

To this point, the authors have dealt only with the basic abstract concepts that they believe define the aesthetic face. However, numerous works have been completed that objectively measure both hard and soft tissue aesthetic characteristics, and these must not go unnoticed. Although numbers cannot completely describe the aesthetic face, they provide useful references when attempting to quantify relationships. This is especially useful to the surgeon who has not yet developed an "aesthetic sense."

In general, when viewed from the front, the face is divided by the midline vertically, and similar structures in the respective halves are symmetrical. The face is normally broken up into "fifths," being five average "eye widths" wide (Figure 23.8).[2] Facial height is proportionally divided into equal thirds by lines drawn horizontally through the junction of the hairline and forehead skin, subnasale, and menton (Figure 23.8). Trauma victims frequently increase or decrease the various facial thirds owing to the displacement or impaction of facial bones. This is also common in congenital maxillomandibular deformities expressed as too much or too little jaw growth.

In profile, the projection and interrelationships of facial aesthetic units such as the forehead, nose, dental structures, and jaws are extremely important. Their "normalization" can greatly enhance facial aesthetics as previously shown.

Beginning with lateral cephalometric analysis of hard tissue structures, the two most important landmarks are the Frankfort horizontal line, defined as a line drawn from the upper part of the external auditory meatus to the infraorbital

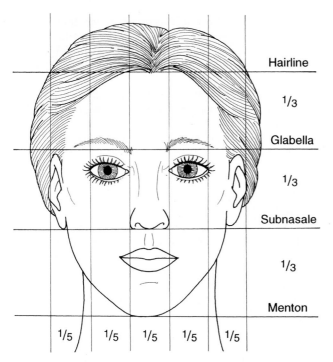

FIGURE 23.8 Facial dimensions divided vertically into fifths and horizontally into thirds.

TABLE 23.1 Cephalometric analysis.

	Range
Mandibular plane angle (FH-MP)	26° ± 4.5
Maxillary depth (FH-NaA)	90° ± 3
Facial depth (FH-NaPO)	87° ± 3
Point A to nasion perpendicular	1 mm
PO to nasion perpendicular	−2 to +4 mm
Overbite	3 ± 1.5 mm
Overjet	1–2 mm
Upper incisor—NaA(mm)	0–8 mm
Lower incisor—NaB(mm)	2–10 mm
Upper incisor to lower incisor	120°–140°
Lower anterior dental height	40 mmF/44 mmM

unfamiliar with dental structures and occlusion, we recommend review of texts dedicated to orthognathic surgery of the jaws.

Soft tissue profile aesthetics have been studied extensively, but several numbers bear remembering. Again, we feel that the two most useful landmarks are the Frankfort horizontal line and the Smith nasion perpendicular (SNP) (Figure 23.10). SNP is defined as a line perpendicular to the Frankfort horizontal line and tangent to the depth of soft tissue nasion and extending through soft tissue pogonion. The aesthetic nasal dorsum takes off from SNP at approximately 35°.[3,9] The height of the nasal dorsum measured from the medial canthus area is approximately 15 mm according to Goldman.[10] The

rim, and MacNamara's line, which is a line that begins at nasion and is dropped perpendicular to the Frankfort horizontal (Figure 23.9).[6–8] Using only these two reference lines, the surgeon may identify anomalies of jaw and teeth position using the normal values listed in Table 23.1. For surgeons who are

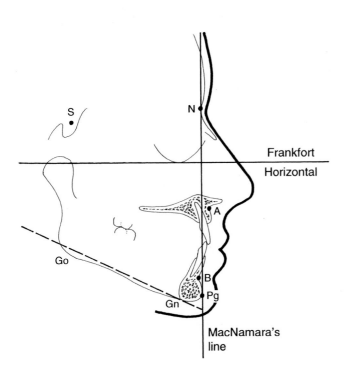

FIGURE 23.9 Lateral cephalometric radiographic references for Frankfort horizontal and MacNamara's line.

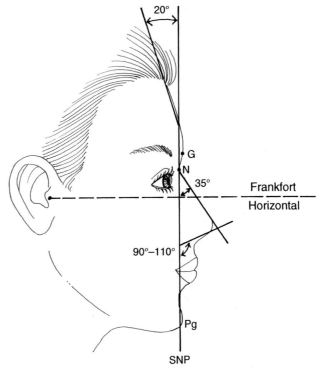

FIGURE 23.10 Smith nasion perpendicular (SNP) and Frankfort Horizontal SNP extends through soft tissue nasion and pogoion which differs by these defined landmarks from the zero meriden of Gonzalez-Ulloa.[3]

nasolabial angle should be in the range of 90° for men and up to 110° for women.[3,9,11]

The aesthetic forehead slopes away from the SNP at an angle of 20°.[12] The glabella is slightly rounded in the midline, not flat, and it projects 2 to 3 mm anterior to SNP.[13] This point must be considered during craniofacial reconstruction.

Summary

Although the list of "numbers" presented here is by no means exhaustive, it represents a starting point for an objective assessment of the face as it relates to craniomaxillofacial surgery. When it is used in conjunction with the abstract concepts of beauty previously presented, the surgeon should be able to effectively analyze the individual patient's face and formulate a surgical plan that will maximize the aesthetic outcome.

References

1. Beeson WH. Facial analysis in aesthetic surgery of the aging face. Beeson WH, McCollough EG, eds. St. Louis: C.V. Mosby Co.; 1980.

2. Bell WH, Proffitt WB, White RP. *Surgical Correction of Dentofacial Deformities.* Philadelphia: WB Saunders Co.; 1980:115–123.

3. Powell N, Humphreys B. *Proportions of the Aesthetic Face.* New York: Thieme-Stratton Inc.; 1980:1–9;1984:15–39.

4. Binder WJ, Schoenrock LD, Terino EOL. Augmentation of the malar-submalar/midface. *Facial Plastic Surg Clin.* 1994;2(3):265–284.

5. Mittleman H. The anatomy of the aging mandible and its importance to facelift surgery. *Facial Plastic Surg Clin.* 1994;2(3): 301–310.

6. Tweed CA. The Frankfort-mandibular plane angle in orthognathic diagnosis, classification, treatment planning and prognosis. *Am J Orthod Oral Surg.* 1946;32:175–230.

7. Mourvees CFA, Kean MR. Natural head position: a basic consideration for analysis of cephalometric radiographs. *Am J Phys Anthropol.* 1958;16:213–234.

8. McNamara JA Jr. A method of cephalometric analysis. In: McNamara JA Jr, Ribbens KA, Howe RP, eds. *Clinical Alteration of the Growing Face.* Monograph No. 14, Craniofacial Growth Series. The Center for Human Growth and Development, The University of Michigan, Ann Arbor, MI; 1983.

9. Sheen JH, Sheen AP. *Aesthetic Rhinoplasty,* Vol 1, 2nd ed. St Louis, MO: C.V. Mosby; 1987:67–127.

10. Goldman IB. *Rhinoplasty Manual.* NY Restricted Publication, 1968.

11. Aiach G, Levignac J. *Aesthetic Rhinoplasty.* Edinburgh: Churchill Livingstone; 1991:21–23.

12. Bon M. L'Esthetic Face a la Chirurgie Esthetique. Private Publication. Paris 1977.

13. Tessier P. Personal Communication, 1989.

Section IV
Craniomaxillofacial Reconstructive Bone Surgery

24
Considerations for Reconstruction of the Head and Neck Oncologic Patient

Douglas W. Klotch and Neal D. Futran

The history of treatment of head and neck cancer has been one of continual applications of new techniques in the hope of improving cure rates and functional rehabilitation after tumor ablation. Before the 1960s the drive to resect head and neck cancer (seemingly at all costs) frequently resulted in radical ablation with horrendous deformities and often significant morbidity. During the 1960s and 1970s combination therapy, using radiotherapy and surgery, yielded higher cure rates than aggressive ablative surgery alone in many circumstances. At that same time, several surgeons established the concept that less tissue could be removed in many cases without compromising the cancer cure rates.[1–12] Since the 1970s, however, there has been a virtual plateau in the cure rates for tumors of most regions of the head and neck.

Modern head and neck surgery is characterized by its emphasis on reconstruction and rehabilitation. Over the past two decades there have been steady advances in the available surgical techniques for reconstruction of the head and neck. The 1970s introduced the pectoralis major myocutaneous flap, which rapidly became the "work horse" flap in head and neck reconstruction.[13,14] Although microvascular transfer of free-tissue grafts to the head and neck were performed as early as 1959 by Sidenberg et al.,[15] it was not until the 1970s that microvascular free-tissue transfer became recognized as a versatile tool in head and neck reconstruction.[16–20]

The 1980s and 1990s have seen continued refinement in surgical techniques, particularly in the area of microvascular surgery.[21–31] With microvascular free-tissue transfer achieving rates of graft viability greater than 95% in many centers, the reconstructive emphasis is to tailor these free flaps to create the best form and function possible.[32–39] Many investigators continue to look for new and improved donor sites for free-tissue transfer as well.

Currently, head and neck surgeons find themselves paying much more attention to reconstruction and rehabilitation in their treatment of the patient with head and neck cancer. The surgeon can perform major resection of neoplasms in the head and neck without the degree of concern for restoration of form and function experienced by clinicians in earlier decades. The surgeon no longer views the often horrendous deformities cre-ated by radical ablative surgery of the head and neck region as an inevitable consequence of tumor control. Presently, the focus is oriented toward obtaining the ideal reconstruction whenever possible.

The criteria by which we judge outcomes in the reconstruction of the craniomaxillofacial skeleton are related to function, aesthetics, and satisfactory quality of life. Ideally, the techniques used to achieve these goals should minimize the tissue damaged or removed, and they must imitate the form, geometry, and quality of the injured structures. Normal function should also be restored as completely as possible.

All patients, however, may not be suitable candidates for the "ideal" reconstruction. Patient age, associated medical problems, diet, performance status, the individual's motivation, and family dynamics are all factors that must be considered when planning the surgical complexity of the reconstruction.[23–25,34,38] The extent of the disease dictates the extent of surgical resection although the size and location of soft tissue defects, as well as concomitant partial or total loss of adjacent nervous, muscular, vascular, and skeletal tissues are a few of the anatomic variables that must also be considered.

Many of these patients undergo radiation therapy to the head and neck as part of the overall treatment plan.[1–5,8–12] The decreased vascularity of radiated tissue limits the use of alloplastic materials alone to successfully reconstruct soft tissue and bony defects. Regional or distant vascularized flaps are usually necessary to promote adequate healing, especially when any contamination is present.[24,31,34,40–42]

Physician factors also play a role in determining the materials and techniques utilized in head and neck reconstruction. Although microvascular free flaps allow for the transfer of a variety of tissue types to the head and neck, many centers do not have physicians and support personnel with the necessary microvascular skills. These procedures require longer operative time than many traditional reconstructive techniques. The surgeon must be cognizant of the potential morbidity associated with each donor flap harvested. The expected success rate of the transposition must be weighed against the difficulty of performing each procedure, which translates into operative time for the surgeon and the patient. This is particularly dependent on the patient's general medical status. On the other hand, distant donor sites far removed from the head and neck provide an opportunity for synchronous double team surgery and actual shortening of operative time, which is often not possible with many regional flaps.[21–25,28,31–34,42]

The availability of a qualified maxillofacial prosthodontist also may determine the type of reconstruction used, especially in midface defects. Precisely fabricated prostheses can provide an excellent and sometimes superior method of reconstruction with much less morbidity than many tissue transfer techniques.

The craniomaxillofacial skeleton can be divided into thirds: lower, middle, and upper. Most bony defects from extirpation of head and neck cancers involve the lower oromandibular complex and midface structures. Considerations for reconstruction of each region will now be delineated.

Oromandibular Complex Reconstruction

The goals of reconstructing the oromandibular complex are to reconstitute its three-dimensional shape, preserve or restore lower facial contour, provide a denture-bearing surface, and maintain or re-create occlusal relationships and oral continence. The oral cavity is unique in that several host factors come into play when considering which techniques will be used to achieve these goals. The problem of salivary contamination must be addressed in every case, particularly in radiated patients. The area of mandible to be reconstructed is a significant factor in the timing of definitive bony reconstruction. Immediate bony reconstruction of the denture-bearing surface may allow primary placement of osseointegrated implants and earlier dental prosthetic rehabilitation than delayed techniques.[26,30]

Resection of the anterior mandibular arch produces the "Andy Gump" deformity, a debilitating functional and aesthetic problem. Oral competence suffers from the patient's inability to manage oral secretions, speak, eat, or swallow. This is, therefore, the most important mandibular defect to reconstruct primarily. The need for bone, intraoral soft tissue, and external skin coverage must be assessed carefully, with attention paid to the relative amounts of each tissue required. Reconstruction of this defect with a microvascular, bone-containing free flap is the optimal method for achieving the best result.[17,19,21–24,26–28,30,31,33–36,40,42] Bony stabilization can be achieved before initial resection. In those cases where the neoplasm has not penetrated through the buccal cortex of the mandible, an AO reconstruction plate may be adapted to the mandible prior to resection of the tumor. Holes are drilled, screws are placed, and then the plate and screws are removed. Early fixation maintains essentially perfect contours. Futran et al.[43] recently showed fewer long-term plate complications when using the titanium hollow screw reconstruction plate (THORP) or titanium AO reconstruction plate than with the AO stainless steel plate. After tumor resection, the plate is reapplied to the mandible. The surgical specimen is then available as a visualized reference for graft shaping as well as serving as a template for graft size and length. Although this is our preferred method, some cases dictate and authors advocate the use of miniplates to fixate the graft to the residual mandible.[22,28] Once the composite graft is revascularized, primary placement of osseointegrated implants allows more rapid dental rehabilitation. They provide the most rigid form of stabilization to withstand the forces of mastication. In situations in which soft tissue reconstruction or the height of the alveolar ridge is not sufficient for a tissue-borne denture, implants offer the most suitable alternative.[26,30] Four to 6 months after surgery, when the integration process has occurred and postoperative radiation therapy has been completed, the implants are uncovered, loaded, and ready for prosthetic placement.

Immediate restoration of the mandible prevents the development of muscle contracture. In postresection situations, scarred masticatory muscles pull the mandibular segments upward and medially, distorting occlusion. Once this process has occurred, restoration of a normal configuration is difficult. Graft shaping in secondary reconstruction is a mystery at best, as a result. It is also not in the patient's best interest to live with a devastating aesthetic and functional deformity and to be subjected to two long operative procedures instead of one.

When the posterior lateral mandible, the angle, and the ascending ramus are removed, the defect can be dealt with in a variety of ways with equal restoration of form and function.[34,40–42,44–51] Free flaps have no demonstrable superiority in the reconstruction of this defect. In fact, not all of these patients need to be reconstructed. Simple collapse of the segments often allow closure of the soft tissue defect primarily. Although facial contour is slightly disturbed by shift of the anterior mandible to the affected side, these patients maintain very adequate speech and swallowing. This technique is especially suitable for the medically compromised patient and will minimize operative time.

Intraoral tissue concerns are a higher priority than immediate restoration of the bony defect in these areas of the mandible.[32,52] The use of reconstruction plates in conjunction with soft tissue free flaps or pedicled flaps allow an expedient method to obtain an excellent cosmetic and functional result with minimal donor site disability.[41,42,47,48,52,53] It is best for lateral and posterior lower volume defects in the debilitated, the elderly, and in patients with a poor prognosis. This method is no panacea. Failure usually requires rescue with a vascularized bone graft. With the proper selection of patients, however, this will rarely be necessary. A major weakness in the plating systems available at present is their tendency to fracture if they remain in place too long, although the newer THORP plates appear to be more resistant to this problem than their stainless steel predecessors.[43,49] Complications including fistulae, late plate extrusions, and required plate removals are also reportedly higher for reconstructions in irradiated fields.[41,48]

Restorations of coexistent temporomandibular joint (TMJ) and mandibular defects is a challenging undertaking. Ideally, this joint is necessary for unencumbered function. Realistically, immediate restoration with the articulation of the glenoid fossa may not significantly contribute to cosmetic or functional improvement following radical ablative surgery.

Several approaches are available to synchronous reconstruction of the TMJ and auxiliary mandibular defects. Initially, intermaxillary fixation is applied to the preexisting dentition to maintain occlusion. The use of reconstruction plates with a condylar head (AO-titanium, THORP) allows for a hemijoint reconstruction in conjunction with skeletal fixation of a vascularized bone graft or residual mandible.[49] The surgeon must be aware that condylar head alloplastic devices are now FDA approved. Soft tissue arthroplasty using temporalis tissue or other tissue during bony transfer has facilitated TMJ reconstruction, especially in older patients. In younger patients, and especially in children, costochondral grafts can be used along with the vascularized bone technique. Any technique must address the risk to the facial nerve both during the procedure and with subsequent mandibular function. Fortunately, very few oral cancers other than sarcomas involve the TMJ and require resection of the condyle. When squamous cell cancers involve the jaw joint, removal of the meniscus and even the glenoid fossa may be required. These patients usually require high-dose radiotherapy. The senior author does not advocate the use of alloplastic condylar reconstruction for these situations.

When the neoplasm extends anteriorly through the mandibular buccal cortex and into the soft tissues, contouring the reconstruction plate to maintain ideal mandibular form is impossible prior to resecting the tumor. To maintain proper position of the condyles in the glenoid fossae, external fixation devices such as the Joe-Hall-Morris or Anderson biphasic splint may be applied.[45,47] The AO condylar positioning device is also available to provide positioning of the mandible stumps and the condyles with the unobstructed ability to resect tumors with anterior extension. Following resection of the mandible a bridging plate and/or bone flap can be precisely applied, with preservation of the precise occlusal and condylar relationships. Alternatively, a universal reconstruction plate may be used to achieve the same result. Adequacy of the anterior mandibular projection is determined by the judgment of the surgeon as the bone grafts and plates are placed in relation to the anterior maxillary arch.

One other method that deserves mention has occurred with the advent of three-dimensional computed tomography (CT) imaging. Special software packages allow three-dimensional reconstruction of the oromandibular complex. An alloplastic mandible can then be generated and used as a template or temporary spacer prior to definitive reconstruction.

The primary advantage of delayed reconstruction is the avoidance of wound contamination by saliva.[46,50] Lateral and posterior defects are the simplest to repair. In 1982 Lawson et al.[46] found that reconstruction of the mandible with allo-plastic materials and free bone grafts achieved an improved rate of restoring mandibular continuity in the delayed setting, than when using these techniques primarily. Few patients, however, achieved a significant functional benefit or used dental appliances.

The presence of scar contracture after tumor extirpation causes malalignment of the remaining mandibular segments, if not initially maintained by an AO reconstruction plate or external fixation device. Realignment and precise reconstruction of the defect become a more formidable task in this setting.

Many patients who undergo delayed reconstruction will have had radiation therapy immediately after extirpative surgery. The resultant decreased tissue vascularity and fibrosis dictates the need for vascularized tissue transfer to achieve the desired reconstructive goals. Invariably, the results are not as optimal as reconstruction in the primary setting. Although restoration of mandibular continuity can be achieved, these factors indicate an inevitable delay in functional dental rehabilitation. Reconstructive problems are similar to those in delayed reconstruction when repairing oromandibular defects created by salvage surgery. Frequently, these patients have extensive scarring from previous procedures and/or radiation therapy reducing the host tissue's ability to support alloplastic materials. Free vascularized tissue transfer is almost always necessary in this type of patient if definitive reconstruction is to be undertaken.[27,31,36,54]

Whenever possible, therefore, immediate single-stage reconstruction is always preferable to delayed reconstruction when the former can be achieved with acceptable success rates and low morbidity. This is especially important for patients who have advanced neoplasms, for whom prognosis is poor, and for whom early palliation is crucial to maintain the quality of life.

Midface and Skull Base Defects

The midface can be characterized as the juxtaposition of three cavities in complex bony mucosal units: the oral cavity, nasomaxillary complex, and the orbital cavity with its contents. Many neoplasms in this area extend to the skull base and may enter the cranial cavity. A broader spectrum of approaches to the skull base with improved exposure has permitted safer and more complete ablative procedures in this area. The goal of reconstruction is to restore to normal the physical and functional relationship of these massive defects.

The complexity of immediate reconstruction is largely dependent on the defect created. Conventional management of maxillectomy defects when the globe is spared includes resurfacing the inner cheek with a skin graft and obturating the palate and sinus defect with a maxillofacial prosthesis.[55] This allows functional reconstruction for mastication, swallowing, and speech. Recurrence of tumor is readily identified by visualization of the maxillary cavity. The globe may be supported by a variety of autologous or alloplastic materials. These defects are also easily managed by the patient and require only gentle irrigation of the cavity when fully healed.

Some authors do advocate free tissue transfer reconstruction of this defect, citing problems of crusting, infection, or osteoradionecrosis in a skin-grafted cavity.[22,25,29,38,39,56-59] Although the palate may be sealed with soft tissue, fitting of a dental prosthesis may require further soft tissue revision surgery to achieve a successful result.

The radical orbitomaxillectomy results in communication of the oral cavity, nasal cavity, maxillary sinus space, and orbit. Abnormal airflow is created and saliva or food bolus can escape through the nose/sinus cavities. The support of the globe (if present) and nasal support may be undermined. Extension to the overlying skin may result in more severe food and airway flow disorders. In addition, contraction of the lips and soft tissues of the face may occur, resulting in grossly abnormal speech and appearance. The three-dimensional complexity of these skin-covered, mucosa-lined areas of bone is ordinarily much too demanding for perfect reformation.

The nasomaxillary region may be considered as the transitional zone, and can be replaced with well-vascularized tissue (with or without bone). The most relevant functional areas are determined and the main volume is obliterated. Support of the globe is provided. The hard palate, lateral nasal wall, and infraorbital rim can be recreated. In selected cases, primary or secondary placement of osseointegrated implants will allow improved support and stability of maxillofacial prostheses. When the orbit is exenterated, preservation of the eyelids allows for improved cosmetic results with an orbital prosthesis than if the eyelids are sacrificed with the tumor.[25,29,34,56]

The most important goal of reconstructing most defects of the skull base, especially when dura is exposed or the cranial cavity entered, is to provide coverage with vascularized tissue.[38,58,59] The risk of cerebrospinal fluid leak, and even more importantly the risk of a secondary infection, necessitate the anatomic and functional separation of extracranial and intracranial cavities. Delayed reconstruction is usually reserved for the improvement of aesthetics and function not attainable by maxillofacial prosthetics. Vascularized soft tissue with bone grafts (vascularized or nonvascularized) or alloplastic materials may be used to re-create the orbital components, nasal dorsum, and/or palate.

Frequently, these tissues have been irradiated, and the presence of scar tissue and fibrosis limits the ability to provide optimal aesthetics and function.

The issue of oncologic surveillance has been raised regarding the use of free-tissue transfer to reconstruct skull base defects. The placement of any flap to fill a defect certainly inhibits the physician's ability to detect recurrent disease by physical examination. However, the repeated use of sophisticated imaging techniques helps to detect changes postoperatively, which may direct further diagnostic studies.[59] The use of free-tissue transfer for reconstruction of the skull base

should be reserved for situations in which vascularized tissue is required and when regional flaps are not suitable. In addition, when the application of a free flap holds the promise of a better quality of life than can be achieved with alternative techniques, then this, too, represents a worthy indication. Arguments based on the philosophy that patients should be forced to live with their deformity for a finite period of time prior to definitive reconstruction hearken back to similar arguments regarding primary mandibular reconstruction. These arguments should be deplored for two reasons: the results of secondary reconstruction are almost always inferior to primary reconstruction, and in many patients with skull base malignancies the detection of recurrent disease is often a theoretical exercise. Many of our patients have exhausted other therapeutic modalities, including prior surgery, when they are referred for skull base surgery. The anatomic areas where these patients are most likely to recur are those that are least amenable to safely achieving clear margins. It is unlikely, in most cases, that salvage surgery or meaningful alternative therapy would be feasible or beneficial. It therefore seems unreasonable to condemn such patients to an inferior quality of life for the time that they have remaining.

Although advances in technology, physician training, and sophisticated surgical techniques have broadened our ability to extirpate advanced neoplasms and provide functional and aesthetic reconstruction, the buzzword in medicine for the remainder of the decade and beyond is "cost-effectiveness." Each patient and defect to be reconstructed must be evaluated and treated individually. Surgeons must use those techniques that are best suited to their abilities, or that reconstructive goals can be achieved in a timely, efficient manner. Morbidity and patient hospitalization must be minimized to meet the demands of economic medicine.

References

1. Million RR, Fletcher GH, Jesse RH. Evaluation of elective irradiation of the neck for squamous cell carcinoma of the nasopharynx, tonsillar fossa and base of tongue. *Radiology.* 1963;80:973–978.

2. Leonard JR, Litton WB, Latourette HB. Combined radiation and surgical therapy: tongue, tonsil and floor of mouth. *Ann Otol Rhinol Laryngol.* 1968;77:514–533.

3. Biller HF, Ogura JH, Davis WH, Powers WE. Planned preoperative irradiation for carcinoma of the larynx and laryngopharynx treated by total and partial laryngectomy. *Laryngoscope.* 1969;79:1387–1395.

4. Strong EW. Preoperative radiation and radical neck dissection. *Surg Clin North Am.* 1969;49:271–276.

5. Million RR. Elective neck irradiation for TxNo squamous carcinomas of the oral tongue and floor of mouth. *Cancer* (Phila). 1974;34:149–155.

6. Lingeman RE, Helmus C, Stephens R, Ulm J. Neck dissection: radical or conservative. *Ann Otol Rhinol Laryngol.* 1977;86: 737–744.

7. Jesse RH, Ballantyne AJ, Larson D. Radical or modified neck dissection: a therapeutic dilemma. *Am J Surg.* 1978;136:516–519.

8. Wang CC. Radiation therapy in the management of oral malignant disease. *Otolaryngol Clin North Am.* 1979;12:73–80.

9. Shumrick DA, Quenelle DJ. Malignant disease of the tonsillar region, retromolar trigone, and buccal mucosa. *Otolaryngol Clin North Am.* 1979;12:115–124.

10. Rabuzzi DD, Chung CT, Sagerman RH. Prophylactic neck irradiation. *Arch Otolaryngol.* 1980;106:454–455.

11. Panje WR, Smith BS, McCabe BF. Epidermoid carcinoma of the floor of the mouth: surgical therapy vs. combined therapy vs. radiation therapy. *Otolaryngol Head Neck Surg.* 1980;88:714–720.

12. Decroix Y, Ghossein NA. Experience of the Curie Institute in treatment of cancer of the mobile tongue. I. Treatment policies and results. *Cancer* (Phila). 1981;47:496–502.

13. Ariyan S, Krizek TJ. Reconstruction after head and neck cancer. *Cine Clinics Clinical Congress of the American College of Surgeons,* Dallas, Oct. 1977.

14. Biller HF, Baek SM, Lawson W, Krespi YP, Blaugrund SM. Pectoralis major myocutaneous island flap in head and neck surgery: analysis of complications in 42 cases. *Arch Otolaryngol Head Neck Surg.* 1981;107:23–26.

15. Sidenberg B, Rosenah SS, Hurwitt ES, et al. Immediate reconstruction of the cervical esophagus by a revascularized isolated jejunal segment. *Ann Surg.* 1959;149:162–171.

16. Taylor GI, Miller GH, Ham FJ. The free vascularized bone graft: clinical extension of the microvascular techniques. *Plast Reconst Surg.* 1975;55:533–539.

17. Daniel RK. Mandibular reconstruction with free tissue transfers. *Ann Plast Surg.* 1978;1:346–371.

18. Panje WR, Krause CJ, Bardach J. Reconstruction of intraoral defects with the free groin flap. *Arch Otolaryngol.* 1977;103:78–83.

19. Panje WR. Free compound groin flap reconstruction of anterior mandibular defect. *Arch Otolaryngol Head Neck Surg.* 1981;107:17–22.

20. Baker SR. Free lateral thoracic flaps in head and neck reconstruction. *Arch Otolaryngol.* 1981;107:409–413.

21. Silverberg B, Banis JC, Acland RD. Mandibular reconstruction with microvascular bone transfer: Series of 10 patients. *Am J Surg.* 1985;150:440–446.

22. Swartz WM, Banis JC, Newton D, et al. The osteocutaneous scapular flap for mandibular and maxillary reconstruction. *Plast Reconstr Surg.* 1986;77:530–545.

23. Baker SR. Microvascular free flaps in soft-tissue augmentation of the head and neck. *Arch Otolaryngol Head Neck Surg.* 1986;112:733–737.

24. Sullivan MJ, Baker SR, Crompton R, Smith-Wheelock M. Free scapular osteocutaneous flap for mandibular reconstruction. *Arch Otolaryngol Head Neck Surg.* 1989;115:1134–1340.

25. Jones NF, Hardesty RA, Swartz WM, et al. Extensive and complex defects of the scalp, middle third of the face, and palate: the role of microsurgical reconstruction. *Plast Reconstr Surg.* 1988;82:937–952.

26. Riediger D. Restoration of masticatory function by microsurgically revascularized iliac crest bone grafts using endosseous implants. *Plast Reconstr Surg.* 1988;81:861–877.

27. Jewer DD, Boyd JB, Manktelow RT, Zukor RM, et al. Orofacial and mandibular reconstruction with the iliac crest free flap: a review of 69 cases and a new method of classification. *Plast Reconstr Surg.* 1989;84:391–403.

28. Hidalgo DA. Fibula free flap: a new method of mandibular reconstruction. *Plast Reconstr Surg.* 1989;84:71–79.

29. Coleman JJ. Microvascular approach to function and appearance of large orbital maxillary defects. *Am J Surg.* 1989;158:337–342.

30. Urken ML, Buchbinder D, Weinberg H, Vickery C, et al. Primary placement of osseointegrated implants in microvascular mandibular reconstruction. *Otolaryngol Head Neck Surg.* 1989;101:56–73.

31. Urken ML, Vickery C, Weinberg H, Buchbinder D, Biller HF. The internal oblique-iliac crest osseomyocutaneous microvascular free flap in head and neck reconstruction. *J Reconstr Microsurg.* 1989;5:203–216.

32. Urken ML, Weinberg H, Vickery C, Biller HF. The neurofasciocutaneous radial forearm flap in head and neck reconstruction: a preliminary report. *Laryngoscope.* 1990;100:161–173.

33. Sanger JR, Matloub HS, Yousif NJ. Sequential connection of flaps: a logical approach to customized mandibular reconstruction. *Am J Surg.* 1990;160:402–404.

34. Harii D. The free flap in head and neck reconstruction. In: Fee WE, Goepfert H, Johns ME, Strong EW, Ward PH, eds. *Head and Neck Cancer, Vol. 2.* Philadelphia: B.C. Decker; 1990:33–35.

35. Lukash FN, Tenebaum NS, Moskowitz G. Long-term fate of the vascularized iliac crest bone graft for mandibular reconstruction. *Am J Surg.* 1990;160:399–401.

36. Hoffman HT, Harrision N, Sullivan MJ, et al. Mandible reconstruction with vascularized bone grafts. *Arch Otolaryngol Head Neck Surg.* 1991;117:917–925.

37. Aviv JE, Urken ML, Vickery C, et al. The combined latissimus dorsi-scapular free flap in head and neck reconstruction. *Arch Otolaryngol Head Neck Surg.* 1991;117:1242–1250.

38. Jones TR, Jones NF. Advances in reconstruction of the upper aerodigestive tract and cranial base with free tissue transfer. *Clin Plast Surg.* 1992;19(4):819–839.

39. Coleman JJ. Osseous reconstruction of the midface and orbits. *Clin Plast Surg.* 1994;21(1):113–124.

40. Gullane PJ, Holmes H. Mandibular reconstruction: new concepts. *Arch Otolaryngol Head Neck Surg.* 1986;112:714–719.

41. Klotch DW, Gump J, Kuhn L. Reconstruction of mandibular defects in irradiated patients. *Am J Surg.* 1990;160:396–398.

42. Gullane PJ. Primary mandibular reconstruction: analysis of 64 cases and evaluation of interface radiation dosimetry on bridging plates. *Laryngoscope.* 1991;101(suppl 54):1–24.

43. Futran ND, Urken ML, Buchbinder D, Moscoso JF, Beller HF. Rigid fixation of vascularized bone grafts in mandibular reconstruction. *Arch Otol.* 1995;121(1):70–76.

44. Parel SM, Drane JB, Williams EO. Mandibular replacements: a review of the literature. *J Am Dent Assoc.* 1977;94:120–129.

45. Adamo A, Szal RJ. Timing, results, and complications of mandibular reconstructive surgery: report of 32 cases. *J Oral Surg.* 1979;37:755–763.

46. Lawson W, Baek S, Loscalzo L, et al. Experience with immediate and delayed mandibular reconstruction. *Laryngoscope.* 1982;92:5–10.

47. Komisar A, Shapiro BM, Danziger E. The use of osteosynthesis in immediate and delayed mandibular reconstruction. *Laryngoscope.* 1985;95:1363–1366.

48. Klotch DW, Prein J. Mandibular reconstruction using AO plates. *Am J Surg* 1987;154:384–388.

49. Raveh J, Sutter F, Hellem S. Surgical procedures for reconstruction of the lower jaw using the titanium coated screw re-

construction plate system: bridging defects. *Otolaryngol Clin North Am.* 1987;20:535–558.

50. Komisar A, Warman S, Danziger E. A critical analysis of immediate and delayed mandibular reconstruction using A-O plates. *Arch Otolaryngol Head Neck Surg.* 1989;115:830–833.

51. Tucker HM. Nonrigid reconstruction of the mandible. *Arch Otolaryngol Head Neck Surg.* 1989;115:1190–1192.

52. Boyd B, Mulholland S, Gullane P, et al. Reinnervated lateral antebrachial cutaneous neurosome flaps in oral reconstruction: are we making sense? *Plast Reconstr Surg.* 1994;93(7):1350–1359.

53. Saunders JR, Hirata RM, Jaques DA. Definitive mandibular replacement using reconstruction plates. *Am J Surg.* 1990;160: 387–389.

54. Kiener JL, Hoffman WY, Mathes SJ. Influence of radiotherapy on microvascular reconstruction in the head and neck region. *Am J Surg.* 1991;162:404–407.

55. Thanley SE, Panje WR, Batsquis JG, Linberg RD. Comprehensive management of head and neck tumors. Philadelphia: WB Saunders; 1987:408–460.

56. Shestak CK, Schusterman MA, Jones NF, et al. Immediate microvascular reconstruction of combined palatal and midfacial defects. *Am J Surg.* 1988;156:252–255.

57. Sadove RC, Powell LA. Simultaneous maxillary and mandibular reconstruction with one free osteocutaneous flap. *Plast Reconstr Surg.* 1993;92:141–146.

58. Jones NF, Sekhar LN, Schramm VL. Free rectus abdominis muscle flap reconstruction of the middle and posterior cranial base. *Plast Reconstr Surg.* 1989;78:471–479.

59. Urken MD, Catalano PI, Sen C, Post M, Futran ND, Biller HF. Free tissue transfer for skull base reconstruction. Analyses of complications and a classification scheme for defining skull base defects. *Arch Otol Head Neck Surg.* 1993;119:1318–1328.

25
Autogenous Bone Grafts in Maxillofacial Reconstruction

Michael Ehrenfeld and Christine Hagenmaier

Bone grafts in maxillofacial surgery are used to correct or replace missing bone. Bone defects can either be the consequences of congenital and developmental malformations or originate from tumor surgery, trauma, or infections. There are many indications for bone grafts in cosmetic surgery as well.

So far as the biological qualities of bone substitutes are concerned, fresh autogenous bone still represents the gold standard among all available grafting materials.[1,2] Nonresorbable ceramic materials are prefered only for contour augmentation procedures because they do not have the unpredictable initial remodeling and resorption seen with free autogenous bone grafts.

Fresh autogenous bone grafts can be transplanted in three principally different techniques: free bone grafts, pedicled bone grafts, and microvascular bone grafts.[3–19] For microvascular revascularized tissue transplants, some authors prefer the term "flap," such as "the osteomusculocutaneous fibula flap."

Free Bone Grafts

Free bone grafts are usually harvested from certain preferred donor site areas. During harvesting, tissue connections between bone graft and surrounding tissues are transected. In the recepient site the bone must be revitalized mainly via tissue ingrowth, although it is also known that osteocytes within free bone grafts are able to survive after transplantation.[1,2,20–26] The revitalization goes along with a process of initial remodeling and bone resorption, which is associated with a loss of bone volume. This process is generally called resorption. The amount of resorption depends on many factors, such as the dimensions of the bone graft (it takes longer to revitalize large bone grafts, and therefore they show a greater percentage of bone loss), the quality of the bone (cortical, cancellous), tissue qualities at the recipient site (vascularization), biomechanical properties (functional loading), and bone graft fixation to surrounding bone.[7,27–32] A serious problem for the clinician is the fact that the amount of bone loss after free bone transplantation is unpredictable. From various donor sites, free bone grafts with different bone qualities can be harvested.

Indications for Free Bone Grafts

Free bone grafts are generally indicated for the filling of bone defects, for example, after extirpation of large cysts. They are also used for ridge augmentation procedures in preprosthetic surgery and dental implantology. Small mandibular or maxillary continuity defects can be reconstructed with free bone grafts; other examples include osteotomy gaps in orthognathic surgery, defect zones in fractures, facial clefts, and small continuity defects in tumor surgery.[33] Free bone grafts are also used for augmentation procedures in esthetic surgery (malar augmentation, chin augmentation), but because of a potential loss of bone volume, grafting materials with less resorption (nonresorbable ceramic implants, homogeneous cartilage) should be taken into consideration on a case-by-case basis.[34,35]

Donor Sites

The choice of the donor site depends on the amount as well as the desired quality of the bone and potential donor site morbidity. The patients also must be informed about alternatives.

Chin

From the chin of mandibles of normal height, cortical bone grafts and also some cancellous bone can be taken in an amount of 3 cm^3.[36,37] The exposure of the chin region is performed from an intraoral incision. Depending on the patient's dentition, the incision is made in the nonattached vestibular mucosa or at the junction of the gingival margin. Under the apices of the lower incisors and canines and laterally to the mental foramina, the vestibular cortical plate is cut with a small round bur or a microsaw and taken with the use of a chisel (Figure 25.1). Under the cortical plate, some cancellous bone is also available. The amount of bone is sufficient for smaller regional grafting procedures such as cleft osteo-

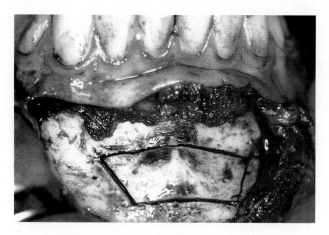

FIGURE 25.1 Harvesting of bone grafts from the chin.

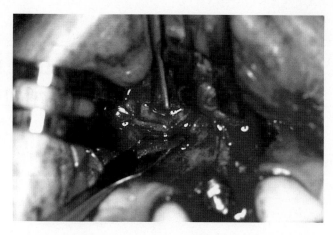

FIGURE 25.3 After a small incision in the upper vestibule, free bone graft can be taken from the nasal aperture.

plasties, filling of osteotomy gaps, and regional augmentation procedures in implantology. If a large bone graft has been taken, the defect in the chin region should be filled with resorbable ceramics or covered with a semipermeable membrane (guided bone regeneration) to prevent supramental soft tissue depression. The harvesting of too much cancellous bone can result in a permanent devitalization of the anterior mandibular dentition.

Retromolar Area

From the retromolar regions of both mandible and maxilla, small cortical and corticocancellous bone grafts can be taken via intraoral incisions and without significant donor site mor-

bidity (Figure 25.2).[38] The access is not as easy compared to the chin, and the amount of bone is somewhat smaller. It can be used for the same indications as bone grafts from the chin. One should consider the retromolar regions if the patient's wisdom teeth need to be removed.

Nasal Aperture

A small amount of cortical bone can be taken from the nasal aperture via an intraoral incision in the upper vestibular mucosa (Figure 25.3). Other than swelling and pain for a few days, there is no donor site morbidity. The bone is sufficient for small defects such as localized ridge augmentations in dental implantology.

Skull

From the skull, full-thickness free bone grafts as well as split-thickness cortical bone grafts from the outer table can be harvested.[39-41] Full-thickness bone grafts are taken for skull reconstruction. They are harvested using a template and then split with the help of a saw and a chisel in two grafts, one representing the outer and the other the inner table. One is used to reconstruct the missing bone, and the other is replanted into the donor site defect to reestablish normal contours and brain protection.

Outer table bone grafts can be harvested as cortical bone grafts of varying thickness, and as thicker corticocancellous bone grafts as well. Especially in craniofacial traumatology, calvarial bone grafts have become widespread in use, but they are also used in preprosthetic and esthetic surgery. The skull is exposed through a coronal or hemicoronal incision; the patient's head is not shaved (Figure 25.4). The bone is usually taken posteriorly from the coronal and laterally from the sagittal suture. To avoid injury to the sinuses and massive hemorrhage, care must be taken to place the donor site in such a way as to prevent perforation of the inner table in these areas.

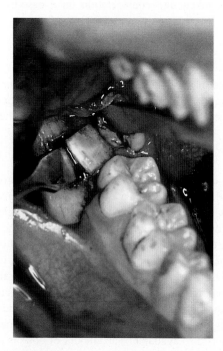

FIGURE 25.2 Retromolar area of the mandible is exposed for harvesting of free nonvascularized bone grafts.

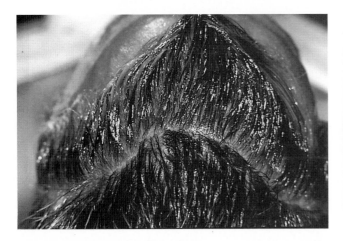

FIGURE 25.4 Planning of a coronal incision. The patient's hair has been treated with a gel, and then the incision line is defined with a comb. After that the head is washed with a local disinfectant.

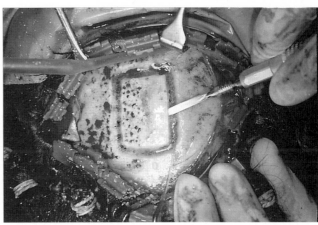

FIGURE 25.6 A microsaw is introduced between cortex and diploe to separate the table.

After exposure of the bone surface the desired size and shape of the bone graft are marked with a round bur (Figure 25.5). Drilling is performed through the outer table until a decreasing resistance indicates that the bur has reached the diploe. After that, a microsaw is inserted underneath the cortical bone to free it from the diploe (Figure 25.6). The osteotomy is then completed with a small chisel (Figures 25.7, 25.8). The use of a microsaw before introducing the chisel significantly reduces the risk of unpredictable fractures of the bone graft. Significant bleeding from the well-perfused diploe is prevented using bone wax to seal the donor site vessels. Harvesting of outer table bone grafts can result in a palpable depression, which is usually hidden to the observing eye. Nevertheless, the donor site defects can be filled with a pericranial galeoperiosteal rotation flap or alloplastic materials (ceramic implants, GoreTex sheets). Serious complications may arise from perforations through the inner table with subsequent hemorrhage and all the possible sequelae of epidural or, in extreme cases with dural laceration, subdural hemorrhage.

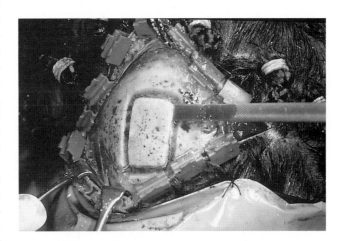

FIGURE 25.7 The bone graft is mobilized with the help of a small chisel.

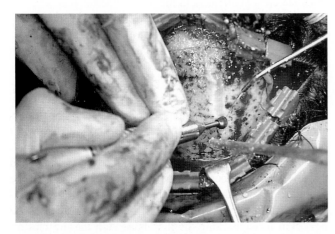

FIGURE 25.5 The desired amount of bone is marked. With a bur, the outer cortex is divided until the diploe is reached.

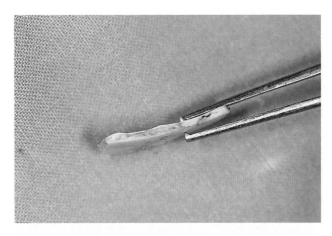

FIGURE 25.8 Isolated bone graft from the outer table for reconstruction of facial walls.

Rib

A free rib graft was among the first autogenous bone grafts to reconstruct the continuity of a mandible.[6,7,42] Because of the insufficient amount of bone and unpredictable resorption, a free rib graft today is not among the bone grafts of choice for mandible reconstruction in adults. Free rib grafts can be harvested at full thickness or split thickness and as composite costochondral grafts. Today we rarely see an indication for a full- or split-thickness rib graft, whereas costochondral grafts are used for reconstruction of the ascending ramus in children and for the condylar process in adults. A rib segment is harvested from a slightly curved incision in the anterior chest wall on the right side (Figure 25.9). Normally the fifth, sixth, or seventh rib, and in special cases also more than one rib, are taken. The incision is performed through skin and subcutaneous tissue and through the attached muscles to the anterior rib surface. After that the periosteum is stripped and the

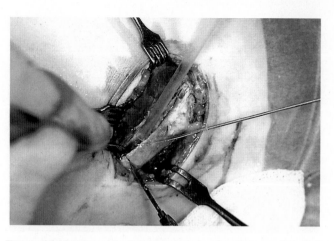

FIGURE 25.10 After stripping of muscles and periosteum the rib is osteotomized, in this pediatric patient with a help of a microsaw. The underlying soft tissues and the pleura must be protected.

osteotomies are performed with a saw or a special rib cutter (Figure 25.10).

Care must be taken not to harm the pleura. If a pleural laceration occurs, the defect must be sutured and a control x-ray must be taken after the operation because a pneumothorax may result. In the treatment of a possible pneumothorax, a thoracic surgeon should be consulted. Another possible complication is the development of pleuritis. The left side of the chest wall should be avoided to prevent penetration of the pericardium. After harvesting a rib graft, patients often complain of uncomfortable pain associated with movements of the chest wall while breathing.

Iliac Crest

The iliac crest is a donor site of outstanding importance for all kinds and shapes of free bone grafts and vascularized bone flaps.[9,43–45] Bone from the hip can be taken as cancellous, thin cortical, corticocancellous, and bicorticocancellous (full-thickness) bone grafts. The bone can be taken from the anterior iliac crest posteriorly to the anterosuperior iliac spine or the posterior ilium. The anterior iliac crest is the donor region of choice in most cases because during maxillofacial operations patients are usually in a supine position. To approach the posterior ilium a patient must be turned and thus the operation is prolonged; also, two-team operations are not possible. The size and the form of the ilium permits creating bone grafts in different shapes and sizes. The different bone grafts and bone qualities from the hip cover all the indications for free bone grafts as listed here.

Cancellous bone can be harvested as particulate bone and marrow and as cancellous bone blocks. To avoid donor site complications, cancellous bone and marrow are best taken utilizing a fenestration technique. The iliac crest is approached by a skin incision along the iliac bone with the muscles attached to the lateral side of the ilium remaining untouched.

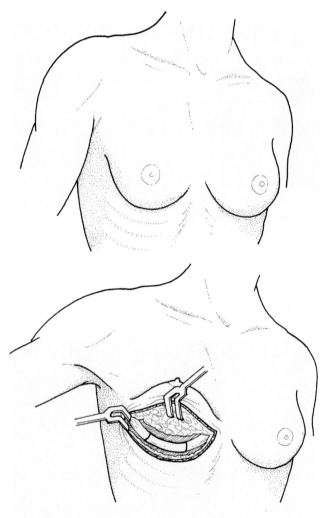

FIGURE 25.9 Free rib grafts are taken after a slightly curved incision overlying the fifth, sixth, or seventh rib on the right side of the chest wall. In female patients, the incision line can be hidden in the breast fold.

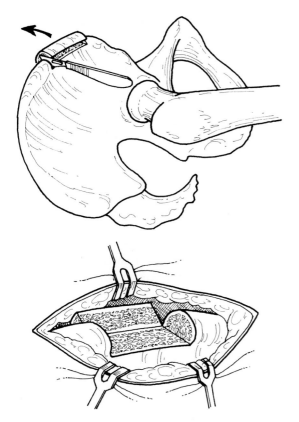

FIGURE 25.11 In pediatric patients the cartilage overlying the bony part of the ilium is separated from the bone with a scalpel. No osteotomy is needed for harvesting of cancellous bone and marrow.

In an adult, the fascia overlying the iliac crest is incised including the periosteum, with the periosteum and the muscles stripped only from the upper border of the iliac crest. With a saw, the cortical plate is cut but remains attached to the medial periosteum and the attached muscles. The marrow is harvested with a sharp spoon curette. After that, the cortical plate

is repositioned and fixed with a strong resorbable suture. With this technique the lateral and medial muscles stay in place and the bony contour is not affected. In pediatric patients, the cartilaginous growth area overlies the bony iliac crest and should be preserved to avoid growth disturbances and deformations of the hip. After exposure of the hip as described, the cartilage is separated from the bone with a knife (Figure 25.11). The bone under the cartilage is soft and can be harvested without any problems. Then, the cartilage is repositioned and fixed with a resorbable suture. Generally the wounds must be closed layer by layer.

Cancellous bone blocks are harvested with a similar technique, but in addition the periosteum on the inner surface of the hip must be elavated to allow an osteotomy of the inner cortex. The cortex on the lateral surface of the ilium is usually thin and is included in a cancellous bone block (Figure 25.12). The segment is then mobilized with a saw and a chisel and subsequently removed. The inner cortex is drilled down if a purely cancellous block is desired. A small amount of cancellous bone can also be taken through a stab incision laterally or above the iliac crest with the help of a trephine.

Cancellous bone and marrow are used to fill bone defects after extirpation of bone cysts, for alveolar clefts, and for smaller continuity defects such as defect fractures or osteotomy gaps. For reconstruction of larger continuity defects, cancellous bone and marrow were used in the past in tray systems such as titanium or dacron meshes or even in homogeneous mandibular cribs. Recent publications report significant complication rates after continuity reconstructions with cancellous bone and marrow in titanium trays.[46,47] In the authors' experience microvascular bone flaps are far superior to cancellous bone in tray systems, especially for reconstruction of larger continuity defects and in donor sites of poor quality.

In preprosthetic surgery, cancellous bone from the hip is used for sinus augmentation procedures and in combination with semipermeable membranes for localized ridge augmen-

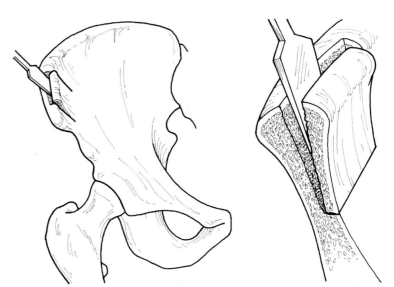

FIGURE 25.12 Cancellous bone blocks from the hip are removed from the inner surface with the inner cortex in place during harvesting.

tations. Cancellous bone blocks are frequently used for onlay and interposition osteoplasties in preprosthetic surgery and for reconstruction of (smaller) mandibular or maxillary continuity defects in jaw reconstruction or in complex orthognathic operations. Some authors prefer cancellous bone blocks versus corticocancellous bone grafts because for new bone formation the cortical layer-barrier is missing; other authors prefer corticocancellous grafts because of fixation reasons. Screws tend to have more primary stability if they engage at least one cortex, although the cortical part of the graft primarily is not vital bone.

Corticocancellous bone grafts are best taken from the inner surface of the hip, because the stripping of the inner periosteum is not as painful as the stripping of the outer periosteum, especially during walking on the first postoperative days. The approach is similar to that described for cancellous bone and marrow. In addition, the periosteum on the medial aspect of the ileum is elevated, including the attached muscles of the abdominal wall. With the help of a saw and a chisel, corticocancellous bone grafts can be harvested without contour deformations. As described, corticocancellous bone grafts mainly cover the same range of indications as cancellous bone blocks.

If a bicorticocancellous bone graft is needed, the periosteum and muscles must be stripped on both the inside and outside of the hip. Contour deformations can be avoided if the iliac crest itself is preserved (Figure 25.13). Bicortical grafts are sometimes used for mandibular reconstruction because they are more easily fixed with plates and screws than are cancellous blocks. After the fixation of a bicortical graft, the cortex areas not used for bone graft fixation should be

perforated with multiple bur holes or drilled down for better tissue ingrowth.

The hip is not the donor site of first choice for cortical bone grafts. Cortical bone grafts are mainly used in complex craniofacial surgery. These cases are frequently approached via a coronal incision, and thus the outer table of the skull, which is an excellent donor site for bone grafts, is already exposed. Also, the cortical plates of the hip are very thin and sometimes very soft. Complex craniofacial osteotomies sometimes require cancellous bone and cortical bone grafts as well, and in these rare cases both can be taken from the hip.

Tibia

In adult individuals, cortical and corticocancellous bone grafts can be harvested from the anterior surface of the tibial plateau without significant donor site complications. Bone grafts from the tibia have been used mainly for ridge augmentation and cleft palate procedures.

Pedicled Bone Grafts

In contrast to free bone grafts, pedicled bone grafts remain connected with the donor site by a vascular pedicle or attached soft tissues. This requires that the donor and recipient sites be located close to each other.

Pedicled Rib Grafts

Vascularized rib grafts can be harvested together with a pectoralis major muscle flap (vascular pedicle: superior thoracoacromial vessels) and in combination with a latissimus dorsi flap (vascular pedicle: branches from the thoracodorsal vessels to the serratus anterior muscle and the anterior chest wall). Both types of combined musculocutaneous-osteocutaneous flaps have been used for simultaneous reconstruction of large soft tissue defects in combination with continuity defects of the mandible.[17,18,48] Because of the limited range of these flaps, their indication is mainly limited to tissue defects in the lower third of the face and the neck with accompanying defects of the mandible. Today pedicled rib grafts together with soft tissue flaps from the pectoralis major or latissimus dorsi muscle are not the grafts of first choice, especially for mandible reconstruction, because the perfusion of the rib is unpredictable and pedicled rib grafts are often lost because of infection or partially lost because of resorption. Besides that, a rib usually does not give enough volume for functional mandible reconstruction. The placement of dental implants is virtually impossible.[49] In the authors' opinion, the current indications for combined pedicled flaps are limited to special problems in reconstruction, which in our hands consist mostly of large soft tissue defects in patients who have had radical cancer operations in the lower facial third and neck with full-dose irradiation therapy.

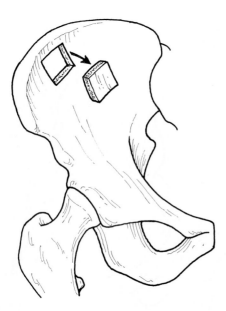

FIGURE 25.13 Harvesting of a bicorticocancellous bone block should be performed with preservation of a bony bridge in the region of the iliac crest to prevent contour deformations.

Temporalis Osteomuscular Flap

Together with the well-known temporalis muscle (better, musculofascious) flap, pedicled on the deep temporal vessels, a split- or even full-thickness portion of underlying temporal bone can be harvested. In connection to the temporal vessels the composite flap has a limited range and limited freedom of orientation as well, but it has been used to reconstruct maxillary and hard palate defects and even segments of the ascending mandibular ramus. The composite flap has also been advocated for use as a free microvascular flap, but poor results have been reported, especially for mandible reconstruction.[50]

Harvesting of temporal muscle and composite flaps may have a significant donor site morbidity. Among the unwanted side effects are a temporary or even permanent reduction in mouth-opening capacity and an unpleasant cosmesis known as temporal hollowing. The latter can be camouflaged by implanting alloplastic material (silastic, Gore Tex, ceramics, or other) into the temporal region.

Microvascular Bone and Composite Flaps

Microvascular bone flaps are always combined hard and soft tissue composite grafts, with bone, periosteum, and attached muscles, the so-called osteomuscular flaps. These composite flaps can be harvested from several donor areas; most frequently used in craniomaxillofacial reconstructive bone surgery are flaps from the iliac crest, scapula, fibula, and forearm. Composite bone grafts with a skin island are called osteomusculocutaneous flaps. In contrast to free nonvascularized grafts, microvascular bone flaps are nourished over a vascular pedicle containing a supplying artery and at least one draining vein, which in the recipient site must be connected to an artery and one or two accompanying veins. Under ideal conditions a microvascular flap therefore remains viable tissue directly after transplantation and does not need to be revascularized from the surrounding tissues. As an important consequence, almost no initial bone resorption and bone loss are observed after transplantation. A microvascular flap is by far more independent from the tissue qualities in the recipient site (scar formation, previous irradiation) compared to nonvascularized grafts. The possibility of transferring soft tissues together with bone for combined one-stage bone and soft tissue reconstruction has advantages in tumor surgery.

In contrast, a microvascular bone transplantation is technically much more demanding than a free bone transfer. It requires special surgical training and special equipment. Microvascular tissue transplantations are usually lengthy operations and can be problematic for patients in poorer general condition.

Indications for Microvascular Boneflaps

Microvascular bone flaps are indicated for the reconstruction of large bone defects, defects in recipient sites of poor quality, and when a simultaneous bone and soft tissue reconstruction is desired.

Combined Iliac Bone and Soft Tissue Flaps

Osteomuscular bone flaps from the hip contain iliac bone, periosteum, and at least a small strip of iliac muscle. Additional larger muscle islands from the internal oblique muscle are also possible. Both types of transplants can be harvested pedicled at the superficial circumflex iliac artery and vein (SCIA, SCIV) and the deep circumflex iliac vessels as well (DCIA, DCIV). The DCIA and DCIV are the more reliable vessels as far as the blood supply of the various iliac flap modifications is concerned.[16]

Iliac bone flaps are raised with the patient in a supine position and the donor site hip is elevated with the help of a cushion. The superior iliac spine, the iliac ligament, the pubic bone, and the femoral artery are palpated and marked on the patient's skin (Figure 25.14). The DCIA leaves the external iliac artery on its medial aspect normally 1 to 3 cm cranially to the inguinal ligament. The venous blood is usually drained by two accompanying veins, which mostly form one venous trunk 1 to 2 cm before the external iliac vein is reached. The two veins have complex connective branches and sometimes resemble a network of more than two distinct vessels. Therefore, both veins must be preserved during dissection. The DCIA and accompanying veins run superior to the inguinal ligament in a duplication of the fascias of the thigh and the abdominal wall, and reach the inner aspect of

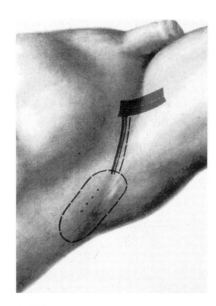

FIGURE 25.14 The femoral artery, the inguinal ligament, and the iliac crest are palpated and marked. The supplying vessels (DCIA, DCIV) leave the external iliac artery superior to the inguinal ligament toward the medial aspect of the iliac crest. The axis of the skin portion should be parallel to the crest; two-thirds of the skin island is located superiorly to the bone margin. The level of the perforators is outlined with dots.

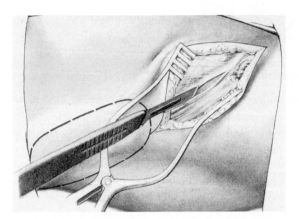

FIGURE 25.15 The femoral artery and vein are identified. After that the skin overlying the inguinal ligament is incised and the junction of the fascias of the abdominal wall and the thigh is exposed. The inguinal ligament is cut parallel to the axis of the DCIA and DCIV.

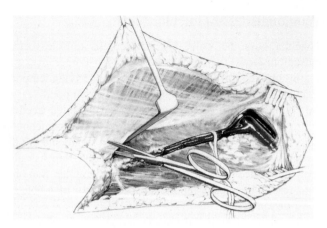

FIGURE 25.17 The edges of the skin island are cut down to the underlying fascia after the vascular pedicle has been isolated. The three layers of the abdominal muscles are divided leaving a muscle strip 3 cm wide attached to the bone and the overlying skin. The vascular pedicle lies in the junction of the iliacus and the transversalis fascia.

the ilium in the fascia of the iliac muscle 1 to 3 cm from the inner cortex of the iliac crest.

Overlying and superior to the iliac crest a skin island can be harvested. The skin portion is nourished by perforating vessels from the DCIA and DCIV, which reach the surface on the medial aspect of the iliac crest at a distance of 1 to 2 cm. The axis of the skin flap lies between the superior inferior iliac spine and tip of the scapula. Dissection starts with the exposure of the femoral artery, which can be easily palpated caudally to the inguinal ligament. Further dissection in the proximal direction leads to the DCIA, which leaves on the lateral aspect of the vessel, now called the external iliac artery, normally 1 to 3 cm cranially to the inguinal ligament (Figure 25.15). After that the DCIA and frequently the two accompanying veins are dissected as a bundle in a craniolateral direction. Dissection comes to a stop at 2 to 3 cm from the anterior superior iliac spine (Figure 25.16).

To raise an osteomuscular bone flap with a skin island, the desired skin portion is now dissected free. The incision divides skin and subcutaneous tissues down to the underlying abdominal fascia. Medially to the anterior superior iliac spine,

the lateral cutaneous femoral nerve should be exposed and preserved. The external and internal oblique as well as the transverse abdominal muscles are now incised 3 to 4 cm cranially to the iliac crest (Figure 25.17). The muscle portion of the flap must remain attached to the fascia and the skin so as not to harm the blood supply of the skin. The strip of abdominal muscle attached to the medial aspect of the iliac crest contains the perforating vessels, which are very sensitive and may be harmed even by shearing the different soft tissue layers against each other. At 3 to 4 cm superior to the iliac crest, the transverse abdominal muscle is represented through the transverse fascia, which is also incised. The abdominal wall is retracted medially, and the junction between transversal fascia and the fascia of the iliac muscle is identified (Figure 25.18). The vascular pedicle lies in the duplication of the two fascias and can be palpated at this stage.

The muscles on the lateral aspect of the ilium are then stripped. The periosteum can either be elevated or left in place if additional soft tissue coverage of the bone is desired. The

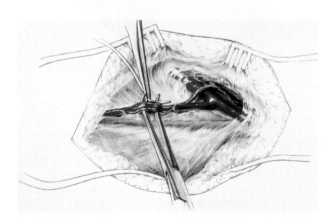

FIGURE 25.16 The vascular pedicle containing the DCIA and in most cases two accompanying veins is dissected.

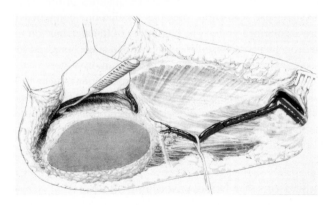

FIGURE 25.18 The fascia of the iliacus muscle together with a 2- to 3-cm strip of muscle must also be included in the flap. The iliacus muscle can be divided by blunt dissection.

bone is then osteotomized with an oscillating saw in the desired size and shape (Figure 25.19). The osteotomy site is sealed with bone wax (Figure 25.20). The iliac bone flap is completely freed from all surrounding tissues and remains only connected to the vascular pedicle. If there is any delay in the craniofacial part of the operation (tumor ablation, preparation of the recipient site), the flap is deposited in a subcutaneous pocket. Shortly before transplantation, the DCIA and then the DCIV are ligated and transected. The flap may be irrigated with saline solution but is not routinely rinsed with anticoagulants.

For raising of an osteomuscular iliac bone flap without a skin or a separate muscle island, the dissection is performed very similarly to the procedure just described. Because no skin is taken, the abdominal skin overlying the iliac crest is incised parallel to the bone. On the medial aspect of the ilium, the transverse and oblique abdominal muscles are cut close to the bone; only a strip of iliac muscle and fascia containing the vascular pedicle is left attached to the medial aspect of the ilium.[16,51,52]

A special consideration, in obese patients, is that the composite osteomusculocutaneous iliac bone flap provides too much bulk for intraoral soft tissue reconstruction. As an important variation, a osteomuscular flap with a large fasciomuscular soft tissue island from the internal oblique muscle can be harvested.[53] Therefore, the fascia of the transverse abdominal and external oblique muscles is cut close to the iliac crest. The internal oblique, underlying the external fascia and muscle, is now exposed. A nonconstant separate branch of the DCIA, which leaves the artery on its way between the internal iliac artery and anterior superior iliac spine, may go directly to the internal oblique muscle in a mediocranial direction and should be preserved when present. The internal oblique muscle and its fascia are dissected in the desired length and remain attached to the medial aspect of the iliac crest. A strip of iliac muscle containing the vascular pedicle is also included in the flap. The result is a compound flap of solid iliac bone with a potentially large soft tissue island of

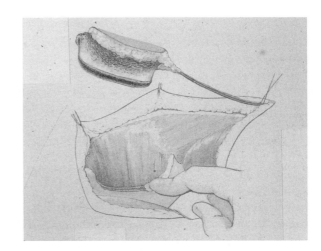

FIGURE 25.20 The vascular pedicle is ligated and divided after complete isolation of the flap. After sealing the iliac bone with bone wax, the abdominal wall is closed layer by layer.

internal oblique muscle and fascia (Figure 25.21), which can be used to replace resected intraoral mucosa (Figure 25.22). Therefore, the intraorally placed muscle and fascia are left to granulation (Figure 25.23) and subsequent secondary epithelialization from the surrounding mucous membrane. Despite a certain amount of shrinkage, usually good functional results can be obtained (Figure 25.24).

Flap Contouring

Especially in chin reconstruction, the only slightly curved iliac bone must be bent to adapt it to the shape of a mandible. For this purpose, the outer cortex (lateral cortex) of the flap's bony portion is osteotomized with an oscillating saw (Figure 25.25). The bone cut goes through the outer cortex and the cancellous portion of the flap. Care must be taken not to penetrate the medial cortex, because in so doing the attached segment of iliac muscle, the periosteum, and the vascular pedi-

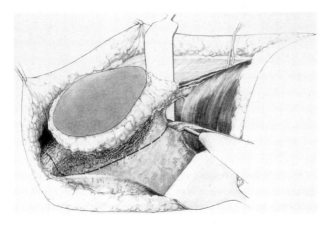

FIGURE 25.19 After stripping of muscles and periosteum attached to the lateral aspect of the iliac crest, the bony portion is cut with an oscillating saw.

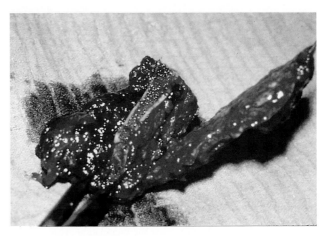

FIGURE 25.21 Osteomuscular bone flap from the hip with attached internal oblique muscle.

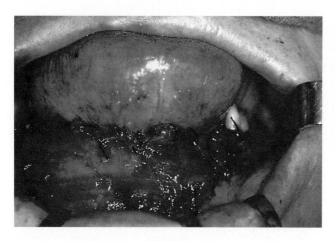

FIGURE 25.22 The internal oblique muscle can be used to cover defects of the oral mucosa, in this clinical case, of the anterior floor of the mouth.

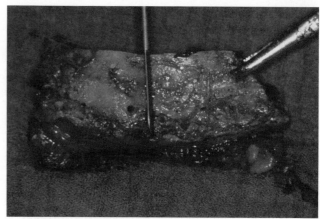

FIGURE 25.25 An osteotomy of the former lateral cortex of the hip now included in osteomuscular iliac bone flap is necessary if the bone must be bent to adjust it to a special clinical situation.

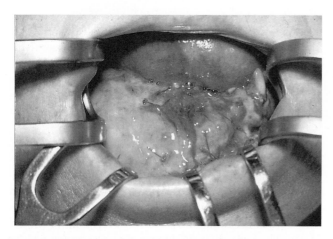

FIGURE 25.23 The muscle granulates after transplantation and is secondarily epithelialized from the surrounding mucosa.

cle may be injured, thus compromising the blood supply. After that the bone can be bent in the desired fashion (Figure 25.26).

Scapular Bone and Combined Flaps

The scapula is a triangular-shaped bone with a very thin center portion, whereas the borders of the scapula are composed of more solid bone. The lateral border of the scapula provides sufficient bone for craniomaxillofacial reconstruction purposes. Pedicled on the circumflex scapular artery and frequently two accompanying veins, bone flaps with a thickness of approximately 1.5 cm, a height of approximately 3 cm, and a length of 10 to 14 cm can be harvested. Although the

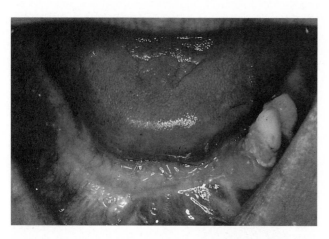

FIGURE 25.24 Clinical situation after the granulation process is finished.

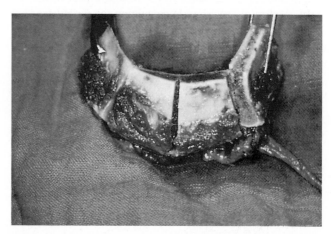

FIGURE 25.26 Bone flap after multiple monocortical osteotomies. Depending on the desired length of the flap, the bone can either be contoured by removing wedges from the lateral aspect of the hip or by monocortical osteotomies and bending to the medial aspect as shown. The bone gaps at the osteotomy sites are then filled with cancellous bone and marrow.

absolute amount of bone depends very much on the individual patient's condition, the lateral border of the scapula is usually composed of enough bone even for mandible reconstruction.

The vascular axis containing the circumflex scapular artery can be elongated in dissecting the subscapular vessels up to the axilla. Through this technique a long vascular pedicle of approximately 12 to 14 cm can be created, which has advantages for special indications, among them reconstruction of the maxilla or mandible in a compromised vessel situation. On the common subscapular vascular pedicle, the scapular bone flap can be combined with a scapular or parascapular fasciocutaneous and a musculocutaneous flap from the latissimus dorsi muscle. Various flap combinations are also possible.

Flap dissection is usually performed with the patient turned on their side. Important anatomic landmarks are the scapular spine, the lateral border of the scapula, and the muscle gap between major and minor teres muscles on one side and the long triceps head on the other side. This muscle gap lies cranially to the middle portion of the lateral margin of the scapula. The bone is supplied via vessels running in a deep plane parallel to the lateral margin of the bone, whereas two other small terminal branches of the circumflex scapular artery nourish the scapular and parascapular flaps, respectively (Figure 25.27). The scapular flap is raised over a vascular axis that runs parallel to the scapular spine approximately in the middle between scapular tip and scapular spine. The parascapular flap vessel axis also lies parallel to the lateral margin of the scapula, but in a subcutaneous plane.

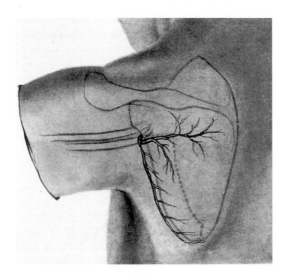

FIGURE 25.27 Bone grafts from the glenoid fossa to the tip can be taken from the lateral aspect of the scapula. Pedicled on the cutaneous branches of the circumflex scapular artery, a scapular or parascapular skin flap (or both) can be harvested in addition. Before dissection of the lateral border of the scapula, the crista scapulae and the muscular gap between teres minor and major muscles and the long head of the triceps muscle are palpated and marked.

To make microvascular anastomoses easier, it is advisable to include the subscapular artery and vein in the pedicle and therefore prepare as much vessel length as possible. The dissection of the axillary and subscapular vessels starts with a skin incision over and parallel to the anterior axillary fold. In the loose subcutaneous tissues, the junction between axillary and subscapular vessels is exposed. The circumflex scapular artery leaves the subscapular artery normally 2 to 4 cm caudally to the axillary vessels. As an important variation, sometimes both arteries leave the axillary artery separately. Two veins normally run with the circumflex scapular artery; both should be dissected and preserved. The vascular pedicle is further dissected medially into the lateral muscular gap. Careful ligation of small vessels to the surrounding muscles is mandatory. To gain better access, the skin overlying the vascular pedicle can be incised. The muscle gap beside the lateral scapular border is palpated and localized. After retraction of the latissimus dorsi and teres major muscles, the vascular pedicle can be seen in the muscle gap. There the subscapular vessels divide into three terminal branches, one to the bony portion and the remaining two to the scapular and parascapular skin islands.

If a combination of a bone flap together with a scapular or a parascapular flap is desired, the size of the soft tissue island must be defined at that stage of the operation. This is usually performed with the help of an individual template. Then, an incision is made through skin and underlying fascia and the soft tissue flap is raised from the muscle. This is performed from medially to laterally in the case of the scapular and in a caudal-cranial direction so far as the parascapular flap is concerned. Lateral to the bony border, in the region of the muscle gap, both skin flaps must remain in connection with the circumflex scapular vessels.

If a osteomuscular bone flap without additional skin flaps is desired, the skin overlying the scapula is simply incised parallel to the lateral bone margin from the scapular spine to the tip. On the lateral aspect of the scapula, the teres minor muscle inserts cranially and the teres major muscle inserts caudally. The muscles are cut leaving a muscle strip at least 1 cm wide attached to the bone. The vascular pedicle is thus protected. Osteotomy of the bone is now performed from posterior with a saw (Figure 25.28). The upper osteotomy line must remain approximately 2 cm from the glenoid fossa. Now the one strut, which is still connected to the underlying muscles, is elevated.

The subscapular muscle, which has its origin on the costal aspect of the scapula, is incised leaving a muscle strip of approximately 1 cm attached to the bone. The bone or combined bone and soft tissue flap is now completely isolated on its vascular pedicle, and the latter is ligated in the desired length (Figure 25.29). If the subscapular vessels are included in the vascular axis, the thoracodorsal artery and vein must also be ligated. Preserving these vessels allows various flap combinations potentially including a scapular bone flap, scapular and parascapular soft tissue flaps, and

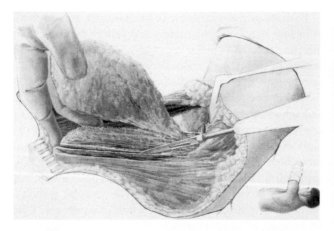

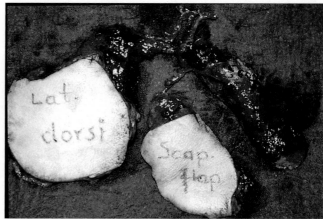

FIGURE 25.28 After dissection of the circumflex scapular vessels, and, if a long vascular pedicle is required the subscapular vessels as well, the desired fasciocutaneous flap is elevated first. The muscles attached to the lateral border of the scapula are then divided leaving a strip of muscle approximately 2 cm wide attached to the bone. The muscles inserting on the posterior aspect of the scapula are also divided, leaving a thin muscle cuff in place. The bone is cut with a saw and elevated. After access is given to the costal surface of the scapula, the subscapular muscle is divided.

a musculocutaneous latissimus dorsi flap,[19,51,52] (Figure 25.30).

FIGURE 25.30 Combination of osteomuscular and fasciocutaneous scapula and a musculocutaneous latissimus dorsi flap on the common subscapular vascular pedicle.

Fibula Bone and Combined Flaps

The fibula is a source for long bone flaps with a compact bone structure. The flap can be harvested with the patient lying on the back, side, or abdomen. A two-team approach in max-

illofacial reconstructive surgery can usually only be achieved with the patient in a supine position. The patient's leg is flexed in both hip and knee with the hip joint in inward rotation. In this position the complete fibula can normally be palpated through the skin from the fibula head to the lateral malleolus (Figure 25.31).

The supplying vessel of the fibula bone and combined flap is the peroneal artery, which rarely is also the dominant vascular supply for the foot. Therefore, before flap harvesting an angiogram is mandatory. The vascular axis of the bone flap lies medial to the fibula. The bone itself is nourished mainly via perforators to the medial periosteum. As a consequence, stripping of the medial periosteum during dissection or flap fixation must be avoided. Dissection of the bone flap starts with the incision of the skin on the lateral aspect of the fibula.

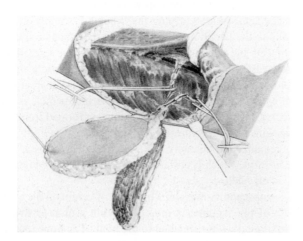

FIGURE 25.29 The osteomuscular and the fasciocutaneous portions of the combined flap are isolated and pedicled on the common vascular axis represented by the circumflex scapular vessels. The latissimus dorsi muscle is elevated. Now the flap can be transposed anteriorly into the axilla, and the subscapular vessels can be dissected to gain a longer vascular pedicle. An additional portion of a latissimus dorsi flap pedicled on the thoracodorsal vessels can also be included in the flap.

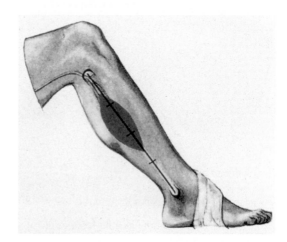

FIGURE 25.31 For harvesting of a fibula flap, the patient's leg is flexed in both hip and knee with the hip joint in inward rotation. In this position the complete fibula is palpated through the skin from the fibula head to the external malleolus and marked. An ovally shaped skin island can be harvested parallel to the bone axis and overlying the proximal two-thirds of the bone.

The common popliteal nerve, which runs in a subcutaneous plane lateral to the fibular head, is exposed and preserved. The subcutaneous tissues are separated down to the deep muscular fascia. After that, the so-called posterior intermuscular septum between the anteriorly (long and short peroneal muscles) and posteriorly located muscles (soleus muscle, long and short flexor hallucis muscles) is dissected (Figure 25.32). Blunt dissection of the anteriorly and posteriorly located muscles gives good access to the lateral surface of the fibula. The peroneal muscles are freed from the fibula, whereas the periosteum should remain attached to the bone because stripping of the lateral periosteum may lead to an elevation of the periosteum on the medial side, thus separating the vascular pedicle from the bone. Preservation of the periosteum is essential for the blood supply to the bony portion of the flap.

This first step of the dissection ends when the anterior edge of the fibula is reached. Adherent to the anterior edge is the anterior intermuscular septum. It is cut close to the bone, and then the long and short extensor digitorum muscles are also separated from the bone again in an epiperiosteal plane. Directly in front of the fibula, the anterior tibial artery and vein can be palpated and inspected after the extensor muscles have been cut. These vessels must be preserved; together with the extensor muscles they are retracted to the side. The interosseous membrane is exposed over and cut shortly above the fibula. The vascular axis of the fibula flap containing the peroneal vessels, lying on the medial aspect close to the bone, must be handled with great care. Now the fibula is osteotomized in the desired length to allow sufficient access to the soft tissues on the posteromedial side of the bone (Figure

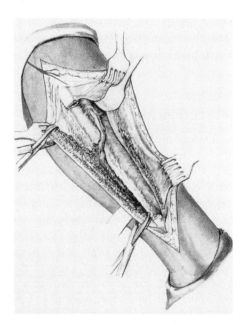

FIGURE 25.33 Harvesting of a bone-only flap. After detaching the muscles on the lateral and anterior surface of the fibula, the bone is divided and transposed laterally. After that the peroneal vessels are easily identified. A strip of the posterior tibialis and hallucis longus muscles together with the periosteum remains attached to the bone.

25.33). The bony segment is mobilized laterally and posteriorly. Behind the distal osteotomy line the peroneal vessels are identified and ligated. The vascular pedicle lies posterior to the interosseous membrane embedded in loose connective tissues. In this stage of the dissection, care must be taken to not separate the vessels from the periosteum. Finally, the peroneal vessels are dissected proximally up to the popliteal vessel and then ligated.

If a fibula flap with a skin paddle is required, the planning starts with the definition of the desired amount of skin. The axis of the skin portion overlies the lateral border of the fibular bone and the posterior intermuscular septum. Blood supply to the skin is brought by septocutaneous or musculocutaneous perforators out of the peroneal vessels, which are located in the posterior intermuscular septum and sometimes in the soleus muscle close to the muscle surface. To make perfusion of the skin island safer, it is recommended that a strip of soleus muscle adjacent to the intermuscular septum be included in the flap.

The posterior and anterior edges of the flap are incised and the skin is elevated on both sides together with the deep fascia. Via the posterior intermuscular septum, the center of the flap always remains in close contact to the lateral aspect of the bone. The skin portion is now elevated anteriorly and the dissection is directed toward the posterior crural septum, until the perforators can be identified in the subcutaneous layer. The bone is now divided into the desired lengths, after which further soft tissue dissection is easier. The soleus muscle is separated from the fibula, leaving a thin strip of muscle (about 1.0 cm) attached to the bone. The flexor hallucis longus mus-

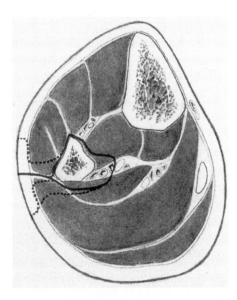

FIGURE 25.32 Cross cut through the lower leg. The supplying peroneal vessels are lying on the medial aspect of the bone. The skin island is nourished by perforators from the peroneal vessels, which come around the posterior surface of the fibula into the posterior intermuscular septum. Sometimes they are lying in the soleus muscle close to the muscle surface. Therefore, some authors recommend including a strip of soleus muscle in the flap.

cle is separated, and then the peroneal vessels are ligated and cut at the distal end of the flap. The final steps of the dissection are similar to the dissection of a bone-only flap.[51–53]

Radial Forearm Osteomuscular-Fasciocutaneous Flap

The fasciocutaneous distal radial forearm flap today seems to be one of the most popular flaps for intraoral reconstruction.[54] The thin and pliable flap is pedicled on the radial artery and the deep venae commitantes. For venous drainage of the soft tissue flap, subcutaneous veins from the forearm are also sufficient. The radial artery and the accompanying veins lie in a duplicate of the antebrachial fascia. From there small vessels ascend to the overlying skin, and other vessels descend to the brachioradialis muscle. Together with a part of this muscle, a segment of the radius can be taken, thus turning the fasciocutaneous soft tissue into a fasciocutaneous-osteomuscular radial forearm flap.

Harvesting of the composite radial forearm flap has quite a significant donor site morbidity; radius fractures in up to 20% of the cases have been reported. The available bone is very small in width, height, and length. Therefore, the radial forearm bone and soft tissue flap is not a flap of first choice for functional mandible reconstruction.

References

1. Axhausen W. Die Bedeutung der Individual- und Artspezifität der Gewebe für die freie Knochenüberpflanzung. *Hefte Unfallheikunde.* 1962;72:1.
2. Schweiberer L. Experimentelle Untersuchungen von Knochentransplantaten mit unveränderter und denaturierter Knochengrundsubstanz. Hefte Unfallheilk 103. Berlin: Springer; 1970.
3. Bardenheuer B. Über Unter- und Oberkieferresektion. *Verh Dtsch Ges Chir.* 1892;21:123–130.
4. Sykoff V. Zur Frage der Knochenplastik am Unterkiefer. *Zentralbl Chir.* 1900;27:81.
5. Krause F. Unterkiefer-Plastik. *Zentralbl Chir.* 1907;34:1045–1046.
6. Axhausen G. Histologische Untersuchungen über Knochentransplantationen am Menschen. *Dtsch Z Chir.* 1908;91:388–428.
7. Lexer E. Die Verwendung der freien Knochenplastik nebst Versuchen über Gelenkversteifung und Gelenktransplantation. *Arch Klin Chir.* 1908;86:939.
8. Rydygier LRV. Zum osteoplastischen Ersatz nach Unterkieferresektion. *Zentralbl Chir.* 1908;35:1321–1322.
9. Lindemann A. Über die Beseitigung der traumatischen Defekte der Gesichtsknochen. In: Bruhn C, Hrg. *Die gegenwärtigen Behandlungswege der Kieferschußverletzungen.* Hefte IV–VI. Bergmann Wiesbaden: 1916.
10. Matti H. Über freie Transplantation von Knochenspongiosa. *Langenbecks Arch Clin Chir.* 1932;168:236.
11. Converse JM. Early and late treatment of gunshot wounds of the jaw in French battle casualities in North Africa and Italy. *J Oral Surg.* 1945;3:112–137.
12. Conley JJ. Use of composite flaps containing bone for major repairs in the head and neck. *Plast Reconstr Surg.* 1972;49:522.
13. Boyne P. Methods of osseous reconstruction of the mandible following surgical resection. *J Biomed Mat.* 1973;4:195.
14. Taylor GI, Miller G, Ham F. The free vascularized bone graft. A clinical extension of microvascular techniques. *Plast Reconstr Surg.* 1975;55:553–554.
15. O'Brien B McC. *Microvascular Reconstructive Surgery.* Edinburgh: Churchill Livingstone; 1977.
16. Taylor GI, Townsend P, Corlett R. Superiority of the deep circumflex iliac vessels as the supply for free groin flaps. *Plast Reconstr Surg.* 1979;64:745.
17. Quillen CG. Latissimus dorsi myocutaneous flap in head and neck reconstruction. *Plast Reconstr Surg.* 1979;63:664.
18. Ariyan S. The viability of rib grafts transplanted with the periostal blood supply. *Plast Reconstr Surg.* 1980;65:140–151.
19. Swartz WM, Banis JC, Newton ED, Ramasastry SS, Jones NF, Acland R. The osteocutaneous scapular flap for mandibular and maxillary reconstruction. *Plast Reconstr Surg.* 1986;77:530–545.
20. Axhausen W. Die Quellen der Knochenneubildung nach freier Transplantation. *Langenbecks Arch Klin Chir.* 1951;279:439–443.
21. Axhausen W. Die Knochenregeneration—ein zweiphasiges Geschehen. *Zentralbl Chir.* 1952;77:435–442.
22. Chalmers J. Transplantation immunity in bone homografting. *J Bone Joint Surg.* 1959;41B:160–179.
23. Williams RG. Comparison of living autogeneous and homogeneous grafts cancellous bone heterotopically placed in rabbits. *Anat Rec.* 1962;143:93.
24. Heiple KG, Chase SW, Herndon CH. A comparative study of the healing process following different types of bone transplantation. *J Bone Joint Surg* 1963;45A:1593.
25. Ray RD, Sabet TY. Bone grafts: cellular survival versus induction. *J Bone Joint Surg.* 1963;45A:337.
26. Burwell RG. Osteogenesis in cancellous bone grafts: considered in terms of cellular changes, basic mechanisms and the perspective of growth control and its possible aberrations. *Clin Orthop.* 1965;40:35–47.
27. Lentrodt J, Höltje WJ. Tierexperimentelle Untersuchungen zur Revaskularisation autologer Knochentransplantate. In: Schuchardt K, Scheunemann H, eds. *Fortschriffe der Kiefer-und Gesichts-Chirurgie,* Vol. 20. Stuttgart: Thieme; 1976:17–21.
28. Eitel F, Schweiberer K, Saur K, Dambe LT, Klapp F. Theoretische Grundlagen der Knochentransplantation: Osteogenese und Revaskularisation als Leistung des Wirtslagers. In: Hierholzer G, Zilch H, eds. *Transplantatlager und Implantatlager bei verschiedenen Operationsverfahren.* Berlin: Springer, 1980.
29. Schweiberer L, Brenneisen R, Dambe LT, Eitel F, Zwank L. Derzeitiger Stand der auto-, hetero- und homoplastischen Knochentransplantation. In: Cotta H, Martini AK, eds. *Implantate und Transplantate in der Plastischen und Weiderherstellungschirurgie.* Berlin: Springer; 1981:115–127.
30. Lentrodt J, Fritzemeier CU, Bethmann I. Erfahrungen bei der osteoplastischen Unterkieferrekonstruktion mit autologen freien Knochentransplantaten. In: Kastenbauer E, Wilmes E, Mees K, eds. *Das Transplantat in der Plastischen Chirurgie.* Rotenburg: Sasse; 1987:59–61.
31. Steinhäuser EW. Unterkieferrekonstruktion durch intraorale

Knochentransplantate—deren Einheilung und Beeinflussung durch die Funktion—eine tierexperimentelle Studie. *Schweiz Monatsschr Zahnheilk.* 1968;78:213.

32. Reuther JF. *Druckplattenosteosynthese und freie Knochentransplantation zur Unterkieferrekonstruktion.* Berlin: Quintessenz; 1979.

33. Bell WH. *Modem Practice in Orthognathic and Reconstructive Surgery.* Philadelphia: WB Saunders; 1992.

34. Sailer HF. *Transplantation of Lyophilized Cartilage in Maxillo-Facial Surgery.* Basel: Krager; 1983.

35. Wolford LM. The use of porous block hydroxyapatite. In: Bell WH, ed. *Modern Practice in Orthognathic and Reconstructive Surgery.* Philadelphia: WB Saunders; 1992:854–871.

36. Hoppenreijs TJM, Nijdam ES, Freihofer HPM. The chin as a donor site in early secondary osteoplasty: a retrospective clinical and radiological evaluation. *J Craniomaxillofac Surg.* 1992;20:119–124.

37. Sailer HF, Pajarola GF. Plastische Korrekturen an Weichteilen und Knochen. In: *Orale Chirurgie.* Stuttgart: Thieme; 1996:308–309.

38. Schliephake H. Entnahmetechniken autologer Knochentransplantate. *Implantologie* 1994;4:317–327.

39. Tessier P. Autogenous bone grafts from the calvarium for facial and cranial application. *Clin Plast Surg.* 1982;9:531–538.

40. Maves MD, Matt BH. Calvarial bone grafting of facial defects. *Otolaryngol Head Neck Surg.* 1986;95:464–470.

41. Frodel JL, Marentette LJ, Quatela VC, Weinstein GS. Calvarial bone graft harvest: techniques, considerations, and morbidity. *Arch Otolaryngol Head Neck Surg.* 1993;119:17–23.

42. Payr E. Über osteoplastischen Ersatz nach Kieferresektion (Kieferdefekten) durch Rippenstücke mittels gestielter Brustwandlappen oder freier Transplantation. *Zentralbl Chir.* 1908;35:1065–1070.

43. Klapp R. Über chirurgische Behandlung der Kieferschußbrüche. *Z Ärztl Fortbild.* 1916;13:225–232.

44. Rehrmann A. Das freie Knochentransplantat zum Unterkieferersatz unter besonderer Berücksichtigung der Kinnrekonstruktion. In: Schuchardt K, Schilli W, eds. *Fortschritte der Kiefer- und Gesichts Chirurgie,* vol. 23. Stuttgart: Thieme; 1978:39.

45. Riediger D, Ehrenfeld M. Der vaskularisierte Knochenspan, experimentelle Grundlagen und klinische Anwendung. In: Kastenbauer E, Wilmes E, Mees K, eds. *Das Transplantat in der Plastischen Chirurgie.* Rotenburg: Sasse; 1987:4–9.

46. Esser E, Mrosk T. Langzeitergebnisse nach Unterkieferrekonstruktionen mit avaskulärem Spongiosatransfer und Titangitter. In: Schwenzer N, ed. *Fortschritte der Kiefer- und Gesichts Chirurgie,* vol. 39. Stuttgart: Thieme; 1994:90–92.

47. Michel C, Reuther J, Meier J, Eckstein T. Die Differentialindikation mikrochirurgischer und freier autogener Knochentransplantate zur Rekonstruktion des Unterkiefers. In: Schwenzer N, ed. *Fortschritte der Kiefer- und Gesichts Chirurgie,* vol. 39. Stuttgart: Thieme; 1994:96–100.

48. Riediger D, Schmelzle R. Modifizierte Anwendung des myokutanen Latissimus dorsi-Lappens zur Defektdeckung im Mund-KieferGesichtsbereich. *Dtsch Z Mund Kiefer Gesichts Chir.* 1986;10:364–374.

49. Jack U. Vergleichende Untersuchung zahnärztlicher Implantatsysteme auf ihre Eignung zur Implantation in Rippentransplantate. Thesis. Germany: University of Tübingen; 1994.

50. Hammer B, Prein J. Differentialindikation mikrochirurgischer Knochentransplantate für die Rekonstruktion des Unterkiefers. In: Bootz F, Ehrenfeld M, eds. *Aktuelle Ergebnisse des mikrovaskulären Gewebetransfers im Kopf-Hals-Bereich.* Stuttgart: Thieme; 1995:149.

51. Strauch B, Yu HL. *Atlas of Microvascular Surgery.* New York: Thieme; 1993.

52. Riediger D, Ehrenfeld M. Mikrochirurgie. In: Hausamen JE, Machtens E, Reuther J, eds. *Kirschnersche allgemeine und spezielle Operationslehre. Mund-, Kiefer- und Gesichtschirurgie.* Heidelberg: Springer; 1995:559–615.

53. Urken ML, Weinberg H, Vickery C, Buchbinder D, Lawson W, Biller HF. The internal oblique-iliac crest free flap in composite defects of the oral cavity involving bone, skin, and mucosa. *Laryngoscope.* 1991;101:257–270.

54. Soutar DS. The radial forearm flap in intraoral reconstruction. In: Riediger D, Ehrenfeld M, eds. *Microsurgical Tissue Transplantation.* Chicago: Quintessence; 1989:31–38.

26
Current Practice and Future Trends in Craniomaxillofacial Reconstructive and Corrective Microvascular Bone Surgery

Hubert Weinberg, Lester Silver, and Jin K. Chun

The introduction of vascularized bone grafting has dramatically improved the potential for reconstruction of complex defects of the mandible, and it has improved the results of surgical restoration of the midface and cranial regions following tumor ablation or severe trauma. The reconstruction of the mandible in particular had been fraught with many difficulties, especially by the unfavorable milieu caused by oral contamination. The requirements of the reconstructed mandible include the maintenance of structural integrity for mastication, the successful union of adjacent bone segments, and the continued mobility of the jaw.[1] Reconstruction of the midface and cranium, on the other hand, has different requirements for accurate three-dimensional stable bony replacement. The replacement bone in this region must often be thin and pliable to provide the proper shape and size.[2]

The first vascularized bone grafts (VBGs) were described for lower-extremity reconstruction by Taylor et al.[3] and Buncke et al.[4] Shortly thereafter, McKee[5] described the microvascular rib transposition for mandibular reconstruction. Since then, there have been numerous studies both of the head and neck and of the extremities, which have examined the relative merits of vascularized and nonvascularized bone grafts. While nonvascularized bone heals by resorption and creeping substitution, vascularized bone maintains live cells that are capable of regeneration and provides immediate structural support.[6-8] In addition, vascularized bone has been shown to continue to survive in a radiated bed with evidence of callus formation and a fully viable bone marrow with new bone formation in the subperiosteal and endosteal layers.[9]

Mandibular Reconstruction

Absolute indications for reconstructing the mandible with VBGs were given by Chen et al.[10] and include: (1) osteoradionecrosis of the mandible or an irradiated tissue bed; (2) hemimandibular reconstruction with a free and facing glenoid fossa; (3) long segment mandibular defect, especially across the symphysis; (4) inadequate skin or mucosal lining; (5) defects demanding sandwich reconstruction; (6) inability to ob-

tain secure immobilization on the reconstructed unit; (7) failure of reconstruction by other methods; and (8) near-total mandibular reconstruction. The advantages of VBGs in these settings have been clearly demonstrated in extensive clinical studies. The early success rate in these studies has exceeded 90%, further demonstrating the safety and reliability of mandibular reconstruction with vascularized bone.[11,12]

The ideal qualities of the vascularized bone graft for mandibular reconstruction have been described by Urken.[13] It should be well vascularized; of sufficient length, width, and height; easily shaped without compromise to its vascularity; accessible for a simultaneous two-team approach; and have minimum donor site morbidity. Particularly for the mandible, the ideal qualities of the composite soft tissue requirements also need to be considered. The soft tissue component should be again well vascularized, thin, pliable, abundant, sensate if possible, and well lubricated. Often it is the soft tissue component and not solely the restoration of bony continuity that will determine the ultimate success of the mandibular reconstruction. The soft tissue may be needed to restore external neck or facial skin, and it may be required for mucosal replacement of the mandible, tongue, or pharynx. Soft tissue reconstruction should maintain tongue mobility and allow unimpeded swallowing and articulation.

The choice of donor sites available for mandibular reconstruction includes the iliac crest, fibula, scapula, metatarsus, cranium, rib, radius, ulna, and humerus. At present, in the vast majority of mandibular reconstructions, the iliac crest, fibula, or scapula is used. The iliac crest has proven to provide the best bone stock, especially for primary placement of endosseous dental implants (Figure 26.1).[14] A modification of the iliac crest osteomyocutaneous free flap including the internal oblique muscle has been described.[15-17] This latter muscle provides thin, well-vascularized soft tissue that upon denervation atrophy approximates the appearance of mucosa. The fibula provides the greatest bone length of all the VBGs and can be contoured to that of a mandible with numerous osteotomies (Figure 26.2).[18] The height of the fibula is, however, somewhat restrictive in its capacity to accept an endosseous implant, although it can be sectioned and double-

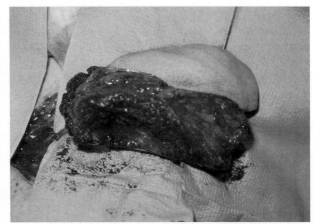

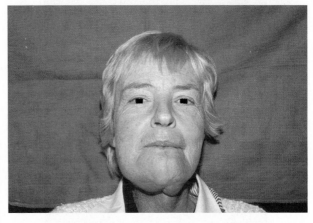

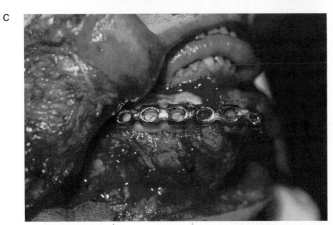

FIGURE 26.1 Deep circumflex iliac artery osteocutaneous flap. (a) Flap design. (b) Harvested flap in situ. (c) Flap inset with rigid fixation. (d) Postoperative result.

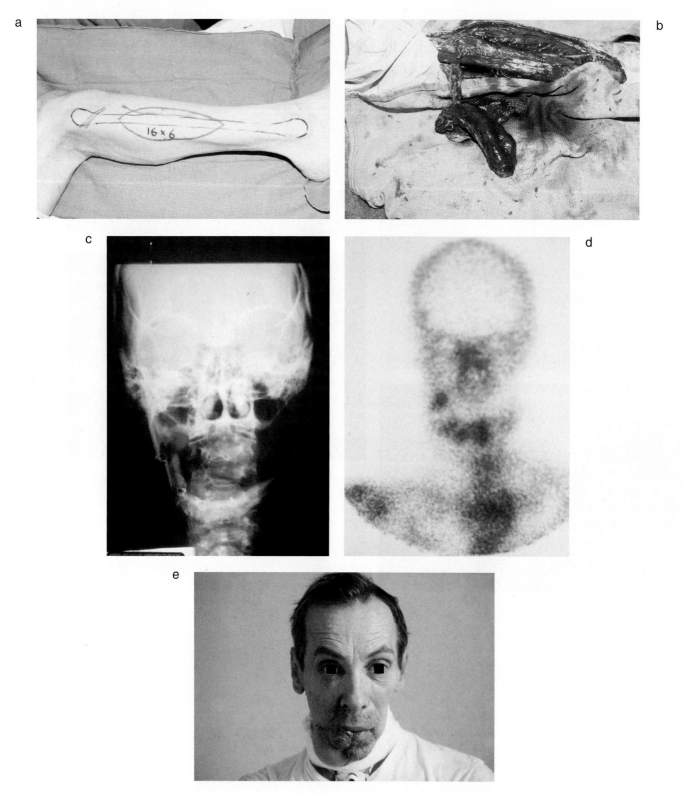

FIGURE 26.2 Fibula osteocutaneous flap. (a) Flap design. (b) Harvested flap with osteotomized segments and miniplate fixation in situ. (c) Postoperative posterior-anterior radiograph. (d) Postoperative technetium-99 bone scan demonstrating vascular uptake. (e) Postoperative result.

layered to increase its height, as in the double-barrel technique.[19,20] The cutaneous segment of the fibula flap may also at times prove to be unreliable. The scapula flap has an excellent soft tissue component that makes it ideal for soft tissue restoration in the mandibular region.[21] However, the bone stock available is again fairly limited as is bone length. Furthermore, because of patient positioning, a two-team approach is often needed, thereby increasing the difficulty of this procedure.

Craniofacial Reconstruction

The indications for use of vascularized bone grafts for craniofacial reconstruction are less well defined than in the mandible.[26] The soft tissue bed in this region is well vascularized, and often autogenous, nonvascularized bone grafts and alloplastic substitutes do quite well. Furthermore, well-described pedicled bone flaps based on the temporoparietal fascia can be rotated into adjacent regions with little difficulty (Figure 26.3).[22,23] Should the recipient bed, however, be scarred with poor vascularization and the required bony reconstruction quite large, then certainly VBGs are indicated and have been used successfully.[24] Vascularized bone grafts in these circumstances have been noted to maintain contour and size very well when followed for periods ranging from 3 to 8 years.[25]

The choice of bone graft donor sites will depend on careful analysis of the characteristics of the defect and the corresponding characteristics of the flap. An analysis must therefore be made of the extent of bone loss, the soft tissue deficit, whether skin, mucosa, or both, and the nature of the functional derangement. Computer-generated templates have also been used to accurately predict size, contour, and orientation of the VBG.[27] The choice of flap in turn must address the length of the vascular pedicle, the thickness of the soft tissue component, the mobility of the soft tissue, the dimensions and configuration of the bone in relation to the defect, and finally the associated donor site morbidity.[2] Unlike the mandible, with a number of recipient blood vessels from which to choose, in the craniofacial region strong consideration must be given to the selection and location of a recipient pedicle. The facial artery and vein are often the best suited for vascular anastomoses in reconstruction of the midface, but they will probably not be of sufficient length for reconstructions of the nose and orbit. The superficial temporal vessels, while at times suitable as recipient vessels, will often be of small caliber and prove to be inadequate for microvascular anastomoses. Vein grafts may be required to achieve a sufficiently long pedicle, but this will certainly add to the time and complexity of the surgical endeavor.

Probably the most versatile VBG for reconstruction of the craniomaxillofacial region has been the scapula flap.[19] The circumflex scapular artery, a branch of the subscapular supplies either a horizontal, vertical, or a combination skin pad-dle, and also supplies the lateral border of the scapula (Figure 26.4). An angular artery, a branch of the thoracodorsal artery, can also be included in the design of the scapular flap to allow two separate vascularized bone grafts to be harvested using a single vascular pedicle.[26]

The iliac crest and the fibula, while useful under certain circumstances, rarely are ideal for reconstruction where thin bone and skin of good quality and color match are essential for an optimal result. Recently, reconstruction of small, thin defects of the orbital region has been accomplished with vascularized cortex taken from the medial supracondylar region of the femur.[28]

Current Research

To reduce the very substantial donor site morbidity inherent in most vascularized bone graft transfers, attention has recently focused on the prefabrication of vascularized bone flaps. Based on the preliminary studies of Hirase,[29,30] most of these studies use a principle of staged flap reconstruction. In the initial phase of this reconstruction vascularized tissue with a large identifiable pedicle is induced to perfuse the selected bone graft donor site. The bone remains in situ until sufficient vascularization has occurred from its new pedicle that a successful transfer can be accomplished. The great advantage of this technique is that bone can be harvested from almost any site in exactly the dimensions that are required without regard to its native blood supply. The disadvantage is the necessity for two stages and the possibility that despite staging, the bone donor will still be inadequately vascularized by its new vascular pedicle.[31]

Another intriguing possibility was initially suggested by Nettelblad et al.[32] and then more recently revised by Mitsumoto et al.[33] A vascularized bone graft was formed by placing bone marrow into cylindrical hydroxyapatite chambers to which allograft demineralized bone matrix powder had been added. Those chambers that were implanted subcutaneously with implantation of a vascular bundle showed accelerated neovascularization and early bone formation. The possibility that such prefabricated and preshaped vascularized bone grafts could be used clinically for elective craniofacial reconstruction is certainly worth contemplating.

Summary

Microvascular surgery has opened numerous possibilities for single-stage reconstruction of complex deformities of the craniomaxillofacial region. Newer techniques will undoubtedly further advance the reconstructive options of the surgeon, perhaps simplifying the sometimes difficult procedures or allowing more refinement in the everlasting pursuit of perfect form and function. Surgery and creativity must continue to form a close alliance to further refine the

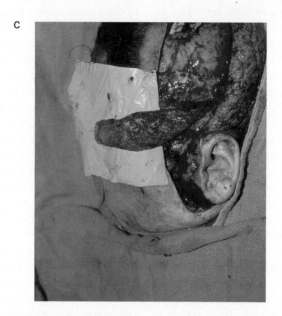

FIGURE 26.3 Temporoparietal osteofascial flap-superficial temporal artery. (a) Preoperative mandibular contour defect. (b) Harvested flap in situ. (c) Transposition of flap prior to inset and rigid fixation.

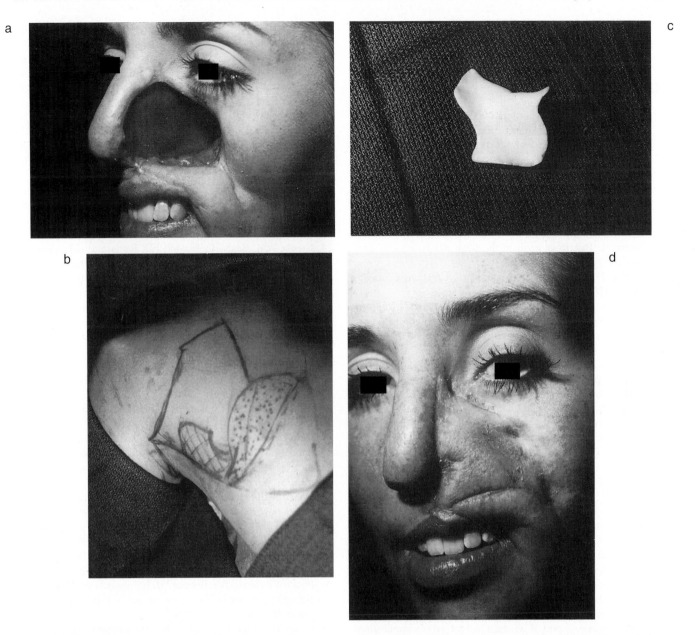

FIGURE 26.4 Scapula osteocutaneous flap-circumflex scapular artery. (a) Preoperative composite soft tissue and bony defect. (b) Flap design demonstrating inferior medial deepithelized paddle to be used for mucosal lining, inferior lateral bone segment, and superior skin paddle. (c) 3-Dimensional CT imaging computer-generated template of bony defect. (d) Postoperative result. (Reprinted with permission: Rose EM, Norris MS, Rosen JM: Application of high-tech three dimensional imaging and computer-generated models in complex facial reconstructions with vascularized bone grafts. *Plast Reconstr Surg*. 1993;91:252–264)

art and science of reconstruction of the craniomaxillofacial region.

References

1. Finseth F, Kavarana N, Antia N. Complications of free flap transfers to the mouth region. *Plast Reconstr Surg.* 1975;56: 652–653.
2. Coleman J. Osseous reconstruction of the midface and orbits. *Clin Plast Surg.* 1994;21:113–124.
3. Taylor GI, Miller GD, Ham FJ. The free vascularized bone graft. A clinical extension of microvascular techniques. *Plast Reconstr Surg.* 1975;55:533–544.
4. Buncke HJ, Furnas DW, Gordon L, Achauer BM. Free osteocutaneous flap from a rib to the tibia. *Plast Reconstr Surg.* 1977;59:799–804.
5. McKee DM. Microvascular bone transplantation. *Clin Plast Surg.* 1978;5:283–292.
6. Berggren A, Weiland AJ, Dorfman H. Free vascularized bone grafts: factors affecting their survival and ability to heal to recipient bone defects. *Plast Reconstr Surg.* 1982;69:19–29.
7. Berggren A, Weiland AJ, Dorfman H. The effect of prolonged ischemia time on osteocyte and osteoblast survival in composite bone grafts revascularized by microvascular anastomoses. *Plast Reconstr Surg.* 1982;69:290–298.
8. Moore JB, Mazur JM, Zehr D, Davis PK, Zook EG. A biomechanical comparison of vascularized and conventional autogenous bone grafts. *Plast Reconstr Surg.* 1984;73:382–386.
9. Altobelli DE, Lorente CA, Handren JH, Young J, Donoff RB, May JW. Free and microvascular bone grafting in the irradiated dog mandible. *J Oral Maxillofac Surg.* 1987;45:27–33.
10. Chen YB, Chen HC, Hahn LH. Major mandibular reconstruction with vascularized bone grafts: indications and selection of donor tissue. *Microsurgery.* 1994;15:227–237.
11. Jewer DD, Boyd JB, Manktelow RT, Zuker RM, Rosen IB, Gullane PJ, et al. Orofacial and mandibular reconstruction with the iliac crest free flap: a review of 60 cases and a new method of classification. *Plast Reconstr Surg.* 1989;84:391–403.
12. Urken ML, Weinberg H, Buchbinder D, Moscoso JF, Lawson W, Catalano PJ, et al. Microvascular free flaps in head and neck reconstruction. Report of 200 cases and review of complications. *Arch Otol Head Neck Surg.* 1994;120:633–640.
13. Urken ML. Composite free flaps in oromandibular reconstruction. *Arch Otol Head Neck Surg.* 1991;117:724–732.
14. Moscoso JF, Keller J, Genden E, Weinberg H, Biller HF, Buchbinder D, et al. Vascularized bone flaps in oromandibular reconstruction: a comparative anatomic study of bone stock from various donor sites to assess suitability for enosseous dental implants. *Arch Otol Head Neck Surg.* 1994;120:36–43.
15. Ramasastry SS, Tucker JB, Swartz WM, Hurwitz DJ. The internal oblique muscle flap: an anatomic and clinical study. *Plast Reconstr Surg.* 1984;73:721–733.
16. Ramasastry SS, Granick MS, Futrell JW. Clinical anatomy of the internal oblique muscle. *J Reconstr Microsurg.* 1986;2:117–122.
17. Urken ML, Vickery CB, Weinberg H, Buchbinder D, Lawson W, Biller HF. The internal oblique-iliac crest osseomyocutaneous free flap in oromandibular reconstruction. Report of 20 cases. *Arch Otol Head Neck Surg.* 1989;115:339–349.
18. Hidalgo DA. Fibula free flap: a new method of mandible reconstruction. *Plast Reconstr Surg.* 1989;84:71–79.
19. Jones NF, Swartz WM, Mears DC, Jupiter JB, Grossman A. The "double-barrel" free vascularized fibula bone graft. *Plast Reconstr Surg.* 1988;81:378–385.
20. Stoll P. Fibula double barrel technique. In: Greenberg AM, Prein J, eds. *Craniomaxillofacial Reconstructive and Corrective Bone Surgery: Principles of Internal Fixation Using the AO/ASIF Technique.* New York: Springer-Verlag; 2002.
21. Swartz WM, Banis JC, Newton ED, Ramasastry SS, Jones NF, Acland R. The osteocutaneous scapular flap for mandibular and maxillary reconstruction. *Plast Reconstr Surg.* 1986;77:530–545.
22. McCarthy JG, Zide BM. The spectrum of calvarial bone grafting: introduction of the vascularized calvarial bone flap. *Plast Reconstr Surg.* 1984;74:10–18.
23. Rose EH, Norris MS. The versatile temporoparietal fascial flap: adaptability to a variety of composite defects. *Plast Reconstr Surg.* 1990;85:224–231.
24. Yaremchuk MJ. Vascularized bone grafts for maxillofacial reconstruction. *Clin Plast Surg.* 1989;16:29–39.
25. Stal S, Netscher DT, Shenaq S, Spira M. Reconstruction of calvarial defects. *South Med J.* 1992;85:812–819.
26. Rose EH, Norris MS, Rosen JM. Application of high-tech three-dimensional imaging and computer-generated models in complex facial reconstructions with vascularized bone grafts. *Plast Reconstr Surg.* 1993;91:252–264.
27. Coleman JJ, Sultan MR. The bipedicled osteocutaneous scapula flap: a new subscapular system free flap. *Plast Reconstr Surg.* 1991;87:682–692.
28. Kobayashi S, Kakibuchi M, Masuda T, Ohmori K. Use of vascularized corticoperiosteal flap from the femur for reconstruction of the orbit. *Ann Plast Surg.* 1994;33:351–357.
29. Hirase Y, Valauri FA, Buncke HJ. Neovascularized bone, muscle, and myo-osseous free flaps: an experimental model. *J Reconstr Microsurg.* 1988;4:209–215.
30. Hirase Y, Valauri FA, Buncke HJ. Prefabricated sensate myocutaneous and osteomyocutaneous free flaps: an experimental model. Preliminary report. *Plast Reconstr Surg.* 1988;82:440–446.
31. Khouri RK, Upton J, Shaw WW. Prefabrication of composite free flaps through staged microvascular transfer: an experimental and clinical study. *Plast Reconstr Surg.* 1991;87:108–115.
32. Nettelblad H, Randolph MA, Leif T, Ostrup LT, Weiland AJ. Molded vascularized osteoneogenesis: a preliminary study in rabbits. *Plast Reconstr Surg.* 1985;76:851–856.
33. Mitsumoto S, Inada Y, Weiland AJ. Fabrication of vascularized bone grafts using ceramic chambers. *J Reconstr Microsurg.* 1993;9:441–449.

27

Considerations in the Fixation of Bone Grafts for the Reconstruction of Mandibular Continuity Defects

Peter Stoll, Joachim Prein, Wolfgang Bähr, and Rüdiger Wächter

Treatment of malignant tumors of the oral cavity frequently requires resection of bone that is infiltrated by the tumor. Particularly, if sections of the mandible are resected, this causes problems as far as form and function are concerned. Serious and life-threatening sequelae can occur, especially following resection of the anterior part of the mandible.[1] The goal of mandibular reconstruction, however, is not only restitution of continuity and form but the reestablishment of masticatory function. The repair of soft tissue defects is highly dependent on the underlying supporting structures.

A decisive step in the improvement of quality of life in patients suffering from loss or partial loss of the mandible due to malignant tumors was the development of reconstruction plates to bridge the bony defects as shown in our patient (Figure 27.1). They fulfill special biomechanical and anatomic requirements.[2-6]

Temporary or permanent reconstruction of the mandible after continuity resection by using alloplastic materials has to take the following conditions into consideration:

1. Stability under function
2. Fixation of the remaining bone stumps in the anatomically correct position
3. Preservation of the possibility of primary or secondary bone grafting
4. Preservation of the possibility of adjuvant radiotherapy

Recent investigations have confirmed the clinical experience that despite the use of those metallic "foreign bodies" an adjuvant, fractionated radiotherapy is feasible (see Chapter 34).[7-11]

Bridging osteosynthesis by using reconstruction plates, however, represents only one step in the patient's rehabilitation after continuity resection of the mandible. The low perioperative morbidity rate is overshadowed by a high long-term morbidity rate.[11-16] In addition, if no bony reconstruction is performed the result may be poor, especially so far as function is concerned.

Pressure of the plate against the bone may interfere with the blood circulation within the bony cortex and cause demineralization (Figure 27.2). Experimental studies with over-sized plates used for the fixation of mandibular fractures in sheep have shown this phenomenon.[17] After injecting ink into the sheep's carotid arteries at the time of sacrifice of the animal, it was clearly visible that the area underneath the plate was less well supplied (Figures 27.3 and 27.4). This finding should not be called *stress protection*.[18,19] The consequences are loss of contact between plate and bone, eventually leading to instability of the entire system. When the plate has lost its contact with the bone surface, it exerts uncontrolled forces upon the screws during masticatory function. Primarily well-fixed screws become overloaded, and the result is loosening of the screws with further bone loss in the screw holes (Figure 27.5).

Plate fractures (Figure 27.6) as well as hardware extrusion (Figure 27.7) may also occur following bridging osteosynthesis, even if the soft tissue conditions are adequate.[11]

Reconstruction of the bony continuity with alloplastic material alone can only be a temporary measure for the majority of the cases. Although 70% of our patients aged 60 or more years do not want further and/or extensive surgery after bridging osteosynthesis, the surgeon has to insist and do a bony reconstruction by using free or microanastomosed vascularized bone graft in a second procedure.

Keeping this in mind, one has to consider whether bone grafting after continuity resection either by using free or microvascular grafts should be performed primarily to make a second operation unnecessary.

The choice of the graft depends on these points:

1. The size and location of the bony defect
2. The type and size of the soft tissue defect ("composite defect")
3. The question of preoperative or postoperative radiation therapy, or both
4. The type of tumor and prognosis for the patient
5. The condition of the recipient area
6. The timing of the reconstruction
7. The donor site morbidity
8. The patient's compliance[20]
9. The question of cost-effectiveness

317

a

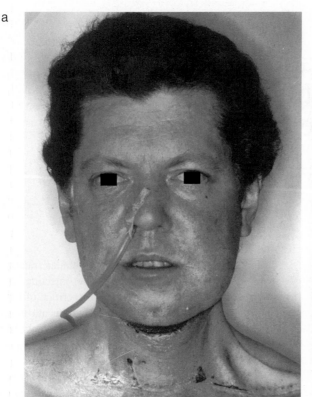

b

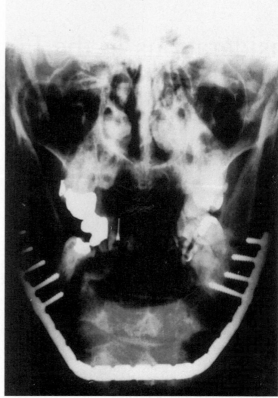

FIGURE 27.1 (a,b) A 34-year-old patient 12 days after resection of the anterior segment of the mandible and immediate alloplastic reconstruction of the chin area using an AO reconstruction plate [three dimensionally bendable reconstruction plate (3-DBRP)]. Percutaneous radiation therapy has already started.

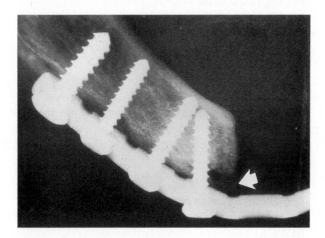

FIGURE 27.2 Resorption underneath a conventional AO reconstruction plate (3-DBRP) due to pressure against the bone surface (arrow).

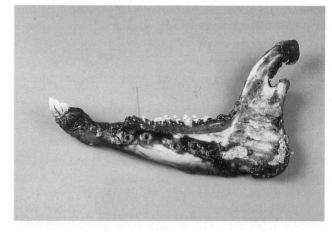

FIGURE 27.3 Sheep mandible, left side. Red area indicates zone of disturbance of circulation. The reason was pressure caused by an oversized plate.

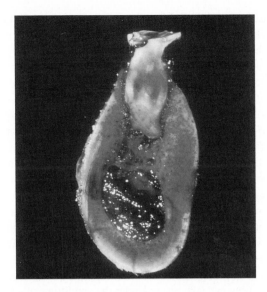

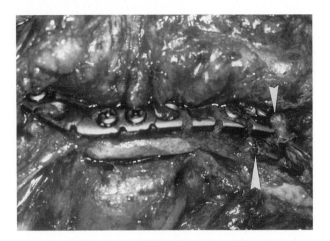

FIGURE 27.6 Clinical site of a plate fracture in a case of alloplastic repair (arrows).

FIGURE 27.4 Cut section through a sheep mandible after fracture fixation with an oversized plate. Zone of demineralization on the left side where the plate was pressed against the cortex.

Full rehabilitation, however, is achieved only after the reestablishment of masticatory function with osseointegrated dental implants (Figure 27.8) and prosthetic suprastructures. Therefore, the bone grafts should be suitable for this procedure.[21]

In recent years, microvascular reconstruction of the mandible has reached enormous popularity.[22] Not only the number but the success rate of those reconstructions has increased dramatically. In this context, however, it has to be stressed that the free nonvascularized iliac bone graft still has its importance as a "workhorse" in the majority of the cases.

The most common donor sites for microvascular bone grafts are iliac crest, scapula, fibula, and radius.[23] We now use mainly grafts taken from the fibula or the scapula. As far as the quality of the bone, the amount of soft tissues, and the length of the vascular pedicle are concerned, each flap has specific characteristics.

Problems

The pros and cons of different bone grafts and their indications have been widely discussed (see Chapter 25),[22,24–32] but little attention has been given to the various fixation techniques available.[32–36]

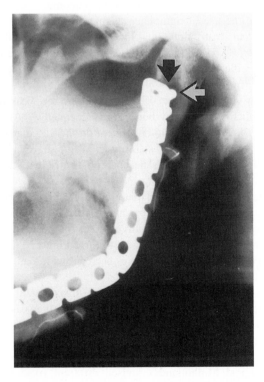

FIGURE 27.5 Loosening of screws and osteolysis (arrows).

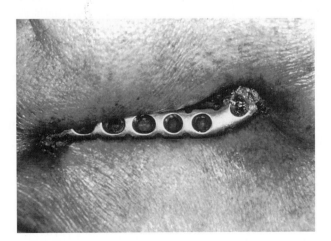

FIGURE 27.7 Lateral extrusion of a reconstruction plate 12 months after surgery.

a

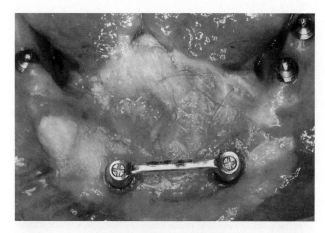

b

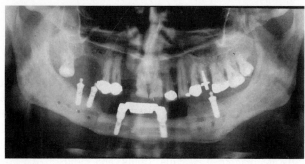

FIGURE 27.8 (a,b) Clinical and radiographic situation after insertion of dental implants (Bonefit®, ITI Strauman, Waldenberg, Switzerland) in the case of a patient with a squamous cell carcinoma as well in the original mandibular bone as in the fibula bone graft. The intraoral soft tissue defect was covered by a skin paddle.

For understanding the possibilities of graft fixation, the knowledge of their anatomy and pathophysiology is mandatory.

Fresh autogenous avascular grafts contain all the components of living tissue. A certain percentage of osteoblasts is initially nourished by diffusion until vascularization is completed. In the first days after grafting these osteoblasts proliferate and start building up a woven bone. Primary osteogenesis is achieved by the surviving bone cells and not by the surrounding soft tissue (osteoblast theory). The breakdown of the graft's bone matrix by osteoclasts runs parallel to the composition of new woven bone. The leftover mucopolysaccharides induce undifferentiated mesenchymal cells of the ingrowing surrounding tissue to become osteoblasts (induction theory).

Therefore, the basic prerequisites of a secure integration of a free avascular bone graft are these:

1. Good vascularization of the surrounding soft tissue
2. Mechanical stability for the transplant
3. Close contact between surface of the bone transplant and the surrounding soft tissue[4]

Avascular bone grafts for the replacement of mandibular bony substance show a high failure rate when they are inserted in an unstable surrounding environment. Creeping substitution through neovascularization is not possible if the bone graft is not adequately stabilized.

It takes 8 to 12 weeks for the bony transformation at the contact areas to occur. After primary integration of the transplant it is supposed that further remodeling depends on the functional load. One has to take into account the expected loss of bone volume of approximately 25% of the original free graft, for which the surgeon needs to overcompensate.[37] Cancellous bone has a higher osteogenic potency than compact bone, but as a free iliac crest graft it does not withstand the mechanical stress when bridging mandibular defects.

In contrast to free avascular grafts, there is no progressive transformation in microanastomosed grafts, and little bone resorption may occur.[24,34] The bone repair at the contact area between vascularized graft and mandible resembles the well-known phenomenon of fracture healing, where even primary bone healing can take place. Under the conditions of adequate stability, screws for the fixation of metal plates are osseointegrated totally and are not likely to come loose due to remodeling processes as in avascular grafts.

In this context it has to be stressed that the grafts have to be inserted atraumatically. Compression osteosynthesis between graft and bone remnant is not an issue, but adequate stability has to be achieved to avoid movement between the microvascular graft and the bone stump.

Vascularized bone grafts (e.g., iliac crest or fibula) do survive under unstable conditions as long as their vascular pedicle is intact, but malunion, nonunion, or even displacement of the bone graft can greatly limit a patient's masticatory rehabilitation and overall postoperative outcome.

While the use of miniplates or microplates is propagated to prevent restriction of blood supply of vascularized grafts,[34,38,39] on the other hand, stable fixation of the grafts without the possibility of micromovement is emphasized.[15,32,33,35,40,41]

In our view miniplates or microplates are too weak to stabilize microvascularized bone grafts adequately. Although their survival is definitely dependent on the vascular supply and not on the amount of stability as in free grafts, we have seen dislocations of grafts because of insufficient stabilization with miniplates.[42]

In general, it can be stated that vital bone grafts transplanted with microvascular techniques can be fixed with either a reconstruction plate or several universal fracture plates or sometimes with miniplates. In contrast to this, it must be said that free avascular grafts must always be fixed with load-bearing reconstruction plates.

This fixation technique is also most successful in *microvascular* defect reconstruction.[43] Particularly in cases with secondary microvascular bone grafting, when a reconstruction plate is already in place, the plate can be used as a safe pattern for adaptation of the graft in the desired shape.

Boyd and Mulholland[36] revised different fixation techniques in vascularized bone grafts. They found a 75% failure rate by using several 4- to 6-hole dynamic compression plates for fixation of iliac crest grafts, whereas the success rate was 100% when using reconstruction plates for bridging osteosynthesis. This is logical because dynamic compression plates may exert too much compression at the wrong place, e.g., within the graft.

Methods

In our unit, bony defects up to a length of 6 cm are usually reconstructed by using corticocancellous grafts taken from the iliac crest. Cases exhibiting a compromised recipient site due to previously performed radiation therapy or for whom further radiation therapy is planned are excluded from transplantation of avascular grafts, although the bony defect may be relatively small. Nevertheless, the use of free corticocancellous hip bone is still a valuable help in the majority of minor defects, as stated before.[28,44] On the other hand, larger defects, particularly after irradiation, require microvascular repair.[45]

In the case of defects that require only the replacement of bone without soft tissues, we prefer the fibula[34] as the graft of choice. Its architecture is, unlike iliac crest or scapula, similar to that of the mandible. Defects up to a length of 25 cm can be repaired. The graft can be easily adjusted to the shape of the mandible by using the intersection technique. It is associated with very low postoperative donor site morbidity, and last but not least, it allows insertion of dental implants due to its mandibular-like width.[22,46] The main disadvantage—the limited height—can be overcome by using the "double-barrel" technique.[47]

Since the skin paddle of the fibula is relatively thin and sometimes exhibits a limited reliability,[48] we use the fibula osteocutaneous flap or the supramalleolar composite graft[49] only in cases with small soft-tissue defects.

In cases with large soft tissue defects, scapula bone and parascapular flaps are more appropriate. The scapula, however, seems to be unfavorable as far as length and diameter are concerned. Frequently, especially in females,[31] secondary insertion of dental implants is not possible. In addition, time in surgery is extended because a simultaneous two-team approach is not possible. On the other hand, like fibula grafts, scapula grafts present a low postoperative donor site morbidity rate.[50,51]

It is important to understand the appropriate possibilities for the fixation of different grafts. In our experience, adequate internal fixation by using reconstruction plates combined with autogenous bone grafts seems to be most satisfactory. Corticocancellous iliac crest bone as well as microanastomosed fibula or scapula grafts can easily be adjusted to the given curvature of the plate.

Bridging osteosynthesis guarantees stability during the healing phase (Figure 27.9). Generally, nonvascularized corticocancellous iliac crest grafts should not be fixed with screws to the plate. During the remodeling phase, the screws may come loose and act as a foreign body because the bone

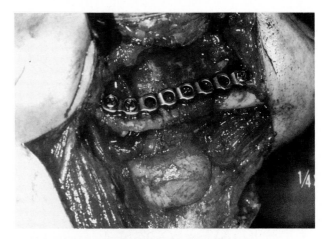

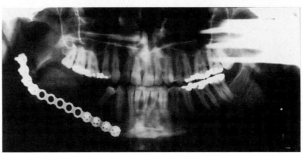

FIGURE 27.9 (a,b) Clinical and radiographic situation after immediate bone repair using a free nonvascularized iliac crest bone graft in a case of an ameloblastoma.

is not vital and is subsequently replaced by newly formed woven and lamellar bone. Infection and loss of bone can occur.

In those cases fixation of the bone grafts to the remnants is achieved, for example, by using the AO-3-Dimensionally Bendable Reconstruction Plate system (3-DBRP), which can provide compression between the graft and the bone stumps (Figure 27.10).

Since 1984, we have used the AO-Titanium Hollow Screw Reconstruction Plate system (THORP). With this system one cannot exert compression, but because its anchoring device between the screwhead and plate acts as an "internal fixator," it is possible to avoid bone resorption underneath the plate and secondary instability of the entire osteosynthesis.[5,52–55] By using this system, screw fixation of an avascular graft may be possible since the screwhead does not move inside the screw hole. Nevertheless, we intend not to interfere with the bone's remodeling and prefer adaptation of the graft to the plate by using resorbable sutures.

Statistical evaluation of our patient sample, however, has shown that since we have abandoned fixation of avascular grafts to the plate by using screws, the infection rate could be dramatically reduced (screw fixation, $N = 97 = 32\%$; without screw fixation, $N = 82 = 4\%$).

Today we generally do not use nonvascularized bone grafts in an irradiated bed or when postoperative external radiation

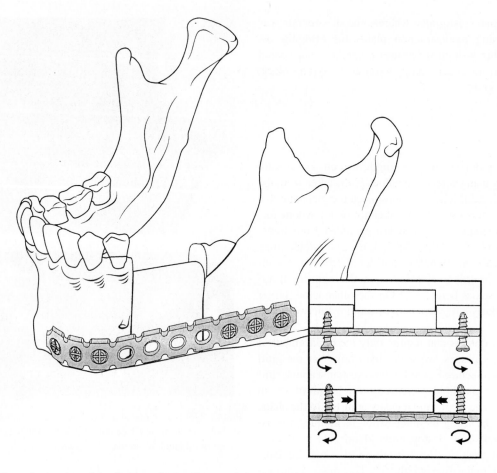

FIGURE 27.10 Schematic drawing of the fixation of a free bone graft for the replacement of a defect in the lateral mandible. The inset shows loose screws (above) at the time of placement of the graft. By tightening of the screws (below) the graft is fixed via compression.

therapy is planned. This may contribute to the better results.

On the other hand, microanastomosed bone grafts can be fixed to reconstruction plates with metal screws. It should be emphasized though that those screws serve only to hold the graft in position between the rigidly fixed mandibular segments.

Since microvascular grafts consist of living tissue and behave like an edentulous mandible, osseointegration of the screws can be expected. Compression of the bone grafts between the bone remnants is not necessary for fixation but can carefully be exerted. Impairment of the blood supply of the graft has to be avoided. Gaps between the bone graft and the remnant, if any, are filled with bone dust and/or bone slices or cancellous bone from the iliac crest.

In our hands blood supply of microvascular grafts is not impaired when using functionally stable AO-reconstruction-plates (3-DBRP or THORP). On the contrary, this procedure seems to protect the anastomosis and promote uneventful healing. Loosening of plate and screws, pseudoarthrosis, and infection, which can occur from using functionally unstable fixation devices like miniplates, are unusual in our sample. Sometimes, however, the use of reconstruction plates is not possible, especially in cases with composite grafts. Here, sev-

eral smaller plates like universal fracture plates may avoid impairment of the blood supply of the skin paddle.

Conclusion

Various types of bone graft fixation are used in oral and maxillofacial surgery. It is important to understand that adequate stability favors the incorporation of the transplant. Generally, alloplastic restitution of the mandibular continuity is performed by using a reconstruction plate.

This plate preserves the distance between the bone stumps. Bone grafts can be adjusted and fixed to the plate either primarily or secondarily. The plate acts like a template for the shaping of the bone graft because it follows the original mandibular arch.

Two main types of grafts or flaps are available for autogenous reconstruction of mandibular defects. In general, either an avascular free-bone graft or a bone graft that is reanastomosed with microvascular technique and therefore vital is used.

While free avascular grafts must always be stabilized with the help of complete bridging osteosynthesis, there may be an option for fixation of microvascular grafts by using smaller plates. Particularly in cases with large soft tissue defects where the repair has to be performed by using composite grafts, a reconstruction plate may hinder the vascular supply of the soft tissue compartment of the graft. In the majority of the cases, however, the application of a reconstruction plate is a comfortable measure to insert a bone graft. Nevertheless, a microvascular graft with several intersections, which are necessary to achieve a natural curvature, may be further stabilized by using smaller plates, preferably universal fracture plates (Figures 27.11 and 27.12).

In the case of secondary bone repair, a primarily applied reconstruction plate preserves the distance between the bone stumps during the postoperative follow-up period and facilitates the placement of a graft.

The AO-THORP system offers a long-term reliable fixation that will not fail due to micromovement or bone remodeling. The locking-screw plate design makes it possible to achieve a stable reconstruction by using only three or four screws per bone stump. The new 2.4 mm Unilock reconstruction plates with special locking screws have been designed to be similar in function to the AO-THORP system to prevent screw loosening after graft healing has occurred and may be used for nonvascular and vascularized grafts (see Chapter 41 for 2.4 Unilock module specifications). These newer plates are less thick and may be used in situations where the AO-THORP system and AO3-DBRP are considered for use, with caution concerning the size of the graft and defect.

Conventional reconstruction plate systems as the AO-3-DBRP, where the plate is pressed against the bony surface during tightening of the screws, may become loose with time due to bone resorption underneath the plate. Therefore, they are less suitable for long-term alloplastic repair alone. This kind of reconstruction device is used preferably in combination with primary bone repair (Figure 27.13). Then, bony restitution takes place before the plate loses its stability. In addition, a bone graft can be compressed between the stumps and fixed by using compression.

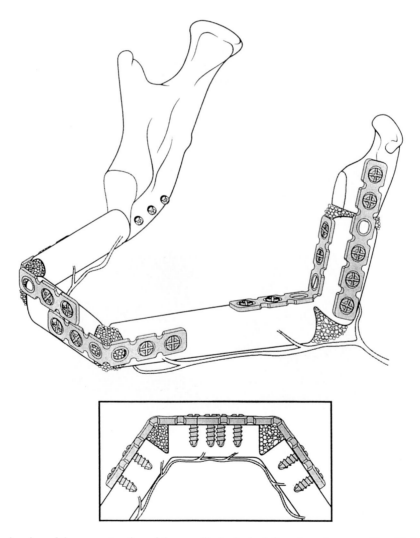

FIGURE 27.11 Schematic drawing of the reconstruction of the mandibular body, left angle and ramus with a fibula. Fixation was performed with several universal fracture plates. The bone gaps at the osteotomy site were filled with cancellous bone.

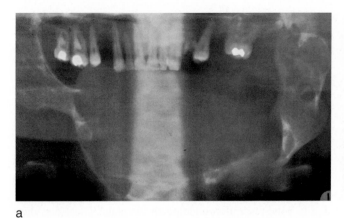

a

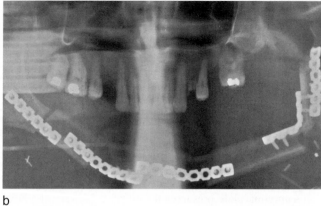

b

FIGURE 27.12 (a,b) Radiographic situation with an extensive ameloblastoma within the mandible preoperatively and postoperatively after resection and reconstruction of the defect with a mi- crovascular fibula graft fixed with universal fracture plates as shown schematically in Figure 27.11.

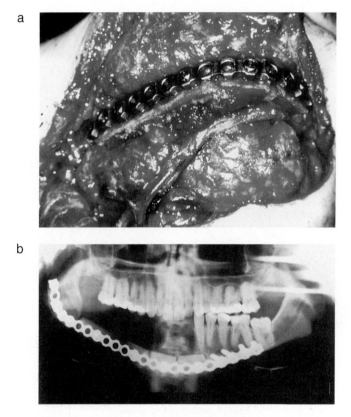

a

b

FIGURE 27.13 (a,b) Clinical and radiographic situation of a vascularized fibula bone repair after extensive resection of an osteosarcoma.

Generally it can be said that primary bone repair by using free or vascularized bone grafts is easier to perform. Secondary repair after the formation of scars and soft tissue shrinkage has taken place is more difficult. This is also due to the deficiency of the soft tissue layer and compromised vascular supply (especially after radiation), which may limit the desired treatment.

References

1. Stoll P. Lebensqualität nach radikaler Tumorchirurgie im Mund-Kiefer-Gesichtsbereich. *Aktuel Inf Arzt.* 1992;6:2–3.
2. Luhr HH. Ein Plattensystem zur Unterkieferrekonstruktion einschliesslich des Gelenkersatzes. *Dtsch Zahnärztl Z.* 1976;31: 747.
3. Ewers R, Joos U. Temporäre Defektüberbrückung bei Unterkieferresektionen mit osteosynthese-methoden. *Dtsch Zahnärztl Z.* 1977;32:332–333.
4. Spiessl B. Die Unterkieferresektionsplatte der AO. Ihre Anwendung bei Unterkieferdefekten in der Tumorchirurgie. *Unfallheilkunde.* 1978;81:389–405.
5. Raveh J, Stich H, Schawalder P, Sutter F, Straumann F. Konservative und chirurgische Massnahmen zur Herstellung der Kiefergelenksfunktion und neue Möglichkeitn und Methoden zur Defektüberbrückung am Unterkiefer. *Schweiz Monatsschr Zahnheilk.* 1980;90:932–948.
6. Schmoker R. *Die funktionelle Unterkieferrekonstruktion.* Berlin: Springer; 1986.
7. Stoll P, Wächter R, Hodapp N, Schilli W. Radiation and osteosynthesis? Dosimetry on an irradiation phantom. *J Craniomaxillofac Surg.* 1990;18:361–366.
8. Klotch DW, Gump J, Kuhn L. Reconstruction of mandibular defects in irradiated patients. *Am J Surg.* 1990;160:396.
9. Gullane PJ. Primary mandibular reconstruction analysis of 64 cases and evaluations of interface radiation dosimetry on bridging plates. *Laryngoscope.* 1991;101:1–24.
10. Maurer J, Kirschner H, Halling F, Duhmke E. Klinische und strahlenphysikalische Untersuchungen über den Einfluss von Unterkieferrekonstruktionsplatten (MRS) auf die Dosisverteilung von ultraharten Photonen. *Strahlenther Onkol.* 1993; 169:279–284.
11. Stoll P, Wächter R. Tumorbestrahlung und Überbückungsosteosynthese? *Dtsch Z Mund-Kiefer-Gesichtschir.* 1993;15:224–229.
12. Komisar A, Warman S, Danziger E. A critical analysis of immediate and delayed mandibular reconstruction using AO plates. *Arch Otolaryngol Head Neck Surg.* 1989;115:830–833.
13. Davidson J, Birt BD, Gruss J. AO plate mandibular reconstruction: a complication critique. *J Otolaryngol.* 1991;20:104–107.
14. Freitag V, Hell B, Fischer H. Experience with AO reconstruction plates after partial mandibular resection involving its continuity. *J Craniomaxillofac Surg.* 1991;19:191–198.
15. Schusterman MA, Reece GP, Kroll SS, Weldon MA. Use of the AO plate for immediate mandibular reconstruction in cancer patients. *Plast Reconstr Surg.* 1991;88:588.
16. Kim MR, Donoff RB. Critical analysis of mandibular reconstruction using AO-reconstruction plates. *J Oral Maxillofac Surg.* 1992;50:1152–1157.
17. Rahn B, Prein J. Unpublished experiment. AO Research Institut, Clavadelerstrasse, CH-7270 Davos/Switzerland, 1973.

18. Predieri M, Gautier E, Sutter F, Tepic S, Perren SM. Vermeidung der Porose unter Osteosyntheseplatten. *Acta Med Austraca.* 1990;17:49.
19. Schiller K, Wolf I, Kessler SB. Die Bedeutung der Knochengrösse für das Ausmass der plattenbedingten Zirkulationsschäden. *Acta Med Austrica.* 1990;17:444–447.
20. Wächter R, Lauer G, Fabinger A, Stoll P. Zur Compliance von Tumorpatienten mit dentalen Implantaten. In: *Jahrbuch der Gesellschaft für Orale Implantologie.* Berlin: Quintessenz; 1994;299.
21. Wächter R, Stoll P, Bähr W, Lauer G. Osseointegration of ITI-dental implants (Bonefit) in non-vascularized and vascularized mandibular bone grafts. Proceedings of the 1st World Congress of Osseointegration, Venice, Sept. 29–Oct. 2, 1994.
22. Urken ML. Composite free flaps in oromandibular reconstruction. Review of the literature. *Arch Otolaryngol Head Neck Surg.* 1991;117:724–732.
23. Frodel JL, Funk GF, Capper DJ, Fridrich KL, Blumer JR, Haller JR, et al. Osseointegrated implants: a comparative study of bone thickness in four vascularized bone flaps. *Plast Reconstr Surg.* 1993;92:449–455.
24. Riediger D. Restoration of masticatory function by microsurgically revascularized iliac crest bone grafts using enosseous implants. *Plast Reconstr Surg.* 1988;81:861–877.
25. Kärcher H, Penkner K. Ergebnisse der freien und gefässgestielten Knochenrekonstruktion nach Unterkieferkontinuitätsdefekten. *Dtsch Z Mund-Kiefer-Geischtschir.* 1991;15:285–291.
26. Kuriloff DB, Sullivan MJ. Mandibular reconstruction using vascularized bone grafts. *Otolaryngol Clin North Am.* 1991;24: 1391–1418.
27. Divaris M, Goudot P, Princ G, Lalo J, Vaillant JM. Reconstruction mandibulaire par lambeaux libres osseux microanastomoses. Nos indications actuelles. *Ann Chir Plast Esthetique.* 1992;37:297–308.
28. Lindqvist C. Mandibular reconstruction with free bone grafts. *Curr Opin Dent.* 1992;2:25–37, Review.
29. Mayot D, Perrin C, Lindas P, Dron K. Reconstruction de la symphyse mandibulaire par transferts osseux vascularises libres iliaques et scarpulaire. *Ann Otolaryngol Chir Cervico-faciale.* 1992;109:123.
30. Ferri J, Piot B, Farah A, Gaillard A, Mercier J. Notre experience des lambeaux libres vascularises osseux dans le reconstructions mandibulaires. Le lambeau brachial extreme, le lambeau fibulaire, le lambeau parascapulaire. *Rev Stomatol Chir Maxillofac.* 1993;94:74.
31. Bekiscz O, Adant J, Denoel C, Lahaye T. Mandibular reconstruction. An anatomical study of bone thickness in three donor sites. 12th Congress of the European Association for Cranio-Maxillofacial Surgery, The Hague, 5–10 September 1994.
32. Komisar A, Shapiro BM, Danziger E, Szporn M, Cobelli N. The use of osteosynthesis in immediate and delayed mandibular reconstruction. *Laryngoscope.* 1985;95:1363–1366.
33. Gullane PJ, Holmes H. Mandibular reconstruction. New concepts. *Arch Otolaryngol Head Neck Surg.* 1986;112:714–719.
34. Hidalgo DA. Titanium miniplate fixation in free-flap-mandible reconstruction. *Ann Plast Surg.* 1989;23:498–507.
35. Buchbinder D, Urken ML, Vickery C, Weinberg H, Biller HF. Bone contouring and fixation in functional, primary microvascular mandibular reconstruction. *Head Neck.* 1991;13:191–199.

36. Boyd JB, Mulholland RS. Fixation of the vascularized bone graft in mandibular reconstruction. *Plast Reconstr Surg.* 1993;91:274.

37. Hausamen JE, Neukam FW. Transplantation von Knochen. *Eur Arch Otorhinolaryngol I Suppl.* 1992:163–177.

38. Hidalgo DA. Aesthetic improvements in free-flap-mandible reconstruction. *Plast Reconstr Surg.* 1991;88:574–585.

39. Barnard NA, Vaughan ED. Osteosynthetic titanium miniplate fixation of composite radial forearm flaps in mandibular reconstruction. *J Craniomaxillofac Surg.* 1991;19:243–248.

40. Wenig BL, Keller AJ. Microvascular free-tissue transfer with rigid internal fixation for reconstruction of the mandible following tumor resection. *Otolaryngol Clin North Am.* 1987;20:621–633.

41. Wenig BL, Keller AJ, Shikowitz MJ, Stern JR, Casino AJ, Pollack JM, et al. Anatomic reconstruction and functional rehabilitation of oromandibular defects with rigid internal fixation. *Laryngoscope.* 1988;98:154–159.

42. Prein J, Ettlin D, Hammer B. Vor- und Nachteile unterschiedlicher Fixationstechniken für mikrovaskuläre Transplantate bei der Unterkieferrekonstruktion. IV. International Symposium on Microsurgery in Reconstructive and Plastic Surgery, Microsurgery '95. Jena 1995; Publication 1998.

43. Stoll P, Bähr W, Wächter R. Die Wertigkeit des Fibulatransplantates bei der Rekonstruktion von Unterkieferdefekten. Proceedings of the IV International Symposium on Microsurgery in Reconstructive and Plastic Surgery. Jena 1995; Publication 1998.

44. Tidstrom KD, Keller EE. Reconstruction of mandibular discontinuity with autogenous iliac bone graft: report of 34 consecutive patients. *J Oral Maxillofac Surg.* 1990;48:336–346.

45. Fossion E, Boeckx W, Jacobs D, Ioannides C, Vrielinck L. La reconstruction microchirurgicale de la mandibule irradiée par le lambeau circonflexe iliaque profond. *Ann Chir Plast Esthetique.* 1992;37:246–251.

46. Huryn JM, Zlotolow JM, Piro JD, Lenchewski E. Osseointegrated implants in microvascular fibula free flap reconstructed mandibles. *J Prosthet Dent.* 1993;70:443–446.

47. Bähr W, Stoll P, Wächter R. "Fibuladoppeltransplantat" als gefässgestielter Unterkieferersatz. *Dtsch Z Mund-Kiefer-Gesichtschir.* 1994;18:219–223.

48. Schusterman MA, Reece GP, Miller MJ, Harris S. The osteocutaneous free fibula flap: is the skin paddle reliable? *Plast Reconstr Surg.* 1992;90:787–793.

49. Wolff KD, Stellmach R. The osteoseptocutaneous or purely septocutaneous peroneal flap with a supramalleolar skin paddle. *Int J Oral Maxillofac Surg.* 1995;24:38–43.

50. Sullivan M, Baker S, Crompton R, Smith-Wheelock M. Free scapular osteocutaneous flap for mandibular reconstruction. *Arch Otolaryngol Head Neck Surg.* 1989;115:1334–1340.

51. Thomassin JM, Bardot J, Inedjian JM. Le lambeau osteocutane scapulaire dans reconstruction mandibulaire. *Rev Stomatol Chir Maxillofac.* 1990;91, Suppl. 1:15.

52. Raveh J, Stich H, Sutter F, Greiner R. Use of titanium-coated hollow screw and reconstruction system in bridging of lower jaw defects. *J Oral Maxillofac Surg.* 1984;42:281–294.

53. Sutter F, Raveh J. Titanium-coated hollow screw and reconstruction plate system for bridging of lower jaw defects: biomechanical aspects. *Int J Oral Maxillofac Surg.* 1988;17:267–274.

54. Stoll P, Wächter R, Bähr W. Bridging lower jaw defects with AO plates: comparison of THORP and 3-DBRP systems. *J Craniomaxillofac Surg.* 1992;20:87–90.

55. Wächter R, Stoll P. Komplikationen nach primärer Unterkieferrekonstruktion mit THORP-Platten. In: *Ästhetische und plastisch-rekonstruktive Gesichtschirurgie.* Neumann H-J, Hrsg. Reinbek: Einhorn-Presse-Verlag; 1993;259.

28

Indications and Technical Considerations
of Different Fibula Grafts

Peter Stoll

Bridging osteosynthesis using reconstruction plates represents only one step in the patient's rehabilitation following continuity resection of the mandible. The low perioperative morbidity rate is overshadowed by a high long-term morbidity rate.[1–6] In addition, functional outcome is relatively poor in many cases.

Bone resorption underneath the plate, loosening of screws, plate fractures, and hardware extrusion frequently occur.[6] For the patients' comfort and to avoid long-term hardware complications, primary or secondary reconstruction using free-tissue or microanastomosed vascularized bone grafts is therefore desirable.

The choice of the grafts depends on the following:

1. The size of the bony defect
2. The amount of resected soft tissue
3. Radiation therapy considerations

Full rehabilitation, however, is achieved only after the reestablishment of masticatory function with osseointegrated dental implants and prosthetic suprastructures.[7–9] Therefore, the bone grafts should also be suitable for this purpose.

Avascular bone grafts for the reconstruction of mandibular continuity defects demonstrate a high failure rate when they are placed in an unstable surrounding environment. Creeping substitution through neovascularization is impossible without stable fixation of the bone graft to the remaining bone segments. This is in contrast to vascularized bone grafts, which will often survive even under unstable conditions, as long as their vascular pedicle is intact. However, malunion, nonunion, or even displacement of the bone graft can greatly limit a patient's masticatory rehabilitation and overall postoperative outcome.

Nevertheless, the use of free cancellous hip bone is still a valuable technique in the treatment of most minor defects. The bone graft height and width can be shaped to the remaining bone segments. Overcorrection with excess bone is often helpful, as nonvascularized bone grafts have a higher resorption rate.[10,11]

Cases exhibiting a compromised recipient site owing to previous radiation therapy or when additional radiation therapy is planned usually should be excluded from transplantation of avascular grafts (even for small bony defects).

Since microanastomosed bone grafts consist of living tissue, they are capable of independent survival within a compromised recipient site. Furthermore, vascularized grafts are able to improve the local wound regenerative situation[12,13] and should therefore be considered more suitable than avascular grafts.

In strictly osseous defects, vascularized fibula grafts present numerous advantages. Their bony architecture is similar to that of the mandible, unlike iliac crest or scapula, and they are capable of restoring defects up to a length of 25 cm. The grafts can be easily adjusted to the curvature of the mandible using the intersection technique (Figure 28.1). They are associated with very low postoperative donor site morbidity and facilitate the insertion of dental implants owing to fibular similarity to mandibular width and marble-like bone structure[14,15] (Figure 28.2). Since vascularized grafts behave like an edentulous mandible, osseointegration can generally be expected[9] (Figure 28.3).

Owing to their shape, fibula grafts are better suited to the insertion of dental implants than scapula or hip bone. Scapula also seems to be limited as far as length and diameter is concerned. Frequently, especially in females, the insertion of dental implants is not even possible.[16–18]

In this context, it is important to note that the harvesting of fibula grafts can be performed using a two-team approach. This procedure saves considerable operating time. The harvest of scapula grafts requires lateral positioning of the intubated patient, which prevents simultaneous surgery by a second team.

Since the skin paddle of the fibula is relatively thin and sometimes exhibits limited reliability,[19] use of the fibula osteocutaneous flap is indicated in cases with smaller soft tissue defects. For large defects it is better to use the supramalleolar skin paddle[20] together with the fibula. This is owing to a relatively long vascular pedicle, which allows the application of a reconstruction plate for fixation of the bone graft.

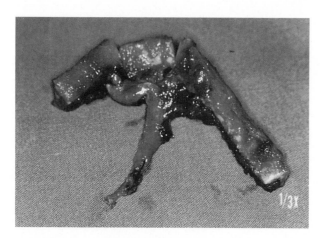

FIGURE 28.1 Single strut fibula graft sawed into three sections with adherent soft tissue prepared for microvascular anastomosis.

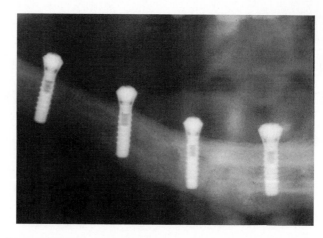

FIGURE 28.3 Radiograph demonstrating osseointegration of ITI-dental-implants (Bonefit®, ITI Strauman, Waldenberg, Switzerland) in a vascularized fibula graft.

The main disadvantage of conventional fibula grafts is their limited height. This especially causes problems in dentate patients, in whom the residual bone segments are normal size. The use of a single strut fibula bone graft with its height of approximately 1.5 cm produces a considerable step between the graft and residual bone segment (Figure 28.4).

Recently interest in the placement of osseointegrated implants into these bone grafts to facilitate improved functional dental rehabilitation has grown dramatically. Although enormous efforts have been made concerning the osseointegration of dental implants in bone grafts, the placement of an adequate prosthesis and return to function have fallen short of ideal goals.[8,21] This is often owing to scarred intraoral tissues, induration, loss of vestibule, altered muscle function, loss of

sensation, mucosal changes from irradiation,[22] and last but not least limited compliance.

In addition to other surgical measures (i.e., vestibuloplasty), prosthetic rehabilitation and fabrication of an acceptable denture may be improved by enlarging graft height. By reducing the distance between the upper rim of the graft and the occlusal plane the vertical dimension of the dental suprastructure can be reduced, and the reverse. Thus unfavorable forces upon buttressing teeth or dental implants caused by long lever arms can be avoided.

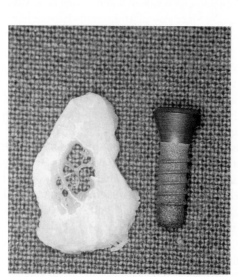

FIGURE 28.2 Cross section of the fibula with a marble-like bone structure of the thick compact layer giving an excellent anchorage for dental implants (left). Diameter-reduced ITI-dental implant (Bonefit®, ITI Strauman, Waldenberg, Switzerland) 8 mm in length (right).

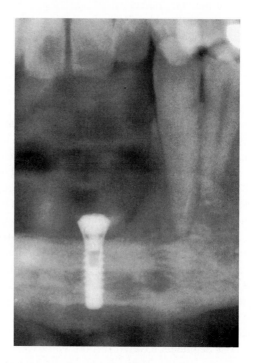

FIGURE 28.4 Radiograph demonstrating a considerable step between the remaining dentate mandible (right) and the fibula bone graft (left).

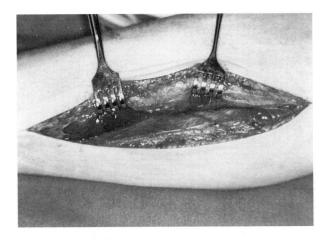

FIGURE 28.5 Lateral access to the fibula after separation of the crural fascia, the long lateral peroneous muscle, and the soleus muscle.

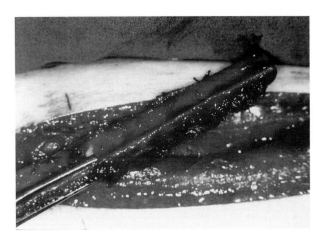

FIGURE 28.6 The diaphysis of the fibula is osteotomized proximally and distally. The size of the graft has to be taken double as long as the mandibular defect.

Owing to its extensive periosteal vascular network, the diaphysis of the fibula can be transversally osteotomized into different segments without danger of necrosis (Figure 28.1).[11] The principle of setting one fibular segment beside the other was primarily used for reconstruction of the tibia.[23,24] This reinforced "double barrel" served as a strong buttress.

In 1994, Bähr et al.[25] were the first to introduce this method for the repair of mandibular defects.

After angiographic imaging of the tibial and peroneal vessels, the fibula is dissected by using a lateral approach (Figure 28.5).[26] At first, the crural facia is separated and then the fibula is degloved between the long lateral peroneal muscle

and the soleus muscle. The diaphysis is osteotomized proximally and distally so that the removed bone segment is at least twice as long as the resected section of the mandible (Figure 28.6). Then the vascular pedicle, which is maintained for as long as possible, is severed and the graft is divided into sections. The intersection technique can also be used when the bone graft is still connected to its original blood supply.

Cases exhibiting a straight mandibular bony defect (i.e., the horizontal ramus) require only one osteotomy to obtain two equal pieces. One of the two pieces is now rotated 180° and is laid on the other (Figure 28.7).

Cases with arched mandibular defects (i.e., comprising the

a

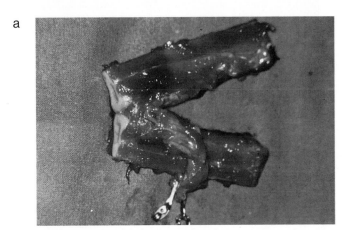

b

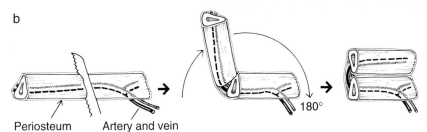

Periosteum   Artery and vein

180°

FIGURE 28.7 (a,b) Double barrel for straight mandibular defects. After cutting the bone graft into two equal pieces without damaging the vascular pedicle, one of the two pieces is rotated 180° and placed over the other.

a

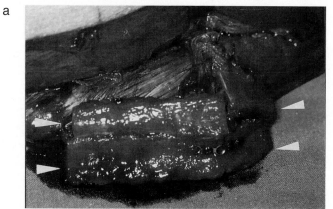

b

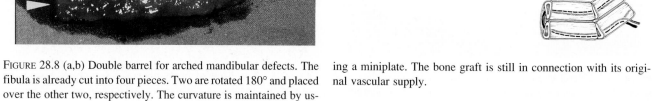

FIGURE 28.8 (a,b) Double barrel for arched mandibular defects. The fibula is already cut into four pieces. Two are rotated 180° and placed over the other two, respectively. The curvature is maintained by us-

ing a miniplate. The bone graft is still in connection with its original vascular supply.

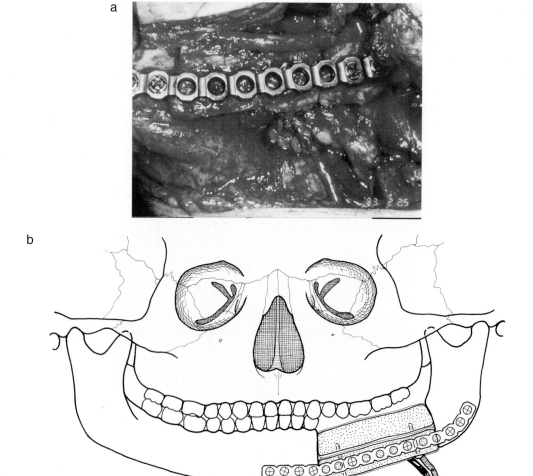

FIGURE 28.9 (a,b) Insertion and fixation of a fibula double barrel into a straight mandibular defect.

horizontal ramus and the anterior part) require three intersections to gain four pieces of bone. Following the same procedure as described earlier, two of the bone pieces are now rotated 180° and laid upon the other two. Thus the graft can later be adjusted to the mandibular curvature. Adaptation of the graft segments can be accomplished by using miniosteosynthesis plates (Figure 28.8).

It is mandatory that during this procedure the peroneal vessels must not be compromised. The original dorsal surfaces of the bone graft are now put together, with the peroneal vessels in a lateral position.

The artery and the two accompanying veins of the vascular pedicle of the graft are now anastomosed at the recipient site. Since this vascular pedicle is relatively long (6 to 8 cm) and the diameter of the vessels relatively large (1.5 to 4 mm),[27,28] the anastomosis can be accomplished with a high margin of safety.

Finally the fibula double-barrel bone graft is inserted into the resection defect, which was maintained by using a reconstruction plate (Figures 28.9 and 28.10). The reconstruction plate ensures, during the postoperative period, stable fixation of the remaining bone stumps under function in either primary or secondary vascular bone repair. This procedure seems to protect the anastomoses and promote uneventful healing. Loosening of plates and screws, pseudoarthrosis and infection, which can occur using functionally unstable fixation devices (i.e., miniplates), are unusual.

If necessary, final adjustment of the graft by shortening or sloping of the ends can be easily performed. The lower part of the double barrel is now rigidly fixed to the reconstruction

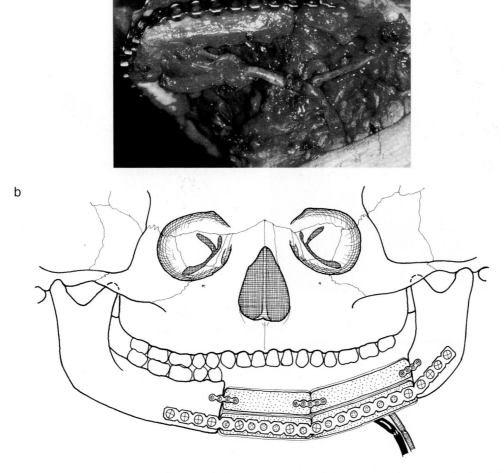

FIGURE 28.10 (a,b) Insertion and fixation of a fibula "double barrel" into an anterolateral mandibular defect.

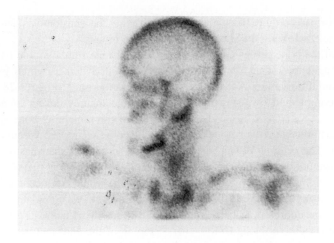

FIGURE 28.11 Positive technetium scintigraphy 3 days after mandibular bone repair using a fibula double-barrel vascularized graft.

a

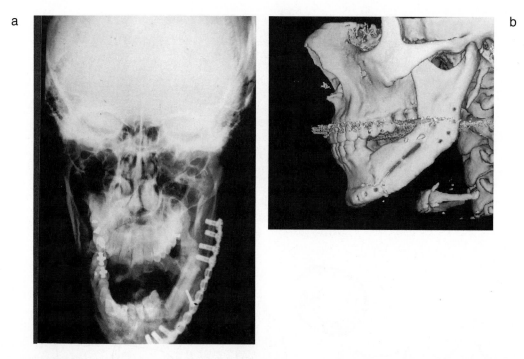

b

FIGURE 28.12 (a) X-ray showing the double-barrel fibula bone graft prior to removal of the reconstruction plate. (b) Three-dimensional CT scan showing the double-barrel fibula bone graft after the removal of the reconstruction plate. The height of the bone graft is approximately the same as the neighboring mandible.

plate using metal screws. It should be emphasized that these lag screws are not load-bearing, but serve only to hold the graft in position between the rigidly fixed mandibular segments. Gaps between the bone graft and the remnant, if any, are filled with bone dust, bone wedges, or both.

Black ink injections in human cadavers[23] and intraoperative findings have demonstrated that the perfusion of fibula struts is maintained despite the 180° rotation of one bone strut.

Postoperatively, the vascular anastomosis is checked by conventional Doppler sonography and technetium scintigraphy (Figure 28.11). Blood flow and immediate accumulation of the radionucleotide can be registered if the vessels are patent.

In the case of a nonvascularized bone graft, accumulation of technetium owing to vascular invasion[29] can be detected only after the 11th postoperative day.

Because the periosteum and the vascular periosteal network must not be stripped to preserve the blood supply of the graft, the two bone struts interface only with the residual bone segments and not with each other. Functionally, this is not important because bony consolidation between the segments and the double barrel is sufficient. The height of the bone graft is equal to that of the adjacent mandible (Figure 28.12).

Six months after vascular bone repair, the reconstruction plate is removed. The bone graft is now ready for insertion of dental implants (Figure 28.13).

At our institution we have abandoned simultaneous dental implant placement during bone repair for two reasons. The first is possible impairment of the graft's blood supply, and

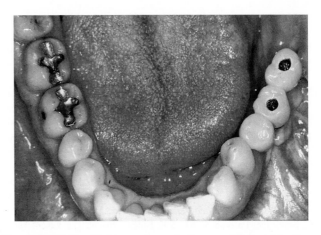

FIGURE 28.14 Fixed bridgework attached to two ITI dental implants (Bonefit®, ITI Strauman, Waldenberg, Switzerland) 3 months after insertion.

the second is inability to control correct implant position during placement and adaptation of the graft.

Three months after insertion of endosseus dental implants, the prosthetic suprastructure can be fabricated (Figure 28.14).

References

1. Komisar A, Warman S, Danziger E. A critical analysis of immediate and delayed mandible reconstruction using AO-plates. *Arch Otolaryngol Head Neck Surg.* 1989;115:830.

2. Davidson J, Birt WD, Gruss J. AO-plate mandibular reconstruction: a complication critique. *J Otolaryngol.* 1991;20:104.

3. Freitag V, Hell B, Fischer H. Experience with AO-reconstruction plates after partial mandibular resection involving its continuity. *J Craniomaxillofac Surg.* 1991;19:191.

4. Schusterman MA, Reece GP, Kroll SS, Weldon MA. Use of the AO-plate for immediate mandibular reconstruction in cancer patients. *Plast Reconstr Surg.* 1991;88:588.

5. Kim MR, Donoff RB. Critical analysis of mandibular reconstruction using AO-reconstruction plates. *J Oral Maxillofac Surg.* 1992;50:1152.

6. Wächter R, Stoll P. Komplikationen nach primärer Unterkieferrekonstruktion mit THORP-Platten. In: Neumann H-J, Hrsg. *Ästhetische und plastisch-rekonstruktive Gesichtschirurgie.* Rheinbek: Einhorn-Presseverlag; 1993:259.

7. Wächter R, Diz Dios P. Zur oralen funktion von tumorpatienten nach operation und versorgung mit Bonefit-implantaten. Erste qualitative und quantitative ergebnisse. *Z. Zahnärztl Implantol.* 1993;9:134.

8. Wächter R, Stoll P, Schilli W. Possibilities and limits of endosteal implants for the oral rehabilitation of tumor patients after radiotherapy. 5th International Congress On Preprosthetic Surgery, Vienna. April 15–18, 1993.

9. Wächter R, Stoll P, Bähr W, Lauer G. Osseointegration of ITI-dental implants (Bonefit) in non-vascularized and vascularized mandibular bone grafts. Proceedings 1st World Congress of Osseointegration, Venice. Sept. 29–Oct. 2, 1994.

10. Riediger D. Restoration of masticatory function by microsurgically revascularized iliac crest bone grafts using enosseous implants. *Plast Reconstr Surg.* 1988;81:861.

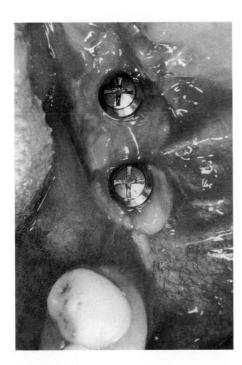

FIGURE 28.13 Insertion of two ITI dental implants (Bonefit®, ITI Strauman, Waldenberg, Switzerland) 6 months after bone repair.

11. Hidalgo DA. Fibula free flap: a new method of mandible reconstruction. *Plast Reconstr Surg.* 1989;84:71.

12. Duncan MJ, Manktelow RT, Zucker RM, Rosen IB. Mandibular reconstruction in the radiated patient: the role of osteocutaneous free tissue transfer. *Plast Reconstr Surg.* 1985;76:829.

13. Ioannides C, Fossion E, Boeckx W, Herrmans B, Jacobs D. Surgical management of the osteoradionecrotic mandible with free vascularized composite flaps. *J Craniomaxillofac Surg.* 1994;22:330.

14. Urken ML. Composite free flaps in oromandibular reconstruction. Review of the literature. *Arch Otolaryngol Head Neck Surg.* 1991;117:724.

15. Huryn JM, Zlotolow JM, Piro JD, Lenchewski E. Osseointegrated implants in microvascular fibula free flap reconstructed mandibles. *J Prosthet Dent.* 1993;70:443.

16. Serra JM, Paloma V, Mesa F, Ballesteros A. The vascularized fibula graft in mandibular reconstruction. *J Oral Maxillofac Surg.* 1991;49:244.

17. Frodel JL, Funk GF, Capper DT, Fridrich KL, Blumer JR, Haller JR, et al. Osseointegrated implants: a comparative study of bone thickness in 4 vascularized bone flaps. *Plast Reconstr Surg.* 1993;92:449.

18. Bekiscz O, Adant J, Denoel C, Lahaye T. Mandibular reconstruction. An anatomical study of bone thickness in three donor sites. Proceedings from the 12th Congress of the European Association for Cranio-Maxillofacial Surgery, The Hague, Sept 5th–10th, 1994.

19. Schusterman MA, Reece GP, Miller MJ, Harris S. The osteocutaneous free fibula flap. Is the skin paddle reliable? *Plast Reconstr Surg.* 1992;90:787.

20. Wolff K, Herzog K, Ervens J, Hoffmeister B. Experiences with the osteoseptocutaneous fibula-flap. 12th Congress of the European Association for Cranio-Maxillofacial Surgery, The Hague, Sept. 5th–10th, 1994.

21. Bundgaard T, Tandrup O, Elbrond O. A functional evaluation of patients treated for oral cancer. A prospective study. *Int J Oral Maxillofac Surg.* 1993;23:28.

22. Lukash FN, Sacks SA. Functional mandibular reconstruction. Prevention of the oral invalid. *Plast Reconstr Surg.* 1989;84:227.

23. Jones MF, Swartz WM, Mears DC, Jupitter JB, Grossman A. The "double barrel" free vascularized bone graft. *Plast Reconstr Surg.* 1988;81:379.

24. O'Brian B, Gumley GJ, Dooley BJ, Pribaz JJ. Folded free vascularized fibula transfer. *Plast Reconstr Surg.* 1988;82:311.

25. Bähr W, Stoll P, Wächter R. "Fibula Doppeltransplantat" als gefäßgestielter Unterkieferersatz. *Dtsch Z Mund-Kiefer-Gesichtschir.* 1994;18:219.

26. Gilbert A. Vascularized transfer of the fibula shaft. *Int J Microsurg.* 1979;1:100.

27. Manktelow RT. *Mikrovaskuläre Wiederherstellungschirurgie. Anatomie, Anwendung und chirurgische Technik.* Berlin: Springer Verlag; 1988.

28. Wood MB. *Atlas of Reconstructive Surgery.* Rockville, MD: Aspen; 1990.

29. Berggren A, Weiland A, Östrup L. Bone scintigraphy in evaluating the viability of composite bone grafts revascularized by microvascular anastomoses, conventional autogenous bone grafts, and free non-vascularized periosteal grafts. *J Bone Joint Surg Am.* 1982;64:799.

29

Soft Tissue Flaps for Coverage of Craniomaxillofacial Osseous Continuity Defects with or Without Bone Graft and Rigid Fixation

Barry L. Wenig

Mandibular continuity defects arising from trauma, infection, or tumor resection can often lead to serious and crippling disabilities. Loss of hard tissue (i.e., bone) will result in the inability to support the soft tissues of the oral cavity and oropharynx. This, in turn, will translate into significant deficiencies in the functions of swallowing, chewing, and talking as well as creating a disfiguring facial appearance.

The multitude of reconstructive options that have appeared in the literature attest to the difficulties that are associated with reconstruction of these continuity defects. Regardless of the technique that is chosen, the premise behind the reconstructive effort is based on the reestablishment of continuity while maintaining a normal maxillary-mandibular relationship. Structural support obtained in this manner will result in satisfactory return of form and function.

Mandibular resection following tumor ablation clearly results in the most challenging of all continuity defects. The significant soft tissue deficit and oral contamination associated with this type of treatment as well as advancing age, malnutrition, and prior radiation therapy that often accompany this patient population makes reconstruction of these individuals extremely complicated.

Decision Making in Reconstruction

The major issue confronting the surgeon faced with a mandibular continuity defect is the timing of the reconstruction. Is it in the best interest of the patient to perform the procedure at the time of tumor resection or would a secondary reconstruction be more advantageous?

Primary reconstruction at the time of ablative surgery has several distinct advantages. The most obvious advantage is that it allows for the restoration of mandibular continuity which, in turn, enables the patient to obtain immediate functional and cosmetic results. By avoiding multiple surgical procedures, the need to dissect in a previously operated or radiated field is eliminated. The patient is not faced with a radically altered appearance or disfigurement, which could

have a potentially devastating psychological effect. The ability to tolerate an oral diet or to verbally communicate limits the self-perception of the handicap that is often associated with individuals undergoing mandibular resection.

Secondary or delayed reconstruction offers the advantage of time. Allowing a certain interval to pass affords the surgeon and patient the knowledge that local and/or regional tumor control has been obtained. This option is certainly not unreasonable in an individual with very advanced disease, who may be in poor medical condition. On the other hand, secondary reconstruction is carried out in a scarred operative field that has often been subjected to radiation therapy. The chance of obtaining a very satisfactory cosmetic and functional result under these circumstances is certainly reduced in comparison with a primary repair.

Other variables that factor into the decision-making process include the use of radiation therapy and the location of the defect. The sacrifice of bone generally indicates an advanced-stage tumor. As such, radiation therapy is incorporated into the treatment plan in either a presurgical or postsurgical role. If radiation is administered in a preoperative manner, the surgeon is forced to contend with bone that is, by definition, hypoxemic. Surgical trauma may result in decreased vascularity, which will negatively impact on healing. Increased infection and fistulization can be anticipated. Delivery of radiation in an adjunctive, postoperative manner will have some impact on the mandible within the operative field. In this setting, it is imperative that vascularized tissue of some sort be transferred to the area if rigid fixation is being used. Despite this precaution, osteoradionecrosis, with resultant infection and extrusion, may ensue.

Location of defects similarly plays a role in the decision-making process. The anterior mandible remains the critical issue in any discussion of reconstruction. Owing to the devastating potential functional and cosmetic sequelae associated with sacrifice of the mandibular symphysis and arch, primary reconstruction in this area appears to be imperative. Reports indicate that in this region vascularized bone has a distinct advantage over any other technique.[1–11] Lateral defects, however, serve as an area of greater controversy since both cosmetic and functional deficits are neither as apparent nor as debilitating. Here, questions arise as to whether reconstruction is necessary at all.

Approaches to Reconstruction

The recent trend toward mandibular preservation has changed the approach of many physicians. Traditionally, the mandible was sacrificed if tumor even approximated the periosteum for both oncologic and practical reasons. As a result of the work of McGregor et al.[12–14] and Carter et al.,[15] it appears that two patterns of spread of squamous cell carcinoma within the mandible can be identified. The first involves spread in relation to the inferior alveolar nerve, while the second relates to spread in spaces between cancellous bony trabeculae. Based on these data, it appears that the extent of bone resection required can be estimated on the basis of tumor extent on the occlusal surface of the mandible regardless of whether only the upper border is being removed or a segmental resection is being undertaken. Furthermore, an adequate margin of safety can be considered to be 5 to 10 mm of apparently normal bone on either side of the main tumor mass. These concepts have radically altered opinion on the need to resect full segments of mandible, thereby eliminating much of the disability associated with extirpation and reconstruction. However, in cases where prior radiation has been administered, rim resection appears to be unsafe because of the variable and unpredictable routes of tumor entry.

Once the decision to resect has been reached, the degree or extent of resection then factors into the reconstruction decision-making process. Will it be necessary to reconstitute bone, lining, coverage, or a combination of these? Will the defect involve the symphysis and arch, body, or hemimandible?

As previously mentioned, the mandibular arch remains the most difficult region to reconstruct. Gravitational and muscular forces effectively eliminate the possibility of using any tissue other than vascularized bone as a free microvascular transfer. Although other methods have been successful in this area, the literature bears out the clear advantage enjoyed by this technique.[5,11,16] Decisions regarding reconstruction of ramus and/or body mandibular defects, however, are clinically based and relate to the functional and cosmetic goals that are desired.

Bone Substitutes

Numerous bone substitutes for mandibular defects have been tried. Irradiated[17,18] or cryopreserved mandible,[19] standard autologous bone grafts, particulate corticocancellous grafts with and without tray alloplasts (Figure 29.1),[20–22] and combinations of these techniques all were used in an attempt to replace the bone that was removed. These were generally done as secondary procedures for fear of contamination and infection or eventual tumor recurrence. While mandibular conti-

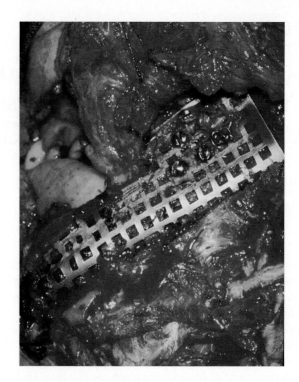

FIGURE 29.1 Corticocancellous bone graft within a vitallium tray alloplast.

nuity may have been reconstituted, large, pedicled flaps were often added to restore soft tissue defects.

Rigid Fixation

Early methods of stabilizing bony defects of the mandible have included Kirschner wires and their variations (Figure 29.2)[23–25] and extraskeletal fixation.[26,27] Metal impants were initially extensively described by Conley[28,29] and have been employed in numerous forms and ways since that time.[30]

Approximately 20 years ago, Schmoker et al.[31] introduced the concept of the reconstruction plate for the bridging of a mandibular defect. The major advantage offered by this plate was stability of the remaining mandibular segments following local trauma. The principles that developed from the treatment of traumatic injuries were then applied to patients undergoing mandibulectomy for malignancy.[32,33] Although initially made of steel, the current versions are fabricated from vitallium, or more commonly, titanium. The ability to contour and adapt these plates intraoperatively makes them ideal as replacement materials where large discontinuity defects are created during surgery.

The technique employed for placement has been fairly standardized. Before resection, the mandible is exposed and the anticipated sites of osteotomy are delineated. Using a template, the contour of the bone is marked, and the plate is then adapted to the form of the template. Drilling is then carried out followed by measurement of the holes. If a non–self-tapping screw system is used, the holes are then tapped, while tapping becomes unecessary in systems using self-tapping

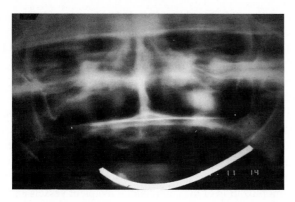

FIGURE 29.2 Kirschner wire used to reconstruct mandibular defect.

screws. The plate is then fixed to the bone with the screws and removed at which point the osteotomies are carried out. Following completion of the resection, the plate is fixed in position using the appropriate screws and mandibular continuity is reestablished maintaining the contour and rigidity of the fragments.

When contouring is performed prior to resection the potential for prognathism exists because the plate is contoured to the outer mandibular cortex. This is particularly true in anterior defects and much less of a problem in lateral ones. Alternatively, the plate may be contoured and applied after resection. In patients who are dentulous, intermaxillary fixation may be used to maintain normal occlusion of the residual dentition and removed at the end of the procedure. In the edentulous patient, a splint may be fabricated in advance to hold the upper and lower jaws in position until the plate can be applied.[26] Similarly, screws can be individually drilled in the upper and lower jaws and wired together to simulate occlusion until the plate is fixed in position. The fixation device can then be removed.

The Titanium Hollow-Screw Reconstruction Plate (THORP) is based on the osseointegration of titanium screws and the rigid fixation of the head of the screws to the plate.[34,35] The system combines the advantages of an external fixation device and those of internal osteosynthesis. Unlike standard reconstruction plates, THORP stability comes primarily from osseointegration of the hollow screws. Although the steps used to place the plate are similar to those used with standard reconstruction plates, the holes that are drilled and the screws that are placed are wider. Following neutral placement of the hollow screws, a conical expansion bolt is inserted into the free end of the hollow screw. The purpose of this bolt is to expand the flanges on the hollow screw so that it compresses the bone screw to the plate to achieve plate stability.

Soft Tissue

The principles originally developed for trauma were successfully applied to individuals undergoing mandibulectomy for tumors. This technique proved to be successful when the mandibulectomy was not combined with extensive soft tissue resection, as in the case of benign lesions (e.g., ameloblastoma). In instances where extensive resection of the oral or oropharyngeal mucosa was necessary, success has been less consistent.[11,36,37] These findings imply that under these conditions rigid fixation alone is insufficient and that soft tissue coverage is essential if a successful reconstruction is to be achieved. If the issue were simply a matter of stability, a high failure rate even in the absence of soft tissue defects would be expected, yet this has not proven to be the case. Additionally, information garnered from the vast orthopedic literature supports the idea that prolonged rigid fixation of long bones requires coverage with healthy tissue to reduce the risk of exposure and increase the probability of healing. With intraoral exposure, additional factors of contamination, such as constant exposure to saliva and oral bacteria, further complicate matters.

If no flap is employed in the closure of an oral or oropharyngeal defect and only rigid fixation is used following the removal of a significant volume of soft tissue, a primary closure of the wound may be tenuous. Under these circumstances, in the presence of a metal foreign body, any suture-line breakdown will predictably lead to plate exposure (Figure 29.3). This, in turn, may result in screw loosening, infection, and the ultimate extrusion or rejection of the plate.

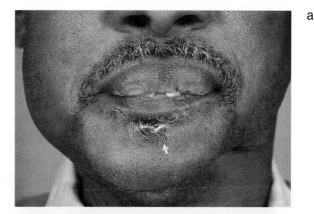

a

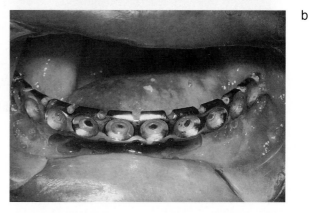

b

FIGURE 29.3 (a) External plate exposure following jaw resection and reconstruction without the use of a flap. (b) Intraoral plate exposure resulting from excessive tension on the suture line despite the use of a pectoralis major flap.

Vascularized, pedicled soft tissue flaps and microvascular free-tissue transfer have dramatically altered concepts relating to soft tissue reconstruction. The pectoralis major muscle as well as the latissimus dorsi and other bulky, pedicled flaps have been successfully employed in mandibular reconstruction (Figures 29.4 and 25.5).[38–43] Although extremely effective in lateral defects,[44] this technique is not without complications. Success rates vary in the literature yet, with the average approximating the 75% range.[38,45] Complications such as plate exposure, extrusion, flap breakdown, wound dehiscence, and others range from 23% to 65%.[38] Despite these statistics, this technique is effective in restoring immediate mandibular continuity and function. This is particularly important since the vast majority of these patients experience a recurrence of their disease, suggesting that an effective reconstruction with a minimum amount of difficulty may be in the best interest of the patient.

As microvascular techniques have advanced, many options have become available for free-tissue transfer. Differences exist with each flap regarding such things as the maneuverability and bulkiness of the soft tissue, the availability of a sensory nerve for reinnervation, the length of the vascular pedicle, the level of difficulty in harvesting and insetting, and donor-site morbidity. Although the flap can be customized, no one ideal flap exists.

When selecting a free-tissue donor flap to repair a defect involving resection of the mandible, the surgeon must take into account the size of the defect and the nature of the tissue that needs to be replaced. The rectus abdominis donor site has been well documented.[33,46–48] It offers the ability to reconstruct very complex three-dimensional head and neck deformities where soft tissue is required. The myocutaneous flap has been used for coverage of very large composite defects, particularly when sufficient skin for reconstruction of the mucosal and cutaneous defects is not available.

The rectus abdominis free flap is often chosen because of its long reliable vascular pedicle, versatile skin paddle, and favorable donor site, which offers the ability to elevate the flap simultaneously with the resection of the head and neck tumor. Additionally, with proper orientation of the skin paddle, mobilization of the contralateral recipient vessels and dissection of the flap vessels to their origin, anastomoses can be effectively and safely accomplished on the contralateral neck vessels, obviating the need for vein grafts. While the flap offers sufficient muscle to envelop the rigid fixation device, it has the drawback of being quite bulky and not easy to fit and contour into a relatively small defect. Without some type of neck dissection that includes removal of the sternocleidomastoid muscle, the flap is difficult to inset and undue pressure may be placed on the pedicle in an attempt to "squeeze" it into the proper position.

Less commonly, combination flaps such as the serratus anterior muscle (SAM) together with the latissimus dorsi have been described to repair composite oromandibular defects.[49] These composite flaps offer both lining and external coverage yet are often difficult to elevate and very time consuming.

The radial forearm flap (Figure 29.6)[50–52] and the lateral

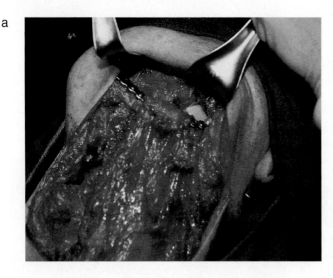

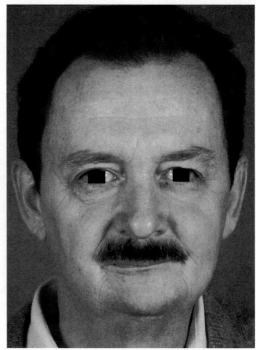

FIGURE 29.4 (a) Pectoralis major flap used to reline and cover defect. THORP plate employed to reconstruct the mandible. (b) Five-year result following surgery and postoperative radiation therapy.

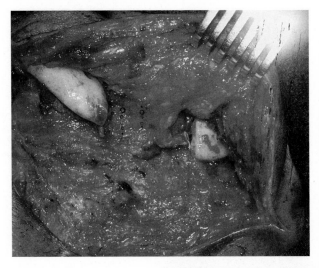

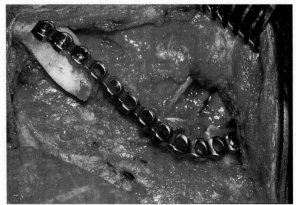

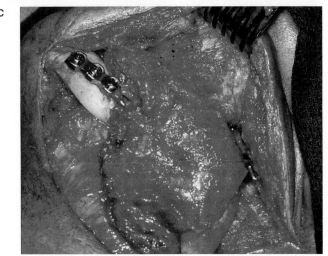

FIGURE 29.5 (a) Secondary defect of lateral mandible and soft tissue. (b) THORP plate used to span defect and hold stumps in position. (c) Pectoralis major flap to cover plate and fill in soft tissue.

arm free flap (Figure 29.7)[53–55] offer excellent alternatives to the bulkier rectus abdominis or attached pectoralis major flaps. By positioning the radial forearm or lateral arm flaps intraorally, the oral contents can be separated from the reconstruction plate and the chance of plate loosening or exposure can be decreased. The flap sits up high within the oral cavity and offers a thin, pliable mucosal substitute. The difficulty associated with either of these flaps results when a large resection is performed requiring more coverage and bulk than can be supplied by either of these fasciocutaneous flaps.

Bone Grafts

Autogenous free, nonvascularized bone grafts have been used to reconstruct mandibular defects since 1900.[56] Although rib, tibia, and clavicle all have been reported as donor sites, it appears that the best results are associated with grafts taken from the iliac bone. Corticocancellous autogenous bone from the

ilium provides viable cellular and osteoconductive capacity.[57] Blocks of this bone or particulate cancellous bone and marrow in an allogeneic bone tray are considered more acceptable than alloplastic replacements. This technique is, however, associated with a high morbidity due to complications such as infection (Figure 29.8), necrosis, or functional impairment. High donor-site morbidity, bone resorption, poor contour, lack of tissue bulk, and unpredictable results[1] all raise serious doubt as to the efficacy of this approach.

Several factors must be taken into consideration when bone grafting is contemplated. If significant bone stress shielding results from the rigid internal fixation device or if the period of healing is prolonged, then the graft may undergo undue bone resorption. Furthermore, the grafted bone must come into contact with the mucous membrane on its inner surface and the skin on its outer. These surfaces contain bacteria that can infect and destroy a graft. Additionally, the grafted bone must contain enough cortex to help it withstand the forces of

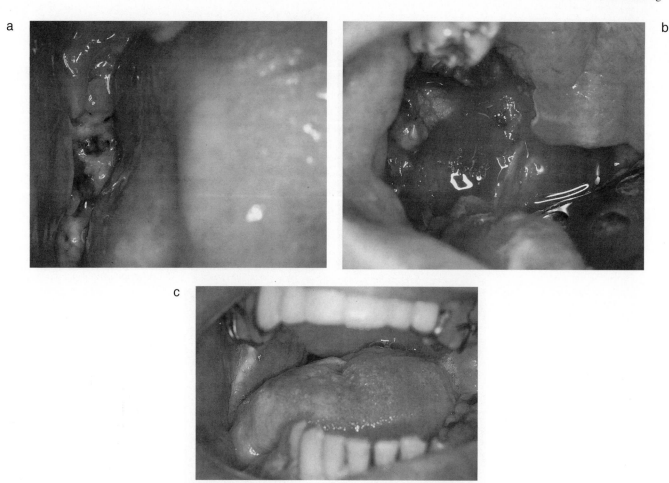

FIGURE 29.6 (a) T4N0M0 SCC of the right retromolar trigone. (b) Soft tissue and bone defect following resection. (c) Radial forearm flap inset over mandibular reconstruction plate. Five-year result.

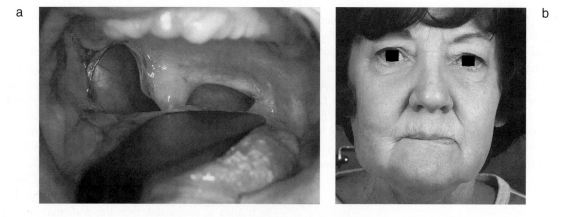

FIGURE 29.7 (a) Lateral arm flap inset over mandibular reconstruction plate in a patient with recurrence following radiation therapy. (b) Five-year result.

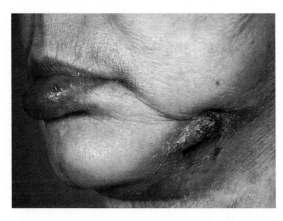

FIGURE 29.8 Exposure and infection following bone graft and alloplastic tray.

jaw function and provide a barrier to soft tissue ingrowth, which limits bone regeneration. The graft must also contain sufficient cancellous bone, with its nutrient-rich cellular components, to assist in rapid graft incorporation.[56]

With the deleterious effects of radiation therapy, which is commonly used following surgical extirpation, it seems reasonable to conclude that primary grafting is at best a risky adventure. Bone grafting appears to be most successful in the patient who has had surgery and has received postoperative radiation therapy and who requires a secondary reconstruction. Here, the factors noted earlier play a much smaller role. Primary internal stabilization of the remaining segments using mandibular reconstruction plates followed by delayed, secondary reconstruction appears to be the most widely accepted treatment option.[32,35,58–60]

Conclusions

Mandibular continuity defects continue to challenge the technical skills of surgeons involved in the care of these patients. The goals remain to reestablish bony and soft tissue contour, to provide proper occlusion, to allow sufficient mobility of the oral and oropharyngeal tissues, and to create an optimal situation to allow for dental rehabilitation.

As described here, any of several alternatives may be employed in the repair of such a defect. The correct choice will depend on the skill, experience, and judgment of the physician. The method chosen in any particular case should endeavor to achieve the stated goals with the least morbidity and the greatest chance for success.

References

1. Kuriloff DB, Sullivan MJ. Mandibular reconstruction using vascularized bone grafts. *Otolaryngol Clin N Am.* 1991;24:1391–1418.
2. Boyd JB, Morris S, Rosen IB, et al. The through-and-through oromandibular defect: rationale for aggressive reconstruction. *Plast Reconstr Surg.* 1994;93:44–53.
3. Urken ML, Vickery C, Weinberg H, et al. The internal oblique-iliac crest osseomyocutaneous microvascular free flap in head and neck reconstruction. *J Reconstr Microsurg.* 1989;5:203–214.
4. Moscoso JF, Keller J, Genden E, et al. Vascularized bone flaps in oromandibular reconstruction. *Arch Otolaryngol Head Neck Surg.* 1994;120:36–43.
5. Kroll SS, Schusterman MA, Reece GP. Immediate vascularized bone reconstruction of anterior mandibular defects with free iliac crest. *Laryngoscope.* 1991;101:791–794.
6. Buchbinder D, Urken ML, Vickery C, et al. Bone contouring and fixation in functional, primary microvascular mandibular reconstruction. *Head Neck.* 1991;13:191–199.
7. Hidalgo DA. Fibula free flap: a new method of mandible reconstruction. *Plast Reconstr Surg.* 1989;84:71–79.
8. Baker SR, Sullivan MJ. Osteocutaneous free scapular flap for one-stage mandibular reconstruction. *Arch Otolaryngol Head Neck Surg.* 1988;114:267–277.
9. Hoffman HT, Harrison N, Sullivan MJ, et al. Mandible reconstruction with vascularized bone grafts. *Arch Otolaryngol Head Neck Surg.* 1991;117:917–925.
10. Urken ML, Weinberg H, Vickery C, et al. Oromandibular reconstruction using microvascular composite free flaps. *Arch Otolaryngol Head Neck Surg.* 1991;117:733–744.
11. Wenig BL, Keller AJ. Microvascular free tissue transfer with rigid internal fixation for reconstruction of the mandible following tumor resection. *Otolaryngol Clin N Am.* 1987;20:621–633.
12. McGregor AD, MacDonald DG. Patterns of spread of squamous cell carcinoma within the mandible. *Head Neck.* 1989;11:457–461.
13. McGregor IA, MacDonald DG. Spread of squamous cell carcinoma to the non-irradiated edentulous mandible—a preliminary report. *Head Neck.* 1987;9:157–161.
14. McGregor AD, MacDonald DG. Routes of entry of squamous cell carcinoma into the mandible. *Head Neck.* 1989;11:457–461.
15. Carter RL, Pittam MR. Squamous cell carcinomas of the head and neck: some patterns of spread. *J R Soc Med.* 1980;73:420–427.
16. Shockley WW, Weissler MC. Reconstructive alternatives following segmental mandibulectomy. *Am J Otolaryngol.* 1992;13:156–167.
17. Hamaker RC. Irradiated autogenous mandibular grafts in primary reconstruction. *Laryngoscope.* 1981;91:1031–1051.
18. Hamaker RC, Singer MI. Irradiated mandibular autografts update. *Arch Otolaryngol Head Neck Surg.* 1986;112:277–279.
19. Cummings CW, Leipzig B. Replacement of tumor involved mandible by cryosurgically devitalized autograft. *Arch Otolaryngol Head Neck Surg.* 1980;106:252–254.
20. Lawson W, Biller HF. Mandibular reconstruction: bone graft techniques. *Otolaryngol Head Neck Surg.* 1982;90:589–594.
21. Maisel RH, Hilger PA, Adams GL. Reconstruction of the mandible. *Laryngoscope.* 1983;93:1122–1126.
22. Lowlicht RA, Delacure MD, Sasaki CT. Allogenic (Homograft) reconstruction of the mandible. *Laryngoscope.* 1990;100:837–843.
23. Lee KY, Lore JM, Perry CJ. Use of the Kirschner wire for mandibular reconstruction. *Arch Otolaryngol Head Neck Surg.* 1988;114:68–72.

24. Gaisford JC, Hanna BC, Gutman D. Management of the mandibular fragments following resection. *Plast Reconstr Surg.* 1968;28:192–206.

25. Reyneke JP, Wilcock VE. Immediate mandibular reconstruction after resection using a modified Kirschner wire splint. *J Oral Surg.* 1979;37:415–418.

26. Reece GP, Martin JW, Lemon JC, et al. Mandible fragment fixation during reconstruction: the splint and plate technique. *Ann Plast Surg.* 1993;31:128–133.

27. Fleming ID, Morris JH. Use of acrylic external splint after mandible resection. *Am J Surg.* 1969;118:708–715.

28. Conley JJ. The use of vitallium prosthesis and implants in the reconstruction of the mandibular arch. *Plast Reconstr Surg.* 1951;8:150–162.

29. Conley JJ. A technique of immediate bone grafting in the treatment of benign and malignant tumors of the mandible and review of 17 cases. *Cancer.* 1953;6:568–577.

30. Söderholm A-L, Lindqvist C, Laine P, et al. Primary reconstruction of the mandible in cancer surgery. *Int J Oral Maxillofac Surg.* 1988;17:194–197.

31. Schmoker R, Spiessl B, Mathys R. A total mandibular plate to bridge large defects of the mandible. In: *New Concepts in Maxillofacial Bone Surgery.* New York: Springer-Verlag, 1976: 156–166.

32. Kellman RM, Gullane PJ. Use of the AO mandibular reconstruction plate for bridging mandibular defects. *Otolaryngol Clin N Am.* 1987;20:519–533.

33. Wenig BL, Keller AJ, Shikowitz MJ, et al. Anatomic reconstruction and functional rehabilitation of oromandibular defects with rigid internal fixation. *Laryngoscope.* 1988;98:2154–2159.

34. Vuillemin T, Raveh J, Sutter F. Mandibular reconstruction with the titanium hollow screw reconstruction (THORP) system: evaluation of 62 cases. *Plast Reconstr Surg.* 1988;82:804–814.

35. Hellem S, Olofsson J. Titanium-coated hollow screw and reconstruction plate system (THORP) in mandibular reconstruction. *J Craniomaxillofac Surg.* 1988;16:173–183.

36. Gullane PJ, Holmes H. Mandibular reconstruction: new concepts. *Arch Otolaryngol Head Neck Surg.* 1986;112:714–719.

37. Papel ID, Price JC, Kashima HK, et al. Compression plates in the treatment of advanced anterior floor of mouth carcinoma. *Laryngoscope.* 1986;96:722–725.

38. Disher MJ, Esclamado RM, Sullivan MJ. Indications for the AO plate with a myocutaneous flap instead of revascularized tissue transfer for mandibular reconstruction. *Laryngoscope.* 1993; 103:1004–1007.

39. Murphy JB, Weisman RA, Kent K. The use of stabilization plates in the immediate repair of defects following mandibular resection. *Oral Surg Oral Med Oral Pathol.* 1989;68:380–384.

40. Klotch DW, Gump J, Kuhn L. Reconstruction of mandibular defects in irradiated patients. *Am J Surg.* 1990;160:396–398.

41. Lehtimaki K, Pukander J. Primary mandibular reconstruction after ablative cancer surgery. *Acta Otolaryngol.* 1992;Suppl. 492: 160–163.

42. Lindqvist C, Söderholm AL, Laine P, et al. Rigid reconstruction plates for immediate reconstruction following mandibular resection for malignant tumors. *J Oral Maxillofac Surg.* 1992; 50:1158–1163.

43. Margarino G, Scala M, Gipponi M, et al. Mandible reconstruction with metallic endoprosthesis following Commando's operation for advanced head and neck cancer. Personal experience. *Eur J Surg Oncol.* 1993;19:320–326.

44. Schusterman MA, Reece GP, Kroll SS, et al. Use of the AO plate for immediate mandibular reconstruction in cancer patients. *Plast Reconstr Surg.* 1991;88:588–593.

45. Shockley WW, Weissler MC, Pillsbury HC. Immediate mandibular replacement using reconstruction plates. *Arch Otolaryngol Head Neck Surg.* 1991;117:745–750.

46. Meland NB, Fisher J, Irons GB, et al. Experience with 80 rectus abdominis free tissue transfers. *Plast Reconstr Surg.* 1989; 83:481–487.

47. Jones NF, Sekhar LN, Schramm VL. Free rectus abdominis muscle flap reconstruction of the middle and posterior cranial base. *Plast Reconstr Surg.* 1986;78:471–477.

48. Taylor GI, Corlett R, Boyd JB. The versatile deep inferior epigastric inferior rectus abdominis flap. *Br J Plast Surg.* 1984; 37:330–350.

49. Ioannides C, Fossion E, Boeckx W. Serratus anterior muscle in composite head and neck flaps. *Head Neck.* 1992;14:177–182.

50. Davidson J, Gullane PJ, Freeman J, et al. A comparison of the results following oromandibular reconstruction using a radial forearm flap with either radial bone or a reconstruction plate. *Plast Reconstr Surg.* 1991;88:201–208.

51. Soutar DS, Scheker LR, Tanner NS, et al. The radial forearm flap: a versatile method for intraoral reconstruction. *Br J Plast Surg.* 1983;36:1–8.

52. Kawashima T, Harii K, Ono I, et al. Intraoral and oropharyngeal reconstruction using a de-epithelialized forearm flap. *Head Neck.* 2989;11:358–363.

53. Wenig BL. The lateral arm free flap for head and neck reconstruction. *Otolaryngol Head Neck Surg.* 1993;109:116–119.

54. Matloub HS, Larson DL, Kuhn JC, et al. Lateral arm free flap in oral cavity reconstruction: a functional evaluation. *Head Neck.* 1989;11:205–211.

55. Kuek LBK, Chuan TL. The extended lateral arm flap: a new modification. *J Reconstr Microsurg.* 1991;7:167–173.

56. Tidstrom KD, Keller EE. Reconstruction of mandibular discontinuity with autogenous iliac bone graft. *J Oral Maxillofac Surg.* 1990;48:336–346.

57. Kim MR, Donoff RB. Critical analysis of mandibular reconstruction using AO reconstruction plates. *J Oral Maxillofac Surg.* 1992;50:1152–1157.

58. Kudo K, Fujioka Y. Review of bone grafting for reconstruction of discontinuity defects of the mandible. *J Oral Surg.* 1978; 36:791–795.

59. Kruger E, Krumholz K. Results of bone grafting after rigid fixation. *J Oral Maxillofac Surg.* 1984;42:491–494.

60. Vuillemin T, Raveh J, Sutter F. Mandibular reconstruction with the THORP prosthesis after hemimandibulectomy. *J Craniomaxillofac Surg.* 1989;17:78–87.

30
Mandibular Condyle Reconstruction with Free Costochondral Grafting

Christian Lindqvist

Reconstruction of the temporomandibular articulation is one of the most demanding challenges in maxillofacial surgery. The goals include not only rehabilitation of the complex mechanism of the normal joint, but restoration of facial symmetry, occlusion, and mastication. As advanced temporomandibular joint (TMJ) disease can lead to disturbances in these features and functions, this often constitutes major indications for arthroplastic procedures. The alleviation of pain is also of great importance, especially in the considerations for surgical treatment of degenerative joint disease. In children, mandibular growth imposes additional constraints on the reconstructive process.

Indications

The most common indications for TMJ arthroplasty are various forms of ankylosis, which cause restriction of mouth opening and disturbed masticatory function (Table 30.1). In most cases, trauma or rheumatoid disease is responsible for the development of ankylosis.[1–3] Today, middle-ear infections and osteomyelitis are infrequent causes of ankylosis. Various forms of dysplasia and mandibular deformity can also constitute indications for joint arthroplasty, but with such conditions additional mandibular and maxillary surgery is often necessary.[4] Tumors of the mandibular condyle are rare indications for TMJ arthroplasty. Oral cancer operations that require disarticulation of the condyle may necessitate combined extracapsular mandibular and joint reconstruction.

Several methods have been advocated for the treatment of restricted TMJ mobility. The most common method has been interposition arthroplasty. This was the mainstay of the treatment of ankylosis for more than 100 years. However, problems associated with interpositional arthroplasty can have an adverse effect on the results. When alloplastic materials have been used, the problems of articulation, stabilization, and fixation of the graft and foreign-body reactions have sometimes had detrimental effects.

Autogenous Arthroplasty

Several autogenous tissues have been used for replacement grafting of the mandibular condyle. Iliac bone, fibular head, metatarsal bone, metatarsophalangeal joint, clavicle, and sternoclavicular joints, together with orthoptic allografts, have all proved to be successful in restoring lost function of the temporomandibular articulation.[5–11]

Costochondral Arthroplasty

Gillies was probably the first to use a costochondral graft for this purpose in 1920.[12] Since then, a number of authors have recommended autogenous costochondral grafts for congenital dysplasia, ankylosis, osteoarthritis, neoplastic disease, and posttraumatic dysfunction of the TMJ.[12–19]

Advantages

The advantages of costochondral grafting are the biological and anatomic similarities to the condyle, low morbidity and regeneration of donor sites, and a demonstrated growth potential in juveniles.[19,20] Several experimental studies have demonstrated that rib cartilage has characteristics similar to those of the mandibular condyle.[19,21,22] This makes it more likely that growth adaptation and function in the new site will occur.

Disadvantages

In spite of the ideal intrinsic and adaptive growth characteristics of the costochondral junction, there are also difficulties associated with rib grafting, the most commonly encountered of which have been pneumothorax and hemothorax, pain, infection, and uncontrolled and unpredictable growth.[12,18,20,23]

Radiology

Preoperative radiologic evaluation of the joint usually includes panoramic images and two- and three-dimensional computed tomographic (CT) reconstructions (Figure 30.1).[24]

TABLE 30.1 Indications for arthroplasty.

Ankylosis
   Traumatic
   Rheumatoid
   Arthritic
   Postinfection
Tumors
   Benign
   Malignant
Dysplasia
   Hypoplasia
   Hyperplasia
Osteomyelitis

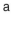
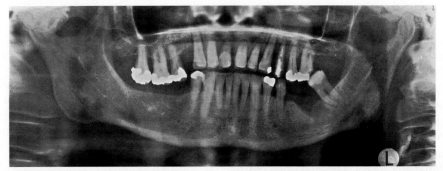

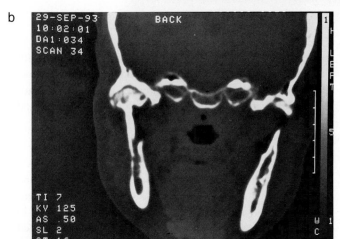
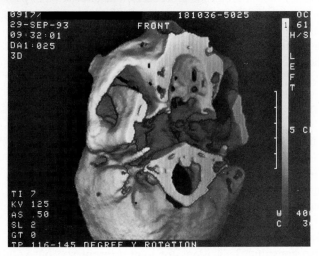

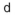
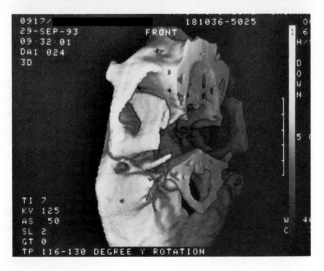

FIGURE 30.1 (a) Panoramic image of 57-year-old woman with anky-losis of right TMJ due to unknown reason. (b) Two-dimensional CT. (c,d) Three-dimensional CT. The extent of the ankylotic process is clearly shown in the CT scans.

a

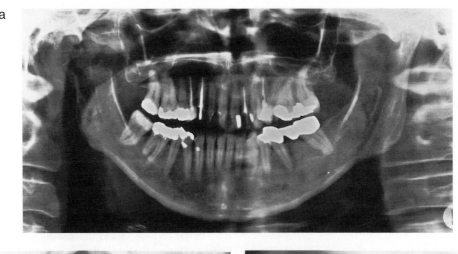

b

c

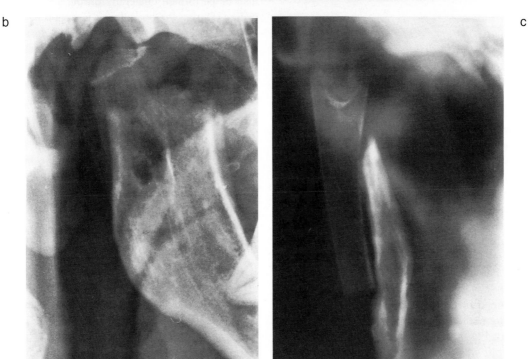

FIGURE 30.2 (a) Postoperative radiograph of patient with costochondral arthroplasty to the right. Graft fixed with polylactide screws. (b) Detailed lateral view. (c) Detailed posteroanterior view. These examinations are useful in follow-up.

Panoramic examinations taken with image layer programs designed especially for the temporomandibular joint in lateral and posteroanterior projection are useful (Figure 30.2).[1,25,26] Examinations that include imaging both joints at the same exposure (Zonarc Instrumentarium, Finland) or detailed images of a single joint (Scanora Orion Corp., Soredex, Finland) can be used. A conventional panoramic radiograph is also usually included in the examination.

Condylar translation can be measured on the TMJ lateral panoramic images taken with the mouth closed and open, and the rotational movement can also be evaluated.[25]

Plain films and conventional tomography are of limited value in preoperative evaluation of the joint.[24]

Our experience is limited regarding magnetic resonance imaging (MRI). Its use should be limited to patients not operated upon earlier because even minute metal debris from tools (e.g., drills), produce large artifacts that deteriorate the image over a large area.

Operative Procedure

During operation, the TMJ is exposed, usually by a submandibular or retromandibular and/or a preauricular (extended in some cases to a bicoronal) approach, and the condylar head (ankylotic segment) is resected. This is the most important and usually most difficult stage of the operation, because often when ankylosis is present the bone mass can be very large and to attempt complete removal might be dan-

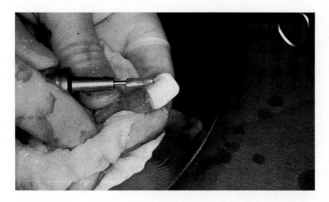

FIGURE 30.3 The cartilaginous end of the rib is shaped to match the temporal fossa.

gerous.[1] Because of the medial vascular anatomy, severe bleeding can be encountered. Great care must be taken to preserve the neurovascular bundle of the mandible. In ankylosis cases, coronoidectomy is often performed, sometimes bilaterally. Occasionally, the fossa is lined with the temporal muscle, including fascia. The length of the required graft is determined, and a portion of rib (usually from the sixth or seventh rib) is removed via a submammary incision. The pectoral muscles and underlying periosteum are divided, and the required length of bone with cartilage is exposed and removed. It is very important not to traumatize the costochondral junction, which in children is often quite fragile and easily separates. After confirming that the parietal pleura is intact, the wound is closed in layers. The rib is preserved in moistened swabs until the mandible has been prepared to receive the transplant.

The glenoid fossa is judiciously recontoured with burs and the cartilaginous end of the rib shaped to fit into the fossa (Figure 30.3). Prior to the advent of rigid fixation, the rib was usually decorticated to fit into the mandible as an inlay (Figure 30.4). The graft was then fixed with two 0.5-mm stainless steel wires. Today, decortication of the rib is unneces-

sary. It is fixed laterally with two or three 2.7-mm steel, titanium, or polylactide (PLLA) lag screws (Figure 30.5). Sometimes the rib is very soft and washers have to be used to enlarge the area of pressure (Figure 30.6).[1] Particularly in cases where the mandible is retrognathic and advanced forward with simultaneous arthroplasty, the rib can be positioned transversally to the dorsal side of the ramus (Figure 30.7),[27] and graft fixation is obtained with miniplates. It is also possible to fix the graft laterally by one miniplate and 2.0-mm bicortical screws (Figure 30.8).[28] Because the rib can occasionally be very soft and thin, fixation (either screw or miniplate) does not always provide enough stability for immediate mandibular mobilization. Intermaxillary fixation (IMF) might be necessary in some cases for 2 to 3 weeks. TMJ arthroplasty can also be performed bilaterally during a single operative procedure. During the operation it is important that IMF maintains the desired occlusion, usually with elastics. The fixation has to be released occasionally to check the bite, to confirm that interferences do not exist and that sufficient maximal interincisal opening has been achieved.

Complications

Operative complications are infrequent. In our series on 66 arthroplasties[1] the external carotid had to be ligated in one patient because of severe bleeding. In one case, pneumothorax occurred and had to be treated by pleural suction. No chest infections or wound breakdowns were recorded.[1]

Patient Material

Between 1969 and 1987, 41 female and 31 male patients underwent 82 nonvascular costochondral arthroplasties at the Department of Oral and Maxillofacial Surgery, Helsinki University Central Hospital, Helsinki, Finland. The mean age of the patients was 32 years. In nearly half of the cases, ankylosis was the main indication for the operation. The next most frequent indications, in descending order, were dysplasia, tu-

a 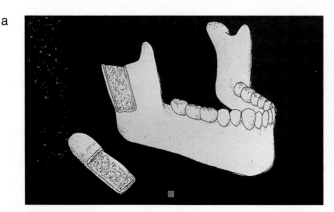 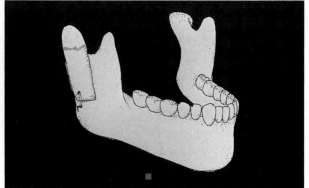 b

FIGURE 30.4 (a) The decorticated rib and ramus of the mandible. (b) The rib fits into the mandible as an inlay. The graft is fixed with two 0.5-mm stainless steel wires.

a
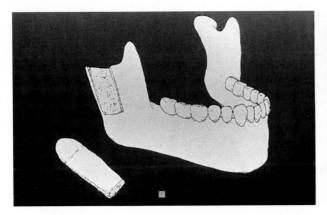
b
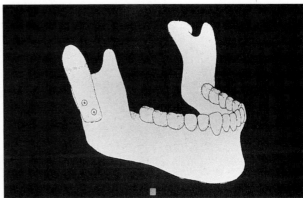

FIGURE 30.5 (a) When screws are used for fixation there is no need for decortication of the rib. (b) Rib fixed with two bicortical stainless steel or polylactide screws.

mors, and osteomyelitis. In 8 patients the arthroplasty was performed bilaterally.

Results

Maximal mouth opening increased on average by 13 mm.[29] The great majority of the patients (67%) were relieved of their preoperative pain and were able to chew without difficulty. In 56% of the cases with ankylosis, function of the mandible was considered to be good or excellent. Five patients (6.9%), however, suffered subjectively from restricted mouth opening and had difficulties in eating. Two relapses required further opera-

tions, and in one case, total patient neglect of the postoperative training program led to an unsatisfactory result. Very little donor site or recipient site morbidity was observed. Three cases exhibited auriculotemporal syndrome, six had slight weakness of the mandibular branch of the facial nerve, and seven exhibited paresthesia of the lower lip on the operated side. In no case was a pseudoarthrosis between the graft and ramus diagnosed.

Reankylosis after costochondral arthroplasty is rare. However, it is possible that an overgrowth of the cartilagous part with ossification can occur. We have observed this in two patients. In these cases, the joint region can exhibit signs of tumor growth both clinically and radiologically (Figure 30.9). Reoperation is usually indicated.

a
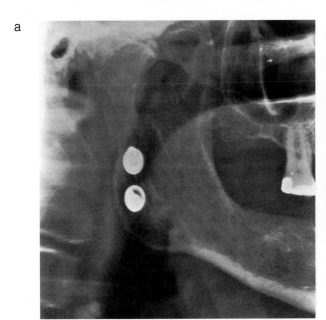
b
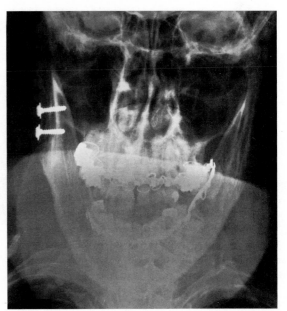

FIGURE 30.6 (a) Costochondral graft fixed with 2.7-mm bicortical screws together with washers. (b) Anteroposterior view showing the lateral fixation.

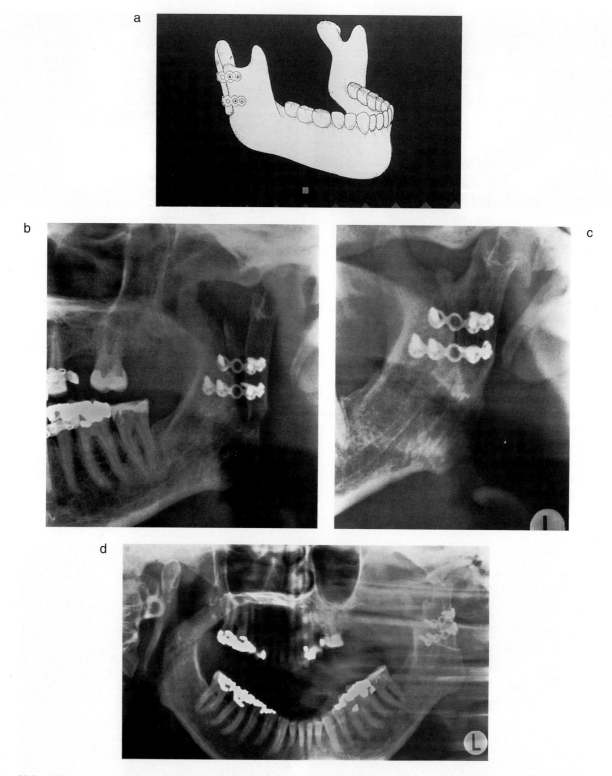

Figure 30.7 (a) Transverse fixation of rib with miniplates. (b) Post-operative radiograph of transversely fixed costochondral graft in 44-year-old female patient. (c) JLA of the situation 4 years later. Partial ossification of the chondral part can be observed. (d) Maximal mouth opening shows normal rotation and fairly good translation at the left side.

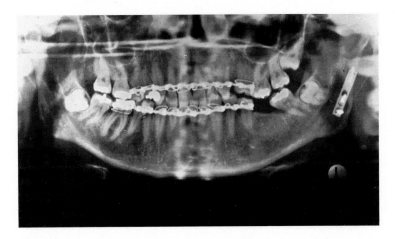

FIGURE 30.8 Lateral fixation of rib with miniplate and bicortical screws.

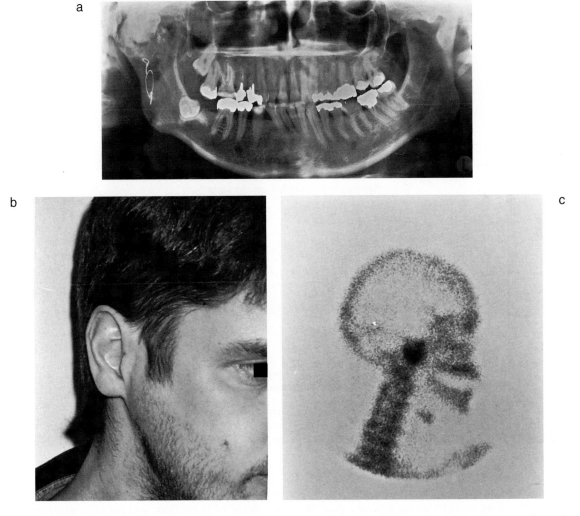

FIGURE 30.9 (a) Radiograph of 38-year-old man who underwent costochondral TMJ arthroplasty to the right 15 years earlier owing to post-traumatic TMJ ankylosis. (b) Note preauricular swelling. MIO 12 mm. (c) Bone scan shows extensive uptake.

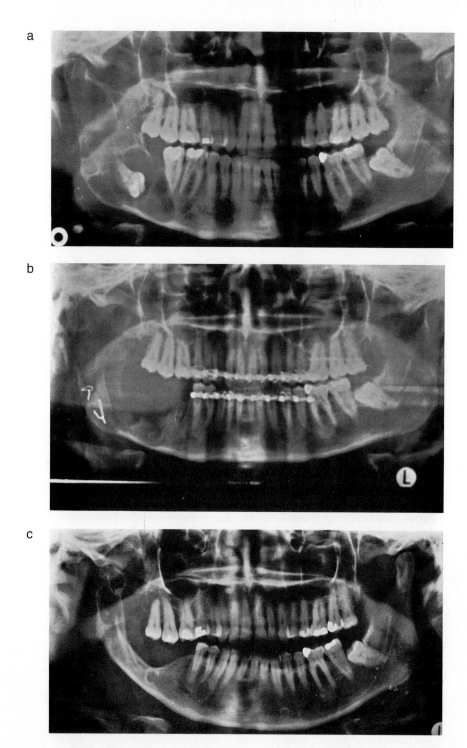

FIGURE 30.10 (a) Keratocyst in right mandible. (b) Reconstruction with costochondral graft after cyst removal. (c) Recurrence in the rib and mandibular body 14 years later. (d) The removed rib with tumor. (e) Radiograph of removed rib shows cystic tumor. (f) Reconstruction with titanium condylar plate (note two incisions). (g) Panoramic image showing the final result.

Recurrent disease can develop in certain cases within a costochondral graft. Figure 30.10 shows the case of a 38-year-old female patient. She had a keratocyst in her right mandible 14 years earlier. This was extirpated and the ra- mus reconstructed with a costochondral graft. A recurrence was noted 14 years later, and the graft was removed and re- placed with a titanium reconstruction plate with condylar head.

d

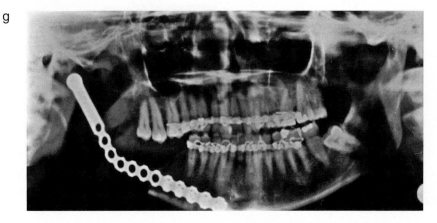

e

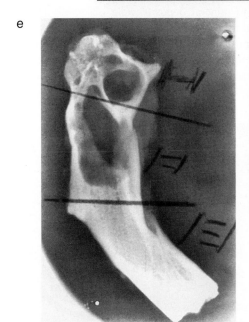

f

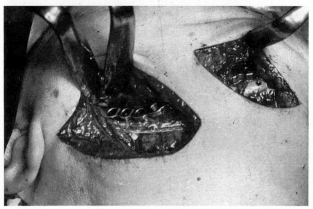

g

FIGURE 30.10 *Continued.*

Late Results

Sixteen patients who underwent operation in our unit before 1982 were followed up clinically and radiologically.[25] All of these patients have had unilateral grafts. The mean follow-up time was 9.9 years. Patients were questioned regarding general satisfaction, chewing ability, and facial or joint pain. Other items recorded related to facial motor and sensory function, TMJ clicking or crepitus, joint pain on palpation, maximum mouth opening, lateral excursions, and protrusion of the mandible. The TMJs were radiographed in lateral and posteroanterior projections using a Zonarc (Zonarc, Instrumentarium, Finland) device for panoramic radiography with the patient in the supine position. After the follow-up time, which extended for nearly a decade on average, the mean mouth opening for these 16 patients was 39.4 mm.[25] Opening increased postoperatively with time. During the follow-up period, contralateral excursion also increased by an average of 3.1 mm.[25] All patients had a symmetrical facial appearance, with the teeth in centric occlusion. On maximal opening, however, 8 patients exhibited a mean deviation of the chin point of 3.5 mm.[25]

Calcification (ossification) of the transplanted cartilage was graded as follows:

1. Sharp osteochondral margin, similar to postoperative situation with no calcification of the cartilage: 0
2. Slightly noticeable calcification: +
3. Considerable calcification but no apparent formation of a condyle: ++
4. Total or almost total calcification, ossification of the cartilaginous part with joint surface formation, or both: +++

Radiologically, good bony healing was seen in all patients and no postoperative displacement of the grafts were observed. In six patients, calcification of the cartilaginous region of the rib was total or subtotal, with joint surface formation. In five patients, calcification was considerable but no condyle had been formed during the follow-up period. Only slight calcification was recorded in three patients. In two patients, no mineral deposits were observed. The osteocartilaginous margin was still sharp. As seen on the radiographs, the average translation movement of the rib condyle was 5.0 mm on the operated side and 7.0 mm on the opposite side. The mean angle of rotation was 10°.[25] The extent of condy-

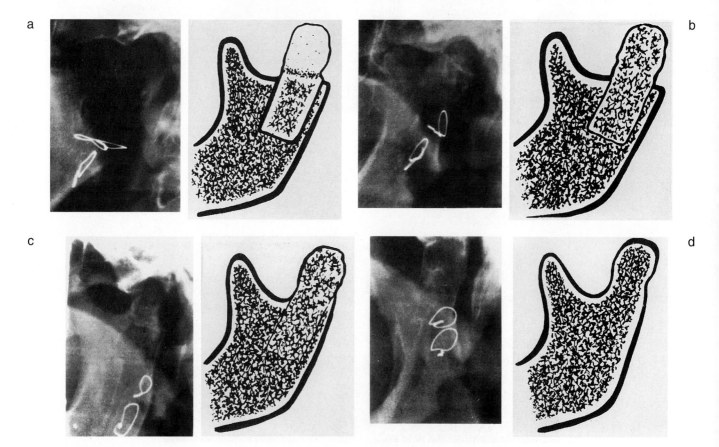

FIGURE 30.11 Different degrees of radiologic calcification and remodeling (adaption) of costochondral grafts to the TMJ. Example of representative radiograph (left). Corresponding schematic drawing (right). (a) Sharp osteochondral margin with no calcification of cartilage: 0 (−). (b) Slight calcification: +. (c) Considerable calcification without formation of condyle: ++. (d) Almost total calcification of cartilaginous part with joint surface formation: +++.

lar translation was significantly greater in the grafts that showed complete adaptation, but no other correlations were found (Figure 30.11–13, Table 30.2).

Several methods have been advocated for the treatment of restricted mobility of the TMJ. The most common method has been interposition arthroplasty, which has been the method of choice for more than 100 years.[30] However, there seem to have been several problems with interpositional arthroplasties that may compromise the result. Later when alloplastic

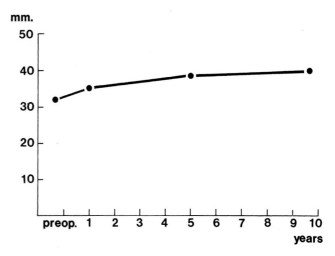

FIGURE 30.13 Average maximal mouth opening in 16 patients before and 1, 5, and 10 years after autogenous costochondral TMJ grafts.

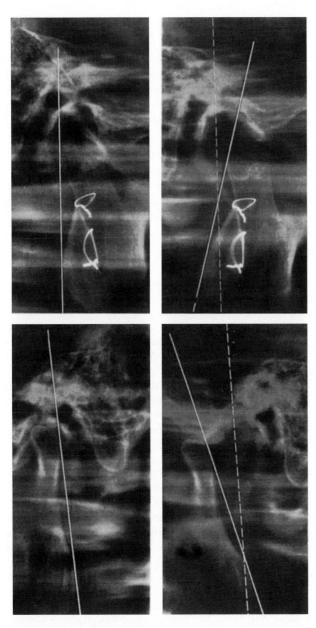

FIGURE 30.12 TMJ lateral panoramic films taken with mouth closed (top and bottom left) and open (top and bottom right). Slight calcification of the cartilage is seen 12 years after reconstruction (top). Translation is 6 mm on operated side and 17 mm on contralateral side. Rotation is 15° on both sides.

materials have been used, problems with articulation, stabilization, and fixation of the polymer, together with foreign-body reactions have had detrimental effects on the results.[30] The problem of finding a suitable interpositional autogenous graft still needs to be solved.[31] High incidences of postsurgical recurrence of the ankylosis have also been reported.[32]

Several physical, biomechanical, and animal experiments followed by clinical series have been presented concerning metallic or ceramic joint prostheses.[30,33–37] A wide range of commercially available condylar prostheses have produced satisfactory results in the rehabilitation of adult patients suffering from ankylosis. Particularly in severe cases, simultaneous correction of the dental-skeletal problem has been considered an indication for the use of metallic condylar prosthesis. Additionally, there is no need for postsurgical intermaxillary fixation, which must be considered a clear advantage during the early postoperative phase. The use of alloplastic condyles should, however, be restricted to adult patients. Several studies have shown that in children and young adolescents, the costochondral graft has the possibility of responding to the dynamic morphologic changes present during the growth period.[14,16,19,20] In patients with rheumatoid arthritis, a costochondral graft is also probably safer, owing to the resorption of the glenoid fossa seen in patients reconstructed with bilateral metallic condyles.[30,36] Whether this holds true for patients with ankylosing spondylitis or osteoarthritis of the TMJ is unclear.

As early as 1951[38] osteoarthritis was suggested as an indication for costochondral grafting. It seems that in severe cases the disease leads to a restriction of mouth opening and total deformity of the mandibular condyle. In these cases, when conservative treatment methods have failed, arthroplasty should be considered. It must, however, be emphasized that dysfunction of the TMJ without radiological changes, various

TABLE 30.2 Various signs and symptoms in 16 patients with costochondral TMJ arthroplasties according to degree of radiologic adaptation of graft.

Degree of adaptation	Patients	Mean age (years)	Mean follow-up (years)	Pain	Joint noises	Mean opening (mm)	Mean translation (mm)	Mean rotation (degrees)
0	2	36	10.6	1/2	1/2	38	3.0	7.5
+	3	31	9.1	1/3	—	48	4.3	13.3
++	5	22	11.8	1/5	1/5	39	4.9	9.0
+++	6	37	7.0	2/6	1/6	36	7.8	10.2
Totals	16	31	9.6	5/16	3/16	40	5.0	10.0

"internal derangements," and atypical facial neuralgias should not be considered as indications for costochondral arthroplasty. The same holds true for malignant tumors in the condylar region, when disarticulation is performed during the primary ablative procedure. However, when there is no recurrence of tumor within 2 to 3 years after the primary treatment, a costochondral graft can be used for the reconstruction of the condyle. With respect to benign tumors, there do not appear to be any contraindications for costochondral grafting at the primary operation.[12]

Congenital dysplasia has been a common indication for grafting.[12] The term has been used to characterize either excessive or inadequate growth of the condyle. It has been recommended that in cases of hypoplasia or aplasia of the condyle the patients should be operated on at an early age. Also, with respect to hyperplasia, a resection with or without grafting has been advocated.[39] In young persons, however, continued growth of the transplant is unpredictable.[40] The intrinsic growth potential in transplanted costochondral junction growth centers has been reported several times.[20,41,42] Therefore, undercorrection may be justified in juvenile cases.

Primary chronic osteomyelitis of the mandible remains a therapeutic problem. In our patients, the process involved the mandibular condyle and led in some cases to a disturbance of joint function. In fact, osteomyelitis seemed to cause ankylosis of the TMJ in a number of patients.[43,44] All these patients also suffered from severe pain, which was refractory to conservative treatment. Costochondral arthroplasty seems to be a solution for these infrequent but problematic cases as good mandibular function was achieved with disappearance of pain. The osteomyelitic process did not appear to affect the transplanted rib during the observation period.

The frequency of early or late complications is rather low and through further refinement of surgical technique, the neurological sequelae (i.e., dysfunction of fifth or seventh cranial nerves) could probably be still further diminished. The harvesting of a rib as a source of bone seems to be safe and relatively easy. The incidence of pneumothorax is low and does not represent a major problem. Proper postoperative physiotherapy is probably important in avoiding chest infections.

Conclusions

Excellent functional and aesthetic results seem to add support to the contention that costochondral grafting is a reliable method for the treatment of TMJ ankylosis owing to several different etiologies. The same seems to hold true with respect to dysplasia of the condyle, deformities of the mandible, and ascending osteomyelitic processes in the mandibular ramus. The results with respect to cases with TMJ dysfunction or atypical facial neuralgia are, however, disappointing.

Similarly, it does not seem advisable to perform costochondral grafting in patients with malignant tumors of the condyle during the primary operation. The frequency of operative complications is rather low at both the donor and the recipient sites.

References

1. Lindqvist C, Pihakari A, Tasanen A, et al. Autogenous costochondral grafts in temporomandibular joint arthroplasty. A survey of 66 arthroplasties in 60 patients. *J Maxillofac Surg.* 1986;14:143–149.
2. Politis C, Fossion E, Bossuyt M. The use of costochondral grafts in arthroplasty of the temporomandibular joint. *J Craniomaxillofac Surg.* 1987;15:345–354.
3. Kaban LB, Perrott DH, Fisher K. A protocol for management of temporomandibular joint ankylosis. *J Maxillofac Surg.* 1990;48:1145–1151.
4. Posnick JC, Goldstein JA. Surgical management of temporomandibular joint ankylosis in the pediatric population. *Plast Reconstr Surg.* 1993;91:791–798.
5. Smith AE, Robinson M. A new surgical procedure in bilateral reconstruction of condyles utilizing iliac bone grafts and creation of new joints by means of nonelectrolytic metal: a preliminary report. *Plast Reconstr Surg.* 1952;9:393–409.
6. Entin MA. Reconstruction in congenital deformity of the temporomandibular components. *Plast Reconstr Surg.* 1958;6:461–469.
7. Ware WH, Taylor RC. Growth centre transplantation to replace damaged mandibular condyles. *J Am Dent Assoc.* 1966;73:128–137.
8. Snyder CC, Levine GA, Dingman DL. Trial of a sternoclavicular whole joint graft as a substitute for the temporomandibular

joint. *Plast Reconstr Surg.* 1971;48:447–452.

9. Matukas VJ, Szymela J, Schmidt JF. Surgical treatment of bony ankylosis in a child using composite cartilage-bone iliac crest grafts. *J Oral Surg.* 1980;38:903–905.

10. Siemssen SO. Temporomandibular arthroplasty by transfer of the sterno-clavicular joint on a muscle pedicle. *Br J Plast Surg.* 1982;35:225–238.

11. Plotnikow NA. Personal communication; 1984.

12. MacIntosh RB, Henny FA. A spectrum of application of autogenous costochondral grafts. *J Maxillofac Surg.* 1977;5:257–267.

13. Obwegeser HL. Simultaneous resection and reconstruction of parts of the mandible via the intraoral route in patients with and without gross infections. *Oral Surg.* 1966;21:693–705.

14. Kennett S. Temporomandibular joint ankylosis: the rationale for grafting in the young patient. *J Oral Surg.* 1973;31:744–748.

15. Freihofer HP, Perko MA. Simultaneous reconstruction of the area of the temporomandibular joint including the ramus of the mandible in a posttraumatic case. *J Maxillofac Surg.* 1976; 4:124–128.

16. Tasanen A, Leikomaa H. Ankylosis of the temporomandibular joint of a child. Report of a case. *Int J Oral Surg.* 1977;6:95–99.

17. Tasanen A, Rissanen H. Costochondral grafting in temporomandibular joint arthroplasty (Abstract). *Proc Finn Dent Soc Suppl,* II. 1980;76:24.

18. James DR, Irvine GH. Autogenous rib grafts in maxillofacial surgery. *J Maxillofac Surg.* 1983;11:201–203.

19. Figueroa AA, Gans BJ, Pruzansky S. Long-term follow-up of a mandibular costochondral graft. *Oral Surg Oral Med Oral Pathol.* 1984;58:257–268.

20. Ware WH, Brown SL. Growth center transplantation to replace mandibular condyles. *J Maxillofac Surg.* 1981;9:50–58.

21. Durkin JF, Heeley JD, Irving JT. The cartilage of the mandibular condyle. *Oral Sci Rev.* 1973;2:29–99.

22. Poswillo D. Experimental reconstruction of the mandibular joint. *Int J Oral Surg.* 1974;3:400–411.

23. Ware WH, Taylor RC. Cartilaginous growth centers transplanted to replace mandibular condyles in monkeys. *J Oral Surg.* 1966;24:33–43.

24. Westesson P-L. Diagnostic imaging of oral malignancies. *Oral Maxillofac Surg Clin North Am.* 1993;5:207–227.

25. Lindqvist C, Jokinen J, Paukku P, et al. Adaptation of autogenous costochondral grafts used for temporomandibular joint reconstruction: a long-term clinical and radiologic follow-up. *J Oral Maxillofac Surg.* 1988;46:465–470.

26. Hallikainen D, Paukku P. Panoramic zonography. In: DelBalso A, ed. *Maxillofacial Imaging.* Philadelphia: W.B. Saunders; 1990:1–33.

27. Obeid G, Guttenberg SA, Connole PW. Costochondral grafting

28. Mosby EL, Hiatt WR. A technique of fixation of costochondral grafts for reconstruction of the temporomandibular joint. *J Maxillofac Surg.* 1989;47:209–211.

29. Lindqvist C. TMJ reconstruction and rehabilitation using costochondral and alloplastic grafts. Abstract. SFOMK 25th Anniversary Conference, Nyborg Strand, Denmark. 1990:16–17.

30. Kent JN, Misiek DJ, Akin RK, et al. Temporomandibular joint condylar prosthesis: a ten year report. *J Oral Maxillofac Surg.* 1983;41:245–254.

31. Moorthy AP, Finch LD. Interpositional arthroplasty for ankylosis of the temporomandibular joint. *Oral Surg Oral Med Oral Pathol.* 1983;55:545–552.

32. Scheunemann H, Schmidseder R. Gibt es bei der Kiefergelenkankylose eine Standardoperation? In: Schuchardt K, Schwenzer N, eds. *Fortschritte der Kiefer- und Gesichtschirurgie.* Stuttgart: Thieme; 1980:25–109.

33. Fuchs M, Rolffs J, Voy E-D. Tierexperimentelle Untersuchungen zu einer Kiefergelenkendoprothese aus Aluminiumoxidkeramik. In: Schuchardt K, Schwenzer N, eds. *Fortschritte der Kiefer- und Gesichtschirurgie.* Stuttgart: Thieme; 1980:25–142.

34. Sonnenburg I, Sonnenburg M, Fethke K. Totalersatz des Kiefergelenkes durch alloplastisches Material. *Stomatol DDR.* 1982;32:178–185.

35. Raveh J, Stich H, Sutter F, et al. Use of the titanium-coated hollow screw and reconstruction plate system in bridging of lower jaw defects. *J Oral Maxillofac Surg.* 1984;42:281–294.

36. Lindqvist C, Söderholm A-L, Hallikainen D, et al. Erosion and heterotopic bone formation after alloplastic TMJ reconstruction. *J Oral Maxillofac Surg.* 1992;50:942–949.

37. Kent JN, Block MS, Halpern J, et al. Update of the Vitek partial and total temporomandibular joint system. *J Oral Maxillofac Surg.* 1993;51:408–415.

38. Longacre JJ, Gilbey RF. Further observations on use of autogenous cartilage grafts in arthroplasty of temporomandibular joint. *Plast Reconstr Surg.* 1952;10:238–247.

39. Steinhäuser EW. Kondylektomie oder korrektive Osteotomie bei der kondylären Hyperplasie. In: Schuchardt K, Schwenzer N, eds. *Fortschritte der Kiefer- und Gesichtschirurgie.* Stuttgart: Thieme; 1980;25:132–135.

40. Peltomäki T. Growth of a costochondral graft in the rat temporomandibular joint. *J Oral Maxillofac Surg.* 1992;50:851–857.

41. Ware WH, Taylor RC. Replantation of growing mandibular condyles in rhesus monkeys. *J Oral Surg.* 1965;19:669–677.

42. Peltomäki T, Isotupa K. The costochondral graft: a solution or a source of facial asymmetry in growing children. A case report. *Proc Finn Dent Soc.* 1991;87:167–176.

31
Microsurgical Reconstruction of Large Defects of the Maxilla, Midface, and Cranial Base

Rainer Schmelzeisen

Compared to reconstructive procedures in the mandible, bone and soft tissue reconstruction of the maxilla, the midface, and the cranial base often necessitates more complex surface reconstructions. In addition to functional restrictions, extensive defects in that area also lead to changes in the appearance of the patient as the zygomatic or maxillary complex provide the characteristic sagittal and transverse projection of a face.[1] The surgical strategies vary, depending on size and location of the defect. In contrast to the mandible, where significant functional loading also has to be taken into consideration, the biomechanical aspects of maxillary and midface reconstructions are of minor importance. Nevertheless, the multiform morphology of the maxilla and midface contributes to important functions such as deglutition, mastication, breathing, and speech.

Localized bony defects of the maxilla that occur in patients with cleft lip and palate or severe general atrophy of the maxilla are replaced with free corticocancellous bone grafts. Fresh autogenous bone is the material of first choice for bone replacement in these patients. It has been observed that the transfer of corticocancellous bone results in extensive resorption of the grafts if an early functional load (e.g., by the insertion of dental implants) is not applied.[2]

In cleft lip and palate patients, small amounts of cancellous bone usually provide a sufficient volume for later implant placement. The watertight closure of nasal and oral layers is an essential condition for undisturbed healing of these grafts and maximal bone-mass retention/survival.

In patients with severe atrophy of the maxilla, transplants of unicortical horseshoe-shaped bone grafts taken from the medial aspect of the anterior ilium can be utilized. Repositioning of the laterally pedicled cranial aspect of the iliac crest significantly reduces donor-site morbidity and aesthetic restrictions in that region. Another recognized technique is to use grafts taken from the posterior aspect of the ilium, which can provide a greater quantity of bone, although the patient's position must be changed before the harvest.[3] After reflection of the maxillary mucosa, the grafts are contoured and fixed on the residual alveolar ridge with 2.0-mm positioning screws followed by a two-layer soft tissue closure. Removal of the

positioning screws and insertion of screw-type titanium implants may be performed 4 to 6 months after bone grafting, with bone scintigraphy useful in determining the optimal time for the insertion of dental implants. In posterior aspects of the maxilla, sinus-lift procedures may be considered with regard to the needs of the prosthodontist.

Reconstruction of Extensive Maxillary/Midface Defects

Resection of malignant tumors may cause more extensive, composite defects of the palate, cheek, and orbit, which may also include the cranial base. The possibilities for prosthodontic rehabilitation are limited and depend upon the amount of residual bone and remaining teeth. The isolated use of osseointegrated implants for solid anchoring of prosthetics also may be limited and can only be performed with regard to the residual amount and location of bone. In combined treatment protocols of malignancies, additional radiotherapy may further restrict the possibilities of conventional prosthodontic treatment (Figure 31.1).

Conventional rehabilitation usually performed with obturators may separate oral and nasal cavities effectively and permit adequate speech and deglutition. Nevertheless, the inflow of food into the nose and accumulation of debris at the surfaces of the obturator are severe disadvantages. Also, daily prosthetic care cannot be maintained by all of the patients. Large-size epithetics that also cover external surfaces may be extremely unpleasant to wear, especially in cold environments.

Up to a certain amount and in specific locations, local flaps may be used for the reconstruction of defects with a predominant soft tissue loss. Flaps from the forehead leave an extremely unfavorable donor-site scar and should be regarded as obsolete. Transposition of calvarial bone flaps, vascularized by a pedicle of the temporal muscle, allow for a combined reconstruction of soft tissue and bone defects. Nevertheless, multiple-surface reconstruction or multiple-folding procedures of these local flaps are limited by the pedicle dimension and length. In these one-dimensional reconstructive procedures,

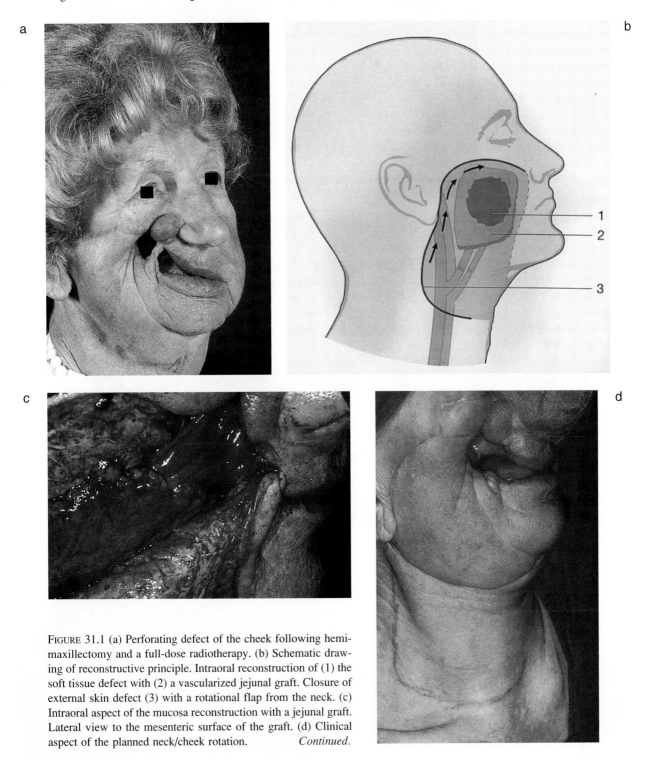

FIGURE 31.1 (a) Perforating defect of the cheek following hemi-maxillectomy and a full-dose radiotherapy. (b) Schematic drawing of reconstructive principle. Intraoral reconstruction of (1) the soft tissue defect with (2) a vascularized jejunal graft. Closure of external skin defect (3) with a rotational flap from the neck. (c) Intraoral aspect of the mucosa reconstruction with a jejunal graft. Lateral view to the mesenteric surface of the graft. (d) Clinical aspect of the planned neck/cheek rotation.   *Continued.*

the amount of bone available is limited, and it cannot be mobilized independently from the adjacent soft tissue. In addition to the possible volume deficit at the donor site, the use of these temporal flaps may be associated with injuries to the frontal branch of the facial nerve; local flaps in general increase the risk for a postoperative limited jaw opening.[1,4–6]

The increasing use of vascularized combined-tissue grafts has offered new possibilities for reconstruction procedures in

the maxillary/midface area. Survival of these grafts is independent of the vascularity of the surrounding tissue and generally permits multidimensional surface reconstruction of complex defects.

In addition to the possibility of a complex first-stage reconstruction, the procedures in the midface remain multiple-step rehabilitations with further minor corrections. It has to be decided, for each individual patient, the level of complexity

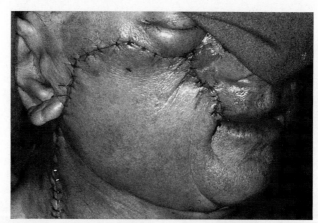

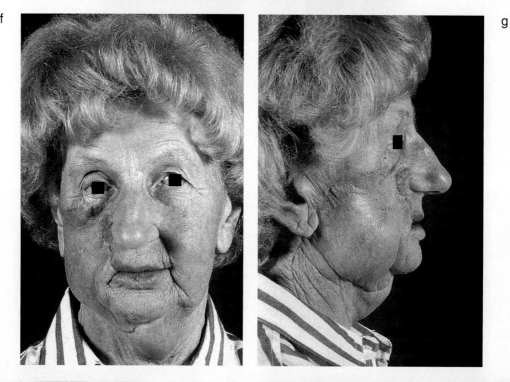

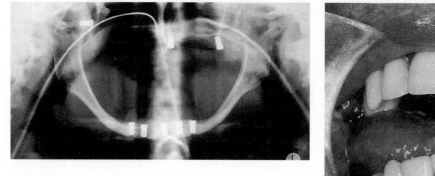

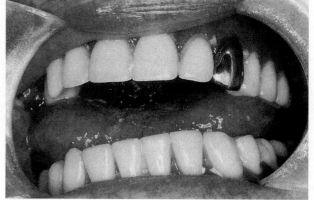

FIGURE 31.1 *Continued.* (e) Immediate postoperative result. (f,g) Extraoral appearance of the patient 6 months following reconstruction. (h,i) Following implant insertion in the residual zygomatic complex and the contralateral maxilla, an implant-borne obturator prosthesis was inserted.

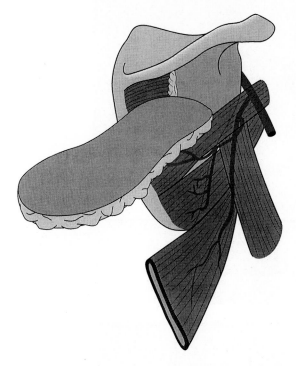

FIGURE 31.2 Schematic drawing of the scapula region. The para-scapula skin flap can be raised together with the lateral border of the scapula. Pedicled to the circumflex scapular vessels, the skin flap can be mobilized relatively independent from the bone graft. Additionally, a scapula flap nourished by the transverse cutaneous branch can be harvested as a second soft tissue pedicle.

to which the primary reconstruction can be performed, especially with regard to an optimal function and safe outcome.

Scapula Grafts

Grafts from the scapula region are most versatile for maxillary/midface reconstructions when both soft tissue and bone defects have to be reconstructed. The grafts offer the advantage of a vascularized thin bone area, which can be combined with one or two soft tissue components, either of which individually or together may be completely or partially deepithelialized (Figure 31.2).[6–9]

The flap designs permit for the reconstruction of complex bony and soft tissue defects with different surfaces to be reconstructed (e.g., palatal mucosa and separation between nasal cavity and maxillary sinus).

Deepithelialized portions may be used for volume augmentation in the midface and offer acceptable volume stability over time as atrophy is unlikely to occur in contrast to muscle flaps.[10] This lower tendency for resorption of the grafts makes combined scapula grafts useful in patients with hemifacial microsomia. In these patients, soft tissue augmentation may be combined with repositioning, reconstruction, or augmentation of the midfacial skeleton (Figure 31.3).

The thin bone of the scapula is ideal for reconstruction of the hard palate or the orbital floor.

It must be decided in the individual case whether de-epithelialization of a parascapular flap is sufficient for surface contouring or whether a bipedicled scapula and parascapular flap is used for the reconstruction of surfaces or volume augmentation in separate locations (Figures 31.4, 31.5).

In maxillary reconstruction, the thicker lateral margin of the scapula, which is suitable for implant insertion, cannot always be positioned in an anatomically correct position for the alveolar process owing to the shortness of the vascular pedicle. This often requires secondary nonvascularized bone grafts as additional augmentation with screw-type implant stabilization into the vascularized scapula bone flap (Figure 31.6).

The fixation of the scapula bone generally is of minor importance. One 2.0-mm plate may be sufficient for fixation of the scapula bone to the residual maxilla or zygoma. It is of crucial importance to provide a good bony contact area between the scapula bone and the residual midfacial skeleton. Therefore, additional free-bone grafts may be inserted in bony discrepancies to provide adequate stability of the graft. Lag-screw techniques may be used if vascularized aspects of the combined scapula grafts are used for onlay grafting [e.g., in the zygomatic region; see Figure 31.4(d,e)].

For vascular anastomosis, the superficial temporal vessels are not always reliable. Therefore, a submandibular incision is chosen. The marginal branch of the facial nerve is identified and elevated. On the surface of the masseter muscle, a tunnel can be dissected toward the maxilla.

This tunnel must be of an adequate diameter not to compress the pedicle vein. No tension must be applied to the anastomosis. The preparation of the tunnel is of crucial importance for the success of the graft, as complications may be due to compression in that tunnel.

Isolated Soft Tissue Grafts

In defects with predominant soft tissue loss, reconstruction may also be performed with musculocutaneous or fasciocutaneous isolated soft tissue grafts. In general, the vascular pedicle of these flaps is longer than in combined bone and soft tissue flaps like scapula, iliac crest, or fibula grafts.

The thin radial forearm flap may be especially useful for closure of maxillary defects with a predominant soft tissue component. For these indications, it may serve as an alternative for jejunal grafts. The minimal flap thickness also makes the flap suitable for reconstruction of combined soft tissue or bone defects of the maxilla when the bone defect is of limited size, and a nonvascularized bone graft can be fixed with a circular good contact to the surrounding bone. The free-bone graft then may be covered with a radial forearm flap, and functional separation between nasal and oral cavity also can be performed by the flap. The length of the vascular pedicle of the radial forearm flap allows for reconstruction of cranially located skin areas (e.g., at the cranial base and the forehead; Figure 31.7).

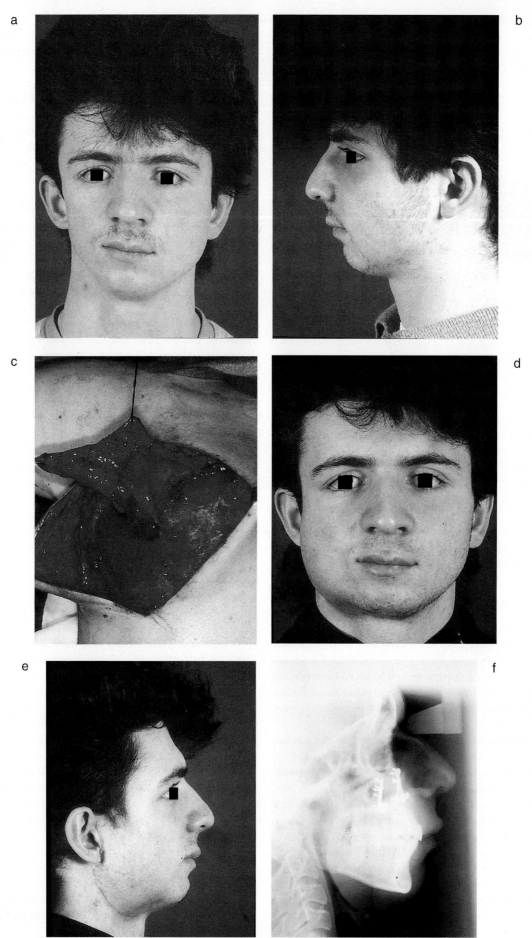

FIGURE 31.3

g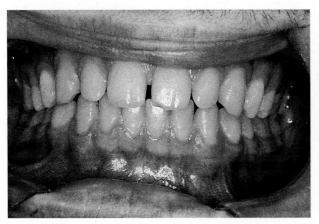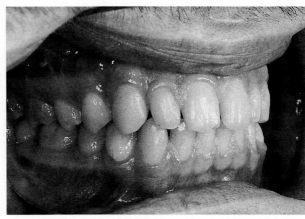h

FIGURE 31.3 (a) Patient with hemifacial microsomia and asymmetry of the maxillary/mandibular complex. Additional significant soft tissue deficit in projection to the right cheek and maxillary/zygomatic region. (b) Profile analysis demonstrates an additional sagittal deficit of the mandibular projection. (c) After bimaxillary osteotomies for correction of the skeletal asymmetry and occlusion, a deepithelialized parascapular flap is harvested for soft tissue augmentation. (d,e) Postoperative aspect of the patient. (f) Postoperative x-ray. (g,h) Postoperative occlusion.

If more soft tissue volume is needed, a latissimus dorsi or rectus abdominis flap may be used. The multiple skin perforators of the latissimus dorsi flap allow for the preparation of several skin paddles for reconstruction of nasal cavity, external skin, palate, or orbit. The muscle volume restores facial contour. Obliteration of the maxillary sinus may be performed with the muscle volume. The length of the vascular pedicle offers various options for the location of the vessel anastomosis.

While the rectus abdominis and latissimus dorsi musculocutaneous flaps are very similar regarding tissue volume, pedicle length, and reliability, harvesting of the rectus abdominis flap offers the advantage of an unchanged patient position.

The disadvantage of these large-volume flaps in the maxilla and midface may be an inferior dislocation of the oral flap surface, which can disturb speech and swallowing function. In general, all vascularized soft tissue flaps used for intraoral surface reconstruction of the maxilla have to be thinned out postoperatively.

Isolated soft tissue grafts may not be suitable for reconstruction of orbital floor defects as they do not provide stable support for the eye.[11–13] Therefore, additional nonvascularized bone grafts (i.e., from the calvarium or iliac crest) may be used for reconstruction of the orbit and the midface.

In children, harvesting vascularized bone grafts may interfere with growth capacity at the donor site. Therefore, vascularized soft tissue reconstruction with free-bone grafting, for example, with split grafts from the ilium, may be primarily considered (Figure 31.8).

Reconstruction of Periorbital/Cranial Base Defects

Whenever possible, localized combined bone and soft tissue defects in the orbital region should be surgically treated with local flaps. Although vascularized grafts offer ideal options for volume augmentation and bony support in the maxillary and midface areas, unsatisfactory aesthetic results often result when external skin areas need to be replaced with flaps from distant sites.

For smaller defects of the orbital frame, including limited external skin replacement, rotational flaps from the scalp may be used for the coverage of alloplastic materials or calvarial split grafts (Figure 31.9).

When complex soft tissue or bone defects are encountered (i.e., trauma or growth inhibition), osteotomies or orbitotomies combined with the use of autologous bone grafts should initially be considered. Tissue expanders are often useful for soft tissue reconstruction in these patients.

Large defects of the orbit and anterior skull base may necessitate again the use of microsurgically vascularized grafts, which allow for the safe coverage of the skull base and duraplasties. Musculocutaneous grafts, such as the rectus abdominis or latissimus dorsi, are used. The consistent vascular anatomy and the length of the vascular pedicle allow for vascular anastomosis with submandibular vessels.

In extensive combined periorbital defects permitting

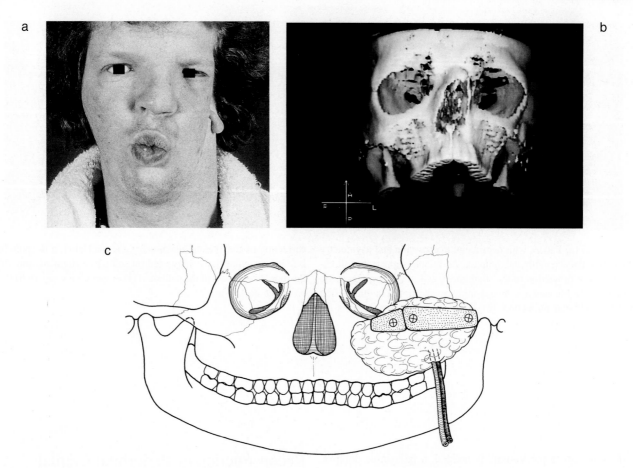

FIGURE 31.4 (a) Preoperative aspect of a 28-year-old patient with hemifacial microsomia. (b) Three-dimensional CT demonstrates hypoplasia of left maxilla, zygoma, and absence of zygomatic arch. (c) Schematic drawing of intended reconstruction.

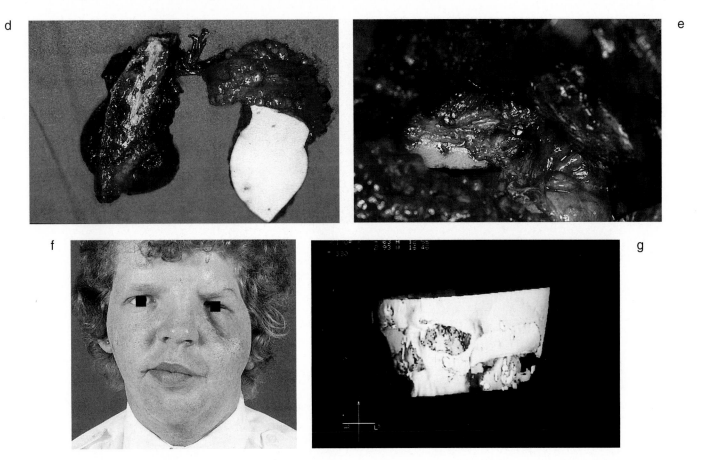

FIGURE 31.4 *Continued.* (d) Harvesting of an osteocutaneous paras-capular flap which was deepithelialized. (e) Lag-screw fixation of the lateral border of the scapula for reshaping the zygomatic arch and the infraorbital region by means of vascularized onlay grafting. (f) Postoperative aspect of the patient with adequate transverse pro-jection of the zygomatic complex. Orbital reconstruction and inser-tion of an orbital prosthesis still to be performed. (g) Postoperative CT scan demonstrates the amount of bony augmentation.

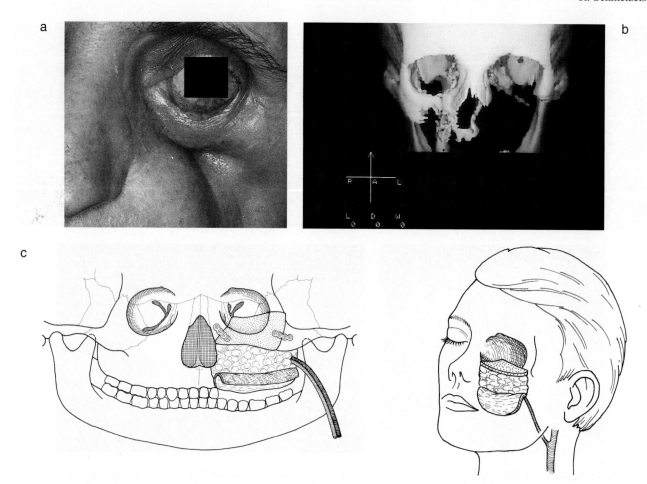

FIGURE 31.5 (a,b) Soft tissue defect following right hemimaxillectomy and resection of the orbital floor in a 50-year-old patient. (b) Postoperative 3-D CT scan demonstrating bony defect. (c) Schematic drawing of reconstructive procedure. (d) Surgical approach to the defect by reopening the preexisting Dieffenbach-Weber incision. (e) Reconstruction of the orbital floor by the thin medial aspect of a scapula graft. Bilateral fixation of the scapula bone by microplates. (f) Partial deepithelialization of the parascapular flap. The deepithelialized part is used for cheek augmentation, and the cutaneous aspect is inserted for oral lining of the maxillary mucosa. The vicinity of the region to be augmented and the area of missing maxillary mucosa allows for harvesting of only one parascapular flap serving both purposes. The necessity to reconstruct separate soft tissue locations would require the preparation of a scapula and a parascapular soft tissue flap. (g) Postoperative aspect of the patient 8 weeks following surgery. Quality of overlying skin often improves with time.

preservation of the eyelids, the vascularized soft tissue graft may provide an adequate aesthetic result. Following large tumor resections, the aesthetic result is often compromised since it is necessary to primarily provide satisfactory coverage of the skull base and a clean skin surface (Figure 31.10).

Also in lateral and posterior skull defects, musculocutaneous flaps may also provide satisfactory coverage of the brain or duraplasties. For primary tumor resection, the skull bone often does not have to be reconstructed.

Radiation therapy should not be considered as a contraindication for the use of vascularized grafts for craniofacial reconstruction.[14,15]

Summary

For complex defects in the maxilla and midface, scapula grafts have to be regarded as reconstruction methods of choice. The vascular anatomy of the scapula region allows for the reconstruction of multiple surface defects, and the thin scapula is ideally suited for reconstruction of the palate and alveolar process.

The thick bone volume of the iliac crest offers better bone volume for the insertion of dental implants. Nevertheless, adequate shaping of the iliac crest for maxillary reconstruction is more difficult, and the soft tissue pedicle cannot be mobi-

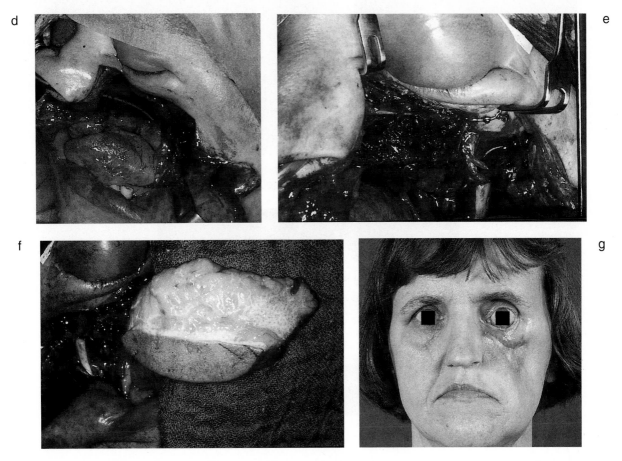

FIGURE 31.5 *Continued.*

lized independently from the bone. The skin paddle is often extremely bulky and is not suitable for reconstruction of multiple surfaces.[16]

Isolated soft tissue grafts are not suitable for orbital support and may undergo gravitational ptosis. However, they may be taken into consideration if maximum safety of a procedure is necessary due to a longer vascular pedicle and a reliable vascular anatomy.

With regard to the maximum safety of reconstruction and possible growth disturbances at the donor site, vascularized soft tissue grafts with secondary bone grafts may be primarily used for reconstructive procedures in children. To our knowledge, the earliest microvascular procedure in the maxilla/midface has been performed by Posnick in a 1-year-old

child with a parameningeal head and neck rhabdomyosarcoma. In that young patient, a radial forearm flap was harvested to reconstruct the skin and the soft tissue defect of the cheek with supply for the lining of the nasal cavity. The flap was anastomosed to the superficial temporal vessels and combined with a split calvarial graft.[17]

The selection of reconstructive methods in the maxilla, midface, and cranial base should be highly individualized. The complexity of reconstruction should be performed with regard to the prognosis of the underlying disease and the expectations of the patient. In general, the increasing use of vascularized grafts from different donor sites has enlarged the reconstructive possibilities in the craniomaxillofacial area, and they are far superior to conventional reconstructive procedures.

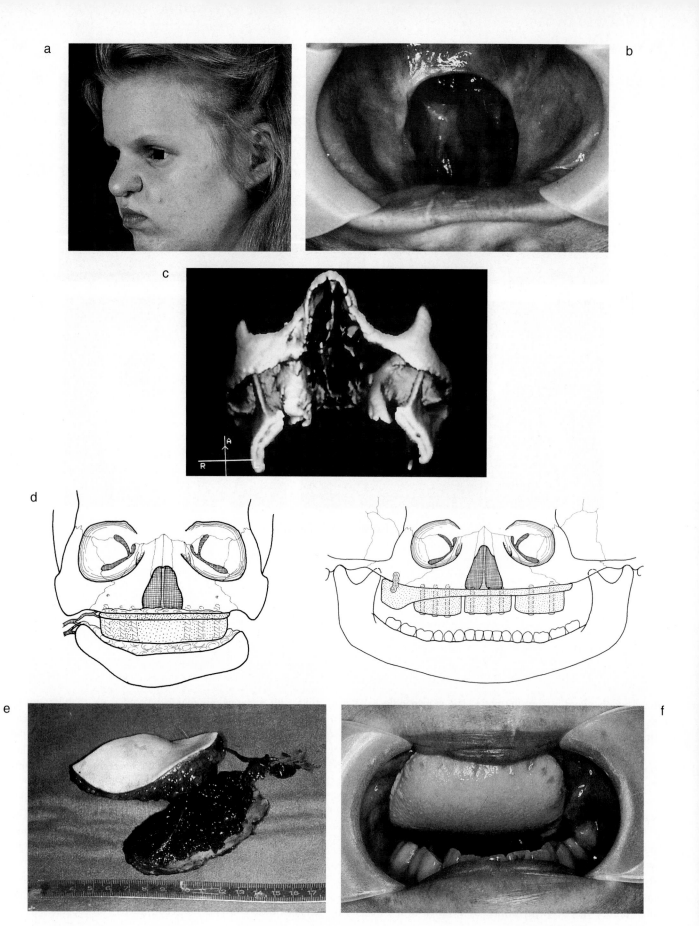

FIGURE 31.6

g
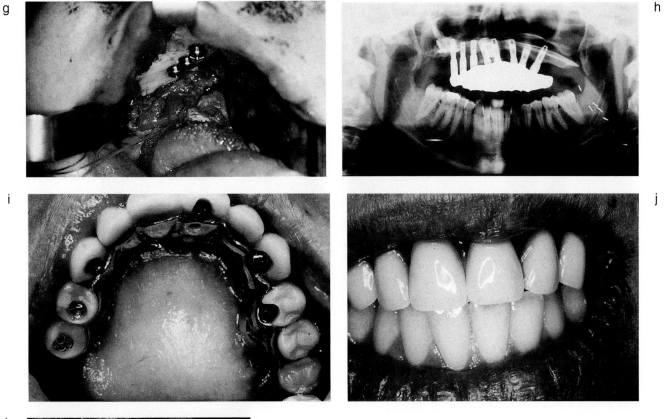

h

i

j

k
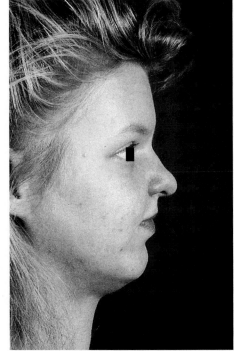

FIGURE 31.6 *Continued.* (a) Fifteen-year-old patient following complete maxillectomy due to a sarcoma of the maxilla at the age of 1 year. Significant soft tissue deficit with inadequate profile of the upper lip. (b) Intraoral aspect with oronasal perforation. (c) Preoperative three-dimensional CT-scan demonstrates amount of bone missing. (d) Parts 1 and 2: Schematic drawing of reconstructive strategy with primary insertion of the osteocutaneous parascapular flap. Secondarily, additional free-bone grafts were fixed to the scapula bone with dental implants acting as positioning screws. (e) Harvested osteocutaneous parascapular flap. (f) Osteocutaneous parascapular flap inserted intraorally, with immediate postoperative significant soft tissue excess. (g) Fixation of additional free bone grafts to the scapula bone with dental implants. Simultaneous volume reduction of the soft tissue flap. (h) Postoperative panoramic radiograph of prosthesis. (i,j) Intraoral views of prosthodontic rehabilitation by means of implant-borne dentures. (k) Postoperative aspect of the patient with adequate upper-lip profile.

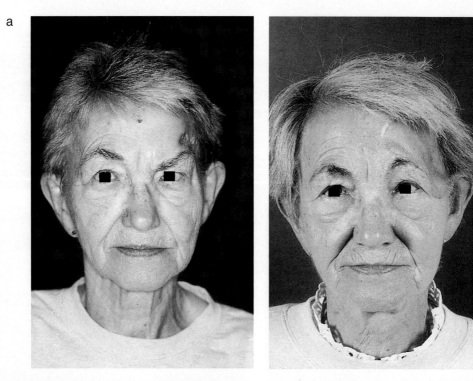

FIGURE 31.7 (a) Patient with basalioma of the left frontal skin. Biopsies proved extensions of the basalioma close to the midline of the forehead without bony invasion. (b) Excision of left forehead skin and coverage of the defect with a radial forearm flap. The length of the pedicle allows for tensionless microvascular anastomosis to the submandibular vessels.

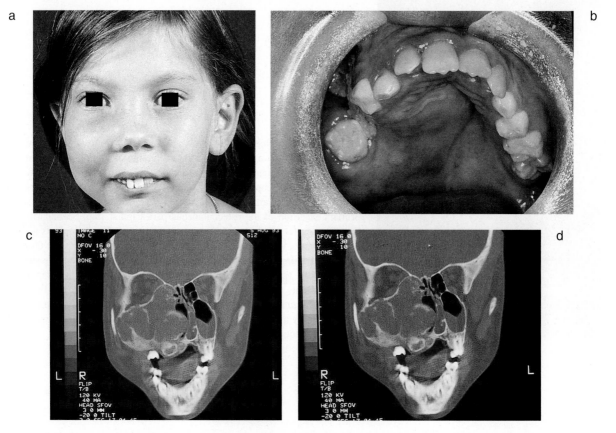

FIGURE 31.8

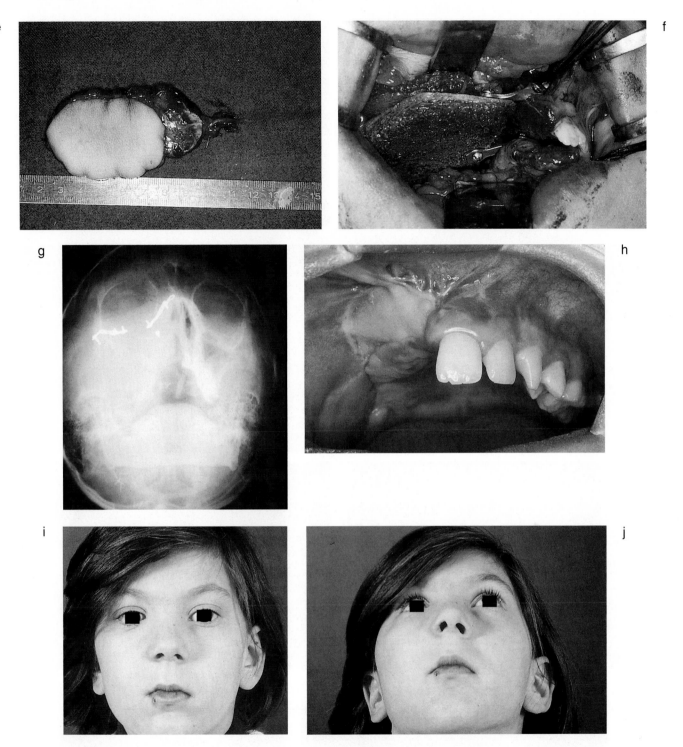

FIGURE 31.8 *Continued.* (a–d) Twelve-year-old girl with large ossifying fibroma of the right maxilla invading the orbit and the ethmoid cells. (e) After resection of the fibroma, a latissimus dorsi muscle flap was harvested to avoid growth disturbances at the donor site of possible combined bone and soft tissue grafts. The latissimus dorsi flap was used for coverage of the skull base, obliteration of the maxillary sinus, and lining of the nasal and oral mucosa. (f) After re-construction of the orbital floor, the palate additionally was reconstructed using a monocortical nonvascularized bone graft from the iliac crest. Miniplate fixation of the two bone grafts. (g) Postoperative x-ray. (h) Intraoral aspect demonstrating isolated skin area of latissimus dorsi flap used for oral lining. (i,j) Postoperative aspect of the patient.

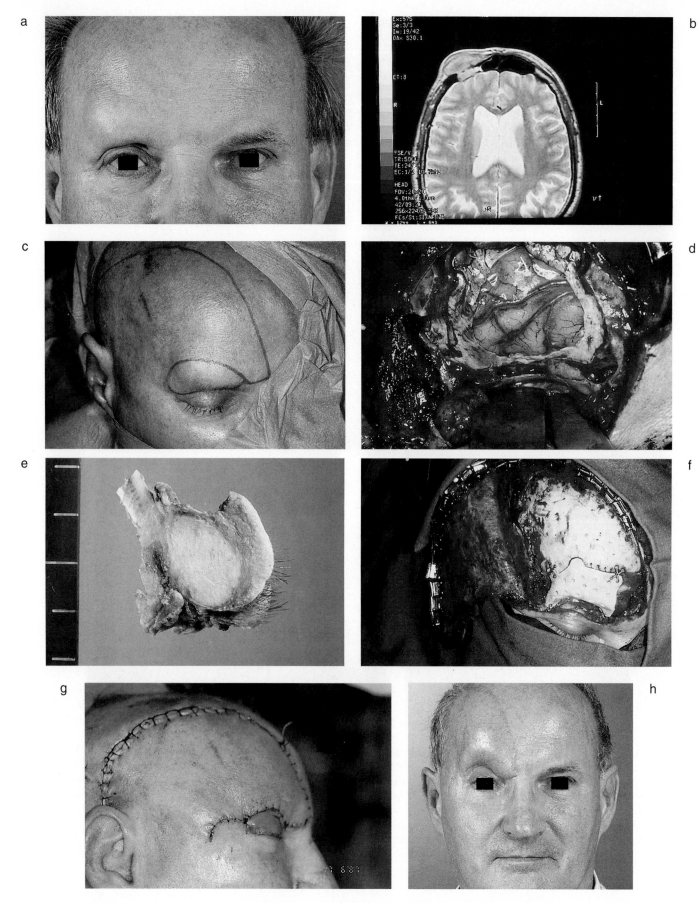

FIGURE 31.9

a
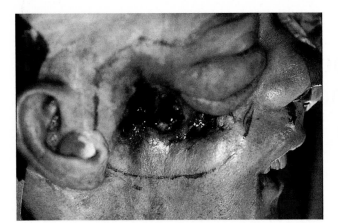

b
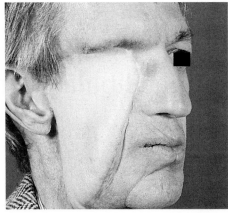

FIGURE 31.10 (a) Amount of palliative resection in a 55-year-old patient with multiple previous operations of recurrent carcinoma of the maxilla. Infiltration of the orbit and the anterior skull base. (b) Following palliatively intended resection, the skull base and orbit were covered with a latissimus dorsi flap.

References

1. Coleman JJ. Microvascular approach to function and appearance of large orbital maxillary defects. *Am J Surg.* 1989;158:337–341.

2. Davis HW, Marshall MW. Effects of osseointegrated implant-supported prosthesis on bone preservation and regeneration in the edentulous mandible. In: Davis WM, Sailer H, eds. *Oral and Maxillofacial Surgery Clinics of North America;* 1994:765–779.

3. Marx RE. Morbidity from bone harvest in major jaw reconstruction: a randomized trial comparing the lateral anterior and posterior approaches to the ilium. *J Oral Maxillofac Surg.* 1988; 48:196–203.

4. Shapiro BM, Komisar A, Silver C, et al. Primary reconstruction of palatal defects. *Otolaryngol Head Neck Surg.* 1986;95:581–585.

5. Colmenero C, Martorell B, Colmenero B, et al. Temporalis myofacial flap for maxillofacial reconstruction. *J Oral Maxillofac Surg.* 1991;49:1067–1073.

6. Kärcher H, Eskici A, Zwittnig P. Oberkieferrekonstruktion mit dem osteokutanen Skapulatransplantat nach Schußverletzung. *Z Stomatol.* 1988;85:371–377.

7. dos Santos LF. *Le Lambeau Scapulaire et L'Artere Cutanee Scapulaire.* Paris, 1980.

8. Nassif T, Vidal L, Bovet J, et al. The parascapular flap: a new cutaneous microsurgical free flap. *Plast Reconstr Surg.* 1982;69: 591–600.

9. Pistner H, Reuther J, Bill J. Skapularegion als potentielles Spenderareal für mikrochirurgische Transplantate. In: Schwenzer N, Pfeifer G, eds. *Fortschritte der Kiefer- und Gesichtschirurgie,* Vol. 35. Stuttgart: Thieme; 1990:87–90.

10. Riediger D. *Mikrochirurgische Weichgewebetransplantation in die Gesichtsregion.* Munich: Hanser; 1983.

11. Hoffman HT, Jalowaysky AA, Robbins KT, et al. Oronasal reconstruction with local mucoperiosteal and free latissimus dorsi flaps. *Arch Otolaryngol.* 1992;118:1238–1241.

12. Peters GE, Grotting JC. Free flap reconstruction of large head and neck defects in the elderly. *Microsurgery.* 1989;10:325–328.

13. Meyer H, Schmidt JW, Terrahe K, et al. Modifikation des mikrovaskulär reanastomosierten Latissimus dorsi Lappens zur Rekonstruktion nach erweiterter Oberkieferresektion. *HNO.* 1991;39:218–223.

14. Fisher J, Jackson IT. Microvascular surgery as an adjunct to craniomaxillofacial reconstruction. *Br J Plast Surg.* 1989;42: 146–154.

15. Robson MC, Zachary LS, Schmidt DG, Faibisoff B, Hekmatpanah J. Reconstruction of large cranial defects in the presence of heavy radiation damage and infection utilizing tissue transferred by microvascular anastomoses. *Plast Reconstr Surg.* 1989;83(3):438–442.

16. Swartz WM, Banis JC, Newton ED, Ramasastry SS, Jones NF, Acland R. The osteocutaneous scapular flap for mandibular and maxillary reconstruction. *Plast Reconstr Surg.* 1986;77(4):530–545.

17. Posnick JC, Polley JW, Zuker RM, Chan HSL. Chemotherapy and surgical resection combined with immediate reconstruction in a 1-year-old child with rhabdomyosarcoma of the maxilla. *Plast Reconstr Surg.* 1992;89(2):320–325.

FIGURE 31.9 (a,b) Patient with adenocarcinoma of the right lacrimal gland with intracranial extension. (c) Planned incision for tumor resection including the overlying skin and eyebrow and closure of the defect with a scalp rotation flap. (d) Extension of the tumor necessitated additional resection of the dura. Duraplasty was performed using a fascia lata graft. (Courtesy of Prof. W Sollmann, MD, Neurosurgery, Braunschweig City Hospital) (e) Tumor specimen demonstrates resection of frontal bone, anterior aspect of orbital roof, and overlying skin. (Courtesy of H Maschek, MD, Institute of Pathology, Medical University of Hannover, Germany) (f) After duraplasty and coverage of the frontal sinus by a galleoperiosteal flap, hard tissue reconstruction was performed with acrylic. (g) Immediate postoperative result. (h) Result 6 months postoperatively.

32
Condylar Prosthesis for the Replacement of the Mandibular Condyle

Joachim Prein

Indications for the application of an alloplastic prosthesis for the replacement of the mandibular condyle are extremely rare. Whenever possible, the reconstruction of the mandibular joint should be performed with autogenous material. Under certain conditions, however, it may be necessary to use a metal prosthesis. During the 20 years between 1974 and 1994, we treated 17 patients with 21 alloplastic prosthesis, mostly made out of steel. At the moment the use of an AO/ASIF alloplastic joint prosthesis is now permitted in the United States because they are FDA approved, currently as a 2.4 mm titanium locking reconstruction plate with condylar head right and left as 3×16, 4×18, and 5×20 hole sizes, and 2.4 mm titanium condylar plates 8 holes right and left (see Chapter 22).[1–11]

Material

In the past, the system consisted of a prosthesis designed to replace the condyle without an artificial fossa. The prosthesis comes in three different sizes. The condylar part is shaped either like a sphere or a barrel. It is connected to a short prebent plate that can be fixed with four-to-six 2.7 screws at the ascending ramus. For those patients in whom part of the lateral mandible together with the joint was replaced, a prebent reconstruction plate with a condyle on top of the vertical part was used (Figure 32.1).

Tests have been made with titanium-coated prostheses and special adaptable condyles in combination with the THORP system. The adaptable version had joints in between the plate and condyle. The purpose was to facilitate the placement of the artificial condyle in the glenoid fossa. Because of technical problems, this version is no longer used.

Method

Generally one distinguishes between a total and a partial arthroplasty. In a total arthroplasty the condyle is replaced together with an artificial fossa. In a partial arthroplasty only the condyle is replaced. In our patient group only partial arthroplasties were performed.

Patients

Between 1974 and 1994 17 patients received 21 prostheses. There were 10 females and 7 males. The mean age was 43.5 years (range 16 to 81). The first prosthesis ever used in our unit was placed in 1974 (surgery performed by Prof. Spiessl). This prosthesis in a young female is now in place for 23 years. The average duration of the 21 prosthesis until 1994 was 8.7 years (range, 13 to 244 months) (Figure 32.2).

Indications

In the majority of our patients (9 of 17) and the majority of all condyles replaced (12 of 21), the procedure was necessary because of an ankylosis. Most of these ankyloses were posttraumatic. One patient suffered from a Morbus Bechterew (spondylarthritis ankylopoetica) and had developed over a period of 18 years a bilateral ankylosis. Her range of motion at the time of surgery was 2 to 1 mm interincisal distance. She now says, 11 years after surgery, that she feels like a newborn person.

In 4 of 21 reconstructed joints, the indication was a tumor or metastasis. In these patients the lateral mandible together with the ascending ramus was replaced by a reconstruction plate with condylar head (Figure 32.3). Since 1994, we have immediately reconstructed the condylar area in severely comminuted fracture situations in several patients (Figure 32.4).

Operative Procedure

In most of the operations, a two-site approach (preauricular and submandibular) was used. In ankylosis operations, the ankylotic mass was removed to create a thicker than normal

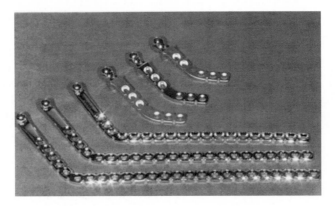

FIGURE 32.1 The top three implants show different sizes of joint prostheses. The bottom three are prebent reconstruction plates with a solid barrel-like condylar head (2.7 system steel AO/ASIF).

a

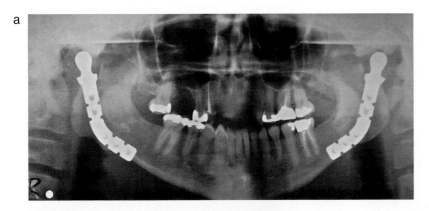

b

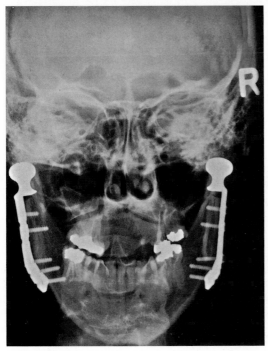

FIGURE 32.2 (a) Panoramic and (b) AP view of a patient with two condylar prostheses. Surgery was performed in 1988. The prostheses are still in place. The position is almost optimal, with satisfactory function.

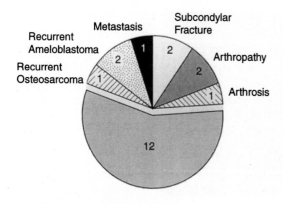

FIGURE 32.3 Indications for surgery for 21 joint replacements between 1974 and 1994.

pseudofossa to prevent the danger of a perforation of the artificial condyle through the base of the skull. An ipsilateral coronoidectomy was usually performed. In all other instances, whenever possible, the disc was left in place as a protection against perforation of the fossa. As a further measure against the danger of perforation we have always tried to place the prosthesis slightly inferior to the fossa. This, of course, is possible only if just for joint replacement. In those patients where

both the joint and the lateral mandible must be replaced, it is especially difficult to place the condyle correctly into the natural fossa and keep it there. However, we have seen postoperative displacements of the condyle into the temporal fossa without clinical consequences (Figure 32.5). Whenever possible, in all patients, intermaxillary fixation was applied during surgery to identify the optimal position for the prosthesis.

Results

Only in one patient with one prosthesis for an ankylosis in 1981 was the prosthesis removed 5 years later in another unit. The precise reasons are not known to us. Originally the patient suffered from an ankylosis with only 2- to 3-mm interincisal distance. One month after surgery his range of motion was 22 mm. He was very uncooperative and did not come back for postoperative control and exercises. As far as we could find out at the time of removal, the distance was 13 mm and no lateral or anterior motion was possible. Several further attempts under general anesthesia were undertaken to improve the range of motion after the removal of the prosthesis.

In general, lateral and anterior motions are almost impossible in patients with two prostheses. In those with one prosthesis, such motion is possible in a limited range.

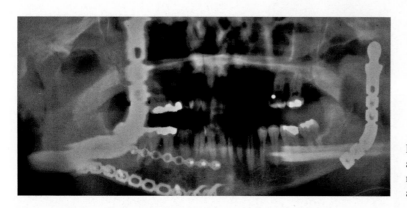

FIGURE 32.4 Replacement of the left mandibular condyle after a comminuted fracture in this area and the mandibular body on the opposite side. The patient was a severe polytraumatized patient and is tetraplegic.

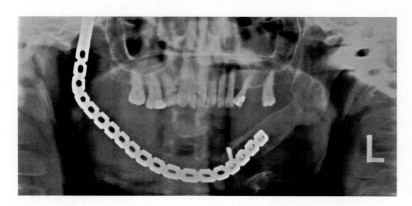

FIGURE 32.5 Replacement of the chin and right side of the mandible because of an osteosarcoma with a 2.7 reconstruction plate with condylar head. The condylar head is displaced laterally out of the fossa. The patient lives with good comfort, and the plate has been in place for over 3 years.

a
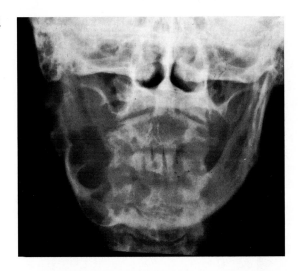

b
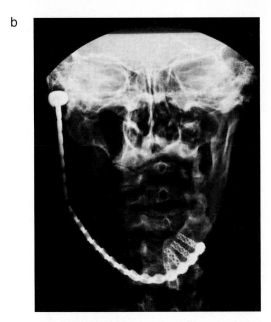

c

d
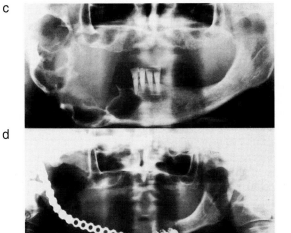

Occlusal problems have been observed, especially in severe trauma cases. In one patient, this problem developed because regular treatment in due time with correct intermaxillar fixation was impossible as a result of the patient's unstable general condition and paraplegia. Her accident occurred in 1985, when immediate repair and stabilization of all facial fractures with plates was not yet a routine procedure. Her facial structure would, without doubt, be much better today with the appropriate application of our treatment protocol for panfacial fractures.

Scars were problematic in only one young patient who developed a broad hypertrophic scar. He had several interventions through his scar because of a laceration of his facial nerve (as a result of an accident) together with a severe fracture of his mandible.

In most of our patients with ankylosis, considerable improvement was achieved. Two patients with three prostheses experienced occasional spontaneous locking with pain, which subsided after appropriate pain medication. In all patients, the range of motion with postoperative exercise was considerably improved. One patient felt some discomfort when it was very cold outside. In all instances, only rotational—and almost no gliding—movements were possible in the area of the artificial joint.

In all patients with wide resections because of tumor invasion and reconstruction with a long plate with a condyle, function was better than in those patients with a condylar prosthesis alone (Figure 32.6). This is remarkable, especially in view of the fact that placement of the artificial condyle in these instances is less accurate than for the patients with only the condylar prosthesis.

Radiology

We observed no screw loosening. On PA views the positioning of the prosthesis was correct in 50% of the cases. In 40% of the patients, the artificial condyle was placed laterally and in 10% dislocation was observed. In 53% of the cases, appositional bone deposition around the head of the prosthesis occurred. To a certain degree this leads to a limitation of motion (Figure 32.7).

In two patients with bilateral prostheses, bony resorption cranially from the condyle was seen without perforation of the middle cranial fossa. Only the two prostheses placed in 1974 and 1975 were positioned slightly too high.

FIGURE 32.6 AP views (a) preoperatively and (b) postoperatively after resection of an extensive ameloblastoma. (c) Preoperative and (d) postoperative panoramic radiographs of the same patient. Surgery was done in 1984. The patient refused a bony reconstruction. The plate has been in place since 1984.

a

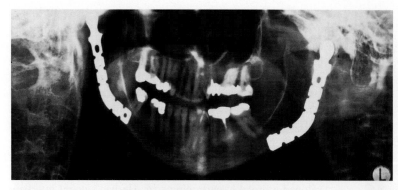

b

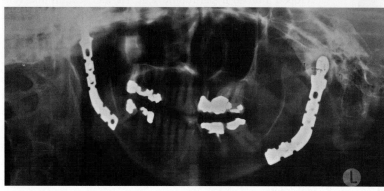

FIGURE 32.7 Bilateral condylar replacement with steel prosthesis because of ankylosis: (a) 10 months postoperatively; (b) 3 years thereafter. Note: Anterior and posterior bony apposition around the artificial condyle.

In summary, indications for an artificial joint with an alloplastic prosthesis are rare. Although in all of our cases partial arthroplasties without fossa replacement were performed, perforation through the glenoid fossa was not observed. Periodic follow-up is necessary because a perforation in the area of the fossa can be asymptomatic. In our view, under certain conditions, the indication for an alloplastic prosthesis is given for ankylosed joints. Additional conditions are severely traumatized joints and patients with tumors invading the mandible or the soft tissues in the area of the joint. If possible, the patients must be well informed and able to be cooperative. Reconstruction with autogenous material, if the local and general conditions permit, is always preferable.

References

1. Kaban LB, Perrott DH, Fisher KA. Protocol for management of temporomandibular joint ankylosis. *J Oral Maxillofac Surg.* 1990;48:1145–1151.
2. Lindquist C, Söderholm A-L, Hallikainen D, et al. Erosion and heterotopic bone formation after alloplastic TMJ reconstruction. *J Oral Maxillofac Surg.* 1992;50:942–949.
3. Poswillo D. Experimental reconstruction of the mandibular joint. *Int J Oral Surg.* 1974;3:400–411.
4. Kent JN, Misiek DJ, Akin RK, et al. Temporomandibular joint condylar prosthesis: a ten year report. *J Oral Maxillofac Surg.* 1983;41:245–254.
5. Kent JN, Block MS, Homsy CA, et al. Experience with a polymer glenoid fossa prosthesis for partial total temporomandibular joint reconstruction. *J Oral Maxillofac Surg.* 1986;44: 520–533.
6. Chassagne JF, Flot F, Stricker M, et al. A complete intermediate temporomandibular joint prosthesis. Evaluation after 6 years. *Rev Stomatol Chir Maxillofac.* 1990;91:423–429.
7. Raveh J, Stich F, Sutter F, et al. New concepts in the reconstruction of mandibular defects following tumor reconstruction. *J Oral Maxillofac Surg.* 1983;41:3–16.
8. Berarducci J, Thompson D, Scheffer R. Perforation into middle cranial fossa as a sequel to use of a proplast-Teflon implant for temporomandibular joint reconstruction. *J Oral Maxillofac Surg.* 1990;48:496–498.
9. Chuong R, Piper M. Cerebrospinal fluid leak associated with proplast implant removal from the temporomandibular joint. *Oral Surg Oral Med Oral Pathol.* 1990;74:422–425.
10. Estabrooks L, Fairbanks C, Collet R, Miller L. A retrospective evaluation of 301 TMJ proplast-Teflon implants. *Oral Surg Oral Med Oral Pathol.* 1990;70:381–386.
11. Moricone E, Popowich L, Guernsey L. Alloplastic reconstruction of the temporomandibular joint. *Dent Clin North Am.* 1986;30:307–325.

33
Problems Related to Mandibular Condylar Prosthesis

Christian Lindqvist, Anna-Lisa Söderholm, and Dorrit Hallikainen

Several different autogenous transplants can be used to restore temporomandibular joint (TMJ) function.[1-4] Whenever possible autogenous grafts are always preferred. There are few relative indications for using a condylar implant in arthroplasty.

For various reasons, autogenous transplantation may be contraindicated. Transplants usually require maxillomandibular fixation (MMF), although fixation of the graft with lag-screw technique can shorten the period of immobilization.[5] When any fixation between the jaws implies a risk because of the patient's general condition, another method of arthroplasty should be chosen. The same holds for situations in which removal of a rib should not be undertaken for the same reason. Other relative contraindications for autogenous arthroplasty might be extremely large osseous ankylotic masses and, in certain cases, reankylosis after costochondral transplantation.

Another type of problem arises when, in addition to the condyle, large segments of the mandible have to be reconstructed. For example, in tumor surgery, when mandibular resection with exarticulation of the condyle is necessary, an allogeneic prosthesis might be the best method for primary reconstruction. The same holds for traumatic cases in which the condyle is avulsed or highly fragmented, and primary restoration of mandible and joint functions by osteosynthesis is impossible.

During the 10-year period 1984–1994, 31 condylar prostheses were placed in 13 male and 11 female patients at the Department of Oral and Maxillofacial Surgery, Helsinki University Central Hospital, Helsinki, Finland. The mean age of the 24 patients was 49 years (range, 39 to 89 years). Two essentially different implant types were used. In 12 patients there was mainly joint pathology (posttraumatic or rheumatoid ankylosis, or condylar tumor), and in 12 the condyle had to be reconstructed along with the extracapsular mandibular segments that had been removed or destroyed because of a malignant tumor or extensive trauma.

In the first group, a condylar prosthesis was used (Figure 33.1a). Four patients with severe posttraumatic osseous ankylosis and four with bilateral ankylosis owing to rheumatoid arthritis had contraindications for an autogenous arthroplasty. In three of these patients, earlier rib arthroplasty had failed and reankylosis developed. A gap arthroplasty was not considered to be sufficient for permanent relief of the ankylotic situation in any of these cases.

In the second group, a reconstruction plate with condylar head was used (Figure 33.1b). In two traumatic cases, both of which represented shotgun injuries, there was no possibility of retaining the multiple bone fragments, including the mandibular condyle. A similar reconstruction was also performed in 11 tumor cases, in which, because of tumor extension, hemimandibulectomy and condylar exarticulation was indicated.

In surgery for TMJ ankylosis, stainless steel AO/ASIF condylar prostheses were used. In the cases in which, in addition to the condylar process, segments of extra-articular mandibular bone also had to be reconstructed, AO/ASIF reconstruction plates including the condylar head were installed.

A combined preauricular, hemicoronal or bicoronal, and retromandibular approach was used in the ankylosis operations. After substantial removal of the ankylotic mass, a new fossa was created in the region of the damaged mandibular condyle. No attempt was made, however, to remove the condylar process totally. Instead, we prefer that some condylar bone is left in the region of the former glenoid fossa (Figure 33.2). A unilateral coronoidectomy at the minimum was always performed. A correctly sized condylar prosthesis was attached to the ramus and angular region with 2.7-mm bicortical screws. Whenever possible, temporary MMF was utilized during insertion of the implant.

In tumor and trauma surgery, MMF must always be applied intraoperatively. In edentulous patients, Erich arch bars can be preoperatively attached to the patients' complete dentures, which are then affixed to the maxilla and mandible by screws and or wires. Thereby, the mandible is immobilized during plate bending and insertion. Effort is taken to remove the condyle carefully to preserve the disk intact within the fossa.

The condylar head might be placed slightly inferior to the fossa (~5 mm) to reduce the risk of glenoid fossa erosion.

a
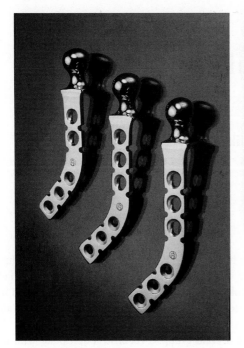

b
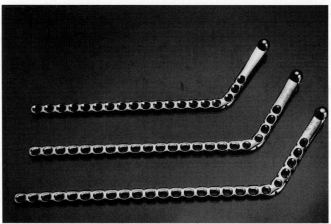

FIGURE 33.1 (a) Three different sizes of AO/ASIF condylar prostheses. (b) Three different sizes of AO/ASIF reconstruction plates including the condylar head. Currently, 2.4 mm titanium plates with condylar heads are available for use (see Chapter 22).

Radiologic Examination

Radiologic evaluation should include a panoramic radiograph and Townes' view. Other images are obtained as appropriate with respect to the diagnostic problem. Lateral panoramic views of both joints (Zonarc, Instrumentarium, Finland), lateral and posteroanterior detailed panoramic views of the operated joint, as well as tomography in the lateral and posteroanterior projection can also be undertaken. We have obtained detailed images and tomograms using Scanora (Orion Corp., Soredex, Helsinki, Finland) equipment.

The radiographs should be evaluated for displacement of the prosthetic condyle and bone resorption in the glenoid fossa and the ramus area (in the region of the screw fixation). Heterotopic bone formation can be recorded and graded according to Brooker (Table 33.1).[6] New bone formation within the fossa is recorded separately and not considered as heterotopic bone (Figure 33.3).

The prosthesis can be regarded as displaced from the glenoid fossa when more than two thirds of its articular surface is incongruent with the joint groove (lateromedially or anteroposteriorly).

Ankylosis

In 1992 we published a follow-up on 19 patients with a total of 23 condylar prostheses[7]). The follow-up time was 29 months on average. During this period, two implants had to be removed, one because of reankylosis and the other because

of severe glenoid fossa resorption. In the first case, 21 months after alloarthroplasty undertaken for a benign condylar tumor, radiologic examination revealed large amounts (Gr IV) of heterotopic bone around the metallic condyle. The patient was

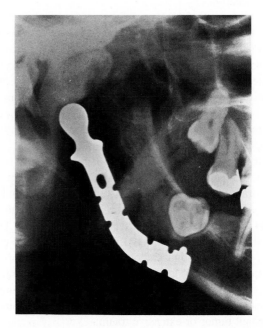

FIGURE 33.2 Postoperative radiograph showing AO prosthesis in place. No attempt was made to remove all the hypertrophic bone from the temporal fossa.

TABLE 33.1 Modified classification of heterotopic bone formation in the temporomandibular joint area according to Brooker.

Class	Description
I	Islands of bone within the soft tissues about the temporomandibular joint.
II	Bone spurs from the condyle or the joint groove leaving at least one third of the joint capsular area free.
III	Bone spurs from the condyle or the joint groove extending over more than two thirds of the joint capsular area.
IV	Apparent bony ankylosis of the temporomandibular joint.

Determination of the classification based on lateral and posteroanterior images.

unable to open her mouth for more than 4 to 5 mm (Figure 33.4a–c). After removal of the implant a costochondral arthroplasty was performed without any subsequent complications (Figure 33.4d). Two years after the second operation, maximal incisal opening (MIO) was 45 mm.

In the other patient, who suffered from severe juvenile rheumatoid arthritis, there was erosion of the glenoid fossa, resulting in perforation of the middle cranial fossa 10 months after arthroplasty. The implant was removed and exchanged for a rib (Figure 33.5). As the dura was exposed the fossa was also reconstructed with a cortical bone transplant. Later, the other joint was also affected and replaced with a rib. The other 9 joints functioned satisfactorily (Table 33.2). The mean MIO for all ankylosis patients was, however, only 22.8 mm. Radiologically, three condyles were not in a correct position with respect to the glenoid fossa. Bone resorption in at least some part of the fossa was diagnosed in 8 of the 11 joints. Heterotopic bone formation was seen in eight cases (Table 33.2). In three of them excessive new bone had been formed in the glenoid fossa and late resorption of the new bony surface was recorded.

Another type of complication has also been noted during later follow-up of three patients. A 63-year-old female patient with severe rheumatic ankylosis (RA) had bilateral TMJ arthroplasty in 1988 (Figure 33.6a,b). Because of the changed

a

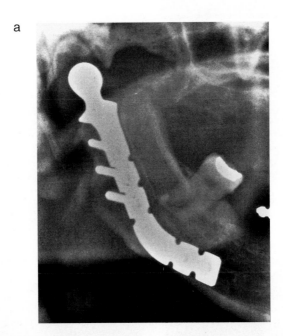

b

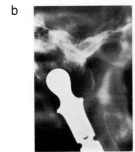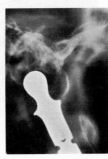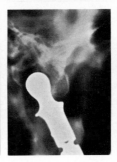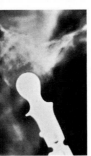

FIGURE 33.3 (a) Right condyle immediately after alloarthroplasty owing to posttraumatic ankylosis. Prosthesis in correct position in the glenoid fossa. Some condylar bone left in fossa. (b) Right lateral tomograms 6 years after alloarthroplasty. Note significant amount of heterotopic bone formation anterior to the condylar head. Restriction of mouth opening.

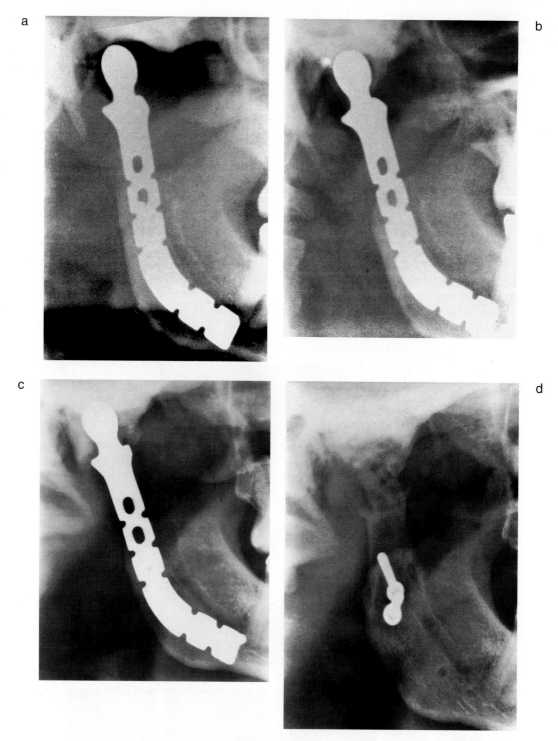

FIGURE 33.4 (a) Panoramic image after right TMJ alloarthroplasty because of benign condylar tumor. (b) Nine months later, signs of heterotopic bone formation around the condylar head. (c) Twelve months later (12 months after arthroplasty) a significant amount of ectopic bone is present. Patient was unable to open her mouth more than 4 or 5 mm. (d) Panoramic image 2 years after removal of prosthesis and costochondral arthroplasty. MIO 45 mm.

form of the mandible combined with the prebent angle of the AO prosthesis, the condylar head was erroneously placed in front of the articular eminence. This led to pain and dysfunction. The prosthesis was changed, and the angle was completely straightened. Only in this position was it possible for the prosthetic head to hit the fossa correctly (Figure 33.6c,d). This consideration for mandibular deformation and standard prosthesis forms should be taken into account when treating patients with RA.

Malignant Tumors and Trauma

The 11 patients who had condylar reconstruction plates placed were followed up for an average of 25 months. Three plates had to be removed because of infection. In 1 patient the plate fractured and was exchanged for a similar one (Table 33.3, patient A). Three patients died during follow-up, 2 of whom had a functional alloplastic joint. The mean MIO for the remaining 6 patients, alive at the end of follow-up with the implant in place, was 31.5 mm.

Radiologically, the condyle was found to be displaced in four cases. The displacement, when occurring, was usually lateral and caudal. In only two patients was the condylar head in an exact position, centered deep within the glenoid fossa (Figure 33.7). In these two, however, there was bone erosion in the skull base. In four joints, heterotopic new bone formation was recorded.

Condylar Position, Resorption, and Heterotopic Bone

Of the total of 23 TMJ half-prostheses, only 16 postoperatively were initially found to be situated in the glenoid fossa. Bone resorption developed during follow-up in 10 cases (43%), and in 1 a perforation to the skull base occurred 10 months after insertion of the implant (initial resorption of the fossa had already been diagnosed 2 months postoperatively). The first evidence of resorption for all 10 cases was recorded between 2 months and 3 years. Late resorption occurred in 3 cases where the condyle was partly incongruent with the joint groove (Table 33.2, patient B; Table 33.3, patients B and D). In 3 cases the resorption did not take place until new bone formation in the fossa had formed a bony surface in close contact with the prosthesis. Bone resorption in the region of the screws was seen in 5 cases (Table 33.2, patients D and E; Table 33.3, patient F). Heterotopic new bone formation was found in a total of 12 joints (52%). In 1 case, this resulted in almost complete restriction of condylar movement, and reoperation was necessary.

In our department the need for alloplastic implants constitute about 20% of cases with indications for TMJ reconstruction. If the pathology is mainly confined to the joint region, costochondral transplantation has been, whenever possible, the primary choice during the last 20 years. Several biological reasons speak for an autogenous transplant,[8,9] and there seem to be few reasons for abolishing this concept.[5] Thus, unlike some authors,[10–12] we do not believe that, for example, rheumatoid arthritis, per se, constitutes an indication for the use of a prosthesis rather than an autogenous graft. Resorption of the fossa with erosion through the skull base secondary to a metallic prosthesis has been reported earlier.[10] This is a serious complication, which occurred in one of our patients with RA. In nearly half of the cases some degree of resorption was noted. It must be emphasized that clinical signs revealed neither the real location of the condyle or the resorption. Therefore, radiologic follow-up examinations are essential in the continued evaluation of the joint replaced with an artificial prosthesis.

We have no experience with a glenoid fossa implant, but bone resorption probably cannot be prevented without the use of one. An artificial socket certainly allows a more even distribution of bite forces over a wide area, but it also involves disadvantages and technical problems.[10,13–15] These problems differ significantly from those encountered in the acetabulum of the hip joint. We believe that a costochondral or any other autogenous graft is still a far better solution than any foreign material in cases with TMJ ankylosis. When using a costochondral graft, there is no need for an artificial fossa, and the risk of heterotopic bone formation is minimal. New bone formation was rarely seen in our series of 16 rib transplants even after a follow-up of more than 10 years.[16]

Heterotopic bone occurs in 70% to 75% of the patients who have undergone total hip arthroplasty.[17–19] However, significant amounts of bone develop in only one fifth of cases (Brooker's classes III and IV). The ectopic tissue limits postoperative motion and causes pain (and need for reoperation) in 2% to 4% of the patients.[19] Nonsteroid antiinflammatory drugs and irradiation have been used to prevent heterotopic bone formation after hip arthroplasty. We are not aware of any corresponding studies with respect to TMJ arthroplasty. Even a fossa implant might not have prevented the formation of new bone, which in our series occurred in 52% of the joints. Grade III or IV bone formation was diagnosed in 22%, and in one patient (4%), it resulted in reoperation. These figures seem to be in accordance with the ones presented in patient materials concerning total hip arthroplasty.[17–19] In tumor surgery there is often no way or reason to try to avoid an alloplastic, albeit temporary, primary reconstruction. Before the introduction of the THORP (titanium hollow-screw reconstruction plate) system by Raveh[20,21] it was difficult to preserve a large enough condylar segment, with space for 4 or 5 screws, without impinging on the extent of resection or ablation. With the development of the THORP system, in which the plate-screw locking principle results in both internal and external fixation, 2 to 3 screws per segment are sufficient to secure plate stability. Even in a small condylar fragment, there is space enough for fixation, and the TMJ can be left intact.[22]

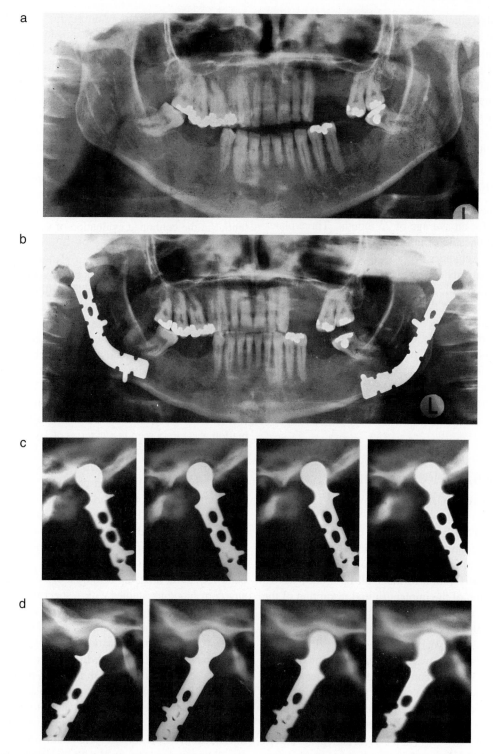

FIGURE 33.5 (a) A 40-year-old woman with rheumatoid arthritis. Note the open bite. (b) Five months after bilateral alloarthroplasty. Panoramic radiograph shows signs of bone destruction to the right. (c) Lateral tomogram of right joint reveals perforation to the cranial base. (d) Left joint has no signs of bone destruction.

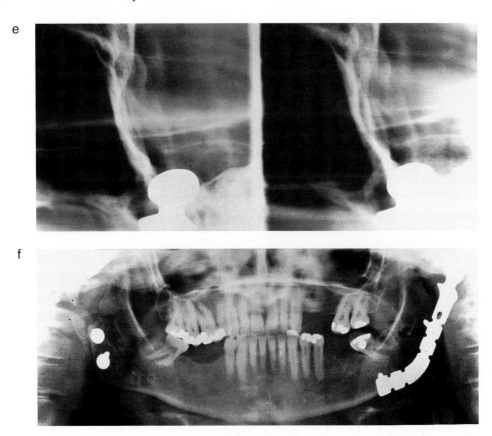

FIGURE 33.5 *Continued*. (e) Anteroposterior detailed image of right joint 10 months after arthroplasty. Perforation is now evident. (f) Situation 4 months after removal of right prosthesis and costochondral arthroplasty. MIO 22 mm. Left side is still unaffected.

TABLE 33.2 TMJ ankylosis. Patient data and follow-up.

Patient	Sex	Age	Diagnosis	Follow-up (months)	Maximum opening (mm)	Position of condyle	Resorption of fossa	Heterotopic bone formation*
A	M	56	PA	3	33	displaced	−	Gr I
B	F	49	tumor	24***	4–5	correct	+	Gr IV
C	M	20	PA	66	27	correct	−	Gr II
D	F	69	RA	22	30			
−left						displaced	−	—
−right						correct	+	Gr II–III
E	F	40	RA	12	15			
−left						correct	+	—
−right				***		correct	+ (perforation)	—
F	F	45	PA	35	25	correct	+	Gr II
G	M	37	PA**	65	30	correct	+	Gr II–IV
H	M	20	RA	48	18			
−left			**			displaced	+	Gr III
−right						correct	+	Gr III–IV

PA = posttraumatic ankylosis
RA = rheumatic ankylosis
*The amount of bone increased with time in three patients
**Reankylosis after costochondral arthroplasty
***Prosthesis removed

a

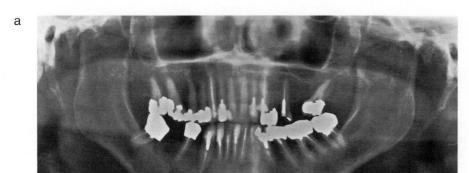

b

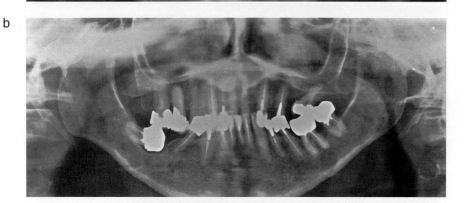

c

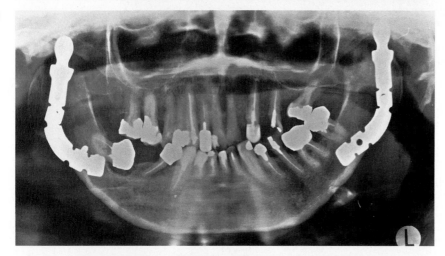

d

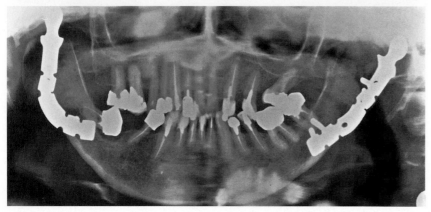

FIGURE 33.6 (a) A 56-year-old woman with severe rheumatoid arthritis. (b) Five years later, total destruction of both condyles. No movement in joints. (c) Bilateral TMJ arthroplasty showing that both condylar heads lie anteriorly to the articular eminence. Significant pain to the left. (d) Situation after left rearthroplasty. Condyle is now in correct position. The prebent angle of the prosthesis was straightened. Because of symptomless right joint, no reoperation has been performed.

TABLE 33.3 Malignant tumors and trauma. Patient data and follow-up.

Patient	Sex	Age	Diagnosis	Follow-up (months)	Maximum opening (mm)	Position of condyle	Resorption of fossa	Heterotopic bone formation
A	M		SCC					
−plate 1		77		26*	40	correct	−	Gr I
−plate 2		79		40	42	displaced	−	Gr I
B	M	45	SCC	18	27	correct	+	Gr I
C	M	56	SCC	57	45	displaced	−	Gr II
D	M	89	SCC	30	38	correct	+	—
E	F	77	SCC	4**	25	correct	−	—
F	M	60	SCC	30	15	correct	−	—
G	F	25	sarcoma	23 DFD	20	correct	−	—
H	F	60	SCC	7 days**	25	displaced	−	—
I	M	67	SCC	6 DFD	20	correct	−	—
J	M	26	gunshot	13***	52	displaced	−	—
K	M	48	gunshot	28**	35	correct	−	—

SCC = squamous cell carcinoma

DFD = dead from disease

*Plate fracture

**Plate removed due to infection

***Plate removed because of reconstruction with bone

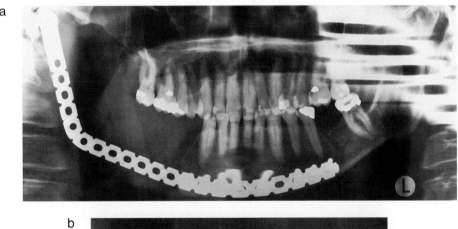

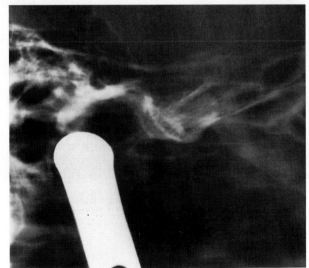

FIGURE 33.7 (a) Hemimandibulectomy reconstructed with alloplast. Condyle in correct position according to panoramic tomogram. (b) Detailed image shows slight resorption dorsally. Condyle is not in exact position.

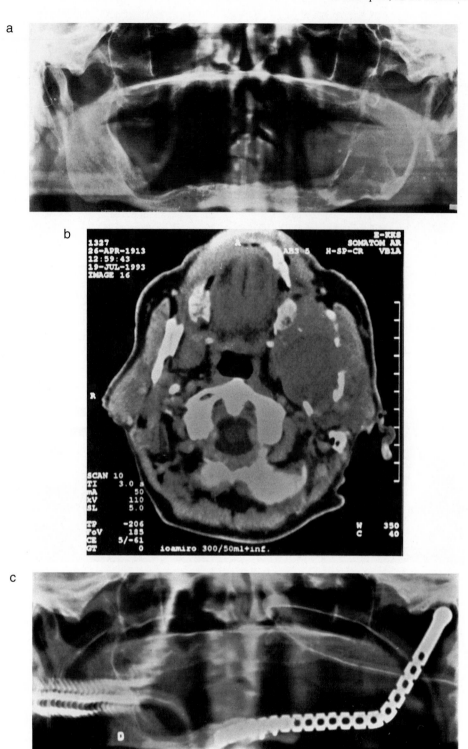

FIGURE 33.8 (a) Panoramic tomogram and (b) CT of 81-year-old male with a large fibrosarcoma in the mandible to the left. (c) Panoramic tomogram showing reconstruction.

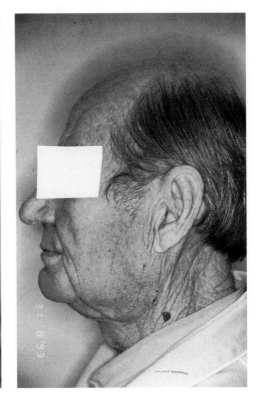

FIGURE 33.8 *Continued.* (d,e) Patient 2 weeks postoperatively.

Large enough safety margins might, however, require condylar exarticulation in radical cancer surgery.[22,23] Especially if the condyle is arthritic, deformed, and poorly functioning, it is probably not worth saving. In such situations, reconstruction of both the condyle and remaining mandible with a plate including the condylar head seems to give good functional and cosmetic results.[24] This is of major importance for the patient with malignant disease (Figure 33.8). A long reconstruction implies considerable stress, and plate fractures have been reported. We had only one such case, and the exchange of the plate was uneventful. Overall, postoperative joint function was far better in the tumor than in the ankylosis patients, and less bone resorption and heterotopic bone formation were seen. One reason for this is probably that the tumor patients did not have any significant joint pathology, and it was possible to leave an intact disc in place in most cases. Although the artificial condyle was found not to be in an exact position in several cases, this did not seem to affect joint function, and most patients were free from pain. Strangely enough, the patients with absolutely correct condyle position displayed more often than the others a resorptive process in the glenoid fossa.

In conclusion, tumor and some trauma patients can benefit from a plate that includes a condylar prosthesis for reconstruction of a large mandibular segmental defect including the condyle. If, however, there is primary joint pathology, as in posttraumatic or rheumatoid ankylosis, artificial implants that do not include a fossa imply a significant risk and do not, at least in our hands, give a satisfactory result. Significant progress has been made during recent years in developing a functioning alloplastic TMJ prothesis for patients with joint ankylosis.[10–12] At the present time, 2.4 mm titanium condylar plates are available for use (see Chapter 22). The special anatomic and functional conditions in the region of the temporomandibular articulation seem to indicate that autogenous materials should still be preferred.

References

1. Smith AE, Robinson M. A new surgical procedure in bilateral reconstruction of condyles utilizing iliac bone grafts and creation of new joints by means of nonelectrolytic metal: a preliminary report. *Plast Reconstr Surg.* 1952;9:393–409.
2. Ware WH, Taylor RC. Cartilaginous growth centers transplanted to replace mandibular condyles in monkeys. *J Oral Surg.* 1966;24:33–43.
3. Ware WH, Taylor RC. Growth centre transplantation to replace damaged mandibular condyles. *J Am Dent Assoc.* 1966;73:128.
4. Matukas VJ, Szymela VF, Schmidt JF. Surgical treatment of bony ankylosis in a child using a composite cartilage-bone iliac crest graft. *J Oral Surg.* 1980;38:903–905.
5. Kaban LB, Perrott DH, Fisher K. A protocol for management of temporomandibular joint ankylosis. *J Oral Maxillofac Surg.* 1990;48:1145–1151.
6. Brooker AF, Bowerman JW, Robinson RA. Ectopic ossification

following total hip replacement. *J Bone Joint Surg (Am).* 1973; 55:1629–1632.

7. Lindqvist C, Söderholm A-L, Hallikainen D, et al. Erosion and heterotopic bone formation after alloplastic TMJ reconstruction. *J Oral Maxillofac Surg.* 1992;50:942–949.

8. Poswillo D. Experimental reconstruction of the mandibular joint. *Int J Oral Surg.* 1974;3:400–411.

9. Ware WH, Brown SL. Growth centre transplantation to replace mandibular condyles. *J Maxillofac Surg.* 1981;9:50–58.

10. Kent JN, Misiek DJ, Akin RK, et al. Temporomandibular joint condylar prosthesis: a ten year report. *J Oral Maxillofac Surg.* 1983;41:245–254.

11. Kent JN, Block MS, Homsy CA, et al. Experience with a polymer glenoid fossa prosthesis for partial total temporomandibular joint reconstruction. *J Oral Maxillofac Surg.* 1986;44:520–533.

12. Kent JN, Carlton DM, Zide MF. Rheumatoid disease and related arthroplasties. *Oral Surg Oral Med Oral Pathol.* 1986;61: 423–439.

13. Chassagne JF, Flot F, Stricker M, et al. A complete intermediate temporomandibular joint prosthesis. Evaluation after 6 years. *Rev Stomatol Chir Maxillofac.* 1990;91:423–429.

14. House LR, Morgan DH, Hall WP. Clinical evaluation of TMJ arthroplasties with insertion of articular eminence prosthesis on ninety patients (an eight year study). *Laryngoscope.* 1977;87: 1182–1187.

15. Rooney TP, Haug RH, Toor AH, et al. Rapid condylar degeneration after glenoid fossa prothesis insertion: report of three cases. *J Oral Surg Maxillofac Surg.* 1988;46:240–246.

16. Lindqvist C, Jokinen J, Paukku P, et al. Adaptation of autogenous costochondral grafts used for temporomandibular joint reconstruction. A long term clinical and radiological follow-up. *J Oral Maxillofac Surg.* 1988;46:465–470.

17. Ahrengart L, Lindgren U. Functional significance of heterotopic bone formation after total hip arthroplasty. *J Arthroplasty.* 1989; 4:125–131.

18. Pedersen NW, Kristensen SS, Schmidt SA, et al. Factors associated with heterotopic bone formation following total hip replacement. *Arch Orthop Trauma Surg.* 1989;108:92–95.

19. Warren SB. Heterotopic ossification after total hip replacement. *Orthop Rev.* 1990;19:603–611.

20. Raveh J, Stich F, Sutter F, et al. New concepts in the reconstruction of mandibular defects following tumor reconstruction. *J Oral Maxillofac Surg.* 1983;41:3–16.

21. Raveh J, Sutter F, Hellem S. Surgical procedures for reconstruction of the lower jaw using the titanium-coated hollow-screw reconstruction plate system: bridging of defects. *Otolaryngol Clin North Am.* 1987;20:535–558.

22. Söderholm A-L, Lindqvist C, Sankila R, et al. Evaluation of various treatments for carcinoma of the mandibular region. *Br J Oral Maxillofac Surg.*1991;29:223–229.

23. Söderholm A-L, Lindqvist C, Hietanen J, et al. Bone scanning for evaluating mandibular bone extension of oral squamous cell carcinoma. *J Oral Maxillofac Surg.* 1990;48:252–257.

24. Lindqvist C, Söderholm A-L, Laine P, et al. Rigid reconstruction plates for immediate reconstruction following mandibular resection for malignant tumors. *J Oral Maxillofac Surg.* 1992; 50:1158–1163.

34
Reconstruction of Defects of the Mandibular Angle

Mark A. Schusterman and Elisabeth K. Beahm

Unrepaired defects of the mandible, including the angle, ascending ramus, and posterior body, leave a significant deformity, both functional and aesthetic. The muscles of mastication pull the remaining mandible into a lingual relationship with the maxillary teeth, rendering the remaining teeth functionless. The soft tissues of the tongue and larynx lose their support, resulting in difficulty with oral competence and intelligible speech (Figure 34.1).

The goals of mandibular reconstruction are to provide a reliable restoration of hard and soft tissue, enhancing both cosmesis and function. Due to its exceptional utility for restoration of the mandible, the three-dimensional reconstruction plate has become the cornerstone of the operative reconstructive strategy for these defects (Figure 34.2). The plate functions as a template of the mandible. It also helps to maintain the orientation and position of the remaining native mandibular segments. Consequently, proper occlusal relationships are preserved. In addition, the plate provides an excellent mechanism for the fixation of vascularized bone grafts.

Vascularized bone transferred by microvascular techniques has become the gold standard for reconstruction of the mandible. Initially, many centers were reluctant to use microvascular transfer, fearing the procedure to be unreliable due to the complex nature of the surgery. Ironically, this "complicated" technique is actually the most dependable method of mandibular reconstruction currently available. Success rates of approximately 95% for microvascular head and neck reconstructions are routinely reported in the literature.[1–3]

There are, however, circumstances in which it may not be imperative to restore bone. This may stem from either the location or extent of the mandibular defect or from variables related to the patient's overall health or prognosis. AO reconstruction plates may be used alone or in combination with soft tissue flaps to provide restoration of the mandible. These alternative techniques allow immediate function with minimal donor deformity in patients whose physical status mitigates against a lengthy surgical procedure. Reconstruction of the mandible solely with an AO plate should likely be limited to lateral or posterior defects due to the excessively high rate of plate exposure when plates are used without vascularized bone on anterior repairs. Reconstruction of 31 patients comparing plate fixation alone to immediate vascularized bone-graft repair demonstrated that while plate reconstruction had an overall success in 15 of 20 patients (75%), the failure rate for anterior plates was 76%. This contrasts with a 100% success rate for the vascularized bone grafts, 6 of 11 of which were for anterior defects.[4]

Types of Flaps in Common Use

Historically, a number of different vascularized bone flaps have been used for mandibular reconstruction, ranging from rib[5,6] to second metatarsal.[7] The most commonly used osteocutaneous flaps include the radial forearm, incorporating a portion of radius, the scapula, iliac crest, and fibula. All these flaps can provide a skin paddle, which may be needed for intraoral lining or external skin coverage. The particular flap used is dependent upon the specific needs of the reconstruction.

The radial forearm flap based on the radial artery and the cephalic vein provides a dependable pedicle and a thin, potentially sensate soft tissue. However, pathologic fractures of the radius and a significant functional and aesthetic donor site deformity can occur.[8–10] The scapular flap has a long pedicle from the circumflex scapular artery, which supplies a large amount of dependable skin for harvest. The skin paddle may be oriented independently of the bone stock, giving added versatility.[11] However, the available bone may be thin and somewhat limited, especially in female patients.[12,13] Most significantly, the lateral positioning of the patient necessary for flap harvest precludes simultaneous dissection with the ablative team, greatly increasing the operative time. We have most commonly employed the fibular flap, which is based on the peroneal vessels. The fibula flap provides excellent bone stock, minimal donor site deformity, and when a small cuff of muscle is included in the dissection, it is a reliable skin paddle as well.[14,15] The iliac crest is a large bone with a bulky skin/soft tissue paddle. The donor site is often painful, but

a

b

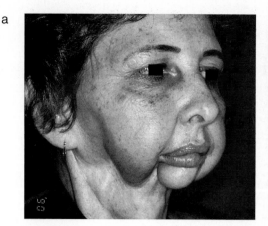
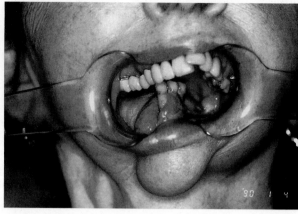

FIGURE 34.1 Residual deformity after posterolateral mandibular resection with primary closure. (a) Oblique view. (b) Intraoral view. Note the tethering of the tongue and the deviation of the mandible.

this flap has shown excellent results for bony restoration in patients with osteoradionecrosis.[16–18]

Preoperative Evaluation

A thorough evaluation of the patient in preparation for the reconstructive surgery is essential in obtaining reliable results. Issues that require assessment include:

1. The size and location of the defect
2. The composition of the defect
3. Status of recipient vessels
4. Overall health and nutritional status of patient
5. History of smoking

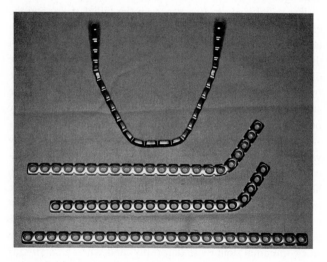

FIGURE 34.2 Reconstruction plates come in a variety of sizes of configurations. They serve as a template for the native mandible and as a fixation device for the vascularized bone flap.

Fibular Free Flap

The fibular flap is our flap of choice for mandibular reconstruction. The operative procedure we employ will be described in detail. The advantages of the fibular flap include:

1. The harvest is straightforward and may proceed simultaneously with the ablative part of the operation
2. The bone stock is of high quality and excellent length
3. The segmental periosteal blood supply allows for multiple osteotomies
4. The skin paddle is reliable if the perforators are protected by including a cuff of soleus muscle in the dissection
5. Donor site morbidity is low

If skin is not required for the reconstruction, the fibula is harvested from the ipsilateral leg. The contralateral leg is used if both skin and bone are needed. A posterior mandibular reconstruction requires creation of a ramus. Use of the proximal fibula mandates pedicle location at the neoangle, which is essential for flap inset and vessel anastomosis. Conversely, the distal fibula is used when a proximal reconstruction is performed, as the vessels are ideally positioned.

Operative Procedure

Occlusion should be set prior to resection, using intermaxillary fixation via arch bars. Both teams begin the operation concurrently. The ablative team is positioned at the patient's head, while the reconstructive team is harvesting the flap from the leg. The ablative surgeon notifies the reconstruction team once the mandible is exposed and ready for resection. The proposed sites for the bone cuts are marked with an oscillating saw penetrating only the outer cortex. Prior to the removal of any bone, the reconstruction plate is bent to precisely match the native mandible. The plate is then fixed into place with screws. The appropriateness of the shape and orientation of the plate is checked. This will allow precise placement of the graft in reference to the existing mandible. The plate is subsequently removed, set aside, and the resection completed.

Fibular Dissection

The patient is positioned supine on the table with a roll under the hip of the donor leg (Figure 34.3a,b). A tourniquet is used to facilitate the dissection.

The course of the fibula is noted. The fibular head is palpated at the knee and marked. The peroneal nerve is palpated and marked in its location just below the fibular head. A skin paddle of the appropriate size is sketched out and centered along the posterior border of the lateral leg. Marks are placed at a distance of 10, 15, 20, and 25 cm from the fibular head. The majority of significant perforators emerge at 10 to 20 cm below the fibular head, thus it is preferable to locate the skin paddle within this location (Figure 34.3c). As the anterior incision is made through the deep fascia, care should be taken to avoid injury to the superficial branch of the peroneal nerve. The dissection continues posteriorly to the posterolateral intermuscular septum, exposing the peroneal muscles (Figure 34.3d). The anterior surface of the septum is then followed down the fibula, and the peroneal muscles are elevated from the lateral and anterior surfaces of the bone. The anterolateral intermuscular septum is divided close to the fibula to preserve the integrity of the anterior tibial neurovascular bundle. The interosseous membrane is then divided as well.

The posterior skin incision is then made through the deep muscle fascia, and the skin paddle is elevated to the edge of the soleus muscle. A 1-cm cuff of soleus muscle is taken from the lateral edge. The fibular cuts are made with an oscillating saw. The proximal cut in the fibula is made first and positioned as superiorly as possible without endangering the peroneal nerve. To ensure stability of the knee the proximal 10 cm of fibula are preserved. However, the majority of the proximal fibula is resected, even if it is not used, to facilitate dissection of the pedicle. Once both cuts are made, the fibula is retracted laterally. The peroneal vessels are located and followed distally where they are ligated and divided. The flap dissection continues in a medial to lateral direction to avoid injury to the perforating vessels of the skin.

After elevation of the flap is complete, the tourniquet is released, the flap perfused, and hemostasis controlled at the donor site (Figure 34.3e).

The previously shaped reconstruction plate is then brought to the leg. Measurements from the mandibular defect are used to determine bone length and location of the osteotomy. To minimize ischemic time, the fibular osteotomies are made in situ while the graft is still being perfused. With the reconstructive plate used as a template, a single closing wedge osteotomy is made to create a neoangle. The bone fragments are then stabilized to the plate with monocortical screw fixation to avoid injury to the underlying vascular pedicle.

Insetting the Flap

The recipient vessels are prepared prior to division of the pedicle and flap transfer. Once the status of the neck vessels is assured, the peroneal vessels are divided, and the flap is transferred to the oral defect. Since fixation of the graft often makes subsequent intraoral repair very difficult, the skin paddle is inset first (Figure 34.3f). The fibula is tailored to fit the defect, placed in anatomic position, and secured to the native mandible by screws placed in the previously drilled holes.

The graft is then revascularized using microvascular techniques. After checking for a watertight intraoral closure, the neck flaps are replaced, and the skin is closed over drains. The leg incision is closed primarily or with a skin graft as needed. Suction drains are placed in the leg and a posterior splint applied.

Postoperative Care

In the immediate postoperative period, the patient is monitored in an intensive care environment by personnel experienced in the evaluation of free-tissue transfers. At a minimum, the flap is checked at hourly intervals. Clinical evaluation is the mainstay of the assessment of flap viability. Mechanical monitoring devices such as Doppler auscultation and laser flow devices may only assist in this endeavor.[19] Any question of flap perfusion must prompt immediate surgical exploration. One may salvage a flap within 2 to 3 hours of occlusion. After 4 hours of secondary ischemia, microcirculatory changes occur in a flap that most often preclude salvage.[20]

If the flap remains healthy, and the patient is stable for 48 to 72 hours, he or she may be transferred to a regular nursing floor. Flap color and perfusion are monitored every 2 to 3 hours until postoperative day 5 or 6.

A feeding tube is placed in all patients requiring any oral or oropharyngeal reconstruction. The patient is not fed by mouth for 1 to 2 weeks to allow adequate healing of the intraoral suture line, thus avoiding fistula formation. Speech and swallowing services evaluate glottic competence and deglutition prior to the introduction of an oral diet.

The patient's activity increases as tolerated after surgery. The patient may begin light "touch-down" weight bearing on day 5 with the aid of a walker, and gradually proceed to unassisted ambulation. Patients should wear a supportive bandage wrap on the donor site for 2 weeks after surgery.

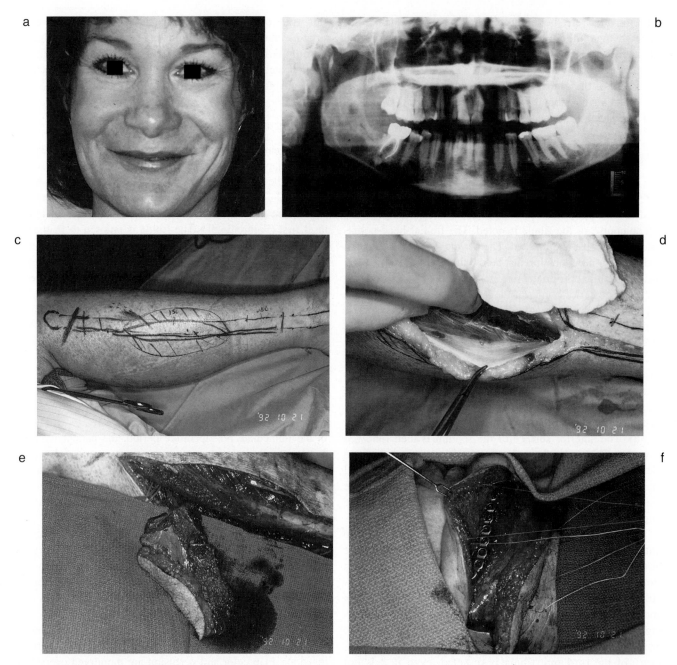

FIGURE 34.3 A 41-year-old female patient with adenoid cystic carcinoma involving the mandibular angle. (a) Frontal preoperative
view of patient. (b) Panorex of mandible. Note cystic lesion of angle on right. (c) Drawing of surgical plan on donor leg. Note proximal location of skin paddle. (d) Elevation of anterior aspect of skin
paddle to the posterolateral intermuscular septum. Note the location
of the perforator vessel providing blood supply to the skin paddle.
(e) Completion of flap elevation. (f) Inset of flap onto reconstruction plate. (g) Panorex of completed surgery. (h) Frontal view of final result. (i) Occlusal view of final result.

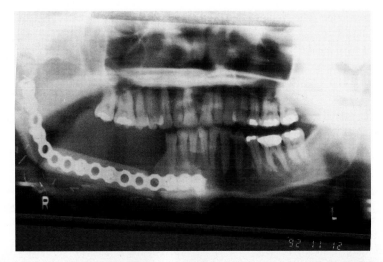

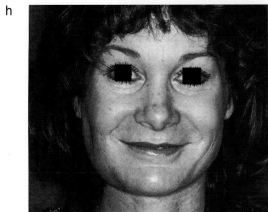

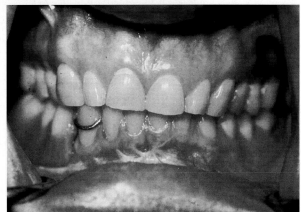

FIGURE 34.3 *Continued.*

Complications

The most feared complication of a free-tissue transfer is loss of a flap. Thrombosis occurs in a small percentage of patients, primarily during the first 24 hours after surgery. Factors such as blood coagulation abnormalities, atherosclerotic vessels, hypotension, and other factors may predispose to thrombosis.[21] However, anastomotic patency rests largely upon the surgical plan and its execution. A well-designed case with meticulous technique, a tension-free anastomosis using large-caliber vessels, and minimal ischemia time is the best way to avert this consequence.

Donor site morbidity from a free fibula is minimal. Complete loss of a skin paddle of a fibular graft is now rare, provided the perforating vessels are preserved by incorporating a small cuff of muscle to protect them. None of our patients have experienced any restriction in their gait or mobility. Partial loss of an iliac crest skin paddle may occur if the bulky flap is compressed too much when it is inset, thereby decreasing flow to the skin. The iliac crest donor site may cause pain, a contour deformity, or abdominal wall herniation.[22] The

lateral femoral cutaneous and ilioinguinal nerves must be protected during harvest to avoid anesthesia and pain in the thigh.

Partial loss of a skin graft, hematoma, seroma, and suture-line infection have an incidence of approximately 6%.[1,2,15] Plate exposure may result whenever there is compromise of the soft tissue cover. This most often occurs in radiated tissues, and as mentioned previously, it is largely a consequence of anterior reconstructions in which vascularized bone is not employed.

Summary

The principles pertinent to mandibular reconstruction in general apply to reconstruction of the defects of the mandibular angle. The critical facet of reconstruction of the posterior mandible is the maintenance of vertical height by accurately restoring the position and orientation of the ramus and angle. The three-dimensional reconstruction plate facilitates reconstruction by acting as a template of the resected mandible, an aid to maintaining proper occlusal relationships, and a fixation device for the vascularized bone. The fibula is our flap of choice due to the ease of dissection, excellent bone quality and length, and the reliable skin paddle it provides for soft tissue replacement.

References

1. Watkinson JC, Breach NM. Free flaps in head and neck reconstructive surgery: a review of 77 cases. *Clin Otolaryngol.* 1991; 16(4):350–353.

2. Urken ML, Weinberg H, Vickery C, et al. Oromandibular reconstruction using microvascular composite free flaps. *Arch Otolaryngol Head Neck Surg.* 1991;117:724–732.

3. Schusterman MA, Miller MJ, Reece GP, et al. A single center's experience with 308 free flaps for repair of head and neck cancer defects. *Plast Reconstr Surg.* 1994;93:472–478.

4. Schusterman MA, Reece GP, Kroll SS, et al. Use of the AO plate for immediate mandibular reconstruction in cancer patients. *Plast Reconstr Surg.* 1991;88:588–593.

5. Serafin D, Riefkohl R, Thomas I, et al. Vascularized rib-periosteal and osteocutaneous reconstruction of the maxilla and mandible: an assessment. *Plast Reconstr Surg.* 1980;66:718–727.

6. Richards MA, Poole MD, Godfrey AM. The serratus anterior/rib composite flap in mandibular reconstruction. *Br J Plast Surg.* 1985;38:466–477.

7. O'Brien BM, Morrison WA, MacLeon AM, et al. Microvascular osteocutaneous transfer using the groin flap and iliac crest and the dorsalis pedis flap and second metatarsal. *Br J Plast Surg.* 1979;32(3):188–206.

8. Corrigan AM, O'Neil TJ. The use of the compound radial forearm flap in oromandibular reconstruction. *Br J Oral Maxillofacial Surg.* 1986;24(2):86–95.

9. Swanson E, Boyd JB, Mulholland RS. The radial forearm osseocutaneous flap: a biomechanical study of the osteotomized radius. *Plast Reconstr Surg.* 1990;85:267–272.

10. Soutar DS, McGregor IA. The radial forearm flap in intraoral reconstruction: the experience of 60 consecutive cases. *Plast Reconstr Surg.* 1986;78:1–8.

11. Swartz WM, Banis JC, Newton ED, et al. The osteocutaneous scapular flap for mandibular and maxillary reconstruction. *Plast Reconstr Surg.* 1986;77:530–545.

12. Thomas A, Archibald S, Payk I, et al. The free medial scapular osteofasciocutaneous flap for head and neck reconstruction. *Br J Plast Surg.* 1991;44:477–482.

13. Gilbert A, Teot L. The scapular crest pedicled bone graft. *Plast Reconstr Surg.* 1981;69(4):601–604.

14. Hidalgo DA. Fibula free flap mandibular reconstruction. *Clin Plast Surg.* 1994;21:25–35.

15. Schusterman MA, Reece GP, Miller MJ, et al. The osteocutaneous fibula flap: is the skin paddle reliable? *Plast Reconstr Surg.* 1992;90:787–793.

16. Fossion E, Boeckx W, Jacobs D, et al. Microsurgical reconstruction of the irradiated mandible with deep iliac circumflex flap. *Ann Chir Plast Esthetique.* 1992;37:246–251.

17. Boyd JB. The place of the iliac crest in vascularized oromandibular reconstruction. *Microsurgery.* 1994;15:250–256.

18. Urken ML, Weinberg H, Vickery C, et al. The combined sensate radial forearm and iliac crest free flaps for reconstruction of significant glossectomy-mandibulectomy defects. *Laryngoscope.* 1992;102:543–558.

19. Mailaender P, Machens H-G, Waurick R, et al. Routine monitoring in patients with free tissue transfer by laser-Doppler flowmetry. *Microsurgery.* 1994;15:196–202.

20. May JW, Chait LA, O'Brien BM, et al. The no-reflow phenomenon in experimental free flaps. *Plast Reconstr Surg.* 1978;61:256–263.

21. Robb GL. Free scapular flap reconstruction of the head and neck. *Clin Plast Surg.* 1994;21:45–58.

22. Jewer DD, Boyd JB, Manktelow RT, et al. Orofacial and mandibular reconstruction with the iliac crest flap: a review of 60 cases and a new method of classification. *Plast Reconstr Surg.* 1989;84:391–403.

35
Mandibular Body Reconstruction

Anna-Lisa Söderholm, Dorrit Hallikainen, and Christian Lindqvist

Mandibular continuity defects are the result of surgery for malignant tumors, large benign tumors of various origins (e.g., dental, mandibular bone, surrounding tissues), or different benign diseases (e.g., extensive fibrous dysplasia, cysts or osteomyelitis, and trauma).

A vast majority of these diseases, including cancer,[1] involve mainly the mandibular body, the angular area, or both. Mandibular reconstruction surgery is, when appropriate equipment and surgical technique are chosen, usually to be considered as reconstruction of the mandibular body. If the hard tissue framework is successfully restored, good function is achieved; that is in contrast to bridging of even restricted continuity defects in the symphysis area. Lost anterior insertion of muscles of the floor of the mouth and tongue, lost soft tissue equilibrium between the floor of the mouth and lower lip, and lost lip support causes major functional problems for the patient, despite successful contouring of the hard tissue frame. Analogous problems may occur if the condyle is lost. Hence, evaluation of adequate extension of the resection to be performed, without unnecessarily large safety margins, is important for the success of the reconstruction.[2]

Rehabilitation of patients with mandibular continuity defects has always been a challenging problem. Without adequate primary reconstruction, loss of mandibular continuity, especially if combined with large soft tissue defects, lead to considerable difficulties with speech, mastication, swallowing, and oral continence,[3–5] as well as psychosocial problems. Previously, free-bone grafting was the only available method for rebuilding the mandible.[3] However, this operation, usually done as a secondary procedure, often led to complications,[6–8] and many patients were never offered such a reconstruction.

Today, immediate postoperative rehabilitation of patients with mandibular defects can be achieved through rigid-plate reconstruction. Bone can be transplanted either primarily or in a secondary procedure.[9,10]

Good early results have been achieved with various plates.[11,12] Several problems, including plate exposure, plate fracture, and infection, however, have occurred during follow-up with the various systems used.[13,14] However, a majority of these problems can, if detected at an early stage, be solved with good results (Tables 35.1 and 35.2).[10,15] Thorough knowledge of the principles and the limits of the system used are essential for good long-term results.[15–18]

In general, all plate systems work on the same basic principles. A conventional reconstruction plate, developed for osteosynthesis, is fixed to the bone by screws, the heads of which press the plate firmly against the bone surface. The screw holes are oval, and the cross-sectional area of the screw is less than that of the hole. Good buccal bone adaption is needed for adequate fixation. In our experimental studies on sheep, however, resorption of the buccal cortex has been observed to occur under the whole length of large reconstruction plates in almost every case, sometimes restricted to the area under individual screws (Figure 35.1). Adequate fixation was found in histological and microradiographic examination in only 26% of the screws (Table 35.3). A similar resorption was also recorded in our follow-up study on patients resulting in 30% screw failures observed on radiologic examination (Figure 35.2, Table 35.4).[15] The plate interferes with blood circulation to the underlying bone, and areas of early osteoporosis are found under rigid plates, corresponding in size to the dimensions of the plate.[9,19,20]

The conventional plates need four to six screws per fragment if stable fixation is to be guaranteed. Owing to a lack of space, placing this number of screws can be difficult to accomplish in tumor surgery, especially in the ramus-condyle area. Accessory approaches may also be needed, increasing risks of nerve damage and/or scar problems. Loosening of screws and an inadequate number of screws often leads to instability, pain, infection, and a need for plate removal (Figures 35.3 and 35.4).[10,14,15]

Conventional reconstruction plates, which were originally developed for fracture ostheosynthesis, are in our opinion hazardous for use in permanent mandibular bridging. In reconstructive surgery, the situation is totally different from that in

TABLE 35.1 Summary of successfully treated late complications (7 of 34 reconstructions).[10]

Patient	Age (years)	Diagnosis (stage of disease)	Resection performed	Plate used at primary surgery	Radiation (dose)	Complications	Interval from primary surgery (month)	Treatment	Current state	Follow-up from diagnosis (months)
1	77	SCC (IV)	Left hemi	AO-RPC	Postoperative (66 Gy)	Plate fracture	24	AO-RPC free bone (iliac crest)	FFD	67
2	66	SCC (IV)	Right body and ramus	AO-ARP	Postoperative (66 Gy)	Screw loosening proximally	12	ARP free bone (iliac crest) + dental implants	FFD	53
3	77	SCC (IV)	Left body and ramus	AO-ARP	Postoperative (66 Gy)	Screw loosening proximally	18	TH-ARP	AWD	44
4	60	SCC (IV)	Symphysis right body	AO-ARP	Postoperative (66 Gy)	Tumor recurrence	12	AO-RPC salvage operation	FFD	41
5	79	SCC (IV)	Symphysis	AO-SRP	Preoperative (64 Gy)	Screw loosening proximally	22	TH-SRP	FFD	30*
6	26	Angiosarcoma (grade II)	Symphysis right body and ramus	W-RPC	Postoperative (66 Gy)	Extraoral plate exposure	3	Sternocleido musculocutaneous flap	DFD	23†
7	45	SCC (IV)	Right hemi	AO-RPC	Postoperative (66 Gy)	Intraoral plate exposure	6	Antibiotics + wound care	FFD	17†

Abbreviations: AO-ARP, classic angular AO plate; AO-RPC, classic AO plate with condylar head; AO-SRP, classic straight AO plate; AWD, alive with disease; D, dead from other reason; DFD, dead from disease; FFD, free from disease; SCC, squamous cell carcinoma; TH-ARP, AO-THORP angular plate; TH-SRP, AO-THORP straight plate; W-RPC, Würzburg plate with condylar head.
*From diagnosis of mandibular metastasis, 50-month follow-up from primary diagnosis of SCC of the tongue.
†Primary plate in place after soft tissue closure.
Source: From ref. 10.

TABLE 35.2 Summary of patient records for late major complications (7 of 34 reconstructions) resulting in plate removal.[10]

Patient	Age (years)	Diagnosis (stage of disease)	Resection performed	Plate	Radiation (dose)	Complication	Interval to removal (month)	State of patient	Follow-up from diagnosis (months)
8	48	SCC (IV)	Symphysis	AO-SRP	Postoperative (66 Gy)	Infection, fistulation	12	FFD	77
9	60	SCC (IV)	Symphysis	AO-ARP	—	Infection, fistulation	10	FFD	66
10	57	SCC (II)	Symphysis	AO-SRP	—	Fistulation Plate exposure (partial flap necrosis)	17	FFD	34
11	69	SCC (III)	Right ramus body	AO-ARP	Postoperative (66 Gy)	Chronic infection, osteoradionecrosis?	6	D	25
12	77	SCC (IV)	Left hemi	AO-RCP	Postoperative (66 Gy)	Chronic infection, fistulation	4	FFD	23
13	78	SCC (IV)	Right ramus body	AO-ARP	Postoperative (66 Gy)	Tumor recurrence, plate exposure	7	DFD	16
14	61	SCC (IV)	Right ramus body	AO-ARP	Preoperative (40 Gy) and postoperative (30 Gy)	Tumor recurrence, infection	2	DFD	6

Abbreviations: AO-ARP, classic angular AO plate; AO-RPC, classic AO plate with condylar head; AO-SRP, classic straight AO plate; AWD, alive with disease; D, dead from other reason; DFD, dead from disease; FFD, free from disease; SCC, squamous cell carcinoma; TH-ARP, AO-THORP angular plate; TH-SRP, AO-THORP straight plate.
Source: From ref. 10.

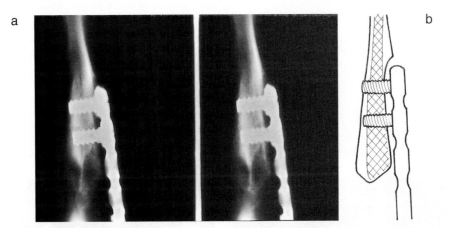

FIGURE 35.1 (a) Resorption under an AO-THORP plate fixed with solid screws for bridging of a continuity defect in a sheep mandible. Detailed image of the plate and the screw fixation in the ramus frag-ment. Slight resorption of the buccal cortex is seen after 8 weeks. Experimental study on sheep (unpublished data). (b) A diagrammatic representation of (a).

fracture treatment, where bone healing at the fracture site en-hances stability after 4 to 6 weeks, before buccal resorption extensive enough to jeopardize plate fixation has developed.

The AO-THORP system was developed by Raveh and coworkers.[21–23] This reconstruction system allows stable fix-ation without compression of the plate against the bone sur-face due to the screw-plate locking principle (Figure 35.5). Good screw adaptation to cortical bone, lingually or buccally, guarantees stability with two or three screws per fragment, as observed in our experimental study on sheep (Figures 35.6 and 35.7)[16,17] and radiologic follow-up study of patients (Fig-ure 35.8).[15] The fixation stability of this system has proved clearly superior to the conventional plate systems both pri-marily and in long-term follow-up (Tables 35.4 and 35.5; Fig-ure 35.9). Although permanent reconstruction with bone, den-tal implants, and bridgework is desirable, plate reconstruction can, for several reasons (e.g., patient's age), be regarded as permanent in many cases. Close monitoring of screw fixation, including adequate radiologic examination, is, however, in such cases required.[15]

Permanent reconstruction of the mandible requires bony continuity to allow rehabilitation of masticatory function with dental implants and/or dental prostheses. In the case of be-nign disease, tumor, or traumatic defect, immediate bone grafting is often indicated. For malignant tumors, the timing of the bone transplantation varies. Some surgeons reconstruct the defect with a vascularized bone graft at primary cancer surgery.[24] Others prefer a secondary procedure using a strictly extraoral approach after primary wound healing.[10,18,25,26] It has also been advocated to wait 1 to 2 years before carrying out the bony reconstruction to ensure early detection of re-currence.[26–29] Whichever procedure is preferred, the rigid-

TABLE 35.3 Screw fixation to cortical bone with classic AO screws.

Sheep	Follow-up (weeks)	Number of screws	Good buccal adaptation	Good lingual adaptation	Adequate fixation
A	5	9	0	0	0
B	9	9	8	4	8
C	9	10	0	4	0
D	14	(10)	(7)	(8)	(7)*
E	14	10	2	7	2
Total		38	10	15	10

*Plate fracture between the screws excluded from the comparison of screw fixation.
Source: From ref. 16.

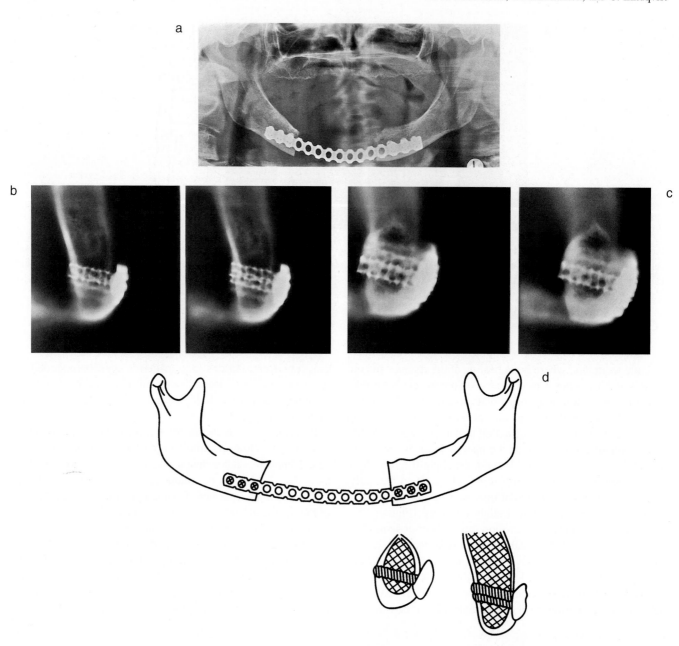

FIGURE 35.2 Reconstruction of the mandibular symphysis area in a 66-year-old woman after cancer ablation surgery. (a) Panoramic view with the plate in place. (b,c) Cross-sectional tomography of the left mandibular body area 5 months postoperatively shows slight re-sorption of the buccal cortex. (Compare buccal and lingual cortex. Normal cortical thickness is preserved lingually.) (d) A diagrammatic representation of (a), (b), and (c).

TABLE 35.4 Radiologic examination of screw fixation and plate stability in nine cases of mandibular reconstruction using classic AO plates.

Case	Resection	Number of screws proximally	Number of screws distally	State of screw fixation	Resorption of cortical bone buccally	Resorption of cortical bone lingually	First signs of screw loosening (months)	Follow-up (months)
A		3	4	2 screws loose	—	—	9	55
B		*	8	good	xx	xx	—	28
C		*	7	1 screw loose	—	—	28	39
D		*	5	good	—	x	—	37
E		4	3	3 screws loose	xxx	xxx	2	4
F		3	4	3 screws loose	xx	—	4	18
G		5	4	4 screws loose	—	—	20	66
H		3	6	3 screws loose	xxx	xxx	5	10
I		4	3	4 screws loose	xxx	xxx	8	10
Total		22	44	20 screw failures	5 cases with resorption	4 cases with resorption		

*Plate with condylar head; x = probable resorption; xx = slight resorption; xxx = moderate resorption.
Source: From ref. 14.

plate reconstruction can successfully bridge the defect during bony healing, and if needed, it can be used to fix the graft in place (Figure 35.9).

Vascularized free-bone grafts are being used increasingly to bridge mandibular defects, especially after large resections in cancer surgery. Vascularized grafts are represented by pedicled rib, scapular, or calvarial bone from the vicinity of the mandibular defect, or distant grafts applied using microvascular techniques. Several different donor sites have been used for free vascularized flaps.[24,30–37] It seems that iliac crest, fibula, and in some cases the scapula are best suited for mandibular functional reconstruction.[35,36,38] However, this technique has limitations with respect to the site and size of the defect, the patient's general condition, the surgical team available, and the facilities of the clinic. The total failure rate reported for vascularized grafts (11%)[35] also has to be taken into account.

Nonvascularized bone grafts are therefore still widely used for mandibular bony reconstruction. Numerous techniques for nonvascularized bone grafting have been presented including

frozen or irradiated autografts from the operation field, alloplastic or bony trays filled with cancellous bone, and compact grafts from the iliac crest.

The introduction of different metal prostheses for primary functional reconstruction has markedly improved the prospects for secondarily performed free-bone grafting.[25,28,39] Nevertheless, failure rates of up to 30% have been reported.[15,25,29] These failures are, however, often due to the use of an inadequate technique. When nonvascularized bone is used in combination with rigid-plate bridging, the plate has to be fixed in the remaining mandible at both ends. If fixed with one end only in the graft, the plate will loosen during rebuilding of the transplanted bone. The requirement of stability when using this technique cannot be neglected without a high complication risk.

The intraoral approach and intraoral contamination of the operation field have been cited as two reasons for the high failure rates of nonvascularized grafts.[25,29,40] Others, however, routinely use the oral approach.[27,41] In our own study we found that one third of the cases where an additional

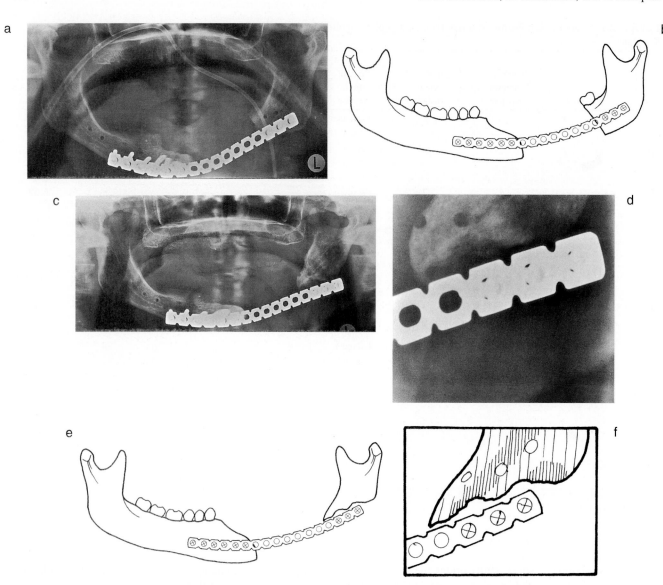

FIGURE 35.3 Recurrent carcinoma of the tongue in the left mandibular area, with resection of the mandibular body and reconstruction of the body defect with a classic AO plate. Fixation was performed with three screws proximally. (a) Immediate postoperative panoramic view. (b) A diagrammatic representation of (a). (c,d) Panoramic detailed images 21 months later shows massive resorption of the angular area. (e,f) A diagrammatic representation of (c) and (d).

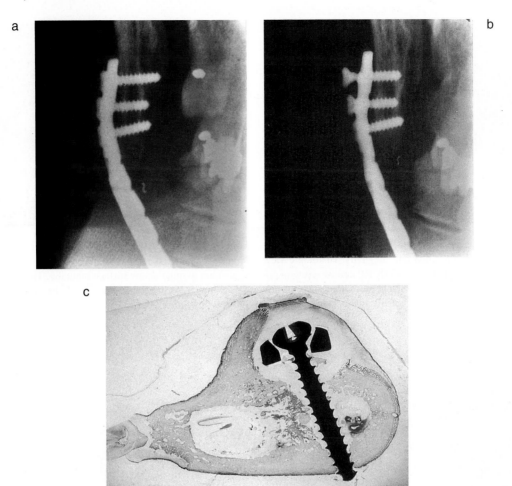

FIGURE 35.4 (a) Postoperative Townes' view of proximal (angular) screw fixation of a plate reconstruction in the body region performed at primary cancer surgery. The straight classic plate was fixed at the angle with only three screws. (b) At check-up, 4 years later loosen-ing of the screws was seen in the x-rays. (c) Histologic view of loose classic AO screw. Buccal cortex resorption under the plate. This screw no longer participates in plate fixation.

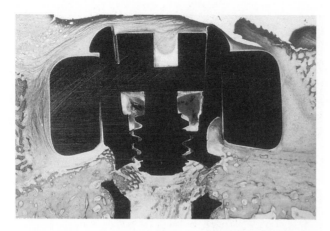

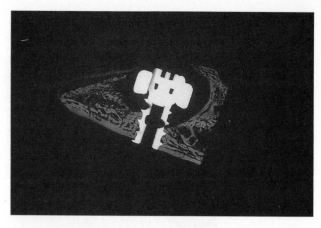

FIGURE 35.5 The screw-plate locking principle ensures adequate plate fixation even with bone apposition only lingually. Histologic view of a section through the head of an AO-THORP hollow screw in position. The expansion bolt presses the head of the screw firmly against the surface of the round plate hole (basic Fuchsin stain, magnification ×16).

FIGURE 35.6 Microradiograph of adequately fixed AO-THORP hollow screw (ramus part). No buccal bone apposition left. Good bone apposition to outer screw surface lingually. This is sufficient for adequate screw fixation with this system because of the screw-plate locking principle.

a

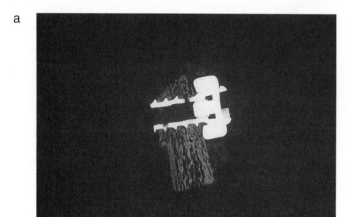

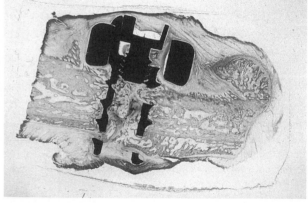

b

FIGURE 35.7 (a) Microradiograph of adequately fixed AO-THORP hollow screw (ramus part). Good bone apposition both buccally and lingually (magnification ×4.4). (b) Histologic view of AO-THORP screw fixed in bone (basic Fuchsin stain; magnification ×12.6).

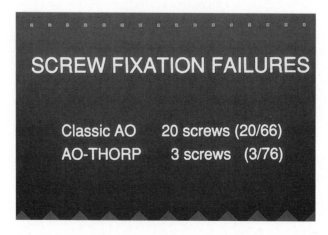

FIGURE 35.8 Comparison of screw fixation failures with classic AO plates and AO-THORP reconstruction in long-term follow-up.[15]

TABLE 35.5 Radiological examination of screw fixation and plate stability in 13 cases of mandibular reconstructions using the AO-THORP system.[15]

Case	Resection	Number of screws (ramus)	Number of screws (body)	State of screw fixation	Resorption of cortical bone buccally	Resorption of cortical bone lingually	First signs of screw loosening (months)	Follow-up (months)
K		3	3	good	—	—	—	6
L		2	2	2 screw fractures	x*	—	1	4
H		3	5	good	xx	—	—	16
M		3	3	good	xx	xx	—	33
N		3	3	good	xx	—	—	5
O		4	4	good	xx	—	—	13
P		2	4	good	xx	—	—	12
Q		2	3	good	—	—	—	9
R		3	3	good	x	x	—	31
S	†	3	3	1 screw loosened	xx†	—	3	9
T		2	3	good	xx	—	—	9
F		3	3	good	—	—	—	35
V		2	2	good	x	—	—	12
Total		35	41	3 screw failures	10 cases with resorption	2 cases with resorption		

*Tumor recurrence at fixation area.
† secondary reconstruction after radiotherapy.
x = probable resorption; xx = slight resorption.

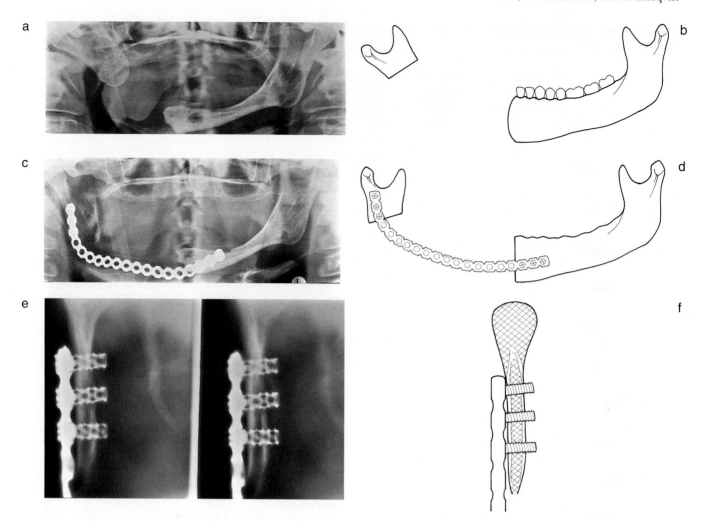

FIGURE 35.9 A segmental resection of the right angle and body was performed due to mandibular cancer in a 55-year-old woman. After postoperative radiotherapy the patient was referred 1 year later to our department for rehabilitation. (a) Panoramic view at referral. (b) A diagrammatic representation of (a). (c) Reconstruction of the mandibular continuity was performed with an angular AO-THORP plate. (d) A diagrammatic representation of (c). (e) Cross-sectional tomography of the condylar neck area 36 months later. The screws are in good position, and no bone resorption has occurred. (f) A diagrammatic representation of (e).

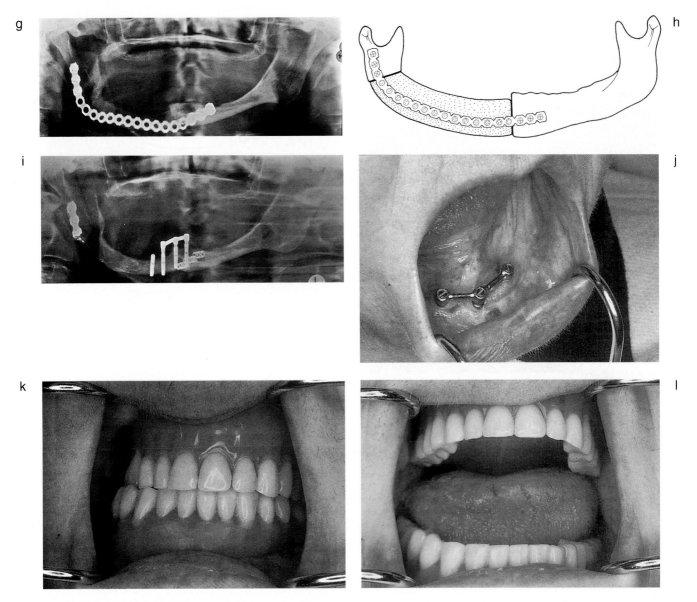

FIGURE 35.9 *Continued.* (g) In a second operation, nonvascular bone from the iliac crest was transplanted to the defect area. Soft tissue shortage was reconstructed by a pectoralis major flap. (h) A diagrammatic representation of (g). (i) Dental implants were thereafter installed in the symphysis area, both in the bone transplant to the right and in the patient's own mandibular bone to the left. The plate was removed from the body area. (j) Intraoral view 4 years later with the dental implants and the connecting bar. (k) The patient's implant based over dentures in good occlusion and (l) mouth opening of the patient. Both speech and masticatory function have improved markedly in consequence of the reconstruction performed.

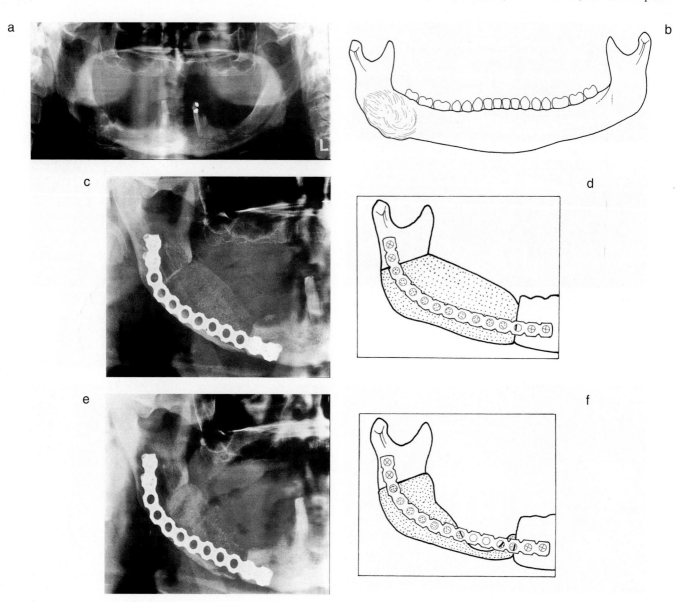

FIGURE 35.10 Because of an ameloblastoma in the right angular area, a segmental resection of the mandible was necessary. Primary reconstruction with an AO-THORP plate and nonvascular bone from the iliac crest was performed. (a) Immediate preoperative panoramic view. (b) A diagrammatic representation of (a). (c) Postoperative detailed image of the plate and the one-piece bone reconstruction. (d) A diagrammatic representation of (c). (e) Due to intraoral wound dehiscence, infection of the resection area and severe resorption of the bone transplant followed. Finally, the transplant was lost. (f) A diagrammatic representation of (e).

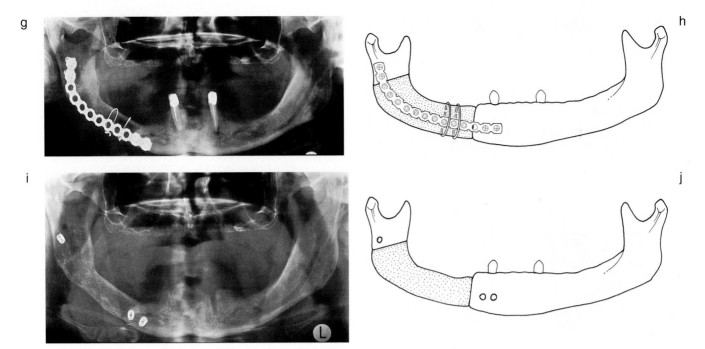

FIGURE 35.10 *Continued.* (g) After revision, antibiotics, and secondary healing, a new similar nonvascular transplant was inserted several months later from a strictly extraoral approach. (h) A diagrammatic representation of (g). (i) The height of the bone trans-plant was unchanged 3 years later. The plate has been removed. Three of the hollow screws were integrated into the bone tissue and could not be removed by a screwdriver and hence were left. (j) A diagrammatic representation of (i).

intraoral approach was needed resulted in postoperative infection and graft failure.[15] In our opinion, these complications stress the importance of extremely good intraoral wound care and the use of an extraoral approach only whenever possible (Figure 35.10).

High plate rigidity has been claimed to enhance graft resorption. Plate removal within 6 months after bone grafting has been recommended.[25,42] This was not confirmed in our own study. The mean interval between bone grafting and plate removal was 26 months for the patients with good bone healing and a resorption of less than 15%.[15]

Nonvascularized bone grafts in combination with rigid-plate reconstruction still play an important role in permanent mandibular reconstruction (Figure 35.11).[15,43] The technique does not require much time or resources and is particularly valuable in trauma and benign tumor cases.

Regular radiologic examination is essential in graft follow-up. Radiologic examination contributes to the evaluation of the possible resorption and resorption rate. Complications can be detected early and rescue therapy initiated wtih adequate time. Special attention must be paid to the imaging technique and image quality (Figure 35.2b,c). Good spatial resolution and good contrast are necessary, and the imaging procedure must be selected according to the specified diagnostic task. Radiologic literature on bone graft evaluation is sparse; especially, experience with computed tomography (CT) and magnetic resonance imaging (MRI) is limited.[44,45] Artifacts originating from metal reconstruction devices may complicate interpretation of CT images. MRI is even more sensitive to minute magnetic metal pieces, such as those originating from drills or other metal tools. We have used panoramic radiography in combination with detailed panoramic images and cross-sectional tomography.[14,18] Close collaboration between clinician and radiologist is beneficial.

Editors Note

Concerning two-screw fixation of segments: Following J. Raveh's initial preference for the fixation of segments with only 2 hollow screws (owing to the possibilities for bone ingrowth), international clinical experience presently indicates the necessity for a minimum of 3 to 4 screws (hollow or otherwise). The exception remains that 2-screw fixation of only the subcondylar segment is acceptable. For further discussion see Chapter 27.

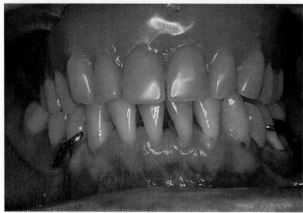

FIGURE 35.11 A large ameloblastoma of the right mandibular angle in a 37-year-old woman was treated by a segmental resection and reconstruction with an AO classic angular plate and multiple nonvascular bone transplants from the iliac crest. (a) A panoramic view of the reconstruction. (b) A diagrammatic representation of (a). (c) The patient's mandible after removal of the plate. (d) A diagrammatic representation of (c). (e,f) Rehabilitation of the dentition was performed by dentures. (g) Excellent occlusion, mouth opening, swallowing, mastication, and speech were achieved.

References

1. Söderholm A-L. Oral carcinoma of the mandibular region. *Br J Oral Maxillofac Surg.* 1990;28:383–389.

2. Söderholm A-L, Lindqvist C, Hietanen J, et al. Bone scanning for evaluating mandibular bone extension of oral squamous cell carcinoma. *J Oral Maxillofac Surg.* 1990;48:252–257.

3. Cohen M, Schoultz RC. Mandibular reconstruction. Symposium on head and neck surgery. *Clin Plast Surg.* 1985;12:411–422.

4. McQuarrie DG. Oral cancer. In: McQuarrie DG, Adams GL, Shons AR, Brown GA, eds. *Head and Neck Cancer. Clinical Decisions and Management Principles.* Chicago: Year Book Medical Publishers, Inc.; 1986.

5. Westin T, Jansson A, Zenckert C, et al. Mental depression is associated with malnutrition in patients with head and neck cancer. *Arch Otolaryngol Head Neck Surg.* 1988;114:1449–1453.

6. Höltje W-J, Lendtrodt J. Infektionen autologer Knochentransplantate nach Defektrekonstruktion des Unterkiefers. *Fortschr Kiefer Gesichtschir.* 1976;20:32–35.

7. Sailer HF. Ergebnisse der gleichzeitigen Resektion und Rekonstruktion des Unterkiefers auf oralem Weg. *Fortschr Kiefer Gesichtschir.* 1976;20:45–46.

8. Duncan MJ, Manktelow RT, Zuker, et al. Mandibular reconstruction in the radiated patient: the role of osteocutaneous free tissue transfers. *Plast Reconstr Surg.* 1985;76:829–840.

9. Spiessl B. *Internal Fixation of the Mandible. A Manual of AO/ASIF Principles.* New York: Springer-Verlag; 1989.

10. Lindqvist C, Söderholm A-L, Laine P, et al. Rigid reconstruction plates for immediate reconstruction following mandibular resection for malignant tumors. *J Oral Maxillofac Surg.* 1992;50:1158–1163.

11. Schmoker RR. Mandibular reconstruction using a special plate. Animal experiments and clinical application. *J Maxillofac Surg.* 1983;11:99–106.

12. Söderholm A-L, Lindqvist C, Laine P, et al. Primary reconstruction of the mandible in cancer surgery. A report of 13 reconstructions according to the principles of rigid internal fixation. *Int J Oral Maxillofac Surg.* 1988;17:194–197.

13. Platz H, Falkensammer G, Hudec M. Zur Problematik der Defektüberbrückung nach Unterkieferresektionen mit Metallimplantaten. *Dtsch Z Mund Kiefer Gesichtschir.* 1987;11:269–275.

14. Komisar A, Warman S, Danzinger E. A critical analysis of immediate and delayed mandibular reconstruction using AO plates. *Arch Otolaryngol Head Neck Surg.* 1989;115:830–833.

15. Söderholm A-L, Hallikainen D, Lindqvist C. Long-term stability of two different mandibular bridging systems. *Arch Otolaryngol Head Neck Surg.* 1993;119:1031–1036.

16. Söderholm, A-L, Lindqvist C, Skutnabb K, et al. Bridging of mandibular defects with two different reconstruction systems: An experimental study. *J Oral Maxillofac Surg.* 1991;49:1098–1105.

17. Söderholm A-L, Rahn BA, Suutnabb K, Lindqvist C. Fixation with reconstruction plates under critical conditions: The role of screw characteristics. *Int J Oral Maxillofac Surg.* 1996;25:469–473.

18. Söderholm A-L, Hallikainen D, Lindqvist C. Radiological follow-up of bone transplants for bridging mandibular continuity defects. *Oral Surg Med Pathol.* 1992;73:253–261.

19. Matter P, Brennwald J, Perren SM. Biologische reaktion des Knochens aus Osteosyntheseplatte. *Helv Chir Acta.* 1974;1:1–40.

20. Gunst MA. Interference with bone blood supply through plating of intact bone. In: Uthoff HK, ed. *Current Concepts of Internal Fixation of Fractures.* New York: Springer-Verlag; 1980: 268–276.

21. Raveh J, Sutter F, Hellem S. Surgical procedures for reconstruction of the lower jaw using the titanium-coated hollow-screw reconstruction plate system: bridging of defects. *Otolaryngol Clin North Am.* 1987;20:535–558.

22. Raveh J. Lower jaw reconstruction with the THORP system for bridging of lower jaw defects. *Head Neck Cancer.* 1990;II:344–349.

23. Sutter F, Raveh J. Titanium-coated hollow screw and reconstruction plate system for bridging of lower jaw defects: biomechanical aspects. *Int J Oral Maxillofac Surg.* 1988;17:267–274.

24. Wenig BL, Keller AJ. Rigid internal fixation and vascularized bone grafting in mandibular reconstruction. *Clin Plast Surg.* 1989;16:125–131.

25. Krüger E, Krumholz K. Results of bone grafting after rigid fixation. *J Oral Maxillofac Surg.* 1984;42:491–496.

26. Esser E, Montag H. Konventionelle Transplantatchirurgie und enosseale Impantate: Ein Behandlungskonzept zur Rehabilation nach radikaler Tumorchirurgie der unteren Mundhölenetage. *Dtsch Z Mund Kiefer Gesichtschir.* 1987;11:77–87.

27. Stoll P, Schilli W. Long-term follow up of donor and recipient sites after autologous bone grafts for reconstruction of the facial skeleton. *J Oral Maxillofac Surg.* 1981;39:676–677.

28. Egyedi P. Wound infection after mandibular reconstruction with autogenous graft. *Ann Acad Med Singapore.* 1986;15:340–345.

29. Krumholz K. Rekonstruktion des Unterkiefers und Oberkiefers mit Knochen: Ein Bericht über 115 Fälle. *Dtsch Z Mund Kiefer Gesichtschir.* 1987;11:408–416.

30. Taylor GI, Townsend P, Corlett R. Superiority of the deep circumflex iliac vessels as the supply for free groin flaps: experimental work. *Plast Reconstr Surg.* 1979;64:595–604.

31. Baker SR. Reconstruction of mandibular defects with the vascularized free tensor fascia lata osteomyocutaneous flap. *Arch Otolaryngol.* 1981;107:414–418.

32. Rosen IB, Mankeltow RT, Zuker RM, et al. Application of microvascular free osteocutaneous flaps in the management of postradiation recurrent oral cancer. *Am J Surg.* 1985;150:474–479.

33. Soutar DS, McGregor IA. The radial forearm in intraoral reconstruction: the experience of 60 consecutive cases. *Plast Reconstr Surg.* 1986;78:1–8.

34. Zuker RM, Mankeltow RT. The dorsalis pedis free flap: technique of elevation, foot closure, and flap application. *Plast Reconstr Surg.* 1986;77:93–102.

35. David DJ, Tan E, Katsaros J, et al. Mandibular reconstruction with vascularized iliac crest: a 10-year experience. *Plast Reconstr Surg.* 1988;82:792–801.

36. Lyberg T, Olstad OA. The vascularized fibular flap for mandibular reconstruction. *J Craniomaxillofacial Surg.* 1991;19:113–118.

37. Urken ML. Composite free flaps in oromandibular reconstruction. Review of the literature. *Arch Otolaryngol Head Neck Surg.* 1991;117:724–732.

38. Fig LM, Shulkin BL, Sullivan MJ, et al. Utility of emission tomography in evaluation of mandibular bone grafts. *Arch Otolaryngol Head Neck Surg.* 1990;116:191–196.

39. Spiessl B. A new method of anatomical reconstruction of extensive defects of the mandible with autogenous cancellous bone. *J Craniomaxillofac Surg.* 1980;8:78–83.

40. Lawson W, Biller HF. Mandibular reconstruction: bone graft techniques. *Otolaryngol Head Neck Surg.* 1982;90:589–594.

41. Obwegeser HL, Häussler F, Ibarra E. Behandlung des infizierten Knochentransplantates bei der Unterkieferrekonstruktion. *Fortschr Kiefer Gesichtschir.* 1984;29:76–77.

42. Lentrodt J, Fritzmeier CU, Bethmann I. Beitrag zur osteoplastischen Rekonstruktion des Unterkiefers. *Dtsch Z Mund Kiefer Gesichtschir.* 1985;9:5–19.

43. Piggot TA, Logan AM. Mandibular reconstruction by "simple" bone graft. *Br J Plast Surg.* 1983;36:9–15.

44. Bowerman JW, Huges LJ. Radiology of bone grafts. *Radiol Clin North Am.* 1975;13:67–77.

45. Kattapuram SV, Phillips WC, Mankin HJ. Intercalary bone allografts; radiographic evaluation. *Radiology.* 1989;179:137–141.

36
Marginal Mandibulectomy

Sanford Dubner and Keith S. Heller

Segmental mandibulectomy has traditionally been the mainstay of surgical therapy for oral squamous cell carcinoma adjacent to or invading the mandible and is the "gold standard" against which all other operations must be compared. Its advantages include adequate margins of resection, excellent exposure, and ease of closure, often without the need for soft tissue flaps. However, the functional and cosmetic consequences of this procedure are devastating to the patient.

Because a tumor does not invade the mandible through periosteal lymphatics,[1,2] surgeons have gradually changed the way in which they manage intraoral cancers. More conservative procedures have been devised to avoid the cosmetic and functional problems arising from segmental mandibulectomy. Mandibulotomy is used to provide access to oral and oropharyngeal malignancies when there is intervening grossly normal tissue between the tumor and bone. Marginal mandibulectomy can be employed to remove a tumor that involves only periosteum or cortical bone. Both techniques, when used appropriately, provide an adequate margin of resection without significantly disrupting mandibular form or function.

The indications for marginal mandibulectomy vary among authors. Gilbert et al.[3] recommended segmental mandibulectomy for alveolar lesions, tumors clinically adherent to the mandible, or for radiographic evidence of bone involvement. Bone involvement did not correlate with tumor location, stage, grade, or extent of metastatic nodal disease. Randall recommended marginal mandibulectomy only when there was no radiographic evidence of bone erosion and less than 50% of the mandibular circumference was involved by tumor.[4] Shaha et al.[5] used marginal mandibulectomy for the treatment of smaller floor of mouth malignancies and segmental mandibulectomy for larger tumors. This resulted in a 21% recurrence rate at the primary site following marginal mandibulectomy. Barttelbort et al.[6] reported a 25% local recurrence rate following marginal mandibulectomy, and a 36% local recurrence rate following segmental mandibulectomy. The local failures all occurred in soft tissue and not in bone.

We reported a 19% local recurrence rate in all patients who underwent marginal mandibulectomy, and a 6% local recurrence rate following segmental mandibulectomy.[7] Our series was a retrospective review of 130 consecutive patients who underwent marginal or segmental mandibulectomy for squamous cell carcinoma of the oral cavity or oropharynx. Seventy-nine patients underwent marginal mandibulectomy and 51 segmental mandibulectomy. The distribution of tumors by site is indicated in Table 36.1. Fifteen of the 79 patients who underwent marginal mandibulectomy had local recurrence of disease, which was independent of the size of the tumor. Two thirds of the patients with locally recurrent disease following marginal mandibulectomy were rendered disease free at the primary site with further surgery, for an ultimate local control rate of 94%. These data suggest that even when marginal mandibulectomy is performed in the presence of superficial bone erosion and invasion, the eventual local control rate is no worse than that following segmental mandibulectomy.

Local recurrence is also independent of nodal status. Our series refutes the concept that tumors that are more likely to metastasize are more likely to recur locally. The lack of correlation of recurrence with degree of bone invasion supports the concept proposed by Pogrel that cortical bone involvement is not a contraindication to preserving mandibular continuity.[8]

Tumor size alone is not a contraindication to marginal mandibulectomy. The local recurrence rate following marginal mandibulectomy in our series is independent of the size of the primary tumor. Other nononcologic factors must be considered when deciding whether marginal mandibulectomy is feasible. Such factors include the patient's dentition and the mandibular height. A postoperative mandibular strut that is inadequate to support a denture or osseointegrated implants, which is almost certain to fracture with mastication, should dissuade one from proceeding with marginal mandibulectomy. In this situation, segmental mandibulectomy with immediate mandibular reconstruction will undoubtedly better serve the patient in the long run.

TABLE 36.1 Distribution by tumor site.

Site	Type of mandibulectomy	
	Marginal	Segmental
Floor of mouth	40	10
Gingiva	24	19
Retromolar trigone	8	9
Buccal	4	3
Base of tongue	3	7
Tonsil	0	3

The accurate preoperative assessment of the extent of bone invasion is a difficult problem. An assortment of techniques have been employed, including clinical evaluation, panoramic radiographs, bone scans, computerized tomography (CT), dental scans, and magnetic resonance imaging (MRI). In a study by Shaha,[9] clinical evaluation was the most accurate, both to determine bone invasion and to decide the type of mandibular resection necessary. The various radiographic techniques are of little help in making the critical decision of the feasibility of marginal mandibulectomy. This is particularly important because cortical invasion may not preclude marginal mandibulectomy. Certainly if CT or dental scan shows deep invasion, a marginal mandibulectomy should not be performed.

The technique of marginal mandibulectomy has been described and modified in several papers.[4,8,10] Sagittal inner table mandibulectomy is ideal for those carcinomas that do not affect the alveolus, but rather the lingual gingiva. This technique preserves the buccal cortex and the buccal edges of the superior and inferior edges of the mandible. The usual marginal mandibulectomy resects the alveolar ridge in conjunction with the lingual cortex, preserving the buccal and inferior cortices. This resection must extend below the mylohyoid line, because preservation of this musculature may result in tumor recurrence within the deep musculature of the floor of the mouth.

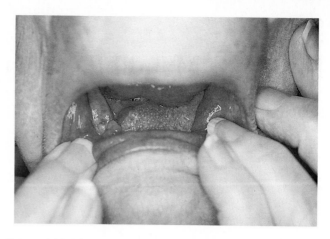

FIGURE 36.2 Bilateral nasolabial flap reconstruction of marginal mandibular defect.

Reconstruction of the resulting defect is determined by multiple factors, including the extent of the defect, its location (anterior or lateral), remaining dentition, the need for prosthetic dental rehabilitation, and any history of prior irradiation. Most surgeons agree that the best time to correct any deformity is at the time of the extirpation. Although primary closure of a defect or leaving an open defect and allowing it to granulate and heal secondarily will achieve a stable wound, this often results in a functionally unacceptable postoperative closure. The tongue will frequently be tethered to the labial mucosa, preventing the patient from adequately maintaining any dental prosthesis. A secondary skin graft vestibuloplasty may be required to restore function and esthetics (Figure 36.1). If postoperative radiation therapy has been employed, skin grafting has a much higher failure rate and may result in osteoradionecrosis of the remaining mandible. Therefore, a skin graft or a mucosal pedicle flap is optimal for resurfacing the anterior floor of mouth defect at the time of the ex-

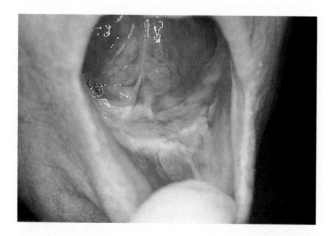

FIGURE 36.1 Split-thickness skin graft reconstruction of marginal mandibular defect.

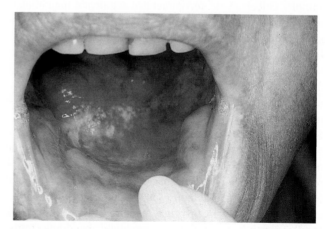

FIGURE 36.3 Pectoralis major myocutaneous flap reconstruction of marginal mandibular defect.

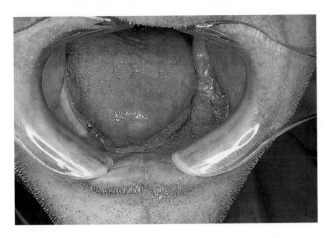

FIGURE 36.4 Radial forearm microvascular flap reconstruction of marginal mandibular defect.

tirpation, obviating any of the serious complications of a secondary reconstructive procedure. Larger defects may require more extensive reconstructions, including pedicled flaps or microvascular tissue transfer.

In the patient who has recurrent tumor or a new primary following irradiation of a prior tumor, a different approach must be used. A skin graft may not heal over a previously irradiated mandible. In this situation, vascularized tissue flaps are preferred (Figure 36.2). Nasolabial flaps, either unilateral or bilateral, can be used to resurface an anterior floor of mouth defect. They have the advantage of bringing vascularized tissue with a defined arterial supply to resurface the exposed mandible. Although these flaps can often be elevated and inset in one procedure, it is occasionally necessary for a secondary procedure to divide the flap pedicles several weeks postoperatively. Platysmal myocutaneous flaps have also been used to reconstruct lateral floor of mouth defects. They can be easily elevated and are fairly reliable, even if performed in conjunction with a radical neck dissection.

More extensive defects, particularly those that include a significant portion of tongue, must be reconstructed with vascularized tissue, either locoregionally or from a distant location (Figure 36.3). The pectoralis major myocutaneous flap has been used frequently in head and neck reconstruction, with varying complication rates. It has the advantage of using nonirradiated tissue to reconstruct a defect, providing muscle to cover and protect the carotid artery in a patient who has undergone a resection in conjunction with a radical neck dissection. We have found the complication rate to be as high as 75% when a pectoralis flap is used to reconstruct anterior floor of mouth defects. In these situations, we prefer to use a microvascular tissue transfer, such as a radial forearm fasciocutaneous flap to reconstruct the tongue and floor of mouth, as well as to resurface the cut edge of the mandible (Figure 36.4). This flap has the advantage of providing supple tissue which can adapt to the contour irregularities of the defect, permit postoperative dental rehabilitation, withstand postoperative radiation therapy without contraction or dehiscence, and even provide a sensate area to assist in nutritional support.[11]

References

1. Marchetta FC, Sako K, Murphy JB. The periosteum of the mandible and intraoral carcinoma. *Am J Surg.* 1971;122: 711–713.
2. McGregor AD, MacDonald DG. Routes of entry of squamous cell carcinoma to the mandible. *Head Neck Surg.* 1988;10:294–301.
3. Gilbert S, Tzadik A, Leonard G. Mandibular involvement by oral squamous cell carcinoma. *Laryngoscope* 1986;96:96–101.
4. Randall CJ, Eyre J, Davies D, Walsh-Waring GP. Marginal mandibulectomy for malignant disease: indications, rationale, and results. *J Laryngol Otol.* 1987;101:676–684.
5. Shaha AR, Spiro RH, Shah JP, Strong EW. Squamous carcinoma of the floor of the mouth. *Am J Surg.* 1984;148:455–459.
6. Barttelbort SW, Bahn SL, Ariyan SA. Rim mandibulectomy for cancer of the oral cavity. *Am J Surg.* 1987;154:423–428.
7. Dubner S, Heller KS. Local control of squamous cell carcinoma following marginal and segmental mandibulectomy. *Head Neck.* 1993;15:29–32.
8. Pogrel MA. The marginal mandibulectomy for the treatment of mandibular tumors. *Br J Oral Maxillofac Surg.* 1987;27:132–138.
9. Shaha AR. Preoperative evaluation of the mandible in patients with carcinoma of the floor of mouth. *Head Neck.* 1991;13(5): 398–402.
10. Collins SL, Saunders VW. Excision of selected intraoral cancers by use of sagittal inner table mandibulectomy. *Otol Head Neck Surg.* 1987;97(6):558–566.
11. Dubner S, Heller KS. Reinnervated radial forearm free flaps in head and neck reconstruction. *J Reconstr Microsurg.* 1992;8(6): 467–468.

37

Reconstruction of Extensive Anterior Defects of the Mandible

Joachim Prein and Beat Hammer

It is well known that reconstruction of lateral mandibular defects is much easier to perform than in the symphyseal area. Although lateral defects of the mandible can be left without reconstruction, symphyseal defects must be reconstructed primarily, whenever possible. Most patients with unreconstructed lateral defects can still function well, although they have a cosmetic disadvantage. This is in sharp contrast to the failure to reconstruct anterior mandibular defects, which results in an oral cripple characterized by disorders of speech, swallowing, and the cosmetic disability known as an Andy Gump deformity (Figure 37.1).

The method of choice for the reconstruction of anterior mandibular defects, even for patients with locally advanced disease, can be considered although it may be palliative, is the free microvascular tissue transfer (usually of composite osteocutaneous flaps). The various publications of the recent years by Schusterman et al., Urken, and others[1–11] show clearly that the introduction of microvascular tissue transfer, especially in the head and neck area has helped considerably to diminish the postoperative morbidity of our patients.

Our experience is that reconstruction with plates alone in the lateral aspect of the mandible for a certain time may be satisfactory, but the rate of complications in the symphysis with this method is considerably higher. Often after reconstruction with plates alone of anterior defects, many plate exposures occur no matter how thick the muscle or skin flap coverage.

We began the reconstruction of major defects in the facial area with microvascular flaps as a routine method in 1989. In the beginning, we preferred to use the iliac crest as a donor site. However, in recent years, and with more experience we now prefer either the fibula or the scapula as a donor site. The advantage of the fibula over the iliac crest is because the fibula can be shaped easier, is longer and the vessels, although shorter, have a larger diameter. The iliac crest on the other hand is larger and meets in a more natural manner the angular shape of the mandible in this region. However, donor site morbidity in the iliac crest is greater than in the lower leg or shoulder area.

Our choice depends on the type of defect (bone only, or bone and soft tissues), the location of the defects (symphysis or lateral aspect), the prognosis for the patient (type of tumor), and the general condition of the patient. In those instances where we use the fibula as a microvascular graft an angiography is performed in all of the patients. Most of our cancer patients are heavy smokers and, owing to severe arteriosclerosis, it may not be possible to harvest the fibula because of the risk of limb loss. As far as the osseous quality, size, and characteristics are concerned, the fibula is superior to the bone that can be harvested from the lateral aspect of the scapula. On the other hand, combined with the bone of the scapula, two soft tissue flaps for an intraoral and extraoral defect closure are available. The scapular myocutaneous flaps are safer than the soft tissue flaps that can be lifted together with the fibula bone.[1,2] Fixation of vascularized bone grafts can either be done with reconstruction plates or with smaller microvascular or mini plates[3] (see chapter 27, Boyd and Mulholland, 1993).

In contrast, it must be emphasized that fixation of nonvital bone grafts must under all circumstances be performed with reconstruction plates. Cosmetically and functionally the results are much better if the reconstruction can be performed primarily. Although the time of surgery may be longer, the overall morbidity of the patients can be lowered considerably when early definitive reconstruction and subsequent rehabilitation with dental implants is performed (Figures 37.2–37.5). Especially in patients who have to undergo combined therapy of surgery and pre- or postoperative radiotherapy, reconstruction with microvascular flaps is mandatory. Depending on the economic system in a country primary microvascular reconstruction that shortens the time of rehabilitation may have a great impact on cost-effectiveness as well. The patients need less time of hospitalization, fewer surgical procedures, and are rehabilitated sooner.

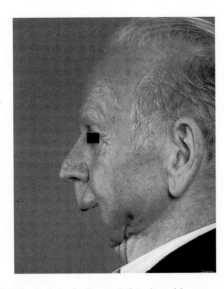

FIGURE 37.1 Typical Andy Gump deformity with a consequent crippling of the patient. In this case primary reconstruction was not performed because of the poor general condition of the patient. Postoperatively it must be said that this was a misjudgment since the general condition of this patient as a consequence of this severe morbidity deteriorated more rapidly.

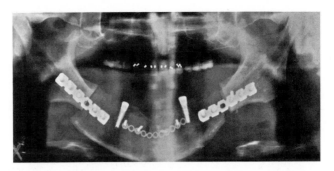

FIGURE 37.3 Orthopantomogram of this patient postoperatively showing reconstruction of the symphyseal area with a microvascular graft taken from the iliac crest. Dental implants in this case were implanted simultaneously. It is no longer performed this way in our institution, since the primary placement of dental implants is often a disadvantage for the prosthodontist. Fixation was obtained with short reconstruction plates. The one necessary osteotomy of the graft itself was fixed with a 2.0 mini-adaption plate.

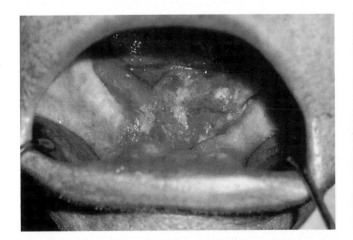

FIGURE 37.2 Squamous cell carcinoma of the floor of the mouth and the alveolar crest in the symphyseal area. The tumor had infiltrated the bone. TNM formula: T4 N0 M0.

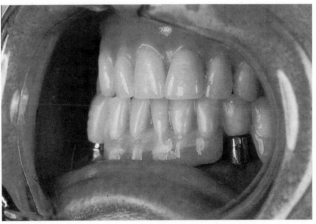

FIGURE 37.4 The patient was provided with new dentures and had an excellent functional result.

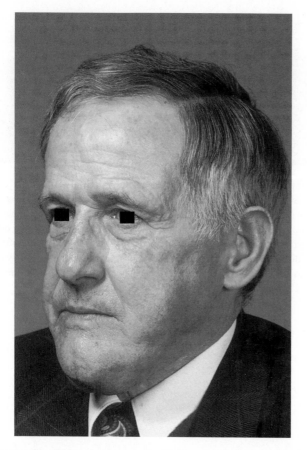

FIGURE 37.5 The patient remained with his original physiognomy including excellent shaping of his chin area. The patient is now 6 years free of disease.

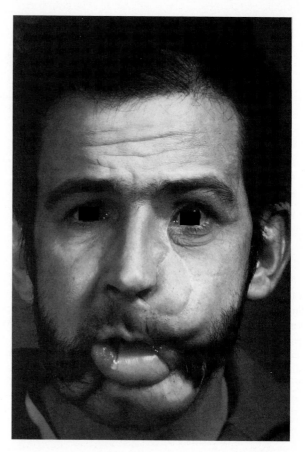

FIGURE 37.6 Frontal view of patient with severe shotgun wound treated between 1973 and 1976. The chin area is inadequately reconstructed with tubular flaps from the shoulder and abdomen. The patient is unable to control his saliva and can not wear dentures, with an Andy Gump deformity.

We have had the opportunity to observe and manage extensive anterior defects of the mandible with a special patient group that we have treated in Basel during the past 25 years. During this period we have seen 33 patients with gunshot wounds of the face. Most of these injuries happened as a consequence of suicidal attempts and mainly caused the loss of the anterior lower and middle facial regions. An example of the considerable progress achieved in facial reconstructive surgery, especially through microvascular techniques and the technique of adequate stable internal fixation with plates and screws, we show two patients from different time periods.

The first patient was treated between 1973 and 1980. This patient had more than 20 operations during 17 hospital stays. Today his hospital bills would amount to 800,000 Swiss francs. Although the cost of treatment in the hospital was much higher than it would be today, the result is absolutely unsatisfactory (Figure 37.6). There is no bony continuity in his symphyseal area, and therefore function of the lips and tongue is insufficient. The patient has considerable problems with eating and was never able to use dentures. In those days, microvascular techniques were not used as a routine and reconstruction plates were still under development. As a result, this patient's facial skeleton was not reconstructed correctly. The soft tissue defects were closed with tubular flaps from the shoulder and abdomen. The patient remained an invalid and received a disability pension, which is a high burden to the state economy. On top of this, his hospital bill was very high. Cost-effectiveness in this case is unacceptable according to today's standards.

In contrast to this, we show a patient of 1997 with a comparable injury that resulted from a self-inflicted shotgun wound. This patient was operated on and underwent complete primary reconstruction 6 days after the accident. His reconstruction included extensive fixation of all facial bones with

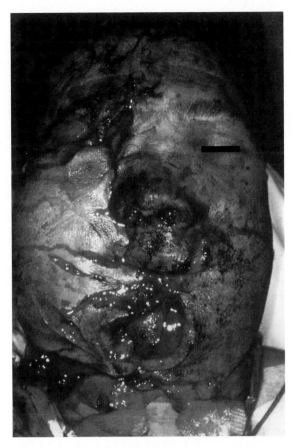

FIGURE 37.7 Severe self-inflicted shotgun wound with extensive panfacial fractures and soft tissue loss.

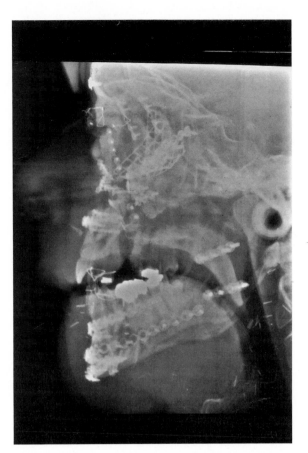

FIGURE 37.8 Extensive reconstruction of the patient's panfacial fractures with good facial projection as a result. No Andy Gump deformity.

AO titanium plates and screws together with a microvascular forearm flap for the reconstruction of his chin area. It also included extensive reconstruction with free bone grafts since the soft tissue coverage of the bones was adequate. Surgery lasted 23 hours (surgeon: Dr. Beat Hammer) (Figures 37.7–37.9). The hospital bill of this patient was 80,000 Swiss francs, one tenth of the bill for the patient treated in 1973 with a similar shotgun wound. In Switzerland, the hospital fee per day is always the same, regardless of the treatment performed, and as a result the hospital incurs a severe financial loss with these types of highly expensive, lengthy, and complicated operations. As a result of primary reconstruction with microvascular tissue transfer, rehabilitation time for this patient is short, and he will not remain a permanent invalid, as did our first patient. The postoperative social costs for this patient are therefore much lower. The ratio of cost-effectiveness is very good, although the surgical costs including the implants are very high.

Our complete results with 43 patients with shotgun lacerations during the last 25 years has been published in a separate paper.[12]

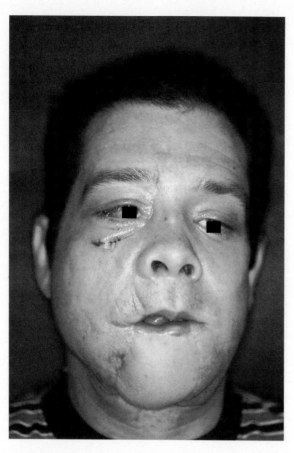

FIGURE 37.9 Patient's view approximately 10 days after surgery. Reconstruction of the soft tissue defect in the chin area with a microvascular forearm flap.

References

1. Schusterman MA, Reece GP, Kroll StS, Weldon ME. Use of the AO-plate for immediate mandibular reconstruction in cancer patients. *Plast Reconstr Surg.* 1991;88:588–593.
2. Schusterman MA, Reece GP, Miller MJ, Harris S. The osteocutaneous free fibula flap: is the skin paddle reliable? *Plast Reconstr Surg.* 1992;90:787–793.
3. Boyd JB, Mulholland RS. Fixation of the vascularized bone graft in mandibular reconstruction. *Plast Reconstr Surg.* 91:274–282 (1993).
4. Buchbinder D, Urken ML, Vickery C, Weinberg H, Biller HF. Bone contouring and fixation in functional, primary microvascular mandibular reconstruction. *Head Neck.* 13:191 (1991).
5. Fu-Chan W, Hung-Chi CH, Chwei-Chin CH, Noordhoff MS. Fibular osteoseptocutaneous flap: anatomic study and clinical application. *Plast Reconstr Surg.* 78:191–199 (1986).
6. Hammer B, Prein J, Ettlin D. Fixation of microvascular grafts for mandibular reconstruction: mini-plate versus reconstruction-plate. *J Craniomaxillofac Surg.* Vol 24 (Suppl. 1):51 (1996).
7. Hidalgo DA. Fibula free flap: a new method of mandible reconstruction. *Plast Reconstr Surg.* 84:71–79 (1989).
8. Riediger D. Restoration of masticatory function by microsurgically revascularized iliac crest bone grafts using enosseous implants. *Plast Reconstr Surg.* 6:861–876 (1988).
9. Swartz WM, Banesi JC, Newton ED, Ramasastry SS, Joes NF, Acland R. The osteocutaneous scapular flap for mandibular and maxillary reconstruction. *Plast Reconstr Surg.* 1986;77:530–545.
10. Taylor G, Townsend P, Coriett R. Superiority of the deep circumflex iliac vessels as the supply for free groin flaps. *Plast Reconstr Surg.* 1979;64:595.
11. Urken ML. Composite free flaps in oromandibular reconstruction. Review of the literature. *Arch Otolaryngol Head Neck Surg.* 1991;117:724.
12. Prein J, Schwenzer N, Hammer B, Ehrenfeld M: Gunshot injuries of the mandible. *Fortschr Kiefer Gesichtschir.* 1996;41:160–165.

38
Radiation Therapy and Considerations for Internal Fixation Devices

Peter Stoll and Rüdiger Wächter

Malignant tumors of the lower oral cavity with infiltration of the mandible frequently require segmental bone resections. The resulting loss of continuity in the mandibular arch causes a significant functional and esthetic deficit. A decisive step in the improvement of quality of life in these patients was the development of alloplastic defect bridging devices. Various techniques and materials can be applied.[1–8]

However, some authors[9] consider subsequent tumor irradiation in the presence of metal implants to be problematic, especially in exposed areas such as the mandible.

As a result of backscatter phenomena, dose enhancement may arise at the interface with denser material. Known as *hot spots,* these areas of increased radiation exposure are considered clinically relevant when in tissue cross section they exceed an area of approximately 2 cm^2 and attain dose values of more than 100% of the intended dosage of the target volume.[10]

The interface problem between more and less radiodense materials has been known for a long time. Measurements for a depth–dose curve at these borderlines of different materials have already been described.[11–25]

The question is whether there exists the danger of increased dosage ("hot spots") when using metal reconstruction plates as mandibular bridging devices during irradiation of head and neck tumors. Are there further differences related to the density of the material that may, as a result, possess other characteristics with respect to transmission and backscatter? Are there differences reflecting the type of radiation used? Furthermore, does the possibility of osseointegration of metal screws used for fixation of reconstruction plates exist at all? How do the covering soft tissues react to external beam radiation, especially with respect to hardware exposure (extrusion) through the skin?

All of these questions are controversially discussed and still open. Since there is a need for reproducible results, it seems prudent to perform simulations by means of an irradiation phantom model. There exist three main measurement designs such as thermoluminescence dosimetry,[26–30] ionization chamber,[30–35] and film dosimetry.[24,27,31,35,36] Also, calculations using the Monte Carlo method are reported in the literature.[34,37] More or less imprecise, however, are the reports on the distance between measuring point and metal (Table 38.1).

The question of whether irradiation can disturb or hinder osseointegration of metal screws, however, cannot finally be answered without animal experimental studies. Schweiger[38] inserted titanium implants into irradiated mandibles (60 Gy) of male beagle dogs. Although statistical significance cannot be related to the results, osseointegration was achieved in half of the irradiated specimens.

Montag[39] reports a study with rabbits, which were irradiated after the insertion of titanium implants (Co^{60}, 60 Gy). His results show a significant reduction of osseointegration, which was normalized after a 150-day survival period compared to a 90-day survival period without irradiation.

Lange et al.[40] report on a study involving female dogs, in which the insertion of titanium implants into the mandible was performed before and after irradiation. The results demonstrate problems with osseointegration when the implants are inserted immediately before or a few months after irradiation. Six months after irradiation, the osteogenic activity has recovered and is sufficient to integrate titanium implants.

To now draw a conclusion concerning radiation therapy and implants, clinical results and experiences have to be compared with the results obtained in phantom measurements and animal studies. Until the present, radiation therapy is consi-dered to diminish the osseointegration process of implanted alloplastic materials owing to its effect on osseous cellular regenerative properties. Since a considerable number of continuity defects bridged with bone plates function well, radiation therapy does not seem to be an absolute contraindication with respect to the presence of implanted metallic foreign bodies.[41–50] It would then appear to be obvious that the reduced regenerative capacity of irradiated bone is not a major risk factor for the long-term osseointegration of screw implants according to the aforementioned studies.

If the assumption that radiation-induced altered bone meta-

TABLE 38.1 Survey of measurements. Dose enhancement as a result of backscatter using different metal implants.

Author	Year	Type of irradiation	Single (S) opposed (O) beam direction	Metal	Relative dose enhancement in front of metal (%)	Distance between measuring point and metal (mm)	Method of measurement
Frössler et al.[26]	1975	cobalt-60	S	titanium	7	In front of the titanium plate	TLD
Gibbs et al.[31]	1976	6-M V photons	S	gold	75	Directly on the plate	ionization chamber and film
				amalgam	55		
			O	gold	30		
				amalgam	20		
Maerker et al.[27]	1976	cobalt-60	S	vitallium	9	Directly in front of the plate	TLD and film ionization chamber
Scrimger[32]	1977	cobalt-60	S	titanium	10	Measured directly at interface	
		8-M V photons		lead	72		
				tin	50		
				brass	32		
				steel	25		
				titanium	12		
Rosendahl and Kirschner[37]	1979	cobalt-60	S	titanium	16 ± 2	0.03	calculation (Monte Carlo method)
Thambi et al.[28]	1979	cobalt-60	S	lead	80	Directly at lead foil	TLD
			O		67		
Sailer[33]	1980	8-M V photons	S	lead	73	Measured directly at interface	ionization chamber
				steel	30		
				aluminum	13		
Hudson et al.[35]	1984	8-M V photons	S	steel	20	Measured at interface	film
				copper	40		
Tatcher et al.[36]	1984	cobalt-60	S	vitallium	43	Measured at the metal plate	film
				steel	33		
				titanium	26		
Farman et al.[29]	1985	cobalt-60	S	gold	21	Region of interproximal gingivae at the phantom	TLD
				amalgam	19		
				aluminum	11		
				steel	8		
Eichhorn et al.[30]	1986	cobalt-60	S	Küntscher-	18–35	At metal implant	TLD and ionization chamber
		10-M V photons		nails: compression plate	45		
Mian et al.[34]	1987	cobalt-60	S	titanium	15	Measured directly at interface	ionization chamber and calculation (Monte Carlo method)
		6-M V photons			14		
		25-M V photons			11		
Stoll et al.[24]	1989	cobalt-60	S	lead	46	0.45	film
				steel	14.5		
				titanium	12.5		
				aluminum	7		
		8-M V photons		lead	58		
				steel	16		
				titanium	12.5		
				aluminum	8		

bolic processes exhibit a dynamic character is true, then the timing of alloplastic reconstruction should not coincide with maximum bone damage (i.e., loss of vitality). This emphasizes the importance of understanding the time course of radiation-induced changes in the bone. The influence of dose, fractionation, and radiation field on bone regeneration, as well as the patient's individual response, need to be taken into consideration.

In the scope of this article phantom measurements, animal studies, and clinical experiences and results are highlighted.

Dosimetry on an Irradiation Phantom

This investigation is performed using four different metals, each subjected to telecobalt-60 irradiation (Philips cobalt device, 1.3-MeV photons) and 8-MeV photon irradiation (Philips Linac SL 75/20). The field size is 20×20 cm^2; the focus surface distances are 80 cm and 100 cm, respectively.

1. Titanium (pure)
2. Steel (DIN 4435)

3. Lead (pure)
4. Aluminum (pure)

The metals used exhibit the form of 2- and 3-mm-thick square plates with an edge length of 5 and 6 cm, respectively. To determine the influence of screw holes, customary stainless steel and titanium AO-reconstruction plates were examined as well. Edge effects were investigated using strips of steel and titanium, which differed from the reconstruction plates only in that they did not have any holes.

In preliminary tests, the angle of the incident beams was varied in order to evaluate any possible effects resulting from a deviation from the perpendicular. The effects to be examined are limited to the immediate vicinity of the metal–tissue interface (i.e., less than 2 mm). This created complications for both the measurements made using ionization chambers and with thermoluminescence dosimeters (TLD)[27–30,51] since the measured volumes in both methods do not correspond to the dimensions of the areas to be measured.

Customary TLDs have a diameter of 1 mm. If these have to be protected from moisture in simulations with a plastic coat, the diameter is increased up to 1.8 mm.

Therefore, we selected an experimental arrangement of the following construction (Figure 38.1). Water and polystyrene were chosen as a tissue substitute since muscle and other soft tissues have the same physical density as these materials. The metal specimens lay in a water bath on a plastic foil 0.1 mm thick. Placed under the water bath one on top of the other were three originally packed Kodak-X-Omat-V2 films on 1- (for cobalt irradiation) or 2-cm-thick (for 8-MeV photon irradiation) polystyrene plates. Irradiation is conducted from below to determine the backscatter effect, whereas the absorption can be measured conducting irradiation from above. The distance in water was also 1 cm for cobalt irradiation and 2 cm for 8-MeV photon irradiation. The film cover and the

plastic foil at the bottom of the water bath leads to measuring points (middle of the film) of 0.45 mm, 1.15 mm, and 1.85 mm either in front or behind the metal test object.

The dose in front of or behind the metal specimens was registered by film blackening. As the metal specimens had enough space between them, there are large enough areas of undisturbed film blackening, which can be compared with the areas at the edges or the holes or with the regions behind or in front of the metal surfaces. Quantification can be obtained when calculating the ratios of the relative dose values on the depth–dose curves of the two irradiation devices, which corresponded to the blackening of films registered in a polystyrene phantom parallel to the beam direction and which has the same optical density as the metal specimen sites of the experimental films. For all optical densities, mean values of several points are taken, which are measured on places where constant dose distribution can be assumed. The mean of several measured values taken independent of the metal test objects is used as a reference value.

Animal Studies

In the scope of an animal study, bilateral mandibular continuity resections were performed between the canines and premolar teeth in 28 full-grown sheep. The defect on the left side was bridged with a conventional AO reconstruction plate, the one on the right with a THORP plate (Figure 38.2). The 3-mm-thick resected bone pieces served as autogenous grafts, were turned 180°, and then reinserted into the gaps.

On the left side, the resected bone was wedged under eccentric compression drilling because of the ovally shaped holes of the AO plate (spherical gliding hole principle). This was not possible on the right side, where the THORP system was used.

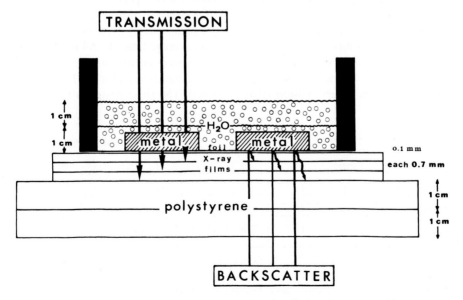

FIGURE 38.1 Schematic cross section of the irradiation phantom model.

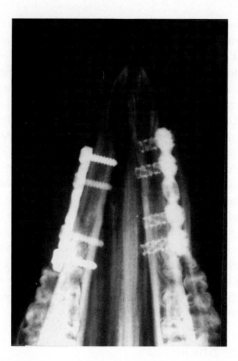

FIGURE 38.2 Basal teleradiography showing the two different plate systems applied (12 weeks postoperatively, the resected bone pieces served as bone grafts and have already healed).

The plates were fixed with plasma-coated hollow screws (THORP system) and solid titanium screws (conventional AO reconstruction plate). Postoperatively, the animals were permitted full masticatory function. To simulate the clinical situation, some of the animals were additionally irradiated with ^{60}Co gamma rays with a dose up to the equivalent of 60 Gy.[52] The observation period was as long as 24 weeks.

The sample was divided into four groups. Three groups (I–III) were subjected to fractionated lateral counterfield irradiation with ^{60}Co gamma rays (Philips cobalt-60 radiation generator). The isocenter of the irradiation was in the mediosagittal plane at a distance of 76 cm between the focus and the skin. The line between the animal's lips served as the cranial boundary. The fractionation schedule (Figure 38.3) shows the different irradiation modifications. Single dose was 4 Gy. Irradiation was performed three times a week. Postoperative

irradiation was not begun until 14 days after bridging osteosynthesis.

According to Ellis[52] the fractionation of 3 × 4 Gy per week selected for the animal experiment corresponds to an effective total dose of 20 Gy (Group I) and 60 Gy (Group II and III) as compared with the 5 × 2 Gy per week fractionation normally used for clinical application. For comparison, a nonradiated control group (Group O) was used.

Incorporation of the implants was demonstrated by means of sequential fluorochrome labeling of the osteogenic activity[53] during the observation period of 24 weeks. After sacrifice of the animals, thin grind sections[54] of the screw-bearing areas were made, and the osteogenic activity indicated by different fluorochrome marker areas was quantified using digital planimetry.

Clinical Studies

In 20 patients with carcinomas of the floor of the mouth, continuity resections of the mandible were necessary. The patient's mandibles were reconstructed immediately by means of a bridging titanium bone plate (AO-3DBRP system). All patients were subjected to postoperative full-dose irradiation therapy (60 Gy) with ^{60}Co.

For various reasons it was possible to harvest bone specimens at different time periods after termination of irradiation therapy. Here, of course, the incorporation of the fixation screws could not be demonstrated by means of any fluorochrome marking. Thin ground sections of the specimens were made, and the vital osteocytes at the interface between the screw and the bone were quantitatively recorded. By means of this method the time period of maximum bone damage could be detected.

In another sample of 140 patients we studied the clinical situation and especially the soft tissue condition using the THORP reconstruction plate. Out of this sample, 64 patients were prospectively evaluated.[55] The plates were left in place for an average time of 13.4 months. Since there has been no standardized documentation sheet available, the Freiburg documentation sheet for the THORP reconstruction plate was created. The sheet designed for entry into a personal com-

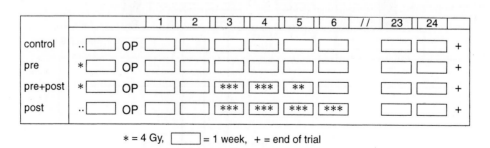

FIGURE 38.3 Fractionation schedule. Group 0 = control group. Group I = preoperative irradiation. Group II = preoperative and postoperative irradiation. Group III = postoperative irradiation.

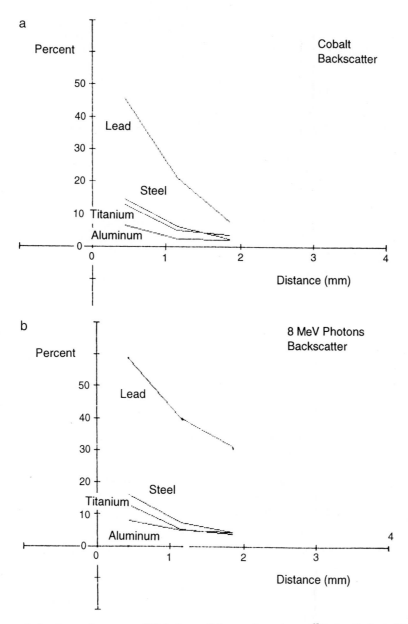

FIGURE 38.4 (a) Backscatter: relative dose enhancement (%) in front of the metal specimen (^{60}Co irradiation). (b) Backscatter: relative dose enhancement (%) in front of the metal specimen (8-MeV photon irradiation).

puter (PC) for statistical analysis comprises a total of six sections (patient data, history, therapy, complications and healing process, function, results) to provide information useful for describing and explaining causal problems.

To understand the entire problem, these three variables—dosimetry, animal, and clinical studies—must be evaluated and their correlations factored together. The question of increased dosage at the interface of bone and metal implant (i.e., screw and plate) can clearly be answered. Quantitative record of backscatter when using plates 2 mm thick at a distance of 0.45 mm for ^{60}Co irradiation (Figure 38.4a) was 46% of the applied dose for lead, 14.5% for steel, 12.5% for titanium, and 7% for aluminum. When using 8-MeV photons (Figure

38.4b) backscattering of 58% for lead, 16% for steel, 12.5% for titanium, and 8% for aluminum could be recorded. At a distance of 1.85 mm from the metal test objects the values dropped to 8%, 2.5%, 3%, and 2.5% for ^{60}Co irradiation and to 31%, 5%, 4%, and 4.5% for 8-MeV photon irradiation respectively. This data obtained from a phantom model, however, do not answer the question as to whether they are important as well in a biological system.

The dose values behind the metal plates (transmission) at a distance between 0.45 mm and 1.85 mm already approached the values determined corresponding to the absorption of the material thickness asymptotically (Figure 38.5).

The type of radiation used—in this case ^{60}Co and 8-MeV

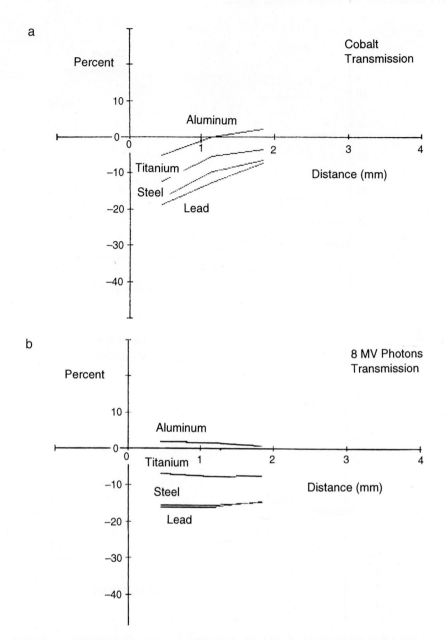

FIGURE 38.5 (a) Transmission: relative dose decrease (%) behind the metal specimen (^{60}Co irradiation). (b) Transmission: relative dose decrease (%) behind the metal specimen (8-MeV photon irradiation).

photons—showed no significant difference regarding backscatter and transmission. The calculations made by Rosendahl and Kirschner[37] and Mian et al.[34] agree with our results[24,56] very closely, although it should be noted that when extrapolating our measurements at a distance of 0.03 mm in front of the metal test object, we would observe greater dose enhancement (>16 ± 2%). Mian et al.[34] found corresponding results in their investigations between calculation and measurements.

There is no essential influence on backscatter exhibit size or perforation of the individual test objects. In preliminary tests, the direction of transmission was seen to depend upon the thickness of the material used. The metal/screw hole in-

terface behaves like the interface at the edges. When varying the angle of the incident beam (deviation from the perpendicular to an angle of 30°) there proved to be no significantly measurable difference in dose increase in front or dose decrease behind the metal specimen.

The differences related to the density of the material are, with respect to backscatter phenomena, clinically irrelevant. Only lead exhibits, both in close proximity to the metal plate and approximately 2 mm far from it, a different behavior as far as backscatter phenomena are concerned.

Under ^{60}Co irradiation, the comparison between titanium and stainless steel plates shows no decisive radiophysical advantage for titanium. As far as irradiation with 8-MeV pho-

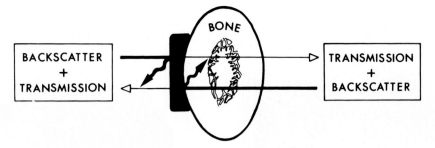

FIGURE 38.6 Backscatter and transmission using the opposing field technique.

tons is concerned titanium (12.5%) provides to be slightly better than steel (16%). With regard to the degree of relative dose enhancement the angle of incident beam appears to be of relatively minor importance, as has already been described by other authors.[17,33,37,57] However, it must be presumed that in the case of irradiation perpendicular to the metal test object, the phenomena of backscatter and decreased transmission at maximum intensity can be measured.[36]

This implies that for postoperative irradiation significant dose enhancement owing to backscatter can be observed in a range of under 1 mm in front of the implanted metal plate. In most cases backscatter is compensated by employing the opposing field technique, which reduces the dose behind the plate (Figure 38.6). Care should be taken, however, in single-field irradiation treatment when the implant is in the region of maximum dose, especially when this lies above the target volume dose, and in fractionated schedules[58,59] in which the biological effect of the dose is greater.

Irradiation damage to the skin as a result of an increased dose due to backscatter has implications when inserting metal implants and can only really occur in this small area. However, even this small area is important for the incorporation and osseointegration of metal screws. Therefore, it is of high interest whether the bone is able to recreate its vitality and within which time period it does so. Regarding the covering soft tissue layer, percutaneous radiation therapy should theoretically—as a result of the phantom experiments—not have any influence on the integrity of the implant, if it is of sufficient thickness.

Concerning the animal studies the comparative group receiving no irradiation (group 0) exhibits bony regeneration progresses smoothly without interruption during the entire observation period (Figure 38.7a). The sample with preoperative irradiation (Group I) presents a low initial osteogenic activity, which is steadily increasing throughout the follow-up period (Figure 38.7b). In our opinion this finding should be interpreted such that the preoperative irradiation has hit a non-injured bone. The osteoblasts apparently respond by reducing their normal activity. Not until the implantation trauma occurs, does the regenerative processes begin to prevail over the irradiation damage. A constant increase in osteogenic activity continues beyond the 24-week observation period.

The same phenomenon just described can initially be observed under preoperative and postoperative irradiation (Group II).

Here, too, increasing osteoblast activity begins after implantation, despite irradiation, but then decreases between the 12th and 16th week before it begins to increase again. It is surprising that in this group, too, there is an overall increase in osteogenic activity throughout the entire observation period (Figure 38.7c). It therefore must be assumed that the regenerative processes induced by the drilling trauma prevails over the irradiation damage.

Another fact that possibly contributes to this phenomenon is that the so-called sandwich technique used for irradiation gives the bone a chance to recuperate for 2 weeks between the sessions. Generally, however, in Group I and II the bone regeneration seems to be sufficient even initially to provide secure anchorage of the fixation screws at the bone/implant interface.

Postoperative irradiation (Group III) shows high osteogenetic activity immediately after the implantation comparable to Group 0 (Figure 38.7d). It decreases only slightly up to the 8th or 10th week, after which time it weakens rapidly. Not until the 20th week is an increase in activity resumed. In other words, when the maximum irradiation response begins, the osteogenic activity slows down after the implant has already healed in. Still, at least in the animal model, recuperation can be observed again after a relatively short period. Figure 38.8a,b shows examples of characteristic fluorescent-optic images of the bone structures around solid titanium screws. To the naked eye, the osteogenic activity in the two samples appears to be nearly identical. The differences described earlier do not show up until the morphometric analysis. Scanning electron microscopic images also exhibit direct contact between the implant and bone with no intermediate tissue in all the groups, independent of the irradiation dose.

No differences within the individual groups with regard to the type of screw, either hollow or solid, are observed in quantitative evaluation of osseointegration (Figure 38.7a–d). Radiographs of the screws in the harvested mandibular segments prior to its embedment confirm these findings (Figures 38.9a,b).

The clinical results correspond well to the results obtained in the animal studies. In the group of the 20 patients we could harvest bone specimens at different times within the follow-

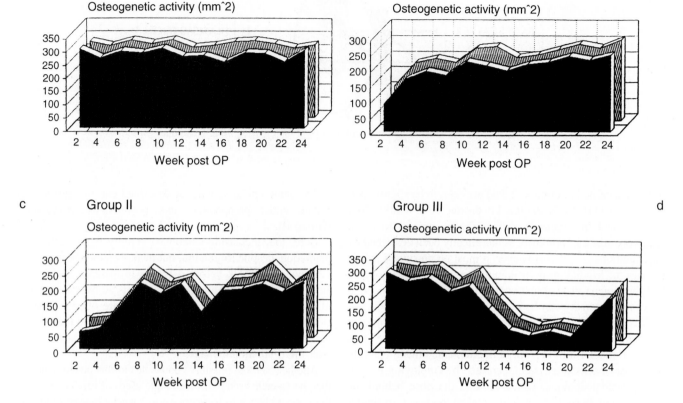

FIGURE 38.7 Osteogenetic activity/mm² over 24 weeks after implantation. Solid titanium screw (in front), hollow titanium screw (behind). (a) Group 0 = control group. (b) Group I = preoperative irradiation. (c) Group II = pre- and postoperative irradiation. (d) Group III = postoperative irradiation.

up period of 600 days after termination of full-dose irradiation (60 Gy ^{60}Co). We could register a minimum of vital osteocytes per square unit at 180 days. At that time the number of vital osteocytes has been diminished to 20% of the initial value. In the following time period, we can observe a slow but constant increase of the rate of vital osteocytes. The initial value, however, is reached only to approximately 80% within the entire follow-up period (Figure 38.10). Nevertheless, osteoneogenesis into the hollow screws is observed even under high irradiation dosage (Figure 38.11).

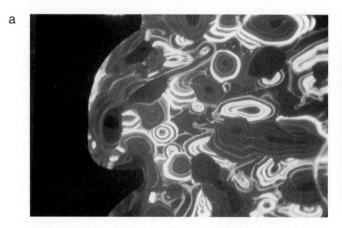
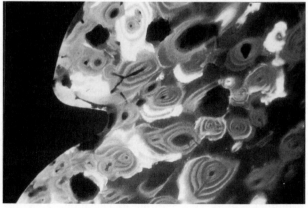

FIGURE 38.8 (a) Bony structure around a solid titanium screw 24 weeks after bone plating (sheep bone specimen, fluorescent microscopy, magnification 60×, control group). (b) Bony structure around a solid screw 24 weeks after bone plating (sheep bone specimen, fluorescent microscopy, magnification 60×, postoperative full dose irradiation 48 Gy, ^{60}Co).

a

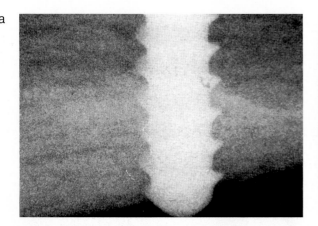

b

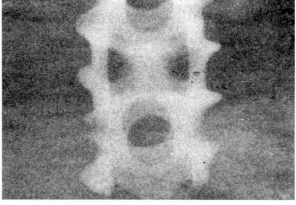

FIGURE 38.9 (a) Radiograph of a solid screw after full-dose irradiation (48 Gy, ⁶⁰Co) 24 weeks after implantation showing osseointegration (sheep). (b) Radiograph of a hollow screw after full-dose irradiation (48 Gy, ⁶⁰Co) 24 weeks after implantation showing osseointegration (sheep).

Soft tissue complications were the main problem. Interesting differences were found with regard to the parameters in the early (<4 weeks postoperatively) and in the late phase (>4 weeks postoperatively). In the early phase the relevant factors were primarily the patient's constitution, so-called mechanical functional factors in conjunction with the operation (i.e. anterior plate location, bridging of large defects, extensive lymph node resections), and factors that interfered with primary wound healing (e.g., alcohol abuse, smoking, poor oral hygiene).

Radiotherapy had the most important influence in the late phase; 39% of the patients exhibited a plate penetration through the surrounding soft tissues. In more than 80% of these patients we observed a skin perforation (Figure 38.12).

We obtained the poorest results following anterior plate bridging in combination with percutaneous irradiation. Under these circumstances 70% of the plates perforated the covering soft tissue. In the lateral (52.4%) and anterolateral area (44.5%) the ratio of perforation and nonperforation was about the same (Figure 38.13a,b). Apparently, irradiation has a major effect on the covering soft tissue in the anterior region. The amount of "tension" tolerated by the soft tissue covering the plate is exceeded when percutaneous irradiation is applied owing to the increase in tissue induration. The soft tissue lying over the plate loses its elasticity and becomes stiff. The rigid plate presses against the altered soft tissue, and after a while perforation results. Extensive lymph node operation (radical neck dissection) also increases the danger of soft tissue perforation. Statistical analysis shows that perforation occurred less frequently when the lymph node operation was more localized (i.e. suprahyoid lymph node removal), despite anterior plate location and postoperative percutaneous irradiation with full-tumor dose (60 Gy).

To solve these problems, two therapeutic procedures may be helpful.

First, to reduce the effect of the percutaneous irradiation therapy, intraoperative radiation therapy (IORT) presents advantages when it is necessary to use a reconstruction plate in the anterior mandible. To date, only few reports on the use of IORT in head and neck surgery have been published.[60–63] IORT makes it possible to apply the necessary dose without irritating skin, vessels, nerves, salivary glands, and bone. The irradiation cone is placed directly upon the tumor bed (Figure 38.14). In this way, the benefit of irradiation can be assured without harm to critical structures, particularly skin and

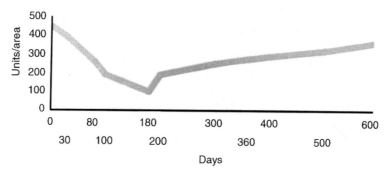

FIGURE 38.10 Osteogenic activity more than 600 days after bone plating (human bone specimen). Note the minimum of vital osteocytes at 180 days.

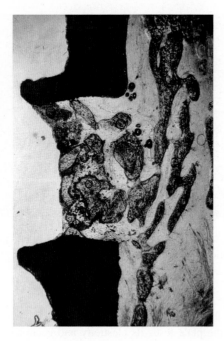

FIGURE 38.11 Growth of newly formed bone into the screw lumen passing the perforations of the side of the screw (human specimen, toluidine blue, magnification 42×, full-dose irradiation 60 Gy, ^{60}Co).

bone. This new therapeutic approach might solve the severe problems of soft tissue complications in these particular cases. Although experience to date with IORT in head and neck surgery does not allow definitive conclusions regarding the

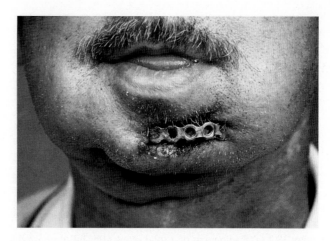

FIGURE 38.12 Skin perforation after anterior alloplastic mandibular reconstruction and full-dose percutaneous radiotherapy.

improvement of survival, the advantages of the method cannot be disputed. When myocutaneous flaps or free vascularized grafts are used to cover defects, the lower dose required for postoperative radiotherapy after IORT means less damage to the transplants. In some cases IORT can result in shorter treatment times, allowing the patient to resume his or her social life sooner. The quality of life is significantly improved. More studies are necessary to show whether the currently applied percutaneous dose of 50 Gy after lymphadenectomy can be reduced any further.

We recommend intraoperative histophathological control of the tumor margins using frozen section evaluation of the

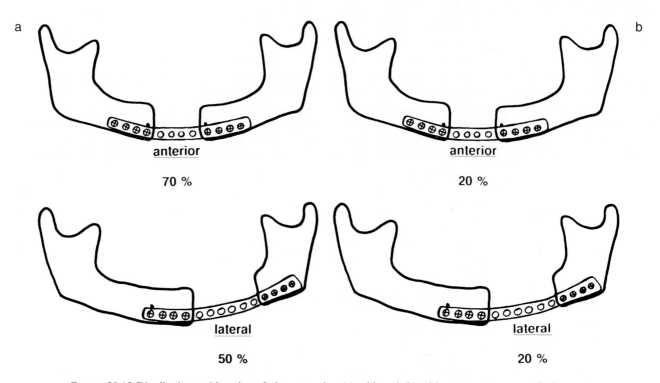

FIGRUE 38.13 Distribution and location of plate extrusion (a) with and (b) without percutaneous radiotherapy.

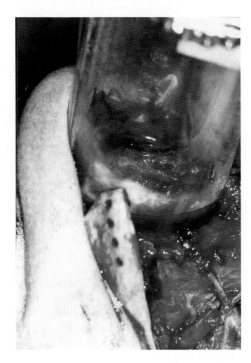

FIGURE 38.14 Irradiation cone is placed directly upon the tumor bed between both mandibular bone stumps.

borders to be able to achieve total tumor removal. Suspicious areas must be resected again during the same operative session.

IORT in conjunction with postoperative percutaneous radiotherapy seems to be an effective treatment of tumors of the head and neck. The disadvantage, however, is that it requires elaborate technical equipment, which will keep restrictions on the method for some time to come.

Second, concerning rehabilitation therapy with osseointegrated dental implants,[64–66] we started to reconstruct the osseous defect primarily. That means that especially in cases with anterior resections of the mandible, there is primary reconstruction using microvascular bone (e.g., fibula bone grafts). Primary bony reconstruction is also favored by many other authors.[25] By means of immediate bone repair, we are able to reduce soft tissue tension across the sharp-edged metal plate. The soft tissue heals to the periosteal and soft tissue surface of the graft. Even plate-wrapping, for example with lyodura, is not sufficient to prevent soft tissue perforation in a long-term follow up. Within a short-term interval, however, this technique may be helpful.

To summarize the data and findings of the three investigation compartments of this study the following remarks can be made.

The question of local enhancement of dosage following implantation of metallic "foreign bodies" can in correlation to other authors[24,26,27,29,30,32–37] be answered in so far that only in a very close distance from the implanted material a mea-

surable increase of dosage is recorded. This finding applies at least to the metallic bone plate material commonly used today. Increased dosage is found as backscattering in front of implanted metal plates (i.e., within the soft tissues), whereas behind the metal plate a slight reduction of dosage, also closely adjacent to the metal surface, is recorded.

The dose values behind the metal plates already reach the values corresponding to the resorption of the material thickness asymptotically at a distance between 0.45 mm and 0.85 mm. A protection of the target volume by means of the relatively thin metal plates is not to be expected. This is at least valid for irradiation using ^{60}Co and 8-MeV photons.

The differences of the radiation quality are of minor importance within this energy range. Since the observed backscatter phenomena already exhibit at a distance of approximately 2 mm from the implanted material a range of less than 5% of the applied dosage, they cannot be made responsible for the often observed extrusions of bridging plates alone.

The animal studies show that under the condition of stable fixation of the implanted material, osseointegration of the fixation screws even under perioperative and postoperative radiation using ^{60}Co gamma rays is possible. It seems plausible to assume that the implantation trauma acts as a stimulus for the osteoblasts and that this stimulus prevails over the irradiation effects upon bone regenerative capacity.

The intensity of the recuperation process is dependent upon the range of the applied dose[42] and the time of irradiation.[67] As our animal study shows, osseointegration can be achieved before the maximum radiation damage of the bone takes place. It remains unclear as to whether that will happen at the time of the lowest osteogenic activity. Usually bridging plate placement is performed immediately after bone resection so that this problem does not really occur.

In the case of a secondary defect bone grafting, we recommend waiting longer than 6 months. It seems more suitable to perform a secondary grafting procedure as early as 1.5 years after the termination of radiation therapy.

In correlating the results of the animal studies to the clinical conditions the difference in tissue response between animals and humans must, of course, be taken into consideration. Bone regeneration is certainly better in 1-year-old sheep than in tumor patients 40 years of age and older. The results of investigations using rabbits[39,67–69] should be interpreted very critically, since these animals have been shown to have a high osteogenic potency per se.

Sheep and dogs, in our opinion, are more suitable for animal models of bone regeneration, implantation of metal screws, and irradiation.

Summary

The application of perioperative or postoperative radiation therapy for malignancies while osteosynthesis material is in place is the subject of much controversy. The reason is that local dose increases in the region of the metallic plates may inadvertently cause damage to the surrounding tissue.

An irradiation phantom was used to measure dose increases concerning backscatter of different metals. We were able to demonstrate that a 12.5% to 16% increase in the radiation dose can be observed for titanium and steel at a distance of 0.45 mm in front of the metal specimen. A comparison between titanium and steel did not demonstrate a relevant advantage for titanium.

In an animal model, mandibular bridging osteosyntheses with autogenous bone grafts were carried out in sheep and the osteogenic activity at the bone/fixation screw interface was assessed qualitatively and quantitatively under perioperative and/or postoperative telecobalt irradiation. The same procedure was followed with human bone sections.

Both the experimental and the clinical results show a reduction in the osteogenic activity that appeared after a time interval depending on the mode and dose of radiation. This reduction appeared at latest after the 12th week concurrently with the radiation-induced vascular lesions. In humans the radiation-induced bone lesions reached the maximum value around 180 days after the end of radiotherapy. A further recovery of the bone cannot be expected until at least 2 years later.

From this it may be concluded that a bridging osteosynthesis should be performed either as a primary procedure (i.e., before the radiolesions of the bone reach the maximum) or as a secondary procedure (i.e., following revitalization of the bone tissue).

Soft tissue complications (i.e., extrusion of the reconstruction plates through the skin) frequently occur in the anterior region. In particular, a thin coverage becomes stiff under full-dose irradiation, and the tension between soft tissue and hard plate can no longer be compensated.

Intraoperative radiation therapy avoids skin damage, since it is directly applied to the tumor bed. Also, immediate microvascular bone repair has a positive influence. Both therapy modifications can help to reduce soft tissue complications.

Acknowledgments The authors would like to thank Prof. Dr. Michael Wannenmacher, former head of the Department of Radiotherapy, University of Freiburg, for his support of this study and Prof. Dr. Herrmann Frommhold, head of the Department of Radiotherapy, University of Freiburg, for his advice in all sorts of questions.

Thanks also to Dr. Norbert Hodapp, Department of Radiotherapy, University of Freiburg, for his extremely valuable help during the phantom measurements.

References

1. Austermann K-H, Becker R, Büning K, Machtens E. Titanium implants as a temporary replacement of mandible. *J Maxillofac Surg.* 1977;5:167–171.

2. Ewers R, Joos U. Temporäre Defektüberbrückungen bei Unterkieferresektionen mit Osteosynthese-Methoden. *Dtsch Zahnärztl Z.* 1977;32:332–333.

3. Reuther J, Hausamen JE. System zur alloplastischen Überbrückung von Unterkieferdefekten. *Dtsch Zahnärztl Z.* 1977;32(4):334–337.

4. Schmelzle R, Schwenzer N. Die Überbrückung von Unterkieferdefekten mit Metallimplantaten. *Dtsch Zahnärztl Z.* 1977;32(4):329–331.

5. Spiessl B. Die Unterkieferresektionsplatte der AO, ihre Anwendung bei Unterkieferdefekten in der Tumorchirurgie. *Unfallheilkunde.* 1978;81:302–305.

6. Raveh J, Stich H, Sutter F, Schawalder P. Neue Rekonstruktionsmöglichkeiten bei Unterkieferdefekten nach Tumorresektion. *Schweiz Monatsschr Zahnheilk.* 1981;91:899–920.

7. Raveh J, Stich H, Sutter F, Greiner R. Use of the titanium coated hollow screw and reconstruction plate system in bridging of lower jaw defects. *J Oral Maxillofac Surg.* 1984;42:281–294.

8. Stoll P, Bähr W, Wächter R. Bridging of mandibular defects using AO-reconstruction plates. 3-DBRP-versus THORP-system. *J Cancer Res Clin Oncol* Suppl. 1990;116:707.

9. Schmelzle R, Schwenzer N. Erfahrungen mit der Tübinger Resektionsplatte in der Tumorchirugie. In: Scheunemann H, Schmidseder R, eds. *Plastische Wiederherstellungschirurgie bei bösartigen Tumoren.* Berlin: Springer-Verlag; 1982.

10. International Commission on Radiation Units and Measurement. *Dose Specification for Reporting External Beam Therapy with Photons and Electrons.* ICRU Report 29.

11. Hine GJ. Scattering of secondary electrons produced by gamma-rays in materials of various atomic numbers. Letter to the editor. *Phys Res.* 1951;82:755.

12. Dutreix A, Bernard M. Études de la dose au voisinage de l'interface entre deux milieux de composition atomique différente exposées aux rayonnements Gamma du 60 Co. *Phys Med Biol.* 1962;7:69.

13. Dutreix J, Bernard N. Dosimetry at interfaces for high energy x and gamma rays. *Br J Radiol.* 1966;39:205–210.

14. Dutreix J, Dutreix A, Bernard M, Bethencourt A. Études de la dose au voisinage de l'interface entre deux milieux de composition atomique different exposées à des RX 11 à 20 MV. *Ann Radiol.* 1964;7:233.

15. Wambersie A, Dutreix J, Bernard M. Variation de la dose au voisinage de l'interface entre le plexiglas et un métal exposées à des RX de 20 MV. *Radiat Biol Ther.* 1965;6:237.

16. Spiers FW. A review of the theoretical and experimental methods of determining the radiation dose in bone. *Br J Radiol.* 1966;39:216–221.

17. Manegold K. Über den Einfluss den Elektronen-Streuung an Inhomogenitätskanten. *Strahlentherapie.* 1970;140:647–650.

18. Wall JA, Burke EA. Gamma dose distributions at and near the interface of different materials. *IEEE Trans Nucl Sci.* 1970;17:305.

19. Berger MJ. *Absorbed Dose near an Interface Between Two Media.* Report 10550. Washington, DC: National Bureau of Standards. 1971:38.

20. Kulkarni RN, Sundararaman V, Prasad MA. The dose across a plane bone-tissue interface. *Radiat Res.* 1972;51:1.

21. Gibbs FA, Palos B, Goffinet DR. The metal/tissue interface effect in irradiation of the oral cavity. *Radiology.* 1977;124:815–817.

22. Murthy MSS, Lakshmanan AR. Dose enhancement due to back-scattered electrons at the interface of two media. *Radiat Res.* 1976;67:215–223.

23. Gagnon WF, Cundiff J-H. Dose enhancement from backscattered radiation at tissue-metal interfaces irradiated with high energy electrons. *Br J Radiol.* 1980;53:466–470.

24. Stoll P, Wächter R, Hodapp N. Radiation and osteosynthesis. Dosimetry on an irradiation phantom. *J Craniomaxillofac Surg.* 1990;18:361–366.

25. Gullane PJ. Primary mandibular reconstruction: analysis of 64 cases and evaluation of interface radiation dosimetry on bridging plates. *Laryngoscope.* 1991;101:1–24.

26. Frössler H, Springer L, Wannenmacher M. Dosismessungen bei Kobalt-Teletherapie-Bestrahlung im Mundhöhlenbereich nach Titanium-Metallimplantation. *ZWR* 1975;84:258–260.

27. Maerker R, Würthner K, Timmermann J. Experimentelle Untersuchungen über die Dosisverteilung bei Co^{60}-Bestrahlung nach Draht- und Plattenosteosynthese. *Fortschr Kiefer-Gesichtschir.* 1976;21:208–210.

28. Thambi V, Murthy AK, Alder G, Kartha PK. Dose perturbation resulting from gold fillings in patients with head and neck cancers. *Int J Radiat Onkol Biol Phys.* 1979;5:581–582.

29. Farman AG, Sharma S, George DI, Wilson D, Dodd D, Figa R, et al. Backscattering from dental restorations and splint materials during therapeutic radiation. *Radiolology.* 1985;156:523–526.

30. Eichhorn N, Gerlach R, Salewski WD, Sommet G. Thermoluminiszenz Dosimetrische Untersuchung zum Absorptions-Verhalten von Knochen ohne und mit Metallimplantaten. *Strahlenther Onkologre.* 1986;262:799–884.

31. Gibbs FA, Palos B, Goffinet DR. The metal/tissue interface effect in irradiation of the oral cavity. *Radiol.* 1984;119:705–707.

32. Scrimger JW. Backscatter from high atomic number materials in high energy photon beams. *Radiology.* 1977;124:815–817.

33. Sailer U. Veränderung der Dosisverteilung ultraharter Röntgenstrahlung durch Ausstreuung aus Inhomogenitäten. *Strahlentherapie.* 1980;156:832–835.

34. Mian TA, Putten van MC Jr, Kramer DC, Jacob RF, Boyer AL. Backscatter radiation at bone titanium interface from high-energy X and gammä rays. *Int J Radiat Oncol Biol Phys.* 1987;13:1943.

35. Hudson FR, Crawley MD, Samaraskera M. Radiotherapy treatment planning for patients fitted with prosthesis. *Br J Radiol.* 1984;57:603–608.

36. Tatcher M, Kuten A, Helman J, Laufer D. Perturbation of cobalt^{60} radiation doses by metal objects implanted during oral and maxillofacial surgery. *J Oral Maxillofac Surg.* 1984;42:108–110.

37. Rosendahl EW, Kirschner H. Änderung der Tiefendosis durch eine Titan-Endoprothese bei der ^{60}CO-Strahlentherapie. *Strahlentherapie.* 1979;155:20–22.

38. Schweiger JW. Titanium implants in irradiated dog mandibles. *J Prosthet Dent.* 1989;60:201.

39. Montag H. Osseointegration of Brånemark Fixtures—an animal study. *XVIII Congress of the European Society for Artificial Organs.* Vienna. 1991.

40. Lange K-P, Laaß M, Retemeyer K. Eine tierexperimentelle Studie zum Einheilverhalten enossaler Implantate im bestrahlten Knochen. *Dtsch Zahnärztl Z.* 1993;48:512–514.

41. Brånemark PI. Einführung in die Osseointegration. In: Brånemark PI, Zarb GA, Albrektsson T, eds. *Gewebeintegrierter Zahnersatz. Osseointegration in Klinischer Zahnheilkunde.* Quintessenz; Berlin; 1985.

42. Jacobsson M, Jönsson A, Albrektsson T, Turesson I. Alterations in bone regenerative capacity after low level gamma irradiation. *Scand J Plast Reconstr Surg.* 1985;19:231–236.

43. Jacobsson M, Tjellström A, Thomsen P, Albrektsson T, Turesson I. Integration of titanium implants in irradiated bone. *Ann Otol Rhinol Laryngol* 1988;97:337–340.

44. Sindet-Pedersen S. The transmandibular implant for reconstruction following radiotherapy and hemimandibulectomy: report of a case. *J Oral Maxillofac Surg.* 1988;46:158–160.

45. Dehen N, Niederdellmann H. Zur postoperativen prothetischen Versorgung von Tumorpatienten. *Z Zahnärztl Implantol.* 1991;7:131–134.

46. Esser E, Dubrawski J. Enossale Implantate bei der Rehabilitation von Tumorpatienten. 32. Congrès Francais de Stomatologie et de Chirurgie Maxillo-Faciale, Strasbourg; 1991.

47. Nishimura RD, Lewis SG, Shimizu KT. Osseointegrated implants and patient's status post radiation therapy. *4th Internat. Congr. Preprosthetic Surg.* Palm Springs, CA; 1991.

48. Stoll P, Wächter R. Tumorbestrahlung und Überbrückungs osteosynthese? *Dtsch Z Mund-Kiefer-Gesichtschir.* 1993;17:224–229.

49. Taylor TD, Worthingthon P. Osseointegrated implant rehabilitation of the previously irradiated mandible: results of a limited trial at 3 to 7 years. *J Prosthet Dent.* 1993;69:60–69.

50. Wächter R, Stoll P. Möglichkeiten und Grenzen enossaler Implantate beider Øralen Rehabilitation von Tumorpatienten nach Bestrahlung. *Z Zahnärztle Implantol.* 1994;10:171–176.

51. Frössler H, Engberding R, Rauba HJ, Schütz J. Erfahrungen mit dem PTW Lithiumfluoridthermolumineszenzdosimeter. *Röntgenpraxis.* 1971;24:242–249.

52. Ellis S. Dose, time and fractionation. A clinical hypothesis. *Clin Radiol.* 1969;20:1.

53. Rahn BA. Die polychrome Sequenzmarkierung des Knochenumbaus. *Nova Acta Leopoldina.* 1976;44:249–255.

54. Donath K. Sägeschlifftechnik. *Fortschr Kiefer Gesichtschir.* 1983;28:97–100.

55. Wächter R, Stoll P. Komplikationen nach primärer Unterkieferrekonstruktion mit THORP-Platten. In: Neumann H-J, ed. *Ästhetische und plastisch-rekonstruktive Gesichtschirurgie.* Einhorn-Presse Verlag, Reinbek; 1993:259.

56. Stoll P, Wächter R, Hodapp N. Tumorestrahlung und Überbückungsosteosynthese. Dosismessungen an einem Bestrahlungsphantom. *Dtsch Z Mund-Kiefer-Gesichtschir.* 1989;13:165–171.

57. Ebbers J, Kürten-Rothes R, Ganzer U. Metallplatten-Osteosynthese und Nachbestrahlung. Eine tierexperimentelle Studie. *Laryngol Rhinol Otol.* 1985;64:32–36.

58. Ellis F, Winston BN, Fowler JS, De Ginder WL. Three or five fractions per week: treated on alternate treatment days. Letter of the editor. *Br J Radiol.* 1969;42:715–716.

59. Ellis F, Sorensen A, Lescrenier C. Radiation therapy schedules for opposing parallel fields and their biological aspects. *Radiology.* 1974:701–707.

60. Garrett P, Pugh H, Ross I, Hamarker R, Singer M. Intraoperative radiation therapy for advanced or recurrent head and neck malignancies In: Dobelbauer R, Abe B, eds. *Intraoperative Radiation Therapy.* Boca Raton, FL: CRC Press; 1989.

61. Freeman SB, Hamarker RC, Singer MI. Intraoperative radiotherapy of head and neck cancer. *Arch Otolaryngol Head Neck Surg.* 1990;116:165–168.

62. Schmitt T, Berbitt N, Puel S, Prodes JM, Martin C, Pinto M. The use of intraoperative radiotherapy in the treatment of T3-T4-carcinomas of the base of the tongue. In: Abe M, Takahashi N, eds. *Intraoperative Radiation Therapy.* New York: Pergamon; 1991.

63. Stoll P, Nilles A. Experience with intraoperative radiation therapy (IORT) in head and neck surgery. In: Schildberg FW, Willich N, Kremling H-J, eds. *Intraoperative Radiation Therapy, Proceedings/4th International Symposium IORT,* Munich; 1992. Essen: Die Blaue Eule; 1993.

64. Wächter R, Diz Dios P. Zur oralen Funktion von Tumorpatienten nach Operation und Versorgung mit Bonefit-Implantaten. Erste qualitative und quantitative Ergebnisse. *Z Zahnärztl Implantol.* 1993;9:134–138.

65. Wächter R, Stoll P. Möglichkeiten und Grenzen enossaler Implantate bei der oralen Rehabilitation von Tumorpatienten nach Bestrahlung. *Z Zahnärztl Implantol.* 1994;10:171–176.

66. Wächter R, Stoll P, Schilli W. Dental implants for the oral rehabilitation in patients with mandibular bone grafts. In: Kärcher H, ed. *Functional Surgery of the Head and Neck.* Graz: RM-Druck u. Verlagsgesellschaft; 1995.

67. Albrektsson T, Jacobsson T, Turesson I. Bone remodelling at implant sites after irradiation injury. Methodological approaches to study the effects of CO^{60} administered in a single dose of 15 Gy. *Swed Dent J.* 1985;Suppl 28:193–203.

68. Sumner DR, Turner TN, Pierson RH, Kienapfel H, Urban RN, Liebner EJ, et al. Effects of radiation from fixation of non-cemented porous-coated implants in a canine model. *J Bone Joint Surg.* 1990;72A:1527–1533.

69. Matsui Y, Ohno K, Michi K-I, Tachikawa T. Histomorphometric examination of healing around hydroxylapatite implants in ^{60}CO-irradiated bone. *J Oral Maxillofac Surg.* 1994;52:167–172.

39
Management of Posttraumatic Osteomyelitis of the Mandible

Robert M. Kellman and Darin L. Wright

As discussed in a previous chapter, there are several different etiologies for mandibular osteomyelitis. Treatment is to a large extent cause specific since the differing pathophysiologies involved require different approaches. Odontogenic osteomyelitis can often be treated medically with a prolonged course of antibiotics. When surgical debridement is necessary, the treatment will still be medical once debridement has been completed unless a pathologic fracture has occurred. On the other hand, if a fracture is present, treatment should be similar to that described here for posttraumatic osteomyelitis (PTOM).

Osteoradionecrosis (ORN) is a term applied to the specific form of osteomyelitis that develops after exposure of the bone to a treatment course of radiotherapy. This particular problem is addressed in a separate chapter.

The specific entity of PTOM refers to the bone infection that develops after a fracture, whether the fracture has been treated or not. As the name implies, PTOM suggests that an infection has developed in the bone at the site of a fracture. It is more than a soft tissue infection, which can generally be treated successfully by drainage combined with systemic antibiotics and stabilization of a nonfixed fracture. Loose hardware must always be removed from an infected wound, although stable appliances will usually withstand a localized wound infection.

PTOM may develop at the site of an unrepaired mandible fracture. Failure to repair a fracture may be due to poor patient compliance, missed diagnosis, or occasionally the presence of severe, life-threatening injuries. In this situation, it is important to differentiate between a localized infection that will respond to drainage, fixation, and antibiotics and a true PTOM, which will require debridement of osteitic bone.

PTOM may also be seen after inadequately or improperly treated fractures. An improperly applied fixation appliance may become a source of infection at the site of an unstable fracture. Swift removal of the appliance and proper stabilization of the fracture fragments may avert progression of infection in the bone.

Finally, teeth in fracture lines have been implicated by many in the later development of PTOM. This remains quite controversial, and in general, it appears that proper fixation of bony fragments overcomes any tendency toward infection provided by teeth in fracture lines.[1-3] The one exception with which most authors will agree is that a preexisting pulp infection in a tooth at the fracture site is highly likely to result in infection and is, therefore, an indication for extraction at the time of fracture repair.[4]

The management of PTOM has evolved slowly over the past three decades. In addition to intravenous antibiotics, surgery often included debridement and packing of wounds open, allowing healing to take place by secondary intention.[5] The advent of transcutaneous suction-irrigation systems has allowed for successful healing using primary closure. The need to stabilize fractures, nonunions, and debridement-created defects has been recognized, and external fixation has been the mainstay for this.[8]

Giordano et al. reported on eight cases of PTOM of which four were treated with decortication and packing and four with debridement and primary closure over a transcutaneous suction-irrigation system.[5] The latter resulted in less patient discomfort and shorter hospital stays. When needed, stabilization was accomplished using external fixators.

In 1985, Adekeye and Cornah reported on 106 cases of mandibular osteomyelitis. Their recommendations for treatment included debridement, drainage, antibiotic therapy, and fixation of mobile fragments.[6] Calhoun et al. advocated the use of judicious debridement, intravenous antibiotics, suction irrigation, and external fixation with the addition of hyperbaric oxygen (HBO) in their study of 60 patients.[7]

The underlying theme in many authors' recommendations for treatment of PTOM is that of staged procedures in which the infection is cleared using debridement, suction-irrigation drains to directly apply an antibiotic irrigant, intravenous antibiotics, and fixation of mobile fragments using intermaxillary fixation, external fixators, or both.[8,9] Reconstruction of mandibular defects is delayed until all signs of infection have been eliminated. Adekeye recommended in 1978 waiting at least 1 month prior to attempting bone grafting for reconstruction.[10] Similarly, in 1991 Mercuri advocated a wait of 2 to 3 months prior to reconstructive attempts.[11]

Not all authors, however, recommend delayed bone grafting. The use of primary bone grafting after debridement of mandibular osteomyelitis was advocated by Obwegeser in 1966.[12] However, while some authors have reported on the occasional use of a primary bone graft, success has been variable, and many authors still decry this procedure. Glahn reported on four cases of mandibular osteomyelitis treated using primary bone grafting at the time of debridement.[13] He recommended the use of a millipore filter to protect the graft from the surrounding soft tissue inflammation. The only case of the four that failed was one in which this filter was not used. Beckers et al. treated 19 patients with PTOM, and 4 of these patients had bone grafts placed primarily.[14] While 2 of the 4 patients developed postoperative infection, both patients went on to osseous union. Obwegeser and Sailer reported on 17 cases of primary reconstruction using rib or iliac bone and stabilization using intermaxillary fixation. Their treatment was successful in 15 patients, with 2 patients requiring removal of necrotic bone.[15]

Equally controversial is the use of rigid internal fixation (RIF) in the treatment of PTOM. In the late 1960s and early 1970s, the use of rigid internal fixation after bony debridement was introduced for the stabilization of PTOM in orthopedic fractures. While advocated occasionally for PTOM of the mandible, resistance has remained strong. In 1984 Rowe stated that many cases of nonunion in infected fractures could be traced to the use of internal fixation.[16] Marx echoed Rowe's recommendations as recently as 1991 stating that ". . . placement of either an internal reconstruction plate or an immediate bone graft is associated with a high incidence of reinfection and is not recommended."[8]

In reviewing reports in the literature, variability in treatments and patient populations make comparative evaluation difficult. The definition of osteomyelitis and particularly acute and chronic osteomyelitis is variable, and criteria for inclusion are quite inconsistent. Most reviews include different types of osteomyelitis including odontogenic, posttraumatic, and osteoradionecrosis as well as less common types in the same series.

In an effort to focus on the particular problem of fixation and PTOM, we have studied the use of rigid internal fixation with or without primary bone grafting in 14 patients. A preliminary report of these patients was presented at the American Academy of Facial Plastic and Reconstructive Surgery meeting in June 1993.[17] This reviews the authors' experience with 14 cases of mandibular osteomyelitis, all of which were associated with persistent nonunions, defects, or both, with a particular focus on the use of RIF and bone grafting. While all cases would fit into the category of chronic osteomyelitis based on the criteria in most reports, the distinction between acute and chronic osteomyelitis is somewhat cloudy and less important than the fact that all patients had failed to resolve on antibiotic therapy of greater than 1 month's duration and osteitic bone was found at surgery in all cases.

Patients

Fourteen patients with PTOM of the mandible were treated surgically using debridement and RIF with an AO mandibular reconstruction plate between 1983 and 1992. The presumed causes of osteomyelitis included unrecognized or untreated fractures in four patients and identifiable treatment errors in seven patients. The remaining 3 patients were treatment failures after RIF of fractures in which the treatment appeared to have been correct and the cause of failure, therefore, could not be identified. Original treatment sites included six body fractures, five angle fractures, and three parasymphyseal fractures.

All patients had evidence of infection involving cortical bone and marrow, with bone loss identified radiologically and/or at surgery in all cases (Figure 39.1). All failed to re-

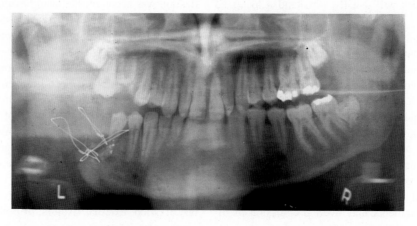

FIGURE 39.1 Panorex of one of the patients included in this series revealing osteomyelitis of an inadequately treated left angle fracture. The fracture is not well reduced, and the surrounding bone is osteopenic.

spond to antibiotic therapy (culture specific or empiric) for 1 month or more. Eleven patients had been treated prior to referral, 7 with courses of antibiotics only and 4 with antibiotics and one or more surgeries in efforts to clear the PTOM.

Prior to surgery, all patients received intravenous antibiotic treatment for 10 to 14 days. Surgery included radical debridement of osteitic bone in all cases without regard for the size of the defect that would result. Defects ranged from 0 to 7 cm after debridement.

Seven patients underwent immediate RIF for stabilization using the AO mandibular reconstruction plate (stainless steel or titanium) at the time of debridement. Five of these patients had bone defects after debridement. Three underwent primary bone grafting at the time of debridement and plate placement and two underwent secondary bone grafting. All grafts consisted of cancellous iliac bone (no cortical component), which was pressed into the defect between the bone ends in the space under the plate. Generous amounts of cancellous bone were used.

Seven patients underwent aggressive surgical debridement without plate placement. In two patients, external fixation was used for stabilization, and in five patients no fixation was used. Secondary plate placement was carried out within 7 to 25 days. At the time of plate placement, five patients had defects grafted using cancellous iliac bone pressed into the space under and around the plate.

Three patients underwent elective plate removal, two of whom had undergone primary placement. At the time of removal, bones showed complete healing and replacement of the grafts with normal-appearing bone. The mandibles were completely stable and tolerated normal masticatory function after plate removal. No plates were removed for any nonelective reasons.

Results

All patients in this series went on to complete bony union without further evidence of infection over a follow-up period of 6 months to 7 years. One patient presented 2 months after secondary repair complaining of pain over the graft site. No clinical evidence of infection was found. Nonetheless, the patient was treated with 4 weeks of intravenous clindamycin using home therapy. No further complaints of pain were made, and clinically normal healing was present at last follow-up. As noted earlier, complete bony union was found in the three patients who underwent plate removal.

Time hospitalized was noted to range from 7 to 43 days (cumulatively, excluding treatment by prior physicians). There was no significant difference between those who had plates placed primarily (range of 7 to 42 days, mean and median of 23 days) and those who had plates placed secondarily (range of 9 to 43 days, mean of 27 days, median of 28 days).

Status of dentition, the presence of teeth in the fractures, and how these were handled were randomly distributed. Cigarette smoking is frequently noted in series to be associated with mandibular osteomyelitis, and this proved true in this series as well (9 of 12 in which it was recorded smoked more than one pack of cigarettes per day); however, this association may well reflect other factors such as socioeconomic status, nutrition, hygiene, etc., and certainly, no causal relationship can be concluded.

Bacteria were cultured from debrided bone material in all but one patient. There was no predominant organism, but anaerobes were most common. Biopsies were consistent with osteomyelitis in eight patients and less definitive in three. In the remaining three, the bone was sent for culture, and no histologic evaluation was performed.

Discussion/Recommendations

While this series certainly does not prove conclusively that RIF with primary placement of a bone graft is the best approach for treatment of PTOM, the success rate of 100% in this series suggests that multistaged approaches may be unnecessary. The authors' current experience includes 17 patients with no cases of nonunion, infection, or bone graft failure. It is the authors' belief that a primary reason for the high success rate is the aggressive use of surgical debridement and the liberal use of preoperative and postoperative intravenous antibiotics, along with the use of a long plate with numerous fixation points (at least three or four per side) placed at a distance from the infected site. As this technique is evaluated further by more surgeons, failures are, of course, inevitable. It is hoped that failures will be critically assessed to determine if they represent failures of RIF or failures of the particular method of application, particularly if the specific technical points noted here are not part of the technique employed.

The early experience involved initial debridement and subsequent plate placement at a secondary procedure. When necessary, bone grafts were placed at this second procedure (thereby avoiding the need for a third procedure in these patients). Complete success in these cases encouraged the author (RMK) to proceed to primary plate placement at the time of debridement, again placing bone grafts when necessary. Successful use of this approach decreases the number of surgeries from three or four to one, even in the presence of a significant bone defect. Cumbersome suction-irrigation systems and external fixators are avoided as well.

As a result of this experience, our current recommendations for the treatment of PTOM include the following important steps:

1. Local incision and drainage (outpatient) if an abscess is present
2. Intravenous antibiotics (can be given as an outpatient) for 1 to 2 weeks or until external signs of local infection (erythema, swelling, drainage) have resolved or diminished

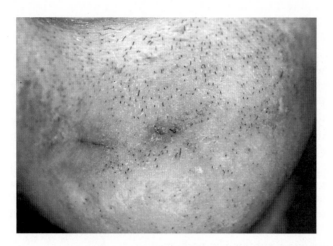

FIGURE 39.2 A patient with osteomyelitis showing resolution of external signs of infection after preoperative antibiotic treatment. Surgical treatment should be delayed until such infection has resolved or has markedly decreased.

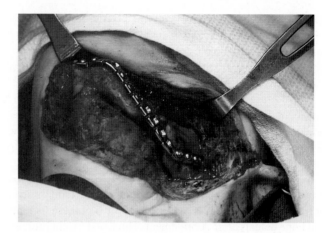

FIGURE 39.4 Positioning of bone fragments and placement of a mandibular reconstruction plate after completion of debridement.

markedly (Figure 39.2). Antibiotics should be culture-specific when cultures can be obtained; otherwise, clindamycin has been the drug of choice

3. Surgery to include:

   a. Aggressive debridement, removing all osteitic and questionable bone, leaving only solid, healthy bone (Figure 39.3). Bone is sent for culture and pathologic examination. Any hardware is removed and cultured.

   b. Placement of a long, strong plate for RIF, taking care to properly reposition the bone fragments prior to fixation. At least three but preferably four screws should be placed into each bone fragment. Note that it is critical to place the screws far enough away from the affected area so that they are not in proximity to the debrided edges or any vaguely questionable bone. This frequently entails wide exposure with the use of a 12- to 14-hole plate (Figure 39.4).

c. Filling the space under the plate between the bone segments with autologous, freshly harvested, cancellous bone packed tightly into the space (Figures 39.5–39.7). Broad-spectrum intravenous antibiotics should be given 1 to 1.5 hours prior to graft harvesting so that the graft bone will be impregnated with antibiotics.

d. Meticulous closure of the soft tissue pocket around the plate and graft, followed by placement of a suction drain and skin closure. The drain is removed after 24 to 48 hours, depending on the amount of drainage.

e. Intravenous antibiotics should be continued for 1 to 4 weeks depending upon the clinical impression at surgery.

f. Later plate removal can be performed after 6 to 12 months (Figure 39.8). The need for removal to prevent stress protection is unclear, but it should be kept in mind. If removal is carried out, it can be done as an outpatient procedure.

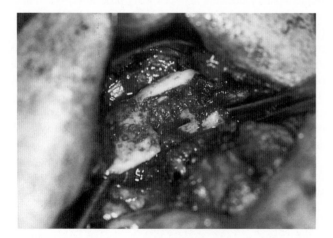

FIGURE 39.3 Exposure of a fracture showing sequestration and involucrum. Debridement must be aggressive to remove all infected bone. Debridement should continue until bleeding bone is seen.

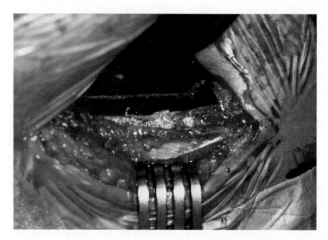

FIGURE 39.5 The iliac crest is uncapped for harvesting of cancellous bone. (The cortical cap is replaced after harvesting of the graft.)

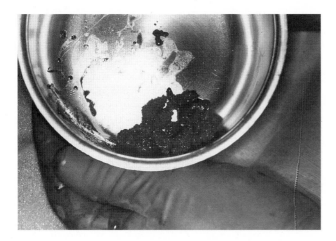

FIGURE 39.6 Harvested cancellous bone.

One of the major advantages using this single-stage approach is the reduction in the number of operative procedures necessary to adequately treat PTOM. With the routine availability of outpatient intravenous therapy, the number of days of hospitalization can be reduced, and consequently an overall reduction in the cost of treating patients with PTOM will result. Furthermore, the high success rate should encourage this approach as well.

Finally, the avoidance of cumbersome appliances such as external fixators and suction-irrigation systems should improve patient satisfaction and compliance. External fixators may be a source of secondary infection, and avoiding their use may help minimize complications.

Conclusion

The use of RIF with and without primary bone grafting for the management of PTOM is advocated. This is combined with perioperative intravenous antibiotic therapy. In the au-

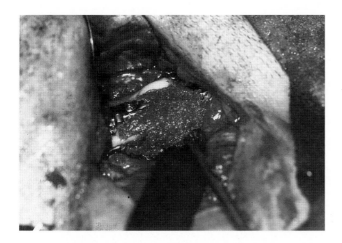

FIGURE 39.7 Another patient showing how cancellous bone is packed tightly into the bone defect under and around the plate.

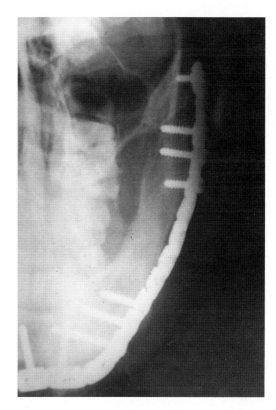

FIGURE 39.8 Postoperative radiograph demonstrating healing of the graft and complete bony union (same patient as in Figure 39.1 and 39.4).

thors' series, primary plate placement at the time of surgical debridement was equal in success rate to secondary plate placement after successful primary debridement. Osteomyelitis resolved in 17 cases, without recurrence or failure of hardware. Aggressive surgical debridement and the use of long, solid fixation plates is believed to contribute to the high success rate.

References

1. Thaller SR, Mabourakh S. Teeth located in the line of mandibular fracture. *J Craniofac Surg.* 1994;5(1):16–19.
2. Kamboozia AH, Punnia-Moorthy A. The fate of teeth in mandibular fracture lines. A clinical and radiographic follow-up study. *Int J Oral Maxillofac Surg.* 1993;22(2):97–101.
3. Berg S, Pape HD. Teeth in the fracture line. *Int J Oral Maxillofac Surg.* 1992;21(3):145–146.
4. Dierks EJ. Management of associated dental injuries in maxillofacial trauma. *Otolaryngol Clin N Am.* 1991;24(1):165–179.
5. Giordano AM, Foster CA, Boies LR, Maisel RH. Chronic osteomyelitis following mandibular fractures and its treatment. *Arch Otol.* 1982;108:30–33.
6. Adekeye EO, Cornah J. Osteomyelitis of the jaws: a review of 141 cases. *Br J Oral Maxillofac Surg.* 1985;23:24–35.
7. Calhoun KH, Shapiro RD, Stiernberg CM, Calhoun JH, Mader JT. Osteomyelitis of the mandible. *Arch Otol Head Neck Surg.* 1988;114:1157–1162.

8. Marx RE. Chronic osteomyelitis of the jaws. *Oral Maxillofac Surg Clin N Am.* 1991;3(2):367–381.

9. Koorbusch GF, Fotos P, Goll KT. Retrospective assessment of osteomyelitis: etiology, demographics, risk factors and management in 35 cases. *Oral Surg Med Pathol.* 1992;74:149–154.

10. Adekeye EO. Reconstruction of mandibular defects by autogenous bone grafts: a review of 37 cases. *J Oral Surg.* 1978;36:125–128.

11. Mercuri LG. Acute osteomyelitis of the jaws. *Oral Maxillofac Surg Clin N Am.* 1991;3(2):355–365.

12. Obwegeser HL. Simultaneous resection and reconstruction of parts of the mandible via the intraoral route. *Oral Surg.* 1966;21:693.

13. Glahn M. The surgical treatment of chronic osteomyelitis of the mandible. *J Maxillofac Surg.* 1974;2:238–241.

14. Beckers HL. Treatment of initially infected mandibular fractures with bone plates. *J Oral Surg.* 1979;37:310–313.

15. Obwegeser HL, Sailer HF. Experiences with intra-oral partial resection and simultaneous reconstruction in cases of mandibular osteomyelitis. *J Maxillofac Surg.* 1978;6:34–40.

16. Rowe N. Nonunion of the mandible. In: Mathog RH, ed. *Maxillofacial Trauma.* Baltimore: Williams & Wilkins; 1984:177–185.

17. Kellman, RM. One stage versus two stage management of post-traumatic mandibular osteomyelitis using the AO mandibular reconstruction plate. Presented at the International meeting of the American Academy of Facial Plastic and Reconstructive Surgery, San Francisco, CA; June, 1993.

40
Bilateral Maxillary Defects: THORP Plate Reconstruction with Removable Prosthesis
Technique/Atlas Case Reports

Christian Lindqvist, Lars Sjövall, Anna-Lisa Söderholm, and Dorrit Hallikainen

Bilateral total maxillectomy is an uncommon surgical procedure. The indication is usually a large malignant tumor extending over the maxillary midline. Few reports can be found in the literature concerning surgical reconstructive procedures.[1,2] Postsurgical prosthetic treatment is another subject that has seldom been discussed. The goal of maxillary reconstruction should always be for a prosthetic solution that makes it possible for the patient to eat, chew, swallow, and speak as normally as possible. It is also important that the aesthetic result should be satisfactory, and the appliance easy to use and clean (especially for disabled and elderly patients).

Following maxillectomy, the palate is often closed with a pedicled or free flap, when the defect is considered to be too large to be obturated only with a prosthetic device. Masticatory rehabilitation after palatal resection may be difficult when a myocutaneous flap has been used for reconstruction. In such cases, the prosthodontist often does not have an underlying stable hard tissue bed for stabilization and retention of the prosthesis. Because of the bulky, often excessive, soft tissue, the use of osseointegrated implants is also difficult. Custom-made abutment extension frameworks are needed, which in turn may transmit undesirable bending forces to the implants.

The lack of retention of the prosthetic replacement is generally agreed to be a major problem. This is particularly true of the postsurgical healing phase, when sufficient adaptation of the intermediate prosthesis is hard to achieve.

The titanium hollow-screw reconstruction plate (THORP) system, originally designed for mandibular reconstruction,[3,4] might in certain cases be considered for use in midfacial reconstruction. Because of the rigid locking of the screw head and the plate, the neutrally loaded device acts as both an internal and external fixator without causing unphysiologic pressure on the bone underneath.

Case 1

A 76-year-old woman had a large squamous cell carcinoma (SCC) of the edentulous maxilla (Figure 40.1). Bilateral total maxillectomy, including both hard and soft tissues, was performed at primary surgery. The dorsal part of the soft palate was left intact. An AO-THORP reconstruction plate was anchored to both zygomatic bones by two hollow screws on each side. A split-thickness skin graft was used to cover the resected soft tissue area. The middle of the reconstruction plate was left exposed (Figure 40.2). The patient's complete upper denture was then used as an interim prosthesis dressing plate, and was temporarily stabilized by bilateral circumzygomatic wiring.

Prosthetic treatment was initiated 5 months later. Using the existing complete upper denture as a tray, an impression of the resected area was obtained. The fairly nonresilient, thin skin graft overlying the hard tissues allowed the use of a putty silicone (Coltoflax, Coltene, Switzerland) instead of a standard impression material. Thus it was possible to place a section of an actual THORP plate accurately in the impression and to have a dental cast made to reproduce the clinical situation (Figure 40.3). The plane of occlusion and the vertical dimension were registered by keeping the denture in the desired position while the impression material was setting. The existing complete lower denture was relined. Two 20-mm hollow screws, similar to those attaching the THORP plate to the zygomas, were then fixed to the exposed part of the plate. Chromium-cobalt sockets were attached to the hollow screws with self-curing composite resin (Figure 40.4). The prosthesis consists of two parts: an obturator and a conventional complete upper denture. The obturator is attached to the sockets by individually cast, chromium-cobalt clips. The denture part again is fixed to the obturator by a dorsal undercut and a screw in the front (Figure 40.5). A two-part construction was chosen to facilitate handling of the prosthesis during daily insertion and removal for cleaning. Later on, the two parts were fused, owing to the patient's improved skill in handling the prosthesis. The clips were adjusted to provide maximal retention while enabling the patient herself to remove the prosthesis (without assistance). The patient is now able to speak clearly and leads a normal social life. She did not lose any weight during the first postoperative year (Figure 40.6).

Five years postoperatively, the plate is completely stable.

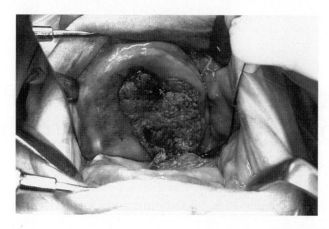

FIGURE 40.1 Case 1. Preoperative view showing extensive squamous cell carcinoma of the patient's upper jaw.

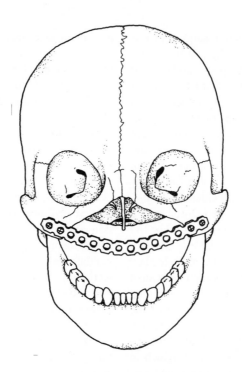

FIGURE 40.2 Drawing of a skull with the AO-THORP plate anchored to zygomas.

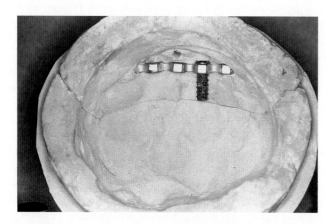

FIGURE 40.3 Stone cast showing the resected undercut free maxillary area with exposed part of plate clearly visible.

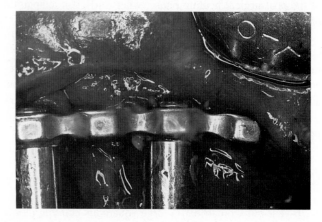

FIGURE 40.4 Chromium-cobalt sockets connected by hollow screws and composite resin to exposed part of palate.

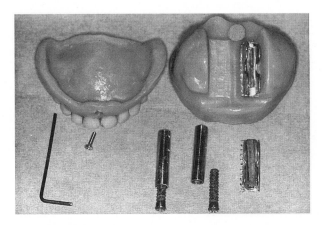

FIGURE 40.5 Prosthetic components. Clips were fixed to the obturator in the mouth by cold-curing acrylic resin.

Radiologically, no osteolysis can be found around the hollow screws (Figure 40.7). It is likely that osseointegration of the fixation screws has occurred.

Case 2

Bilateral subtotal maxillectomy and right orbital exenteration with excision of the right cheek area had been undertaken 12 months earlier in a 74-year-old woman because of an extensive SCC. The palate and skin were reconstructed with a latis-

simus dorsi flap. Postoperatively, 70-Gy radiation therapy was given. No prosthetic rehabilitation was possible, and the patient had significant problems with chewing and swallowing. The aesthetic situation was not satisfactory (Figure 40.8a). The patient was sent to us, and reconstruction was performed with a THORP plate in the same manner as in case 1. Because of a very small area for fixation of the horizontal bar to the right zygoma, a vertical one was attached to the lateral side of the orbit and was connected to the horizontal bar (Figure 40.8b). Three Brånemark implants were also placed in the supraorbital rim. The latissimus dorsi flap was partially re-

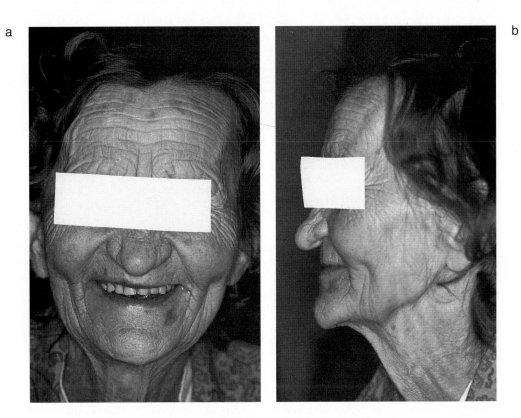

a

b

FIGURE 40.6 (a,b) Patient's appearance 18 months and 36 months after tumor surgery.

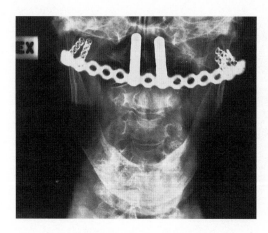

FIGURE 40.7 Radiograph showing plate in place.

moved to create space for the prosthesis. Skin and soft tissues were reconstructed with a pectoralis major musculocutaneous flap. The prosthetic part of the treatment was accomplished by attaching a fixation device to the THORP plate for the one-part acrylic prosthesis. Eight months later, an orbital epithesis was fabricated after attaching the abutments to the three Brånemark fixtures (Figure 40.8c–f). Healing was uneventful, but 27 months postoperatively the vertical THORP bar became exposed through the skin (Figure 40.8g), and this part was removed. The horizontal part of the THORP plate had also become exposed and was covered with a temporal flap (Figure 40.8h). Forty-two months after the primary plate reconstruction, the patient still has the ability to chew and swallow well. Her speech is intelligible and the aesthetic situation is satisfactory (Figure 40.8i).

An excellent description of different methods for retention of maxillary obturators has been presented by Milton et al.[5] They have used, among others, springs attached to the patient's upper and lower dentures, and magnets. Retention can also be achieved by using undercuts created by the scar band. However, this often leads to sore spots and, in some cases,

a
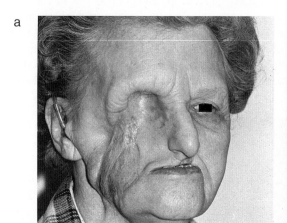

b
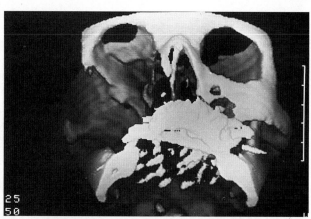

c
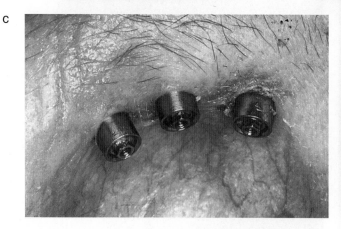

d
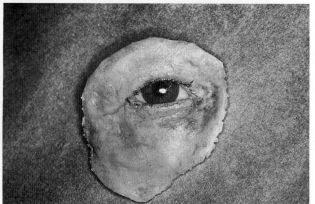

FIGURE 40.8 (a) Case 2. Preoperative photograph before reconstruction. (b) Preoperative three-dimensional CT scan showing the extensive defect. Only the zygomatic process of the temporal bone is left of the whole zygomatic complex. (c) Three abutments in the supraorbital margin. (d) The epithesis. (e) Epithesis in place. (f) Radiograph showing reconstruction. (g) Exposure of the orbital bar. (h) Horizontal part exposed. (i) Final result.

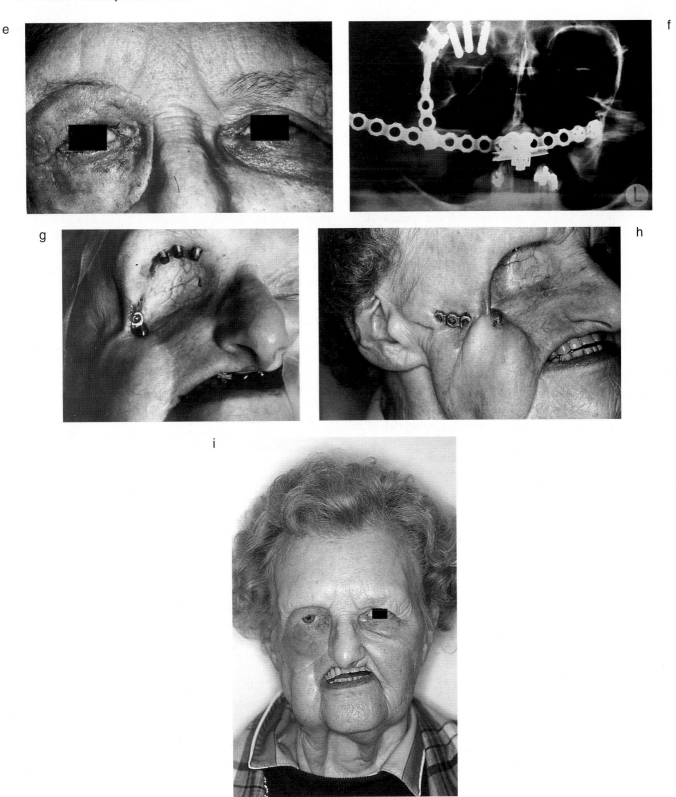

FIGURE 40.8 *Continued.*

pressure ulcers refractory to treatment. One also needs to keep in mind that the thin split-thickness skin graft often used to cover the resection wound is highly sensitive to abrasion and mechanical loading. Coffey[6] presents a technique for obturation of maxillary defects with inflatable balloons. However, there are technical problems, such as puncture of the balloon or leakage through the needle valve system.

The best functional and aesthetic result can probably be achieved with a prosthesis minimally supported by soft tissues and maximally supported by a framework attached to the facial bones by osseointegrated titanium screws. Parel et al.[7] present a case in which a nasal epithesis and a maxillary prosthesis were both attached to an implant-borne framework.

The use of a reconstruction system fixed to the facial bones in the presence of radiation therapy may be considered controversial. Presurgical or postsurgical irradiation of the tumor and adjacent hard and soft tissues is usually part of the treatment of the malignancy. The osteogenetic potential of irradiated bone is markedly lower, perhaps even permanently.[8,9] Still, there are reports of successful treatment with osseointegrated implants in irradiated bone.[9] The success rate, however, is lower than in long-term studies concerning nonirradiated bone. On the other hand, Jacobsson[9] has reported connective tissue growth around the sites of lost fixtures in radiated subjects, without signs of infection or osteoradionecrosis. Thus, there seems to be only a minor risk of severe complications when a titanium implant (or screw) is lost because of nonosseointegration. Accordingly, implantation should be considered in limited cases when the possibilities for rehabilitation are almost impossible from a prosthodontic point of view.

It is generally agreed that exposure of a mandibular reconstruction plate is a complication that often leads to infection of adjacent tissues, necrosis of the underlying bone, and loss of the plate. Although it might have been assumed that this would be the final result in these patients' cases, other factors should be taken into account. When a mandibular reconstruction plate is exposed, the underlying bone is also usually exposed as well. Our two patients have a sufficient soft tissue collar surrounding the entrance of the plate into the tissues, simulating nonattached gingiva around a conventional endosseous titanium implant. Therefore, so long as the ex-

posed part of the plate is kept clean (i.e., free of bacterial plaque), the risk of bone infection is minimized. The survival rate of endosseous titanium implants in edentulous jaws has been shown to be high as long as certain criteria are fulfilled. After osseointegration has occurred, the peri-implant soft tissue has to be kept free of inflammation through strict hygiene, and the biomechanical loading of the implant and associated superstructure must not be excessive. These guidelines can also be applied to a reconstruction of these types of maxillary defects as described earlier. This means that the prosthetic reconstruction should be designed in such a manner that adequate oral hygiene can be maintained. Additionally, unfavorable loading conditions should be avoided by placing the THORP plate in an optimal position from the prosthodontic standpoint. This requires proper presurgical, perisurgical, and postsurgical consultation between the surgeon and prosthodontist.

References

1. Konno A, Togawa K, Iizuka K. Primary reconstruction after total extended maxillectomy for maxillary cancer. *Plast Reconstr Surg.* 1981;67:440–447.
2. Phillips JG, Peckitt NS. Reconstruction of the palate using bilateral temporalis muscle flaps: a case report. *Br J Oral Maxillofac Surg.* 1988;26:322–325.
3. Hellem S, Olofsson J. Titanium-coated hollow screw and reconstruction plate system (THORP) in mandibular reconstruction. *J Craniomaxillofac Surg.* 1988;17:173–176.
4. Raveh J. Lower jaw reconstruction with the THORP system for bridging of lower jaw defects. *Head Neck Cancer.* 1990;2:344–349.
5. Milton CM, Yazdanie N, Bickerton RC. Prosthetic management following bilateral total or subtotal maxillectomy. *J Laryngol Otol.* 1986;100:1145–1154.
6. Coffey KW. Obturation of congenital or acquired intraoral anatomic defects. *J Prosthet Dent.* 1984;52:559–563.
7. Parel SM, Holt RG, Brånemark P-I, et al. Osseointegration and facial prosthetics. *Int J Oral Maxillofac Implants.* 1986;1:12–17.
8. Jacobsson M. On bone behaviour after irradiation. Thesis. University of Gothenburg, Sweden; 1985.
9. Jacobsson M, Tjellström A, Albrektsson T, et al. Integration of titanium implants in irradiated bone. *Ann Otol Rhinol Laryngol.* 1988;97:337–342.

41
AO/ASIF Craniofacial Fixation System Hardware

Alex M. Greenberg and Joachim Prein

Miniplate Fixation Systems

North America: Craniofacial Modular Fixation System (Synthes Maxillofacial)
Europe, Asia, South America, Africa: COMPACT MF (TM) (STRATEC and Mathys)

This system of instrumentation and titanium implants has been developed to address the individual needs of surgeons representing the many head and neck disciplines who perform craniomaxillofacial surgery. This set of implants is divided into different trays based on screw sizes. Each module contains the screws of a specific dimension with corresponding bone plates, mainly for cranial and midfacial locations, with certain mandibular applications. Although the instruments, implants, and screws have the same specifications, there are differences in the way that the modules are configured for North America and other parts of the world. North American instruments are distributed by Synthes Maxillofacial, Paoli, PA, while the rest of the world is supplied by STRATEC Medical, Oberdorf, Switzerland and Mathys LTD Bettlach, Bettlach, Switzerland. All products are AO/ASIF official devices accepted by the special TK (Technical Commission). The Craniofacial Modular Fixation System and COMPACT MF™) instrument modules are organized as separate color-coded trays containing screws of a particular size (1.0 mm, 1.3 mm, 1.5 mm, and 2.0 mm), with corresponding implants and varied stop drill bits (Figures 41.1–41.11). The Craniofacial Modular Fixation System (North American) consists of a graphic case (Figure 41.12), which contains the different tray modules up to a maximum of 4 in. (below) with the Universal Instrument Tray (above). The Craniofacial Modular System consists of 1.0-mm, 1.3-mm, 1.5-mm, 2.0-mm, 1.3-mm/1.5-mm/2.0-mm orthognathic and mesh modules. The COMPACT MF™ System consists of 1.0-mm, 1.3-mm, 1.5-mm, and 2.0-mm modules and has a sterilization tray with the modules stored side by side (Figure 41.13), but they can then be stacked atop the Universal Instrument Tray (Figure 41.14). The 1.3-mm/1.5-mm/2.0-mm orthognathic and mesh modules are only available for the Craniofacial Modular System in North America. Mesh implants are available for the COMPACT MF™ system and can be stored in the auxilliary bin of the modules. The SYNTHES Maxillofacial Craniofacial Modular System and COMPACT MF™ plates, screws, and instruments are exactly the same. The only differences are the ways in which they are arranged in modules or as sets. The 1.3-mm, 1.5-mm, 2.0-mm system drill bits have preset stops at 4 mm, 6 mm, 8 mm, and 12 mm. The micro 1.0-mm system drill bits have preset stops at 3 mm, 5 mm, and 8 mm to prevent the unwanted penetration of associated vital structures. The drill bits are also available as Stryker J-latch, Universal/Hall, Jacob's Chuck and Mini/quick coupling ends. The trays also contain the next size of screws for emergency purposes. A separate Universal Instrument Tray contains the Universal Instruments, which in the Craniofacial Modular System is in the top shelf of the graphic case. The drill bits are held within the lift-out lid that sits inside the auxilliary bin of the Universal Instrument Tray. The auxilliary bin may contain additional instruments. The Universal Instruments consists of the wide-handled screwdriver handle (1 each); narrow-handled screwdriver handle (1 each); plate bending pliers (2 each) (Figure 41.15); right-angle bender (Figure 41.16); plate holding forceps (Figure 41.17); plate cutter; and 1.0/1.3-mm plate holding Castro-Viejo locking forceps (1 each) and 1.5/2.0-mm plate holding Castro-Viejo locking forceps (1 each) (Figure 41.18); and the 3-in-1 plate bender/cutter (Figure 41.19), ratcheting screwdriver (Figure 22.27), and battery powered screwdriver (Figure 22.28).

1.0-mm Module

Color: Green
Indications: Cranium, nasal–orbital–ethmoid.

The 1.0-mm module is a microsystem containing 1.0-mm self-tapping screws in 2-, 3-, 4-, 5-, 6-, and 8-mm lengths (additional lengths available up to 14 mm) and 1.2-mm emergency screws in 2-, 3-, 4-, 5-, 6-, 7-, and 8-mm lengths

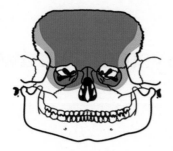
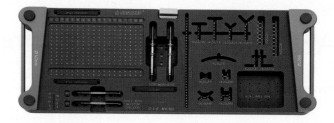

FIGURE 41.1 Craniofacial Modular Fixation System (1.0-mm Module). (Courtesy of Synthes Maxillofacial, Paoli, PA)

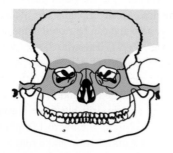
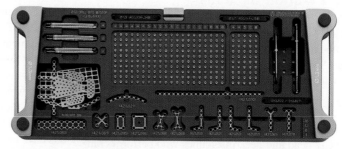

FIGURE 41.2 Craniofacial Modular Fixation System (1.3-mm Module). (Courtesy of Synthes Maxillofacial, Paoli, PA)

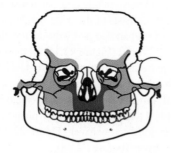
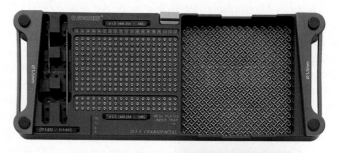
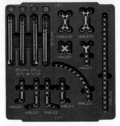

FIGURE 41.3 Craniofacial Modular Fixation System (1.5-mm Module). (Courtesy of Synthes Maxillofacial, Paoli, PA)

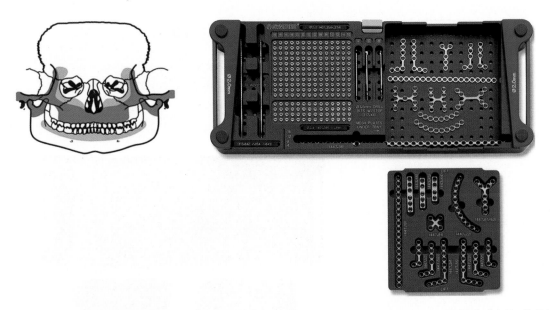

FIGURE 41.4 Craniofacial Modular Fixation System (2.0-mm Module). (Courtesy of Synthes Maxillofacial, Paoli, PA)

(additional lengths available up to 14 mm). Number-embossed markers attach to the top of each modular screw row to indicate the screw length for the customized module in use. The corresponding drill bits for plate fixation are 3 mm × 0.70 mm with stops (2 each) for 2- to 3-mm length screws and 5 mm × 0.76 mm (2 each) for 4-mm and 5-mm length screws and 8 mm × 0.76 mm (2 each) for 6-, 7-, and 8-mm length screws. For lag screw technique, the 1.1-mm × 110-

mm bit contained in the lift-out lid of the auxilliary bin is for the gliding hole; and the 0.76-mm bits are for the threaded hole. These 1.0-mm implants are a variety of X, Y, double Y, H (6 and 11 holes), T, L (left and right) and, curved (orbital rim), straight (adaptation), double row (strut), mesh plates, and burr hole covers (Figure 41.20).

The single and double Y plates are especially useful for nasal fractures and osteotomies. The double Y and H plates

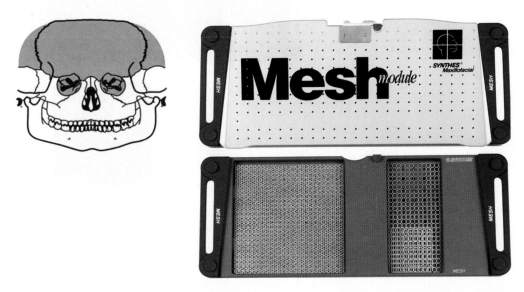

FIGURE 41.5 Craniofacial Modular Fixation System (Mesh Module). (Courtesy of Synthes Maxillofacial, Paoli, PA)

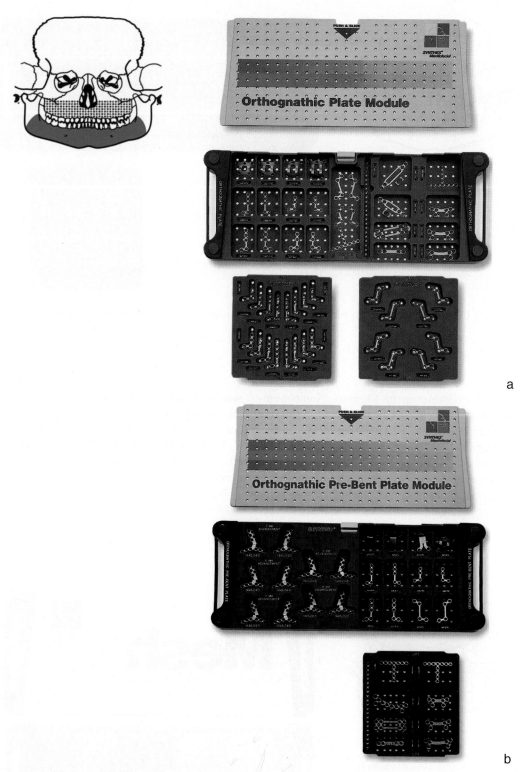

FIGURE 41.6 1.3-mm/1.5-mm/2.0-mm Orthognathic Modular Fixation System. (a) Orthognathic Plate Module. (b) Orthognathic Prebent Plate Module. (c) Orthognathic Screw Module. (Courtesy of Synthes Maxillofacial, Paoli, PA)

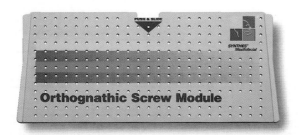

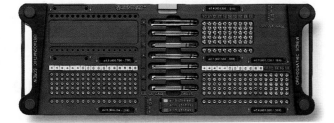

c

FIGURE 41.6 *Continued.*

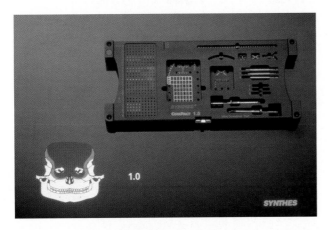

FIGURE 41.7 COMPACT MF(TM) Craniofacial Set (1.0-mm Module). (Courtesy of STRATEC Medical, Oberdorf, Switzerland and Mathys LTD Bettlach, Bettlach, Switzerland)

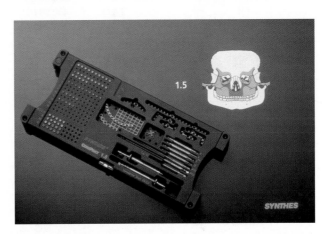

FIGURE 41.9 COMPACT MF(TM) Craniofacial Set (1.5-mm Module). (Courtesy of STRATEC Medical, Oberdorf, Switzerland and Mathys LTD Bettlach, Bettlach, Switzerland)

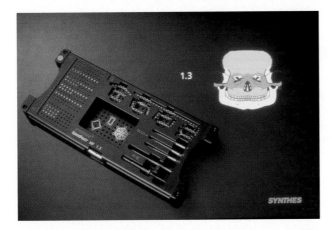

FIGURE 41.8 COMPACT MF(TM) Craniofacial Set (1.3-mm Module). (Courtesy of STRATEC Medical, Oberdorf, Switzerland and Mathys LTD Bettlach, Bettlach, Switzerland)

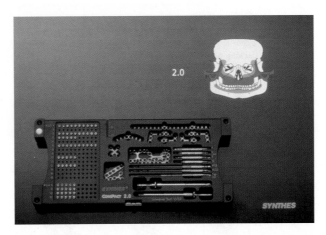

FIGURE 41.10 COMPACT MF(TM) Craniofacial Set (2.0-mm Module). (Courtesy of STRATEC Medical, Oberdorf, Switzerland and Mathys LTD Bettlach, Bettlach, Switzerland)

Screw and Drill Bit Chart

	SCREW INFORMATION		DRILL BIT DIAMETER		
			Threaded Hole	**Gliding Hole / Threaded Hole**	
Screw Size/Thread Dia.	Catalog Number	Emergency Screw Thread Dia./Cat. No.	Plate Technique	Lag Screw Technique For Gliding Hole	For Threaded Hole
1.0 mm	**400.502-.514**	**1.2** mm 400.602-.614	**0.70** mm (3 mm) Use with 2–3 mm length screws **0.76** mm (5,8,14 mm) Use with 4–14 mm length screws	**1.0** mm	**0.76** mm
1.3 mm	**400.623-.638**	**1.7** mm 400.653-.668	**1.0** mm	**1.3** mm	**1.0** mm
1.5 mm	**400.734-.748**	**2.0** mm 400.784-.798	**1.1** mm	**1.5** mm	**1.1** mm
2.0 mm	**401.154-.174**	**2.4** mm 401.306-.318	**1.5** mm	**2.0** mm	**1.5** mm
2.0 mm Coarse Pitch Screws	**401.934-.954**	**2.4** mm 401.306-.318	**1.5** mm	**2.0** mm	**1.5** mm
2.4 mm	**401.506-.540**	**2.7** mm 401.558-.568	**1.8** mm	**2.4** mm	**1.8** mm
2.4 mm Locking Screws	**497.668-.684**	N/A	**1.8** mm	N/A	N/A
3.0 mm Locking Screws	**497.690-.698**	N/A	**2.4** mm	N/A	N/A
4.0 mm THORP Screws (with 1.8 mm Locking Screw)	**497.60-66** Solid screws **497.90-96** Hollow screws **497.78.98** Locking screw	N/A	**3.0** mm	N/A	N/A

a

AO/ASIF

Continuing Education

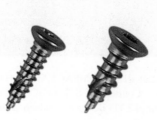

b

FIGURE 41.11 (a) Self-tapping screw and drill bit chart. (b) Self-drilling screws: 1.3-mm, 1.5-mm, and 2.0-mm. (Courtesy of Synthes Maxillofacial, Paoli, PA)

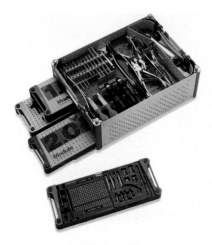

FIGURE 41.12 Craniofacial Modular Fixation System Graphic Case. (Courtesy of Synthes Maxillofacial, Paoli, PA)

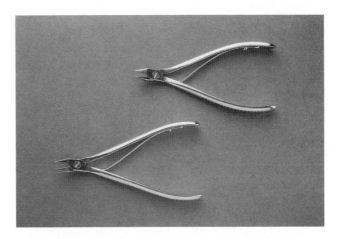

FIGURE 41.15 Plate bending pliers (2). (Courtesy of Synthes Maxillofacial, Paoli, PA)

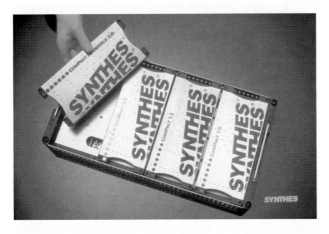

FIGURE 41.13 COMPACT MF™ Sterilization Tray. (Courtesy of STRATEC Medical, Oberdorf, Switzerland and Mathys LTD Bettlach, Bettlach, Switzerland)

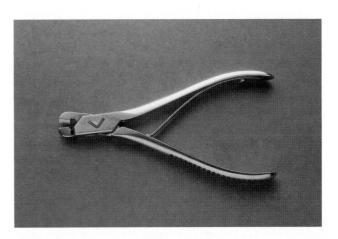

FIGURE 41.16 Right-angle bender. (Courtesy of Synthes Maxillofacial, Paoli, PA)

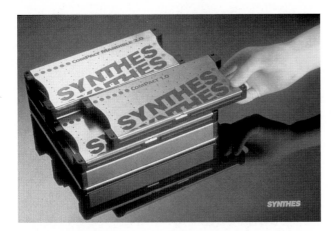

FIGURE 41.14 COMPACT MF™ Modules stacked over the Universal Instrument Tray. (Courtesy of STRATEC Medical, Oberdorf, Switzerland and Mathys LTD Bettlach, Bettlach, Switzerland)

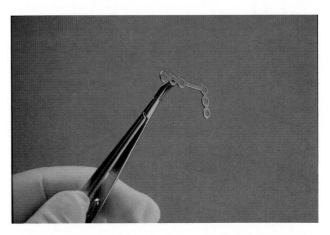

FIGURE 41.17 Plate holding forceps. (Courtesy of Synthes Maxillofacial, Paoli, PA)

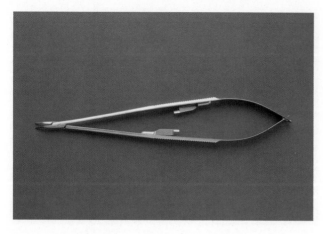

FIGURE 41.18 Plate holding Castro-Viejo locking forceps. (Courtesy of Synthes Maxillofacial, Paoli, PA)

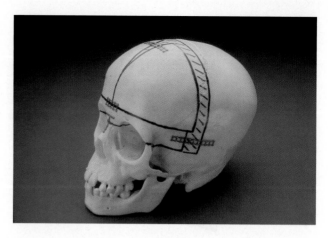

FIGURE 41.21 Strut plates demonstrated in a frontal bone advancement. (Courtesy of Synthes Maxillofacial, Paoli, PA)

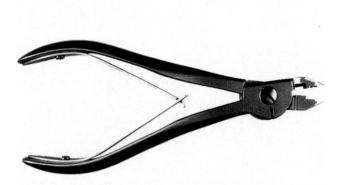

FIGURE 41.19 3-in-1 Plate bender/cutter. (Courtesy of Synthes Maxillofacial, Paoli, PA)

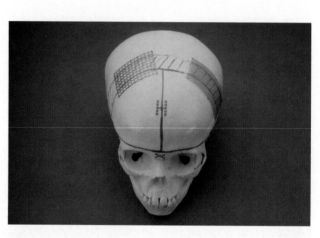

FIGURE 41.22 Mesh plates demonstrated covering cranial defects. (Courtesy of Synthes Maxillofacial, Paoli, PA)

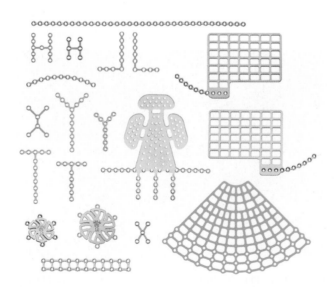

FIGURE 41.20 1.0-mm Module selection of implants. (Courtesy of Synthes Maxillofacial, Paoli, PA)

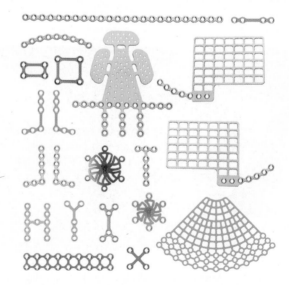

FIGURE 41.23 1.3-mm Module selection of implants. (Courtesy of Synthes Maxillofacial, Paoli, PA)

are designed for fixation of replaced craniotomy segments. T plates are indicated for frontal sinus and naso-ethmoid fractures and pediatric frontal bone advancements. Strut plates (6 × 30 mm and 6 × 42 mm) are useful in pediatric frontal bone advancements, frontal sinus wall fractures, and at the orbital rim (Figure 41.21). The mesh plates (29 × 40 mm, 38 × 42 mm, 50 × 100 mm, and 100 × 100 mm) can be used as a cranioplast for the coverage of cranial bone defects, orbital floor reconstruction, and bridging pediatric maxillary defects (Figure 41.22). The cruciform screwdriver blade with holding sleeve is included (1 to 2 each). In addition the following are available: the 1.0-mm universal orbital floor plate, the 1.0-mm medial wall plates (left and right), the 1.0-mm burr hole covers (12 mm × 6 holes and 17 mm × 6 holes). Drill bits with stop for right-angle drills are also available in 3 mm 0.70 mm), 5 mm, and 8 mm (0.76 mm).

1.3-mm Module

Color: Gold
Indications: Orbito-zygomatic, cranium, nasal–orbital–ethmoid.

The 1.3-mm module is a miniplate system containing 1.3-mm self-tapping screws in 3-, 4-, 5-, 6-, and 8-mm lengths (available in lengths up to 18 mm), 1.3 mm self-drilling screws in 4-, 5-, and 6-mm lengths, and 1.7-mm emergency screws in 3-, 4-, 5-, 6-, and 8-mm lengths (available in lengths up to 18 mm). Number-embossed markers attach to the top of each modular screw row to indicate the screw length for customized module in use. The corresponding drill bits for plate fixation are 1.0 mm in 4-, 6-, and 8-mm lengths with stops. For lag-screw technique, the 1.5-mm bit found in the lift-out lid of the auxilliary bin is for the gliding hole; the 1.0-mm bits are for the threaded hole. The implants are a variety of Y, T, oblique L 6-hole left and right, oblique L 7-hole left and right, curved (orbital rim), straight 24-hole (adaption), universal orbital floor plate, medial orbital wall plates (left and right), strut plate (43 mm × 18 holes), mesh screen (100 mm × 100 mm), mesh plates (38 mm × 53 mm, and 100 mm × 100 mm), box plates (10 mm × 5 mm × 4 holes and 10 mm × 10 mm × 4 holes), 1.3-mm anatomic orbital floor plate, and burr note covers (12 mm × 6 holes and 17 mm × 6 holes) (Figure 41.23). The single Y plates are especially useful for nasal fractures and osteotomies. The burr hole covers are for coverage of craniotome holes. T plates are indicated for frontal sinus and naso-ethmoid fractures and pediatric frontal bone advancements. L plates can be used in fractures of the orbits and cranium, as well as incomplete maxillary fractures. The mesh screen, mesh plates, and box plates are for various cranial applications. The trays also include the 1.3-mm cruciform screwdriver blade with holding sleeve (1 each) and the 1.3-mm cruciform screwdriver blade (self-retaining) (1 each).

1.5-mm Module

Colors: Black (Compact MF for Europe and Worldwide)
Red (Synthes Maxillofacial for North America)
Indications: Orbito-zygomatic, maxillary

The 1.5-mm module is a miniplate system containing 1.5-mm self-tapping screws in 4-, 6-, 8-, 10-, and 12-mm lengths (available up to 18 mm), 1.5-mm self-drilling screws in 4-, 5-, 6-, 7-, and 8-mm lengths, and 2.0-mm emergency screws in 4-, 6-, 8-, 10-, and 12-mm lengths (available up to 18 mm). However, in thick and deep cortical bone it is often necessary to pretap the holes. The 1.5-mm tap (short and long) is contained within the lift-out lid of the auxilliary bin. The proper use of self-stop drill bits is also emphasized to ensure that the screw holes will be sufficiently deep. Number-embossed markers attach to the top of each modular screw row to indicate the screw length for the customized module in use. The corresponding drill bits for plate fixation are 1.1-mm (4-, 6-, 8-, and 12-mm) lengths, with stops (2 each). For lag-screw technique, the 1.5-mm bit is for the gliding hole and is found within the lift-out lid of the auxilliary bin; the 1.1-mm bit is for the threaded hole. The implants are a variety of Y, X, oblique L (5-hold left and right), oblique L (7-hole left and right), curved (8-, 10-, and 12-hole), straight (20-hole) (adaption), universal orbital floor, medial orbital floor (left and right), and the 1.5-mm anatomic orbital floor plate. (Figure 41.24). The single Y plates are especially useful for nasal fractures and osteotomies. The burr hole covers are for coverage of craniotome holes. T plates are indicated for frontal sinus and naso-ethmoid fractures, as well as frontal bone advancements. L plates can be used in fractures of the orbits and cranium and incomplete maxillary fractures. Curved plates are for the orbital rim. Adaption plates, which can be applied to any site, may be especially helpful in bridging defects and

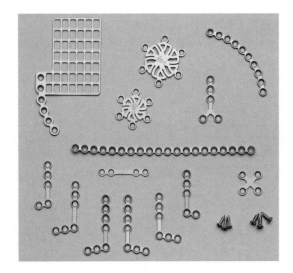

FIGURE 41.24 1.5-mm module selection of implants. (Courtesy of Synthes Maxillofacial, Paoli, PA)

frontal bar fractures. The trays also include the 1.5-mm cruciform screwdriver blade with holding sleeve (1 each) and 1.5-mm cruciform screwdriver blade (self-retaining) (1 each).

2.0-mm Module

Color: Blue.
Indications: Orbito-zygomatic, maxillary.

The 2.0-mm module is a miniplate system containing 2.0-mm self-tapping screws in 4-, 6-, 8-, 10-, 12-, 14-, 16-, and 18-mm lengths (available up to 24 mm), 2.0 mm self-drilling screws 4-, 5-, 6-, 7-, and 8-mm lengths, and 2.4-mm emergency screws in 6-, 8-, 10-, 12-, 14-, 16-, and 18-mm lengths (available up to 24 mm). These screws can also be pretapped when used in thick cortical bone; 2.0-mm taps (long and short) are in the lift-out lid of the auxilliary bin. Number-embossed markers attach to the top of each modular screw row and indicate the screw length for the customized module in use. The corresponding bits for plate fixation are 1.5-mm (4-, 6-, 8-, and 12-mm lengths, with stops). The proper use of the drill bits requires that they are used to drill to the proper depth. For lag-screw technique, the 2.0-mm × 110-mm bit is for the gliding hole and is in the lift-out lid of the auxilliary bin. The 1.5-mm bit is for the threaded hole. The implants are a variety of Y (5 and 8 holes), X, H (8 and 9 holes), oblique L (5-hole left and right), Oblique L (7-hole left and right), Oblique L (10-hole left and right), Curved (8, 10, and 12 holes), adaption plate (20 holes), adaption plate with broad hole spacing (30 holes), and DCP (4, 5, and 6 holes) (Figure 41.25). The single Y and L plates are especially useful for LeFort I fractures and osteotomies, as they allow the placement of screws superior to the root apices of teeth. Adaption plates may be used for LeFort I fractures, bridging of defects, and reconstruction. DCP plates are for the frontozygomatic sites. X, H, and double Y are indicated for naso-orbito-ethmoid region

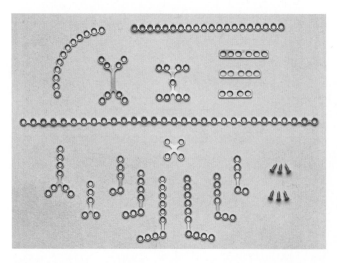

FIGURE 41.25 2.0-mm Module selection of implants. (Courtesy of Synthes Maxillofacial, Paoli, PA)

fractures. The trays also include the 2.0-mm cruciform screwdriver blade with holding sleeve (1 each) and 2.0-mm cruciform screwdriver blade (self-retaining) (1 each). In the Compact MF system the 2.0 mm Midface Plates are stored together with the 2.0 mandible plates in a combined 2.0 module.

1.3-mm/1.5-mm/2.0-mm Orthognathic Modular Fixation System

Color: Black (Synthes Maxillofacial: North America availability only).
Indications: Orthognathic surgery of the maxilla and the mandible.

The Orthognathic Modular Fixation System is a composite 1.3-mm/1.5-mm/2.0-mm system available only in North America. It consists of a graphic case organized with an upper section lift-out standard screwdriver instrument tray or ratcheting screwdriver instrument tray and two separate lower section screw and implant modules. The Orthognathic Screw Module (Figure 41.6c) contains 1.3-mm self-tapping screws in 3-, 4-, 5-, and 6-mm lengths (available up to 18 mm), 1.7-mm self-tapping teal colored emergency in 3-, 4-, 5-, and 6-mm lengths (available up to 18 mm), 1.5-mm StarDrive self-drilling screws (for star shaped screwdriver tip) in 4-, 5-, 6-, 7-, and 8-mm lengths, 2.0-mm StarDrive self-drilling screws with screws in 4-, 5-, 6-, 7-, and 8-mm lengths (available up to 18 mm), 2.0-mm self-tapping gold-colored screws (available up to 24 mm) and 2.4-mm emergency teal-colored screws (available up to 24 mm). Number-embossed markers attach to the top of each modular screw row to indicate the screw length for the customized module. The corresponding drill bits for plate fixation are the 1.0-mm drill bit Stryker J latch (4-, 6-, and 8-mm lengths with self-stops—2 each), 1.1-mm (4-, 6-, 8-, and 12-mm lengths with self-stops—2 each) and 1.5-mm (4-, 6-, 8-, and 12-mm lengths with self-stop—2 each). The proper use of the drill bits requires that they are used to drill the proper depth. For the 1.5-mm lag-screw technique, the 1.5-mm bit is for the gliding hole; the 1.1-mm bit is for the threaded hole. For 2.0-mm lag-screw technique, the 2.0-mm × 110-mm bit is for the gliding hole. The Orthognathic Plate module (Figure 41.6a) contains a variety of maxillary and mandibular implants. The maxillary miniplates (Figure 41.26) consist of L plates 1.5-mm and 2.0-mm left and right (3 × 3 hole in 22-, 24-, 26-, 27-, and 29-mm lengths); oblique L plates 1.3-mm left and right (3 × 3, 3 × 4 holes), 1.5-mm left and right (2 × 3, 3 × 4, 2 × 2 holes short and long), 2.0-mm left and right (2 × 3, 3 × 4, 4 × 6, 2 × 2 short and long); oblique L plates malleable left and right 1.5-mm (2 × 3, 3 × 4, 2 × 2 holes long and short), 2.0-mm (2 × 3, 3 × 4, 2 × 2 holes long and short); adaption plates 1.3-mm (24 holes), 1.5-mm (20 holes) (regular and low profile); 2.0-mm, adaption plates malleable 1.5-mm and 2.0-mm (20 holes) T plates 1.3-mm (3 × 4 holes), 1.5-mm

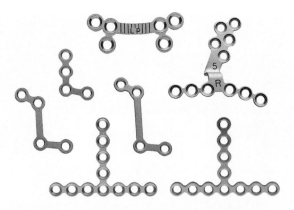

FIGURE 41.26 1.5-mm/2.0-mm Orthognathic Module selection of implants. (Courtesy of Synthes Maxillofacial, Paoli, PA)

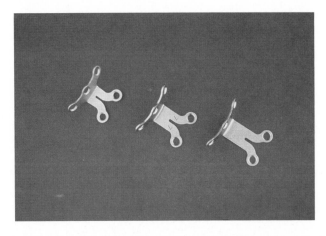

FIGURE 41.28 Chin plates-offset single-bend selection. (Courtesy of Synthes Maxillofacial, Paoli, PA)

(4 × 7 holes), 1.5-mm malleable (4 × 7 holes); Y plates (1 × 3 holes) in 1.3-mm, 1.5-mm, 1.5-mm (low profile) and 2.0-mm (2 × 4 holes); Y plates malleable 1.5-mm (1 × 3 holes) and 2.0-mm (1 × 3 holes); Z plates left and right 1.5-mm short and long, 2.0-mm short and long; Z plates malleable left and right 1.5-mm short and long and 2.0-mm short and long, and pre-bent maxillary plates left and right for 3-, 5-, 7-, 9-, and 11-mm advancement and are available as a separate Pre-Bent Module (Figure 41.6b). The oblique, L, Z, and pre-bent plates are especially useful for LeFort I osteotomies, as they allow the placement of screws superior to the root apices of teeth. Mandibular implants consist of a variety of implants. 2.0 chin plates come in a variety of shapes and lengths, such as the off-set straight (3-, 5-, and 8-mm lengths) (Figure 41.27), the off-set single bend (3-5-, 6-8-, 9-11-mm lengths) (Figure 41.28), and the offset double bend (4-, 6-, 8-, and 10-mm lengths) (Figure 41.29). For mandibular ramus sagittal split osteotomies the 2.0-mm implants include strut (8 holes) (Figure 41.30), curved low profile 6 holes 4-mm bar; 6 holes 8-mm bar; and

6 holes, 12-mm bar, curved 6 holes 4-mm bar; 6 holes 8-mm bar (Figure 41.26), and 6 holes 12-mm bar) (Figure 41.31), curved (10 holes) and straight (4 holes) (Figure 41.32). A special adjustable plate with an adjustable slider for mandibular sagittal split osteotomies is also available (Figures 41.33 to 41.35). Thinner, more malleable, teal-colored implant versions of this system are also available. For the Compact MF system orthognathic plates are ordered separately and can be stored in the auxilliary bin of the 1.5 mm or 2.0 mm modules.

Mesh Module

Color: Black
Indications: Cranium, orbits.

The Mesh Module is designed for use as a cranioplast for the coverage of bony defects of the cranium and for the orbital walls and floor. The implants are 1.0-mm mesh plates (40

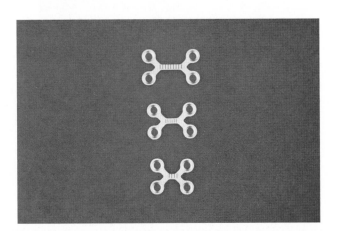

FIGURE 41.27 Chin plates-offset straight selection. (Courtesy of Synthes Maxillofacial, Paoli, PA)

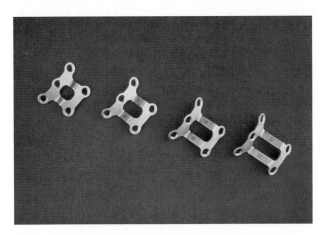

FIGURE 41.29 Chin plates-offset double-bend selection. (Courtesy of Synthes Maxillofacial, Paoli, PA)

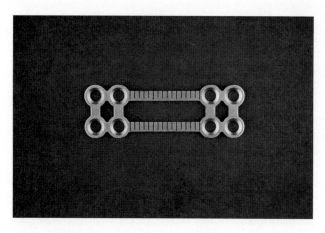

FIGURE 41.30 Sagittal split strut plate. (Courtesy of Synthes Maxillofacial, Paoli, PA)

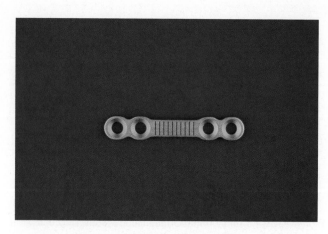

FIGURE 41.32 Sagittal split straight plate. (Courtesy of Synthes Maxillofacial, Paoli, PA)

mm × 29 mm, 42 mm × 38 mm, and 100 mm × 50 mm), mesh screen for 1.0-mm screws (100 mm × 100 mm), mesh plate for 1.3-mm screws (100 mm × 100 mm and 38 mm × 53 mm), and mesh screen for 1.3-mm screws (100 mm × 100 mm) (Figure 41.36), contourable mesh plates rigid and malleable 1.3-mm square (38 × 45 mm), small and large arcs, circular 30-mm, 70-mm, and 100-mm diameters, and 1.5-mm small and large arcs and circular 30-mm, 70-mm, and 100-mm diameters (Figure 41.37). These various implants may be modified to any size and shape with a mesh cutter instrument.

Cranial Modular Fixation System

This is a special modular system organized for use in neurosurgically related procedures only in the cranium. It is composed of a graphic case that can contain two modules with an upper Universal Instrument Tray that lifts out (Figure 41.38). The universal instrument tray consists of universal plate benders (2 each), plate cutter (1 each), and Castro-Viejo locking plate/screw forceps (2 each). There are 1.0-mm, 1.3-mm, and 1.5-mm modules available.

1.0-mm Cranial Modular Fixation System Module

Color: Green
Indications: Cranial bone flap fixation.

The 1.0-mm module (Figures 41.1 and 41.20) is a microsystem containing 1.0-mm self-tapping screws in 3-, 4-, and 5-mm lengths (additional lengths available up to 8 mm) and 1.2-mm emergency screws in 3-, 4-, and 5-mm lengths (additional lengths available up to 8 mm). Number-embossed markers attach to the top of each modular screw row to indicate the screw length for the customized module in use. The corresponding

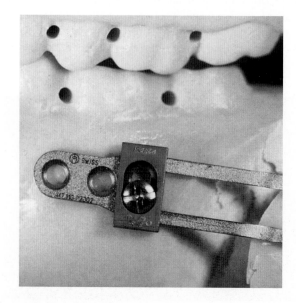

FIGURE 41.33 A 2.0-mm titanium sagittal split plate with adjustable slider (Split Fix) close up of slidably adjustable slot hole. (Courtesy of Synthes Maxillofacial, Paoli, PA)

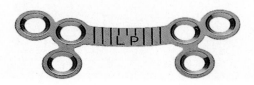

FIGURE 41.31 Sagittal split curved plate. (Courtesy of Synthes Maxillofacial, Paoli, PA)

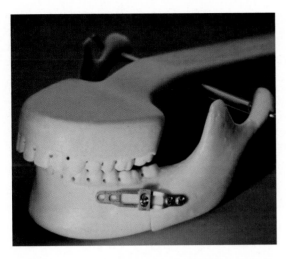

FIGURE 41.34 A 2.0-mm titanium sagittal split plate with adjustable slider (split fix) with osteotomy segments closed together. (Courtesy of Synthes Maxillofacial, Paoli, PA)

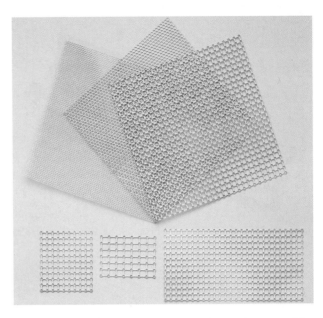

FIGURE 41.36 Mesh module selection of implants. (Courtesy of Synthes Maxillofacial, Paoli, PA)

drill bits for plate fixation are 3 mm × 0.70 mm with stop (2 each) for 2- to 3-mm length screws, 5 mm × 0.76 mm (2 each) for 4-mm and 5-mm length screws, and 8 mm × 0.76 mm (2 each) for 8-mm length screws. For lag-screw technique, the 1.1-mm × 110-mm bit contained in the lift-out lid of the auxilliary bin is for the gliding hole; the 0.76-mm bits are for the threaded hole. These 1.0-mm implants are a variety of X (5 holes), Y (9 holes), adaption plate (34 holes), strut plate (22 holes), burr hole covers (12 and 17 mm). The Y and X plates are designed for fixation of replaced craniotomy segments. Strut plates are useful in pediatric frontal bone advancements, frontal sinus wall fractures, and at the orbital rim. The burr hole covers are used to cover the circular defects left from the use of the craniotome. The cruci-

form screwdriver blade with holding sleeve is also included (1-2 each).

1.3-mm Cranial Modular Fixation System Module

Color: Gold
Indications: Cranial bone flap and cranial fracture fixation.

The 1.3-mm module (Figure 41.39) is a miniplate system con-

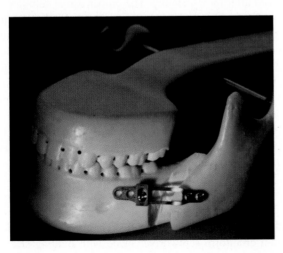

FIGURE 41.35 A 2.0-mm titanium sagittal split plate with adjustable slider (split fix) with osteotomy segments held apart. (Courtesy of Synthes Maxillofacial, Paoli, PA)

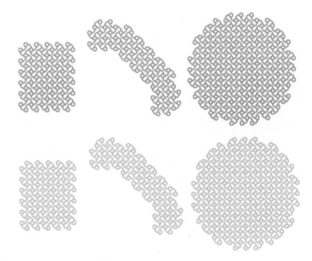

FIGURE 41.37 Contourable mesh implants. (Courtesy of Synthes Maxillofacial, Paoli, PA)

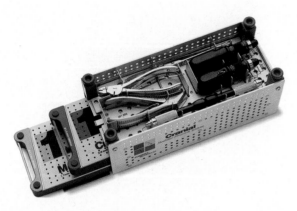

FIGURE 41.38 Cranial Modular Fixation System Graphic Case. (Courtesy of Synthes Maxillofacial, Paoli, PA)

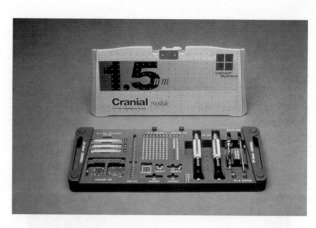

FIGURE 41.40 A 1.5-mm Cranial Module. (Courtesy of Synthes Maxillofacial, Paoli, PA)

taining 1.3-mm cranial StarDrive self-drilling screws in 4- and 5-mm lengths, 1.3-mm cranial self-tapping screws in 3-, 4-, and 5-mm lengths, 1.7-mm cranial emergency self-tapping screws in 3-, 4-, and 5-mm lengths. Number embossed markers attach to the top of each modular screw row to indicate the screw length for the customized module in use. The corresponding drill bits for plate fixation are 1.0 mm in 4-mm and 6-mm lengths with stops. For lag-screw technique, the 1.5-mm × 110-mm bit found in the lift-out lid of the auxilliary bin is for the gliding hole; the 1.0-mm bits are for the threaded hole. The implants are a variety of straight (2 and 4 holes), Y (5 holes), X (4 holes), box plates (4 holes × 5 mm and 10 mm), adaption plate (24 holes), strut plate (18 holes), burr hole covers (12-mm × 6-mm holes and 17-mm × 6-mm holes), and mesh plate (11-mm × 8-mm holes). The trays also include the 1.3-mm cruciform screwdriver blade with hold-

ing sleeve (1 each), 1.3-mm cruciform screwdriver blade (self-retaining (1 each), and 2 black narrow screwdriver handles.

1.5-mm Cranial Modular Fixation System Module

Color: Red.
Indications: Cranial bone flap and cranial fracture fixation.

The 1.5-mm module (Figure 41.40) is a miniplate fixation system containing 1.5-mm cranial StarDrive self-drilling screws in 4-, 5-, and 6-mm lengths, 1.5-mm self-tapping screws in 4-, 5-, and 6-mm lengths, and 2.0-mm emergency self-tapping screws in 4- and 5-mm lengths. Additional 1.5-mm brow lift screws self-tapping (14 mm), and StarDrive self-drilling (14 and 18 mm) are also available for brow lift surgery. They are removed after initial healing. The proper use of self-stop drill bits is also emphasized to ensure that the screw holes will be drilled to a sufficient depth. Number-embossed markers attach to the top of each modular screw row to indicate the screw length for the customized module in use. The corresponding drill bits for plate fixation are 1.1 mm (4-mm and 6-mm lengths with stops—2 each). For lag-screw technique, the 1.5-mm bit is for the gliding hole and is found within the lift-out lid of the auxilliary bin; the 1.1-mm bit are for the threaded hole. The implants are a variety of (5 holes), X (4 holes), adaption (20 holes), box plate (10-mm × 4-mm holes), burr hole covers (12 mm and 17 mm). The burr hole covers (Figure 41.41) are for the coverage of craniotome holes. Adaption plates can be applied to any site and may be especially helpful in bridging defects and frontal bar fractures. The trays also include the 1.5-mm cruciform screwdriver blade with holding sleeve (1 each), 1.5-mm cruciform screwdriver blade (self-retaining) (1 each), and narrow black handles (2 each).

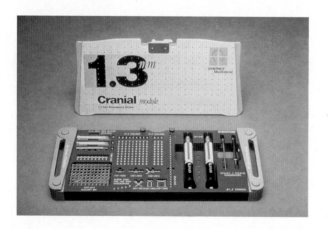

FIGURE 41.39 A 1.3-mm Cranial Module. (Courtesy of Synthes Maxillofacial, Paoli, PA)

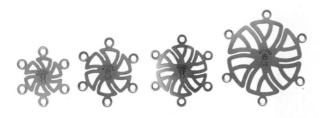

FIGURE 41.41 Cranial Modular System burr hole covers available in different diameters in 1.3-mm and 1.5-mm modules. (Courtesy of Synthes Maxillofacial, Paoli, PA)

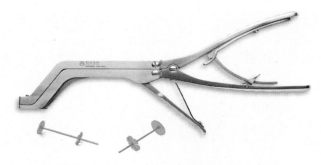

FIGURE 41.43 Titanium cranial flap tube clamps with crimping device. (Courtesy of Synthes Maxillofacial, Paoli, PA)

Cranial Flap Spring Clips and Tube Clamps

The cranial flap spring clips, spring clips with combination burr hole covers, and tube clamps are used for the fixation of cranial flaps (Figures 41.42 and 41.43). The tube clamps are available in 13-mm and 18-mm diameters. For the tube clamps, a crimping device is used to squeeze the clamp disks together to the desired tightness with the solid disk intracranial. The tube is then crimped and sheared by squeezing the second trigger.

Resorbable Fixation System

Indications: Craniofacial, orthognathic, and trauma surgery.

The Resorbable Fixation system is a newly devised plate system (Figures 41.44 and 41.45) for use in craniofacial, orthognathic, and trauma surgery, but not intended for use in the mandible. The system is indicated for fragmented fractures of the naso-ethmoid and infraorbital regions, fragmented frontal sinus wall fractures, midfacial fractures, and reconstructive procedures of the midface or craniofacial skeleton. The plates and screws are manufactured from a resorbable copolymer, in a 70:30 poly(L/lactide-co-D, L-lactide) which resorbs in vivo by hydrolysis into lactic acid and then undergoes metabolism. Resorbable Fixation 1.5-mm and 2.0-mm

screw holes need to be pretapped with self-drilling 1.5-mm and 2.0-mm taps (Figure 41.46).

Use of the Resorbable Fixation system is contraindicated in the presence of active infection, limited vascular supply, insufficient bone quality or quality, and latent infections. The Resorbable Fixation system is not intended for use in mandibular fixation or under conditions of full load bearing. The resorbable implants are shaped through the use of a water bath heater (Figure 41.47) or hot air system (Figure 41.48) that heats the plates or mesh in the operating room environment. The hot air system is for use in North America only. The hot air device is used after it has warmed up to the necessary operating temperature. A plate or mesh implant is held with forceps or by hand within the "U"-shaped nozzle or in front of the narrow nozzle. After approximately 5 to 10 seconds of hot air heating, the plate or mesh can be contoured and molded by hand. The plate is held in the desired form until the material has cooled sufficiently to become rigid. In order to obtain the required shape, a bending template may be utilized. The Hot Air System consists of a hot air device, stand, small nozzle, large nozzle, narrow nozzle interconnect cable, and power supply (Figure 41.48). With the exception of the power supply, the Hot Air System can be steam sterilized. The water bath heater achieves 70°C in 500 cc of water after 15 minutes as indicated by a "ready indicator." As

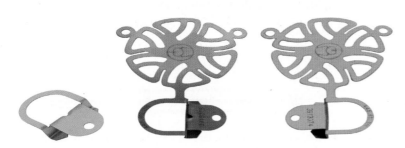

FIGURE 41.42 Cranial Modular Fixation System spring clips and spring clips with burr hole covers. (Courtesy of Synthes Maxillofacial, Paoli, PA)

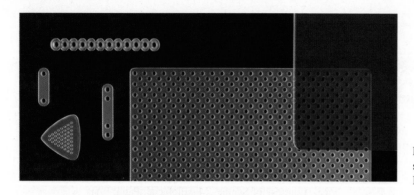

FIGURE 41.44 Selection of 1.5-mm and 2.0-mm resorbable fixation system plates. (Courtesy of Synthes Maxillofacial, Paoli, PA)

with the hot air system, implants heated in the water bath heater must be held with plate holding forceps. Plates may be heated and contoured up to 10 times and can be contoured after 10 seconds of heating. The system contains 2.5-mm emergency resorbable screws (4-, 6-, and 8-mm lengths), 2.0-mm resorbable screws (4.6-, and 8-mm lengths), and 1.5-mm resorbable screws (4-, and 6-mm lengths). The 1.5-mm implants include straight plates (2 and 4 holes), adaption plates (8, 12, and 20 holes), orbital rim plate, oblique L left and right, Y plate, double Y plate, strut plates (2×10 and 2×18 holes), orbital floor plate .5-mm thick, 1.5-mm mesh plates .5 mm thick (50×50 mm, 60×80 mm, 100×100 mm), 1.5-mm mesh plates .8 mm thick (50×50, 75×75, 100×100, and 125×125 mm), 1.5-mm, .5-mm thick sheets (50×50 mm and 75×75 mm), and 1.5-mm, .8-mm thick sheets (50×50 mm and 75×75 mm). The 2.0-mm implants include straight plates (2 and 4 holes), adaption plates (8, 12, and 20 holes), orbital rim plate, oblique L left and right, Y plate, strut plate (2×10 holes), orbital floor plate .5 mm thick, 1.5-mm mesh plates 1.2-mm thick (48×48 mm and 78×78 mm), sheets .5-mm thick (50×50 mm and 75×75 mm), sheets .8-mm thick (50×50 mm and 75×75 mm), burr hole cover, and X plate (Figure 41.44).

Resorbable plates of 1.5 mm are comparable in strength to 1.0-mm titanium plates, and 2.0-mm resorbable plates are comparable in strength to 1.3-mm titanium plates or 1.5-mm malleable titanium plates. The instruments include mesh scissors, plate cutter, plate holding locking forcep, self-drilling 1.5-mm and 2.0-mm taps, 1.5-mm/2.0-mm double drill guide, 2.0-mm/2.5-mm double drill guide, and screwdriver.

Craniofacial Repair System (CRS)

The Craniofacial Repair System (CRS) Figure 41.49 is a self-setting calcium phosphate bone cement. It is used for the restoration or augmentation of defects of the craniofacial skeleton. CRS undergoes hardening to form dahlite, which closely replicates the mineral phase of bone, later gradually remodeling in two phases through osteoclastic resorption and the deposition of new bone by osteoblasts. CRS is an injectable and moldable bone cement that will harden in a warm, wet, or environment. Local tissue injury is not a consideration as it is nonexothermic, and it takes 10 minutes for the material to harden.

The CRS product delivery system reactant packs allow for consistent sterile cement mixing in premeasured amounts. The Reactant packs are available in 3-cc, 5-cc, and 10-cc sizes (Figure 41.49), with premeasured amounts of sodium phosphate and calcium phosphate powder. The reactant packs are mixed in the CRS automated mixer (Figure 41.49). The automatic mixer is powered by a single air hose between 90 to 150 psi operating room supply. If the automated mixer is not being used an alternated mortar, pestle, and spatula can be used.

After mixing the reactant packs are placed in the CRS delivery device (Figure 41.50), which allows ease of handling,

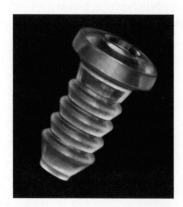

FIGURE 41.45 Example of resorbable screw. (Courtesy of Synthes Maxillofacial, Paoli, PA)

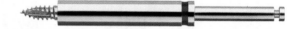

FIGURE 41.46 Self-drilling taps (1.5-mm and 2.0-mm) for resorbable system screws. (Courtesy of Synthes Maxillofacial, Paoli, PA)

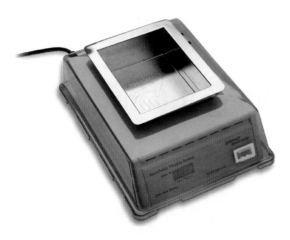

FIGURE 41.47 Water bath system. (Courtesy of Synthes Maxillofacial, Paoli, PA)

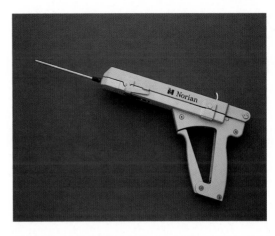

FIGURE 41.50 Craniofacial Repair System delivery device loaded for use. (Courtesy of Synthes Maxillofacial, Paoli, PA)

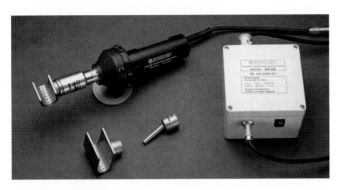

FIGURE 41.48 Hot air system with small, large, and narrow nozzles.

precise cement injection, and access to distant areas. There are different sized delivery needles to meet various surgical requirements. The amounts of CRS material needed to repair or fill various defects vary from 5 cc for a burr hole to 25 cc for a cranial defect or to obliterate the frontal sinus.

Demineralized Bone Matrix (DBX®)

Demineralized Bone Matrix (DBX®) is a 32% in putty and 27% in paste by weight human demineralized allogeneic bone graft for use in a variety of craniomaxillofacial osteoinductive indications and is available as paste 1-cc, 5-cc, and 10-cc syringes, and putty as 1-cc, 5-cc, and 10-cc syringes (Figure 41.51).

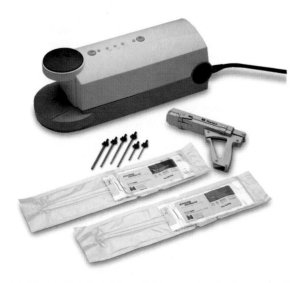

FIGURE 41.49 Craniofacial Repair System (CRS) mixer, 3-cc, 5-cc, and 10-cc reactant packs, delivery device, and delivery needles. (Courtesy of Synthes Maxillofacial, Paoli, PA)

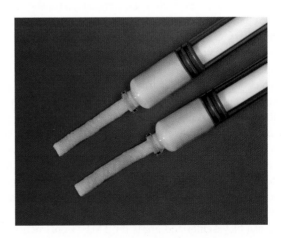

FIGURE 41.51 Demineralized Bone Matrix (DBX®, putty and paste delivery syringes. (Courtesy of Synthes Maxillofacial, Paoli, PA)

42
Microvascular Reconstruction of the Condyle and the Ascending Ramus

Rainer Schmelzeisen and Friedrich Wilhelm Neukam

Today, temporomandibular joint (TMJ), condylar, and ascending ramus reconstruction can be performed with high accuracy as the recent new developments in diagnostic and surgical procedures now offer safe and reliable treatment concepts. Advances in diagnostic imaging facilitate treatment planning and the appropriate selection of reconstructive procedures (Figure 42.1).[1]

In general, nonvascularized grafts including costochondral, metatarsal, fibula, tibia, and iliac crest grafts are used.[2–9] In an unfavorable soft tissue environment and especially in reconstructions of the condyle that also require reconstruction of larger aspects of the ascending ramus, an unpredictable resorption of the grafts may occur (Figure 42.2).

For condylar reconstruction, costochondral grafts are traditionally used. Disadvantages of these rib grafts are poor quality of cortical and medullary bone, flexibility, and elasticity of the bone. Warpage with continuous loading causing a possible separation between cartilage and bone as well as fractures may occur.[10] In contrast to costochondral grafts, sternoclavicular grafts are morphologically and histologically very similar to the condyle throughout the growth process.[11] Grafts used for TMJ reconstruction have a significant influence on mandibular growth, and they also influence maxillary growth processes.[12] Nonvascularized grafts show graft-specific characteristics of growth capacity. Direct exposure of the medullary bone of the sternoclavicular graft to adjacent soft tissues may facilitate integration of the graft to systemic growth-stimulating or -inhibiting processes mediated via blood vessels. In general, growth inhibition or, often more problematic, growth overshoot of nonvascularized grafts cannot be predicted exactly (Figure 42.3).

Therefore, indications for the use of vascularized grafts for condylar and ascending ramus reconstruction may be given in situations of unfavorable soft tissue conditions, the intention to avoid resorption of the graft, and to facilitate easier integration of the graft to systemic growth processes mediated via blood vessels.

The use of vascularized grafts for TMJ reconstruction was first suggested by Siemssen in 1982.[13] He suggested an arthroplasty of the TMJ with a sternoclavicular junction pedicled at the sternocleidomastoid muscle. Reid also reported on a free-flap application of the clavicular head of the pectoralis major muscle as a vascularized clavicular bone graft.[14]

All reconstructive procedures for the ascending ramus including the condyle produce obvious technical challenges with inherent risks of mandibular deviation, malocclusion, ankylosis, and temporal bone erosion. Additional soft tissue deficits pose special problems.[15] In microvascular reconstruction procedures of the mandible, there is an increasing interest in the special role of TMJ reconstruction.[16–18]

Material and Methods

Between 1988 and 1995, vascularized grafts from the iliac crest, the scapula region, and the fibula ($n = 53$) were used for head and neck reconstructions, including reconstruction of the ascending ramus and condyle.

In all patients, preoperative conventional x-ray diagnostics were supplemented by computed tomographic (CT) scans, which in general were also available as three-dimensional reformations. Preoperative three-dimensional soft tissue and bone reconstructions gave valuable information for planning of the surgical procedures. The amount of mandibular repositioning following scar contraction and especially the necessity of repositioning a condylar process in secondary reconstructions prior to insertion of bone grafts could already be assessed preoperatively.

In patients with the condyle and parts of the ascending ramus left in place, the intraoperative repositioning of the condylar segment includes resection of the muscular process to avoid postoperative limitation of mouth opening.

After removal of all scar tissue adherent to the proximal condylar segment, the condyle may be temporarily fixed to the maxilla in its desired position with a long miniplate perforating the oral mucosa. In more complex mandibular reconstruction, additional prosthodontic devices facilitate orientation of the new mandible toward the maxilla if a later insertion of implants for prosthodontic treatment is planned (Figure 42.4).

a

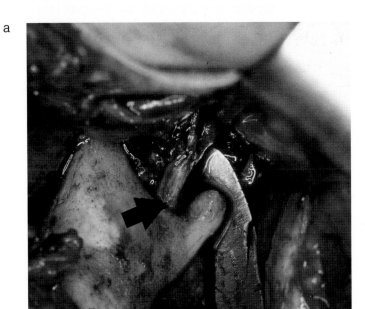

FIGURE 42.1 In a 4-year-old boy with a Goldenhar syndrome, the intraoperative findings confirm the preoperative information about the hypoplastic condyle and the distance between condyle and temporomandibular fossa given by the preoperative three-dimensional image. (Arrow: inferior alveolar nerve). (b) Patient with severe arthrosis of the left condyle before costochondral reconstruction of the left condyle. A three-dimensional CT image reveals additional small-volume ankylosis between the right condyle and the zygomatic arch necessitating also open joint surgery on the right side. (c) Preoperative x-ray of an angle-to-angle defect. (d,e) With a three-dimensional model, fabricated according to CT data, a template facilitating intraoral contouring of the graft can be made.

b

c

d

e

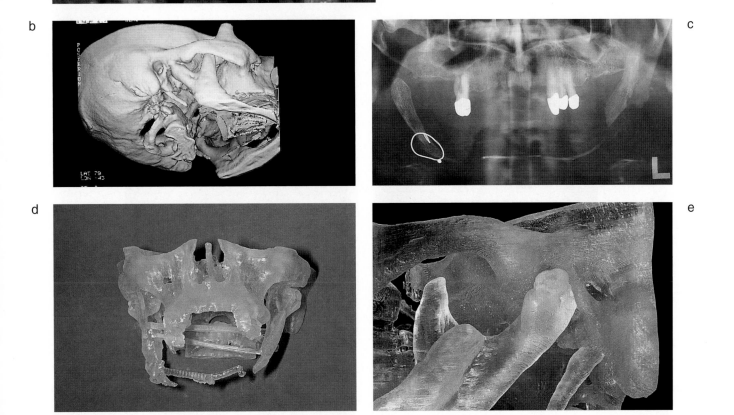

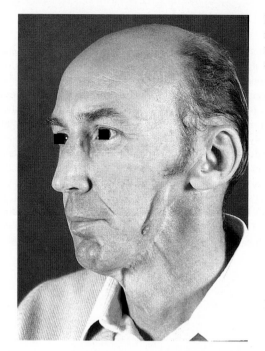

FIGURE 42.2 Severe resorption of a nonvascularized iliac crest graft for reconstruction of the ascending ramus and condyle in a 50-year-old patient. Note the pencil-like shape of the severely atrophic bone graft with additional soft tissue shrinkage.

a

b

c

d

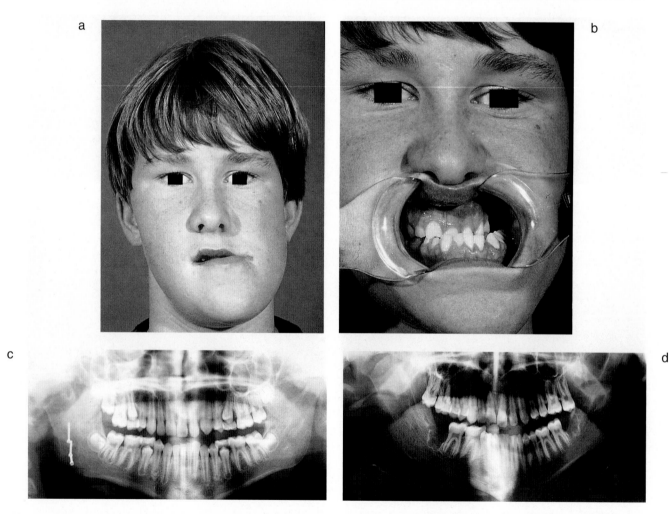

FIGURE 42.3 (a,b) Twelve-year-old boy following reconstruction of the right condyle with a costochondral graft. Excessive growth overshoot 3 years after reconstruction with lateral deviation of the mandible to the left. (c,d) X-ray of the patient immediately and 3 years postoperatively demonstrating the massive mandibular shift.

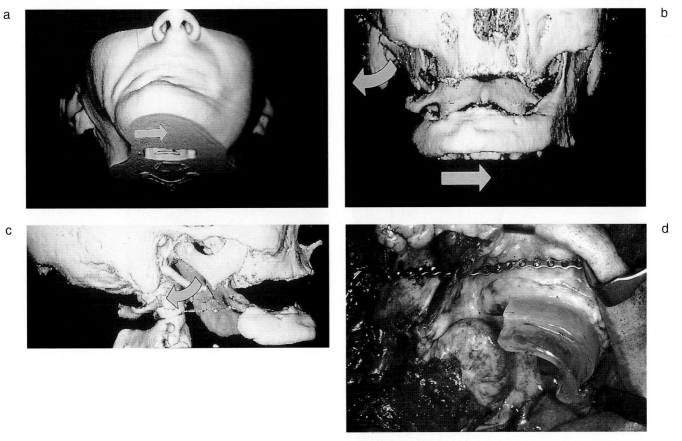

FIGURE 42.4 (a) Three-dimensional soft tissue imaging before reconstruction of a defect of the right ascending ramus demonstrates lateral shift to the left side necessary for symmetrical chin projection. (b,c) Whereas the major mandibular segment has to be repositioned laterally to the left, the condyle has to be repositioned posteriorly and laterally. (d) In cases with the condyle still in situ, the condyle first is mobilized and the muscle process resected. After-ward, the condyle can be kept in its original position with the mini-plate temporarily fixed to the maxilla. Then the length of the ascending ramus and the mandible can be estimated. Additional prosthetic devices fixed to the maxilla with screws in the midline may help to get an orientation for sagittal extension of bone grafts in patients with large mandibular reconstructions.

After positioning of the remaining condyle, plate fixation to the vascular graft should be performed at least with two or three screws at the condyle. Otherwise, removal of the condyle with replacement by the vascularized bone graft must be considered. Alternatively, the remaining condyle may be fixed to the proximal aspect of the vascularized graft according to Hidalgo.[19,20] If a small condyle shows severe signs of osteoporosis with unsecure bone hold, the condyle should also be removed and replaced by the graft. In grafts with sufficient bone volume, an inlay-type osteotomy may facilitate fixation of the remaining short condyle with positioning screws (Figure 42.5).

Several donor sites are useful for reconstruction of the ascending ramus and condyle.

The iliac crest is suitable in cases necessitating reconstruction of larger aspects of the ascending ramus and condyle including potentially tooth-bearing areas of the posterior mandibular body. In these situations, the distal portions of the new mandible allow for insertion of dental implants (Figure 42.6). The grafts are mostly harvested from the ipsilateral hip, if ipsilateral donor site vessels are present. The pedicle then arises at the angle and an appropriate curvature of the graft is given. Defects of the ramus and condyle may be reconstructed with grafts from the contralateral hip, if the recipient vessels are on the contralateral side and the vascular pedicle is to be positioned at the chin area (Figures 42.7 and 42.8).

The ascending ramus may also be reconstructed with grafts from the scapula region which may offer a lower complication rate at the donor site and less graft volume compared to iliac crest grafts.[15,20,21–24] The thin bone with a thicker lateral scapula border can easily be modeled to replace parts of

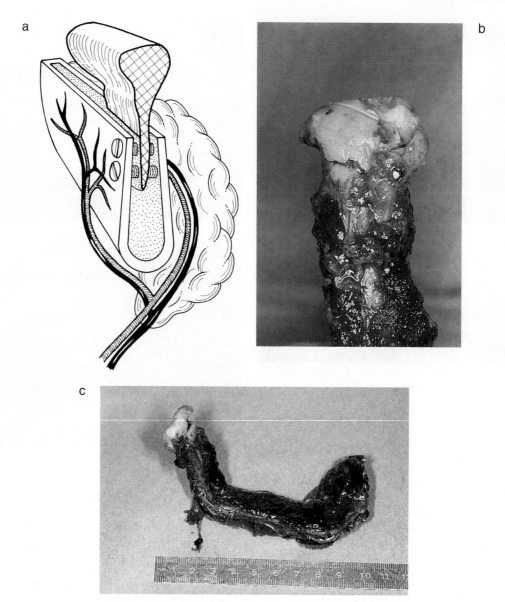

FIGURE 42.5 (a) If the condyle is still in situ, it may be fixed to a vascularized iliac crest graft with positioning screws after preparation of an inlay-like osteotomy. (b,c) The residual condyle is too small to be fixed in situ to a fibula graft. Therefore, the condyle was removed and fixed to the cranial aspect of a vascularized fibula graft. Care must be taken not to fracture thin aspects of the brittle bone during screw osteosynthesis.

the ascending ramus and the condyle. The volume of the necessary soft tissue component can be tailored individually ranging from different amounts of adherent muscle cuffs to a larger portion of deepithelialized soft tissue or even two separate skin flaps for extraoral and intraoral lining (Figures 42.9 and 42.10). The inferior aspect of the scapula tip forms the new condyle with a vascular pedicle located near the mandibular angle (Figure 42.11).

Today, fibula grafts are to be regarded as the grafts of choice for reconstruction even of smaller aspects of the ascending ramus and condyle. They can be harvested simultaneously and without changing the patient's position on the operating table. Due to the segmental vascularization, various osteotomies are possible to match the shape of the original mandible. With experience, the osteotomies can be performed so that the fibula matches the mandibular angle and especially the slight outward deviation of the ascending ramus and the condyle in a cranial direction.

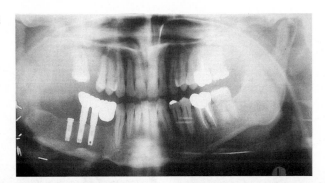

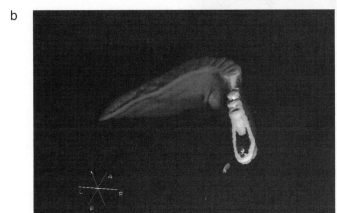

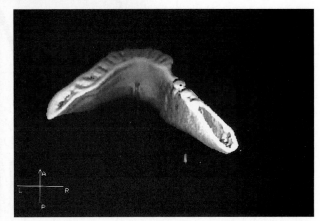

FIGURE 42.6 (a) X-ray following reconstruction of the right body and ascending ramus with a vascularized iliac crest graft, dental implant insertion, and prosthodontic treatment with implant-fixed dentures. (b,c) Three-dimensional CT imaging of the posterior aspect of the newly formed body of the mandible shows sufficient bone volume for insertion of dental implants. This sufficient bone volume with bicortical bone structure and a large volume of medullary bone is also given in the ascending ramus.

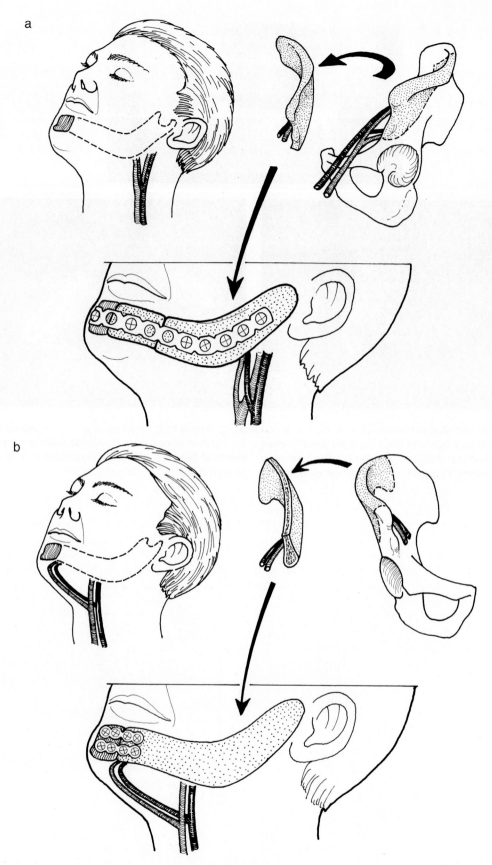

FIGURE 42.7 (a) In situations with a bone defect at the side of the recipient vessels, the iliac crest graft is harvested from the ipsilateral hip. (b) If the vessels are located at the contralateral side, the contralateral hip may be used to locate the vascular pedicle anteriorly.

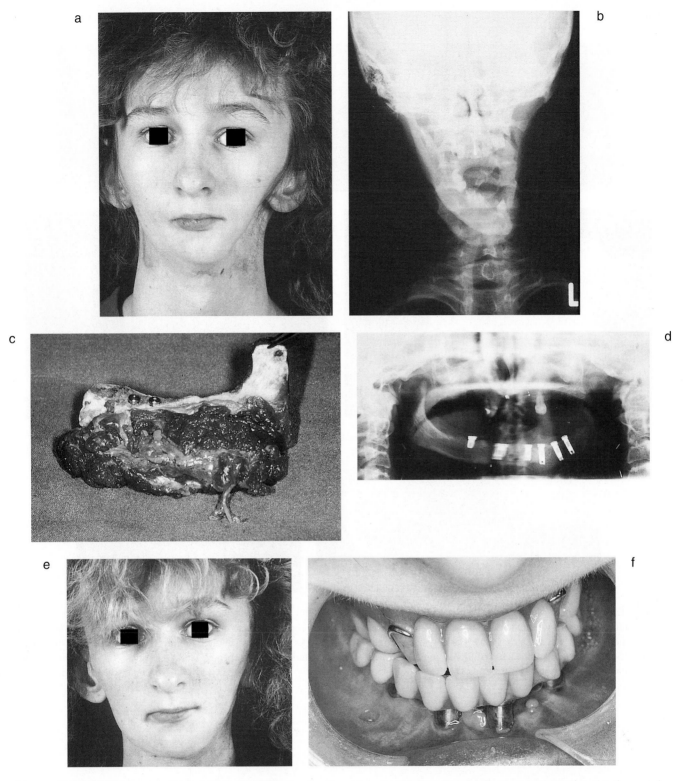

FIGURE 42.8 (a,b) Sixteen-year-old female patient following hemi-mandibulectomy, full-dose chemotherapy, and radiotherapy for os-teogenic sarcoma of the left mandible. (c) For reconstruction, a vas-cularized iliac crest graft was harvested from the ipsilateral hip. At that time, dental implants were inserted primarily. (d) Postoperative x-ray. (e) Situation 1 year following reconstruction showing an ad-equate transverse relationship of the mandibular profile. (f) Intra-oral situation after prosthodontic reconstruction with implant-borne dentures.

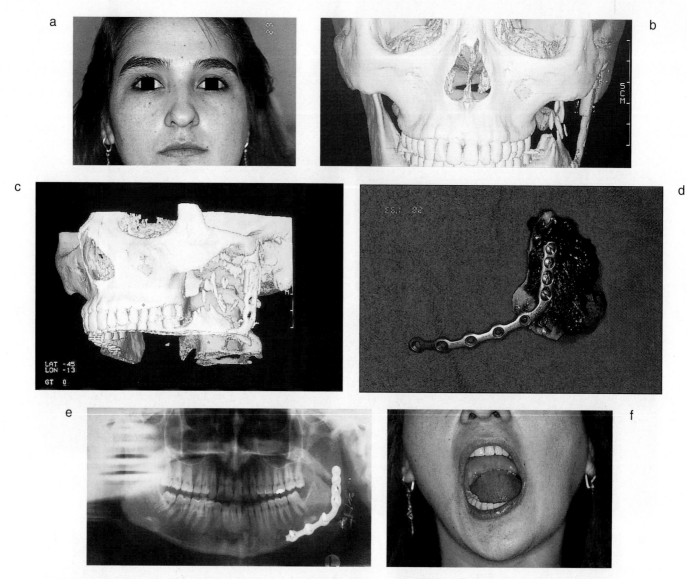

FIGURE 42.9 (a) Clinical view of a patient following resection of a bone tumor necessitating temporary reconstruction of the condyle and ascending ramus with a plate and condylar prosthesis. Slight soft tissue deficit in projection of the left preauricular region. (b,c) Three-dimensional reconstruction of CT scan. (d) The preexisting plate was used for fixation of a vascularized scapula bone graft. (e) Postoperative clinical aspect of the scapula graft for reconstruction of the condyle and the ascending ramus. (f) Postoperative aspect with undisturbed mouth-opening ability. (Patient operated on together with Dr. Hartmann, MD, DDS, at Dortmund City Hospital.)

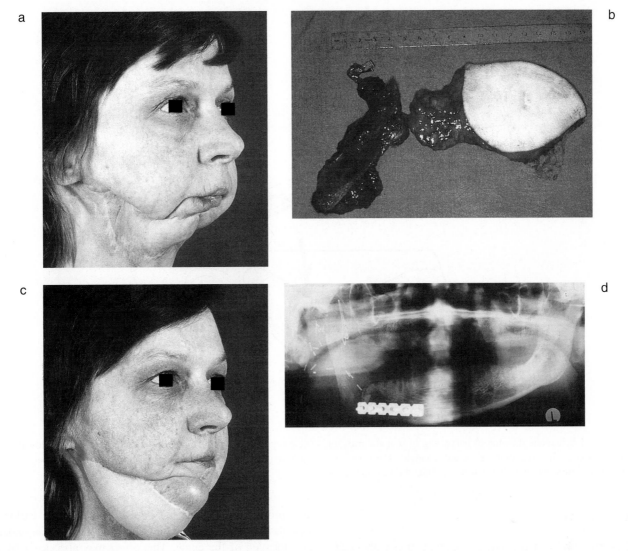

FIGURE 42.10 (a) Clinical situation of a female patient following hemimandibulectomy and postoperative irradiation. (b) Osteocutaneous parascapular flap for reconstruction of the posterior aspect of the mandible and volume augmentation. (c) Postoperative clinical aspect of the patient. (d) Postoperative x-ray. Bone graft fixation was performed with stable reconstruction plate because of the large flap volume.

The fibula must be positioned in such a manner that the vascular pedicle again points toward the donor site vessels in the angular region. The vascular pedicle then runs along the inner or posterior side of the bone. In larger segments of the ascending ramus to be reconstructed, the proximal end of the fibula can be shaped round and placed in the condylar fossa. The desired angle of the mandibular graft is positioned at a region where the pedicle enters the bone.[19] Pedicle length can be increased by removing the proximal part of the fibula subperiostally (Figure 42.12). A resorbable suture or wire positioned at the newly shaped condyle may be helpful for temporary fixation of the fibula in the temporal fossa by fixation of the suture or wire at the zygomatic arch. This type of fixation does not prevent caudal dislocation of the neocondyle postoperatively.

When a fibula graft offers the best solution for bony reconstructions but an additional soft tissue pedicle is needed, the indication may be given to combine a fibula graft with a radial forearm flap, which also allows considerable independence in positioning of the bone and the soft tissues. A precondition for this procedure is an adequate number of recipient vessels. Although it may be considered to anastomose a fibula flap at the distal side of the radial forearm flap or vice versa, there may be an increased risk to lose two flaps with one vascular complication (Figure 42.13).

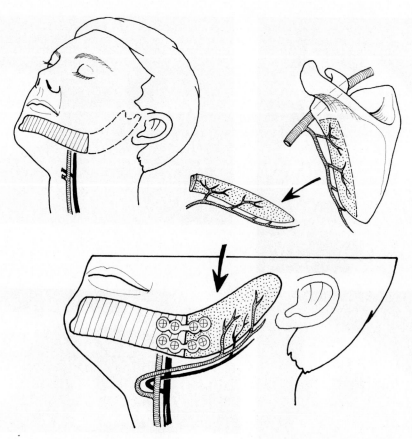

FIGURE 42.11 Schematic drawing of harvesting of scapula graft for reconstruction of the ascending ramus and condyle. The tip of the scapula is positioned in the temporal fossa. Thus the vascular pedi- cle can point toward the angle or may also be positioned toward the midline if the recipient vessels are located on the contralateral side.

Discussion

Indications for isolated condylar reconstruction with vascularized grafts are rare if existent at all. If given indications, microvascular reconstruction of the ascending ramus and condyle is a challenge for the reconstructive surgeon, although the general failure in lateral or posterior mandibular defects is significantly lower compared to anterior mandibular defects.[15]

The graft selection has to be made with regard to the amount of bone necessary and the possible need for additional soft tissues. In our hands, the free fibula graft is to be regarded as the graft of choice for isolated bone defects. Additional soft tissue defects in composite reconstructions may be tailored with flaps from the scapula region. In selected cases and with regard to the patient's general condition and the recipient vessels, a two-flap reconstruction with a fibula and a radial forearm flap may be indicated.

The aesthetic goal of posterior mandibular bone reconstruction is to provide a sufficient symmetrical sagittal chin projection and an adequate contouring of the mandibular angle. It has to be kept in mind that the distance between the condylar head and the angle is about 5 cm in general, and the skin projection of the angle is slightly below the earlobe. Lengthening of the ascending ramus may result in an unnatural location of the angle. This effect may also occur by a gradual caudal displacement of the neocondyle of the bone graft, although in most cases no functional impairment occurs. This effect does not occur if the condyle is still present and grafts can be sufficiently fixed to it. However, efforts should be made for the correct anatomic positioning of the bone graft in the temporomandibular fossa and to provide a bilateral support of mandibular motion.

To overcome the tendencies for dislocation of the neocondyle and the ascending ramus, we more often keep patients in intermaxillary immobilization for 14 days in accordance with other authors.[16,19,20,22] Afterward, postoperative functional therapy in cooperation with the Department of Physiotherapy is performed.

We do not feel it is necessary to fix additional temporomandibular joint prostheses on the cranial aspect of a vascularized graft.[23]

Also, mouth opening does not seem to depend greatly on positioning of the cranial aspect of a posterior bone graft, but rather on scar contraction of the soft tissues. Therefore, the

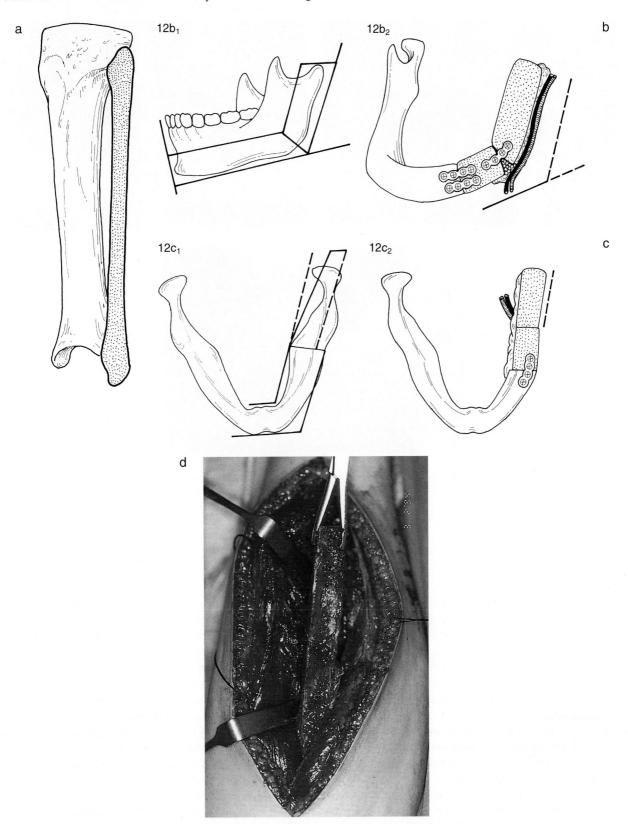

FIGURE 42.12 (a) The ipsilateral leg is chosen for reconstruction of a left-side defect. The vascular pedicle can be elongated by removal of proximal aspects of the fibula bone subperiostally. (b) To resemble the angle of the mandible, an osteotomy at the cranial and lin-gual aspect of the fibula has to be made. The whole length of the ascending ramus averages about 5 cm. (c) Note the outward devia-tion of the ascending ramus. (d) Intraoperative aspect of a fibula af-ter distal and proximal osteotomy.

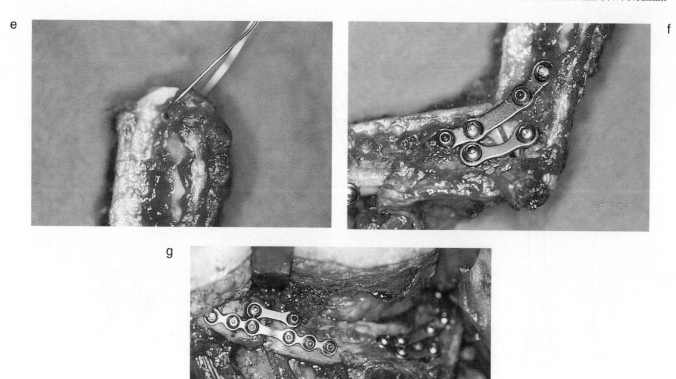

FIGURE 42.12 *Continued.* (e) A wire fixation of the neocondyle in the fibula may facilitate positioning of the graft. (f,g) Fixation of the fibula to the residual mandibular stump and fixation of the osteotomy sites is performed by miniplate osteosynthesis.

indication for resection of scars and, for example, additional intraoral soft tissue reconstructions has to be kept in mind.

Although miniplate fixation is to be regarded as the treatment of choice for fixation of vascularized bone grafts, in patients with free mandibular reconstructions and large graft volumes (i.e., composite grafts), rigid fixation of the graft may help to maintain the position of the bone in the fossa and avoid lateral displacement.[24]

Metatarsal grafts have been used for mandibular reconstruction.[25] Experimental transplantation of vascularized second metatarsal joints show better results than reconstruction of the condyle with nonvascularized joint surfaces and demonstrate a reshaping of the new condyle during functional load.[26] In addition to possible donor site complications, vascularized metatarsal grafts may not demonstrate better clinical results than nonvascularized grafts.[27,28] Concerning the growth capability of vascularized grafts, additional factors, like the age of the patient at the date of operation, may in-

fluence the growth potential, as has been demonstrated for nonvascularized costochondral rib grafts.[29]

Although nonvascularized costochondral grafts have to be regarded as treatment modalities of choice for condylar reconstruction, in selected patients, vascularized bone and composite grafts allow for an individualized reconstruction with special attention to aesthetic and functional components. Perspectives for joint reconstruction also in the temporomandibular joint may be seen in further technical refinements of nonvascularized and vascularized bone grafts. Further investigation of timing of reconstruction and influence of other factors determining growth capacity of different bone grafts is necessary. Histopathological mechanisms of joints allografting in animal experiments are well understood. Clinical application is bound to additional information on duration and adverse effects of immunosuppression or to development of new immunosuppressive agents and may offer interesting perspectives for the future.[30–32]

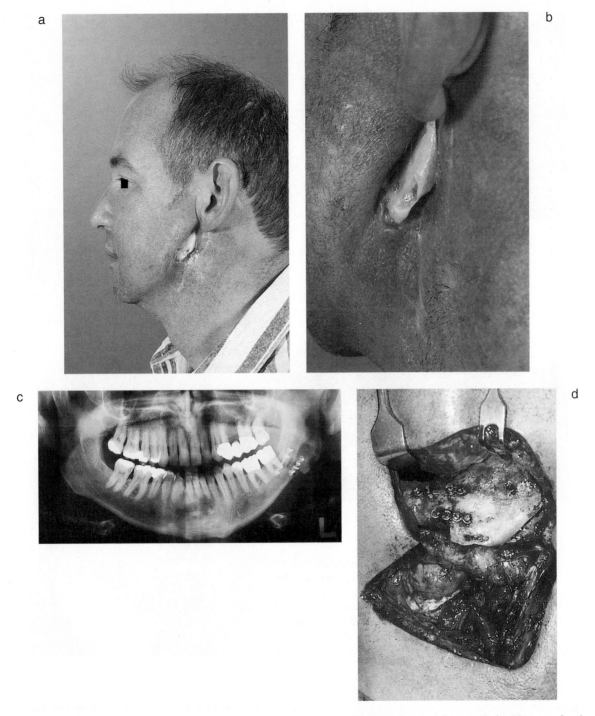

FIGURE 42.13 (a,b) Patient with osteoradionecrosis at the left angle of the mandible. (c,d) X-ray and intraoperative situation of the patient with two microplates for fixation of a temporary osteotomy in situ. In addition to the need for vascularized bone grafts, there also is a lack of soft tissues due to the radiation and previous operations.

Continued.

e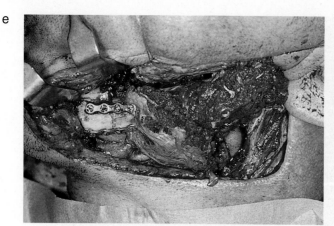

f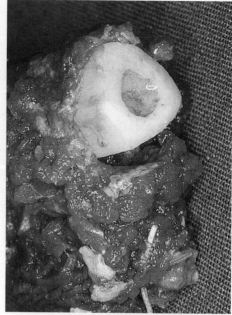

g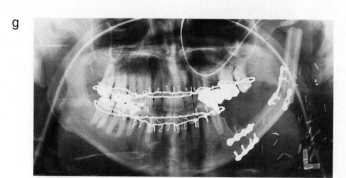

h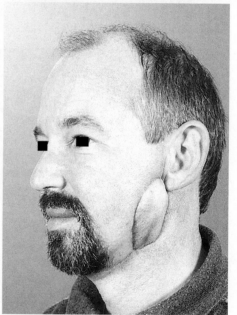

FIGURE 42.13 *Continued*. (e) The fibula graft is fixed anteriorly with two miniplates. (f) The proximal aspect of the mandible is removed subperiosteally. The neocondyle is rounded and placed in the temporal fossa. (g) An intermaxillary immobilization is performed for 2 weeks to keep the condyle in place. (h) Postoperative situation of the patient 6 weeks postoperatively shows adequate projection of the fibula in the soft tissue. The soft tissue was reconstructed by a radial forearm flap.

References

1. van der Kuijl B. Current role of conventional radiography and CT in TMJ treatment planning. Abstract, International TMJ Conference, September 1–3, Groningen, The Netherlands; 1994.
2. Rehrmann A. Osteoplastik am kindlichen Unterkiefer. *Langenbecks Arch Klin Chir*. 1961;299:184–188.
3. Dingmann RO, Grabb WL. Reconstruction of both mandibular condyles with metatarsal bone grafts. *Plast Reconstr Surg*. 1964;34:441–451.
4. Ware WH. Growth centre transplantation in temporomandibular joint surgery. In: Walker RV, ed. *Transactions of the 3rd International Conference on Oral Surgery*. London; 1970:148–157.
5. Kenett S. Temporomandibular joint ankylosis: the rationale for grafting in the young patient. *J Oral Surg*. 1973;31:744–748.
6. Matukas KJ, Szymela VF, Schmidt JF. Surgical treatment of bony anklyosis in a child using a composite cartilage-bone iliac crest graft. *J Oral Surg*. 1980;38:903–905.
7. Kummoona R. Chondro-osseous iliac crest graft for one stage reconstruction of the ankylosed TMJ in children. *J Maxillofac Surg*. 1986;14:215–220.
8. Lindqvist C, Pihakari A, Tasanen A, et al. Autogenous costo-chondral grafts in temporomandibular joint arthroplasty. A sur-

vey of 66 arthroplasties in 60 patients. *J Maxillofac Surg.* 1986; 14:143–149.

9. Svensson B, Feldmann G, Rindler A. Early surgical-orthodontic treatment of mandibular hypoplasia in juvenile chronic arthritis. *J Craniomaxillofac Surg.* 1993;21:67–75.

10. Wolford LM, Cottrell DA, Henry C. Sternoclavicular grafts for temporomandibular joint reconstruction. *J Oral Maxillofac Surg.* 1994;52:119–128.

11. Ellis E III, Carlson DS. Histologic comparison of the costochondral sternoclavicular and temporomandibular joints during growth in *Macaca mulatta*. *J Oral Maxillofac Surg.* 1986;44:312.

12. Guyuron B, Lasa CI. Unpredictable growth pattern of costochondral graft. *Plast Reconstr Surg.* 1992;90(5):880–886.

13. Siemssen SO. Temporomandibular arthroplasty by transfer of the sterno-clavicular joint on a muscle pedicle. *Br J Plast Surg.* 1982;35:225.

14. Reid CD, Taylor GI, Waterhouse N. The clavicular head of pectoralis major musculocutaneous free flap. *Br J Plast Surg.* 1986; 39:57.

15. Boyd JB. Use of reconstruction plates in conjunction with soft-tissue free flaps for oromandibular reconstruction. *Head Neck Reconstr.* 1994;21(1):69–77.

16. Buchbinder D, Urken ML, Vickery C, Weinberg H, Biller HF. Bone contouring and fixation in functional, primary microvascular mandibular reconstruction. *Head Neck.* 1991;13(3):191–199.

17. Shenaq SM, Klebuc MJA. TMJ reconstruction during vascularized bone graft transfer to the mandible. *Microsurgery.* 1994; 15(5):299–304.

18. Shenaq SM, Klebuc MJA. The iliac crest microsurgical free flap in mandibular reconstruction. *Clin Plast Surg.* 1994;21(1):37–44.

19. Hidalgo DA. Fibula free flap mandibular reconstruction. *Head Neck Reconstr.* 1994;21(1):25–35.

20. Hidalgo DA. Condyle transplantation in free flap mandible reconstruction. *Plast Reconstr Surg.* 1994;93(4):770–781.

21. Swartz WM, Banis JC, Newton ED, Ramasastry SS, Jones NF, Acland R. The osteocutaneous scapular flap for mandibular and maxillary reconstruction. *Plast Reconstr Surg.* 1986;77(4):530–545.

22. Urken ML, Weinberg H, Vickery C, Buchbinder D, Lawson W, Biller HF. Oromandibular reconstruction using microvascular composite free flaps. *Arch Otolaryngol Head Neck Surg.* 1991;117:733–744.

23. Lyberg T, Olstad OA. The vascularized fibular flap for mandibular reconstruction. *J Craniomaxillofac Surg.* 1991;19:113–118.

24. Schmelzeisen R, Rahn BA, Brennwald J. Fixation of vascularized bone grafts. *J Craniomaxillofac Surg.* 1993;21:113.

25. Watson DE. Condylar replacement with a metatarsal bone implant. Case report. *Aust Dent J.* 1990;35(4):362–363.

26. Hidding J, Habel G, Becker R. Kiefergelenkersatz durch ein mikrovaskulär reanastomosiertes mittelfußknochen-transplantat. *Fortschr Kiefer Gesichtschir.* 1990;35:25–27.

27. Dattilo DJ, Granick MS, Soteranos GS. Free vascularized whole joint transplant for reconstruction of the temporomandibular joint (a preliminary case report). *J Oral Maxillofac Surg.* 1986; 44:227.

28. Moos KH. The correction of the mandibular defect in hemifacial microsomia. *J Craniomaxillofac Surg.* 1994;22(suppl 1):8.

29. James D. The early management of hemifacial microsomia. *J Craniomaxillofac Surg.* 1994;22(suppl 1):7–8.

30. Goldberg VM. Experimental models for joint allografting. In: Aebi M, Regazzoni P, eds. *Bone Transplantation.* Berlin: Springer-Verlag; 1989:68–75.

31. Goldberg VM, Herndon CH, Lance E. Biology of osteoarticular allografts. In: Aebi M, Regazzoni P, eds. *Bone Transplantation.* Berlin: Springer-Verlag; 1989:52–58.

32. Schmelzeisen R. Experimental reconstruction of mandibular defects with vascularized allogenic bone grafts. PhD thesis; 1991.

43
Orbital Reconstruction

Beat Hammer

Orbital reconstruction may indicate either the replacement of missing segments of the orbital skeleton, reduction of displaced fragments, or both. The indications for surgical intervention are trauma, posttraumatic deformities, defects after tumor resection, and malformations.[1] Despite the considerable differences among these problems, there are commonly applied principles. In this chapter, immediate posttraumatic orbital reconstruction is discussed as a model for orbital reconstruction. The fracture patterns vary considerably in their location as well as in their degree of severity. A formal reconstruction is necessary in the case of severe disruption of the orbital frame or in the presence of a large defect in the orbital walls.

Basic Principles

The orbit is a pyramid-shaped structure containing the ocular globe with its motor apparatus. In all situations, the goal of reconstruction is to restore the normal shape and volume. The orbit is composed of seven individual bones. For surgical purposes however, a differentiation between orbital frame and the orbital pyramid, or internal orbit is adequate (Figure 43.1).

The posterior part of the medial wall is an area of special surgical interest and is called the "key area" for the following reasons:

- It is, together with the lateral wall, the main support for the anterior projection of the globe. The function of the two walls has been compared to a pair of cupped hands holding the globe in its forward position.[2]
- Being a paper-thin structure, it is often damaged in orbital injuries.
- Clinical experience has shown that repair of fractures with an intact "key area" is technically much easier than repair of fractures involving this part of the orbit.[3] Therefore, the first step in repair of complex orbital injuries is repair of the key area as described below.

Orbital reconstruction requires adequate exposure, for which complete subperiostal dissection is a most important aspect.

Diagnosis

CT examination is the cornerstone of orbital fracture diagnosis, permitting an exact and reproducible visualization of every part of the bony orbit as well as the adjacent structures in several planes. The threshold for performing a CT examination should be low, because the clinical signs indicating complex injuries may be discrete. Optimal diagnosis can be made from high-resolution scans in an axial and coronal plane, with a slice thickness of 2 mm. In severely traumatized and unconscious patients, however, coronal scans are often not obtainable because they require retroinclination of the head. Nevertheless, axial scans usually provide sufficient information to clearly identify the injured parts of the orbit and therefore assess the need for orbital reconstruction.

Three-dimensional formatted CT scans give excellent information about the degree of fragmentation to the orbital frame, as well as the position of the fragments. The software available today however is not yet able to correctly provide images regarding the status of the orbital walls. Axial cuts therefore remain indispensable.

Exposure

For major orbital reconstruction, complete subperiosteal dissection up to the apex is necessary. It is done with a combination of a coronal and a mid-lower eyelid incision. The coronal incision can safely be extended far enough to allow visualization of the entire zygomatic body and the arch back to its root.[4]

Subperiosteal dissection of the internal orbit is usually started at the superior lateral part, and is then carried down

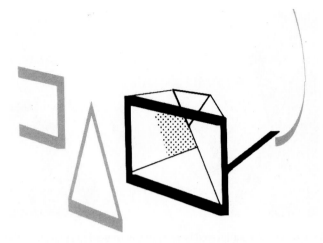

FIGURE 43.1 For surgical purposes, the orbit can be divided into two components: orbital frame (dark black) and orbital pyramid. The shaded area represents the posterior medial wall (key area). (Reproduced with permission from: Hammer, B. *Orbital Fractures: Diagnosis, Operative Treatment, Secondary Corrections.* Hogrefe & Huber, 1995)

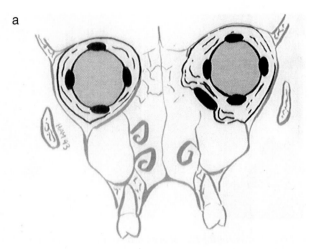

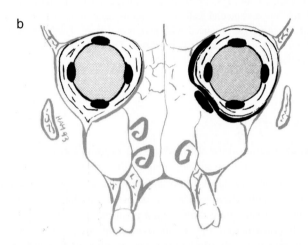

FIGURE 43.2 Schematic drawing of a coronal section through both orbits. The left orbit exhibits a defect involving both the floor and the medial wall. (a) Because of rupture the periorbit, intraperiorbital fat protrudes on both sides of the retractor, making visibility and access difficult. (b) A flexible sheet has been inserted, replacing the ruptured periorbit. It prevents further herniation of fat and improves visibility. (Reproduced with permission from: Hammer, B. *Orbital Fractures: Diagnosis, Operative Treatment, Secondary Corrections.* Hogrefe & Huber, 1995)

along the lateral orbital wall, thus exposing the articulation between the zygoma and the greater wing of the sphenoid. Dissection of the medial wall starts again at the orbital roof and proceeds inferiorly. If the deep part of the medial wall needs to be exposed, a superior marginotomy is advisable.[3,5] Finally, the inferior part of the orbit is exposed through the mid-eyelid incision, thus completing the circular dissection.

Key points to be considered in dissecting the internal orbit are these:

- The lateral canthal ligament is detached, whereas the medial ligament should be left attached to the bone if at all possible.
- Exposure of the posterior medial wall requires transection of the anterior ethmoid artery.
- The connective tissue of the inferior orbital fissure is sectioned to allow visualization of the posterior lower part of the orbit, which forms a triangular groove blending into this fissure.
- Visibility and access to the internal orbit are often a problem, owing to herniation of the intraperiorbital fat which then protrudes on both sides of the retractor. It can be considerably improved by inserting a flexible sheet into the orbit after completion of the dissection (Figure 43.2).[3,6] The sheet is passed from the coronal to the infraorbital incision. We use a resorbable sheet (polydioxanone, PDS Ethicon), which is left in situ as a bridging material for small defects between the bone grafts.
- After completion of the reconstruction, the detached soft tissues and especially the lateral canthal ligament need to be resuspended using subperiosteal face-lift techniques.[7]

Reconstruction Technique

Orbital reconstruction involves two basic steps:

- Reconstruction of the orbital frame and
- Reconstruction of the internal orbit.

The orbital frame is a part of the midface buttress system.[8] It is composed of the two orbital rings and the zygomatic arches, the two components forming a structure resembling the frame of eyeglasses.

Technically the reconstruction is initiated by reducing the zygoma, which constitutes the outer part of the frame (outer facial frame technique).[9] The most important landmark hereby

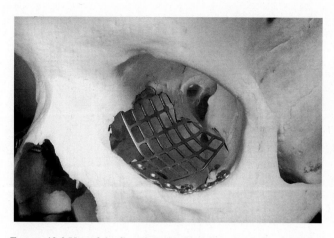

FIGURE 43.3 Use of the flag-shaped orbital floor plate (Synthes Maxillofacial, Paoli, PA) to reconstruct a large defect involving the orbital floor and medial wall and extending back to the posterior third of the orbit. (Reproduced with permission from: Hammer, B. *Orbital Fractures: Diagnosis, Operative Treatment, Secondary Corrections*. Hogrefe & Huber, 1995)

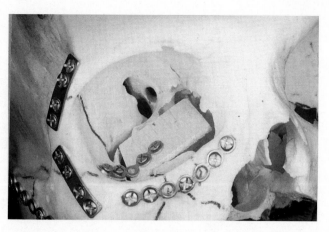

FIGURE 43.4 A cantilevered bone graft can be used to reconstruct the key area. It provides a stable basis for further bone grafts, which can be wedged in without fixation. (Reproduced with permission from: Hammer, B. *Orbital Fractures: Diagnosis, Operative Treatment, Secondary Corrections*. Hogrefe & Huber, 1995)

is the lateral orbital wall, where the zygoma forms a long articulation with the greater wing of the sphenoid.

The second most important landmark is the zygomatic arch.[10] Both sites need to be exposed simultaneously to allow for exact three-dimensional positioning of the zygoma.

Reconstruction of the naso-ethmoid area (inner orbital frame) varies according to the type of injury.[11] Depending on the degree of fragmentation of the canthal ligament-bearing (central) fragment, simple stabilization with plates or a transnasal canthopexy is indicated.

Reconstruction of the internal orbit is indicated in defects extending into the posterior third of the orbit and/or involving two or more orbital walls. These defects are complicated by the following facts:

- The posterior bony ledge is very small and therefore does not offer support for grafts.
- Disruption of the periorbit with fat protruding on both sides of the retractors makes exposure and visibility difficult.

Inadequate reconstruction of these defects results in serious cosmetic and functional defects, of which the secondary correction is difficult if not impossible. It is therefore of utmost importance to identify these defects in CT scans and to perform a meticulous primary repair.

The preferred material for repair is autologous bone (calvaria or iliac crest), eventually combined with a titanium plate to support the grafts. It is important to realize that these large defects cannot be reconstructed with a single graft. With the techniques presently available, it would be very difficult to exactly tailor it to the complex shape of such a defect, not to

mention the difficulties of inserting such a graft into the orbit. To overcome this problem, the defect is reconstructed with several smaller grafts. The first one reconstructs the key area and serves as a platform to support the additional grafts.[1] This first graft is either a specially designed mesh plate (Synthes Maxillofacial, Paoli, PA) orbital floor plate; (Figure 43.3) or a cantilevered bone graft (Figure 43.4). This rigid fixation technique for the internal orbit allows predictable three-dimensional restoration of the orbital shape and volume. Additional bone grafts are inserted to complete the reconstruction. They usually can be wedged in without further fixation.

At completion of the reconstruction, the globe should protrude by about 2 mm to compensate for later volume loss after resolution of the swelling. The procedure is completed by a forced duction test to make sure that no periorbital tissue is entrapped between the grafts, which could cause motility problems.

Case Example (Figure 43.5)

A 21-year-old man was hit in the face by an iron piece of a truck brake, causing a complex fracture of the right orbit involving the floor and the medial wall back to the apex. Inspite of the severe bony destruction, the eye was intact. Reconstruction was performed using a flag-shaped orbital plate (Synthes Maxillofacial, Paoli, PA) in combination with calvarial bone grafts. Healing was uneventful. Diplopia in downward gaze gradually resolved over a period of 9 months without any additional surgery.

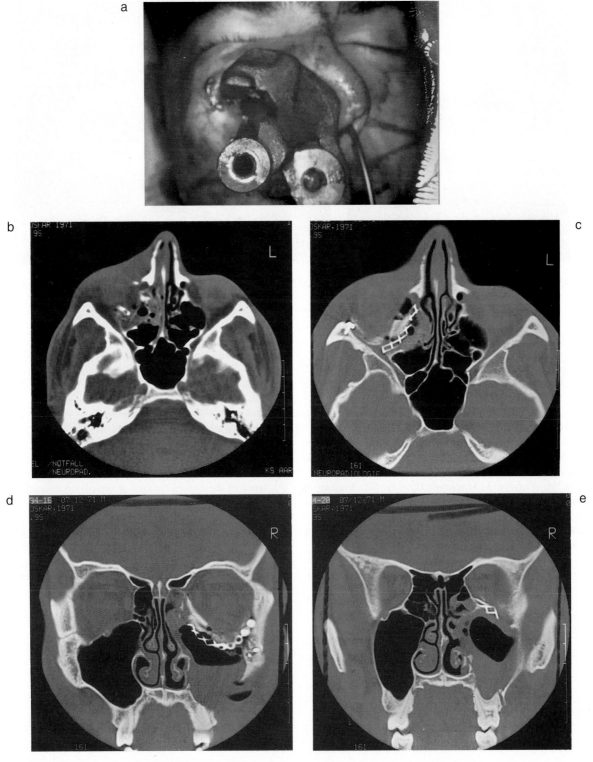

FIGURE 43.5 (a) The patient on admission, with a heavy iron piece impaled in the face. (b) Axial CT scan showing complete destruction of the orbital floor. (c) Axial and (d,e) coronal CT scans show-ing reconstruction of the right orbit with a titanium plate and cal-varial bone grafts.

Continued.

f 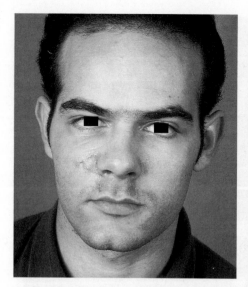 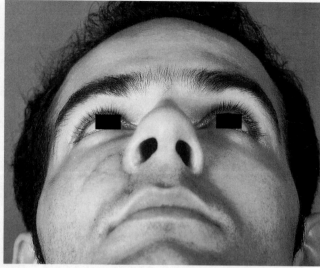 g

FIGURE 43.5 *Continued.* (f,g) The patient 10 months after the accident. Normal eye position and binocular vision have been restored.

References

1. Manson PN, Glassman D, Iliff N, Vanderkolk C, Dufresne C. Rigid fixation of fractures of the internal orbit. *Plast Surg Forum* 1988;11:80–82.
2. Kawamoto HK. Late posttraumatic enophthalmos: a correctable deformity? *Plast Reconstr Surg.* 1982;69:423–430.
3. Hammer B. *Orbital Fractures: Diagnosis, Operative Treatment, Secondary Corrections.* Bern, Göttingen, Toronto, Seattle: Hogrefe & Huber; 1995.
4. Stutzin JM, Wagstrom L, Kawamoto H, Wolfe SA. Anatomy of the frontal branch of the facial nerve: the significance of the temporal fat pad. *Plast Reconstr Surg.* 1989;83:265–271.
5. Sullivan WG, Kawamoto HK. Periorbital marginotomies: anatomy and application. *J Craniomaxillofac Surg.* 1989;17:206–209.
6. Glassmann RD, Petty P, Vanderkolk C, Iliff N. Techniques for improved visibility and lid protection in orbital explorations. *J Craniofac Surg.* 1990;1:69–71.
7. Philips JH, Gruss JS, Wells MD, Chollet A. Periosteal suspension of the lower eyelid and cheek following subciliary exposure of facial fractures. *Plast Reconstr Surg.* 1991;88:145–148.
8. Manson PN, Hoope JE, Su CT. Structural pillars of the facial skeleton: an approach to the management of Le Fort fractures. *Plast Reconstr Surg.* 1980;66:54–61.
9. Gruss JS, Bubak PJ, Egbert MA. Craniofacial fractures. An algorithm to optimize results. *Clin Plast Surg.* 1992;19:195–206.
10. Gruss JS, Van Wyck L, Philips JH, Antonyshyn O. The importance of the zygomatic arch in complex midfacial fracture repair and correction of posttraumatic orbitozygomatic deformities. *Plast Reconstr Surg.* 1990;85:878–890.
11. Markowitz BL, Manson PN, Sargent L, Vanderkolk CA, Yaremchuk M, Glassman D, Crawley WA. Management of the medial canthal tendon in nasoethmoid orbital fractures: the importance of the central fragment in classification and treatment. *Plast Reconstr Surg.* 1991;87:843–853.

44

Nasal Reconstruction Using Bone Grafts and Rigid Internal Fixation

Patrick K. Sullivan, Mika Varma, and Arlene A. Rozzelle

Traditionally, reconstruction of the nasal supporting structure has been achieved with septal or auricular cartilage grafts or a combination of the two. Bone graft nasal reconstruction is advantageous, however, when significant structural support is needed or when cartilage donor sites are inadequate. The technique of bone graft nasal reconstruction has evolved over time.[1–7]

It has often been thought that adequate stabilization of the graft is achieved with complementary shaping of the recipient site, the inner surface of the graft, or both, aided by the compressive forces of the overlying nasal soft tissue.[2,8] The underlying bone may merely be "freshened," it may be smoothed,[2,4,6,8] or it may actually be flattened by resecting the curved surface with an osteotome and applying the flat inner surface of the graft to it.[2,9–11] Complementary grooves and ridges in the graft and recipient site have also been used.[3] The inner surface of the graft may also be somewhat hollowed to fit the convexity of the nasal dorsum.[4,9]

However, wire stabilization[3,4] and screw fixation[5,7,10,12,13] have also been advocated. In the long term, two factors regarding bone graft survival may be applicable in the nose. First, increased bony surface area contact between the graft and the recipient bed improves bone volume conservation.[14] Second, rigid fixation of bone grafts has been shown to decrease resorption and thus theoretically improve long-term maintenance of the results.[15] In addition, rigid fixation of the bone graft in a cantilever fashion allows distant and sometimes multidirectional support.[1,7,16]

Nasal Bone Thickness

To facilitate rigid fixation of nasal bone grafts, we studied the thickness of the nasal bone in cadavers.[7] The nasal bone was thickest superiorly at the nasofrontal angle (an average of 6 mm thick in the midline) and became progressively thinner toward the tip. It was 3 to 4 mm thick in the critical area where screws would be placed for fixation (in the area 5 to 10 mm inferior to the nasofrontal angle). The male nasal bones were significantly thicker than the female nasal bones from the nasofrontal angle to the point 12 mm inferior to the nasofrontal angle (Figure 44.1).

Donor Sites

The commonly used bone donor sites are the cranium, iliac crest, and ribs. Each has advantages and disadvantages.[16] Cranial bone has advantages when only bony support is needed. The donor site is preferred because it is the least conspicuous and least painful, and it is close to the operative site. Membranous bone demonstrates less resorption than endochondral bone when grafted in the face.[17,18] Rigid fixation of a cranial bone graft with screws or plates is more easily accomplished due to the characteristics of the cranial bone, which includes ease of drilling and countersinking for lag screws due to the higher proportion of denser, noncompressible cortical to cancellous bone. Similarly, shaping of the graft is easier. However, when a great deal of bone is needed, it may be advantageous to harvest iliac crest bone or multiple ribs or multiple cranial grafts to form stacked-rib or stacked-cranial grafts. A single rib may be harvested if a relatively small amount of bone is required or if a bone graft with a cartilaginous extension is desired for tip support.

Fixation

Fixation has a number of advantages:[1,5–7,12,13]

1. Along with internal shaping, it controls the position of the graft, assuring that the correct alignment will be retained postoperatively. Without fixation, the exact position of the bone graft cannot always be predicted (Figure 44.2b).
2. Fixation of the cephalic end of the graft provides a true cantilever effect, which can improve tip projection and control.[1,7,12] The thicker soft tissue at the tip of the nose exerts more compressive force on the graft than the thin tis-

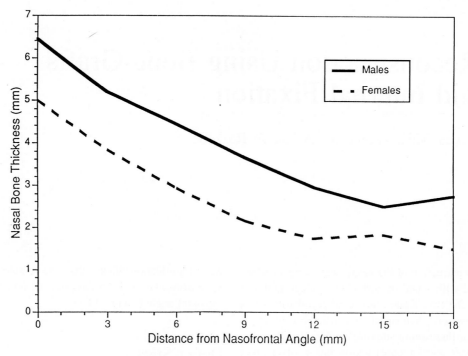

FIGURE 44.1 Nasal bone thickness. The nasal bone is thickest superiorly at the nasofrontal angle (approximately 6 mm) and gradually thins inferiorly. In the critical area where a screw would be placed for fixation (approximately 5 to 10 mm from the nasofrontal angle) it is approximately 3 to 4 mm thick. The nasal bone is significantly thicker in males than in females from the nasofrontal angle to approximately 12 mm inferior.

sue at the cephalic end of the nose (Figure 44.2a), especially if the domes of the alar cartilages are sutured over the tip of the graft. Without fixation, the cephalic end of the graft may be displaced anteriorly, creating a high, obtuse nasofrontal angle (Figure 44.2b).

3. A rib graft can provide lateral and tip soft tissue support by carving an extension on its cartilaginous end. Fixation is necessary to maintain the orientation of such a graft.[7]

4. Tiered rib or cranial grafts can be constructed by securing the grafts to each other with a screw and to the recipient site with screws, thus obviating the need for an iliac crest graft (with its troublesome donor site discomfort) when a large amount of bone is needed.

5. Finally, screw fixation has been shown to decrease graft resorption,[15] and thus, theoretically, it would help maintain the reconstruction in the long term.

Screw fixation has several possible disadvantages, including cost, palpability, the necessity of a stab incision at the fixation site, and possible artifact production on computed tomographic (CT) and magnetic resonance imaging (MRI) scans. The manufacturer's charge for one screw is approximately $35. Palpability can be avoided by using microscrews or carefully countersinking miniscrews. The stab incision has proved to be barely perceptible (Figure 44.3). Artifact production on CT and MRI scans should not be clinically significant if titanium hardware is used.[19]

Technique

We usually place the bone graft via an open rhinoplasty approach, although a closed approach has often been used successfully. A small stab incision, vertically oriented, is made inferior to the nasofrontal angle to allow for screw placement.

We use the lag-screw technique for graft fixation (Figure 44.4). This obliterates the space that may be maintained between the graft and recipient bone by a positional screw. When using a miniscrew, it is necessary to countersink the screw head. Recently, we have been using extra long microscrews that do not require countersinking, as the head will sit flush with the bone graft surface. In the critical area where the screw(s) will be placed for fixation (5 to 10 mm inferior to the nasofrontal angle) the nasal bone is 3 to 4 mm thick (Figure 44.1). Knowing the thickness of the nasal bone here and the thickness of the carved bone graft allows calculation of the correct length of the screw to be used. Optimally, the screw should capture the inner surface of the recipient bone, but not protrude into the nasal cavity.

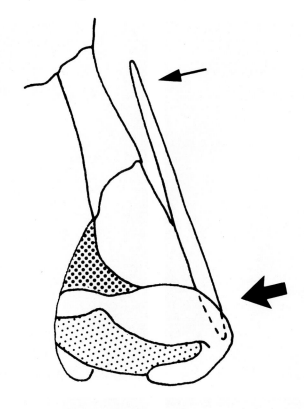

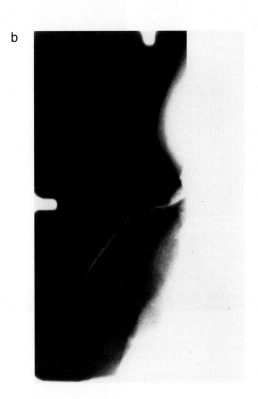

FIGURE 44.2 The nasal soft tissue at the tip is thicker than the cephalic soft tissue. This results in greater soft tissue compressive forces on the inferior end of the graft than on the cephalic end resulting in the situation seen in Figure 44.3a. (b) Lateral radiograph of a nasal bone graft without fixation. The superior end of the graft is not held down by the overlying soft tissue. This may result in a high, obtuse, nasofrontal angle and loss of bone-to-bone contact.

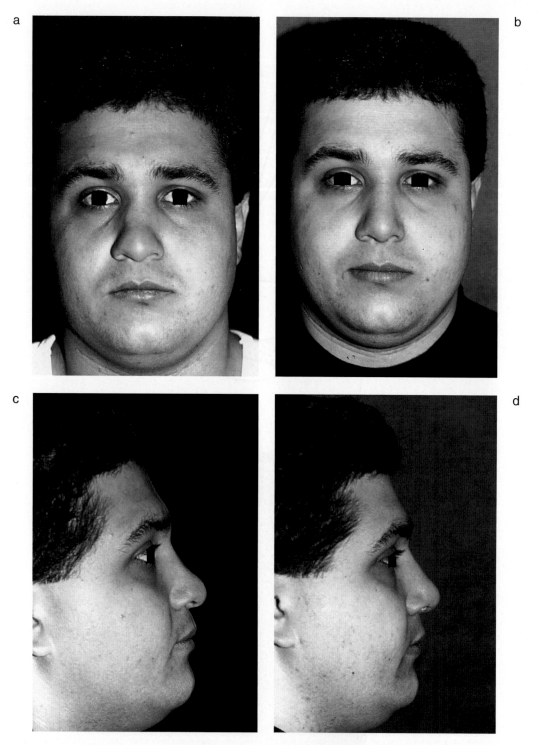

FIGURE 44.3 This patient presented, after multiple nasal injuries, with a lack of support in the middle and lower thirds (tip) of the nose. [Preoperative views on left (a,c,e,g).] A cranial bone graft was shaped and placed as a cantilever via an open rhinoplasty approach with the lag-screw technique. The domes of the alar cartilages were sutured over the inferior tip of the bone graft. Postoperative views are on the right (b,d,f,h). These show an improved nasofrontal angle, a straight, smooth dorsum, and improved tip projection.

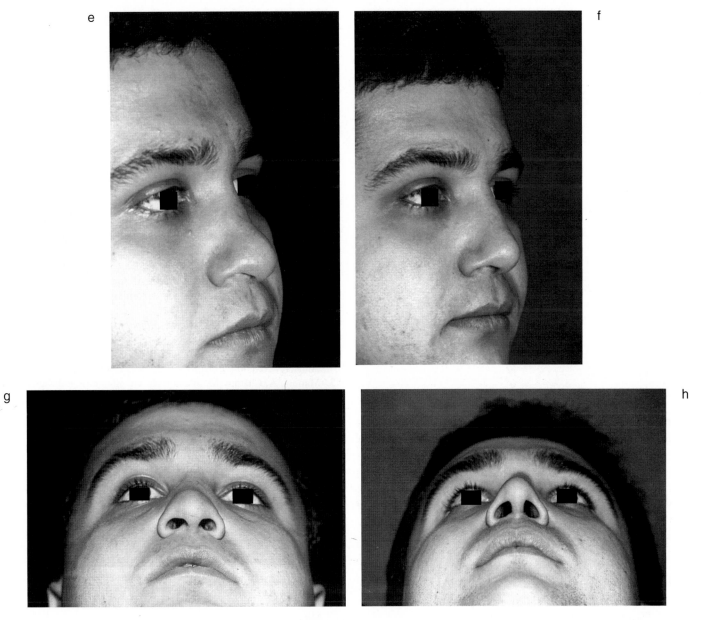

FIGURE 44.3 *Continued.*

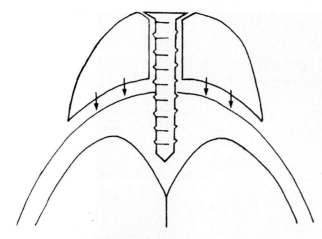

FIGURE 44.4 Lag-screw technique. The screw passes through a channel in the graft larger than the screw diameter, without the threads capturing in the graft, thus compressing it to the recipient bone as the screw threads capture in the recipient bone. The screw head is countersunk, if a miniscrew is used, so that it will not be palpable. Currently, we use microscrews that do not require countersinking.

Summary

Fixation using extra long microscrews and the lag technique is recommended to decrease resorption and to provide graft control with enhanced soft tissue structural support. The length of the screw can be calculated by adding the thickness of the graft to the thickness of the recipient nasal bone, which is 3 to 4 mm thick in the area (5 to 10 mm inferior to the nasofrontal angle) where the fixation screw is usually placed.

References

1. Millard DR. Total reconstructive rhinoplasty and a missing link. *Plast Reconstr Surg.* 1966;37:167.

2. Tessier P. Aesthetic aspects of bone grafting to the face. *Clin Plast Surg.* 1981;8:279.

3. Wheeler ES, Kawamoto HK, Zarem HA. Bone grafts for nasal reconstruction. *Plast Reconstr Surg.* 1982;69:9.

4. Stuzin JM, Kawamoto HK. Saddle nasal deformity. *Clin Plast Surg.* 1988;15:83.

5. Hallock GG. Cranial nasal bone grafts. *Aesth Plast Surg.* 1989;13:285.

6. Posnick JC, Seagle MB, Armstrong D. Nasal reconstruction with full-thickness cranial bone grafts and rigid internal fixation through a coronal incision. *Plast Reconstr Surg.* 1990;86:894.

7. Sullivan PK, Varma M, Rozzelle AA. Optimizing bone graft nasal reconstruction: a study of nasal bone shape and thickness. *Plast Reconstr Surg.* (in press).

8. Ortiz-Monasterio F, Ruas EJ. Cleft lip rhinoplasty: the role of bone and cartilage grafts. *Clin Plast Surg.* 1989;16:177.

9. McCarthy JG, Wood-Smith D. In: McCarthy JG, ed. *Plastic Surgery.* Philadelphia: WB Saunders: *Rhinoplasty.* 3:1886–1890.

10. Mayot D, Perrin C, Haas F, Brunet A. Apport du gresson osseux de voute cranienne dans les septorhinoplasties d'addition. *Ann Oto-Laryngol.* 1990;107:571.

11. Sheen JH, Sheen AP. *Aesthetic Rhinoplasty.* St. Louis: CV Mosby; 1987.

12. David DJ, Moore MH. Cantilever nasal bone grafting with miniscrew fixation. *Plast Reconstr Surg.* 1989;83:728.

13. Mariano A, Champy M. Fixation par vis miniaturisee des greffons osseax d'arete nasale. *Ann Chir Plast Esthetique.* 1986;31:381.

14. Whitaker LA. Biological boundaries: a concept in facial skeletal restructuring. *Clin Plast Surg.* 1989;16:1.

15. Phillips JH, Rahn B. Fixation effects on membranous and endochondral onlay bone-graft resorption. *Plast Reconstr Surg.* 1988;82:872.

16. Motoki DS, Mulliken JB. The healing of bone and cartilage. *Clin Plast Surg.* 1990;17:527.

17. Zins JE, Whitaker LA. Membranous versus endochondral bone: implications for craniofacial reconstruction. *Plast Reconstr Surg.* 1983;72:778.

18. Kusiak JF, Zins JE, Whitaker LA. The early revascularization of membranous bone. *Plast Reconstr Surg.* 1985;76:510.

19. Sullivan PK, Smith J, Rozzelle AA. Cranio-orbital reconstruction: safety and image quality of metallic implants on CT and MR imaging. *Plast Reconstr Surg.* 1994;94:589.

45

Transfacial Access Osteotomies to the Central and Anterolateral Skull Base

Robert B. Stanley, Jr.

Objectives

The transfacial access osteotomies that are discussed in this chapter are not intended for use in treatment of malignant sinus neoplasms that have invaded the skull base. Such tumors require radical resections that frequently produce unavoidable disfigurement and dysfunction. Instead, these osteotomies are designed to maintain form and function of the facial skeleton and overlying soft tissues. They provide wider and more direct access to less aggressive tumors involving relatively inaccessible areas of the skull base itself or beyond to intracranial pathology while reducing or eliminating the need for traction on the brain, brainstem, or cranial nerves. These approaches must be thought of in terms of a surgical funnel, the mouth of which is located at the level of the superficial projections of the facial skeleton and the spout at the skull base. Although the spout size will be increased only slightly or not at all, the mouth of the standard transoral, transnasal, transfrontal, and transtemporal approaches to the skull base will be greatly widened. Thus the working distance from the surgeon's hands to the skull base or intracranial target will be shortened, but the field view angle will be maintained or increased (Figure 45.1).

Preoperative Considerations

The applicability of a transfacial approach is determined by the nature of the pathology, and the choice of approach is determined by the location of the target. Skull-base tumors that are traditionally not treated with an en bloc resection for margin control are ideal candidates for transfacial approaches. Examples range from large juvenile nasopharyngeal angiofibromas, which can be totally resected for cure, to large sphenoid wing meningiomas, which can be subtotally resected for restoration of appearance and maintenance of vision, to clivus chordomas, which can be partially resected for long-term palliation of pain and brainstem compression symptoms. Intracranial targets include suprasellar tumors as well as basi-

lar tip and midbasilar artery aneurysms. Although this broad spectrum of extracranial, junctional, and intracranial pathology occurs within a relatively small area surrounding the sphenoid bone, the complexity of this bone and the multiple structures that course through and around it necessitate the use of different approaches as determined by the exact location of the target.

The location of the target can be described in terms of its relationship to four planes that pass through the pterygoid processes of the sphenoid bone: the sagittal planes through the vertical axis of each process (Figure 45.2a), a coronal plane through the vertical axes of the processes (Figure 45.2a), and an axial plane through the level of the origin of those processes at the connection between the greater wing and body of the sphenoid bone (Figure 45.2b).

In general, targets located between the sagittal pterygoid planes and below the horizontal plane (i.e., the central skull base) can be approached through the mouth (transmandibular or transmaxillary approach). This would include targets within the region of the nasopharynx, posterior ethmoid air cells, sphenoid sinus, clivus, craniocervical junction, or upper cervical spine (Figures 45.3a and 45.4a).[1–3] Additionally, pathology within the pterygoid or retromaxillary space can be reached through a maxillary osteotomy if the target lesion is centered anterior to the coronal pterygoid plane with minimal extension into the infratemporal fossa (Figure 45.5). Targets located between the sagittal planes, anterior to the coronal plane, and above the axial plane can be approached through the frontonasal area (transglabellar approach).[4,5] This would include targets within the anterior cranial fossa and suprasellar area (Figure 45.6a). Any target centered lateral to a sagittal plane or posterior to the coronal plane and above the horizontal plane should be approached through the temporal fossa (transorbitozygomatic approach).[6,7] This would include targets within the posterior orbit, infratemporal fossa, middle cranial fossa, parasellar area, and interpeduncular fossa (Figure 45.7a). Occasionally, a target may overlap planes and the simultaneous use of two approaches may be required. Also, although technically difficult, it is possible to remove the me-

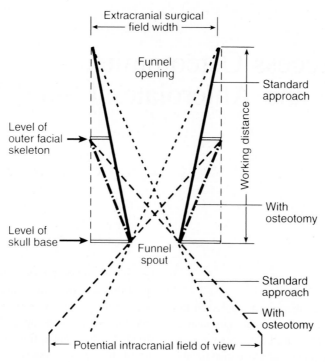

FIGURE 45.1 Surgical funnel. For a given surgical field width (i.e., the space for the surgeon's hands, instruments, and line of sight for binocular vision), the working distance must be increased for a stan-dard approach compared to an approach via an osteotomy. The po-tential intracranial field of view is also reduced for the standard ap-proach if the surgical field width is to be maintained.

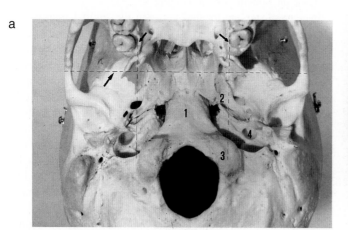

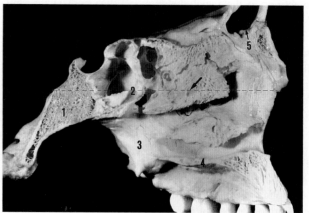

FIGURE 45.2 Pterygoid planes. (a) Sagittal planes (small arrows) and coronal plane (large arrow). Numbered structures are (1) clivus; (2) foramen lacerum; (3) occipital condyle; and (4) carotid canal. (b) Axial plane (arrow). Numbered structures are (1) clivus; (2) sphe-noid sinus; (3) medial pterygoid lamina; (4) hard palate; and (5) frontal sinus.

a
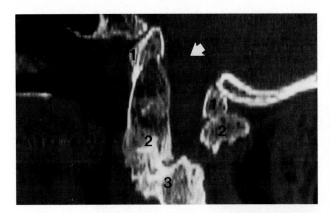

b
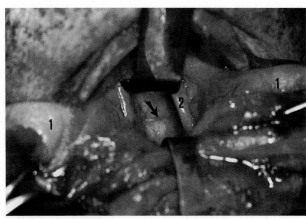

c
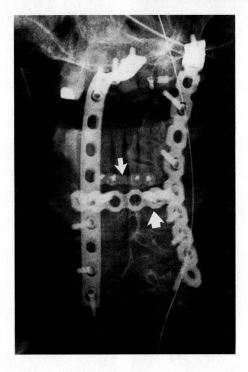

FIGURE 45.3 (a) Preoperative coronal MRI shows basilar invagination of cervical spine into foramen magnum (arrow) in patient with metabolic bone disease. Numbered structures are (1) atlas; (2) axis; and (3) third cervical vertebral body. (b) Intraoperative view of the same patient at level of craniocervical junction (arrow), as seen through midline labiomandibular glossotomy. Numbered structures are (1) bivalved tongue; and (2) retracted soft palate. (c) Postoperative radiograph following removal of odontoid. Because of poor bone quality, a THORP plate (Synthes) (large arrow) with hollow screws and 2.0-mm tension band plate (small arrow) were used to stabilize mandibulotomy. Large vertical plates are part of posterior spinal fusion. (Courtesy of Synthes Maxillofacial Paoli, PA)

dial and lateral laminae of a pterygoid process and reach a lateral target from a transoral approach or a central target from a lateral approach.

Osteotomies

Osteotomies that mobilize tooth-bearing bone or any segment of bone covered by oral mucosa must, of course, maintain the bone as an osteoplastic segment. Osteotomies that mobilize non–tooth-bearing bone, such as through the orbitozygomatic complex and frontal bone, can produce free segments that can be removed from the surgical field and reinserted.

Transmandibular and Transmaxillary

These transoral osteoplastic approaches allow the surgeon to work within limits established by the pterygoid processes cranially and the carotid arteries caudally. The transmandibular approach provides access to only the lowest part of the clivus,

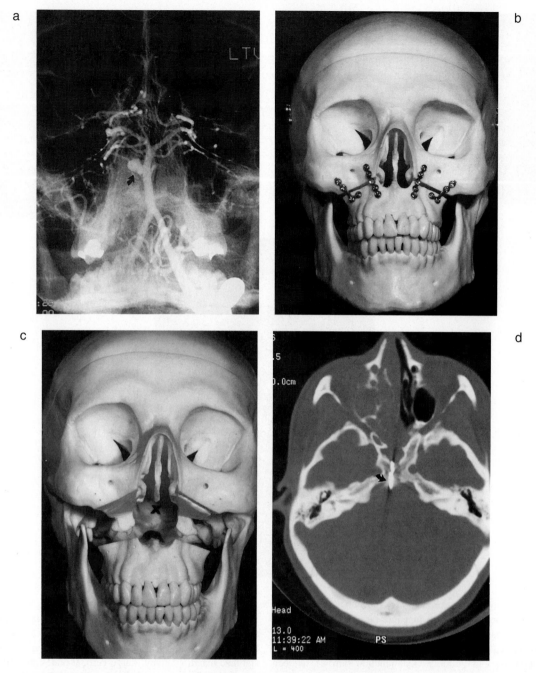

FIGURE 45.4 (a) Preoperative arteriogram that demonstrates a mid-basilar artery aneurysm (arrow). (b) Model showing 1.5-mm plates attached across Le Fort I level osteotomy prior to downfracture of maxilla. (c) Plates removed and maxilla downfractured to expose the clivus. X marks the level of the target aneurysm in relationship to the anterior surface of the clivus. (d) Postoperative axial CT scan shows the transclival successful application of the aneurysm clip (arrow).

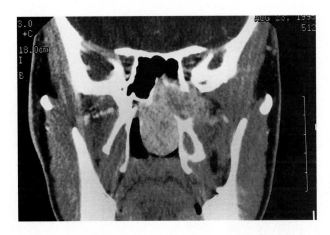

FIGURE 45.5 Coronal CT scan showing large juvenile nasopharyngeal angiofibroma extending through the pterygomaxillary fissure. Total excision was accomplished through maxillotomy approach.

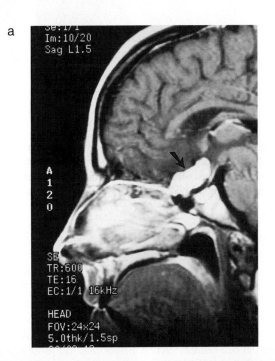

a

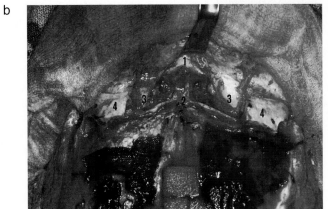

b

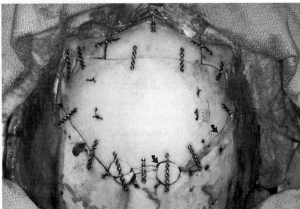

c

FIGURE 45.6 (a) Sagittal MRI demonstrates a large suprasellar schwannoma (arrow). (b) Intraoperative view of osteotomy site from above after dural closure. Numbered structures are (1) nasal bones; (2) area of foramen cecum; (3) orbital soft tissue; and (4) frontal bar lateral to supraorbital formina. (c) Reconstruction with 1.0-mm plates and screws. All craniotome cuts and burr holes have been closed by advancing the bone flap or inserting split cranial grafts (arrows).

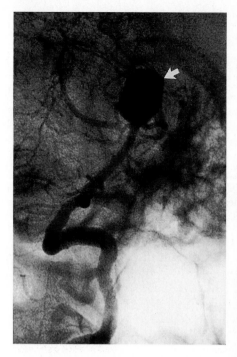
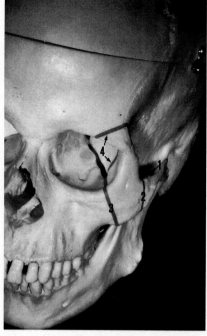
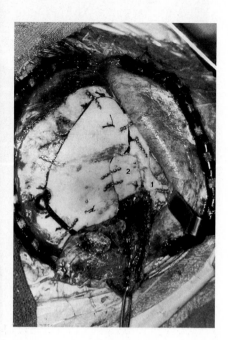

a   b   c

FIGURE 45.7 (a) Preoperative arteriogram demonstrating aneurysm (arrow) of the tip of the basilar artery. (b) Model with lines of four osteotomies marked. See text for details. (c) Reconstruction with 1.0-mm plates and screws. Numbered structures are (1) reinserted zy-goma; and (2) split cranial graft placed to augment floor of temporal fossa where temporalis muscle has been detached deep to lateral orbital rim. This will prevent the temporal hollowing that tends to occur even if muscle is reattached to the rim.

but it is an excellent approach to the upper cervical spine and in most cases the craniocervical junction (Figure 45.3b). A lower lip-splitting incision is required, but the visibility of the healed scar can be minimized by using a stepped or notched course through the vermilion of the lip, then following relaxed skin tension lines around the chin to the level of the hyoid bone. The osteotomy through the anterior mandible can be performed directly in the midline or in a parasagittal stepped fashion. Neither approach should require removal of a tooth if a fine-cutting burr, saw, or osteotome is used between the tooth roots.

The tongue can then be split in the midline or an incision can be directed around the tongue across the floor of mouth to the pharynx. The midline glossotomy requires more time for closure, but the floor-of-mouth incision places the hypoglossal and lingual nerves at risk for injury. Exposure of the craniocervical junction often requires splitting of the soft palate, and this should be done with a "lazy-S" type incision placed to the side of the uvula to reduce the amount of palatal shortening and possible velopharyngeal incompetence that will result. The posterior pharyngeal mucosa can be incised in the midline or an inferiorly based flap can be created, depending on what is to be accomplished when the spout of the surgical funnel has been reached.

Stable fixation of the mandibulotomy, which eliminates the need for postoperative maxillomandibular fixation, can be achieved through a variety of techniques. Theoretically, compression osteosynthesis should not be used to close anterior mandibulotomies made with a saw-cut. It must be remembered that even the finest osteotomy creates a gap between the bone segments, and a change in the occlusal relationship will occur if this gap is closed. Although the successful use of compression osteosynthesis for anterior mandibulotomies done with an osteotome has been described,[8] this type of osteotomy may be more difficult to perform and be of greater risk to the teeth. To ensure that the most accurate realignment of the mandibular segments is achieved during repair of an osteotomy created by a saw-cut, noncompressing fixation plates should be adapted across the line of the proposed osteotomy, and all screw holes should be drilled in an exact neutral position in relation to the plate holes. The plates are then removed and the osteotomy completed. At the time of repair, the preadapted plates are reattached, again with all screws in a neutral position in the plate holes. The type and number of plates and screws used and their points of attachment to the anterior mandible can vary, depending on the status of the dentition, the presence of any metabolic bone disorders, and the experience and preference of the surgeon (Figure 45.3c). In the end, the occlusal patterns should be unchanged, immediate mobilization and early function should be possible, and uncomplicated bony healing should proceed at the osteotomy site.

The transmaxillary approach is a Le Fort I–level maxillotomy with downfracture that provides excellent exposure of the central skull base except at the level of the craniocervical junction.[9] The osteotomy is made through the zygomaticomaxillary buttresses at a level that leaves sufficient bone above the roots of the maxillary teeth for attachment of the transverse limb of an L-shaped minifixation plate (1.3 or 1.5 mm) and through the nasomaxillary buttresses into the nose below the anterior end of the inferior turbinate. Fixation plates should be adapted to the four buttresses, and all screw holes should be drilled before the osteotomy is made or after it is completed but before the maxilla is detached from the posterior pterygomaxillary buttresses (Figure 45.4b).

The nasal septum is managed in a way very similar to a transseptal approach to the sphenoid sinus for adenohypophysectomy. The mucosa is elevated from one side of the cartilaginous portion of the septum, the bony–cartilaginous junction is identified and separated, and then a bilateral submucoperiosteal dissection is completed over the bony septum to the sphenoid rostrum. The bony septum is then removed piecemeal and the cartilaginous septum is elevated off the maxillary crest, which is preserved if possible for later septal reconstruction. After the mucosa of the floor of the nose is elevated bilaterally, an incision is made through the posterior margin of the septal mucoperiosteum and carried out bilaterally through the elevated floor mucosa just anterior to its transition into soft palate. The leaves of septal mucoperichondrium/periosteum are then separated, carrying the septal cartilage to one side still attached to mucoperichondrium. Preservation of the septal cartilage reduces the chance of developing a troublesome anterior septal perforation and maintains support for the nasal dorsum and tip when the cartilage is repositioned onto the retained maxillary crest. Removing the posterior one third to one half of the inferior turbinate will widen the funnel as it approaches the spout, but removing additional turbinate tissue increases the risk of producing atrophic rhinitis symptoms.

Once the maxilla is detached from the pterygoid processes and downfractured, it remains pedicled on the contents of the pterygomaxillary fissure as well as the soft tissues of the palate and faucial pillars. Therefore, it does not move downward evenly to produce a box-like opening, but rather it hinges around the soft tissue pedicles to produce the surgical funnel (Figure 45.4c,d). If further exposure is required, a parasagittal split through the hard palate (maintaining the maxillary crest for reconstruction of the septum) and the soft palate can be performed to create a bivalved maxilla. This maneuver produces unhindered access above and below the craniocervical junction but carries a possible increased risk of aseptic necrosis of the maxillary segments due to kinking of the vascular pedicles. Retraction pressure should be released from time to time to ensure vascular perfusion of both segments in their downward, rotated position. Also, velopharyngeal incompetence may result from the midline split of the soft palate. If the palate is to be split, an additional fixation plate must be adapted across the proposed exit of the osteotomy through the inferior margin of the pyriform aperture and all screw holes drilled. A plate positioned across the posterior extent of the osteotomy should also be considered for maximum stability of the reconstruction. However, application of this plate can sometimes be techni-cally difficult, and a high rate of exposure through the repaired mucosa often necessitates a second surgery for its removal.

Transglabellar

This free-segment approach, when done in conjunction with a frontal craniotomy, facilitates both intradural and extradural dissections by the neurosurgeon along the floor of the anterior cranial fossa. The need for traction on the brain and olfactory nerves is lessened with improved visualization of the suprasellar area. The free segment is removed from the frontal bar of the forehead after dissection of the standard coronal flap is carried over the superior orbital rims and down onto the nasal bones, stopping just short of the medial canthal tendons. The supraorbital neurovascular bundles are then freed from their foramina, and both trochlear tendons are detached from the mediosuperior corner of the orbits. Dissection is carried back along the orbital roofs and down to the frontoethmoidal suture line at the level of the anterior ethmoid artery. Intracranially, the dura is elevated down to the foramen cecum, and the venous channel through this foramen is clipped and transected. After identification of the crista galli, the dura is elevated from both orbits without violating either olfactory tract. Vertical bone cuts are then made through the frontal bar perpendicular to the transverse frontal cut of the craniotomy and into the orbital roofs at the supraorbital notches. These cuts are then connected by a transverse cut across the floor of the anterior fossa at the level of the foramen cecum. The final osteotomy is through the frontonasal suture, angled superiorly toward the foramen cecum. Small cuts with an osteotome in the mediosuperior aspect of the orbit are usually necessary to completely mobilize the central segment of the frontal bar (Figure 45.6b).

Most of the frontal sinus will be contained within the removed segment, and an appropriate form of management of the sinus is cranialization. This is performed by removing the posterior table of the sinus and totally extirpating all mucosa from the anterior wall with round cutting burs. Any sinus that extends into the frontal bone flap or that remains in situ as a lateral extension is treated in a similar fashion. Following completion of the neurosurgical procedure, the frontal segment is replaced and stabilized with microplates and screws (1.0 mm). Split inner table grafts harvested from the frontal bone flap are contoured to fit tightly into the area of the frontonasal orifices and then covered with temporalis fascia to complete the seal between the anterior fossa and the nose and paranasal sinuses. Because a pericranial flap rotated intracranially is usually unnecessary for repair of the dura or skull base in these cases, the frontal bone flap should be advanced to completely close the transverse bone cut made by craniotome (Figure 45.6c). This will prevent a linear depression from developing across the supraciliary and glabellar areas. The widened gap at the superolateral rim of the frontal bone flap, which most likely will be behind the hairline, can be filled with "bone pâté" saved from the craniotomy or strips of split inner table bone from the frontal bone flap.

Transorbitozygomatic

This is a combined osteoplastic-free-segment approach through the temporal fossa. It necessitates complete exposure of the lateral orbit, body of zygoma, and zygomatic arch through an extended hemicoronal dissection. This dissection must be maintained at a level deep to the superficial layer of the deep temporal fascia to avoid damage to the frontal branch of the facial nerve. Two osteotomies through the arch, one placed obliquely through the articular eminence and one placed paralleling the lateral margin of the orbital rim (Figure 45.7b), allow for lateral and inferior retraction of the arch without the need for detachment of the masseter muscle. This prevents the inferior retraction of the muscle and the resultant transcutaneous accentuation of the arch outline that occurs when the arch is removed and replaced as a free segment. The body of the zygoma is then removed as a free segment by first detaching the temporalis muscle from the lateral orbit and temporal fossa, and then creating two additional osteotomies (Figure 45.7b). One osteotomy extends through the body of the zygoma into the lateral end of the inferior orbital fissure, and the other extends from the lateral end of the fissure superiorly along the zygomaticosphenoid suture line to pass obliquely through the base of the zygomatic process of the frontal bone. When used in conjunction with a temporal craniotomy, increased exposure of the junction of the temporal fossa and infratemporal fossa, posterior orbit, middle cranial fossa, parasellar area, and interpenduncular fossa is obtained.

Following completion of the neurosurgical procedure, the posterior orbit is reconstructed as necessary with split cranial bone grafts, and the zygoma and zygomatic arch are repositioned and stabilized (Figure 45.7c). The osteotomy gaps through the body of the zygoma and the anterior arch are closed and stabilized with 1.0- or 1.3-mm plates and screws. The oblique osteotomies through the zygomatic process of the frontal bone and the articular eminence of the arch, which act as sliding osteotomies due to closure of the other gaps, can be stabilized with plates or with lag screws. The temporalis muscle must be firmly reattached to the lateral orbital rim and superior temporal line if temporal hollowing is to be avoided. Additionally, bone grafting to the floor of the temporal fossa should be considered to help maintain overlying soft tissue contours.

Miscellaneous Considerations

A broad-spectrum antibiotic, typically a cephalosporin, is administered to all patients preoperatively and continued for 72 hours postoperatively. For transoral procedures that include exposure of the dura, metronidazole is added. A steroid bolus, usually 12 mg of dexamethasome, is also given preoperatively, and doses of 6 mg are continued every 6 hours for 24 hours postoperatively. The steroids greatly reduce intraoper-

ative edema to further facilitate the approaches, and their short-term administration does not appear to increase the risk of infection, even with the transoral approaches. An attempt should be made to obtain a watertight suture closure of dural and mucosal incisions. However, this may not always be possible at sites deep within the intracranial cavity or high in the nasopharynx. Short-term augmentation of a tenuous closure of either suture line can be obtained with fibrin adhesive, and pressure from cerebrospinal fluid on the dural closure can be reduced with lumbar drainage for a 3- to 5-day period. Alimentation should be given by way of a small-diameter, soft nasogastric feeding tube also for a 3- to 5-day period in patients who undergo transoral approaches. An orogastric tube, which is somewhat more uncomfortable for the patient, or peripheral intravenous alimentation can be used if there is concern regarding the presence of a tube in close proximity to a nasopharyngeal repair. A tracheostomy should not be necessary except in patients who undergo a midline labiomandibular glossotomy or in patients who will likely have airway or aspiration problems related to postoperative lower cranial nerve palsies caused by the neurosurgical portion of the case.

Acknowledgments. The author would like to thank H. Richard Winn, M.D., Professor and Chairman, and M. Sean Grady, M.D., Associate Professor, of the Department of Neurological Surgery, University of Washington School of Medicine, Seattle, WA, for the opportunity to participate in the care of their patients.

References

1. Archer DJ, Young S, Utley D. Basilar aneurysms: a new trans-clival approach via maxillotomy. *J Neurosurg.* 1987;67:54–58.
2. Grime PD, Haskell R, Robertson I, Gullan R. Transfacial access of neurosurgical procedures. I. The upper cervical spine and clivus. *Int J Oral Maxillofac Surg.* 1991;20:285–290.
3. Sasaki CT, Lowlicht RA, Astrachan DI, Friedman CD, Goodwin WJ, Morales M. LeFort I osteotomy approach to skull base. *Laryngoscope.* 1990;100:1073–1076.
4. Raveh J, Vuillemin T. The subcranial-supraorbital and temporal approach for tumor resection. *J Craniofac Surg.* 1990;1:53–59.
5. Shekahr LN, Nanda A, Sen CN, Snyderman CN, Janecka IP. The extended frontal approach to tumors of the anterior, middle, and posterior skull base. *J Neurosurg.* 1992;76:198–206.
6. Grime PD, Haskall R, Robertson I, Gullan R. Transfacial access for neurosurgical procedures. II. Middle cranial fossa, infratemporal fossa, and pterygoid space. *Int J Oral Maxillofac Surg.* 1991;20:291–295.
7. Alaywan M, Sindou M. Fronto-temporal approach with orbito-zygomatic removal. *Acta Reconstr Surg.* 1992;87:362–364.
8. Hale RG, Timmis DP, Bays RA. A new mandibulotomy technique for the dentate patient. *Plast Reconstr Surg.* 1991;87:362–364.
9. Janes D, Crockard HA. Surgical access to the base of skull and upper cervical spine by extended maxillotomy. *Neurosurgery.* 1991;29:411–416.

Section V
Craniomaxillofacial Corrective Bone Surgery

46
Orthognathic Examination

Peter Ward-Booth

It has been estimated that 1.2 million patients in the United States[1] could benefit from surgical orthodontics. It is important therefore that a patient with this potential problem should have a standard careful and complete examination. Orthognathic surgery is no longer a "one-off" surgical procedure, but routine oral and maxillofacial surgery in which patients reasonably expect a safe predictable outcome.

The lifelong functional and aesthetic benefits of orthognathic surgery are enormous in those with severe facial deformity, such as cleft patients, or those less severely afflicted. Poor planning, however, or even worse, failing to discuss orthognathic surgery with the patient, can leave a lifelong legacy of failure (Figures 46.1a–g).

Medical Examination

The medical examination covers two elements. The first concerns the suitability of the patient, both physically and psychologically, to undergo surgery, and the second is a "medical" component of the facial disharmony; for example, a syndromic patient may have associated medical problems. It is however not the role of this chapter to discuss the general medical examination of patients.

Psychologic problems in patients seeking orthognathic surgery are significant. The dysmorphic patient with poor self-esteem and inappropriate body image is unlikely to be happy after orthognathic surgery. These patients do not enter the consultation wearing a large sign warning the surgeon they are dysmorphic personalities. Taking a good history and spending time not only talking to, but more importantly listening to, the patient usually reveals these problems. These dysmorphic patients often seem to have an exaggerated image of what appears to be a minor facial disharmony. They frequently dwell at great length on their problem, which to the surgeon seems minimal. They frequently are introverted with an obsession with the problem, providing on occasion long lists or diagrams of their condition. If surgery proceeds, they expect perfection in the outcome. Frequently they are

older patients and may well have already consulted a number of different specialists about similar cosmetic problems. Such patients must be treated surgically with great caution. Specialist help from interested psychiatrists can be helpful. It should be stressed that if these patients are carefully treated with good support and communications, a satisfied, happy patient is certainly possible. The patient difficult to detect is the dysmorphic patient who actually has a significant facial disharmony.

The available evidence suggests[2] that orthognathic patients are different from patients seeking pure cosmetic surgery, such as a face-lift. They do not seem to have the same degree of poor self-esteem, and their response to orthognathic surgery is generally very positive. As in so many aspects of surgery, good information, including realistic comments on the improvements that are possible as well as the complications and postoperative difficulties, yield handsome dividends in patient satisfaction. Unfortunately, a comprehensive explanation of surgery using very vivid language may "put off" some patients who could have coped well with the surgery.

It certainly is a skill to inform a patient fully yet not engender unnecessary anxiety. It is most important that the surgery be explained to close friends or family of the patient, because in the first days after surgery support of the family can be an invaluable aid to the patient. My personal aid to the delicate balance of "informing not frightening" the patient is to arrange for the patient and relatives to sit and talk, on their own, with a patient who has recently had similar surgery. Those patients who have related medical problems, such as acromegalia,[3] are important from the surgical point of view because of complications that may arise perioperatively. In some syndromes having a genetic element, genetic counseling should be considered.

Orthognathic surgery is, "normally," and there is a good case for stating it should be "always," the second stage of a three-part procedure of orthodontics and surgery. The first stage is orthodontic, the second stage is surgical, and the last stage orthodontic "tidying up." The examination therefore should be a joint orthodontist/maxillofacial surgeon process.

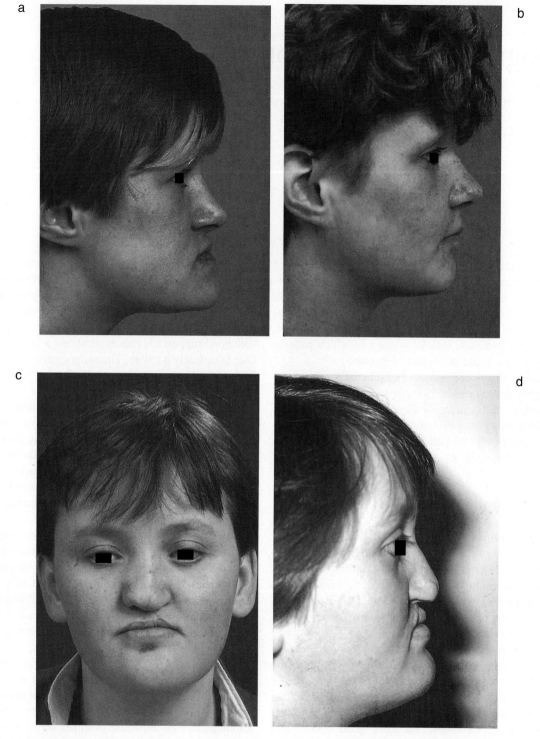

FIGURE 46.1 (a) This patient required a maxillary Le Fort I advancement and bilateral sagittal splint pushback procedure. The acute nasiolabial angle was corrected by inferiorly positioning the maxilla. (b) Postoperative. (c) Cleft patients often display marked maxillary hypoplasia as the result of poor primary surgery. (d) The full-face view displays this maxillary hypoplasia and highlights the three-dimensional hypoplasia with reduced facial height.

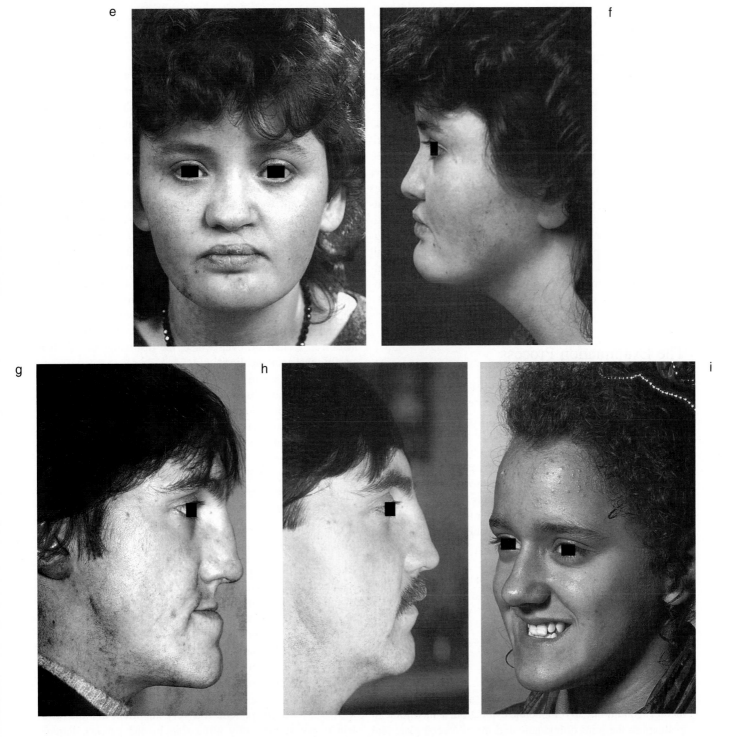

FIGURE 46.1 *Continued.* (e) Postoperative. (f) Postoperative. (g) Clear evidence of failure of planning; too much attention was focused on the dental element of the face. (h) An unsatisfactory postoperative appearance; the mandibular pushback has highlighted the prominent nose and nasion. (i) This patient underwent extensive orthodontic treatment, yet the facial appearance was ignored. The result was a good occlusion but unsatisfactory facial appearance.

The planning for orthognathic surgery is as much art as science.[3] The need for artistic skills, however, can never be used as a reason for "cutting corners," "guessing," or a "that's close enough" type philosophy. The fact that "artistic judgment" is needed for surgery and planning demands even higher and more precise standards of evaluation to provide the data needed to make a treatment decision. The actions of an experienced surgeon when examining or operating can appear to the poorly informed to be intuitive. In reality the experienced surgeon is in fact still working through a careful, well-rehearsed algorithm, but experience allows this to be a faster process. There is no doubt the more precise and meticulous the examination and the surgery, the more artistic the outcome. It is also apparent that while most experienced clinicians agree in broad terms about a diagnosis of an orthognathic case, the plan to the last fraction of a millimeter will vary from clinician to clinician.[4] This is as much about cultural, ethnic "norms," and personal preferences as it is an objective scientific decision.

The Examination Process

The new trainee, faced with the first case to examine, wants a didactic list to work through. Indeed many units provide just that process, and I have outlined my particular process here (Figure 46.2). This however is like a phrase book in a foreign country; you will be able to "get by," but you will not really understand the language or the meaning. A moment's thought shows that examining by a script will miss many subtle features. The examination should thus be seen as a "planning process" in which many items enter the equation but not all will be relevant to this particular patient. There is thus a cycle of activity following the patient's wish to seek treatment, involving questioning, examining, recording data in a variety of ways, collating the data, and planning from that data; the options are then brought back to the patient to complete the cycle.

The Examination Cycle

The examination cycle encompasses the patient's hopes, their medical conditions, an orthodontic evaluation, a maxillofacial evaluation, the joint orthodontic and maxillofacial plan, and the patient's responses to the orthodontic and surgical plans.

After completion of this examination cycle, the patient then moves on to definitive treatment. This may be "no treatment," review and repeat the whole process later, or (and this is the most common outcome) proceed along an orthodontic/surgical/orthodontic route. It is essential that any progress along any of these routes is driven by a fully informed patient who comprehends all the options.

Clinical Examination

General Observations

The gender of the patient is important. For example, the male normally feels comfortable with a slightly prognathic jaw, but the female finds a small degree of prognathism gives an aggressive image. Cultural and racial differences are of course important, even with those races derived from the same ethnic group. From a British perspective (Figure 46.3), it is often noted that in certain parts of the United States a degree of prognathism in a female is attractive. Some British patients may be desperate to have a chin "reduced" that in United States terms would not appear to be a severe problem. Racial variations of "normal" can be much more marked.

The height of the patient can be important. Tall people tend to stoop and mask a prognathism. To what extent prognathism encourages a "head-down" posture is less certain. Examination of the patient standing up is thus extremely important. This is essential in cases of torticollis, which is not infrequently associated with plagiocephaly and scoliosis. Examination in a chair or, even worse, the restricting dental chair easily masks any scoliosis.

It is important to note the patient's soft tissue structure. This may be an observation about obesity, which will certainly affect for example the outcome of a ramus "pushback" procedure, particularly in the chin-neck angle. Similarly, thin delicate nasal skin would certainly affect the outcome of a tip rhinoplasty, where every irregularity of cartilage surgery would be very visible. Thick soft tissues may reduce the amount of anteroposterior movement necessary for good aesthetics, compared with the pure skeletal examination.

Observations of Relevant Systemic Disorders

The age of the patient is important for three reasons. Is the patient mature enough to understand the indications for, and the nature of, the surgery? Will the surgery interfere with the normal facial growth? Will postsurgical growth negate the surgery? The first point is probably the most difficult to discern. The intellectual and emotional maturity of the adolescent is difficult to predict by only the chronologic age of the patient. A careful consultation, preferably at some point with the youngster on their own without a parent, usually reveals the maturity of the patient. It is very important that the problem is not significantly influenced by the parents. Parents normally fall into two clear groups; those who can see no problem with their child's face and those who are trying to impose surgery. Fortunately most parents are in the first category, but are very aware of and understand that their child's views are the most important.

The effects of surgery on facial growth remain confusing. The dramatic adverse effect of surgery in cleft lip and palate patients, particularly bony surgery, on facial growth inhibition

DEPARTMENT OF ORAL & MAXILLOFACIAL SURGERY

DEFINED DATA BASE

PATIENT..   TEL. ....

ADDRESS ....   **SEX**

....   Male   ☐   1 - 2

....   Female   ☐   1 - 3

HOSPITAL NO. .... 1 - 0   **DATE**

SURVEY NO. .... 1 - 1   Month   ☐   1 - 4

    Year   ☐   1 - 5

    D.O.B.   ☐   1 - 6   ☐   1 - 7   ☐   1 -

OCCUPATION ....   REFERRED BY ....

ORTHODONTIST..

1) GENERAL HISTORY AND PHYSICAL

    1. Chief Complaint

    2. General Health History

    3. General Physical Assessment

    4. Patient Motivation

      Poor   ☐   2 - 0

      Average   ☐   2 - 1

      Good   ☐   2 - 2

PLAN FROM EXAMINATION   PLAN WITH CEPHALOMETRICS

PLAN WITH MODELS   FINAL PLAN

FURTHER ORTHO REQUIRED   NEXT APPOINTMENT

FIGURE 46.2 This systematic approach to the clinical appearance is too long for routine use, but provides a guide to planning for trainees.
Continued.

DENTO - FACIAL EXAM

FACIAL CONTOUR

Frontal

Symmetry

Yes ☐ 3 - 0

No ☐ 3 - 1

Facial Height

Normal ☐ 3 - 2

Long ☐ 3 - 3

Short ☐ 3 - 4

Eyes

Normal ☐ 3 - 5

Abnormal ☐ 3 - 6

State:
Intercantha Distance
Interpupillary Distance

Nose

Normal ☐ 3 - 7

Abnormal ☐ 3 - 8

State:
Deviated
Wide alar base
Narrow alar base

Malar

Normal ☐ 3 - 9

Abnormal ☐ 3 - 10

State:
Flat
Prominent

Upper Lip

Normal ☐ 3 - 11

Long ☐ 3 - 12

Short ☐ 3 - 13

Lip to tooth ratio

☐ mm. of maxillary incisors visible 3 - 14

Interlabial gap

☐ mm. between upper and lower lips (relaxed) 3 - 15

Lower lip and chin

FIGURE 46.2 *Continued.*

Normal   3 - 16

Abnormal   3 - 17

State:
Long
Short

Mental Strain (Lips closed)

Yes   ☐   3 - 18

No   ☐   3 - 19

Lateral

Eyes

Normal   ☐   4 - 0

Abnormal ☐   4 - 1

State:
Enophthalmos
Exophthalmos
Exorbitism

Nose

Normal   ☐   4 - 2

Abnormal ☐   4 - 3

State:
Large
Small
Convex
Concave

Malar

Normal   ☐   4 - 4

Abnormal ☐   4 - 5

State:
Large
Small
Convex
Concave

FIGURE 46.2 *Continued.*

Upper Lip

Normal [ ]   4 - 6

Abnormal [ ]   4 - 7

State:
Prognathic
Retrognathic
Acute Naso-labial angle
Obtuse Naso-labial angle

Lower lip and chin

Normal [ ]   4 - 8

Abnormal [ ]   4 - 9

State:
Prognathic
Retrognathic
Deep mental fold
Shallow mental fold

Oral Cavity

Soft Tissues

Normal [ ]   5 - 0

Abnormal [ ]   5 - 1

Hygiene

Good [ ]   5 - 2

Fair [ ]   5 - 3

Poor [ ]   5 - 4

Caries

Minimal [ ]   5 -5

Moderate [ ]   5 - 6

Severe [ ]   5 - 7

Tongue Size

Normal [ ]   5 - 8

Large [ ]   5 - 9

Small [ ]   5 - 10

FIGURE 46.2 *Continued.*

Tongue Thrust

Yes   [   ]   5 - 11

No   [   ]   5 - 12

Maxillary dental midline to facial midline

Matches   [   ]   5 - 13

Deviates   [   ]   mm L R from facial   5 - 14

Mandibular dental midline

Matches   [   ]   5 -15

Deviates   [   ]   mm L R from facial   5 - 16

Occlusal plane to pupillary plane

Parallel   [   ]   5 - 17

Occlusal plane down

                 [   ]   degrees   L   5 - 18

                 [   ]   degrees   R   5 - 19

T. M. J.

Clicking

No   [   ]   6 - 0

L   [   ]   6 - 1

R   [   ]   6 - 2

Pain

No   [   ]   6 - 3

L   [   ]   6 - 4

R   [   ]   6 - 5

FIGURE 46.2 *Continued.*

Sensation

Normal ☐   6 - 6

Abnormal ☐   6 - 7

State:
Paraesthesia
Hyperaesthesia
Anaesthesia

Opening mm $\frac{1/}{1/}$ —☐   6 - 8

Deviation

None ☐   6 - 9

to L ☐   6 - 10

to R ☐   6 - 11

FIGURE 46.2 *Continued.*

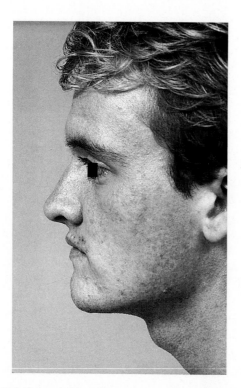

FIGURE 46.3 Although this patient remains somewhat prognathic, his appearance is quite acceptable with a normal occlusion.

has left a tradition that surgery stops facial growth. Orthognathic surgery in young growing teenagers does not, however, appear to have the same effects. Continued postsurgical facial growth may certainly account for "relapse." The difficulty is knowing when facial growth has really finished. The growth curves for patients are known as the rapid growth phases for males and females are available.[5] The problem is that statistics apply to groups of patients, not the individual patient facing the surgeon. Nevertheless, even informal questions to the patient and parents soon give a good indication how rapid the growth phase is and when it started. It is normally possible to be fairly certain in individual patients when the majority of growth has taken place.

Finally, clinically obvious pathology must be detected and identified. It would be essential to identify, for example, temporomandibular joint dysfunction before orthodontics or surgery was undertaken. Similarly, careful neurologic examination must be made.

Detailed Orthognathic Examination

For the examination to be useful, it must be logical and proceed in logical steps. The examination should encompass the following, and preferably in the order listed here.

1. The clinical examination should be of the full face and profile, systematically evaluating:

Soft tissue
Hard tissue
Dentition

2. Radiologic material
3. Articulated models

Clinical Examination

The examination is conveniently divided into *anterior* and *lateral* (*left* and *right*), and the examination should start peripherally and finish at the occlusal level.

Anterior Examination, "Full Face"

There is sometimes a reluctance to examine full face for fear of not detecting the main problems. This is not true, and other features are detected that are often more important to the patient, who normally see themselves in this view (Figure 46.4).

Pure "numbers" or measurements of facial size are not useful as we all come in varying sizes. What is important, however, is "ratios" or facial proportions of the full facial features. The method most frequently used is to divide the full face into those well-rehearsed equal "thirds" (Figures 46.5a–c): *lower third*, from the chin (menton) to base of nose (columella/labial junction); *middle third*, base of nose (columella/labial junction) to bridge of nose (soft tissue nasion); and *upper third*, bridge of nose (soft tissue nasion) to the hairline

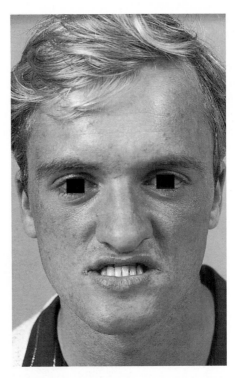

FIGURE 46.4 Full-face examination is often underused. It is the view the patient most frequently sees, and other subtleties may be exposed. This patient felt he looked too aggressive.

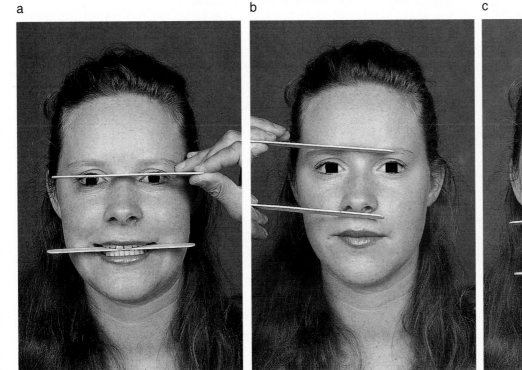
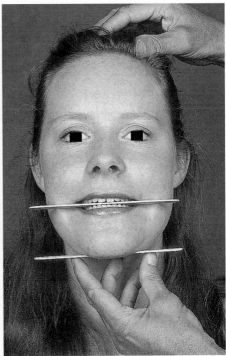

FIGURE 46.5 (a) Division of the face into equal "thirds." (b) The lower two-thirds as divided into the surgically useful upper and lower face heights. (c) Evaluation of the occlusal plane, noting its relationship to the pupils and the lower border of the mandible.

(a very poorly defined point). This approach is fine for trauma in which there can be loose descriptions of fractures (e.g., a mid-third fracture) but is not very useful, especially the upper third, for orthognathic planning. As it is absolutely essential to plan from the whole face, dividing the face into half may be more useful. In this instance, the upper half is from the soft tissue nasion to the top of the calverium, and the lower half from soft tissue nasion to menton; the lower half is then divided into equal thirds as before. This simple approach is very effective in highlighting variations from normal.

Similarly the *width* of the face can be assessed (Figures 46.6a–d). Here it is not quite so easy because the face tapers from its widest point somewhere between the anterior end of the zygomatic arch and the mastoid prominence. The facial shape behind the ears is so influenced by the ears as not to be significant, and thus just anterior to the tragus is a useful "end point" to measure from, as well as along the line of the zygomatic arches, which are normally the widest point of the face. Exceptionally, in marked masseteric hyperplasia the gonial angles may be the widest point. Normally the gonial angles would be 2 to 4 mm medial to a vertical line dropped from the most prominent part of the zygomatic arches.

As with the vertical ratios, the width of the face can be evaluated with a series of linked ratios. The width of the face

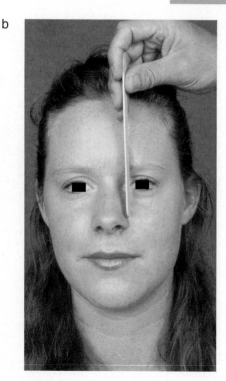
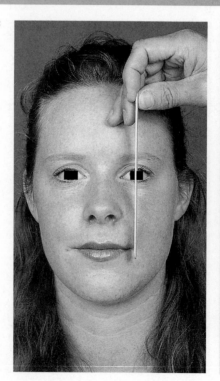
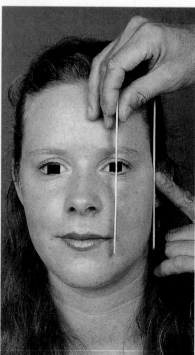

FIGURE 46.6 (a) The center line is fundamental to planning. The widths of the canthii and pupils are best compared to other facial features, such as the lips, rather than relying on absolute measurements. (b–d) Clinical evaluation of facial width.

is normally four times the interalar base width. The interalar base width is the same as the intercanthal. This however is quite varied, being only "correct" in 40% of patients; in about one-third, the interalar distance is 2 or 3 mm greater. Interestingly, in the United States a larger intercanthal than alar distance is considered a sign of attractiveness.

The intercanthal distance is normally equal to the distance between inner and outer canthi. The outer canthus is normally 2 to 4 mm higher than the inner canthus. A vertical line from the center of the pupils should mark the outer limits of the lips at rest (Figure 46.7). The amount of upper incisor visible at rest with the teeth apart is about 2 to 3 mm, and the upper teeth are visible to the first premolar.

Although the malar prominence forms one of the most important aesthetic landmarks in facial attractiveness, it is particularly difficult to define in the full-face view. The malar prominence is ideally broad, being an almost direct projection of the zygomatic arch (Figure 46.8). In the full-face view it is difficult to identify flat malars unless this is severe, as is seen in some cranial base syndromes such as Crouzons, where there may be excessive sclera display. There does however need to be a definable angle between the lower lid and the prominence caused by the malar, at the base of the orbicularis oculi.

The full-face examination is of course critical to document facial asymmetry. In many cases asymmetry is a progressive

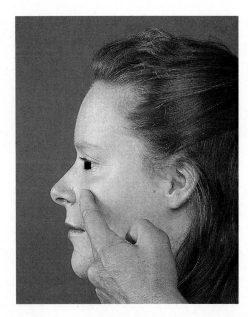

FIGURE 46.8 Malar prominence is difficult to define both clinically and radiologically, yet is most obvious in grossly hypoplastic or prominent malars. This patient needs careful planning, as she has prominent malars yet is hypoplastic in the paranasal area.

feature and even in pure mandibular asymmetry it progresses subtly along the mandible; rarely is it seen as a definable volume of asymmetry. When this progressive asymmetry involves the face and skull, it becomes hard to define the volume that requires correction. A useful way to treat this problem is to take the face in its "thirds" and examine each portion and identify the center, ideally by temporarily covering the other "thirds" to avoid distraction. Thus, the center of the forehead is marked, then the soft tissue nasion and the center of the tip of the nose. Finally, turning to the lower "third," identify the center of the upper and lower lips and chin. A wooden spatula is then placed along the marks to highlight the asymmetry. The dental midlines are noted. The patient with a poorly defined, diffuse asymmetry should be cautioned that complete craniofacial correction can rarely be achieved.

Incisor display is extremely important to note. This should be examined at rest, when smiling, and with a broad smile (Figures 46.9a–c). Evidence of forcing lip competence should be noted because this may invalidate "normal" incisor show. Vertical maxillary excess with a long lower face height and prominent incisors is normally easily detected; the failure to display incisors may be easily overlooked (Figure 46.10a,b).

Profile Examination

The profile observation is a very traditional approach to the examination and, sadly and erroneously, often the only clinical examination to be undertaken. It is important not to sim-

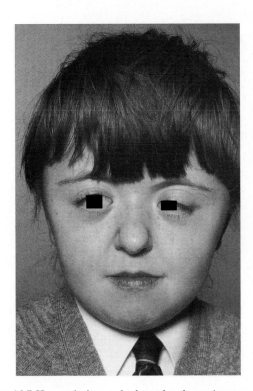

FIGURE 46.7 Hypertelorism and telecanthus in an Aperts patient.

a 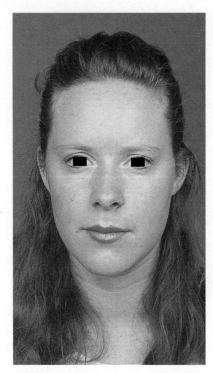 b 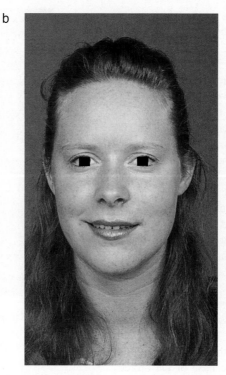 c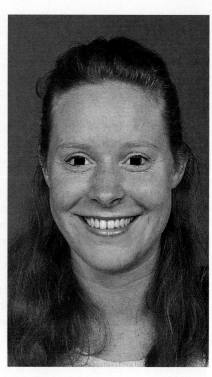

FIGURE 46.9 (a) Assessment of the incisor show is as important as it is difficult. "At rest" to the patient may force an unnatural tension in the muscle. (b) This view, however, represents her normal relaxed incisor show, which is normal at about 2 mm. (c) It is important to get a big smile to ensure that there is not excessive gingival show, as this may have to be built into the surgical plan.

a 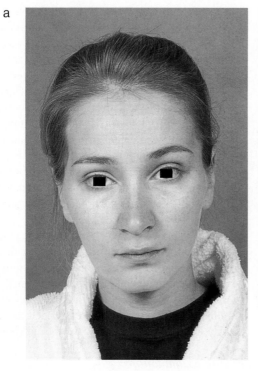 b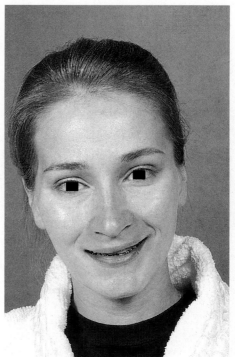

FIGURE 46.10 (a,b) Most surgeons and patients are very aware of the patient with vertical maxillary excess and excessive tooth and gingiva exposure. Care must be taken not to miss the patient like this with minimal incisor show.

ply repeat the lateral cephalogram radiographic examination. It is particularly important to examine the whole face (Figure 46.11), neck, and posture of the head. These data cannot be easily obtained from the lateral cephalogram. The shape and position of the forehead, particularly the non-hair-bearing part, is absolutely critical to successful planning. The appearance of the neck-chin angle and form is again so important in predicting the outcome. Missing a fat bulky submental area and undertaking a mandibular "pushback" that will exaggerate this fold will certainly not remain unnoticed by the patient, who will be very concerned by this new "double chin." Again, the examination can begin with the division of the profile into thirds or quarters, as described in the full-face examination. This should confirm the earlier findings.

Examination of the all-important forehead is difficult because there are few "numbers," "angles," or "projections" to guide the evaluation. The position of soft tissue nasion has an important relationship to menton. Often however it is important to assess the whole forehead up to the hairline, and this is not well documented. It is important to note the shape of the forehead with particular emphasis on a prominent or bossing appearance. Similarly, a steeply receding forehead should be noted. The forehead should incline from the vertical with the head in the natural head position, by 10° to 5°, with that of males being slightly more inclined. The line dropped vertically from soft tissue nasion (Gonzalez-Ulloa)[6,7] meeting a projected Frankfort horizontal at 90° should just touch soft tissue pogonion (Figure 46.12).

The nose, which is so important to aesthetics, has been well defined in the literature. The length of the nose should be contained in the division of the face into thirds and be about twice the height of the nasal tip to the base of the alar. The nose ideally should be 20° from the vertical, and the soft tissue nasion 3 to 4 mm posterior to the glabellar, to give a nasal frontal angle of about 130° (Figure 46.13). The dorsum of the nose is concave from a line from the soft tissue nasion to the tip by about 2 mm.

In orthognathic planning the nasiolabial angle is very important (Figure 46.14). The angle ranges from 95° to 105°, being more acute in females. Similarly, the relationship of the nose to the lower third of the face in profile is very important to planning. Ricketts has projected a line from nasal tip to soft tissue pogonion, and suggested the upper lip be 4 mm and the lower 2 mm behind this line[8–11] (Figure 46.14). Steiner suggests a line from the soft tissue pogonion, at a tangent to upper and lower lips, should bisect the nose[12,13] (Figure 46.15).

Even when armed with all these data on profiles, there still must be a systematic approach. One useful approach is to (1) evaluate the forehead relative to the rest of the face; (2) relate the forehead (soft tissue nasion) to the chin; (3) relate the

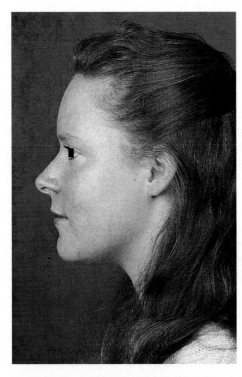

FIGURE 46.11 Profile examination is a chance to examine the whole face, neck, and posture.

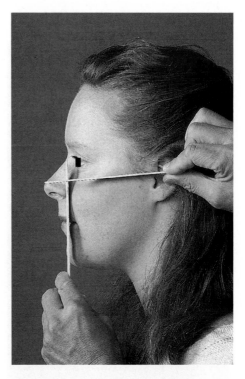

FIGURE 46.12 A vertical from soft tissue nasion at right angles to Frankfort horizontal is a good way to relate the upper face to the lower and midface.

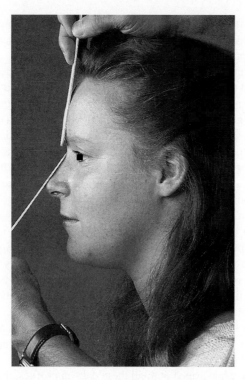

FIGURE 46.13 The frontal nasal angle (130°) is an important angle.

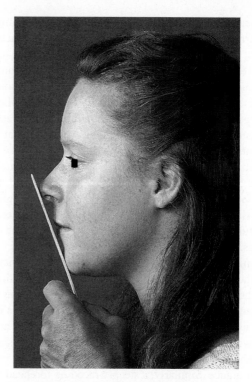

FIGURE 46.15 A line from nasal tip to pogonion relates the lips to nose and chin and is very useful in planning.

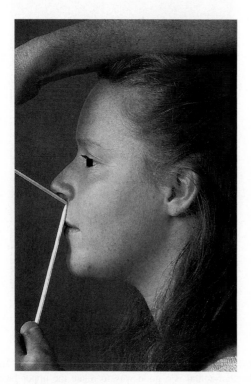

FIGURE 46.14 The nasolabial angle often reflects the relationship between the midface and lower face.

nose to the upper lip (nasolabial angle); (4) relate the lips to the nose; (5) compare the upper facial height to the lower facial height; and (6) evaluate malar prominence.

Dental Examination

From a purely surgical point of view, the dental examination is directed at establishing any dental factors that might impede a surgical plan. The presence of unerupted teeth or inadequate space for segmental procedures must be observed. Clearly, when dental infection or periodontal infection is present, elective surgery is contraindicated.

Because the surgeon does not have the expertise of the orthodontist in alignment or positioning of teeth before surgery, a dialogue must be established. The planned surgical movements, especially changes in occlusal plane angles, must be brought into the orthodontic planning process.

Radiologic Examination

Radiology has three very important roles

1. Identification of bony pathology, including a persistent growth center, for example, at the condyle
2. Record keeping; documenting presurgical, postsurgical, and follow-up positions of the facial bones
3. An aid to planning

Identification of Bony Pathology

Different medical-legal systems in different countries demand different levels of investigation. A thorough medical history and clinical examination must be taken and documented. In a patient undergoing elective surgery, a panoramic radiograph, which scans the teeth, mandible, and lower maxilla and sinus, is necessary. If these examinations suggest other pathology then it may be appropriate to have a more detailed or extensive radiologic examination. In most cases, this type of examination usually reveals no more than impacted third molars. Many surgeons feel these should be removed prophylatically before orthognathic surgery, especially for ramus procedures.

Naturally significant bone pathology such as cysts must be identified. In asymmetric cases, attention should be drawn to the condyles as well as the extent of the asymmetry of the mandible. Diagnosis of persistent and asymmetric growth at the condyle is most certainly made by detecting it on repeat articulated models. The use of bone scans to detect continued growth is not as useful as once declared. In the first instance, the injection of a radionucleotide into any patient who might be pregnant is unacceptable, and unfortunately the results of scans in any patient are frequently equivocal. The problem is that in patients with enlarged condyles there is often some traumatic TMJ dysfunction producing some inflammation, and this will provoke an increased uptake of isotype. Thus, it may be difficult to diagnose continued bone apposition from inflammatory changes.

The panoramic radiograph will normally suggest where the pathology lies by showing either an enlarged condyle or a diffuse enlargement of the mandible. As with the scan, to demonstrate continued activity is much more difficult. The use of sequential study models is the most reliable if slow method of evaluating continued growth.

Record Keeping

It is only good clinical practice to audit the effectiveness and stability of orthognathic surgery. The use of the standard lateral cephalogram to document the position of the facial bones before surgery, immediately postoperatively, and then at subsequent follow-up visits is clearly the best way of documenting the movements achieved and the long-term stability (Figures 46.16a,b). The radiographs must include at least immediate pre- and postoperative films. Immediate postoperative films may be confused by the need to use final occlusal splints. The timing of long-term follow-up films is not as critical, but most surgeons would expect 3-, 6-, and 12-month films. Although it is important academically to document longer-term stability, the majority of the relapse and soft tissue settling occurs early.

The cephalometric landmarks used for auditing stability are usually those used in the planning process, but other landmarks or projections may be useful for specific audits of groups of patients. These cephalometric landmarks will be discussed in the planning section.

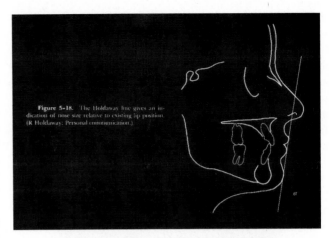

a

Figure 5-18. The Holdaway line gives an indication of nose size relative to existing lip position. (R Holdaway: Personal communication.)

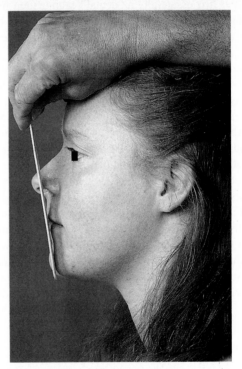

b

FIGURE 46.16 (a) This approach seems more informative. The line bisects the "S" curve of the nose and upper lip. (b) Clinical use.

In patients in whom rigid maxillomandibular fixation (MMF) is used, it is important to ensure the condyles have not been distracted from the fossa. Unfortunately, simple standard x-rays are not reliable and specialized views are needed, like reverse Townes, transpharyngeal, or even CT scans. The use of rigid MMF is however quite rare.

Aid to Planning

It would be naive not to assume that there are some surgeons who use lateral cephalometrics as the only method of planning orthognathic surgery. Some clearly "get away" with this method, but it is less than desirable. Even very well executed films have inherent errors. The film is converting a three-dimensional object to a two-dimensional plane. There is disproportionate magnification, from 15% at one side to 0% where the skin touches the cassette. Any vertical movement of the bones is accompanied by rotation at the condyles, and these structures have the most marked magnification errors. The majority of cephalometric analysis predominately measures the dental structures and rarely considers the head, face, and neck as a whole. Many orthognathic surgical planning programs exclude the forehead in the planning process, a potentially disastrous error. In some patients and particularly in some syndromes, the skull base, which forms the "starting" point of most angular and linear measurements, is not a "standard" shape or position. If the surgical procedure is defined by cephalometric data, the wrong aesthetic result may ensue. It is essentially a "dental" examination for a facial problem. In planning, cephalometrics should thus be used as confirmation of the careful clinical examination and as a guide to the orthodontic movements needed.

This chapter does not provide the data that are available in textbooks on cephalometrics, but it is useful to highlight some of the analyses available. The very basic assessment is the measurement of vertical height ratios, nasion to anterior nasal spine (ANS), and ANS to menton. Angular measurements of SNA and SNB give useful information about the relative positions of the maxilla and mandible. Angular measurements of the occlusal plane angle may be helpful in anterior openbite cases of those with anterior or posterior height discrepancies. Finally, the angulation of the incisors should be noted. The British orthodontists have developed a surgical planning program that provides a relatively simple analysis, with the option for the more commonly used surgical procedures. It takes a small "window" of the face and is limited as a planning device, but is useful in trying some surgical options.

It recognizes that the soft tissue responses to bony movements are very much a "guess." The risks of planning from radiographs only cannot be stressed enough (Figures 46.1g,h). In this case, failure to appreciate the forehead and nasion prominence has produced a distressing result.

The Delaire analysis attempts to overcome many of the shortcomings of conventional analyses.[14–16] This method plans from the whole skull and neck and seeks to establish proportions. It has some disadvantages, particularly the need to have a penetrated view of the whole skull, with use of increased irradiation. It is a little more complex than other procedures, but those routinely using the technique report familiarity renders it no more difficult than most analyses. As with all systems, the Delaire analysis inherently has errors of point recognition, and is converting a three-dimensional head to a two-dimensional film.[14–16] Again, despite its attempt to evaluate the whole head, it fails to document the important relationship of the forehead to the facial skeleton. This analysis is not readily available in a computer system, but a number of analyses are available (Figures 46.17a,b). Some integrated programs like OTP (Ortho Treatment Planner), Pacific Coast Software, Inc. have the option of warping the soft tissue image to reflect the procedure and adjust the image according to the surgical program. All these devices must be carefully explained to the patient because the quality of the printout can easily mislead the patient to believe this will be the final result (Figures 46.18a–f).

The use of "surgical templates," that is, transparencies of Bolton standard heads and faces, seems too easy to be taken seriously.[17] There are three sizes of Bolton standard faces marked on a transparent film, which is simply placed over the cephalometric radiograph. This technique does however have the benefit of giving a good overview of the whole face,

a

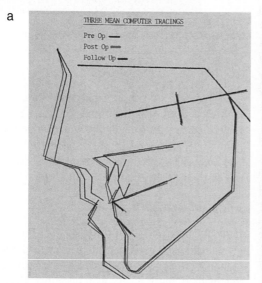

b

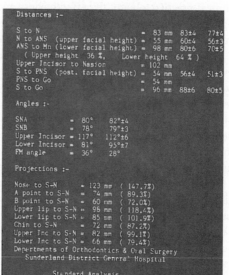

FIGURE 46.17 (a) Record keeping can be done by cephalometric computer storage. (b) Using a variety of measurements.

FIGURE 46.18 (a) Rickett's analysis. (b) McNamara's analysis. (c) A simple analysis. (d) Planning program of UK orthodontists; this ignores the forehead. (e) Digitized points on O.T.P. Planner. (f) Surgical treatment, maxilla impaction, mandible advance and rotate.

Continued.

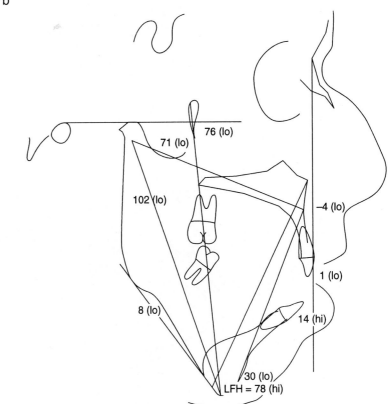

c

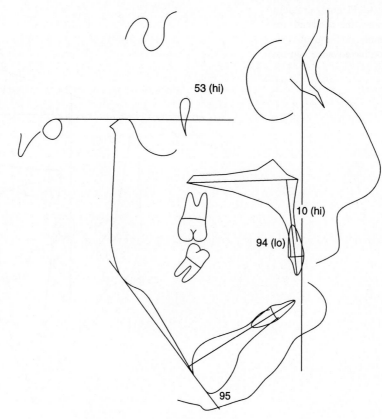

53 (hi)

10 (hi)

94 (lo)

95

d

NAME

SEX
FEMALE

DOB
15-06-79

SUPERIMPOSITION
Sella–Nasion & Sella

20-01-94C (├ ─ ─ ┤) ON 20-01-94 (├────┤)

PRE-OP ORTHODONTICS (PREDICTION)

Incisors decompensated . . .
   Upper incisors tipped −8.0°
   Lower incisors tipped −3.5°
Occlusal plane levelled

SURGICAL PROCEDURES (PREDICTION)

Mandibular ramus osteotomy
   Class I incisors . . .
   10.5 mm →, −2.5 mm ↓

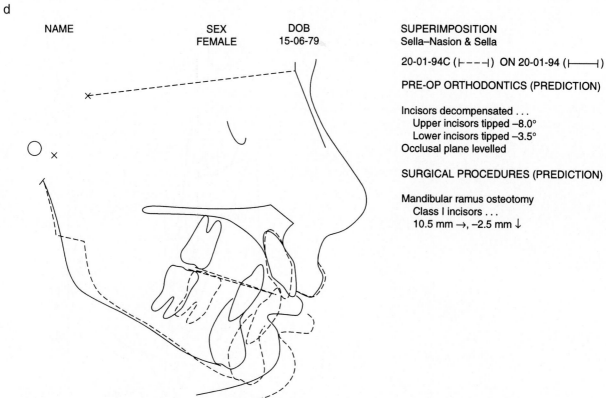

FIGURE 46.18 *Continued.*

e

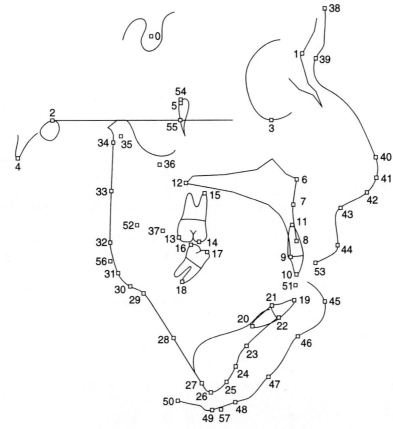

f

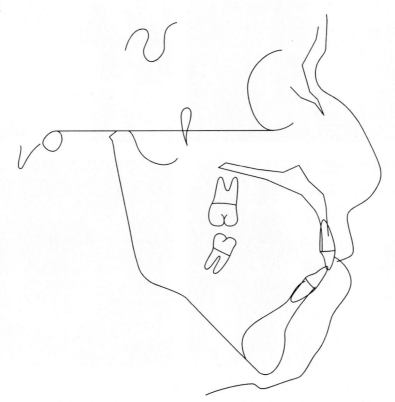

FIGURE 46.18 *Continued.*

often omitted in some of the more sophisticated analyses. Its main disadvantage is its inability to "measure" the movements required to obtain a harmonious appearance. There are many other analyses that provide much more comprehensive data, hopefully leading to a better diagnosis of the clinical problem. The Delaire analysis is particularly interesting as it attempts to find a more stable "starting point" or base to the analysis.[14–16] It also includes a much more complete analysis of the facial skeleton.

Model Surgery and Planning

Although this step is at the end of the planning cycle, it is most important. Good model surgery gives the surgeon more real information about the three-dimensional movements his osteotomy will allow to occur. This is so important with modern rigid internal fixation, because any errors of fixation will be looking at the surgeon the next day!

The aim is to obtain good articulated models with the correct bite. The bite is often erroneously recorded because patients needing osteotomies have malocclusions. This may well produce a slightly postured bite of convenience and comfort that involves a small distraction of the condyle from the fossa. Although it may not be accurate, the use of an articulator does help to establish the occlusal plane angulation and the possible axis of rotation of the mandible (Figures 46.19a–d).

The models should be accurately mounted with adequate measurements, so that the osteotomy cuts can be made and the movements simulated. This identifies any inappropriate or potentially unstable movements. This problem classically occurs in anteroposterior movements that increase the vertical height, and only if the models are cut and moved anatomically can these unstable vertical movements be picked up.

Good model surgery also helps to ensure accurately constructed intermediate and final splints. The "Achilles heel" of model surgery is accurately documenting the position of the condyle and the point of rotation of the mandible. The condylar position almost certainly changes from the awake to the anesthetized to the postoperative positions. Postoperative evaluation of the actual rotations that occur show an unpredictable and wide range of rotation points, making preoperative predictions impossible.

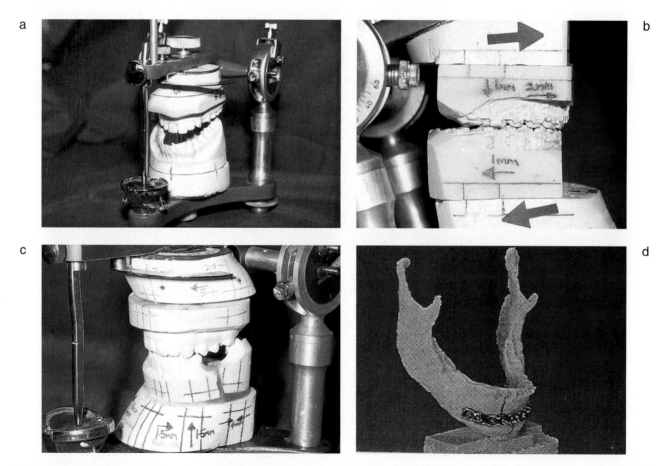

FIGURE 46.19 (a) Model surgery is extremely important in visualizing the presenting position. (b) Planned movements. (c) Great care is required at all stages of preparation; it is not however totally accurate, especially in rotational movements. (d) Computer-generated models from CT give much greater accuracy but the amount of irradiation and cost preclude this as a routine procedure.

Completing the Planning Cycle

Completion of planning entails collating all the data, resolving a definitive plan, and then presenting the options to the patient. In most cases, planning will begin before orthodontic work and so at that stage a provisional plan will be presented to the patient. The patient must be informed that this plan will be reviewed at the end of orthodontic work once the projected tooth movements become a reality. Other supplementary surgery, for example, removal of impacted teeth, may be undertaken during the orthodontic process.

At this consultation it is important to inform the patient about the surgery, its potential complications, and what the patient should expect. Arranging for the patient to see a recently operated patient is an excellent way of "informing" yet not frightening the patient. The patient must however accept there will always be a variation in outcome and in the patient's response to the surgery (Figures 46.20a,b). Warning of possible damage to the infraorbital and particularly the inferior alveolar nerves must be conveyed to the patient.

The stability of the surgery must be discussed briefly with the patient. The current evidence suggests that small movements are more stable than large movements, 7 to 8 mm being the boundary between large and small. The stability of

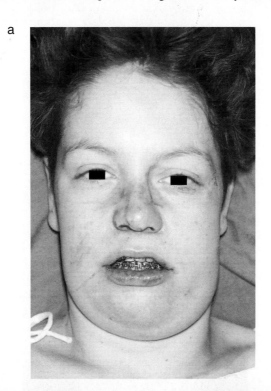

a

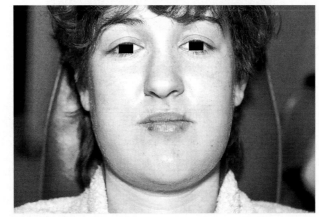

b

FIGURE 46.20 (a) Postoperative complications are important to discuss with the patient. Nerve damage and swelling are always difficult to predict. Both these patients had mandibular procedures by the same surgeon. (b) The patient's response is also difficult to gauge preoperatively; minimal postoperative swelling.

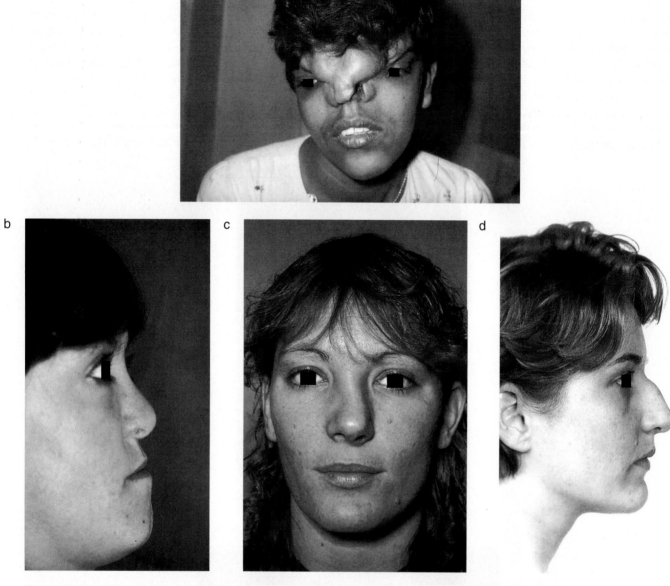

FIGURE 46.21 (a) The surgeon must have the surgical repertoire to give the patient the operation the planning demands, rather than a "favorite" operation. (b) An example of Binders syndrome. (c) Posttraumatic nasal deformity. (d) Congenital nasal deformity.

the soft tissue is equally important but less predictable.[18]

Finally, the surgeon must feel happy to undertake the surgery that the patient needs and not be restricted by surgical convenience or preference. As with all surgery, "the commonest conditions present most commonly" and the majority of patients need standard routine procedures. There will be a small group of patients, however, presenting with more unusual needs, and the maxillofacial surgeon should be able to treat them equally well (Figures 46.21a–d).

References

1. Proffit WR, White RP. Who needs surgical-orthodontic treatment? *Int J Adult Orthod Orthogn Surg*. 1990;5(2):81–89.
2. Flanary CM, Barnwell GM, Van Sickels JE, Littlefield JH, Rugh AL. Impact of orthognathic surgery on normal and abnormal personality dimensions: a two-year follow-up study of 61 patients. *Am J Orthod Dentofacial Orthop* 1990;98 (4):313–22.
3. Serra Payro JM, Vinals Vinals JM, Palacin Porte JA, Estrada

Cuixart J, Lerma Gonce J, Alacron Perez J. Surgical management of the acromegalic face. *J Craniofac Surg.* 1994;5 (5):336–338.

4. Phillips S, Bailey LJ, Sieber RP. Level of agreement in clinicians' perceptions of class II malocclusions. *J Oral Maxillofac Surg.* 1994;52(6):565–571.

5. Tanner JM, Davies PSW. Clinical longitudinal standards for height and height velocity for North American children. *J Paediatr.* 1985;107:317–329.

6. Gonzales-Ulloa, M. Planning the integral correction of the human profile. *Plast Reconstr Surg.* 1961;36:364–373.

7. Gonzales-Ulloa M, Stevens E. The role of chin correction in profile plasty. *Plast Reconstr Surg.* 1966;41:477–486.

8. Ricketts RM. Planning treatment on the basis of the facial pattern and an estimate of its growth. *Angle Orthod.* 1957;27:14–37.

9. Ricketts RM. Cephalometric analysis and synthesis. *Angle Orthod.* 1961;31:141–156.

10. Ricketts RM. Perspectives in the clinical application of cephalometrics. *Angle Orthod.* 1981;51:115–150.

11. Ricketts RM. The value of cephalometrics and computerized technology. *Angle Orthod.* 1972;42:179–199.

12. Steiner CC. Cephalometrics in clinical practice. *Angle Orthod.* 1959;29:8–29.

13. Steiner CC. Cephalometrics as a clinical tool. In: Kraus BS, Reidel RA, eds. *Vistas in Orthodontics.* Philadelphia: Lea & Febiger; 1962.

14. Delaire J. L'analyse architecturale et structurale craniofaciale (de profil); principles théoriques; quelques exemples d'emploi en chirugie maxillo-faciale. *Rev Stomatol Chir Maxillofac.* 1978;79:1–33.

15. Delaire J. Quelques pièges dans les interpretations des téléradiographies cephalometriques. *Rev Stomatol Chir Maxillofac.* 1984;85:176–185.

16. Delaire J, Schendel SA, Tulasne JF. An architectural and structural craniofacial analysis: A new lateral cephalometric analysis. *Oral Surg.* 1981;85:226–238.

17. Broadbent BH Sr, Broadbent BH Jr, Golden WH. *Bolton Standards of Dentofacial Developmental Growth.* St. Louis: CV Mosby Co., 1975.

18. Hack GA, de Mol van Otterloo JJ, Nanda J. Long-term stability and prediction of soft tissue changes after Le Fort I surgery. *Am J Orthod Dentofacial Orthop.* 1993;104(6):544–555.

47

Considerations in Planning for Bimaxillary Surgery and the Implications of Rigid Internal Fixation

Brian Alpert, George M. Kushner, and Gerald D. Verdi

Rigid fixation is one of the latest and indeed one of the most significant advances in the surgery of dentofacial deformities. Although the use of intermaxillary fixation is routine to the surgeons who utilize it, it is often a cause of anxiety to others. Orthodontists, nurses, anesthesiologists, and other health care providers often have great concern, indeed fear, about its use, as do many patients for whom the prospect of being "wired shut" often negatively impacts on their decision to undergo corrective surgery.

The advantages of rigid fixation are obviously an easier and shorter hospital admission, with the elimination of the need for overnight intubation or nasal airways, which are often associated with intensive care unit or transitional care unit stays. The avoidance of intermaxillary fixation has dramatically diminished the perception of, if not the actual existence of, potential airway problems.

Rigid fixation permits an earlier return to function with regard to mastication and speech, which otherwise would be limited during the convalescent period. There is decreased long-term trismus, and by the time a patient who is treated with intermaxillary fixation is allowed to open, a comparable patient with rigid internal fixation is at full function.

Several studies have shown rigid fixation to be at least as stable as conventional skeletal fixation,[1–3] with others indicating that it is more stable.[4,5] There has been a resurgence of attempts to do corrections with rigid fixation that in the past were deemed inherently unstable when wire fixation[6] was utilized. These procedures include maxillary downgrafts as well as closure of open bites at the expense of the mandibular angle. It remains to be seen whether rigid fixation will offer a solution in unstable corrections.

Rigid fixation has certain disadvantages because it is a more difficult procedure and is certainly more technique sensitive, with very little margin for error. Utilizing conventional techniques with wire gives a certain amount of leeway, as adjustments can be made during the convalescent period. The segments themselves will exhibit a degree of movement to offer this potential adjustment, as opposed to the use of rigid fixation in which the segments are absolutely stable with only orthodontic adjustments possible.

The learning curve in the use of rigid fixation is much longer than wire fixation techniques. As experience is gained, however, surgeons can often apply rigid fixation more rapidly than conventional wiring techniques. There is certainly also greater potential for morbidity with rigid fixation. The obvious surgical misadventure of violating a nerve or tooth root with a screw occasionally occurs. The less obvious rigidly fixed error, resulting in malposition of bone fragments, also occasionally occurs with resultant malocclusion, condylar malposition, and contour defects.

One of the major reasons for increased morbidity potential with rigid internal fixation is when it is necessary to perform bilateral sagittal split ramus osteotomies for the correction of mandibular deformities. This particular procedure for the correction of mandibular prognathism has greater inherent potential for morbidity than the oblique subcondylar osteotomy, (which does not readily lend itself to rigid fixation techniques).

Rigid fixation is more costly because specialized equipment and costly hardware are required. However, this increased equipment expense is usually offset by a shorter, less costly hospital stay.

Indications for Bimaxillary Surgery

A discussion of all the intricacies of planning for dentofacial deformity correction is beyond the scope of this review. However, there are a number of indications for two-jaw surgery. Large anteroposterior discrepancies often necessitate two-jaw surgery. The treatment of at least moderate mandibular excess or deficiency in conjunction with open-bite, long or short face deformity almost always requires simultaneous mobilization of both jaws. When significant asymmetries exist in both maxillary and mandibular midlines, two-jaw surgery is often necessary. When discrepancies are present in the orientation of the occlusal plane either in the anteroposterior dimension as in deep bite deformities, or in lateral dimension as in hemifacial microsomia or condylar hyperplasia cases, simultaneous mobilization of both jaws is performed.

Obviously, one can usually find an indication to operate

both jaws. However in the context of a whole face, a 2- to 3-mm correction is insignificant. As such, a two-jaw correction for 4 to 6 mm of total discrepancy in the absence of midline alterations, open bites, or significant discrepancies of the occlusal plane is a great deal of treatment for minimal gain. The surgeon must consider the potential for morbidity with respect to the benefit gained.

There are some basic truths with respect to orthognathic surgery. It is well known that the conventional Le Fort I maxillary osteotomy (downfracture) has minimal potential for long-term morbidity. This differs from the sagittal split ramus osteotomy, which has significant potential for permanent morbidity in the form of paresthesia and regression or relapse. Condylar resorption, TMJ problems, etc. are more unusual complications of this operation. Similarly, segmental osteotomies are not periodontally predictable; 20% of these procedures demonstrate permanent periodontal defects at the osteotomy site. The Le Fort II osteotomy has also been found to be a relatively unstable correction.

Recognition of these "truths" should guide the surgeon and orthodontist in developing a treatment plan that should fit the operation to the patient and not the patient to the operation. The development of a treatment plan is based on establishing a diagnosis from which a list of the patient's problems and the available surgical or orthodontic solutions is formulated. Discussion between the surgeon, orthodontist, and the patient should weigh the potential for morbidity of the solutions to arrive at a treatment plan with a favorable risk-to-benefit ratio. Fundamentally, the benefit gained must outweigh the risk of complications, because minor problems will require minor corrections, while major problems will require major corrections. (One does not need a sledgehammer to drive a tack.) Consideration must also be made of other treatment alternatives, all of which could be valid options. A patient with a dentofacial deformity could be presented to five different surgical-orthodontic teams and get multiple alternative treatment plans, all of which may be acceptable. Beauty and facial form are in the eyes of the beholder.

There are numerous factors to be considered in the development of a surgical treatment plan that will guide the surgeon and the orthodontist. These include nasal form, nasolabial angle, lip to incisal edge relationship, neck drape, facial height and proportion, and dental and skeletal midlines. Nasal form is often a determinant for which the jaw needs to be corrected. For example, if a patient has a large although well-formed nose and an absolute mandibular prognathism, mandibular setback will make the nose seem even larger, and a maxillary advancement may be indicated. Maxillary advancement in an individual with a small nose may create an anthropoid appearance. The nasolabial angle offers a point of reference with regard to maxillary advancement or setback. A setback in an obtuse nasolabial angle will make it even more obtuse. Maxillary advancement with an obtuse nasolabial angle will make it more acute.

Lip to incisal edge is one of the more critical areas of assessment and is a reference for the vertical position of the maxilla. The patient should show 2 to 4 mm of tooth at rest.

Neck drape is critically important in determining mandibular corrections. One needs to be careful in setting back a mandible and creating jowls. Indeed, many patients with true, but moderate mandibular prognathisms are better treated by advancing their maxilla because their neck drape is already optimal. Facial height and proportion need to be assessed along with dental and skeletal midlines. All these considerations must be discussed with the patient and family before surgery so they can participate in the treatment planning.

What Is Needed from the Orthodontist

Once a surgical decision has been made, the orthodontist is responsible for decompensating the dentition. Fundamentally, this means placing the teeth in their optimal position to basal bone. Often the deformity that has dental compensations will become more skeletally apparent following orthodontic treatment. Indeed, changes in the surgical treatment plan often become evident at this point in orthodontic preparation. In any event, the orthodontist needs to decompensate the dentition so that models fit into an appropriate postoperative relationship. Obviously, in a suitably orthodontically decompensated dentition, nonsurgical attempts to close an anterior open bite must be avoided. The orthodontic appliances will also need appropriate surgical hooks for intraoperative intermaxillary fixation and/or postoperative training elastics. At this stage, the surgeon and orthodontist (and patient!) should decide on an optimal lip to incisal edge relationship.

Setting Up the Case

In our view, anatomic articulators and facebow transfers add an aura of precision and mystique to planning and splint fabrication but are unnecessary for precise surgical execution. One needs dental models that can be articulated in both the final occlusal relationship and a preoperative occlusal relationship. The relationship of the teeth (which can be seen and of which we have an exact facsimile) are used to set the case, not areas for osteotomies and ostectomies that can only be imagined.

In bimaxillary osteotomies, either jaw can be mobilized first, but it is preferable to mobilize the maxilla first because it can almost always be rigidly fixed. If a mandibular sagittal split is unfavorable, it may not be possible to perform rigid fixation in a convenient manner. If this occurs, then the ability to relate the maxilla to the mandible is lost. In the technique to be described, a transitional interocclusal splint is used to relate the maxilla in the corrected position to the unoperated mandible. Then a final splint will relate the mandible in the desired position to the corrected (and rigidly fixed) maxilla. The models are articulated and marked in the postoperative position as well as the preoperative position with appropriate vertical and horizontal references lines (Figure 47.1). An interocclusal splint is made relating the models in the final occlusion (Figure 47.2).

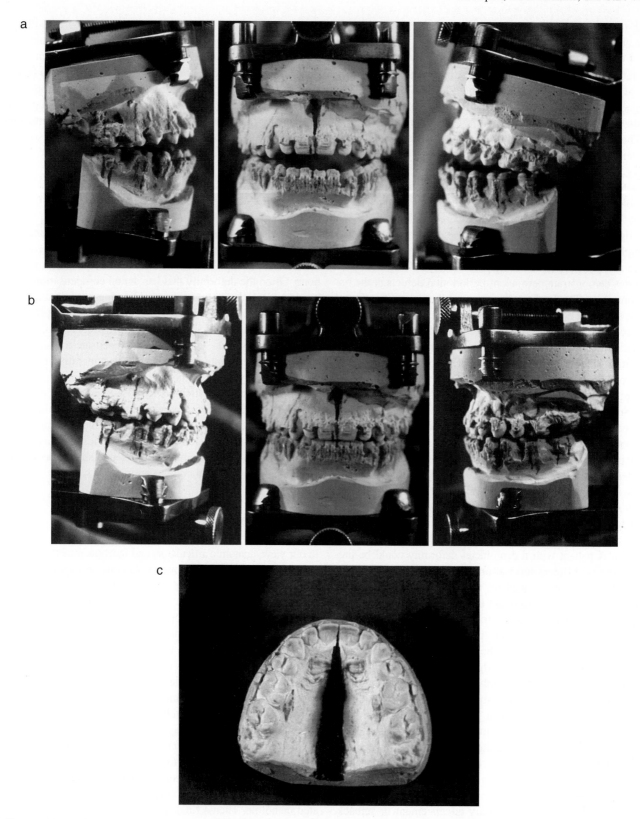

FIGURE 47.1 (a) Models articulated in presurgical relationship. Reference lines are marked. (b) Models articulated in final postsurgical relationship. (c) Note midpalatal split and widening of maxilla are required in this instance.

a

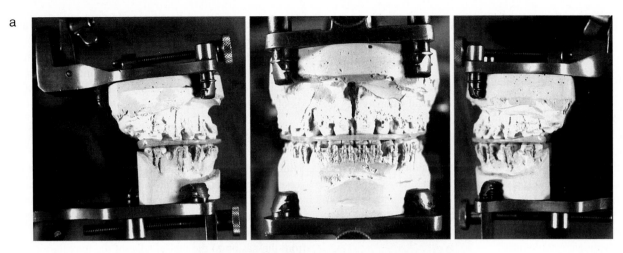

b

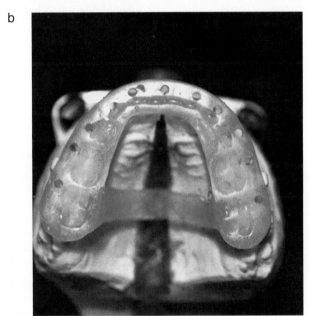

FIGURE 47.2 (a) A final interocclusal splint (index) is made in the postsurgical relationship. (b) Note the palatal strap on the index, which minimizes distortion or bending of the index and supports the expansion of the maxilla during convalescence because maxillomandibular fixation is not used.

The maxillary model in corrected position is now related to the mandibular model in its uncorrected position utilizing the horizontal and vertical reference lines on the teeth as a guide (Figures 47.3a,b). A "transitional" interocclusal splint (index) is made at this point (Figures 47.3c,d). If the maxilla has been segmented, a splint within a "final" splint can be used (Figures 47.4a–c). This allows only one splint to be wired into place (making the segmented maxilla intact) rather than changing splints after the maxilla is rigidly fixed. Thus, only one splint will have to be wired (fixed) to the maxillary arch after it is segmented. The transitional splint carries with it all the anteroposterior (AP), lateral, and occlusal plane corrections that the treatment plan calls for, using the maxillary and mandibular teeth as reference points and the patient's mandible as the articulator. The vertical position (lip to incisal edge relationship) is set at surgery. Thus, an extremely precise treatment plan that utilizes fixed reference points, the teeth, can be incorporated into two interocclusal acrylic splints (indices) (Figure 47.4).

Additional Treatment Planning Considerations

Multiple Segment Le Fort I

As surgical experience has been gained and orthodontics has advanced, we tend to do fewer multiple segment Le Fort I osteotomies. In our institution, we try to achieve single piece Le Fort I osteotomy preparation by having the orthodontist "work harder." An exception is midline or paramidline splits for posterior expansion. In excessive posterior maxillary or transverse hyperplasia, it is not unusual to set the case up with good cuspid-to-cuspid occlusion, but an open bite posteriorly. These posterior open bites close spontaneously, avoiding the need for multiple segment osteotomies.

Cleft Palate Patients

Rather than perform Le Fort I osteotomies with simultaneous closure of fistulae and bone grafting on extensive clefts utilizing anterior soft tissue pedicles (which can pose considerable difficulties), we now simultaneously graft the alveolar clefts and close the fistulae in advance (age 7 to 12). In this way, we can perform a conventional Le Fort I osteotomy on a one- or two-piece maxilla without the anterior pedicles and surgical struggle (with the attendant increased risk of necrosis of flaps and recurrent fistulae).

Setting Facial Height (Lip to Incisal Edge)

Setting proper facial height has been one of the most controversial areas in orthognathic surgery planning. A number of techniques have been advocated for this endeavor. Some have used measured bone removal with internal reference points based on cephalometric prediction. Others have used calipers from the nasion to the incisal edge of the maxillary central incisor.[7,8] Yet others have measured from a screw placed in the nasion to the incisal edge of the central incisor.[9] We utilize the relationship of the inferior margin of the lip to the incisal edge. The salient point of this technique is that the nose must be undistorted by the endotracheal tube so that the lip is not retracted or elongated. (See Figures 47.6a,b later in this chapter.)

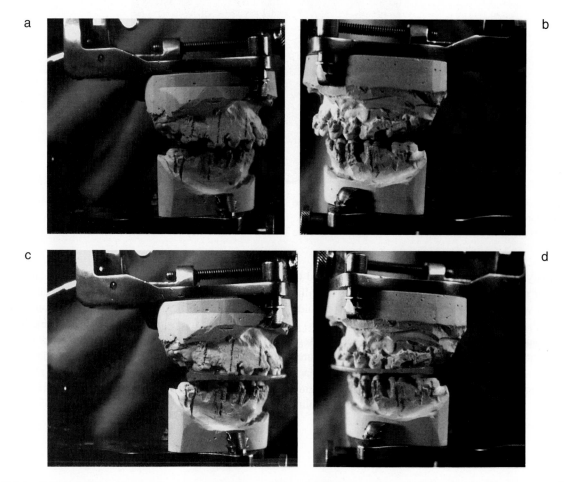

a   b

c   d

Figure 47.3 (a–d) Utilizing the reference lines as a guide, the maxillary model in *corrected* position is related to the *uncorrected* mandibular model. Note that the maxilla has been advanced and the open bite corrected at the expense of the posterior maxilla.

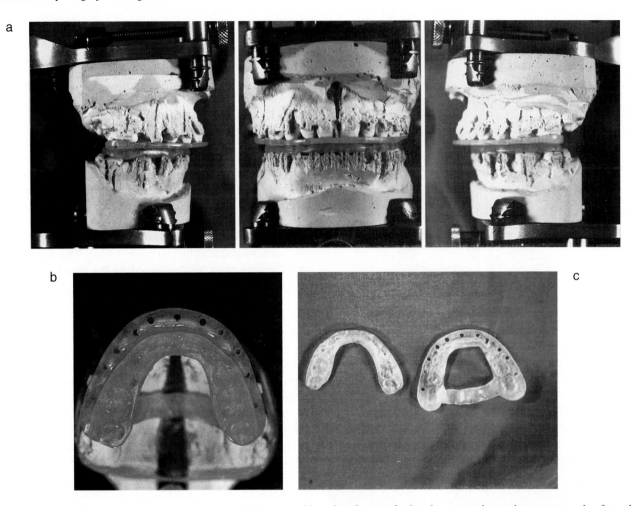

FIGURE 47.4 (a–c). The final splint and transitional splint serve as blueprints for transferring the extremely precise treatment plan from the laboratory to surgery. (c) Note the final splint is right and the transitional splint is left. The final splint is reinforced with a palatal strut.

Setting Condylar Position (Bilateral Sagittal Split Ramus Osteotomy [BSSRO])

The available techniques utilized have been high-low wires,[10,11] various mechanical devices that relate the proximal segment to the maxilla (bone to bone),[12,13] the proximal segment to the maxillary arch wire,[14] the maxillary arch wire to reference points on proximal segments,[15,16] etc. Other techniques have advocated the use of bone clamps, while others utilize screw slots.[17] Our technique uses manual repositioning with a trocar point, which is described later.

Considerations for Rigid Fixation

In maxillary surgery, the surgeon must think of rigid internal fixation when designing the osteotomy. The superior regions of the piriform apertures and zygomatic buttresses need be exposed to find substantial bone that will hold screws. Likewise, the osteotomy should be designed a little higher than normal to allow placement of the plates on the mobilized

segment while avoiding tooth roots (Figure 47.5). Bone should be judiciously trimmed in the maxillary buttress and piriform aperture areas so that contact remains in these areas

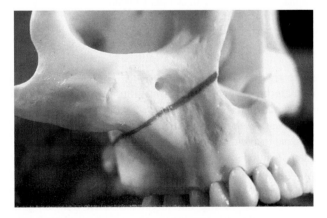

FIGURE 47.5 Ideal lines of Le Fort I osteotomy when the use of rigid fixation is intended. This may be considered somewhat higher than normal to facilitate plate and screw fixation.

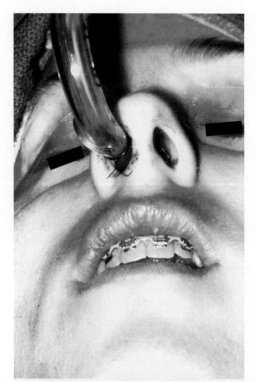

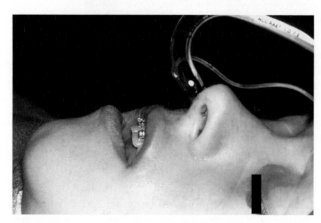

FIGURE 47.6 (a) The endotracheal tube is placed and positioned so that the nose is undistorted, and can be returned to this undistorted position during surgery. (b) Note how the tube is fixed with a heavy suture to the nasal septum.

where rigid fixation is to be placed. The hardware should maintain bone contact in the piriform aperture and buttress regions rather than holding the fragments apart.

Precise, stable intermaxillary fixation cannot be overemphasized to avoid slipping of the occlusion during screw tightening. Position screws should be utilized instead of lag screws to minimize condylar distraction caused by rotation of the segments. The screws should be inserted perpendicular to the bone to avoid sliding the fragments when tightening the screws. In splits that involve rotation of the mandible around the horizontal axis, bone between the splits needs to be trimmed or shims utilized before placement of screws in these

areas of rotation to permit passive fit of segments. Finally, impacted teeth need to be removed in advance (3–6 months if possible) to permit superior quality and quantity of bone for screw fixation.

Executing the Treatment Plan During the Surgical Exercise

The precise treatment plan has been prepared and is transferred to the patient at surgery through the use of the surgical splints. These are the presurgically determined templates or road maps that guide the surgeon during the course of the operation. *One does not plan at surgery but before.*

The first step in the procedure is placement and fixation of the nasoendotracheal tube (Figure 47.6a). This is critical in that the nose must be undistorted by the tube (or able to be repeatedly placed in an undistorted posture) during the course of surgery. This is the key to properly setting facial height. The tube is placed and taped securely to the head so that the nose is undistorted. Tape is not used to fix the tube to the nose. Occasionally the tube may be sewn to the nasal septum for additional security (Figure 47.6b). The position and the reproducibility of this position are checked before draping.

Following the usual prep, drape, throat pack, etc., the areas of surgery are infiltrated with local anesthetic solution for hemostasis (Figure 47.7). Use of 0.5% or 1% lidocaine with epinephrine 1:200,000 is preferred. To reduce hemorrhage during the course of surgery, the anesthesiologist is asked to keep the systolic blood pressure below 100 mmHg. This is usually done with deep inhalation anesthesia, although occasionally formal hypotensive anesthesia is utilized.

Attention is first directed to the mandible where, following exposure, cortical osteotomies are made in standard fashion (Figure 47.8). Burs are utilized although some operators prefer saws. The osteotomies are designed for "chisel access," which later allows the chisel to be directed at the inner aspect of the buccal cortex, attempting to avoid the inferior alveolar

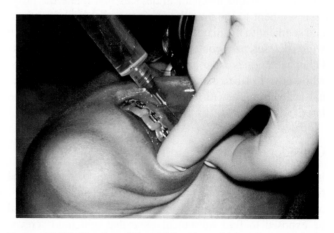

FIGURE 47.7 Infiltration of the incision sites with local anesthesia for hemostasis; 0.5% lidocaine with epinephrine 1:200,000 is preferred.

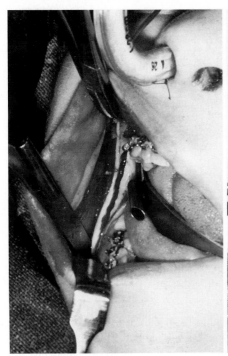
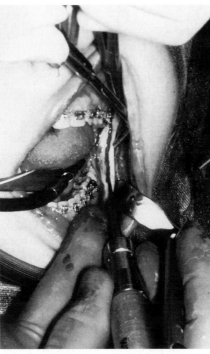

FIGURE 47.8 The mandibular osteotomy sites are exposed and the cortical osteotomy cuts made. The osteotomies are not yet mobilized with osteotomes.

neurovascular bundle during the split (Figure 47.9). The cuts are made bilaterally but the splits are not completed, and then the wounds are packed if necessary and attention directed to the maxilla.

A flattened U-shaped incision is made high in the vestibule from approximately second premolar to second premolar (Figure 47.10). This U-shaped incision is utilized because it allows for a broader buccal mucosal pedicle with ample surgical access and is less likely to tear when retractors are placed in the pterygomaxillary fissure (Figure 47.11). The piriform apertures are exposed to the infraorbital rims and the dissection is carried high on the zygomatic buttress. The nasal mucosa is stripped from the medial and lateral nasal walls and the floor.

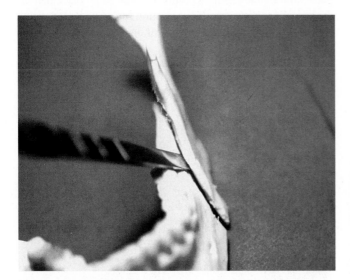

FIGURE 47.9 Model demonstrating the concept of separating the buccal cortex of the proximal fragment from the medullary bone of the distal fragment in an attempt to avoid the neurovascular bundle. This plan necessitates "chisel access," which means designing and contouring the cortical cuts to allow the osteotome to be directed laterally.

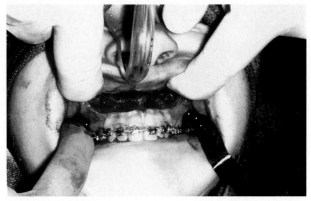

FIGURE 47.10 High, U-shaped incision enhances the buccal pedicle. It also is less likely to tear from retractors.

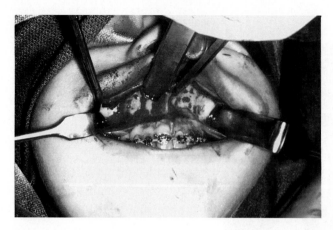

FIGURE 47.11 Excellent exposure of osteotomy site provided by high, U-shaped incision.

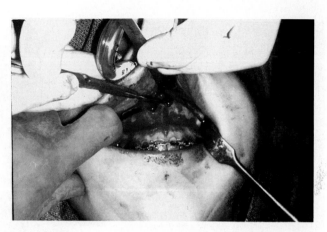

FIGURE 47.13 The lateral nasal walls and septum are sectioned with an osteotome. No attempt is made to preserve or avoid the greater palatine vessels.

The bone cut, with bur or saw, is made from pterygomaxillary fissure to piriform aperture approximately 6 to 8 mm above the apices of the teeth (Figure 47.12). No attempt is made to remove a measured segment of bone. The nasal septum is freed with a specialized osteotome and the lateral nasal walls are sectioned with an osteotome (Figure 47.13). No attempt is made to avoid the greater palatine vessels. Pterygoid osteotomes complete the section in standard fashion.

The maxilla is downfractured with digital pressure, the use of disimpaction forceps rarely being necessary. The maxilla is now thoroughly mobilized so that it can be moved with ease to literally any position. If necessary, hemostasis is achieved with packing and/or electrocautery. With good hypotensive anesthesia, excessive bleeding is unusual. A heavy towel clip is now placed in the nasal spine region and the maxilla is mobilized anteriorly and inferiorly (Figure 47.14).

Bone is now removed in the posterior regions of the maxilla utilizing a rongeur and large bone bur. This maneuver is accomplished at this time because these are the areas that are difficult to access once intermaxillary fixation is in place and the maxilla and the mandible are being autorotated. Significant bone reduction is accomplished in the posterior maxillary wall, the lateral nasal walls, and the region of pterygomaxillary junction. The nasal crest is removed along its entire length and replaced by a groove (Figure 47.15). At this point the maxilla is sectioned if necessary utilizing conventional technique.

The transitional splint is now fixed to the maxillary arch: if the maxilla has been sectioned, the final splint is wired to place, uniting the segments. This is followed by placement of the transitional splint within the splint. Intermaxillary fixation is now placed in this corrected position, which relates the op-

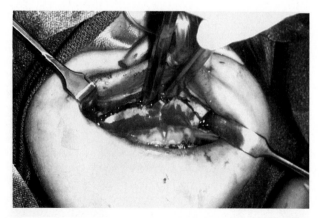

FIGURE 47.12 Buccal bone cuts are made from the pterygomaxillary fissure to piriform apertures. No attempt is made to remove a measured amount of bone; a cut is just made.

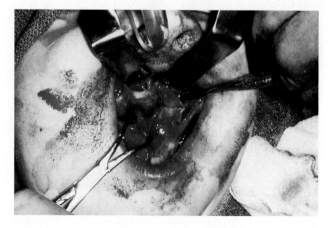

FIGURE 47.14 The maxilla is thoroughly mobilized and pulled forward with a towel clip (through the nasal spine area) for access to the posterior regions.

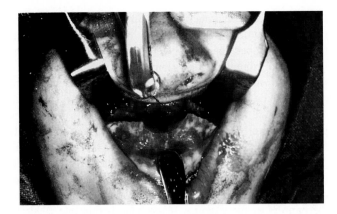

FIGURE 47.15 Bone has been reduced in the posterior maxillary and lateral nasal walls. The piriform aperture has been widened, the nasal crest eliminated, and a midline groove placed.

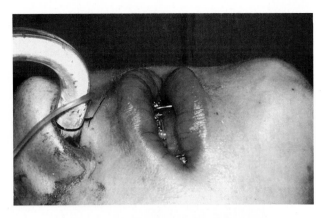

FIGURE 47.17 With the nose maintained in undistorted position, facial height is set using the inferior margin of the upper lip to the maxillary incisal edge. Bone is judiciously reduced from the maxillary buttress to piriform aperture until proper height is achieved. This lip-to-incisor relationship will be maintained after healing is complete.

erated maxilla to the unoperated mandible (Figure 47.16). The maxilla and mandible are now autorotated making sure that the mandibular condyles are properly seated. The inferior margin of the upper lip to the incisal edge relationship is utilized to set facial height (Figure 47.17). It is critical that the nose (and lip) is undistorted and is in the reproducible position. At this point the only areas of bone contact remaining are between the zygomatic buttresses and piriform apertures. These are trimmed under direct vision until a proper lip to incisal edge relationship is obtained. At this point there should be bone contact in the piriform aperture and buttress regions (Figure 47.18). If proper facial height has been achieved and there is no contact at any point, shims of bone graft need be placed (Figure 47.19).

The piriform apertures are now contoured with rotary instrumentation for proper nasal form. If the maxilla is being advanced or intruded, this generally means widening and deepening these piriform apertures so that the nose is undis-

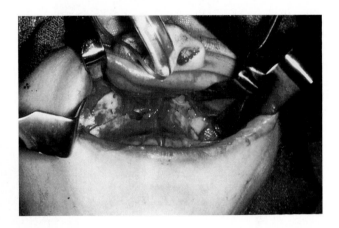

FIGURE 47.18 Bone contact resulting from judicious trimming to achieve proper facial height.

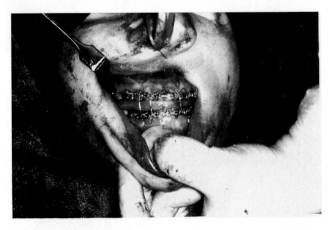

FIGURE 47.16 Utilizing a final splint with a transitional splint, intermaxillary fixation is placed, relating the mobilized maxilla to the intact mandible.

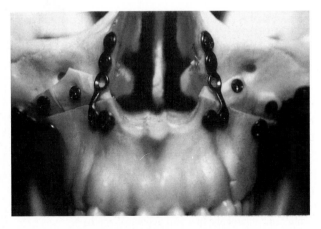

FIGURE 47.19 Model demonstrating placement and lag screw fixation of bone grafts to establish bony continuity of anterior maxillary walls in "downgrafts."

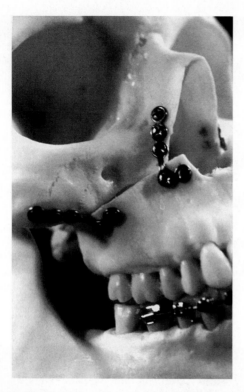

FIGURE 47.20 Model demonstrating proper placement of plate and screw fixation. Note that the double cortex on the lateral margin of the nasal bones is used anteriorly and the relatively thick zygomatic buttress posteriorly for screw fixation.

torted in the alar regions. If this maneuver is done properly, nasal cinch sutures are unnecessary. Indeed, if the bone contour is not proper, the nasal cinch sutures are not helpful. At this point a submucous resection of the septum is performed from below if necessary to avoid buckling the septum. Care must be taken to leave adequate dorsal and caudal supports.

The maxilla is now fixed in this position with four plates placed bilaterally in the piriform aperture and zygomatic buttress regions. The plates are placed in sites that allow for the greatest screw retention (Figure 47.20). Anteriorly, this would be the lateral margin of the nose where the lateral nasal and anterior maxilla walls join. Posteriorly, one should extend to the buttress of the zygoma. If the bone is thin one needs to extend higher. The plates are contoured so that they rest on the bone passively. Screw holes should be placed with low-speed twist drills of appropriate size utilizing drill guides (Figures 47.21a–c). High-speed drills without drill guides tend to whip slightly, making larger holes. Once the maxilla has been fixed in its corrected position, the intermaxillary fixation is released and the occlusion is checked (against the transitional splint). If it is not correct, the plates are removed and the fixation repeated. When the position is proper, intermaxillary

a
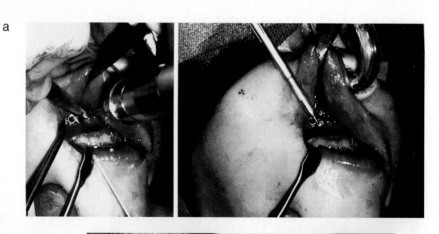
b

c
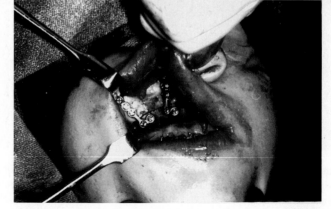

FIGURE 47.21 (a) A drill guide and low-speed twist drill are used to make holes. The drill guide centers the hole and does not allow the drill tip to "whip" and enlarge the hole. (b) Screws of appropriate length (generally 4–6 mm) fix the plate to the bone. (c) Complete fixation at piriform aperture and maxillary buttress.

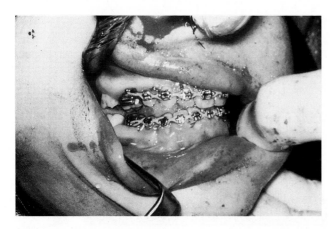

FIGURE 47.22 Intermaxillary fixation has been released and the transitional splint discarded. The maxilla is now in proper postoperative position. Note the lateral open bite in this example, resulting from the correction of a tilted occlusal plane.

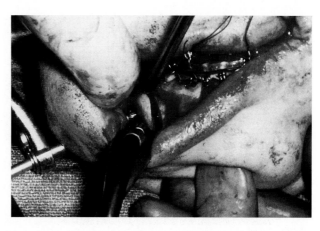

FIGURE 47.24 Use of the transbuccal trocar to place screw fixation of the sagittal osteotomies.

fixation is released and the transitional splint discarded (Figure 47.22).

Attention is now directed to the mandible where the sagittal cuts are now completed and segments mobilized. Care is taken to direct the chisel to the outer cortical plate in an attempt to avoid the inferior alveolar neurovascular triad (Figure 47.23). Once the splits are complete, necessary detachments of pterygoid muscle on the distal fragments are done with a gloved finger. Tight intermaxillary fixation is placed utilizing the final splint as a guide. One has to ensure that the intermaxillary fixation is quite stable because tightening screws can often alter an occlusal relationship that is not rigidly fixed. Bone in and around the osteotomy sites is now contoured, trimmed, or shimmed so that it comes passively together in a position amenable to osteosynthesis.

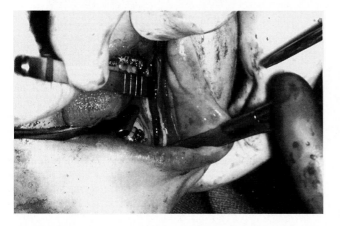

FIGURE 47.23 Splitting of the sagittal osteotomies. Note how the osteotome is directed toward the inner aspect of the lateral cortex to avoid the inferior alveolar neurovascular bundle.

A transbuccal trocar is used to place the screw fixation perpendicular to the osteotomies (Figure 47.24). The point of the trocar is also utilized to control the position of the proximal fragments while screw fixation is being accomplished (Figures 47.25a–f). A 5-mm stab incision is made approximately one finger breadth inferior to the mandible below the osteotomy site. An obturator is placed into the trocar and the trocar is passed through the stab incision into the mouth. The obturator is removed and the trocar sleeve is loosened and adjusted so that the point is in the six o'clock position in relationship to the inferior border of the mandible. The sleeve is tightened. A cheek retractor ring or blade is now fixed to the trocar sleeve.

A hole is drilled in the proximal segment with a 1.8-mm drill through the trocar just above the inferior border of the mandible. The trocar point is now placed into this hole, effectively making the trocar into a "handle" on the proximal fragment. The proximal fragment (and condyle) are now manipulated into proper position, seating the condyle gently in the fossa. The key to this maneuver is that once the proper condylar position is achieved, the surgeon's hand manipulating the trocar is not moved. A drill guide is placed, a bicortical hole drilled, the depth measured, and a screw of appropriate length placed. While the screw is being tightened, it is important to watch the occlusion to make certain it is not being altered by tightening the screw. Two additional screws are placed in triangular fashion. The procedure is repeated on the opposite side, the intermaxillary fixation is removed, and the occlusion checked for accuracy (Figure 47.26). If the occlusion is off, the screws are removed and the procedure repeated. This has rarely been found necessary when utilizing the described trocar point technique to control the proximal fragment. The wounds are closed in standard fashion. Sometimes it is necessary to do a V-Y closure of the maxillary wound. Resorbable sutures are utilized.

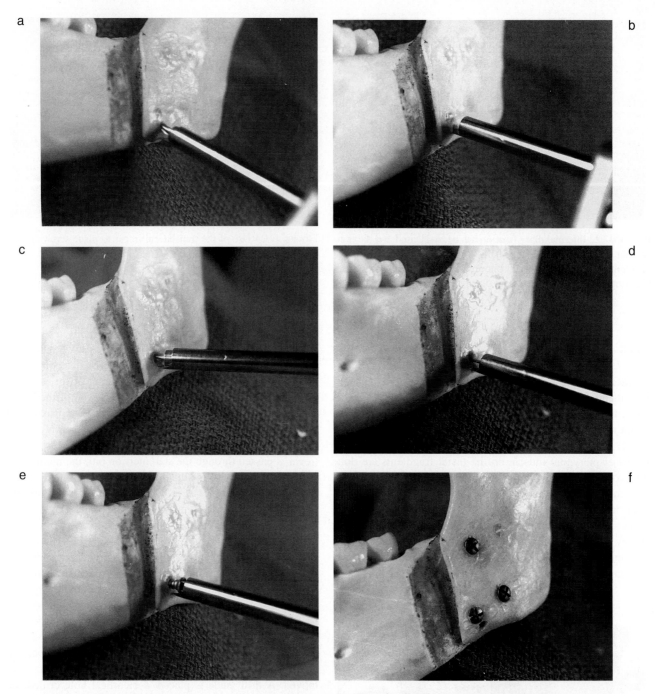

FIGURE 47.25 Technique of screw fixation and proximal segment control utilizing the transbuccal trocar. Note: for photographic purposes, the cheek retractor ring or blade is not in position on the trocar sleeve. (a) A 1.8-mm hole is drilled through the proximal fragment just above the inferior border. (b) The point of the trocar sleeve is placed in the hole, effectively making the trocar into a handle on the proximal fragment. The proximal fragment is positioned appropriately, seating the condyle and lining up the inferior border. This position is maintained by not moving the trocar through the ensuing steps. (c) A drill guide is placed and a bicortical hole is drilled through the proximal and distal fragments (1.8 mm for 2.4 mm screws). (d) The depth is measured with a depth gauge. (e) An appropriate length screw is placed. The proximal fragment is now fixed in place. (f) Two or three additional screws are placed in box or triangular fashion. Note the hole below the anterior inferior screw that served to hold the trocar point. Editor's note: Usually it is desirable to place two or three screws along the superior border of the osteotomy. One or more screws may be placed along the inferior border if the situation requires.

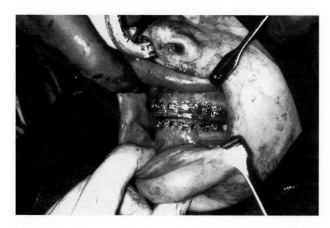

FIGURE 47.26 The mandible is manipulated to ensure correct reproducible occlusion.

During the first postoperative days, the patient is usually unable to completely close into the occlusion because of swelling. One should not be concerned because proper maxillomandibular relationship was appreciated at surgery. Training elastics are placed during the first week or two and then night elastics only. The patient should be on a soft diet for 1 month, advancing to a regular diet at the end of the month. It should be noted that these cases are won and lost through careful postoperative management. Minor adjustments of the occlusion can be managed with training elastics if the patient has been in orthodontic appliances. In these cases the arches are quite "plastic" and will respond to minor movement. If the patient has not been under active orthodontics, minor tooth movement is much more difficult.

Figures 47.27 through 47.29 show examples of various two-jaw osteotomy corrections.

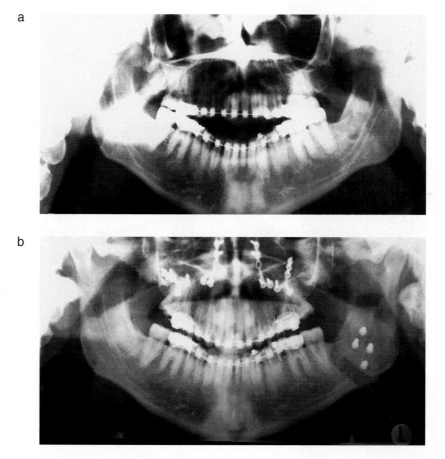

FIGURE 47.27 Preoperative (a) and postoperative (b) x-rays of an asymmetric class II open bite corrected by a unilateral mandibular advancement and closure of the open bite at the expense of the posterior maxilla. Note the combination of L & Y plates used to rigidly fix the maxilla.

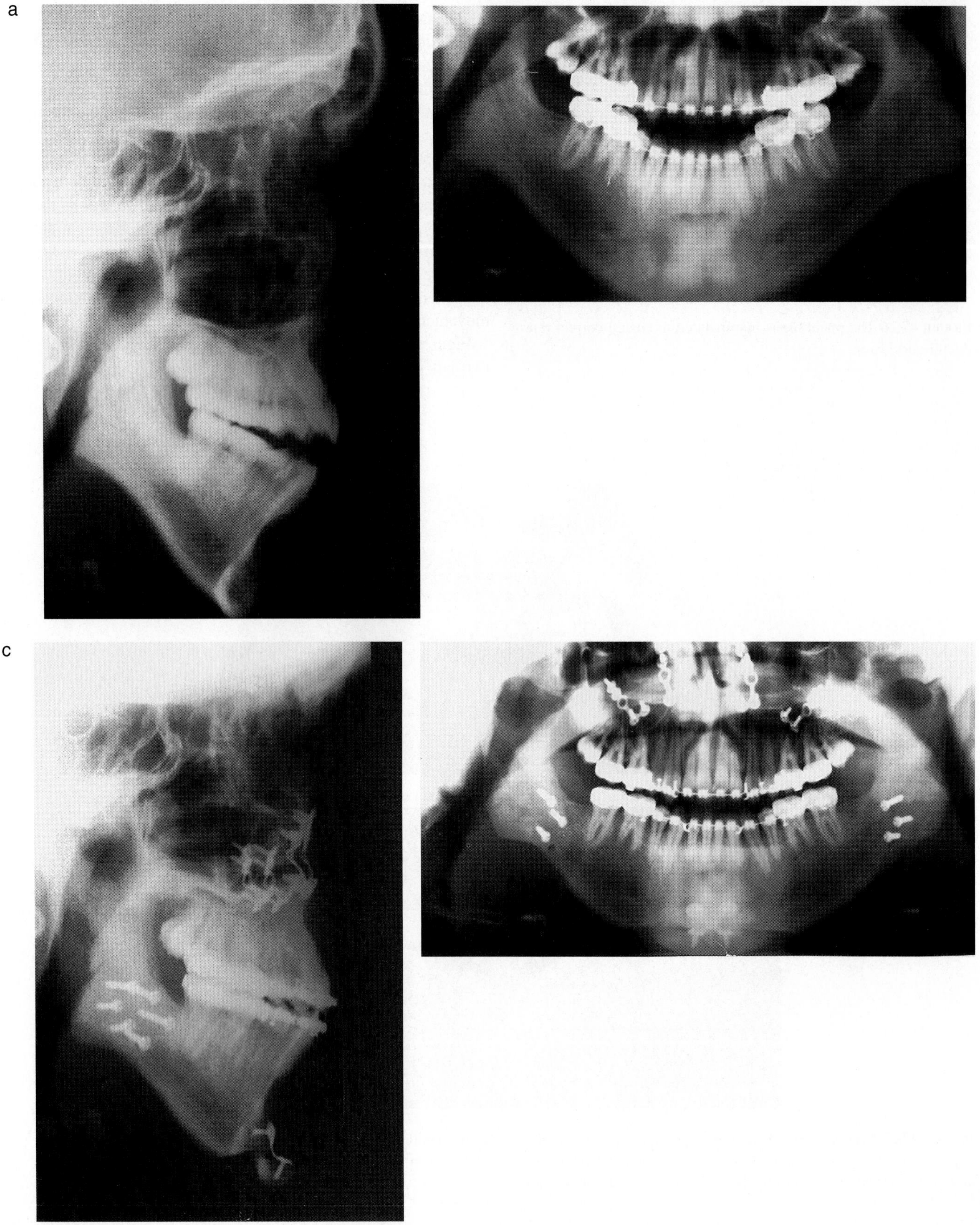

a

b

c

d

FIGURE 47.28 Preoperative (a,b) and postoperative (c,d) x-rays of patient in Figures 47.1 through 47.4. The correction involved closure of a skeletal open bite by impacting the posterior maxilla, and mandibular advancement, and an advancement genioplasty.

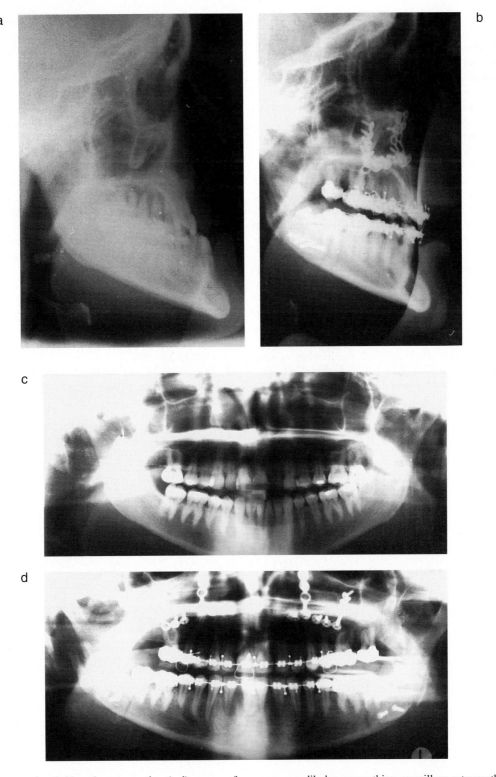

FIGURE 47.29 Preoperative (a,b) and postoperative (c,d) x-rays of a severe mandibular prognathism–maxillary retrognathia corrected by maxillary advancement and mandibular reduction.

References

1. Abeloos J, DeClerq C, Neyt L. Skeletal stability following mini-plate fixation after bilateral sagittal split osteotomy for mandibular advancement. *J Oral Maxillofac Surg.* 1993;51:366–369.

2. Watzke I, Turvey T, Phillips C, Proffitt WR. Stability of mandibular advancement after sagittal osteotomy with screw and wire fixation. *J Oral Maxillofac Surg.* 1990;48:108–121.

3. Horste W. Experience with functionally stable plate osteosynthesis after forward displacement of the upper jaw. *J Oral Maxillofac Surg.* 1980;8:176.

4. Carpenter CW, Nanda RS, Currier GF. The skeletal stability of LeFort I downfracture osteotomies with rigid fixation. *J Oral Maxillofac Surg.* 1989;47:922–925.

5. Kierl M, Nanda RS. A 3-year evaluation of skeletal stability of mandibular advancement with rigid fixation. *J Oral Maxillofac Surg.* 1990;46:587–592.

6. Carlotti A, Schendel S. An analysis of factors influencing stability of surgical advancement of the maxilla by the LeFort I osteotomy. *J Oral Maxillofac Surg.* 1987;45:924–928.

7. Perkins S, Newhouse R, Bach D. A modified Boley gauge for accurate measurement during maxillary osteotomies. *J Oral Maxillofac Surg.* 1992;50:1018–1019.

8. Van Sickels JE, Larsen AJ, Triplett RG. Predictability of maxillary surgery: a comparison of internal and external reference marks. *Oral Surg Oral Med Oral Pathol.* 1986;61:542–545.

9. Nishioka GJ, VanSickels JE. Modified external references measurement technique for vertical positioning of the maxilla. *Oral Surg Oral Med Oral Pathol.* 1987;64:22–23.

10. Booth DF. Control of the proximal segment by lower border wiring in the sagittal split osteotomy. *J Oral Maxillofac Surg.* 1981;9:126–128.

11. Singer R, Bays R. A comparison between superior and inferior border wiring techniques in sagittal split ramus osteotomies. *J Oral Maxillofac Surg.* 1985;43:444–449.

12. Linqvist C, Soderholm AL. A simple method for establishing the position of the condylar segment in sagittal split osteotomy of the mandible. *Plast Reconstr Surg.* 1988;82:707–709.

13. Hiatt W, Schelkun P, Moore D. Condylar positioning in orthognathic surgery. *J Oral Maxillofac Surg.* 1988;46:1110–1112.

14. Rotskoff K, Heubosa E, Villa P. Maintenance of condyle-proximal segment position in orthognathic surgery. *J Oral Maxillofac Surg.* 1991;49:2–7.

15. Fujimara N, Nagova H. New appliance for repositioning the proximal segment during rigid fixation of the sagittal split ramus osteotomy. *J Oral Maxillofac Surg.* 1991;49:1026–1027.

16. Heffez L, Marsik J, Bressman J. A simple means of maintaining the condyle-fossa relationship. *J Oral Maxillofac Surg.* 1987;45:288–290.

17. Mommaerts M. Slot osteosynthesis technique for sagittal ramus split osteotomies. *J Cranio-Maxillo-Fac Surg.* 1991;19:147–149.

48

Reconstruction of Cleft Lip and Palate Osseous Defects and Deformities

Klaus Honigmann and Adrian Sugar

Embryological Development

Primary Embryological Palate (Lip, Alveolus)

Embryologically, a cleft is a non-union of facial growth centers, these being ridges and tubercles conditioned by the growth of mesenchyme.[1,2] At the end of the first month of pregnancy, by the activity of mesodermal cells, the medial nasal tubercle and maxillary tubercle join each other forming the primary embryological palate. This provides the base for the upper lip and the premaxilla. A more recent view suggests that the material for the premaxilla does not come down from the frontal tubercle but comes forward from the base of the skull.[3] In the middle of the second month of pregnancy, fusion takes place between the premaxillary and maxillary centers.[4] Non-union between the premaxilla and the maxillary alveolar process leads to a uni- or bilateral alveolar cleft.

Secondary Embryological Palate (Hard and Soft Palate)

By the end of the second month of pregnancy, the mandible has grown so far that the tongue now finds enough space and can descend to the mandibular level. In consequence the palatal tubercles, at first positioned lateral to the tongue, can rise up, turn medially, and join each other and the downward-growing vomer in the midline. Non-union of the palatal shelves and the vomer results in a palatal cleft. A palatal cleft as a part of cleft lip and palate may be uni- or bilateral. In an isolated cleft of hard and soft palate, the palatal cleft is always bilateral.

Incidence and Etiology

The incidence of clefting in Europeans varies according to source, from 1 cleft child in 500 newborn,[5] 1 in 530,[6] 1 in 580,[7] to 1 in 630.[8] In the Japanese, the incidence varies from 1 in 370[9] to 1 in 470,[10] and in white Americans, from 1 in 530 in Washington,[11] 1 in 750 in Pennsylvania, to 1 in 1050 in Philadelphia.[12] More rare are clefts in the African population, 1 in 2400,[10] and in the black American population, 1 in 3300 to 1 in 4400.[12]

The etiology of cleft lip and palate is explained by a majority of authors as a multifactorial genetic system with additive polygenia and threshold effect.[13,14] This means that the combination of defects in different genes lowers the threshold for a negative influence of environmental factors. As a pathologic principle, these environmental factors cause a deficiency in oxygen supply to the fetus[15,16] just at the time when the facial tubercles are transformed and close the fetal cleft.

Classification and Diagnosis

Davis and Ritchie[17] introduced an anatomic classification with group 1 for prealveolar clefts, group 2 for postalveolar clefts, and group 3 for complete pre- and postalveolar clefts. The cleft extension in these anatomic sections is added in thirds (1/3, 2/3, 3/3). Veau[18] classified into four groups: group A represents clefts of the soft palate, group B clefts of the hard palate, group C complete unilateral clefts of lip, alveolus, and palate, and group D complete bilateral clefts of lip, alveolus, and palate. Based on practical considerations, Fogh-Andersen[19] divided clefts into three groups: group 1 is for cleft lip, group 2 for cleft lip and palate, and group 3 for cleft palate. The Cleft Lip and Palate Subcommittee of the International Confederation of Plastic Surgical Societies supplements this with a group 4 for rare clefts (median, oblique, horizontal, and other very rare clefts).

Kernahan and Stark[20] approach classification from the view of embryological development. They differentiate group 1 for clefts anterior to the incisive foramen (that is, clefts of the primary embryological palate, the anatomic sections of lip and premaxilla), group 2 for clefts posterior to the incisive foramen (that is, clefts of the secondary embryological palate, the anatomic sections of hard and soft palate), and group 3 for clefts that are both anterior and posterior to the incisive foramen (that is, clefts of the primary and secondary embryological palate, the anatomic sections of lip, alveolus, and hard and soft palate). This latter classification has been adopted by the World Health Organization into the International Classification of Diseases.

For clinical practice, Koch[21] proposed division into the four anatomic sections, that is, lip, alveolus, hard palate, and soft palate, and the subdivision of these sections into thirds. He uses the initials of the sections and adds the number of the third to which the cleft extends. Arabic numbers stand for the open cleft parts and Roman numbers for the submucous cleft parts. For visualization of cleft types, Pfeifer[22] introduced a diagram of primary and secondary palate, the cleft extension being given by outfilling of the respective fields. A 90° rotation of this symbol allows the diagnosis to be written. Kernahan[23] permits visualization with a striped Y, modifications of which have been proposed.[24–26] For use on a computer, Kriens[27] introduced LAHSHAL. Honigmann[28] uses the initials of the four sections and adds the number of the third to which the cleft extends. Reflecting the x-ray situation, this method begins with the right side of the lip and ends with the left side. As an example, the diagnosis of a complete right-sided unilateral cleft is written as L3 A3 H3 S3 and that of a complete bilateral cleft L3 A3 H3 S3 H3 A3 L3. Submucous parts of the cleft are written by a Roman number; for example, HI SIII1 is the short diagnosis of a submucous cleft in the posterior third of the hard palate and in the complete soft palate with a bifid uvula. Unfortunately, there is no agreement among these classifications, making comparison of cases between the different centers difficult.

Dysmorphology

Nonseparation of Nasal and Oral Cavity

An alveolar as well as a palatal cleft means no separation of the nasal and oral cavities. A histological examination of the border between these two cavities shows a transition zone of squamous cell epithelium in the mouth and pseudostratified ciliated columnar epithelium in the nose.

Movable Premaxilla in Bilateral Alveolar Cleft

In bilateral alveolar clefts, the premaxilla is fixed only at the nasal septum and the vomer. No osseous connection between the premaxilla and the maxilla exists. As a result, the premaxilla is movable: it can protrude, swing, or descend and end in a malposition.

Variations of Cleft-Adjacent Teeth

The lateral incisor on the cleft side is usually harmed. This can be manifested by an absence of the tooth germ or a malformed tooth. It may be found medial or lateral to the cleft and two lateral incisors may even be present, each on one side

of the cleft. In the second dentition, the canine and central incisor roots may be immediately adjacent to the cleft and the central incisor is commonly rotated and may be ectopic.

Support of Alar

The alveolar crest normally gives support to the overlying soft tissues. In an alveolar cleft, the support for the overlying alar of the nose is lacking, and the alar base tends to drop into the cleft. This contributes to the nasal asymmetry.

A Cleft Palate Is Also a Nasal Malformation

In every case, a palatal cleft means a nasal malformation too. In bilateral cleft palate, the vomer is hypoplastic and both nasal meati are open. In unilateral cleft palate, the vomer deviates to the closed side and one nasal meatus is open.

Is a Cleft a Deficiency?

We are used to considering this birth defect as involving a lack of tissue. Kriens[29] has analyzed plaster models of 251 untreated cleft infants and, especially in 91 of them with a complete unilateral cleft lip and palate, he has found no actual deficiency of tissue. His three-dimensional reflex microscope measurements explain the visible clinical cleft as a displacement and a distortion of the bony cleft segments caused by volume, tonus, and action of the tongue and its imbalance with the action of the facial soft tissues. Thus, there is some reason to question the presence of an actual tissue deficiency, at least in the alveolar cleft.

Functional Consequences

To regard a cleft as a deformity only is inadequate. This malformation causes a number of functional disturbances that indispensably should be taken into consideration in determining appropriate treatment.

Nutrition Difficulties

Nutrition in cleft infants has often been described as difficult because of their incompetence in sucking.[30–32] In reality, babies need to suck only to position the nipple, and for drinking they "milk" the nipple with their tongue.[33] Nutrition difficulties are caused by the tongue position in the cleft palate, occluding the nasal airway.[34,35] Therefore, cleft babies are unable to drink and breathe at the same time.

A palatal obturator, once introduced as an orthopedic device for bringing the maxillary segments into a better position[36] and for steering growth of maxillary segments,[37,38] improves nutrition.[35,39–41] With its separation of nasal and oral cavities, it brings the tongue out of the nasal airway and into a more anterior position in which the tongue can reach the nipple.[34] Based on this knowledge, breast-feeding with all its advantages, especially in cleft infants,[42–44] becomes possible and should be recommended to all who desire to do so.

Hearing Disorders

By swallowing, the Eustachian tubes are opened and the secretions of the middle ear can flow off. In the presence of a cleft palate, however, the velopharyngeal ring muscle system is interrupted[45] and the insertion of the tensor veli palatini muscles at the tube cartilage is abnormal.[46,47] In consequence, the opening mechanism of the Eustachian tubes cannot work. The middle ear secretions become thickened and are congested. The resulting seromucotympanon[48] hinders sound conduction and promotes middle ear infections. Speech development relies on hearing[49,50] and in cleft infants, who usually suffer some speech problems anyway, defective hearing will mean a double handicap. Moreover, in hearing disorders the maturation of the hearing tracts to the central nervous system is retarded.[51]

The management of these problems depends on careful otologic examination of the tympanic membrane with the microscope. In the presence of retraction of the ear drum, paracentesis with suction (myringotomy) of any middle ear secretions is indicated. If seromucous or putrid secretions are present, a tube (gromet) should be inserted. An active approach to early middle ear drainage, as well as closure of the soft palate during the first year of life, is desirable to reduce the incidence of middle ear disease in cleft children.[52,53]

Speech Problems

Nasality, articulation problems, suprapalatal resonance, voice diseases, myofunctional imbalances, and mimic movements may all be manifested in the speech problems of cleft patients. Nasality is the result of velopharyngeal incompetence caused by shortness or inadequate activity of the soft palate, which itself is based on the displaced muscle insertions (Figure 48.1). Articulation problems originate from a posterior tongue position but malposition of teeth and gaps in the dental arches may contribute.

An increase in suprapalatal resonance tends to occur because of a wider nasopharynx, which is caused by interruption of the velopharyngeal ring muscle system by the cleft of the soft palate. Measurement of the distance between the pterygoid processes[54] and its expression in the pterygomandibular index and the pterygoid abduction angle[55] provide evidence for this. Vomerian hypoplasia and unreconstructed nasal meati contribute to the nasopharyngeal width and thus to the increased suprapalatal resonance.

Voice diseases may occur accidentally or following attempts to compensate for speech disturbances. Myofunctional imbalances are the result of the displaced tongue with its dislocated functional pressure and the dysharmonious interaction of tongue and orofacial musculature.[56] Mimic movements are the attempt by cleft patients to compensate for velopharyn-

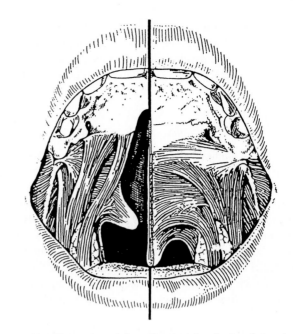

FIGURE 48.1 Shortening of the soft palate by displaced muscle insertions in a cleft.

geal incompetence by grimace with labial, nasal, or frontal muscles. Speech therapy actually starts with breast-feeding, which demands considerable effort by the child and provides practice for the musculature. Later on, stimulation and myofunctional therapy create favorable general conditions for speech development.[57,58] Treatment of articulation problems comes at the end of the speech therapy program. In this way, it is hoped that normal colloquial speech will be achieved by the time of school entry.

Growth Disturbances

Maxillary hypoplasia[59] and scarring from surgery[40,59–62] are said to be responsible for growth disturbances. Often the influence of muscle action on growth of bony structures is not considered, although it plays an important role.[63,64] This was recognized in 1961 by Rosenthal,[65] who described the functional stimulation on the clefted maxilla by early reconstruction of soft palate muscles. In our experience, reduction of scarring after palatal repair is possible if the creation of a dead space between the palatal flaps and the underlying bone surface can be avoided. This can be achieved by a palatal dressing applied at the end of the operation[66,67] and the exact reconstruction of the nasal meati with intact epithelial layers on both sides of the cleft.

Orthodontic supervision, modern methods of orthodontic treatment, and continuous follow-up can help to reduce the incidence of major incongruences of the maxilla and mandible. If it should become necessary, operative correction of dysgnathia can be carried out without major problems, as we describe later. However, the significance of growth disturbances today is much less in comparison to the other problems associated with a cleft (such as speech problems, hearing disorders, and psychological disturbance) in those areas where good primary surgery and careful multidisciplinary follow-up are the norm.

Psychological Problems

A number of studies[68–70,72] have examined the influence that a cleft lip and/or palate has on the affected children themselves, their families, and the general public including health care professionals. It seems clear that children with repaired clefts tend to perceive themselves as being less socially adept and more frequently sad and angry than their peers. On the whole, they tend to identify their problems as relating both to their facial deformity and to difficulties with and abnormalities of speech. This poor self-concept has the potential for influencing performance in school, but not all such children are affected.

As Lansdown[71] put it, it is not that such children are likely to be neurotic or delinquent. Their problems are however likely to lead to increased psychological strain. For them life is just that little bit harder, and those of us looking after such children may help by being constantly aware of this and offering support to children and families when it is needed.

Alveolar Cleft Defect Bone Grafting

Wolff[73] and Veau[74] considered that closure of a cleft lip and palate should involve repair and reconstruction of each of the clefted and abnormal tissues/layers corresponding to normal anatomy. They did not realize this aim themselves. Wassmund[75] in particular emphasized the importance of achieving the complete closure of the alveolar cleft with a nasal and an oral layer. The requirements of Wolff and Veau however were not fulfilled until Schmid[76] in 1951 proposed and carried out bone grafting into the alveolar cleft. Since then a number of surgeons have initiated different methods of alveolar cleft bone grafting, including Nordin and Johansson,[77] Schrudde and Stellmach,[78] and Schuchardt and Pfeifer,[79] as well as Boyne and Sands.[80]

Aims of Bone Grafting

Continuous Maxillary Alveolus

At one time, bone grafting tended to be performed only in bilateral alveolar clefts to fix a mobile premaxilla to the maxilla. This reason remains valid.[81] It has however now been extended to include the achievement of a continuous alveolus in all cleft patients with an alveolar defect. For those patients who will subsequently need a maxillary osteotomy, it creates the possibility of that procedure being carried out more safely, and perhaps with more stability, in one piece.

Tooth Eruption and Support, Orthodontic Alignment, and Prosthetics

In the overwhelming majority of cases, a cleft alveolar osseous defect prevents the normal eruption of teeth adjacent to the cleft. It is therefore one of the principal aims of alveolar bone grafting to enable the eruption of those teeth.[82–84] Such a tooth passing through the graft brings with it its own supporting structures including periodontal membrane and bone, and this is applicable to both dentitions.[85] Not only should an appropriately timed alveolar graft allow teeth to erupt through it, but it should also give improved bony support to other teeth adjacent to the graft, even those which have already erupted. This makes possible what would otherwise be quite difficult orthodontic movements, for example, derotation of incisors or orthodontic alignment of palatally erupted canines,[86] without compromising their support.

The permanent maxillary canine on the side of the cleft is foremost among the teeth concerned.[86] Successful bone grafting carries with it the potential for allowing the eruption of this tooth in such a way that there is a continuous dental arch.[81,87] This may avoid the need for prosthetic rehabilitation. When gaps persist in the maxillary dental arch in the cleft area (either because of hypodontia, failure, or absence of a graft), a graft when inserted should give good support to dental replacements such as a denture or fixed bridge. If it has sufficient volume, it may also make prosthetic rehabilitation possible with titanium implants supporting a crown or fixed bridge in the cleft area.[83] If placed after the maxillary segments have been expanded and moved in other directions, a graft in the alveolar defect(s) will to a considerable degree give support to that orthopedic movement.

Support for Alar Base

The grafted alveolar cleft gives support to the base of the alar on the cleft side.[81,83] Although not a substitute for correction of the cleft nasal deformity, by correcting the skeletal dysplasia it brings the patient closer to normality.

Closure of Oronasal Fistulae

The closure of oronasal fistulae demands the recreation of the original anatomy and tension-free repair of a nasal and oral layer. The presence of a graft between those layers not only restores normal anatomy but assists successful fistula closure.[81,83,88]

General Considerations

Preoperative Orthopedics

The pioneer in the field of preoperative orthopedics in cleft infants is McNeil.[36,89] The stated aims of such treatment are arch alignment with reduction of cleft width before the first surgical intervention, with postoperative retention and stimulation of bone formation through functional impulses. Among the many followers of McNeil's concept, Hotz and Graf-Pinthus[90,91] consider the tongue as a factor of essential influence on the cleft width. For them, the crucial effect of the plate is in keeping the tongue away from the cleft. Up to the present in bilateral clefts, the principal argument for preoperative orthopedics is the movement of the premaxilla and the prolabium to a more favorable position for surgical repair.[92–96] A variety of techniques has been proposed, including extraoral traction[97–100] and oral pinning with traction.[101–103]

Although most clinical reports defend the advantages of presurgical orthopedics, there is reason to doubt whether neonatal orthopedics is worth undertaking in the majority of cases[104] and certainly to question whether it achieves what is claimed. These questions will not be answered satisfactorily until sufficiently large longitudinal studies based on serial dental casts, lateral cephalometric, and photographic records beyond the postpubertal growth period have been published.[105]

In our unit, Honigmann's[107] experience until the mid-1980s had been with preoperative orthopedics in most of the bilateral and some unilateral clefts. Subsequently, this inconvenience for the babies, especially in the treatment with extraoral devices, was abandoned. Today the policy in Basel is to trust in the effect of the repaired labial muscles to approximate the maxillary segments.[106] We have never seen a dehiscence of the repaired lip, even in wide bilateral clefts with extreme protrusion of the premaxilla, nor have the aesthetic results appeared worsened.

General Conditions

The general condition of the patient should be as good as possible before surgical repair is carried out. Local infections, general infections, and vascular and metabolic diseases increase the risk of failures and should be treated before the operation. In the presence of infection, surgery should be postponed. A prophylactic perioperative antibiotic regimen seems to be helpful. Nevertheless, in both primary and secondary cleft repair we apply antibiotics only when the intervention includes bone grafting and/or osteotomy.

Nomenclature

The nomenclature of alveolar bone grafting with regard to timing is quite confusing. The terms 'primary,' 'secondary,' and 'tertiary' osteoplasty are in use, as well as 'early' and 'late' as a supplement. Some authors are referring to dental age, others to a surgically operated or unoperated alveolar cleft.

Honigmann proposed in 1992 an alternative nomenclature.[107] Accepting the terms "plasty" for primary repair and "correction" for secondary repair, one can call a first alveolar bone grafting an 'alveolo-osteoplasty' and a repeated grafting an 'alveolo-osteocorrection.' By adding the patient's age at operation, a clear basis for comparison with other centers is possible.

At the congress of the German Association for Oral and Maxillofacial Surgery in 1992 at Munich, a nomenclature commission recommended the following terms:

Primary osteoplasty: bone grafting during the first dentition, independently of a one- or two-stage intervention
Secondary osteoplasty: bone grafting during the mixed dentition
Tertiary osteoplasty: bone grafting after the end of the second dentition.[108,109]

Operating Technique

Recipient Site

The condition of the recipient site is far more important than the type of graft material used. Criteria for the quality of the recipient site are blood supply and complete coverage of the graft by soft tissue.

For a good blood supply, the recipient site should ideally be free of scars. This situation exists only in a surgically unoperated cleft. Delayed closure of the alveolar cleft after previous repair of the lip or the hard palate certainly involves dissection in a scarred area. The graft should have close contact to surrounding tissues, which means to the alveolar process stumps as well as to the soft tissue cover. Dead space around the grafted material will fill with hematoma, which through its organization by connective tissue leads to a thicker scar.

Complete coverage of the graft by soft tissue is an important factor for achieving a good blood supply and is essential for the protection of the graft against infection. Infection produces necrosis and with it graft failure. The ideal soft tissue cover is that which corresponds completely to the normal anatomy of this area. The nasal mucosa should be horizontal (axial) without any transposed oral mucosa. The palatal mucosa should be adjacent to the alveolus at its palatal inclination, and the buccal mucosa should similarly lie on the inclination of the buccal alveolus. Over the alveolar crest, there should be fixed gingivae, with mobile mucosa away from the crest.

Bone Grafts

A wide variety of materials has been proposed for alveolar grafting including homologous bone, allogeneic freeze-dried bone marrow, homologous cartilage, and various bone substitutes. Good, or at least satisfactory, results with these materials have been claimed. However, there is widespread acceptance that autologous bone grafts have the lowest risk in primary healing and give the best results.[110,111] We therefore limit ourselves to considering them only.

Different donor sites for autologous bone grafts have been proposed and used including anterior and posterior iliac crest,[112,113] rib,[113] mandible,[114–117] calvarium,[82,118] tibia,[83] periosteal flaps,[119–121] and periosteal grafts.[120,122,123] The decision in favor of one or other of the different donor sites depends among other things on the age of the patient at operation, that is, the quantity of cancellous bone at the different donor sites in different ages. In an optimal recipient site, one can obtain good results with every graft, although autologous cancellous bone is the most proven successful graft. With it one can fill out the defect completely. It allows vessels to grow into the graft from the recipient site and to transform the graft into the locally adapted bone in the easiest and most rapid way. Moreover, cancellous bone has the highest resistance against infection.

In patients older than 2 years, cancellous bone can be harvested from the iliac crest with the help of a trocar (Figures 48.2 and 48.3). This procedure diminishes the extension of the secondary intervention and the pain at the donor site, and the resulting graft is compressed. Alternatively, and especially when large quantities are required, the iliac crest itself can be raised as an osteoplastic flap, cancellous bone chips removed, and the lid replaced. The key to prevention of postoperative morbidity at this site is the avoidance of any muscle stripping in particular on the lateral aspect of the crest and the use of a long-acting local anesthetic agent (e.g., bupivicaine) titrated over 24 hours postoperatively into the wound via an epidural cannula.

Adequate stability is always important especially in bilateral alveolar clefts. During the first postoperative weeks, bone grafting cannot abolish the mobility of the premaxilla. Indeed, mobility of the fragments may well prevent bone union between the fragments and across the cleft(s). Some form of fixation of the fragments is needed, for example, by external devices such as dentally fixed splints or arch wires. Internal fixation methods such as plates and screws can be applied in a simultaneous osteotomy of the premaxilla or in a secondary intervention with the need for bigger grafts (Figures

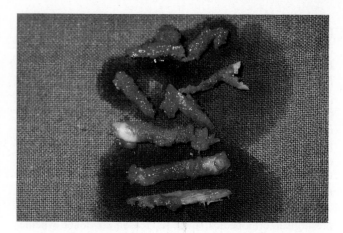

FIGURE 48.3 Bone harvested from the iliac crest by trocar.

48.4–48.6). Some authors describe a simultaneous palato-osteoplasty. Their intention is to reconstruct all the layers corresponding to the normal anatomic situation. We have no personal experience with this procedure because we cannot see the functional need.

The Basel Approach

In 1983, Honigmann described a method that had been adopted in 1980.[124] This technique involved closure of the soft palate and the lip in one stage in uni- and bilateral complete clefts at the age of 6 months. The alveolar and the hard palate cleft were closed in a second intervention at the age of 3 to 5 years with bone grafting into the alveolar cleft. The bone graft was harvested from the iliac crest, and from 1985 onward using a trocar. In some cases the bone chips were mixed with a granulate of tricalcium phosphate.[125] The aims of the timing were to construct the labial and velar muscle systems as soon as possible for optimal functional development, to re-

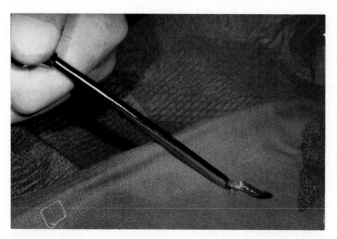

FIGURE 48.2 Bone collection from the iliac crest by trocar.

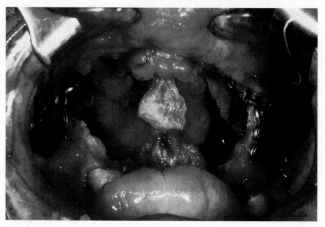

FIGURE 48.4 A bilateral cleft lip and palate with a big bone defect; status after Le Fort I osteotomy and fixation with 2.0-mm plates and screws.

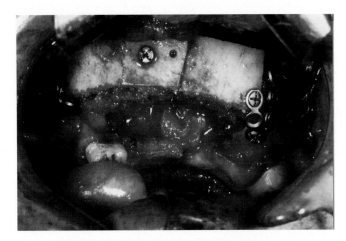

FIGURE 48.5 Same patient as in Figure 48.4 grafted with cortico-cancellous bone from the iliac crest; fixation with 2.0-mm plates and screws.

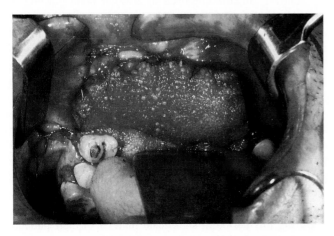

FIGURE 48.6 Same patient as in Figure 48.6; oral cover of the graft with a tongue flap.

duce the number of interventions for primary cleft repair, and to enable the children to enter school with a completely closed cleft and normal colloquial speech. The failure rate in bone grafting at that time was 11.3%. Normal colloquial speech at school entrance was achieved in 91.6% of the children.[28]

In 1991, this concept was changed with the aim of obtaining a completely closed cleft at the end of the first year of life for a better functional and psychological development of the cleft child. Based on the aim of reducing the number of surgical interventions and thus hospitalizations, an attempt was made to try to close all forms of clefts in one stage at least by the age of 6 months. Because of modern methods of pediatric anaesthesia, there were no significant problems even in a 4-hour operation, which was needed in complete bilateral clefts. Subsequently it was found that this all-in-one procedure for unilateral cleft lip and palate patients had been proposed in 1966.[126] The late results of that work were reported at the 7th International Congress on Cleft Palate and Related Craniofacial Anomalies in 1993 at Broadbeach, Australia.[127] The operative steps in detail are as follows.

The child's head is placed in the 'Rose' position, that is, the surgeon is seated with the child's head on his/her knees. The mouth is opened by a Rosenthal retractor (the widely used Dingman retractor covers the lip and the alveolar cleft with its extraoral frame, so it is impossible to get the view needed for the alveolo-osteoplasty). The incision of the soft palate edges continues with the dissection of pedicled palatal flaps including the preparation and mobilization of the palatal vessels (Figure 48.7). This provides a good view for the intravelar muscle dissection. With the aid of mucoperiosteal vomerine flaps and the mobilized lateral nasal mucoperiosteum, the nasal meatus can be formed in the complete alveolar and palatal cleft (Figure 48.8), and in bilateral clefts the two nasal meati can be separated (Figure 48.9).

Suture of the mobilized and posteriorly directed soft palate muscle stumps and pushback of the totally mobile palatal soft

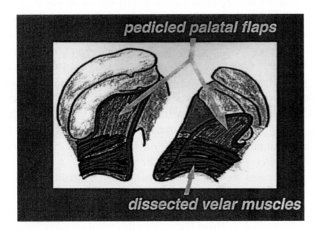

FIGURE 48.7 Dissection of the soft palate muscles and the pedicled palatal flaps.

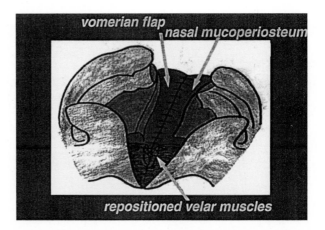

FIGURE 48.8 Formation of the nasal meatus in the unilateral alveolar and palatal cleft.

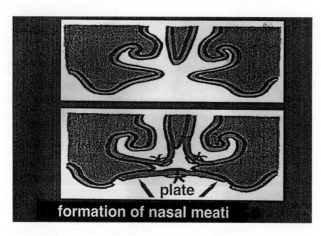

FIGURE 48.9 Separation of the two nasal meati in a bilateral cleft.

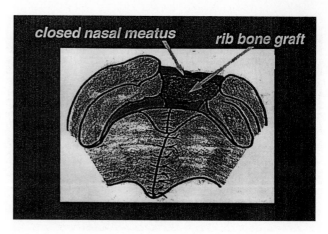

FIGURE 48.11 Primary alveolar cleft bone grafting.

tissues lengthens the soft palate into a normalized anatomic situation (see Figure 48.1). The palatal flaps are sutured only in the midline and then lightly pressed against the palatal bone with the aid of a palatal dressing. Thus a dead space between the palatal bone and soft tissues can be avoided, and with it a hematoma and the resulting thicker scar. After repositioning the child onto the table, a rib bone graft is harvested (Figure 48.10) and the alveolar cleft(s) filled with the cancellous bone (Figure 48.11). Integrated into the final lip repair is cover of the bone graft by mucoperiosteum advanced from the vestibular side of the lesser maxillary segment and its suturing with the tips of the palatal flaps.

In this manner, alveolar bone grafting is a part of an all-in-one closure of all clefts. More than 80 complete uni- and bilateral clefts have been closed in this all-in-one procedure (case 1: Figure 48.12 and case 2: Figure 48.13). At this time, the rate of healing complications is 5.9% (3 partial hard palate dehiscences, 2 bone graft losses), and the first functional results with regard to speech development and hearing disorders are very encouraging.

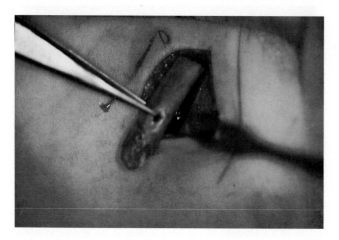

FIGURE 48.10 Rib graft resection.

The Swansea Approach

By contrast, Sugar's approach to alveolar bone grafting in Swansea (and until 1994 in Chepstow) has been unchanged since 1985. Grafting has been carried out ideally in the mixed dentition shortly before the eruption of the permanent maxillary canine teeth, the classic secondary graft. This approach has varied little from the method proposed by Boyne and Sands[80] and reported by Abyholm and colleagues.[81] However, in our patients, operating on children whose primary surgery has been carried out by a number of surgeons, there has been a clear need for a significant amount of orthodontics, primarily to correct collapsed or misplaced alveolar segments, before grafting can take place. Only cancellous bone harvested from the anterior iliac crest has been used and with consistently good results.

During this period, a significant number of cleft patients presented who had, for various reasons, missed the opportunity of receiving a graft into their alveolar clefts during the mixed dentition phase. In most cases these have been managed with careful orthodontic preparation with fixed bands and tertiary alveolar grafting in exactly the same way as mentioned.[128] This has applied equally to those patients who have not required orthognathic surgery, the graft not only facilitating closure of fistulae but also giving support to dental restorations with or without osseointegrated implants. Whenever grafting is carried out during orthodontic therapy, the orthodontist places in advance either lateral retaining arms from molar bands or rigid arch wires to maintain arch width. This is usually reinforced by a transpalatal bar, positioned sufficiently far posteriorly and relieved from the mucosa to enable any required palatal surgery to be performed.

In all cases the complete alveolar cleft is identified. Any labial fistula is excised and this excision incorporated into the mucoperiosteal flap(s) of the lesser segment(s) (see Figures 48.14a–g–48.22). These flaps critically include keratinized gingivae. In unilateral cases, a mucoperiosteal flap is also raised up to one unit on the greater segment. In bilateral cases, virtu-

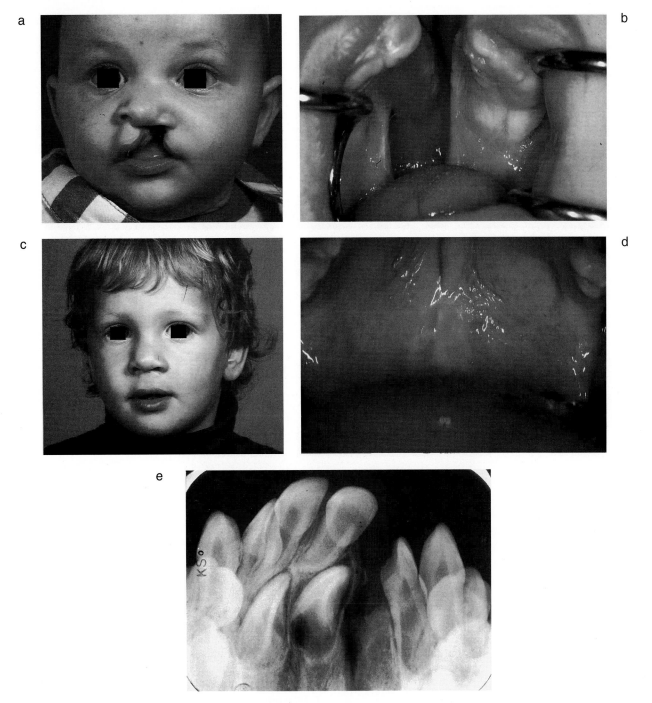

FIGURE 48.12 Case 1. (a) Five-month-old boy with a unilateral cleft lip and palate (CLP). (b) Intraoral aspect. (c) Two years old, after the one-stage closure. (d) Intraoral aspect. (e) X-ray of the grafted alveolar cleft, 18 months postoperative.

a
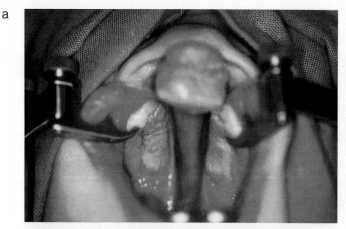

b
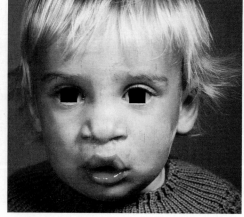

c
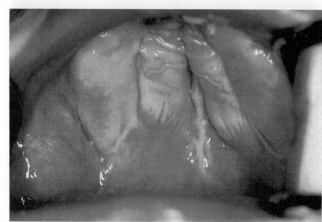

FIGURE 48.13 Case 2. (a) Bilateral complete CLP in a 6-month-old boy. (b) Same boy, aged 1 year and 6 months, after the one-stage closure. (c) Intraoral aspect.

ally no dissection is permitted on the premaxilla, whose blood supply is perilous. The closure of anterior palatal fistulae in two layers at this stage is mandatory. The repair of posterior palatal fistulae away from the alveolar cleft is optional, but the opportunity to do this simultaneously is difficult to resist.

Scar tissue within the alveolar cleft is excised and the nasal mucosa repaired. It is important that this repair is carried out in such a way that the nasal floor lies at the same height as the normal side. This, together with excision of the scar tissue in the cleft, redefines the complete alveolar deficit into which are then packed the cancellous bone chips. The lateral flaps are then advanced, aided by appropriate division of periosteum, and closed with keratinized fixed gingivae over the alveolar crest. These flaps are sutured across the crest to the palatal oral mucosa. The posterior deficits of mucoperiosteum over the alveolus buccally from where the flaps have been advanced are allowed to heal by secondary epithelialization. Antibiotics are administered intravenously during the operation. Even when large fistulae have been present we have always been able to use local flaps, although on occasion the palatal flaps have had to be 'islanded' (i.e., Millard island flaps) when advancement has been required. We have never needed or used a Burion flap in this situation.

Case 3 (Figure 48.14)

A 10-year-old with left unilateral complete cleft of lip and alveolus.

Treatment:

1. Raising of mucoperiosteal flaps
2. Excision of sinus and scar tissue within cleft
3. Removal of supernumerary tooth
4. Repair of nasal mucosa at level of normal nasal floor
5. Harvesting of cancellous bone from anterior iliac crest
6. Insertion of graft into alveolar defect
7. Flap advancement and closure over graft

The Role of Osseointegrated Implants

Although modern cleft surgery aims to create a dentition without gaps, this aim is not always achieved. The incidence of hypodontia in cleft patients is higher than in the noncleft population, and it is not always possible for this to be disguised with the help of grafting, orthodontic treatment, and orthognathic surgery alone. There are also many patients who have not received alveolar bone grafts and also those who have lost

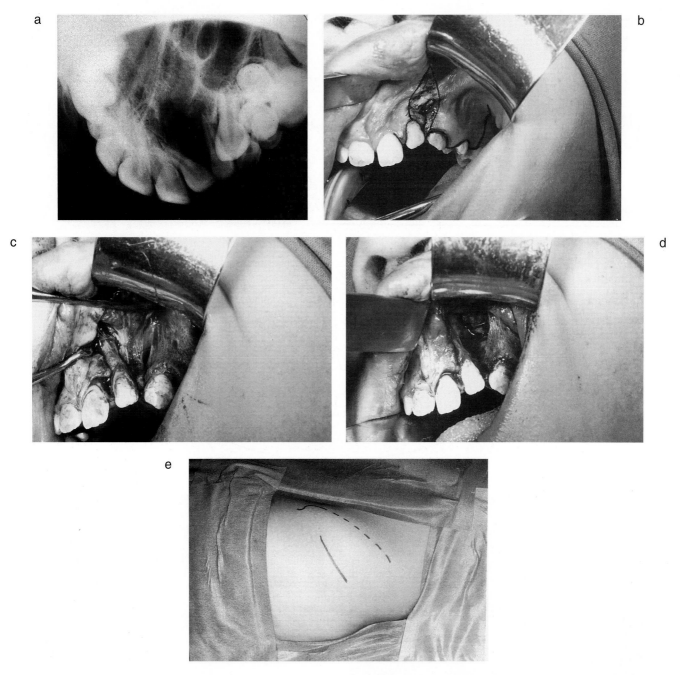

FIGURE 48.14 Case 3. (a) X-ray of secondary alveolar defect. (b) Incisions for alveolar bone grafting outlined with excision of labial fistula. (c) Scar tissue within the alveolar cleft. (d) Alveolar defect after excision of scar tissue and repair of the nasal mucosa. (e) Incision (continuous line) marked lateral to the left anterior iliac crest (interrupted line) for harvesting of cancellous bone.

Continued.

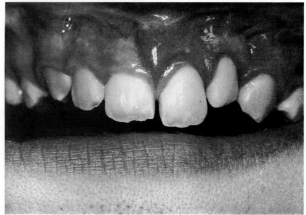

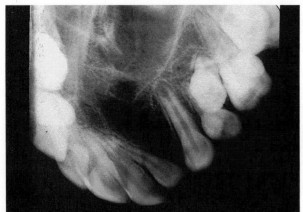

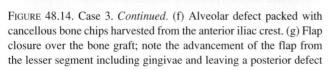

FIGURE 48.14. Case 3. *Continued.* (f) Alveolar defect packed with cancellous bone chips harvested from the anterior iliac crest. (g) Flap closure over the bone graft; note the advancement of the flap from the lesser segment including gingivae and leaving a posterior defect over the lateral maxilla, which is left to epithelialize by secondary intention. (h) Diagram of procedure. (i) X-ray of the alveolus in the grafted area in the same patient 6 months after surgery. (j) Oral view of the same patient 6 months after surgery.

teeth early and whose conventional dental restorative treatment is problematic.

The restoration of gaps in the dentition is ultimately the responsibility of the restorative dentist. Their options include dentures and fixed bridgework supported by teeth. The availability of titanium osseointegrated implants now adds to this repertoire the possibility of crowns or bridges supported by implants, as well as implant-supported overdentures.

Case 4 (Figure 48.15)

A 25-year-old with left unilateral complete cleft lip and palate, not having received an alveolar bone graft and missing the left maxillary lateral incisor.

Treatment:

1. Alveolar bone grafting with autogenous cancellous iliac bone as described in Figure 48.14
2. Orthodontic arch alignment
3. Insertion of Brånemark titanium fixture into grafted area with additional small bone graft for labial defect provided from suction filter during the drilling process and covered with resorbable membrane (two-stage implant procedure)
4. Construction of implant-retained crown

(*Restorative treatment courtesy of Will McLaughlin, Consultant in Restorative Dentistry, University Dental Hospital, Cardiff, Wales*)

Case 5 (Figure 48.16)

A 16-year-old with bilateral complete cleft lip and palate assessed following orthodontics and bilateral alveolar bone grafting and with regard to two missing teeth in the left cleft.

Treatment:

1. Insertion of two Brånemark titanium fixtures (two-stage procedure) into maxillary alveolus, previously grafted in conjunction with orthodontics
2. Construction of implant-retained bridge

(*Restorative treatment courtesy of Arshad Ali, Consultant in Restorative Dentistry, Morriston Hospital, Swansea, Wales*)

Maxillary Osteotomies

Secondary deformities in patients with repaired cleft lip and palate present an interesting, if not difficult, surgical challenge. Careful assessment of the patient in the years following primary repair needs to take into consideration speech, hearing, facial growth, and dental development. The presence of fistulae, lip scars, and poor lip function, as well as residual nasal deformity and nasal resistance, needs to be assessed for correction. Alveolar defects and occlusion should be considered along with dental overcrowding, missing, malformed

and misplaced teeth, caries, and periodontal health. The ability and desire of the patient (and in the case of children, their family) to comply with what can often be prolonged treatment needs to be determined and taken into account.

This heterogeneity of problems requires the cooperation of a number of different specialties, foremost of which are a surgeon, speech therapist/pathologist, hearing specialist, and orthodontist, all preferably with a special interest in cleft problems. In late adolescence, a specialist in restorative dentistry is a valuable addition to the team. It is particularly useful to attempt to identify at as early an age as possible those children with significant midface hypoplasia that may require later surgical correction. If orthognathic surgery is to be delayed until approximately 16 years of age when most jaw growth is complete, early identification of those children is helpful.

Timing

In most cases speech patterns will have developed by the age of 4, and it should be possible to assess the need for a pharyngoplasty to correct velopharyngeal incompetence. Speech assessment and recording, anenometry, nasendoscopy, and video-fluoroscopy all assist in that decision. Ideally this should be carried out before school entry.

At the age of 8 years, and with the aid of orthopantomogram (OPT) and oblique occlusal and lateral cephalometric radiographs, it is useful to start to consider the need for dental extractions for orthopedic alignment of displaced and collapsed arches and for grafting of alveolar defects. When facial growth appears to be essentially normal, definitive orthodontics can then continue.

A clinical evaluation of facial form, noting the presence or absence of midface hypoplasia, a class III malocclusion, and dental compensation, may lead the team to the conclusion that jaw osteotomies are indicated in due course. This in turn allows the decision that orthodontics should be limited at that stage to the orthopedic alignment of segments and perhaps the correction of minor anterior incisal discrepancies. Definitive presurgical fixed-band orthodontics can then be delayed until the approximate age of 14 years when the patient can be prepared for orthognathic correction by osteotomies at 16. This has the merit of saving the child from 6 to 8 years of continuous orthodontic treatment with the inconvenience and almost inevitable lack of compliance that can result.

The Role of Alveolar Bone Grafting

Primary Grafting

We have described in our previous section the purpose of considering and carrying out alveolar bone grafting as well as a number of different approaches to it. Primary alveolar bone

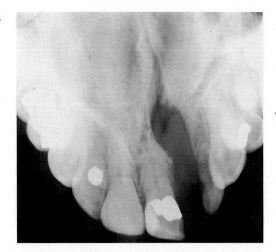

a

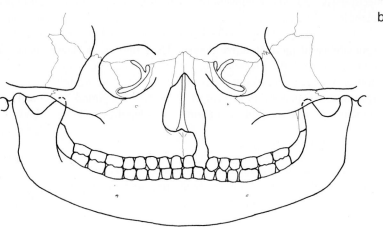

b

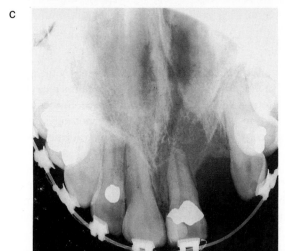

c

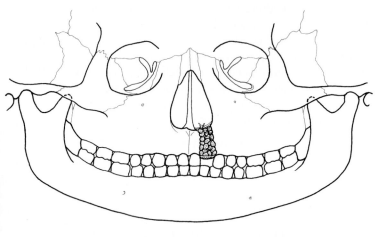

d

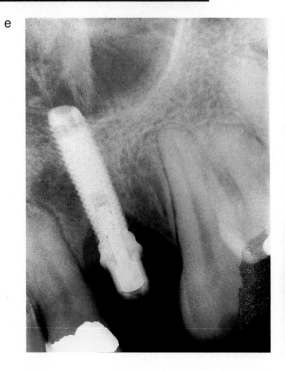

e

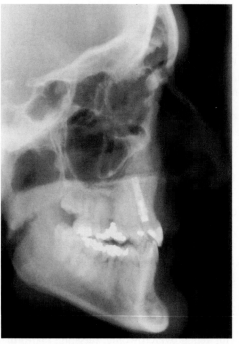

f

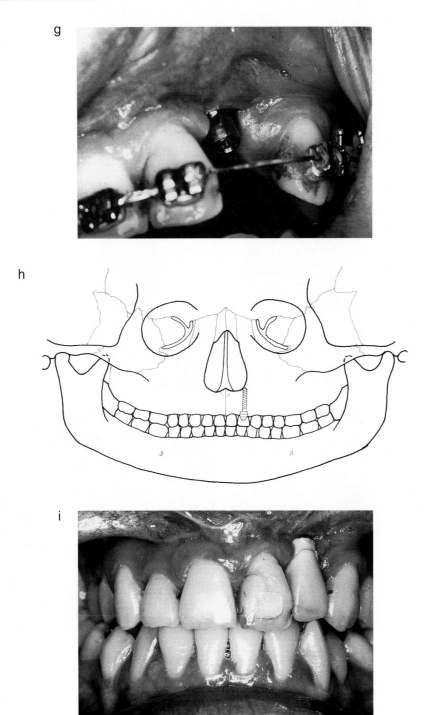

FIGURE 48.15 Case 4. (a) X-ray of alveolar defect. (b) Diagram of alveolar defect. (c) X-ray of grafted alveolar defect. (d) Diagram of grafted alveolar defect. (e) Intraoral x-ray of implant in grafted alveolar defect. (f) Lateral cephalogram showing position of implant. (g) Oral view with implant/abutment in situ. (h) Diagram showing implant in situ. (i) Oral view showing implant retained crown in situ.

a

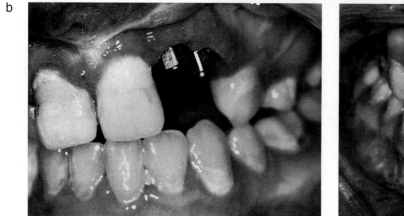

b

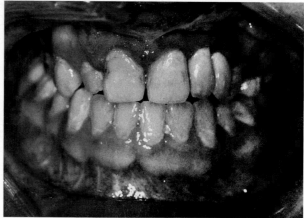

c

FIGURE 48.16 Case 5. (a) X-ray of implants in grafted alveolus. (b) Oral view of abutments. (c) Implant-retained bridge in situ.

grafting is that which is carried out during the primary dentition or even before the eruption of the deciduous teeth. We do not yet have available from Basel medium- or long-term results of this approach, and much of the hostility to primary grafting has come from the apparently poor effect on maxillary growth.[129] However, others[130] have reported very encouraging results in this respect more recently. Rosenstein et al.[130] have presented the long-term results in a regimen of cleft repair that has included primary bone grafting of the alveolar cleft at 4 to 6 months of age. This remains an area of considerable controversy.

Secondary Grafting

Secondary alveolar bone grafting, by which we mean grafting shortly before the eruption of the permanent maxillary canine teeth, has by contrast become very widely accepted. The method described by Boyne and Sands[80] was popularized by the reporting of large series by Abyholm and his colleagues.[81] It has undoubtedly made an important difference to the management of cleft patients. It makes the simultaneous repair of residual fistulae easier and by producing a one-piece maxilla facilitates a future maxillary osteotomy if needed. The production is facilitated by well-aligned and continuous dental arches, with good bone support for the maxillary permanent canine and adjacent teeth. If there are gaps in the dental arch, it produces a stable base for the construction of fixed bridgework and implant-retained crowns and bridges. The overwhelming majority of compliant cleft children with an alveolar defect that has not been previously grafted will benefit from secondary alveolar bone grafting provided that the preparation and timing are carefully considered and the surgery well executed.

The popularizing of this technique in Norway was based, in the main, on children who did not have grossly collapsed dental arches. It has been the experience of the authors that secondary bone grafting of alveolar clefts without prior correction of misplaced segments creates significant difficulties. The segments may become fixed in an abnormal position with orthopedic movement no longer possible or at best very difficult (Figure 48.17).

Case 6 (Figure 48.17)

Patient with bilateral complete cleft lip and palate.

Treatment:

1. The alveolar clefts had been bone grafted before orthopedic expansion and alignment of segments.
2. The premaxilla was thus fixed in its position significantly displaced inferiorly and to the right as were the lateral segments in their contracted position.
3. Later orthodontics was thus made very difficult. In some cases the problem can only be resolved with the help of multipiece osteotomies (see case 8, Figure 48.19).

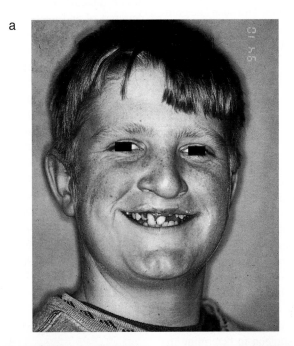

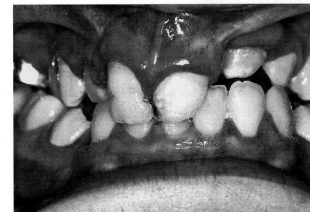
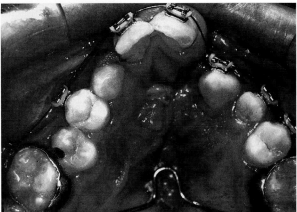

FIGURE 48.17 Case 6. (a–c) Result of grafting of bilateral alveolar clefts before orthopedic alignment of the segments.

Careful assessment with an orthodontist experienced in the management of clefts is therefore essential to determine the presurgical needs, which should include alignment of any misplaced segments. After this, the orthodontist will design an appliance that will both retain the parts which have been moved and not impede surgery. Because the latter may well involve the repair of residual palatal oronasal fistulae, the appliance in situ during surgery must not cover any part of the palate to which access is required.

Tertiary Grafting

Patients who present after the eruption of the permanent canine teeth and at the end of the mixed dentition phase of development sometimes have not received any form of alveolar bone graft. Others have poor results from earlier grafting attempts and have inadequate bone for orthodontic movement of teeth, for support for prostheses, or for carrying out a maxillary osteotomy in one piece. In these cases, and notwithstanding the allegedly poor results that have been claimed for such late grafting by some authors (relative to secondary grafting), it has been our reported experience that excellent results can still be obtained.[128] We therefore always consider, in conjunction with our multidisciplinary team, tertiary grafting in such cases.

Investigation

Facial Appearance

The principal tool in the diagnosis of residual facial deformity is clinical evaluation by an experienced surgeon. It is useful to document those parts of the upper, middle, and lower face that show anteroposterior, vertical, and transverse deficiencies or excesses. Dysmorphology and abnormality should be noted in all areas and in particular of the nasal bones, septum, tip, columella, and alar bases, as well as of the philtrum and upper lip.

Measurement of some aspects of the face in both frontal and profile views and comparison with norms is of value. The exposure at rest and when smiling of the upper incisor teeth, as well as measurement of the clinical crown height, are just a few examples. These enable the surgeon to determine the vertical movements needed of the anterior maxilla to create an ideal relationship with the upper lip, but consideration needs to be given to the need for lip revision in this respect and any of the resultant effects on lip–tooth relationship.

The interalar distance needs to be known if only to avoid making it worse after maxillary advancement; sometimes simultaneous revision of this distance needs to be built into the treatment plan. The intercanthal distance and nasofrontal angle may also increase in Le Fort II or Le Fort III osteotomies and should be recorded. The relationship between the maxillary and mandibular dental centers and the facial midline and chin needs to be known so that attempts at creating symmetry may be made. The presence of missing teeth in the cleft patient may make this particularly difficult.

Many forms of cephalometric measurement are available,

some of which are particularly designed for analysis of the patient with a jaw deformity. While these can be useful, allowance does need to be made for the different values that are observed in cleft patients. A particularly relevant example is the cranial base to which the position of the maxilla and mandible is usually related. When the cranial base angle is abnormal (that is, it is outside the normal range of values), the angles of SNA and of SNB also vary widely, and this needs to be taken into consideration.

Occlusion

Dental study casts are essential in the overall analysis. In this way, the precise needs of presurgical orthodontics can be determined and results monitored.

Speech

It is always desirable that the cleft patient should be managed in coordination with a speech therapist/pathologist with experience of and interest in cleft patients. Children should be assessed at regular intervals during their development. The axiom that treatment should aim at producing an individual who "looks well and speaks well" remains valid today.

In relation to midface osteotomies, it is well recognized that these have the significant potential for improving the articulatory aspects of speech by correcting malocclusion and skeletal disproportion. However they also carry the unwanted risk of producing, or making worse, velopharyngeal incompetence (VPI). Consequently all cleft patients should have a thorough speech assessment immediately before undergoing midface advancement. This should involve a standard form of assessment with speech recording and anenometry. Nasendoscopy and videofluoroscopy may be valuable but can usually be reserved for those cases with problems postoperatively. The experienced speech therapist/pathologist, especially working in the same team and with the same surgeon, should be able to identify those patients most at risk of developing VPI.

Deformities/Diagnosis

Maxillary hypoplasia in cleft patients has a clear relationship to both the original deformity and the consequences of early surgical repair. We now describe the principal forms.

Unilateral Complete Cleft Lip and Palate (UCLP)

In this cleft defect, when midfacial hypoplasia is present it is manifested predominantly by an anteroposterior deficiency of the maxilla with lack of support to the nasal tip. There is often a vertical deficiency producing a lack of exposure of the upper incisor teeth at rest, influenced by any distortion of the upper lip. There will usually be an alveolar defect on the side of the cleft unless it has been grafted previously. Even without a previous periosteoplasty,[119] bone bridging across the alveolar defect is sometimes seen. Transverse collapse of the alveolar segments may also occur, perhaps the most common being displacement inward (palatally) and upward (cranially) of the lesser segment.

Several studies have shown that the mandible often lacks some forward growth in the repaired UCLP patient. In relation to surgery, it is questionable whether this usually requires correction. There is, however, often a lack of chin prominence but an excess of chin height. These contribute to an unesthetic and often drooping or ptotic appearance of the lower lip and warrant intervention.

Although the principal secondary nasal deformities are predominantly cartilage and soft tissue, the lack of support to the nasal tip may be severe. The dorsum of the nose is usually described as being essentially normal, but cases are seen where it is retropositioned and asymmetry is not uncommon. Labial or palatal fistulae may be present, communicating with the nasal cavity. The septum is usually deviated to the non-cleft side and is often quite wide. In the authors' experience, septa more than 1 cm wide can occur with complete blockage of the nasal airway. The inferior turbinate on the cleft side is usually hypertrophied.

Bilateral Complete Cleft Lip and Palate (BCLP)

Although class III malocclusions are seen in BCLP patients, very much depending on the method of primary repair, the principal finding is prominence of the premaxilla (and prolabium), especially vertically. In ungrafted cases, the premaxilla is usually mobile, poorly inclined (retroclined), and to one side or the other. The patient will often have, or with the aid of orthodontics be capable of having, a class I incisor relationship.

Class II-based deformities with mandibular retrognathia or retrogenia are seen in BCLP patients (Figure 48.18), and sometimes this is the only skeletal defect that requires correction. Occasionally bimaxillary advancement is indicated.

Case 7 (Figure 48.18)

Patient with bilateral complete cleft lip and palate and anteroposterior deficiency of the mandible.

Treatment:

1. Fixed-band orthodontics commenced in both arches to remove dental compensation, align teeth, and produce compatible arches on the basis of three-point contact following orthognathic surgery.
2. Before the movement of teeth adjacent to the alveolar clefts, these clefts were bone grafted in the way that we have described.
3. Following completion of the presurgical phase of orthodontics, mandibular advancement was carried out using bilateral sagittal split osteotomies of the mandibular rami, fixation being by four 2.7-mm titanium position screws (two on each side) inserted transbuccally.
4. Orthodontics was then completed.

(Orthodontics courtesy of Jeremy Knox, Dept. of Child Dental Health, University Dental Hospital, Cardiff, Wales)

It is common for teeth in the premaxilla of bilateral cleft patients to be poorly formed and prone to caries or crumbling; such teeth are not a good support for orthodontic devices. Nevertheless, malposition of the premaxilla and lateral segments can usually be corrected by the orthodontist before cleft bone grafting. Jones and Sugar[128] have reported one case in whom this was carried out with an orthodontic device when the patient had no teeth on the premaxilla. There are, however, instances in which repositioning of the premaxilla can be difficult or impossible. In such occasional cases, surgical repositioning of the premaxilla before grafting should be considered (see case 9, Figure 48.20). The nose in the bilateral cleft patient may be broad at the alar bases and often also at the bridge with a short columella. Anteroposterior deficiency of the dorsum is rare.

Cleft Palate (CP)

The patient with a repaired isolated cleft of the palate may also exhibit anteroposterior and sometimes vertical deficiency of the maxilla. It has been argued that many deformities of this kind in these and complete cleft lip and palate patients are not necessarily cleft related. Undoubtedly instances of class III skeletally based malocclusion of familial rather than cleft origin do occur, but the relative rarity of class II deformities in cleft patients is food for thought. The patient in case 8 (Figure 48.19a) has a repaired cleft palate with maxillary hypoplasia. Figure 48.19(c) shows her "identical" twin sister who has no cleft.

Case 8 (Figure 48.19)

Patient in Figure 48.19(a) has a repaired cleft of the secondary palate with anteroposterior and vertical deficiency of the maxilla. Figure 48.19(c) shows her identical twin sister who had no cleft, the photographs being taken on the same day as those of her sister. The principal difference noticeable between the sisters is the maxillary hypoplasia exhibited by the sister with a repaired cleft.

Surgery:

1. One-piece Le Fort I maxillary advancement and downward movement
2. Fixation using four L-shaped titanium 2-mm miniplates
3. Augmentation of the anterior maxillary bone steps only with corticocancellous blocks harvested from the medial aspect of the anterior iliac crest

Indications for Orthognathic Surgery

The principal indications for carrying out orthognathic surgery in patients with repaired cleft lip and/or palate are as follows.

1. To improve facial aesthetics and in particular the appearance of the midface, including the upper lip and nose

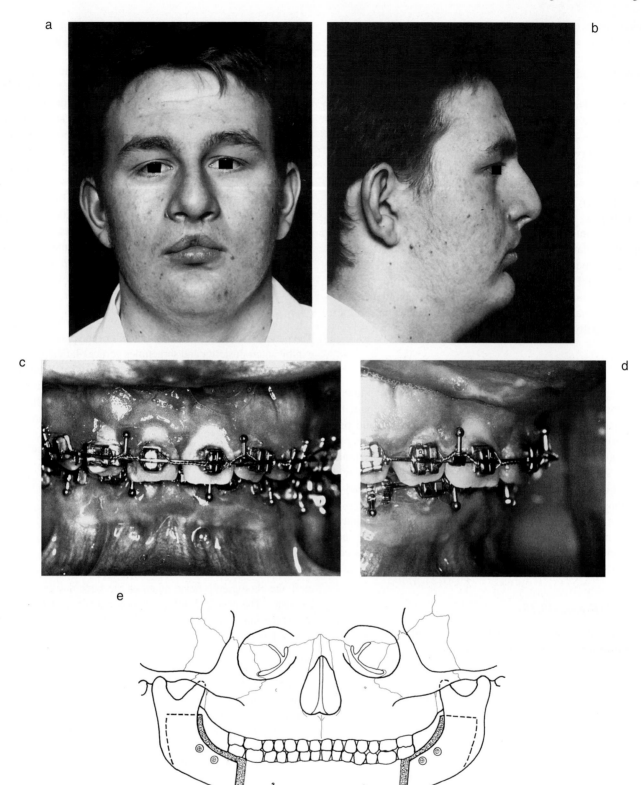

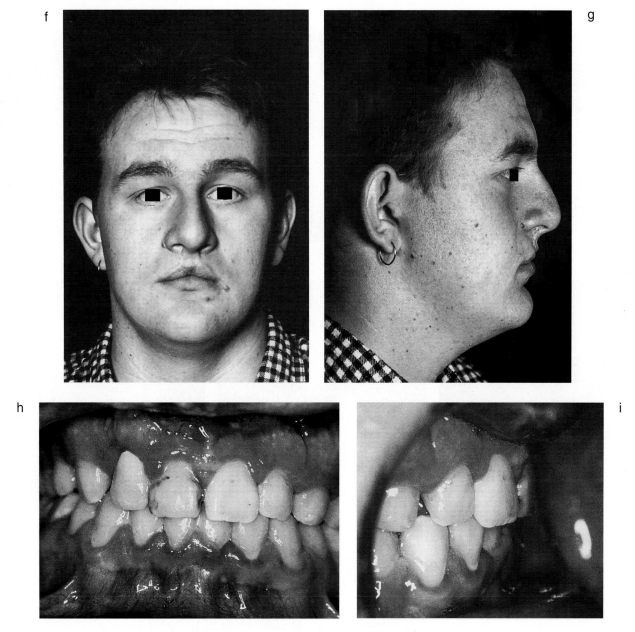

FIGURE 48.18 Case 7. Anteroposterior mandibular deficiency in a patient with bilateral cleft lip and palate (BCLP). (a–d) After orthodontic preparation but before surgery. (e) Diagram of surgical procedure (sagittal split advancement). (f–i) Following surgery and completion of orthodontics.

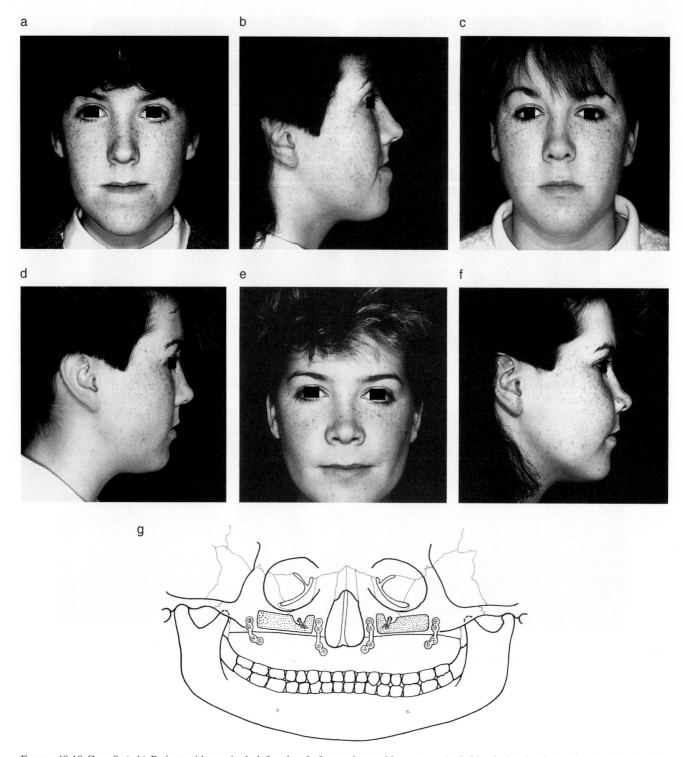

FIGURE 48.19 Case 8. (a,b) Patient with repaired cleft palate before orthognathic surgery. (c,d) Identical twin sister of patient in a,b who had no cleft. (e,f) Patient in a,b after Le Fort I maxillary advancement and correction of vertical deficiency. (g) Diagram of procedure.

2. To permit the full correction of skeletally based malocclusions
3. To improve the nasal airways by reducing nasal resistance
4. To improve speech, especially the articulatory aspects

Orthodontic Requirements

To achieve these aims optimally, orthodontic management is required to accomplish these aims:

1. Correct major displacement of segments by orthopedic movements
2. Permit the ideal choice of timing for alveolar bone grafting
3. Correct crowding and adopt a rational approach to tooth position where teeth are missing (hypodontia)
4. Remove dental compensation, especially abnormal inclinations of upper and lower incisors
5. Produce well-coordinated dental arches that will be compatible after surgery
6. Fine-tune tooth positioning and occlusion following surgery

Planning, Soft Tissue Effects, and Predictions

Planning in orthognathic surgery[131] is the process by which the assessment, investigation, and resulting diagnosis are translated into a coherent treatment plan. It should be based predominantly on a clinical determination of treatment objectives. In the typical case with moderate to severe anteroposterior and vertical deficiency of the maxilla, and provided that the alveolar segments were aligned before bone grafting, it will probably involve the advancement of the maxilla at the Le Fort I level. Although every patient needs to be assessed individually, there is a tendency in some quarters to avoid large maxillary advancements by "splitting the difference" and moving the mandible back simultaneously. There are undoubtedly cases of true mandibular prognathism in which this is called for, but it is still necessary to carry out full correction of a retropositioned maxilla. Advancements of more than 2 cm may be necessary.

Model surgery is an absolute requirement in all cases. Models should be set up on a semiadjustable anatomic articulator after face bow recording. Reference lines are drawn and various distances in three planes are recorded. The desired movements are then carried out and the measurements retaken and recorded. These movements need to relate to the clinical treatment objectives, and it is valuable to test the achievement of those objectives against a predictive computer program. Once the movements have been finalized, acrylic occlusal wafers should be constructed, one in the case of a single-jaw osteotomy and two (including an intermediate position) in the case of bimaxillary procedures. These at least will remove some of the guesswork from the operating room, although vertical determinations will still need to be made.

Most computer packages for orthognathic surgery planning are based on surgery on a digitized lateral cephalometric radiograph. They are not infallible but can be a remarkably valuable indication of what will happen. We have analyzed two of the most commonly used such packages in the United States and U.K. specifically for internally fixed Le Fort I osteotomies including clefts.[132,133] Soft tissue changes in cleft patients have a tendency to differ from those in noncleft patients, probably because of the lack of elasticity of the enveloping tissues. It is hoped that in the future such programs will be able to take this into consideration and thus give more accurate predictions. It is questionable whether more sophisticated (and expensive) techniques of three-dimensional prediction are of much value in the average case. However, video capture techniques with color print predictions of the result of surgical movements allow the patient to see a reasonable simulation of what surgery can achieve. They may also be helpful to the surgeon.

Treatment planning should take into consideration the views of the speech therapist or speech pathologist on the likelihood of the development or worsening of velopharyngeal incompetence. When very large advancements are considered, this may dictate a modification of surgical technique.

Surgical Procedures

Premaxillary Osteotomy

Osteotomies of the maxilla of cleft patients have to be tailored to the different anatomy, to the blood supply of the different parts of the maxilla, and to the nature and effects of previous surgery. This is especially the case when the part to be moved is the premaxilla. In the bilateral cleft patient, the bone of the premaxilla is attached very narrowly to the nasal septum. Its blood supply is derived principally from the labial mucoperiosteum. These need to be taken into consideration when designing the surgical approach and osteotomy technique if the premaxilla is not to become a free graft.

Premaxillary osteotomies will be needed only rarely because orthodontic methods are quite good at guiding this bone into the correct position. When needed, it will usually be because the bone would not move in this way. The bony attachment of the premaxilla may be approached from the palatal side or laterally (Figure 48.20), in both cases from within the cleft. It is also possible to use a midline labial vertical mucoperiosteal incision. Following osteotomy of the narrow attachment, the bone may then be moved digitally and fixed in its new position with the guidance of an occlusal wafer.

Fixation is best achieved with a strong arch wire within preexisting fixed orthodontic bands. It is unlikely, however, that this premaxilla will then become stable without the arch wire. It will eventually be stabilized by bilateral alveolar bone grafting, and the authors consider that this is visually best carried out as a separate procedure a few months later.

Case 9 (Figure 48.20)

A 10-year-old girl with bilateral complete cleft lip and palate. The premaxilla is misplaced and would not move with orthodontic appliances.

Treatment:

1. Model surgery to reposition the premaxilla and fabricate an occlusal wafer
2. Noted that this was only possible with the surgical removal of part of the premaxilla including a developing supernumerary (or abnormal lateral incisor) tooth germ
3. Securing of orthodontic fixed bands and fabrication of a strong arch wire that would support the premaxilla in its new position
4. Surgery in which the premaxilla was approached through a small lateral incision, permitting the removal of both the required amount of the premaxilla and division with a small osteotome of its bony attachment
5. Digital movement of the premaxilla into its new position, temporary fixation into the preformed occlusal wafer, and stabilization with a strong arch wire. The wafer was then removed
6. Three months later, bilateral alveolar bone grafting was carried out with simultaneous repair of the palatal fistula
7. Continued orthodontics

(*Orthodontics courtesy of Prof. Malcolm Jones, Consultant Orthodontist and Head of Department of Child Dental Health, University Dental Hospital, Cardiff, Wales*)

Le Fort I Osteotomy

The Le Fort I osteotomy is the most valuable procedure in cleft adolescents with maxillary hypoplasia. We consider that the most important aims must be full mobilization and good fixation.

Nasal airway obstruction, a severely retropositioned maxilla, and previous pharyngoplasty may all conspire to make nasal endotracheal intubation in these patients difficult. However, it is most unusual for the nares to prevent passage of an endotracheal tube at least on one side. Forewarning of the problem of the tube hitting the posterior pharyngeal wall enables the anesthetist to carefully redirect it inferiorly. This can sometimes be helped by a finger placed in the mouth above and behind the soft palate, where the tube can be palpated and brought forward and downward. Pharyngoplasties, especially superiorly or inferiorly based pharyngeal flaps, may limit access for intubation. The presence of such flaps should be noted preoperatively; most can be bypassed without damage but the patient should be warned of the risk of the pharyngoplasty being damaged or in extreme cases of it having to be divided and repaired. Fortunately, dynamic pharyngoplasties have become more popular and they present much less restriction to intubation.

In the past, multipiece and segmental procedures were effectively forced on surgeons with what was then the stage of development of orthodontic support and before the common use of alveolar bone grafting. The work of Tideman et al. is particularly recognized in this context,[134] with his innovative use of substantial closure of the alveolar cleft by advancement of the lesser or lateral segments. Posnick[135] has also developed a closely related approach based on orthodontics and multipiece osteotomies in the ungrafted cleft patient. Case 10 (Figure 48.21) demonstrates an adaptation of these techniques in a previously bone-grafted bilateral cleft patient where presurgical orthodontic preparation could not be completed to permit a one-piece osteotomy.

Case 10 (Figure 48.21)

An 18-year-old with bilateral complete cleft lip and palate. The occlusion was mildly class III with the premaxillary teeth proclined. Further orthodontic preparation was not possible because of the very short roots on the upper central incisors. Successful bilateral alveolar bone grafting had been carried out elsewhere.

Treatment:

1. Following presurgical orthodontics, sectional arch wires were placed
2. Le Fort I osteotomy carried out from a lateral approach attempted to preserve the maximum mucoperiosteal attachment to the premaxilla both palatally and labially
3. Ostectomies carried out in the previously grafted clefts bilaterally
4. Positioning of the three bone segments of the maxilla into a preformed occlusal wafer and wiring of a prefabricated arch wire across all segments fixed to the orthodontic brackets. The proclined premaxilla was retroclined, and the lateral segments advanced to close off the gaps in the dental arch coinciding with the alveolar clefts
5. Internal bone fixation with titanium 2-mm L-shaped miniplates was followed by removal of the wafer and intermaxillary fixation (IMF)
6. Grafting of the anterior bone steps with corticocancellous blocks harvested from the medial aspect of the anterior iliac crest, and of the interdental bone cuts with cancellous bone chips

(*Orthodontics courtesy of David Howells, Consultant Orthodontist, Morriston Hospital, Swansea, Wales*)

With these particular methods, special care is required for blood supply, and tunneling incisions are usually advisable anteriorly. Difficulty may be encountered because of the presence of scar tissue from the primary palate repair and poor access to break it down; this can be a particular problem for large advancements. Loss of part of the maxilla is rarely reported but is not unknown when carrying out maxillary osteotomies in cleft patients, and it is arguable that segmental procedures increase the risk. Although demonstrating good results, it has been shown[136] that grafting the cleft at the time

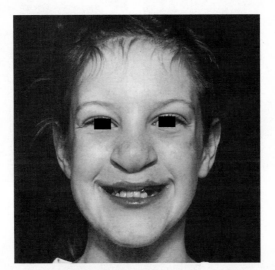

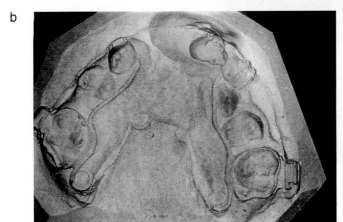

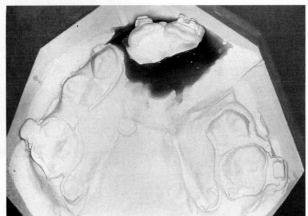

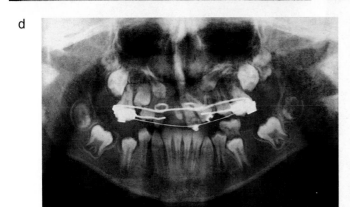

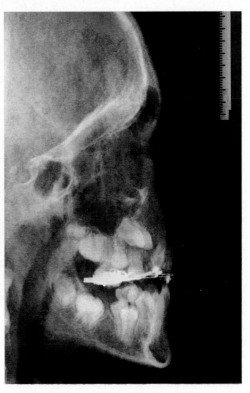

FIGURE 48.20 Case 9. (a) A 10-year-old girl with BCLP and a malpositioned premaxilla. (b) Model of maxillary arch. (c) Model surgery to reposition the premaxilla. (d) OPT before premaxillary surgery. (e) Lateral cephalogram before premaxillary surgery.

Continued.

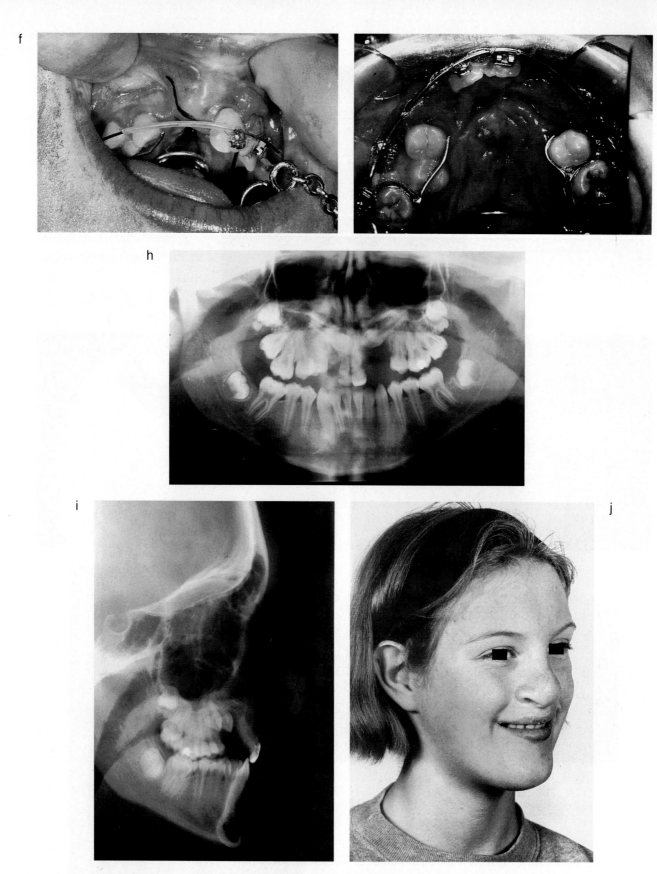

FIGURE 48.20 Case 9. *Continued*. (f) Surgical approach to the pre-maxilla marked. (g) Repositioned premaxilla after osteotomy. (h) OPT of repositioned premaxilla with bilateral alveolar bone grafts. (i) Lateral cephalogram taken at same time as h. (j) Patient follow-ing this treatment.

a

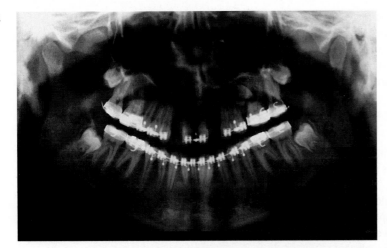

b

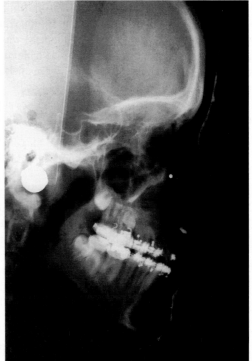

c

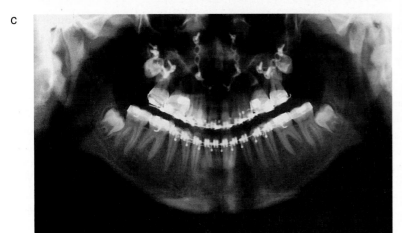

d

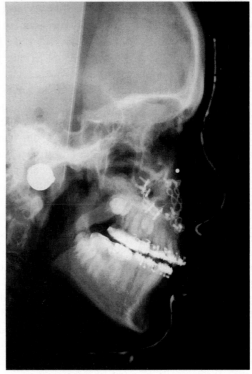

FIGURE 48.21 Case 10. Multipiece maxillary Le Fort I osteotomy in a bilateral cleft lip and palate (CLP) patient using a modified Tideman/Posnick technique. This patient had been grafted previously elsewhere, but the proclination of the premaxilla and condition of the roots of the upper incisor teeth prevented complete orthodontic decompensation and correction of the position of the premaxilla (a,b). Consequently, osteotomies were carried out through the grafted alveolus on each side. The premaxilla was then retroclined, the lateral segments advanced to close off the alveolar clefts, and the whole maxilla advanced. Fixation was aided by a temporary acrylic wafer and intermaxillary fixation (IMF), both during surgery only, and was maintained with an arch bar wired to the orthodontic brackets and four 2-mm titanium L-shaped miniplates (c,d).

of osteotomy is not quite as effective as grafting as a separate procedure. Our own experience in South Wales (before 1985 when the present approach was adopted) was of a much greater difference in the results with much more successful graft take in the alveolar cleft when this was performed as a procedure separate from maxillary osteotomy.

Three developments have permitted us to change our approach:

1. Improved primary surgery, leaving the maxilla in a better developed condition with less hypoplasia and less arch collapse.
2. Improved dental health and sophisticated orthodontics so that cleft patients can now expect to have a complete dentition (with the exception of those teeth that have not developed) with oral hygiene and tooth condition such that they can be offered fixed-band orthodontics.
3. Alveolar bone grafting which, in a good multidisciplinary team, can be timed to fit in with bone and tooth development and with other procedures, and will usually produce a continuous maxillary dental arch.

It is the view of the authors, therefore, that segmental osteotomies in the cleft maxilla can usually be avoided. Most maxillae will present in one piece following successful secondary (or primary) alveolar grafting. In those rare cases when the grafting has been less than totally successful, it can be repeated and other patients who have not received a primary or secondary graft at all can be prepared for tertiary grafting in the way that we have described.[128] Having taken this approach, it is not very logical or sensible to follow with sectioning of the maxilla into multiple pieces. Consequently, we try to carry out all cleft osteotomies with a one-piece maxilla using a downfracture approach. To date only one case (a BCLP case bone grafted in another unit) has shown signs of the maxilla failing to remain in one piece, and the minor cracks that occurred in the grafted area did not compromise the result, the segments being held in a strong arch wire.

The incision is placed anteriorly (Figure 48.22), being modified from the standard Le Fort I approach. It commences high in the cheek, just above and anterior to the openings of the parotid ducts. It is then continued down across the inside of the upper lip. This permits a broader posterolateral pedicle to supplement the palatal supply and still gives good access to the pterygoid area. This incision is used for grafted unilateral and bilateral cases alike, and since it was adopted 11 years ago not a single instance of compromised blood supply has been encountered.

The osteotomy is carried out using saws and fine osteotomes and with separation of tuberosities from pterygoid plates with a chisel. The cuts are placed high to facilitate internal miniplate fixation. Mobilization is carried out digitally and with disimpaction forceps and mobilizers. The nasal mucosa is preserved on both sides but in places may have to be cut to separate it from the oral (principally palatal) mucosa.

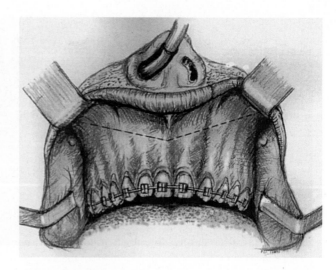

FIGURE 48.22 Modified incision for one-piece Le Fort I osteotomies in all grafted cleft patients.

There is often very little space for disimpaction forceps in the palate, especially with rubber protection for the blades. There is also a small risk of damaging previous palate repairs. We therefore always use a purpose-constructed metal palatal coverage plate (Figure 48.23) first designed in our unit by Ross and Bocca that permits use of the forceps without rubber covers and protects the palate effectively during mobilization. We always break down digitally the palatal scar tissue holding the maxilla back, and we do this from above through the opening created by the downfracture.

With the maxilla displaced downward, it is then possible to assess the internal nasal structures. A broad septum may be reduced, and inferior (partial) turbinectomy carried out if indicated. A preformed acrylic wafer is attached to the teeth by orthodontic powerchain and intermaxillary fixation (IMF) placed with more powerchain.[137] The maxilla is fixed using

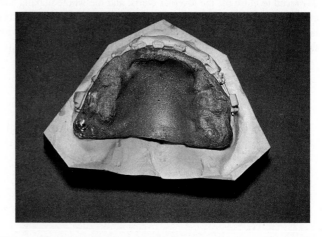

FIGURE 48.23 Palatal protection plate for mobilizing cleft maxillae with disimpaction forcep (Designed by Ross and Bocca).

L-shaped 2-mm miniplates, long L-shaped plates being particularly valuable for large advancements (Case 11, Figure 48.24).

Case 11 (Figure 48.24)

A 17-year old with bilateral complete cleft lip and palate and treated hypertelorbitism.

Treatment:

1. Orthopedic expansion and alignment of segments
2. Bilateral alveolar bone grafting and palatal fistula repair
3. Presurgical orthodontic preparation
4. One-piece Le Fort I osteotomy as described in the text, internally fixed with long L-shaped titanium 2-mm miniplates and bone grafted. The advancement in this case was 22 mm and the downward movement anteriorly was 10 mm
5. Completion of orthodontics. The stability of the result is demonstrated in the lateral cephalometry in Figure 48.24(h) 2 years after surgery

(*Orthodontics courtesy of Prof. Malcom Jones, Consultant Orthodontist and Head of Dept. of Child Dental Health, University Dental Hospital, Cardiff, Wales, and David Bachmeyer, Sydney, New South Wales, Australia*)

We always bone graft these cleft osteotomies, using autogenous corticocancellous blocks harvested from the medial aspect of the anterior iliac crest. The grafts are placed anterolaterally and occasionally are fixed with screws. Grafts are never placed into the region behind the maxilla, where they are in any event unstable. The wounds are closed primarily and without tension with no attempt to use the so-called V to Y single or multiple advancements. We consider that these closures, designed to produce vertical lip lengthening, actually produce increased anteroposterior lip projection and a tight wound and lip. In our hands, IMF is always removed at the end of the operation and before extubation. We have never encountered instability in these cases, even for the largest maxillary advancements (more than 2.5 cm in some cases), and have never had to resort to later IMF.

Case 12 (Figure 48.25)

A 21-year-old with repaired complete unilateral cleft lip and palate, anteroposterior and vertical midface deficiency and retrogenia, and secondary alveolar bone graft having been inserted previously.

Treatment:

1. Presurgical orthodontics
2. One-piece Le Fort I maxillary osteotomy as described above with miniplate fixation
3. Advancement genioplasty (horizontal sliding osteotomy) with 2-mm miniplate fixation
4. Completion of orthodontics

(*Orthodontics courtesy of Russell Samuels, Consultant Orthodontist, Glenfield Hospital, Leicester, England*)

Case 13 (Figure 48.26)

A 16-year-old with right unilateral complete cleft lip and palate. Secondary alveolar bone graft inserted after arch expansion at the age of 9 years with simultaneous closure of a large palatal fistula. Presented with significant anteroposterior and vertical maxillary deficiency.

Treatment:

1. Presurgical orthodontic preparation
2. Le Fort I maxillary advancement (1.5 cm) and downward movement (5 mm) as described above, fixation being with 2-mm titanium L-shaped miniplates and anterior maxillary grafting with corticocancellous blocks harvested from the medial aspect of the anterior iliac crest
3. Completion of orthodontics

(*Orthodontics courtesy of Simon James, Consultant Orthodontist, Withybush General Hospital, Haverfordwest, Wales*)

This approach has of course made these procedures much more popular with our anesthetic colleagues with safer postoperative airway management. Expensive intensive or high dependency care management in the immediate postoperative period can almost always be avoided. It has also made the postoperative period much more comfortable for the patient, who has often had to endure many operations.

The downfracture approach has been criticized in some quarters because of the risk of making velopharyngeal function worse. Using the technique described here, this has not been our experience. Velopharyngeal incompetence only seems to be present postoperatively in patients in whom it was present before surgery. It has been reported that the development of VPI can be avoided if a palatal approach to the osteotomy is adopted, the intention being to leave the palatal musculature and soft palate behind when the maxilla is advanced.[138–141] This certainly has merit but unfortunately also has some disadvantages. Intraoperatively, there is reduced access anteriorly to the nose and for fixation, and among the postoperative complications there is a high incidence of residual oronasal fistulae that require further surgery. Average skeletal relapse in the position of the maxilla anteroposteriorly has been reported as high as 29% in one series.[140]

The literature and experience indicate that Le Fort I osteotomies in cleft patients can be associated with particularly high incidences of relapse in the opposite direction to the movements carried out. It is our clear impression that this is no longer the case with our approach.[142] This is discussed further later.

a

b

c

d

e

f

g

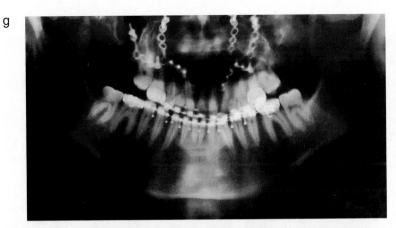

i

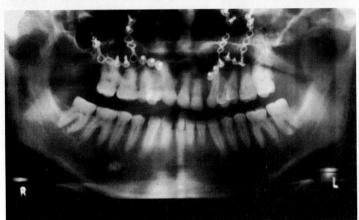

h

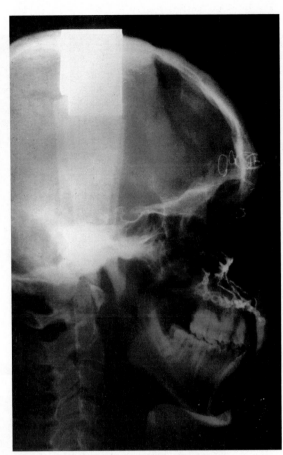

FIGURE 48.24 Case 11. Use of long cantilevered L-shaped 2-mm miniplates to fix and maintain a large one-piece maxillary advancement (22 mm) and anterior downward movement (10 mm) in a patient with bilateral complete cleft lip and palate. (a) Maxillary dental arch before orthodontics and grafting. (b) Maxillary dental arch after orthodontics and bilateral alveolar bone grafting. (c) Profile of this patient before maxillary advancement. (d) Lateral cephalogram before maxillary advancement. (e) Profile after large maxillary advancement (22 mm) and downward movement (10 mm). (f) Lateral cephalogram demonstrating the use of long cantilevered titanium L-shaped miniplates for fixation of this large movement. (g) OPT taken at the same time as f. (h) Lateral cephalogram showing stability of the movement 2 years later. (i) OPT taken at the same time as (h).

a

b

c

d

e

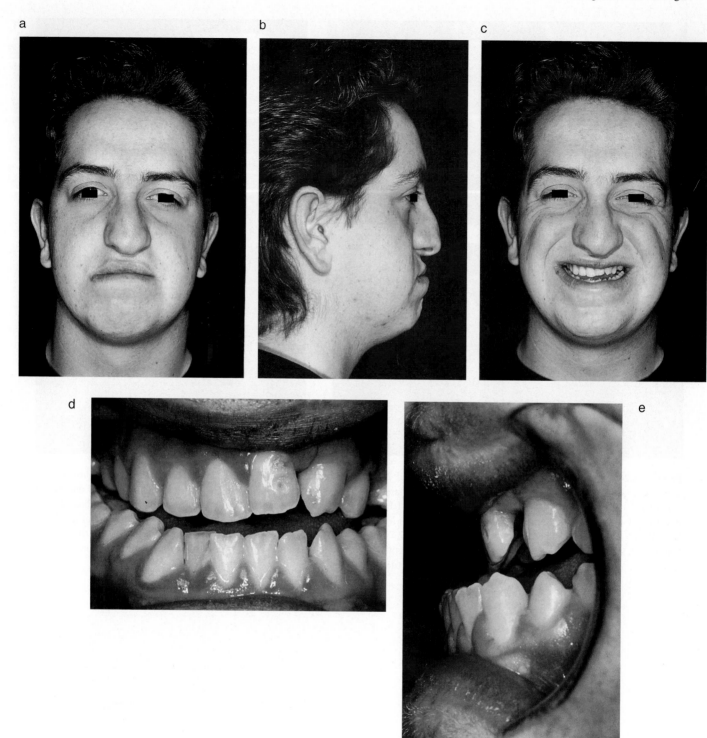

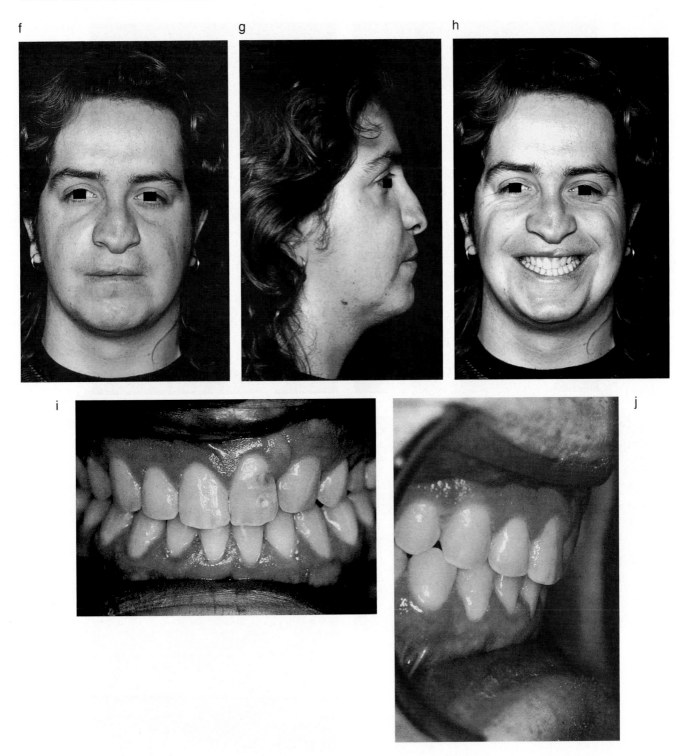

FIGURE 48.25 Case 12. One-piece maxillary and chin advancement osteotomies in a patient with a repaired unilateral complete cleft lip and palate. (a,b,c) Facial views before orthognathic surgery. (d,e) Occlusion before surgery. (f–h) Facial views after Le Fort I one-piece maxillary advancement osteotomy fixed internally with four 2-mm titanium L-shaped miniplates, grafting anteriorly with corticocancellous autogenous bone blocks from the medial aspect of the anterior iliac crest placed, and advancement genioplasty also fixed with miniplates. Views taken before rhinoplasty. (i,j) Occlusion after the surgery.

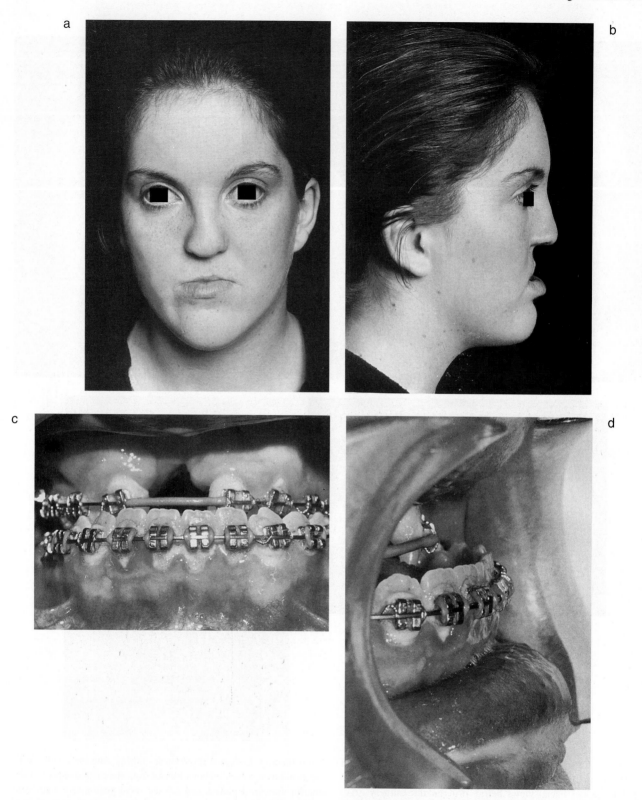

FIGURE 48.26 Case 13. One-piece maxillary advancement and down-ward movment in a patient with a repaired unilateral complete cleft lip and palate. (a,b) Facial views before orthognathic surgery. (c,d) Occlusion before surgery. (e,f) Facial views after large Le Fort I ad-vancement osteotomy, with fixation by four 2-mm titanium L-shaped miniplates, and bone grafting anteriorly with bone harvested from the anterior iliac crest. (g,h) Occlusion after the surgery with tem-porary prosthesis in situ.

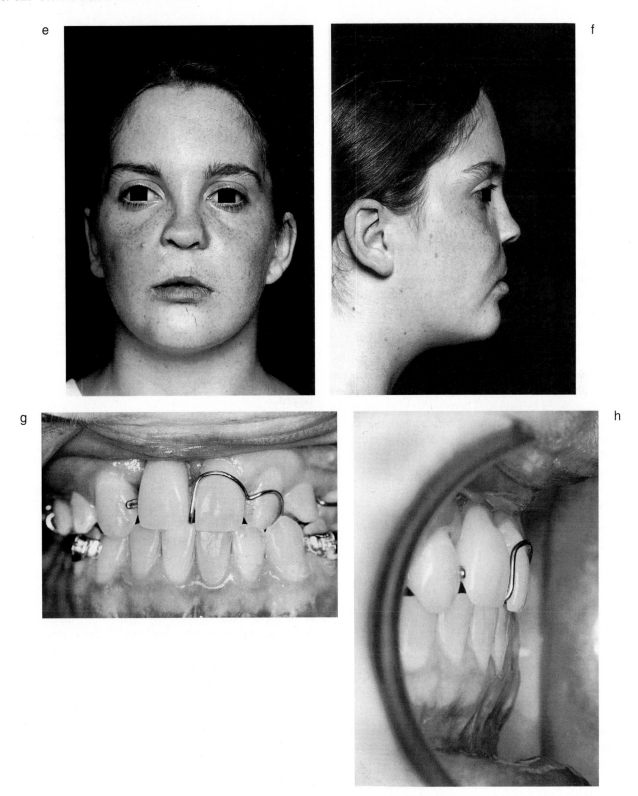

FIGURE 48.26 Case 13. *Continued*.

Le Fort II Osteotomy

Nasomaxillary hypoplasia is seen in some cleft patients with genuine retroposition of both the maxilla and entire nose. When the shape of the nose is otherwise normal, Le Fort I osteotomies may well make nasal appearance worse. The best approach is to carry out a Le Fort II osteotomy as described by Henderson and Jackson.[143]

We carry out this procedure through coronal and oral incisions because this gives the best access for the osteotomy, fixation, and grafting, and avoids further scars on the face. It is never possible to achieve the same degree of mobility as with the Le Fort I downfracture osteotomy. This seems to be compensated by the much larger block of bone tissue mobilized and the good opportunity for rigid fixation. Miniplate fixation is always used, usually with 2-mm plates and screws, and we prefer two L-shaped plates across the sides of the nose and two at the zygomatic buttress. The gaps are filled with autogenous corticocancellous or cancellous blocks of bone harvested from the anterior iliac crest.

When carrying out Le Fort II osteotomies it is important to consider carefully the nasofrontal angle, which can become too obtuse, and the intercanthal distance, which can increase with displacement anteriorly of the canthi. The former can be avoided by judicious bone removal to reduce the nasofrontal angle at osteotomy. The latter often requires transnasal canthopexy through the osteotomy gap so that the ligaments can be approximated and moved into a more posterior position.

Case 14 (Figure 48.27)

An 18-year-old with unilateral complete cleft lip and palate and nasomaxillary hypoplasia.

Treatment:

1. Presurgical orthodontics
2. Le Fort II osteotomy carried out through combined coronal and oral approaches
3. Fixation at four sites (nasofrontal and malar-maxillary) on both sides with 2-mm L-shaped titanium miniplates
4. Completion of orthodontics
5. Result also shown 6 years postoperatively with complete stability

(*Orthodontics courtesy of Prof. Malcolm Jones, Consultant Orthodontist and Head of Department of Child Dental Health, University Dental Hospital, Cardiff, Wales*)

A related approach to these nasomaxillary problems in cleft patients has been described by Tideman[144] and is only really feasible because of internal plate fixation. The different needs in terms of advancement of the nose and maxilla are addressed in appropriate cases by carrying out a Le Fort II osteotomy to place the nose in its correct position and a few weeks later a Le Fort I to reposition the maxilla for the occlusion.

Malar Maxillary Le Fort III Osteotomy

Occasionally the nature of the midface deformity suggests the need for a Le Fort III or modified Le Fort III procedure. It is rare that these can be accomplished at one level, the needs for malar advancement usually being different from those at a dentoalveolar and occlusal level. We have therefore carried out these procedures at two levels at the same operation (i.e., simultaneous Le Fort III and Le Fort I).

Genioplasty

Retrogenia and increased chin height are common in cleft patients and are very amenable to correction. We favor a horizontal genioplasty osteotomy, sometimes with the excision of a slice of bone above the osteotomy to permit upward positioning. The attachment of the periosteum and suprahyoid musculature to the chin point is preserved, and the mental nerves carefully identified and avoided. Fixation is with two L-shaped 2-mm miniplates, one being placed on each side. Plates placed in the midline in this area are often palpable later. Although we have tried to use smaller plates and screws in this site, we have found that the titanium screw heads tend to shear off in this quite dense bone unless the holes are pre-tapped.

Bimaxillary Procedures

True mandibular prognathism is rare in cleft patients but when present needs to be corrected in a conventional orthognathic manner. Even more rarely, and predominantly in bilateral cleft patients, there is an indication for bimaxillary advancement. We favor, for the mandibular movement in whichever direction, bilateral sagittal split osteotomies with fixation using bicortical 2.4-mm screws. Where bone is in contact we will sometimes insert lag screws but in most cases, and especially where there are gaps, position screws are more appropriate. We used to insert three on each side but two good rigid screws at the upper border are probably sufficient. A transbuccal approach is used as we have described[145] and is greatly facilitated by more recent improved instrumentation. Incisions of only 3 to 5 mm are required and, perhaps surprisingly, we have never seen a poor scar in more than 200 patients treated in this way.

Stability

It is widely recognized that midfacial advancement osteotomies in cleft patients are potentially less stable than in noncleft patients. Much of the responsibility for this has been ascribed to the presence of scar tissue in the region of the previous palate repair posteriorly, the common need for very large advancements, and the difficulty in achieving good fixation.

We therefore decided to study[140] a carefully controlled group of our cleft patients. These all underwent consecutive

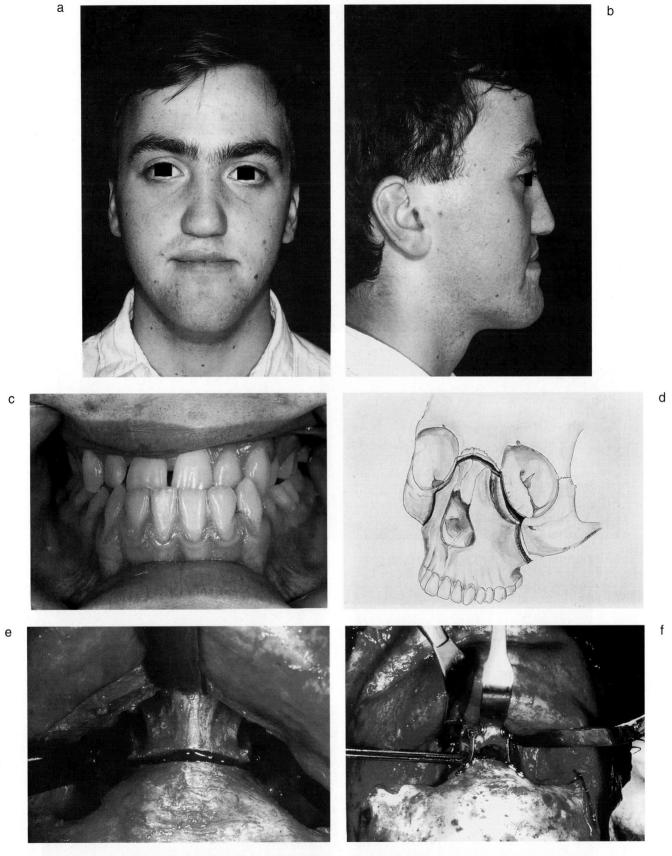

FIGURE 48.27 Case 14. Patient with repaired unilateral complete cleft lip and palate and nasomaxillary hypoplasia managed by a Le Fort II osteotomy. (a–c) Facial and occlusal views before surgery. (d) Drawing of the Le Fort II nasomaxillary osteotomy. (e) The nasofrontal exposure and osteotomy. (f) The nasofrontal fixation before grafting.

Continued.

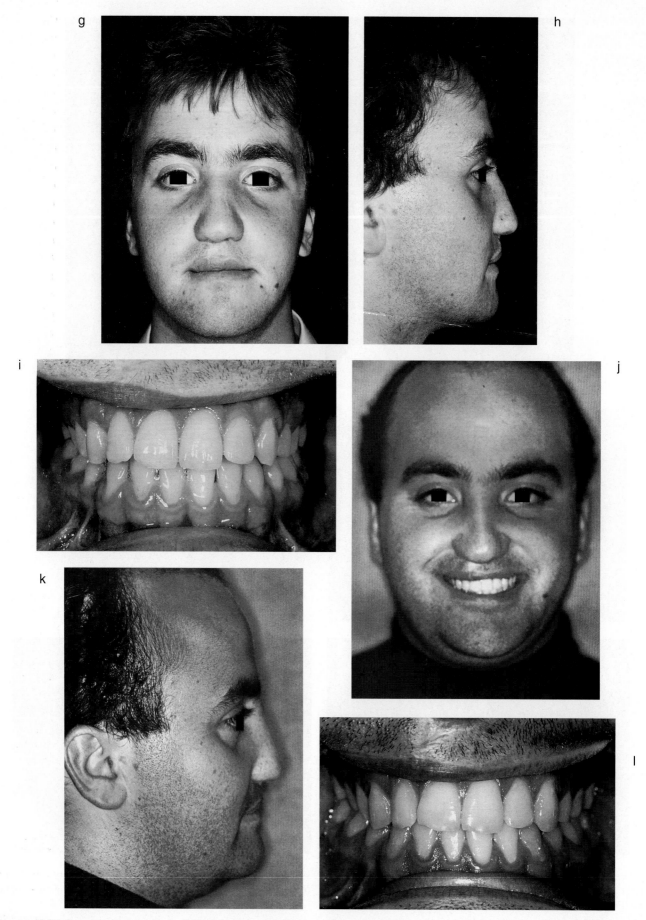

Figure 48.27 Case 14. *Continued*. (g–i) Facial and occlusal views after surgery and orthodontics. (j–l) Facial and occlusal views 6 years after surgery.

Le Fort I osteotomies to our prescribed protocol as described. Presurgical fixed-band orthodontics was always carried out, with secondary or tertiary bone grafting of any alveolar defect before or during that orthodontic phase. One-piece osteotomy from an anterior downfracture approach with anterior maxillary grafting using autogenous corticocancellous blocks and internal fixation was carried out by the same surgical team. Neither intermaxillary fixation nor external fixation was used in any case.

We have compared this test group with a control group of noncleft patients being treated by the same surgeons and to the same protocol. The study has been carried out with serial lateral cephalometric radiographs taken on the same machine by the same radiographer and at the same time intervals up to a minimum of 1 year. These were digitized by the same calibrated individual on two occasions, with at least 2 months between determinations, using Dentofacial Planner 4.32 software. Error measurement using paired t-tests showed no statistically significant difference between the two digitizations for both hard and soft tissue points.

The mean maxillary hard tissue advancement was similar in both groups (10.3 mm with a SD of 3.4 in the cleft group, and 10.5 with a SD of 2.9 in the nonclefts). The mean vertical movements were downward in the cleft group and upward in the nonclefts. The hard tissue changes up to 1 year, reflecting relapse or remodeling, were very small in both groups. The clefts moved posteriorly by 1.2 mm or 11.5% (SD 0.7) and the nonclefts by 0.7 mm or 6.5% (SD 0.8). The difference between the operated cleft and noncleft relapse rates was not statistically significant. The vertical changes were barely measurable and were all less than 0.5 mm. There was no statistically significant difference in the horizontal surgical soft tissue changes between the two groups, but the vertical soft tissue changes were different. The upper lip tended to go up in the nonclefts and down in the clefts. Upper-lip thickness decreased in both groups.

This study continues, and is presently based on relatively small numbers (10–15) in each group. However, there is good reason to believe at this stage that there is little difference in the way that cleft and noncleft osteotomies heal up to 1 year later after they have been performed in the way described. The one-piece cleft maxillary osteotomies also seem to be quite stable, and relapse or remodeling is well within clinically acceptable limits.

References

1. Streeter GL. Developmental horizons in human embryos. *Contrib Embryol (Carnegie Inst Wash)*. 1951;11:165–196.
2. Töndury G. Über die Genese der Lippen-, Kiefer- Gaumenspalten. *Fortschr Kiefer Gesichts Chir*. 1955;1:1–8.
3. Kriens O. Kommt der Zwischenkiefer vom Stirnfortsatz oder? Vortrag 7. *Symposium Interdiszipl. Arbeitskreis LKG-Spalten*, 1994, Mainz.
4. Jirasek JE. The development of the face and mouth cavity. *Acta Chir Plast*. 1966;8:237–248.
5. Klaskova O. An epidemiological study of cleft lip and palate in Bohemia. *Acta Chir Plast*. 1973;15:258–262.
6. Jensen BL, Kreiborg S, Dahl E. Cleft lip and palate in Denmark, 1976–1981: epidemiology, variability, and early somatic development. *Cleft Palate J*. 1988;25:258–269.
7. Saxen I, Lahti A. Cleft lip and palate in Finland: incidence, secular, seasonal, and geographical variation. *Teratology*. 1974;9:217–223.
8. Muehler, G. Die Bedeutung der Humangenetischen Beratung von Gesichtsspaltraegern und ihren Familien. *Stomatol DDR*. 1982;32:861–867.
9. Neel JK. A study of major congenital defects in Japanese infants. *Am J Hum Genet*. 1958;10:398–403.
10. Coerdt I. Erkrankungen der Kiefer und der Zaehne. In: Betke K, Kuenzer W, Schaub J, eds. *Keller/Wiskott. Lehrbuch der Kinderheilkunde*. Stuttgart: Thiemes; 1991.
11. Emanuel I, Culver BH, Erickson JD, Guthrie B, Schuldberg D. The further epidemiological differentiation of cleft lip and palate: a population study of clefts in King County, Washington, 1956–1965. *Teratology* 1973;7:271–282.
12. Ivy RH. The influence of race on the incidence of certain congenital anomalies, notably cleft lip–cleft palate. *Plast Reconstr Surg*. 1962;30:581–585.
13. Jörgensen G. Zur Aetiologie der Lippen-, Kiefer- und Gaumenspalten. *Med Heute*. 1969;18:293–298.
14. Fraser FC. The multifactorial/threshold concept—uses and misuses. *Teratology*. 1976;14:267–280.
15. Poswillo D. Mechanisms and pathogenesis of malformation. *Br Med Bull*. 1976;32:59–64.
16. Millicovsky G, Johnston MC. Hyperoxia and hypoxia in pregnancy: simple experimental manipulation alters the incidence of cleft lip and palate in CL/Fr mice. *Proc Natl Acad Sci USA*. 1981;78:5722–5723.
17. Davis JS, Ritchie HP. Classification of congenital clefts of lip and palate. *JAMA*. 1922;79:1323–1328.
18. Veau V. *Division Palatine*. Paris: Masson et Cie, 1931.
19. Fogh-Andersen P. Documentation. Discussion by invitation. In: Schuchardt K, ed. *Treatment of Patients with Clefts of Lip. Alveolus and Palate*. Stuttgart: Thieme; 1966.
20. Kernahan DA, Stark RB. A new classification for cleft lip and cleft palate. *Plast Reconstr Surg*. 1958;22:435–441.
21. Koch J. Zur Diagnostik der Lippen-, Kiefer-, Gaumenspalten. *Dtsch Stomatol*. 1963;13:660–666.
22. Pfeifer G. Classification of clefts of lip, alveolus and palate. Discussion by invitation. In: Schuchardt K, ed. *Treatment of Patients with Clefts of Lip, Alveolus and Palate*. Stuttgart: Thieme; 1966:224–226.
23. Kernahan DA. The striped Y. *Plast Reconstr Surg*. 1971;47:469–470.
24. Elsahy NI. The modified striped Y—a systematic classification for cleft lip and palate. *Cleft Palate J*. 1973;10:247–50.
25. Millard DR. *Cleft Craft*. Vol. I. Boston: Little, Brown; 1976.
26. Friedman HI, Sayetta RB, Coston GN, Hussey JR. Symbolic representation of cleft lip and palate. *Cleft Palate Craniofac J*. 1991;28:252–259.
27. Kriens O. LAHSHAL. A concise documentation system for cleft lip, alveolus and palate diagnosis. In: Kriens O, ed. *What Is a Cleft Lip and Palate?* Stuttgart: Thieme; 1989:30–34.
28. Honigmann K. *Die Pirmärbehandlung von Lippen-Kiefer-Gaumen-Segelspalten*. Basel: Habil.-Schrift University; 1995.

29. Kriens O. Data-objective diagnosis of infant cleft lip, alveolus, and palate. Morphologic data guiding understanding and treatment concepts. *Cleft Palate Craniofac J.* 1991;28:157–168.

30. Paradise JL. Primary care of infants and children with cleft palate. In: Bluestone CD, Stool SE, Arjona SK, eds. *Pediatric Otolaryngology*: Philadelphia: WB Saunders; 1983.

31. Schmitt BD, Berman S. Ear, nose & throat. In: Kempe CH, Silver HK, O'Brien D, Fulginiti VA, eds. *Current Pediatric Diagnosis & Treatment*. Norwalk: Appleton & Lange; 1987.

32. Biesalski P, Collo D. *Hals-Nasen-Ohren-Krankheiten im Kindesalter.* Aufl. 2. Stuttgart: Thieme; 1991.

33. Clarren SK, Anderson B, Wolf L. Feeding infants with cleft lip, cleft palate, or cleft lip and palate. *Cleft Palate J.* 1987; 24:244–249.

34. Koppenburg P, Leidig E, Bacher M, Dausch-Neumann D. Die Darstellung von Lage und Beweglichkeit der Zunge bei Neugeborenen mit oralen Spaltfehlbildungen durch transorale Ultraschallsonographie. *Dtsch Zahnärztl Z.* 1988;43:806–809.

35. Kriens O. Neuere Aspekte in der Behandlung von Lippen-Kiefer-Gaumenspalten. *Spaltträger Forum.* 1990;2:25–30.

36. McNeil CK. Orthodontic procedures in the treatment of congenital cleft palate. *Dent Rec.* 1950;70:126–132.

37. Hotz M. Pre- and early postoperative growth guidance in cleft lip and palate cases by maxillary orthopedics. *Cleft Palate J.* 1969;6:368–372.

38. Gnoinski WM. Early maxillary orthopedics as a supplement to conventional primary surgery in complete cleft lip and palate cases—long-term results. *J Maxillofac Surg.* 1982;10:165–172.

39. Behrman RE, Vaughan VC. *Nelson Textbook of Pediatrics.* 13th ed. Philadelphia: WB Saunders; 1987.

40. Gnoinski WM. Third international symposium on the early treatment of cleft lip and palate. Zürich 1984. *Schweiz Monatsschr Zahnmed.* 1985;95:462/18–469/25.

41. Saunders IDF, Geary L, Fleming P, Gregg TA. A simplified feeding appliance for the infant with a cleft lip and palate. *Quintessence Int.* 1989;20:907–910.

42. Weatherly-White RCA, Kuehn DP, Mirrett P, Gilman JI, Weatherly-White CC. Early repair and breast-feeding for infants with cleft lip. *Plast Reconstr Surg.* 1987;79:879–885.

43. Duncan B, Ey J, Holberg CJ. Exclusive breast-feeding for at least 4 months protects against otitis media. *Pediatrics.* 1993; 91:867–872.

44. Honigmann K, Herzog C. Stillen von Kindern mit einer Lippen-Kiefer-Gaumen-Segelspalte. *Paediatrica.* 1993;4:16–22.

45. Tasaka Y, Kawano M, Honjo I. Eustachian tube function in OME patients with cleft palate. *Acta Otolaryngol Suppl (Stockh).* 1990;471:5–8.

46. Moss ALH, Piggott RW, Jones KJ. Submucous cleft palate. *Br Med J.* 1988;297:85–86.

47. Matsune S, Sando I, Takahashi H. Insertion of the tensor veli palatini muscle into the eustachian tube cartilage in cleft palate cases. *Ann Otol Rhinol Laryngol.* 1991;100:439–446.

48. Stool SE, Randall P. Unexpected ear diseases in infants with cleft palate. *Cleft Palate J.* 1967;4:99–103.

49. Fria TJ, Paradise JL, Sabo DL, Elster BA. Conductive hearing loss in infants and young children with cleft palate. *J Pediatr.* 1987;111:84–87.

50. McMillan JA, Oski FA, Stockman JA, Nieburg PI. *Pädiatrische Daten und Fakten.* Stuttgart: Ferdinand Enke Verlag; 1988.

51. Koch J, Schiel H, Koch H. Neue Gesichtspunkte zur kausalen Therapie der Hör- und Sprachentwicklungsstörungen durch Gaumenspalten. *Monatsschr Kinderheilkd.* 1987;135:75–80.

52. Godbersen GS. Die mechanische Verlegung der Tubenostien. *Folia Phoniatr.* 1990;42:105–110.

53. Braganza RA, Kearns DB, Burton DM, Seid AB, Pransky SM. Closure of the soft palate for persistent otorrhea after placement of pressure equalization tubes in cleft palate infants. *Cleft Palate Craniofac J.* 1991;28:305–307.

54. Malek R, Psaume J, Mousset MS, Trichet CH. A new sequence and a new technique in complete cleft lip and palate repair. In: Hotz M, Gnoinski W, Perko M, Nussbaumer H, Hof E, Haubensack R, eds. *Early Treatment of Cleft Lip and Palate.* Stuttgart: Hans Huber; 1986.

55. Oesch IL, Looser C, Bettex MC. Influence of early closure of soft palatal clefts on the pharyngeal skeleton: Observation by CT scan. *Cleft Palate J.* 1987;24:291–298.

56. Garliner D. *Myofunctional Therapy.* Philadelphia: WB Saunders; 1976.

57. Codoni S. Anwendung der myofunktionellen Diagnostik und Therapie bei de Behandlung des LKG-Spalten-Kindes. *Spaltträger Forum.* 1992;4:22–28.

58. Graf-Pinthus B, Campiche M. Die Suche nach einem holistischen Behandlungskonzept bei Lippen-Kiefer-Gaumen-Spalten. *Myofunktion Ther.* 1994;1:58–66.

59. Obwegeser H. Chirurgische Behandlungsmöglichkeiten von Sekundärdeformierungen bei Spaltpatienten. *Fortschr Kieferorthop.* 1988;49:272–296.

60. Markus AF, Smith WP, Delaire J. Primary closure of cleft palate: a functional approach. *Br J Oral Maxillofac Surg.* 1993;31:71–77.

61. Henderson D, Poswillo D. *A Colour Atlas and Textbook of Orthognathic Surgery.* London: Wolfe; 1985.

62. Bardach J, Salyer KE. *Surgical Techniques in Cleft Lip and Palate.* St. Louis: Mosby-Year Book; 1991.

63. Fränkel R. Die Bedeutung der Weichteile für die Induktion und Formorientierung des Kieferwachstums unter Zugrundelegung der Behandlungsergebnisse mit Funktionsreglern. *Fortschr Kieferorthop.* 1964;25:413.

64. Koch J. Jährige Erfahrungen mit der primären Knochentransplantation beim Verschluss der Kiefer- und Gaumenspalte im 4. Lebensjahr. In: Pfeifer G. ed. *Lippen-Kiefer-Gaumenspalten.* 3. Internationales Symposium, Hamburg 1979. Stuttgart: Thieme; 1982.

65. Rosenthal W. Die primäre orthopädische Beeinflussung des Spaltkiefers beim Säugling. *Dtsch Stomatol.* 1961;11:622–630.

66. Rosenthal W. Spezielle Zahn-, Mund- und Kieferchirurgie. Leipzig: Johann Ambrosius Barth; 1951.

67. Honigmann K. The celluloid-acetone-dressing in palatoplasty. *Cleft Palate Craniofac J.* 1994;31:228–229.

68. Kapp-Simon K. Self-concept of primary-school-age children with cleft lip, cleft palate, or both. *Cleft Palate J.* 1986;23: 24–27.

69. Strauss RP, Broder H, Helms RW. Perceptions of appearance and speech by adolescent patients with cleft lip and palate and by their parents. *Cleft Palate J.* 1988;25:335–342.

70. Broder H, Strauss RP. Self-concept of early primary school age children with visible or invisible defects. *Cleft Palate J.* 1989;26:114–117.

71. Lansdown R. Psychological problems of patients with cleft lip and palate: discussion paper. *J R Soc Med.* 1990;83:448–450.

72. Eliason MJ, Hardin MA, Olin WH. Factors that influence ratings of facial appearance for children with cleft lip and palate. *Cleft Palate Craniofac J.* 1991;28:190–193.

73. Wolff J. *Das Gesetz der Transformation der Knochen.* Berlin: Hirschwald; 1892.

74. Veau V. Plastie palatine. *J Chir.* 1936;48:465–481.

75. Wassmund M. Der Verschluss des Kieferspaltes und Nasenbodens bei vollständiger Spaltbildung—Zeitpunkt und Methoden. *Fortschr Kiefer Gesichts Chir.* 1955;1:27–36.

76. Schmid E. Die Annäherung der Kieferstümpfe bei Lippen-Kiefer-Gaumenspalten; ihre schädlichen Folgen und Vermeidung. *Fortschr Kiefer Gesichts Chir.* 1955;1:37–39.

77. Nordin KE, Johansson B. Freie Knochentransplantation bei Defekten im Alveolarkamm nach kieferorthopädischer Einstellung der Maxilla bei Lippen-Kiefer-Gaumenspalten. *Fortschr Kiefer Gesichts Chir.* 1955;1:168–171.

78. Schrudde J, Stellmach R. Die primäre Osteoplastik der Defekte des Kieferbogens bei Lippen-Kiefer-Gaumenspalten beim Säugling. *Zentrabl Chir.* 1958;83:849–859.

79. Schuchardt K, Pfeifer G. Erfahrungen Über primäre Knochentransplantationen bei Lippen-Kiefer-Gaumenspalten. *Langenbecks Arch Klin Chir.* 1960;295:881–884.

80. Boyne P, Sands N. Secondary bone grafting of residual alveolar and palatal clefts. *J Oral Surg.* 1972;30:87–92.

81. Abyholm FE, Bergland O, Semb G. Secondary bone grafting of alveolar clefts. A surgical orthodontic treatment enabling a non-prosthodontic rehabilitation in cleft lip and palate patients. *Scand J Plast Reconstr Surg.* 1981;15:127–140.

82. Wolfe SA, Berkowitz S. The use of cranial bone grafts in the closure of alveolar and anterior palatal clefts. *Plast Reconstr Surg.* 1983;72:659–671.

83. Kalaaji A, Lilja J, Friede H. Bone grafting at the stage of mixed and permanent dentition in patients with clefts of the lip and primary palate. *Plast Reconstr Surg.* 1994;93:690–696.

84. Dado DV. Primary (early) alveolar bone grafting. *Clin Plast Surg.* 1993;20:683–689.

85. Holtgrave EA. Die osteoplastische Versorgung des Kieferspaltes—ein Fortschritt für die kieferorthopädische Behandlung des Spaltpatienten? *Fortschr Kieferorthop.* 1991;52:237–244.

86. Müssig D. Die Einstellung spaltnaher Eckzähne in Abhängigkeit vom Zeitpunkt der spätprimären Osteoplastik. *Fortschr Kieferorthop.* 1991;52:245–251.

87. Blanchard-Moreau P, Breton P, Lebescond Y, Beziat JL, Freidel M. L'osteoplastie secondaire dans les fentes congenitales du palais primaire. Technique et resultats a propos de 43 observations. *Rev Stomatol Chir Maxillofac.* 1989;90:84–88.

88. Witsenburg B, Remmelink H-J. Reconstruction of residual alveolo-palatal bone defects in cleft patients. *J Cranio-Maxillo-Fac Surg.* 1993;21:239–244.

89. McNeil CK. *Oral and Facial Deformity.* London: Pitman & Sons; 1954.

90. Hotz R, Graf-Pinthus B. Zur kieferorthopädischen Frühbehandlung der Lippen-Kiefer-Gaumenspalten nach McNeil. *Schweiz Monatsschr Zahnheilkd.* 1960;70:1–9.

91. Hotz R, Graf-Pinthus B. Weitere Erfahrungen mit der präoperativen kieferorthopädischen Frühbehandlung von totalen Lippen-Kiefer-Gaumenspalten. *Schweiz Monatsschr Zahnheilkd.* 1962;72:583–590.

92. Peat JH. Early orthodontic treatment for complete clefts. *Am J Orthodont.* 1974;65:28–38.

93. Larson O, Nordin KE, Nylen B, Eklund G. Early bone grafting in complete cleft lip and palate cases following maxillofacial orthopedics. II. The soft tissue development from seven to thirteen years of age. *Scand J Plast Reconstr Surg.* 1983;17:51–62.

94. Reisberg DJ, Figueroa AA, Gold HO. An intraoral appliance for management of the protrusive premaxilla in bilateral cleft lip. *Cleft Palate J.* 1988;25:53–57.

95. Asher-McDade C, Shaw WC. Current cleft lip and palate management in the United Kingdom. *Br J Plast Surg.* 1990; 43:318–321.

96. Cutting C, Grayson B. The prolabial unwinding flap method for one-stage repair of bilateral cleft lip, nose, and alveolus. *Plast Reconstr Surg.* 1993;91:37–47.

97. Cronin TD, Penoff JH. Bilateral clefts of the primary palate. *Cleft Palate J.* 1971;8:349–363.

98. Hellquist R. Early maxillary orthopedics in relation to maxillary cleft repair by perioplasty. *Cleft Palate J.* 1971;8:36–55.

99. Vargervik K. Growth characteristics of the premaxilla and orthodontic treatment principles in bilateral cleft lip and palate. *Cleft Palate J.* 1983;20:289–302.

100. Rutrick R, Black PW, Jurkiewicz MJ. Bilateral cleft lip and palate presurgical treatment. *Ann Plast Surg.* 1984;12:105–117.

101. Georgiade NG, Mladick RA, Thoren FL. Positioning of the premaxilla in bilateral cleft lips by oral pinning and traction. *Plast Reconstr Surg.* 1968;4:240–243.

102. Georgiade NG, Latham RA. Maxillary oral alignment in the bilateral cleft lip and plate infant, using the pinned coaxial screw appliance. *Plast Reconstr Surg.* 1975;56:52–60.

103. Latham RA. Orthopedic advancement of the cleft maxillary segment: a preliminary report. *Cleft Palate J.* 1980;17:227–233.

104. Stassen LFA. The management of patients with a cleft lip and palate deformity. *Br J Oral Maxillofac Surg.* 1994;32:1–2.

105. Berkowitz S. Commentary. *Cleft Palate J.* 1990;27:423–424.

106. Stellmach R. Discussion by invitation. In: Schuchardt K, ed. *Treatment of Patients with Clefts of Lip, Alveolus and Palate.* Stuttgart: Thieme; 1966.

107. Honigmann K, Prein J. Nomenklaturvorschlag zur Knochentransplantation in eine Kieferspalte. *Dtsch Z Mund Kiefer Gesichts Chir.* 1992;16:272.

108. Stellmach R. Historische Entwicklung und derzeitiger Stand der Osteoplastik bei Lippen-Kiefer-Gaumen-Spalten. *Fortschr Kiefer Gesichts Chir.* 1993;38:11–14.

109. Mühling J. Die Osteoplastik bei Lippen-Kiefer-Gaumen-Spalten und zum Lasereinsatz in der Mund-Kiefer-Gesichts-Chirurgie. *Schweiz Monatsschr Zahnmed.* 1993;103:82–84.

110. Witsenburg B. The reconstruction of anterior residual bone defects in patients with cleft lip, alveolus and palate. A review. *J Maxillofac Surg.* 1985;13:197–208.

111. Mullerova Z, Brousilova M, Jiroutova O. The use of bone grafts in orofacial clefts. *Acta Chir Plast.* 1993;35:3–4.

112. Koch J. The closure of the bony part of the cleft lip and palate malformation: the problem of primary osteoplasty. In: Hjorting-Hansen E, ed. *Proceedings from the 8th International Conference on Oral and Maxillofacial Surgery.* Chicago: Quintessence; 1985.

113. Helms JA, Speidel TM, Denis KL. Effect of timing on long-term clinical success of alveolar cleft bone grafts. *Am J Orthod Dentofac Orthop.* 1987;92:232–240.

114. Bosker H, van Dijk L. Het bottransplantaat van de mandibular voor herstel na de gnatho-palatoschisis. *Ned Tijdschr Tandheelkd.* 1980;87:383–389.

115. Koole R, Bosker H, van der Dussen FN. Late secondary autogenous bone grafting in cleft patients comparing mandibular (ectomesenchymal) and iliac crest (mesenchymal) grafts. *J Craniomaxillofac Surg (Suppl)*. 1989;17:28–30.

116. Borstlap WA, Heidbüchel KLWM, Freihofer HPM, Kuijpers-Jagtman AM. Early secondary bone grafting of alveolar cleft defects. A comparison between chin and rib grafts. *J. Craniomaxillofac Surg*. 1990;18:201–205.

117. Sindet-Pedersen S, Enmark H. Reconstruction of alveolar clefts with mandibular or iliac crest bone grafts. *J Oral Maxillofac Surg*. 1990;48:554–558.

118. Maviglio P, De Santis P, Mavilio D, Fiume D. Cranial bone graft in treatment of alveolar cleft. *Riv Ital Chir Plast*. 1990; 22:335–340.

119. Skoog T. The use of periosteal flaps in the repair of clefts of the primary palate. *Cleft Palate J*. 1965;24:332–339.

120. Rintala AE, Ranta R. Periosteal flaps and grafts in primary cleft repair: a follow-up study. *Plast Reconstr Surg*. 1989;83:17–22.

121. Smahel Z, Mullerova Z. Facial growth and development in unilateral cleft lip and palate during the period of puberty: comparison of the development after periosteoplasty and after primary bone grafting. *Cleft Palate Craniofac J*. 1994;31:106–115.

122. Stricker M, Chancholle AR, Flot F, Malka G, Montoya A. Periosteal grafting for the repair of complete primary cleft repair. *Ann Chir Plast*. 1977;22:117–125.

123. Azzolini A, Riberti C, Bertani A. Tibial periosteal graft in the repair of the primary cleft palate: preliminary report of a new technique. *Ateneo-Parmasense Acta Biomed*. 1980;51:473–480.

124. Honigmann K. Die kombinierte Segel- und Lippenplastik als neues Behandlungskonzept in der Spaltchirurgie. *Dtsch Zahn Mund Kieferheilkd*. 1983;71:600–604.

125. Honigmann K, Prein J. Die Kieferosteoplastik als Teil des operativen Gesamtkonzeptes zum LKG-Spaltenverschluss. *Fortschr Kiefer Gesichts Chir*. 1993;38:69–70.

126. Davies D. The one-stage repair of unilateral cleft lip and palate: a preliminary report. *Plast Reconstr Surg*. 1966;38:129–136.

127. Fernandes D, Davies D. The radical one-stage repair of cleft lip and palate in the neonate. Presentation at the 7th International Congress on Cleft Palate and Related Craniofacial Anomalies, Broadbeach, Australia, 1993.

128. Jones ML, Sugar AW. The late management of cleft lip and palate problems: a joint orthodontic surgical approach. *J R Coll Surg Edinb*. 1990;35:376–386.

129. Jolleys A, Robertson NR. A study of the effect of early bone grafting in complete clefts of the lip and palate. *Br J Plast Surg*. 1972;25:229–237.

130. Rosenstein S, Dado DV, Kernahan D, Griffith BH, Grasseschi M. The case for early bone grafting in cleft lip and palate: a second report. *Plast Reconstr Surg*. 1991;87:644–654.

131. Sugar AW. Orthognathic surgery. In: Jones ML, Oliver RG, eds. *Walther and Houston's Orthodontic Notes*. London: Wright (Butterworth-Heinemann Ltd.); 1994: ch 19.

132. Eales EA, Newton C, Jones ML, Sugar AW. The accuracy of computerized prediction of the soft-tissue profile: a study of 25 patients treated by the Le Fort 1 osteotomy. *Int J Adult Orthod Orthognath Surg*. 1994;9:141–152.

133. Eales EA, Jones ML, Newton C, Sugar AW. A study of the accuracy of predicted soft tissue changes produced by a computer software package (COG 3.4) in a series of patients treated by the Le Fort I osteotomy. *Br J Oral Maxillofac Surg*. 1995;33:362–369.

134. Tideman H, Stoelinga P, Gallia L. Le Fort I advancement with segmental palatal osteotomies in patients with cleft palates. *J Oral Surg*. 1980;38:196–199.

135. Posnick JC, Tompson B. Modification of the maxillary Le Fort I osteotomy in cleft-orthognathic surgery: the unilateral cleft lip and palate deformity. *J Oral Maxillofac Surg*. 1992;50:666–675.

136. Samman N, Cheung LK, Tideman H. A comparison of alveolar bone grafting with and without simultaneous maxillary osteotomies in cleft palate patients. *Int J Oral Maxillofac Surg*. 1994;23:65–70.

137. Smith AT. The use of orthodontic chain elastic for temporary intermaxillary fixation. *Br J Oral Maxillofac Surg*. 1993;31:250–251.

138. Converse JM, Shapiro HH. Treatment of developmental malformations of the jaws. *Plast Reconstr Surg*. 1952;10:473–510.

139. Wake M. Paper read to the British Association of Oral Surgeons, April 1976, Royal College of Surgeons of England, London.

140. Poole MD, Robinson PP, Nunn ME. Maxillary advancement in cleft lip and palate patients. A modification of the Le Fort I osteotomy and preliminary results. *J Maxillofac Surg*. 1986; 14:123–127.

141. James DR, Brook K. Maxillary hypoplasia in patients with cleft lip and palate deformity—the alternative surgical approach. *Eur J Orthod*. 1985;7:231–247.

142. Samuels R, Sugar AW, Jones ML, Newton C. Hard and soft tissue changes of internally fixed cleft and non-cleft Le Fort I osteotomies. In: Abstracts of the 12th Congress of the European Association for Cranio-Maxillo-Facial Surgery, The Hague, The Netherlands, September 5–10, 1994. *J Craniomaxillofac Surg*. 1994;22(suppl 1):abstract 127, 44.

143. Henderson D, Jackson IT. Naso-maxillary hypoplasia: the Le Fort II osteotomy. *Br J Oral Surg*. 1973;11:77–93.

144. Tideman H. Staged Le Fort II/Le Fort I osteotomies in cleft patients with naso-maxillary hypoplasia. Norman Rowe Lecture, Conference of British Association of Oral and Maxillofacial Surgeons, Cardiff, Wales, April 1993.

145. Llewelyn J, Sugar AW. Lag screws in sagittal split osteotomies—should they be removed? *Br J Oral Maxillofac Surg*. 1992;30:83–86.

49
Maxillary Osteotomies and Considerations for Rigid Internal Fixation

Alex M. Greenberg

As a result of basic research and clinical advances, maxillary osteotomies have been a predictable method for the management of various maxillary deformities for more than 30 years.[1] Fixation methods have undergone as much change as the development of the surgical procedures. Maxillomandibular fixation and skeletal wire fixation were the mainstay techniques in orthognathic procedures until the availability of rigid fixation in maxillofacial surgery in the 1970s. With the development and refinements of rigid internal fixation, the advantages in maxillofacial surgery continue to be the avoidance of maxillomandibular fixation, superior stabilization and positioning of segments, and the fixation of bone grafts. Rigid internal fixation offers considerable advantages with regard to postoperative airway management, feeding, and a more rapid rehabilitation of the patient.

Historically, various attempts at the movement of the maxilla have been described in the international literature for a variety of surgical indications since von Langenbeck's initial report in 1859.[2] The levels of maxillary and high midfacial osteotomies (Figure 49.1) have been named according to the fracture classification developed by Le Fort in 1901.[3–5] The history of the Le Fort I osteotomy has been well documented by Drommer.[6] In his paper, he reported that the Le Fort I osteotomy evolved from early attempts by Cheever (1867)[7] for excision of a nasopharyngeal polyp, Pincus (1907)[8] for nasopharyngeal polyp removal, and Lanz's (1893)[9] description of Kocher's earlier procedure for access to the pituitary fossa, which included splitting of the upper lip, through the early 1900s when there was an increasing number of reports related to tumor and sinus surgery.[10–15] The beginning of the correction of jaw deformities with Le Fort I level maxillary osteotomies began with Loewe (1905),[16] who described in his text the Patsch procedure (which was a modification of Kocher's method without dividing the upper lip) as a useful technique for the correction of cleft palate deformities. Loewe included descriptions of wire fixation and difficulties with the control of hemorrhage.[16]

The concept of the modern Le Fort I osteotomy did not develop until 1927, when Wassamund performed such a procedure for the correction of a midfacial deformity. Because the osteotomy did not include separation at the pterygoid plates, only limited success was achieved as a result of incomplete mobilization and elastic traction.[17] Incomplete mobilization was performed because of concerns regarding the vascular supply to the dentosseous segment. Axhausen in 1934 described the management of a maxillary fracture malunion managed with a Le Fort I osteotomy that included a paramedian splitting of the palate via a palatal flap,[18] with other similar cases reported in 1936 and 1939.[19,20] Later, in the 1940s Köle and Schuchardt introduced a two-stage procedure with the initial horizontal osteotomy followed by pterygoid plate separation and weight traction.[21] Gillies, Rowe, Converse, and Shapiro also described movement of the maxilla via a transverse palatal osteotomy along the palatine-maxillary junction.[22,23] Schmid in 1956 first described the use of a curved osteotome for the separation of the pterygoid plates.[24] Because of continued concerns related to vascular supply, maxillary osteotomies were being performed as solitary segmental procedures via pedicle flaps or tunneled flaps and later as combined anterior and posterior segmental osteotomies to avoid altering the nasal airway or nasal septum displacement.[25–27] In 1976, Hall and West described the use of combined anterior and posterior maxillary osteotomies for the treatment of maxillary alveolar hyperplasia.[28]

The modern Le Fort I osteotomy downfracture techniques (Figure 49.2) for complete mobilization and segmentalization were not possible until the work of Bell et al. Bell performed microangiography following the sacrifice of rhesus monkeys in which the microcirculation of the mucosal pedicles was demonstrated with the identification of a system for collateral circulation (Figures 49.3a–c).[29] This would have broad implications in terms of the total Le Fort I osteotomy. Bell's later work included the revascularization of the dentosseous segments following Le Fort I osteotomy and transection of the greater palatine arteries.[30] It was Bell's conclusion that, following the total Le Fort I osteotomy downfracture technique, there was a transient vascular ischemia associated with minor osteonecrosis at the osteotomy segment margins. It was concluded that an adequate vascular supply was available from the palatal, buccal, and gingival mucosa to permit

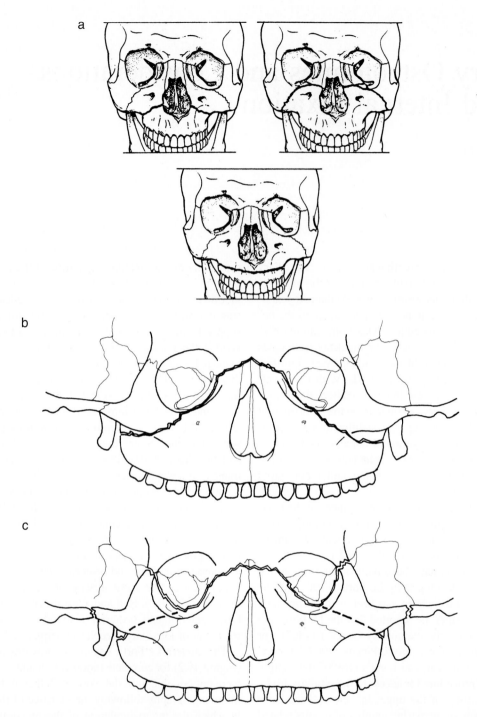

FIGURE 49.1 (a) Examples of maxillary fracture patterns at the Le Fort I levels. *Left:* separation through the piriform aperture. *Right:* separation through the zygomaticomaxillary sutures (high Le Fort I). *Bottom:* separation along the alveolar process (low Le Fort I). (b) Example of Le Fort II fracture that is a combination high Le Fort I involving the bilateral zygomaticomaxillary sutures, the complete nasal bones, and the ethmoid and lacrimal plates. (c) Example of Le Fort III fracture (complete craniofacial dysjunction) involving the bilateral zygomatic, lacrimal processes of the maxillae, nasal and ethmoid bones. (Reprinted with permission from Greenberg AM (ed) *Craniomaxillofacial Fractures: Principles of Internal Fixation Using the AO/ASIF Technique*. New York: Springer Verlag; 1993:14)

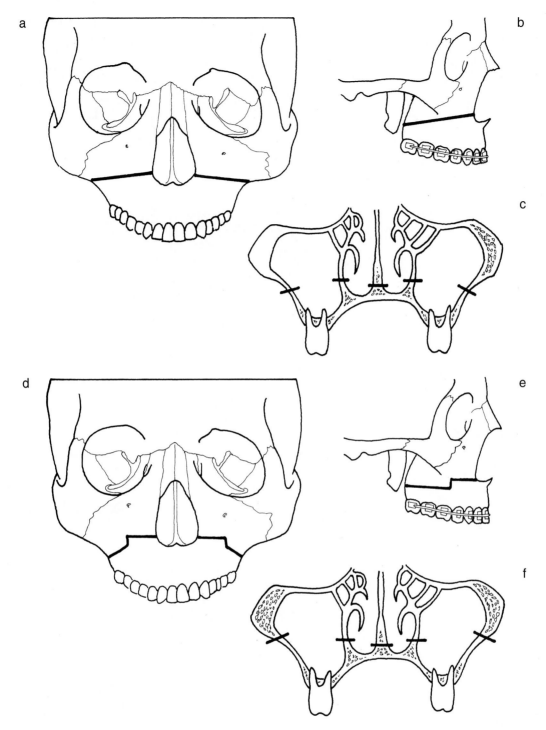

FIGURE 49.2 Various types of Le Fort I osteotomies, ranging from the standard (nonstepped), to the step Le Fort I to the stepped high Le Fort I. (a) original Le Fort I straight-line osteotomy of Bell. (b) Lateral view. (c) Coronal section view demonstrating medial and lateral antral wall and nasal septal cuts. (d) Step Le Fort I osteotomy. (e) Lateral view with superior stepping anterior to the zygomaticomaxillary buttress. (f) Coronal sectional view demonstrating medial and lateral antral wall and nasal septal cuts. (g) Stepped Le Fort I osteotomy with lateral extensions into the zygomatic body lateral to the zygomaticomaxillary sutures. (h) Lateral view demonstrating step anterior to the zygomaticomaxillary buttress. (i) Coronal sectional view demonstrating medial antral and nasal septal cuts, with lateral antral wall cuts high in the zygomatic bodies. (j) High Le Fort I osteotomy with lateral extensions into the zygomatic body lateral to the zygomaticomaxillary sutures. (k) Lateral view demonstrating lateral extensions into the zygomatic body. (l) Coronal sectional view demonstrating the medial antral wall cuts at levels superior to the described osteotomies, with lateral antral cuts high in the zygomatic bodies.

Continued.

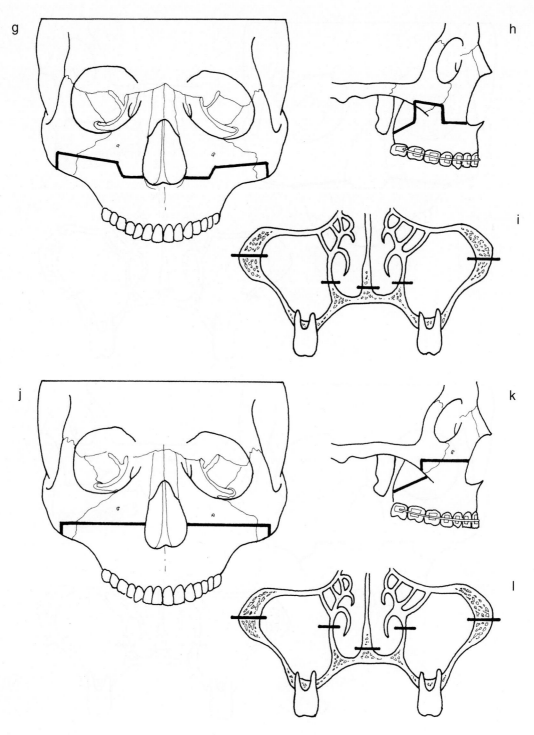

g

h

i

j

k

l

FIGURE 49.2 *Continued.*

FIGURE 49.3. (a) Schematic illustration of the various labiobuccal and palatal vascular sources supplying the inferior osteotomy segment. (Reprinted with permission from Bell WH. *Modern Practice in Orthognathic and Reconstructive Surgery.* Philadelphia: WB Saunders; 1992.) (b) Microangiogram of 1-mm coronal section of nonosteotomied control animal demonstrating normal vascular patterns: buccal (B), palatal (Pa), maxillary sinus (MS), and nasal cavity (NC) blood vessels penetrating bone and anastamosing with intramedullary blood vessels (I) and periodontal vascular plexus (Pe), molar tooth (T), turbinate (Tu), and nasal septum (NS). (Reprinted with permission from Bell WH, Proffitt WR, White RP Jr. *Surgical Correction of Dentofacial Deformities.* Vol. I. Philadelphia: WB Saunders; 1980:250,252.) (c) Microangiogram of 1-mm coronal section of operated experimental animal 1 week after Le Fort I osteotomy demonstrates increased filling of periosteal (P) vascular bed and endosteal (E) circulatory bed in the margins of the osteotomized bone. OS, osteotomy site; Pa, palate; NC, nasal cavity; M, maxilla. (Reprinted with permission from Bell WH, Proffitt WR, White RP Jr. *Surgical Correction of Dentofacial Deformities.* Vol. I. Philadelphia: WB Saunders; 1980:250,252)

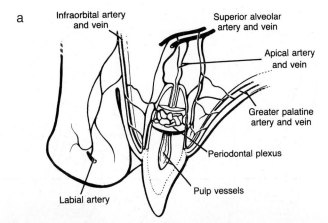

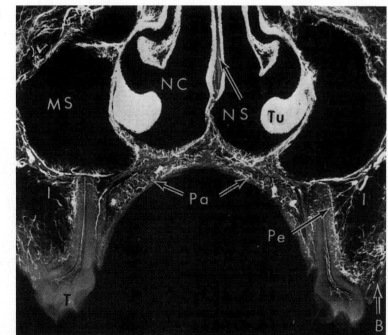

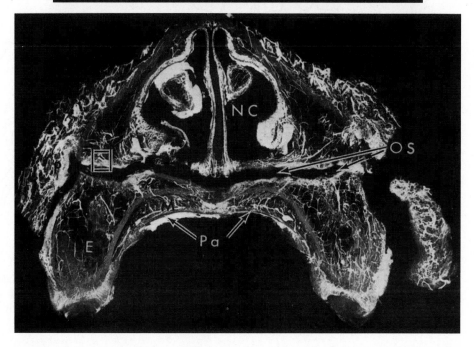

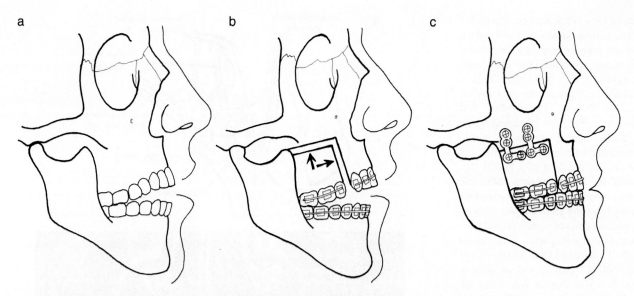

FIGURE 49.4 (a) Anterior apertognathia secondary to posterior maxillary vertical hyperplasia. (b) Posterior maxillary osteotomy between canine and first premolar. (c) Mandibular rotation with anterosuperior repositioning of the segment with closure of the anterior apertoganthia.

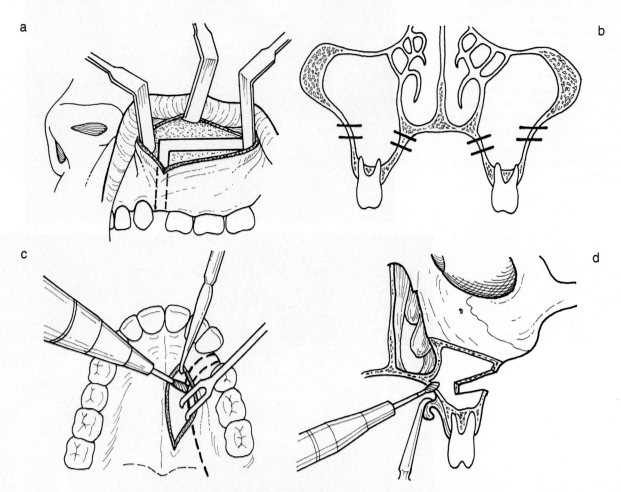

FIGURE 49.5 Schuchardt technique for posterior maxillary osteotomies. (a) Limited buccal incision with combined horizontal and anterior vertical osteotomies. (b) Coronal sectional view indicating bone cuts. (c) Limited palatal incision located medial to planned lateral palatal osteotomy. (d) Coronal view of subnasal palatal alveolar and lateral sinus wall osteotomies.

complete mobilization of the maxillary dentosseous segment. Furthermore, it was elucidated that the preservation of the palatine vessels was unnecessary to maintain viability of the mobilized maxilla.

You et al. demonstrated that in animal models there was a 50% reduction in the postoperative vascular flow, which returns to normal after 1 week and will increase by 70% above normal after the second week.[31] You et al. also performed vascular studies in human cadavers, which demonstrated that there is a centrifugal blood flow arising from the alveolar medullary arterial vascular system.[32,33] Drommer reported selective angiographic studies in 12 adult patients with cleft lip and palate before Le Fort I osteotomy that demonstrated decreased descending palatine artery caliber in 10 of 24 vessels, which was an aid in planning the degree of movement or advancement in those patients. The risks of routine angiography for routine patients could not be justified.[34]

There have been considerations over time regarding the instability of maxillary osteotomies and whether bone grafting would be indicated for routine-type movements. For example, in 1969 Obwegeser advocated bone grafting of the pterygoid plate to stabilize Le Fort I osteotomies and prevent posterior relapse,[35] which did not become generally accepted. Henderson in his text in 1985 advocated that lateral osteotomy bone grafting resulted in improved stability following Le Fort I osteotomy.[36] It could be concluded that, in response to the problems associated with wire fixation of osteotomies, the addition of bone grafts was postulated to assist in the appropriate healing and long-term stability of Le Fort I osteotomies.

Clinical studies have demonstrated that there is excellent healing of osteotomy segments, even with significant bony gaps. Frame et al. studied the effects of autogenous bone grafts on the healing of Le Fort I osteotomies in 12 adult female rhesus monkeys, and demonstrated that there were no significant differences in healing between animals with and without bone grafts.[37] Through the refinement of techniques, extensive clinical experience (e.g., Bell[1] has reported more than 2000 maxillary osteotomies performed at his institution), and basic research, the Le Fort I osteotomy downfracture technique has become a predictable procedure, with low morbidity. Today, the Le Fort I osteotomy is utilized for the management of many varieties of skeletal malocclusion involving single- or double-jaw surgery, whether as a one-piece or multiple-segmented maxilla.

Secondary bone healing has been recognized as the pathophysiologic mechanism in the management of the maxillary fracture patient and is attributed to the large periosteal surface areas in contact with the maxillary region.[38] This has been applied to the fixation of maxillary fractures, whereby direct wire, skeletal suspension, and occlusal stents have been the mainstay of techniques. With the advent of rigid internal fixation and the understanding of the effects of absolute stability of bone segments in fracture healing,[38,39] the same techniques were then applied to maxillary os-

teotomies.[40] In the early phases of healing it appears, on a short-term basis, that with rigid internal fixation there is superior stabilization of segments with rapid healing because the functional aspects of strain on the new ingrowth of tissues are avoided. With wire fixation, the maxilla will continue to have mobility until fixation is released, and under the functional loading of masticatory forces, swallowing, and speech, callus ossification will begin. Internal fixation has permitted many new developments and refinements in the Le Fort I osteotomy techniques.

With the same type of research, improvements in the performance of segmental osteotomies also occurred. In this manner surgeons have the availability of numerous options regarding the performance of maxillary segmental surgery, whether it is as a multisegmented total Le Fort I osteotomy or a single segment. Schuchardt in 1959 first reported posterior segmental osteotomies in which bilateral posterior segmental osteotomies in two stages were employed as a method for the treatment of anterior open-bite deformities[41] (Figures 49.4a–c). Today, the Schuchardt procedure is performed in a single stage via combined buccal and parasagittal palatal incisions (Figures 49.5a–d). Kufner described a posterior segmental maxillary osteotomy via a single buccal incision with combined buccal and palatal osteotomies (Figures 49.6a,b).[42] Perko[43] and Bell[44] have also described techniques for combined buccal and palatal incisions for the performance of posterior maxillary segmental osteotomies for the management of transverse maxillary hyperplasia in low palatal vaults (Figures 49.7a–c). Trimble et al.[45] have also reported posterior maxillary segmental ostetomies. There are also numerous reports related to the management of segments in cleft palate patients, for whom it was not until the early 1980s, such as in the work of Tideman et al.,[46] Poole et al.,[47] and Stoelinga et al.,[48] that segmental osteotomy design could be predictably and safely performed.

There have been many reports regarding anterior maxillary segmental osteotomies, which are indicated for the management of anterior maxillary hyperplasia as either an isolated procedure, usually with the bilateral removal of first premolars (Figures 49.8a–c), or combined with an anterior mandibular segmental osteotomy for the treatment of bimaxillary protrusion. The first anterior segmental maxillary osteotomy was performed by Cohn-Stock in 1921.[49] Wassmund[50] reported in 1935 a type of anterior segmental osteotomy based on both buccally and palatally based flaps (Figures 49.9a–e).[50] Wunderer technique involves a buccally based pedicled dentosseous flap (Figures 49.10a–c).[51] A palatally based and transverse buccal pedicle downfracture technique was advocated by Cupar[52] in 1955 (Figures 49.11a,b).

Maxillary osteotomies have not been without significant complications for many patients who have undergone these procedures. Many earlier reports in the literature have described these complications, which included loss of teeth, bone, bone segments, and even entire maxillae. Several factors

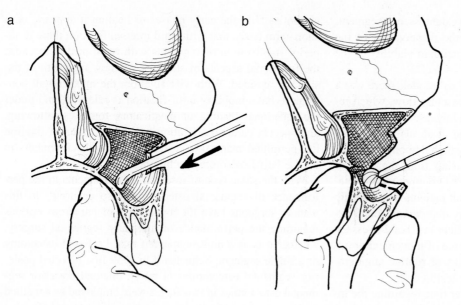

FIGURE 49.6 Kufner technique for posterior maxillary osteotomies. (a) Coronal sectional view of transantral palatal osteotomy via chisel following lateral sinus wall osteotomy. (b) Coronal view of transantral palatal osteotomy trimming of bone segment.

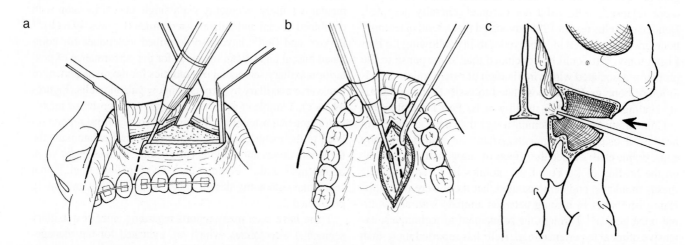

FIGURE 49.7 Perko–Bell technique for posterior maxillary osteotomies. (a) Limited buccal incision with combined horizontal and vertical osteotomies. (b) Limited palatal incision located medial to planned lateral palatal osteotomy. (c) Coronal sectional view indicating bone cuts with transantral medial nasal wall osteotomy.

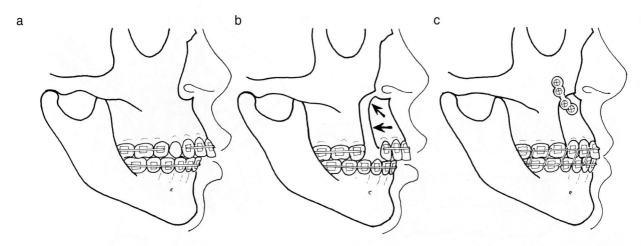

FIGURE 49.8 Anterior maxillary segmental osteotomy. (a) Lateral profile view demonstrating class II skeletal malocclusion secondary to anterior horizontal maxillary hyperplasia with normal mandible. (b) Removal of first premolars with ostectomies through the tooth sockets extending through the piriform rim. (c) Retropositioned anterior maxillary segment into planned surgical stent with miniplate fixation at the piriform rim.

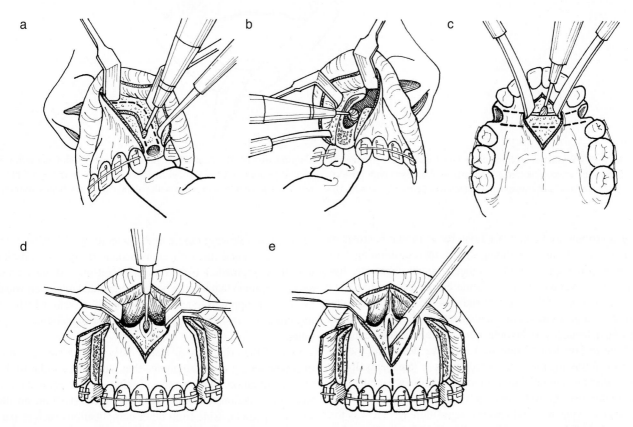

FIGURE 49.9 Wassmund technique for labial and palatal pedicle-based anterior maxillary segmental osteotomy. (a) Creation of ostectomy through tooth sockets following removal of first premolars with vertical incision distal to canine. (b) Extension of ostectomy through the labial aspect along the palate. (c) Midline palatal incision to permit completion of the palatal ostectomy. (d) Midline labial incision with interdental osteotomy between central incisors, incomplete to the alveolar crest. (e) Completion of midline osteotomy through the alveolar crest via osteotome.

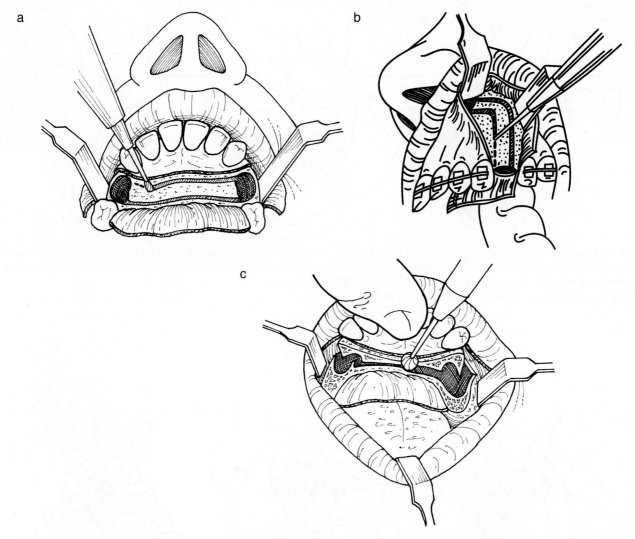

FIGURE 49.10 Wunderer technique for labial pedicle-based anterior maxillary segmental osteotomy. (a) Horizontal incision with posteriorly reflected flap and transpalatal ostectomy being performed. (b) Continuation of ostectomy through tooth sockets following removal of first premolars with vertical incision distal to canine. (c) Anteriorly retracted dentosseous flap with palatal ostectomy bone trimming.

may contribute to the increased risk for avascular necrosis in Le Fort I osteotomies, including significant repositioning, soft tissue flap design, multiple segments, small segments, hypotension, severance of the palatine blood vessels, and tears and perforations of the mucosal pedicles. These complications can also range from simple devitalization of a tooth to periodontal defects, loss of alveolar bone, tooth loss, segment loss, and entire jaw loss. Lanigan et al. have described aseptic necrosis following maxillary osteotomies in 36 patients. It was found that this complication occurred mainly in patients who had undergone multiple segment Le Fort I osteotomies with transverse expansion and superior repositioning.[53] It was the conclusion of Lanigan et al. that ligation of palatal arteries, horizontal palatal mucosa tears, and buccal pedicle compression were the main causes of segment necrosis and dentosseous segment morbidity. Nelson et al. have studied complications through the use of microsphere quantitation of blood flow following the Le Fort I osteotomy.[54] Nelson et al. have also studied three different pedicle designs in anterior maxillary segmental osteotomies.[54] Nelson's studies have also determined that it is the buccal and palatal mucoperiosteal pedicles, as opposed to any specific blood vessels, which are the principal vascular supply to the anterior maxillary segment.

One of the criticisms of Bell's early studies was the lack of repositioning of the segments that would be similar to the clinical situation. During repositioning of the segments in a superior direction, this may have the greatest strain on the vascular pedicle, aside from other complications such as partial or complete transection of the pedicles. The quantification studies of Nelson have shown that there is excellent maintenance of blood flow, except to the areas of the alveolar bone and attached gingiva. These are areas usually supplied by the superior alveolar arteries, and it would appear there is a short-

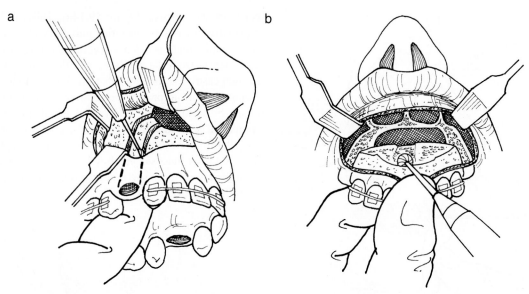

FIGURE 49.11 Cupar technique for palatal and transverse buccal pedicle-based anterior maxillary osteotomy downfracture technique. (a) Vertical ostectomy through tooth sockets to the piriform rim. (b) Following completion of the osteteomies through the transverse labial vestibular incision, downfracture of the anterior segment is performed with direct access to complete the ostectomy and bone trimming of the segment.

term intraosseous ischemia that has a minimal effect upon the rapid healing which is clinically noted. However, these animal studies do not appear to take into account the effects of stretching vascular pedicles during certain types of movements of the maxillary segments. Meyer and Cavanaugh[55] have demonstrated that tooth vitality may be an important and sensitive indicator in the diagnosis of aseptic bony necrosis at an early stage. Electrical pulp testing would not be a test for tooth vitality in osteotomy patients because the branches of the trigeminal nerve have been cut. It is of course also a very important aspect of these procedures that root apices not be severed or injured. Perhaps one of the helpful aspects of internal fixation is the requirement for more superior osteotomy cuts to provide adequate bone for fixation, which helps to avoid direct root apex damage. At the same time the placement of screws requires care to avoid this potential complication. Superior osteotomy cuts may also reduce telescoping effects as the result of better bone contact.

Treatment planning for the management of maxillary deformities should include workups for physical examination of the patient based on facial measurements and proportions, cephalometric analysis, and the evaluation of study casts. Various methodologies for cephalometric analysis are available today, which include the use of computer software programs. Various anatomic articulators are also available for the mounting of these cases. Patients can even have a hinge axis analysis. Luhr and Kubein-Meesenburg[56] have described the use of intraoperative control of condylar position as a presurgical determination that can then be utilized with the patient under general anesthesia while the maxilla is manipulated into final position, which has implications for rigid fixation. Most authors do not advocate special devices, other than care with manual manipulation. This of course becomes a problem for patients with condylar deformities or internal derangements in whom manipulation would be difficult and inaccurate for rigid internal fixation. For further information regarding the presurgical evaluation, see Chapters 2, 4, 23, and 46.

Surgical Technique

Le Fort I Osteotomy

The Le Fort I osteotomy is performed under general anesthesia in the operating room, with special requirements for the availability of hypotensive anesthesia to reduce blood loss, blood for transfusion (which is routinely available today at many centers in elective cases as an autologous donation), and special instrument sets.[1] The patient is brought into the operating room and after induction of general anesthesia, prepared and draped with special requirements as per the surgeon. The administration of antibiotics and steroids is dependent upon the preferences of the surgeon and anesthesiologist. External reference marks are preferred by many surgeons, with a marker placed at nasion in the form of K wires, screws, or pin (Figure 49.12).[1] The throat should be packed, and care should taken to orient the incision so as to provide an adequate buccal pedicle to ensure an ample vascular supply. When adequate attached gingiva are present this should be as a minimum of 5 mm superior to the junction of the attached and free mucosa. Local anesthesia with epinephrine 1:100,000 should be generously injected with a minimum of 15 min before the incision to permit hemostasis.

The incision can be created with either a #15 scalpel blade

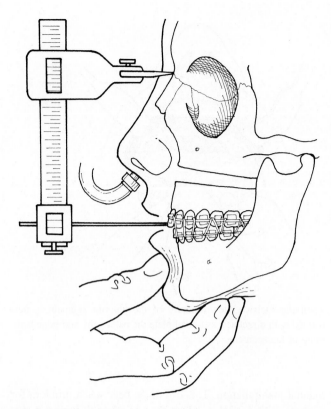

FIGURE 49.12 Example of externally based reference mark utilizing a K wire placed at the nasofrontal suture (nasion) with a measuring device that attaches to it and reference mark on the maxillary appliance.

or a needle bovey, and carried through periosteum to bone, extending from first molar to first molar, so as to leave an adequate posteriorly based buccal pedicle (Figure 49.13). Utilizing a periosteal elevator, the mucoperiosteal flap should be reflected to the level of the pterygoid plates, with care not to

perforate the mucosa (Figure 49.14a). This can be difficult, especially in cases of posterior maxillary alveolar hyperplasia in which there is often a severe curvature of the alveolus as it merges from the junction, with thinning of this mucosa. In such cases, the tissue needs to be elevated judiciously and gradually so as to prevent perforation. At this time exposure of the bilateral anterior and lateral maxillary sinus walls is completed with identification of the piriform foramen (Figure 19.14b). Local anesthesia may be injected directly into the nasal floor mucosa, which will dissect the periosteum free from the nasal floor. The nasal floor mucosa is then elevated from the nasal floor.

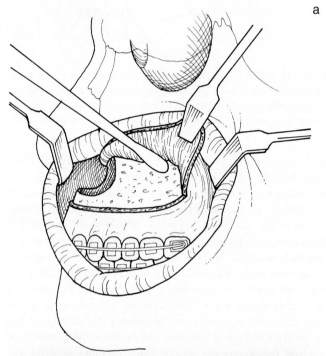

a

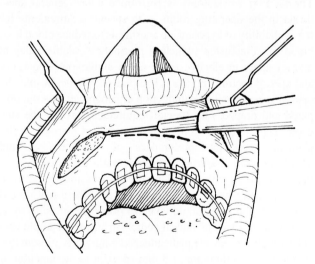

FIGURE 49.13 Example of retracted upper lip with exposure of labial vestibule for an incision to be placed at a minimum of 10 mm superior to the attached gingiva from first molar to first molar. Here a needle bovey is utilized to create the incision.

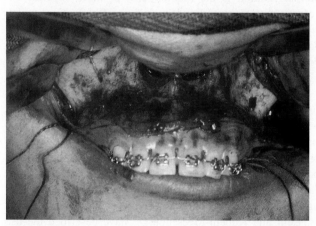

b

FIGURE 49.14 (a) Reflection of the mucoperiosteal flap so as to expose the bilateral piriform rims, lateral maxillary sinus wall, and extension of the subperiosteal dissection to the level of the pterygoid plates. (b) Clinical example of surgical exposure of the maxillary anterior and lateral sinus walls.

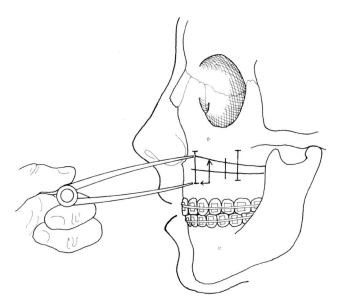

FIGURE 49.15 External reference marks made at the piriform rim and zygomatic buttress should permit adequate space for ostectomy.

It is often the custom of surgeons to place internal reference lines along the anterior maxillary sinus walls in the regions of the piriform rim and zygomatic buttresses, although these are considered to be less accurate in superior repositioning than external reference marks (Figure 49.15). At this time, utilizing a reciprocating saw, an osteotomy is created beginning at the zygomaticomaxillary buttress and oriented toward the piriform rim (Figure 49.16). Depending on the type of correction to be performed, considerations are needed as to a straight osteotomy or wedge ostectomy. There are several good techniques for performing bone trimming for the type of movement to be made. Some surgeons advocate precise removal of wedges (Figures 49.17a,b), others advocate

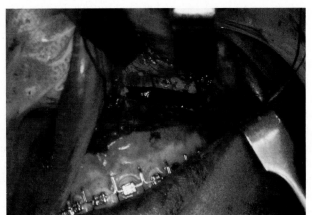

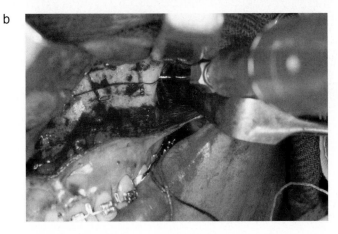

FIGURE 49.16 (a) Use of a reciprocating saw to create an osteotomy through the lateral sinus wall extending to the piriform rim. (b) Use of the reciprocating saw to complete the lateral sinus wall cut to the level of the pterygoid plate.

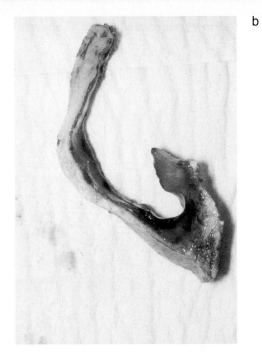

FIGURE 49.17 (a) Maxillary ostectomy with complete wedge removal before completion of pterygoid separation. (b) Example of removed complete bone wedge with intact lateral and medial sinus walls.

a

b

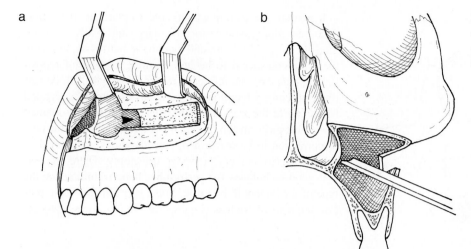

FIGURE 49.18 (a) Safeguarded nasal septal chisel is used to cut the medial sinus wall (arrow). (b) Coronal sectional view of medial sinus wall cut.

trimming after the jaws are placed in intermaxillary fixation with seating of the jaw until satisfactory placement.

Presently, as compared to the original Le Fort I osteotomy, the horizontal bone cut should be performed so as to permit adequate bone superior to the root apices and allow room for the placement of screws. This also has implications in terms of the high Le Fort I[57] and quadrangular osteotomy.[58] Indeed, there has been an evolution in the development of the osteotomy lines for Le Fort I osteotomy, including the step osteotomy,[59] which provides superior bone interfaces for healing (see Figures 49.2d–f). The medial antral walls are then fractured with safeguarded nasal chisels [Figures 49.18(a,b)],

and the nasal septum is separated from the nasal floor with a double-guarded nasal septal chisel (Figure 49.19). At this time the pterygoid plates are separated from the maxilla (Figure 49.20), and the maxilla can then be downfractured with digital pressure or with broad osteotomes. Before the downfracture, hypotensive anesthesia should be obtained with a mean pressure about 50 mmHg.[60] Extensive hemorrhage can be encountered at this stage, and the surgeon must be prepared to control bleeding. Complete mobilization of the maxilla needs to be attained, which should include manipulation not only in a superoinferior direction but also in a lateral to lateral direction. The dissection of the nasal floor mucosa should be

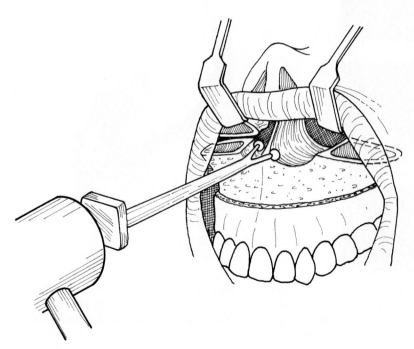

FIGURE 49.19 Separation of nasal septum from the palate via a double-sided safeguarded nasal septal chisel.

FIGURE 49.20 Separation of the pterygoid plate from the posterior sinus wall with a curved osteotome and a finger placed on the palatal mucosa to prevent perforation and tearing.

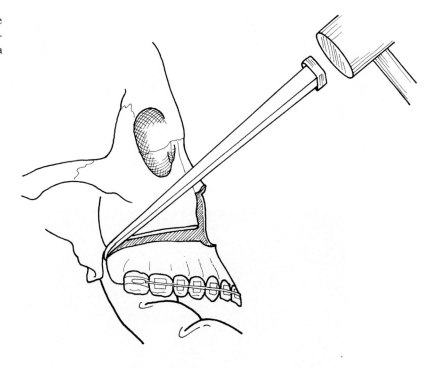

completed. The downfracture of the maxilla is then complete, with the dentosseous segment pedicled only to the mucoperiosteal flaps (Figure 49.21). Segmentalization of the downfractured maxilla can then proceed, depending on the type of correction necessary, with two, three, or four sections created safely.

There is the increased chance for loss of segments with increase in the number of segments created. It is best to begin with anterior segmentation because of the thickness of the anterior palate and interdental osteotomies (Figure 49.22a). Bell[1] has advocated the individualization of osteotomies when segmentalization is performed, so as to reduce the possibilities of complications by ensuring the best possible vascular supply. This is achieved by altering the bone cuts in a way to maximize the soft tissue pedicle. For example, rather than using the typical chevron type of anterior maxillary osteotomy, it is possible to prepare a larger anteroposterior bone segment, and thus allow for a larger surface of palatal mucosa attachment and a better vascular supply (Figure 49.22a). This has an effect on the requirements of internal fixation by creating larger anterior segments, which require more precise geometric bone trimming and fitting. Precise orientation can be achieved, with the exact maintenance of the desired position of anterior maxillary segments through the use of rigid internal fixation. In the case of posterior segmentalization, this proceeds easily because of the ease in cutting through the nasal floor from an anteroposterior direction (Figures 49.22b–d). It is helpful to keep a finger on the palate while creating interdental osteotomies during segmentalization because this will help to avoid perforation of the palatal mu-

cosa. The midline osteotomies should be within the nasal floor, and not within the sinus floor (Figure 49.22e). Upon completion of the maxillary osteotomy and segmentalization, the surgical stent should be placed and wired to the orthodontic appliances. If combined maxillary and mandibular osteotomies are being performed, an intermediate stent is often utilized as well.

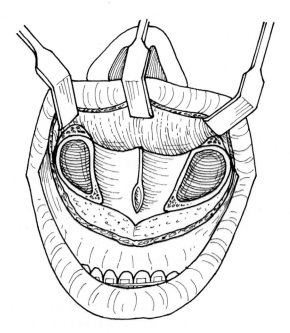

FIGURE 49.21 Downfractured and completely mobilized maxilla pedicled to mucoperiosteum.

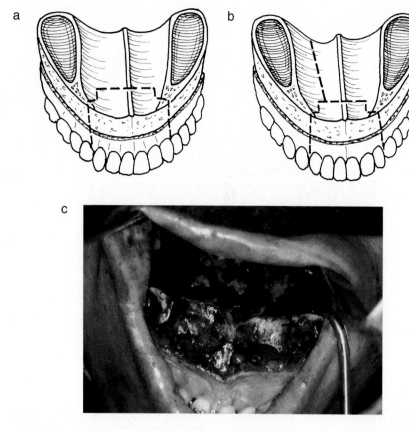

FIGURE 49.22 Maxillary segmentalization techniques. (a) Anterior maxillary segmental osteotomy with nasal floor extension to increase mucoperiosteal attachment and vascular supply. (Adapted from Bell WH. *Modern Practice in Orthognathic and Reconstructive Surgery.* Philadelphia: WB Saunders; 1992.) (b) Three-piece segmental maxillary osteotomy technique with combined anterior and midline segmentalization. (Adapted from Bell WH. *Modern Practice in Orthognathic and Reconstructive Surgery.* Philadelphia: WB Saunders; 1992.) (c) Example of downfractured three-piece segmented maxilla with paramidline osteotomy within the nasal floor, lateral to the bony nasal septum. Note higher osteotomy level to better permit bone plating. (d) Four-piece segmental maxillary osteotomy technique with bilateral paramidline combined with anterior segmentalization. (Adapted from Bell WH. *Modern Practice in Orthognathic and Reconstructive Surgery.* Philadelphia: WB Saunders; 1992.) (e) Midline maxillary osteotomy through nasal floor paramidline. (Adapted from Bell WH. *Modern Practice in Orthognathic and Reconstructive Surgery.* Philadelphia: WB Saunders; 1992)

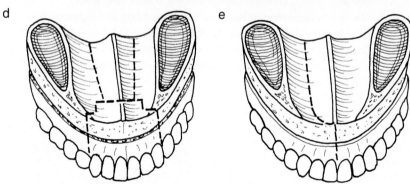

At this time the maxilla needs to be mobilized into maxillomandibular fixation; depending on the type of movement, bone trimming or bone grafting and the application of internal fixation will then proceed. When performing surgery in the maxilla, positioning of the segment(s) depends on preplanned bone trimming and the ability to manipulate the mandible as an anatomic guide. Maxillary repositioning may involve movements in superior, inferior, differential, asymmetric, anterior, and posterior directions. Anterior and inferior movements are the least difficult. Regardless, caution must be exercised so as to adequately trim bone, as a false position can be obtained in spite of proper condylar seating (Figures 49.23 and 49.24). Careful attention must be paid to the manner in which manipulation of the mandible is performed because of mandibular instability under anesthesia with the patient's head rotated backward. It can be easy to falsely position the condyles in the fossae, resulting in an inadequately positioned maxilla despite proper bone trimming (Figure 49.25). It is undesirable to perform positioning of the maxilla in maxillomandibular fixation by forcing the mandibular condyles into a posteriorly retruded position simply by placing force at the chin. An unacceptable occlusion may result, which is regretted later when the patient is awake. With bivector seating of the condyles with downward pressure at the chin and upward pressure at the angles, a more reliable and accurate position can be obtained (Figure 49.26).

It is important for the clinician to recognize that there are two central issues related to this technique. Either there is a

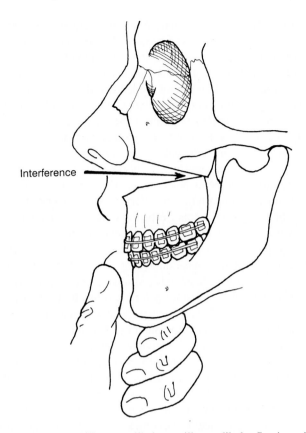

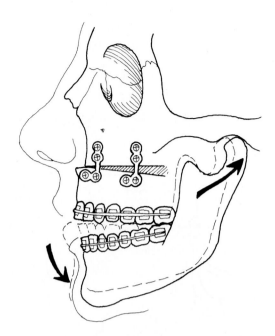

FIGURE 49.25 Inadequate seating with maxilla placed too forward despite proper bone trimming because of improper condylar positioning during fixation, with immediate relapse following appropriate condylar seating.

FIGURE 49.23 Mobilized maxilla in maxillomandibular fixation with manual manipulation demonstrating posterior bony interferences preventing desired positioning.

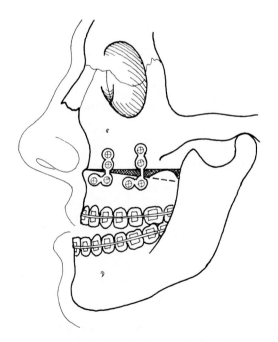

FIGURE 49.24 Incomplete posterior bone trimming with unsatisfactory maxillary positoning and resultant posterior occlusal premature contacts.

problem with correct mandibular manipulation and positioning of the maxilla relative to the condyle–fossa relationship, or there has been inadequate bone trimming in the posterior antral wall, tuberosity, and medial antral wall regions, and the horizontal plate of the palatine bone (especially the posterior medial antral wall as it overlies the greater palatine artery) (Figure 49.27), or combinations of these.[61,62] Bone trimming of segments often is performed with the patient placed in maxillomandibular fixation, using repeated attempts at correct maxillary positioning against the intact superior osteotomy margins. When the maxilla is retracted again inferiorly, this will permit further bone trimming of the antral walls, and nasal septal adjustment, with either osteoplasty of the palatal bony septum (Figure 49.28) or excision of inferior nasal septal cartilage. This cartilage should be saved as it may be used as a nasal graft, especially as a shield graft, or for dorsal nasal augmentation when simultaneous rhinoplasty is performed.

These procedures can be extremely difficult in the adult temporomandibular disorder patient, which usually requires occlusal splint therapy for a minimum of 6 months to reduce cartilaginous and ligamental instability. Some of these patients may not be candidates for rigid fixation and should undergo traditional wire suspension to achieve correct occlusion and with settling of the maxilla relative to the mandible.

It is the management of posterior maxillary hyperplasia and asymmetric and segmental movements that poses the greatest difficulties. Especially in patients with posterior maxillary hyperplasia with anterior apertognathia, a false position can be obtained because of hinging at the posterior maxillary

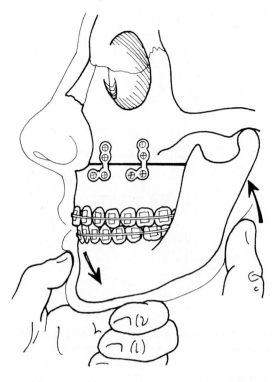

FIGURE 49.26 Appropriately positioned maxilla through proper bone trimming and bimanual mandibular positioning with downward and posterior pressure on chin and upward forward pressure on the ramus.

tuberosity and posteromedial antral wall regions until adequate bone removal has been attained. This becomes critically important in the posterior impaction of the maxilla where seating of the mandible, combined with extensive bone trimming in the tuberosity and posterior medial antral walls, leads to a satisfactory position for bone plating. It is critically important in these situations to achieve the adequate removal of bony interferences that can create premature contacts. Therefore, overreduction in the buttress and tuberosity regions will permit the adequate repositioning of the maxilla to allow correct maxillomandibular positioning, with particular care directed toward the posterior maxillary region at the horizontal plate of the palatine bone, especially the posterior medial antral wall as it overlies the greater palatine artery.

Posterior movements of the maxilla can be performed with alteration of the transverse dimension. This has proven over time to be one of the least stable of movements, especially in the management of anterior open bite. It has been suggested by various authors that a variety of techniques can applied to try to improve the long-term stability of widened maxillary dimensions.[63] These have included internal fixation, bone grafting of the palatal osteotomy sites, and soft tissue releases to improve the mobilization of the segments and reduce soft tissue tension.[58]

Posterosuperior movements result in problems related to the telescoping of segments, which was a greater problem with skeletal wire fixation. Maxillary osteotomies that undergo superior repositioning have the bony segments dis-

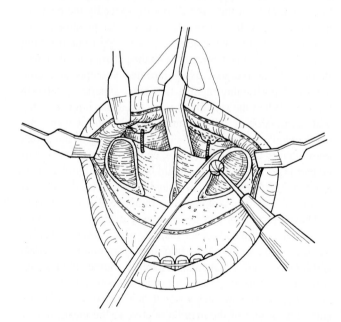

FIGURE 49.27 Bone trimming of the posterior maxillary sinus wall and posterior medial sinus wall, with periosteal elevator in use to protect the greater palatine arteries.

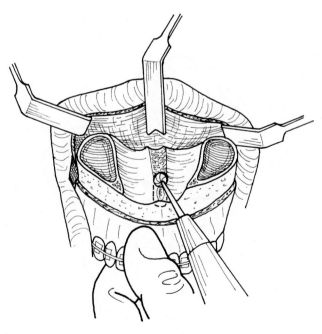

FIGURE 49.28 Bone trimming of the remaining medial and lateral sinus walls, nasal septum, and piriform rims.

placed into the nasal and sinus cavities. These have been difficult to manage with wire fixation because of the lack of bone contact and the dependence on callus formation for the ultimate stabilization of these segments. Changes in osteotomy design such as the stepped and quadrangular osteotomies have improved this situation greatly. Rigid fixation also permits the immediate stabilization of these osteotomies with the avoidance of dependence on callus formation for the stabilization of these segments. Bone grafting is also a more predictable procedure with internal fixation and may be indicated in these movements to improve healing and long-term stability. Bone may be obtained from autogenous sites such as the ilium, calvarium, tibia, maxilla, or mandible.[64–67] Allografts from tissue banks or synthetic materials may also be used. Corticocancellous struts can be used as onlays and in conjunction with lag screw techniques in the place of miniplates (Figure 49.29). This is commonly employed in the management of cleft maxillary Le Fort I osteotomies, as struts across the alveolar cleft defect in addition to the cancellous bone graft (Figure 49.30). Aside from improving the stabilization of the defects, such grafts increase the bone volume for later dental implant placement and improved nasal columella and alar support.

Once the bone trimming is completed and the surgeon is satisfied with the position of the maxilla based on his presurgical workup and choice of internal or external reference points as they pertain to the establishment of the lip-to-tooth relationship, the application of internal fixation may proceed. With the development of hardware specifically sized for midfacial stabilization, internal fixation of maxillary osteotomies has become a routine technique. Hardware systems available for fixation include the 1.3-mm, 1.5-mm, and 2.0-mm craniofacial system miniplates in a variety of straight, Y, and L shapes (Figure 49.31). The advantage of the Y- and L-shaped plates (Figure 49.32) is that they can be used along the su-

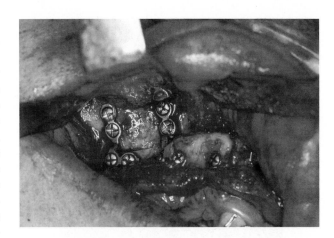

FIGURE 49.30 Onlay bone grafting bridging a unilateral alveolar cleft in a two-piece Le Fort I osteotomy with miniplate fixation at the piriform rim and buttesses.

perior margin of the downfractured maxilla (Figure 49.33) to avoid damaging tooth roots. The microsystem 1.0-mm plates have limited indication for segmental osteotomies, unfavorable antral wall osteotomy fractures, and small bone grafts.

Maxillary osteotomy rigid fixation is a demanding procedure, and special care must be taken to place the segments in their correct position. This requires proper bone trimming and jaw positioning as described (Figure 49.34). The correct application of the hardware generally begins with the placement of plates at the buttresses, which maintains the vertical dimension, followed by the piriform rim (Figures 49.35–49.37). Manual support of the maxillomandibular complex is still required while plating the piriform rim to maintain the desired maxillary position. If the piriform rim plates were placed first, this would permit slippage of the posterior position inferiorly

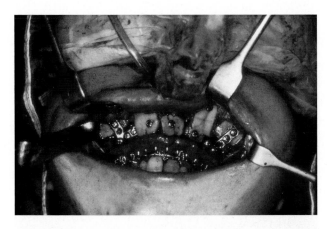

FIGURE 49.29 Le Fort I osteotomy with miniplate at the bilateral buttresses and onlay grafts at the bilateral piriform rims and anterior nasal spine.

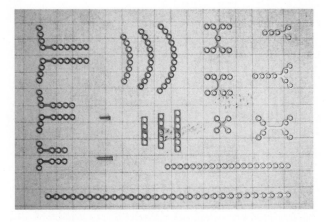

FIGURE 49.31 Selection of craniofacial system miniplates. (Courtesy of Synthes Maxillofacial, Paoli, PA, USA)

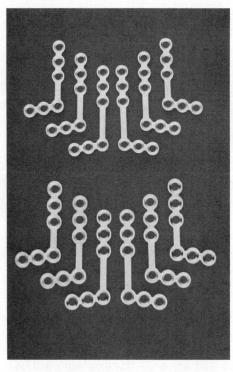

FIGURE 49.32 Examples of 1.5-mm and 2.0-mm L-shape miniplates from the orthognathic system.

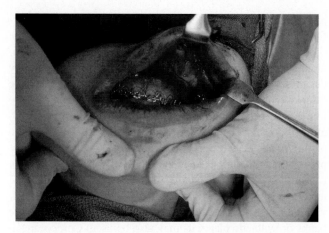

FIGURE 49.34 Bivector seating of the maxillomandibular complex with precise fit of trimmed osteotomy site following ostectomy for the management of posterior maxillary hyperplasia with anterior open bite.

and an anterior open bite postoperatively. If the plates are placed unilaterally in the buttress and piriform regions first, this may cause an asymmetric positioning, which is usually seen as telescoping superiorly on the contralateral side. When segmentation is performed, the buttress plate should still be placed first, which often facilitates positioning of the anterior segment. Following the completion of internal fixation and any bone grafting, the wound is irrigated and closed with continuous resorbable sutures, with many surgeons preferring V to Y closure of the midline.[68–70]

Maxillary anterior and posterior segmental osteotomies are performed for a variety of situations, either isolated or in combination. Rigid fixation has made these procedures extremely stable with fewer complications. Patient comfort is achieved with the earlier removal of stents and reliance on fixed orthodontic appliances.

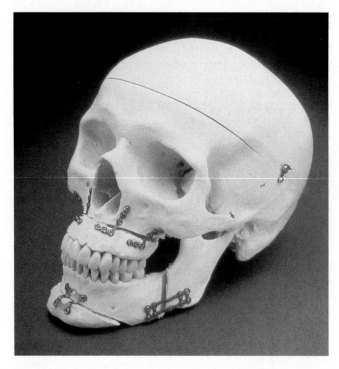

FIGURE 49.33 L-shaped miniplates along the osteotomy of a skull model.

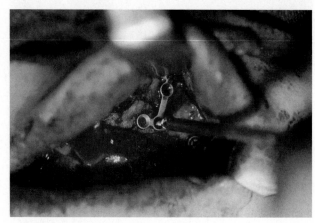

FIGURE 49.35 Following initial placement of a miniplate at the buttress, a miniplate is applied to the piriform rim.

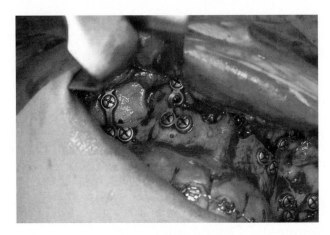

FIGURE 49.36 L-shaped miniplates at the bilateral buttresses and piriform rims.

Anterior Maxillary Segmental Osteotomies

Various methods have been described concerning approaches for the performance of anterior maxillary osteotomies. These include the Wassmund (Figure 49.9), Wunderer (Figure 49.10), and Cupar (Figure 49.11), each distinguished by the types of incisions and surgical access. Osseous segment design is essentially the same among these various surgical approaches, with preferences based on the choice of the surgeon and his experience. Incisions may also play a role in these procedures, based on access to sites that may have rigid fixation applied. Anterior maxillary osteotomies may be bodily moved posteriorly without tipping, or may have tipping movements with rotations. Movements have generally been in the posterior direction. There are limitations reported regarding the management of deep overbites with this technique.[71]

For example, anterior maxillary segmental osteotomies are commonly performed for the patient with class II skeletal an-

terior maxillary horizontal hyperplasia (Figures 49.8a–c). Typically these patients are managed via the removal of the bilateral first premolars when edentulous spaces are not pre-existing. The movement of these segments is in a tipping type of direction posteriorly following the shape of the extraction sockets, which may incorporate some degree of bodily movement. When two planes of occlusion are present, this may require an inferior or superior positioning as well. Sometimes leveling of the occlusal plane may require a total Le Fort I segmental osteotomy to "split the difference" and avoid both excessive movement of a segment and tension on the mucoperiosteal pedicle, with the inherent increased risk of necrosis and tissue loss. Anterior maxillary segmental osteotomies are also indicated for use in patients with bimaxillary protrusion, often in conjunction with an anterior mandibular segmental osteotomy or bilateral mandibular ramus osteotomies (Figures 49.38 and 49.39).

Surgical Technique

The maxillary anterior segmental osteotomy is performed under general anesthesia in the operating room, with special requirements for the availability of hypotensive anesthesia to reduce blood loss, blood for transfusion, and special instrument sets. The patient is brought into the operating room and after induction of general anesthesia, prepared and draped with special requirements as per the surgeon. The administration of antibiotics and steroids is dependent upon the preferences of the surgeon and anesthesiologist.

It is the author's preference to utilize bilateral buccal vertical incisions overlying the distal aspect of the first premolar extending through the interdental papilla to provide a

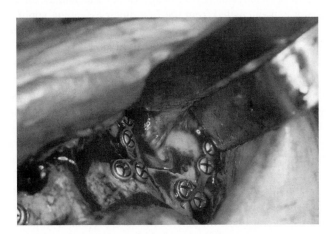

FIGURE 49.37 Close-up view of L-shaped miniplates at the buttress and piriform rim.

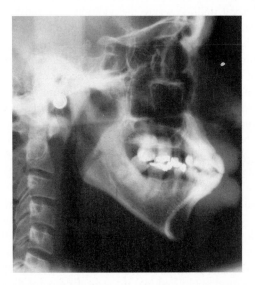

FIGURE 49.38 Preoperative lateral cephalometric radiograph of bimaxillary protrusion.

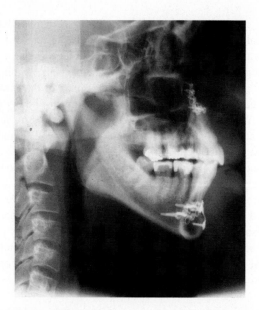

FIGURE 49.39 Postoperative lateral cephalometric radiograph of combined anterior maxillary and mandibular segmental osteotomies with removal of four first premolars and miniplate fixation after completion of orthodontic treatment.

broader pedicle to the anterior segment following Wunderer (Figure 49.9a), without trimming of this flap as it will shrink during healing. Mucoperisoteal flaps are then reflected anteriorly to expose the planned ostectomy site. If the first premolar teeth are still present they should be removed, and preplanned ostectomies are performed via a high-speed bur or reciprocating saw (see Figures 49.8b and 49.9b). Usually the shape of the ostectomies will follow the shape of the tooth socket. Presurgical orthodontics can influence the orientation of the tooth and its socket, as well as the alignment of the dentition of the anterior segment. Attention is then turned to the buccal midline where the addition of a midline vertical incision is created (with preservation of the interdental gingiva between the central incisors) for disengaging the nasal septum from the premaxilla and to provide access for additional nasal floor osteoplasty, and if necessary a midline interdental osteotomy is performed (see Figures 49.9d,e).

Attention is then directed to the palatal mucosa where a midline incision is created (with preservation of the interdental gingiva between the central incisors) to provide access to complete the transverse palatal osteotomy (Figure 49.9c). In this way broad mucosal pedicles are maintained with preservation of the vascular supply. Multiple maxillary segments may be mobilized into a variety of positions for widening in a transverse dimension, anteroposterior shortening with extractions, and leveling of occlusal planes (generally with a differential impaction). The segments are typically moved into a splint fabricated from simulated models. Once the anterior segment is satisfactorily mobilized into the stent, fixation of the segment is performed (Figure 49.8c). Rigid fixation of the segments also permits the wedging of bone grafts into the osteotomy sites, which can then be malletted into position. In performing the

initial osteotomy, it is desirable to leave a minimum of 5 mm of bone superior to the canine bilaterally. In this way damage to the root apices while placing the screws can be avoided. L-shaped plates are particularly advantageous as they run vertically superior to the osteotomy along the piriform rim and horizontally inferior to the osteotomy. Y-shaped plates provide similar fixation. When the anterior segment is divided, a single microplate can be placed across the midline osteotomy site. After the completion of fixation, the wounds are irrigated and closed with resorbable sutures.

Posterior Maxillary Segmental Osteotomies

Posterior maxillary osteotomies are generally performed for either vertical, transverse, or anteroposterior movements. Various techniques are possible depending on the morphology of the posterior palate as either a high vault with alveolar hyperplasia, or a low vault with a transverse arch deformity. The Kufner, Schuchardt, and Perko–Bell techniques permit approaches to these many problems.

Surgical Technique

The posterior maxillary segmental osteotomy is performed under general anesthesia in the operating room, with special requirements for the availability of hypotensive anesthesia to reduce blood loss, blood for transfusion, and special instruments sets. The patient is brought into the operating room and after induction of general anesthesia, is prepared and draped with special requirements as per the surgeon. Administration of antibiotics and steroids is dependent upon the preferences of the surgeon and anesthesiologist. Attention is then directed toward the posterior maxillary vestibular mucosa where local anesthesia is infiltrated. Following Kufner's technique, an incision is then created from the first molar extending approximately to the right maxillary canine or midline (Figure 49.5a). Exposure of the right maxillary lateral sinus wall to the level of the pterygoid plates is performed. In cases of posterior maxillary alveolar hyperplasia, often the mucosa overlying the pterygoid plates is thinned and subperiosteal dissection can be difficult, with care required to avoid perforating the mucosa.

Depending on the type of movement, whether it is either a superior and anterior movement, or a tipping type of movement, an ostectomy design should be contemplated with a bony window created along the lateral aspect of the maxillary sinus wall, as well as a vertical osteotomy. At this time, via the lateral bony window, a curved osteotome can be inserted and an osteotomy through the medial palatal wall created (see Figure 49.6a). Complete mobilization is then obtained by the separation of the pterygoid plate or ostectomy through the tuberosity region/third molar site with a curved osteotome. When the segment is fully mobilized, positioning can take place into a surgical stent that has been created from precut surgical models. Bone trimming can then proceed until satisfactory alignment is achieved. This is often aided by rotating the segment medially to expose the medial antral wall for trimming with a rotary bur or ronguers (Figure 49.6b). The segment is then secured into position with wiring of the orthodontic appliances into a surgical stent, which may also include maxillomandibular fixation. Internal fixation can then be applied with straight, Y, or L plates at the piriform rim (Figure 49.4c). When this is completed, the wound is irrigated and the incision closed with resorbable sutures.

If maxillary widening or narrowing is to be performed with a low palatal vault, owing to the thickness of the bone a palatal incision may be necessary to complete the osteotomy (Figure 49.7b). This would follow the technique of Perko–Bell, and the incision should be created along the medial aspect of the planned osteotomy site. In this way the incision can be closed over sound bone to reduce the possibility of an oroantral communication. Following the completion of the palatal osteotomy (Figure 49.7b), the transantral medial nasal wall osteotomy (Figure 49.7c) is performed. The pterygoid plate or tuberosity region is separated with a curved osteotome, and the segment may then be mobilized, trimmed, and set into desired position.

In all these segmental procedures, rigid fixation offers different advantages. In maxillary widening, additional support to the maxillary stent is supplied by the hardware. In maxillary narrowing, bone-to-bone contact with direct healing is promoted across the palatal process. There are times when occlusal leveling may require palatal pedicle stretching, for which it may be advantageous to use rigid fixation with overbent plates providing internal traction.

There are many controversies regarding the use of maxillary osteotomies for the correction of anterior apertognathia, with the varied experience of clinicians determining their choice of procedures. This range includes considerations for the transverse discrepancy, which is accompanied by the highest rate of relapse. Many authors describe various attempts at managing the transverse width, including single versus double paramidline osteotomies, and even mucosal-releasing incisions to decrease tension across the osteotomy.[57] Rigid fixation has certainly offered an important additional source of stability of these osteotomies. Long-term studies concerning stability reveal that a substantial improvement is obtained in segmental maxillary osteotomies with the advantage of rigid fixation compared to wire fixation. Orthodontic preparation is also very significant in these cases, and must be built into treatment planning regarding the possibilities of segment design and concerns for rigid fixation. Consideration for orthodontic wires and appliance design is also very significant to maintain as much three-dimensional rigidity of the skeletodental complex as possible.

Numerous studies have been performed to determine the effects of rigid internal fixation on the long-term stability of maxillary osteotomies relative to the traditional methods of skeletal wire fixation. Kahnberg et al.[72] studied the correction of open bite by maxillary osteotomy, comparing plate to wire fixation, finding no statistically significant difference between the two groups with regard to relapse. Denison et al., however, indicated that simply the performance of maxillary surgery for the management of open bite is not desirable because of the high rate of relapse.[73] Larsen et al. studied postsurgical maxillary movement: it would appear that serial studies of cephalometric radiographs show there is little difference statistically between the two groups.[74]

Rigid internal fixation has also made the possibility of outpatient orthognathic surgery a reality by removing the concerns for postoperative airway management that exist when patients are placed in maxillomandibular fixation.[75] Knoff et al.[75] reported that of all the outpatient orthognathic procedures they performed, the Le Fort I osteotomy had the greatest potential for severe complications, owing to hemorrhage, nausea, and vomiting. With the changes in health care delivery, outpatient maxillary surgery as individual or combined jaw osteotomies may become more common. This has certainly become possible with the advent of rigid fixation and improved postoperative airway management when compared to the potential for complications that are associated with patients in maxillomandibular fixation.

Distraction Osteogenesis

New techniques for distraction osteogenesis permit greater and more stable maxillary movements in highly retruded cleft palate and craniofacial syndrome patients.[76–80] Extensive bone grafting can also be avoided in these patients through these bone lengthening procedures.[81] An added benefit is the increase in soft tissue volume as the bone lengthening takes place. A variety of intraoral and extraoral devices have been utilized and continue to be developed.[82–84] In the future, combined traditional osteotomies with distraction osteogenesis techniques will change and improve the treatment of maxillary deformities.

Conclusion

There has been an evolution in the techniques associated with the Le Fort I osteotomy since the initial report of von Langenbeck in 1859.[2] Along with the progress in anesthesia and instrumentation, osteotomy design has changed to provide optimal support of the soft tissues to create pleasing esthetic facial appearance, and advances in internal fixation have permitted superior functional results. Internal fixation provides the patients with an easier postoperative course and more rapid return to work without the accompanying dietary difficulties and weight loss, communication problems, and airway compromise. Long-term stability appears to have improved with time, and the complications from these operations are less troublesome. Resorbable plates and screws can be utilized in selected cases with the avoidance of hardware removal.[85,86]

References

1. Bell WH. *Modern Practice in Orthognathic and Reconstructive Surgery*. Philadelphia: WB Saunders; 1992.

2. von Langenbeck B. Betrage zur Osteoplastick—Die osteoplastische Resektion des Oberkiefers. In: Goschen A, ed. *Deutsche Klinik*. Berlin: Reimer; 1859.

3. Le Fort R. Etude experimentale sur les fractures de la machoire superieure. *Rev Chir*. 1901;23:208–227.

4. Le Fort R. Etude experimentale sur les fractures de la machoire superieure. *Rev Chir*. 1901;23:360–379.

5. Le Fort R. Etude experimentale sur les fractures de la machoire superieure. *Rev Chir*. 1901;23:479–507.

6. Drommer RB. The history of the Le Fort I osteotomy. *J Maxillofac Surg*. 1986;14:119–122.

7. Cheever DW. Naso-pharyngeal polypus attached to the basilar process of the occipital and body of the sphenoid bone successfully removed by a section, displacement, and subsequent replacement and reunion of the superior maxillary bone. *Boston Med Surg J*. 1867;8:162.

8. Pincus W. Beitrag zur Klinik und Chirugie des Nasen-Rachenraumes. *Arch Klin Chir*. 1907;82:110.

9. Lanz O. Osteoplastische Resektion beider Oberkiefer nach Kocher. In: Lücke R, ed. *Deutsche Zeitschrift fur Chirugie*. Leipzig: Vogel; 1893.

10. Winkler H. Zur Chirugie de Oberkieferhohlenerkrankungen. *Int Zentralbl Ohrenheilk*. 1903;1:435.

11. Hertle J. Uber einen Fall von temporarer Aufklappung beider Oberkiefer nach Kocher zum Zwecke der Entfernung eines Grossen Nasenrachenfibromes. *Arch Klin Chir*. 1904;73:75.

12. Payer E. Uber neue Methoden zur operativen Behandlung der Geschwulste des Nasenrachenraumes mit besonderer Berucksichtigung der Kocher'schen osteoplastischen Resektion beider Oberkiefer. *Arch Klin Chir*. 1904;72:285.

13. Borchardt M. Zur temporaren Aufklappung beider Oberkiefer. *Zentralbl Chir*. 1908:25:755.

14. Vorschut W. Zwei Falle von exstirpierten malignen Tumoren der Keilbeinhole. In: Bier, ed. *Deutsche Zeitschrift fur Chirurgie*. Leipzig: Vogel; 1908.

15. Kocher T. Ein Fall von Hypophysis—Tumor mit operativer Heilung. In: Bier, ed. *Deutsche Zeitschrift fur Chirugie*. Trendelenburg: Wilms, Leipzig 1909.

16. Loewe L. *Chirugie der Nase*. Berlin: Coblentz; 1905.

17. Wassmund M. *Lehrbuch der Praktischen Chirugie des Mundes und der Kiefer*. Bd I. Leipzig: Meusser; 1935.

18. Axhausen G. Zur Behandlung veralteter disloziert verheilter Oberkieferbruche. *Dtsch Zahn Mund Kieferheilk*. 1934;I:334.

19. Axhausen G. Uber die korrigierende Osteotomie am Oberkiefer. *Dtsch Z Chir*. 1936;248:515.

20. Axhausen G. Die operative Orthopadie bie den Fehlbildungen der Kiefer. *Dtsch Zahn Mund Kieferheilk*. 1939;6:582.

21. Schuchardt D. Ein Betrag zur chirugischen Kieferorthyopadie unter Berusksichtigung ihrer Bedeutung fur die Behandlung angeborener und erworbener Kieferdeformitaten bei Soldaten. *Dtsch Zahn Mund Kieferheilkd*. 1942;9:73.

22. Gillies HG, Rowe NL. L'osteotomie du maxillaire superieur envisagée essentiellment dans les cas de bec-de-liévre total. *Rev Stomatol*. 1954;55:545.

23. Converse JM, Shapiro HH. Treatment of developmental malformations of the jaws. *Plast Reconstr Surg*. 1952;10:473.

24. Schmid E. Zur Wiederherstellung des Mittelgesichtes nach Entwicklungsstorungen und Defekten des knochernen Unterbaues. In: Schuchardt K, ed. *Fortschritte Kiefer- und Gesichtschirurgie*. Stuttgart: Thieme; 1956.

25. Hall HD, Roddy SC. Treatment of maxillary alveolar hyperplasia by total maxillary alveolar osteotomy. *J Oral Surg*. 1975;33:180–188.

26. West RA, Epker BN. Posterior maxillary surgery: its place in the treatment of dentofacial deformities. *J Oral Surg*. 1972;20:562–575.

27. West RA, McNeill RN. Maxillary alveolar hyperplasia, diagnosis, and treatment planning. *J. Maxillofac Surg*. 1975;3(4):239–249.

28. Hall HD, West RA. Combined anterior and posterior maxillary osteotomy. *J Oral Surg*. 1976;34:126–141.

29. Bell WH, Levy BM. Revascularization and bone healing following total maxillary osteotomy. *J Dent Res*. 1973;82: abstract 96 (special issue).

30. Bell WH, Finn RA, Scheideman GB. Wound healing associated with Le Fort I osteotomy. Abstract. *AADR J Dent Res*. 1980;59: special issue A, p 459.

31. You ZH, Zhang ZK, Zhang XE. Le Fort I osteotomy with descending palatal artery intact and ligated: a study of blood flow and quantitative histology. *Contemp Stomatol*. 1991;5(2):71–74.

32. You ZH, Zhang ZK, Zhang XE, Xia JL. The study of vascular communication between jaw bones and their surrounding tissues by SEM of resin casts. *West China J Stomatol*. 1990;8:235–237.

33. You ZH, Zhang ZK, Zhang XE. A study of maxillary and mandibular vasculature in relation to orthognathic surgery. *Chin J Stomatol*. 1991;26(5):263–266.

34. Drommer R. Selective angiographic studies prior to Le Fort I osteotomy in patients with cleft lip and palate. *J Maxillofac Surg*. 1979;7:264–270.

35. Obwegeser HL. Surgical correction of small or retrodisplaced maxilla: the "dish-face deformity." *Plast Reconstr Surg*. 1969;43:351.

36. Henderson D. *A Colour Atlas and Textbook of Orthognathic Surgery*. London: Wolfe; 1985:241–243.

37. Frame JW, Brady CL, Browne RM. Effect of autogenous bone grafts on healing following Le Fort I maxillary osteotomies. *Int J Oral Maxillofac Surg*. 1990;19:151–154.

38. Greenberg AM, Prein J. Considerations for bone healing in the craniomaxillofacial trauma patient. In: Greenberg AM, ed. *Craniomaxillofacial Fractures: Principles of Internal Fixation Using the AO/ASIF Technique*. New York: Springer-Verlag; 1993.

39. Spiessl B. *Internal Fixation of the Mandible: A Manual of AO/ASIF Principles*. New York: Springer-Verlag; 1989.

40. Luyk NH, Ward-Booth RP. The stability of Le Fort I advancement osteotomies using bone plates without bone grafts. *J Maxillofac Surg*. 1985;13:250–253.

41. Schuchardt K. Experiences with the surgical treatment of deformities of the jaws: prognathia, micrognathia, and open bite. In: Wallace AG, ed. *Second Congress of International Society of Plastic Surgeons*. London: E & S Livingstone; 1959.

42. Kufner J. Experience with a modified procedure for correction of open bite. In: Walker RV, ed. *Transactions of the Third International Conference of Oral Surgery*. London: E & S Livingstone; 1970.

43. Perko M. Maxillary sinus and surgical movement of maxilla. *Int J Oral Surg*. 1972;1:177.

44. Bell WH. Total maxillary osteotomy. In: Archer WH, ed. *Oral Surgery: A Step by Step Atlas of Operative Techniques.* Philadelphia: WB Saunders; 1975.

45. Trimble LD, Tideman H, Stoelinga PJW. A modification of the pterygoid plate separation in low-level maxillary osteotomies. *J Oral Maxillofac Surg.* 1983;41:544–546.

46. Tideman H, Stoelinga PJW, Gallia L. Le Fort I advancement with segmental palatal osteotomies in patients with cleft palates. *J Oral Surg.* 1980;38:196–199.

47. Poole MD, Robinson PP, Nunn ME. Maxillary advancement in cleft palate patients. A modification of the Le Fort I osteotomy and preliminary results. *J Maxillofac Surg.* 1986;14: 123–127.

48. Stoelinga PJ, v.d. Vijver HR, Leenan RJ, Blijdorp PA, Schoenaers JH. The prevention of relapse after maxillary osteotomies in cleft palate patients. *J Craniomaxillofac Surg.* 1987;15:326–331.

49. Cohn-Stock G. *Die Chirugische Immediateregulierung der Kiefer speziell die chirugische Behandlung der Prognathie.* Berlin: Vjschr Zahnheilk; 1921;37:320–354.

50. Wassmund M. *Lehrbuch der pratischen Chirugie des Mundes und der Kiefer.* Bd. I. Liepzig: Meusser; 1935.

51. Wunderer S. Die Prognatieoperation mittels frontal gestieltem maxillafragment. *Oest Z Stomatol.* 1962;59:98–102.

52. Cupar I. Die chirurgische Behandlung der Form-und Stellungs-Verandungen des oberkiefers. *Ost Z Stomat.* 1954;51:565–577.

53. Lanigan DT, Hey JH, West RA. Aseptic necrosis following maxillary osteotomies: report of 36 cases. *J Oral Maxillofac Surg.* 1990;48:142–156.

54. Nelson RL, Path MG, Ogle RG. Quantification of blood flow after anterior segmental osteotomy: investigation of three surgical approaches. *J Oral Surg.* 1978;36:106.

55. Meyer MW, Cavanaugh GD. Blood flow changes after orthognathic surgery: maxillary and mandibular subapical osteotomy. *J Oral Surg.* 1976;35:495–501.

56. Luhr H, Kubein-Meesenburg D. Rigid skeletal fixation in maxillary osteotomies: intraoperative control of condylar position. *Clin Plast Surg.* 1989;16:157–163.

57. Obwegesser HL. Surgical correction of small or retrodisplaced maxillae: the "dish-face" deformity. *Plast Reconstr Surg.* 1969;43:351–365.

58. Keller EE, Sather AH. Quadrangular Le Fort I osteotomy. *J Oral Maxillofac Surg.* 1990;48:2–11.

59. Bennett MA, Wolford LM. The maxillary step osteotomy and Steinmann pin stabilization. *J Oral Maxillofac Surg.* 1985;43:307–311.

60. Bell WH. *Modern Practice in Orthognathic and Reconstructive Surgery.* Philadelphia: WB Saunders; 1992:135.

61. Mavreas D, Athanasiou AE. Tomographic assessment of alterations of the temporomandibular joint after orthognathic surgery. *Eur J Orthod.* 1992;14:3–15.

62. Athanasiou AE, Yucel-Eroglut. Short term consequences of orthognathic surgery on stomatognathic function. *Eur J Orthod.* 1994;16:491–499.

63. Arnett WG. Maxillary surgery for the correction of open bites Abstract. *J Oral Maxillofac Surg.* (Suppl 2) 1994;52:21–22.

64. Marx RE, Morales MJ. Morbidity from bone harvest in major jaw reconstruction: a randomized trial comparing the lateral anterior and posterior approaches to the ilium. *J Oral Maxillofac Surg* 1988;46(3):196–203.

65. Tessier P. Autologous bone grafts taken from the calavarium for facial and cranial applications. *Clin Plast Surg.* 1982;9:531–540.

66. Phillips JH, Rahn BA. Fixation effects on membranous and endochondral onlay bone-graft resorption. *Plast Reconstr Surg.* 1988;82:872–877.

67. Zins JE, Whitaker LA. Membranous versus endochondral bone: implications for craniofacial surgery. *Plast Reconstr Surg.* 1985;76:510–514.

68. Stella JP, Streater MR, Epker BN, Sinn DP. Predictability of upper lip soft tissue changes with maxillary advancement. *J Oral Maxillofac Surg.* 1989;47:697–703.

69. Guymon M, Crosby DR, Wolford LM. The alar base cinch suture to control nasal width in maxillary osteotomies. *Int J Adult Orthod Orthognath Surg.* 1988;3:89–95.

70. Hackney FL, Nishioka GJ, Van Sickels JE. Frontal soft tissue morphology with double V-Y closure following Le Fort I osteotomy. *J Oral Maxillofac Surg.* 1988;46:850–855.

71. Rosenquist B. Anterior segmental osteotomy: a 24-month follow-up. *Int J Oral Maxillofac Surg.* 1993;22:210–213.

72. Kahnberg KE, Zouloumis L, Widmark G. Correction of open bite by maxillary osteotomy. A comparison between bone plate and wire fixation. *J Cranio-Maxillo-Fac Surg.* 1994;22: 250–255.

73. Denison TF, Kokich VG, Shapiro PA. Stability of maxillary surgery in open bite versus non open bite malocclusions. *Angle Orthod.* 1989;59(1):5–10.

74. Larsen AJ, Van Sickels JE, Thrash WJ. Postsurgical maxillary movement: a comparison study of bone plate and screw versus wire osseous fixation. *Am J Orthod Dentofacial Orthop.* 1989; 95:334–343.

75. Knoff SB, Van Sickels JE, Holmgreen WC. Outpatient orthognathic surgery: criteria and review of cases. *J Oral Maxillofac Surg.* 1991;49:117–120.

76. Rachmiel A, Aizenbud D, Ardekian L, et al. Surgically assisted orthopedic protraction of the maxilla in cleft lip and palate patients. *Int J Oral Maxillofac Surg.* 1999;28:9–14.

77. Swennon G, Colle F, De May A, et al. Maxillary distraction in cleft lip and palate patients: a review of six cases. *J Craniofac Surg.* 1999;10:117–122.

78. Tate GS, Tharanon W, Sinn DP. Transoral maxillary distraction osteogenesis of an unrepaired bilateral alveolar cleft. *J Craniofac Surg.* 1999;10:369–374.

79. Ko EW, Figueroa AA, Guyette TW, et al. Velopharyngeal changes after maxillary advancement in cleft patients with distraction osteogenesis using a rigid external distraction device: a 1 year cephalometric follow up. *J Craniofac Surg.* 1999;10:312–320.

80. Cohen SR. Midface distraction. *Semin Orthod.* 1999;5:52–58.

81. Toth BA, Kim JW, Chin M, et al. Distraction osteogenesis and its application to the midface and bony orbit in craniosynostosis syndromes. *J Craniofac Surg.* 1998;9:100–113.

82. Figueroa AA, Polley JW, Ko EW. Maxillary distraction for the management of cleft maxillary hypoplasia with rigid external distraction system. *Semin Orthod.* 1999;5:46–51.

83. Chin M, Toth BA. Distraction osteogenesis in maxillofacial surgery using internal devices: review of 5 cases. *J Oral Maxillofac Surg.* 1996;54:45–53.

84. Ahn JG, Figueroa AA, Braun S, et al. Biomechanical considerations in distraction of the osteotomized dentomaxillary complex. *Am J Orthod Dentofacial Orthop.* 1999;116:264–270.

85. Edwards RC, Kiely KD. Resorbable fixation of Le Fort I osteotomies. *J Craniofac Surg.* 1997;9:210.

86. Edwards RC, Kiely KD, Eppley B. Fixation of bimaxillary osteotomies with resorbable plates and screws: experience in 20 consecutive cases. *J Oral Maxillofac Surg.* 2001;59:271–276.

50
Mandibular Osteotomies and Considerations for Rigid Internal Fixation

Victor Escobar, Alex M. Greenberg, and Alan Schwimmer

Introduction

Since the mandibular osteotomy described by Hullihen,[1] maxillomandibular fixation (MMF) during the healing period has been the fixation method of choice (Figure 50.1). New surgical techniques include the use of rigid internal fixation (RIF) with plates[2] and/or screws[3,4] (Figure 50.2). The avoidance of MMF allows increased stability and improved postoperative care[4,5] and accelerates psychological recovery.[6]

Over time, clinicians have critically reviewed their results, and as techniques have developed, it has been suggested that immobilization of the mandible is accompanied by a decrease in mandibular range of motion[7–9] secondary to degenerative changes in the temporomandibular joint (TMJ).[10] Rigid internal fixation shortens immobilization time[11–13] and minimizes the reduction in mandibular range of motion after orthognathic surgery.[7–9,14] Improvements in diagnosis, treatment planning, and osteotomy techniques[15,16] allow patients to open and close the mandible immediately after surgery[17] and to maintain oral nutritional uptake, and reduce postoperative apprehension caused by respiratory limitation, nausea, and vomiting.[18,19]

Mandibular Osteotomies

Historical Review

Mandibular osteotomies for the correction of dentofacial deformities have been performed since the first report of an anterior subapical mandibular osteotomy by Hullihen in 1849 (Figure 50.3). For the remainder of the century, management of malocclusion secondary to prognathism was mainly a transcutaneous resection of a piece of mandibular bone[20] (Figure 50.4) to achieve shortening of the mandible.[21,22] A variation of Hullihen's procedure[1] was used to advance the anterior lower segment[23] and to close anterior open bites.[24] These procedures resembled the anterior mandibular segmental subapical osteotomy in use today.[25] Two other modifications are still in use—single tooth osteotomies[26] and total mandibular alveolar osteotomy[27] (see Figure 50.5).

Over the years, many modifications to mandibular osteotomies have been reported,[20,28–30] but the most stable was the step osteotomy[30] (Figure 50.6) used for advancement of the body of the mandible. During this time, the procedures have shifted from the body to the ramus. It was Blair in 1907[31] who first performed a subcondylar vertical ramus osteotomy (Figure 50.7). Since then, many variations of this osteotomy have been described including several types of sliding osteotomies for the repositioning of segments in multiple planes of space.[20,32–34] A transcutaneous approach was used until 1964[33] despite Ernst's[35] description in 1938 of a transoral approach. As with the anterior mandibular segmental osteotomy,[36] the subcondylar osteotomy has undergone many changes that finally resulted in the intraoral vertical ramus osteotomy (IVRO) which is used today for the treatment of mandibular prognathism (Figure 50.8).[37] The intraoral vertical ramus osteotomy was performed originally at the neck of the condyle[21,33,38] (Figure 50.8e). Because of the lack of stability of this osteotomy postoperatively (presumably because of the lack of medial pterygoid attachment), longer cuts were suggested beginning at the sigmoid notch and ending at different levels behind the angle of the mandible[39,40] close to the gonial notch.[41] In patients requiring mandibular advancement, an anterior iliac crest bone graft block was inserted between the segments[42,43] and in many cases wire osteosynthesis was utilized.[44] Other variations of the subcondylar osteotomy have included the inverted L osteotomy[45] and its modifications,[46,47] including the C osteotomy[48,49] (Figures 50.8b,c).

As pointed out by Bloomquist,[29] perhaps the greatest development in mandibular osteotomies of the vertical ramus is the sagittal split ramus osteotomy (SSRO),[50] which was introduced by Perthes in 1924 and later popularized by Obwegeser[36] and Trauner in 1955 for the management of prognathism (Figure 50.9). Two years later, the same authors[51] proposed correction of both prognathic and retrognathic mandibles with the sagittal split ramus osteotomy and simultaneous genioplasty. With time, several modifications and improvements to the SSRO have been developed[52,53] (Figure 50.9). While Dal Pont[54] suggested that the lateral cut be made

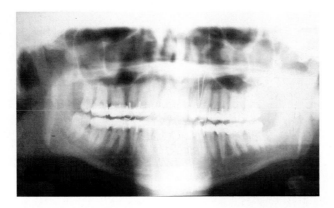

FIGURE 50.1 Panoramic radiograph reveals bilateral mandibular intraoral vertical ramus osteotomies with maxillomandibular fixation. Note circumandibular and piriform rim skeletal wire fixation to prevent extrusion of orthodontically treated teeth.

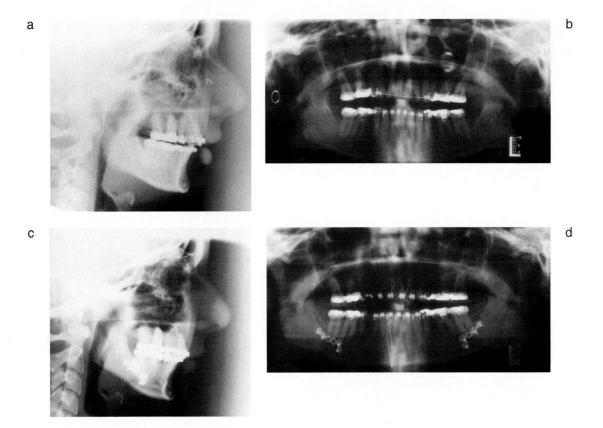

FIGURE 50.2 Patient with skeletal class II malocclusion having undergone bilateral mandibular sagittal split ramus osteotomies with miniplate fixation. Note circumandibular and piriform rim skeletal wire fixation to prevent extrusion of orthodontically treated teeth: (a) preoperative lateral cephalometric radiograph; (b) preoperative panoramic radiograph; (c) postoperative lateral cephalometric radiograph; (d) postoperative panoramic radiograph.

Continued.

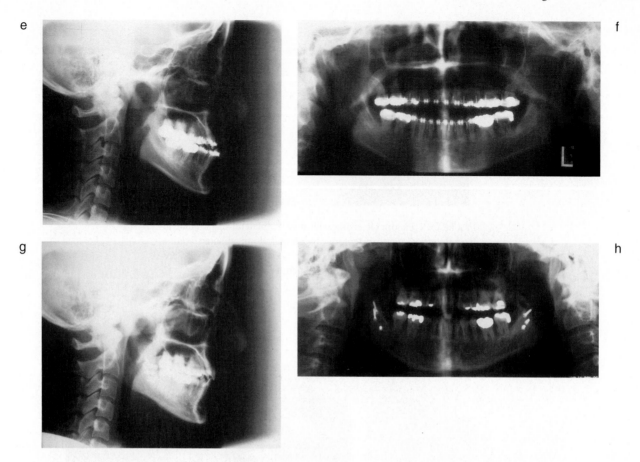

FIGURE 50.2 *Continued*. Patient with skeletal class III malocclusion having undergone bilateral mandibular sagittal split ramus osteotomies with three bilateral superior border 2.0-mm lag screws. (e) Preoperative lateral cephalometric radiograph; (f) preoperative panoramic radiograph; (g) postoperative lateral cephalometric radiograph; (h) postoperative panoramic radiograph.

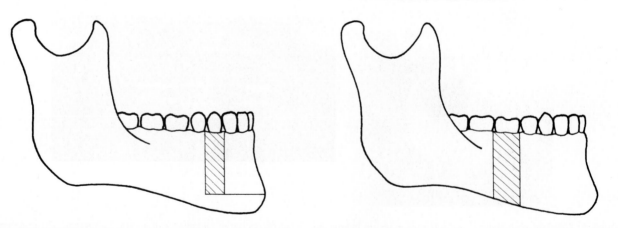

FIGURE 50.3 Subapical osteotomy similar to the one performed by Hullihen in 1849. (From Bell[102])

FIGURE 50.4 Body osteotomy as performed by Blair.[21] (From Bell[102])

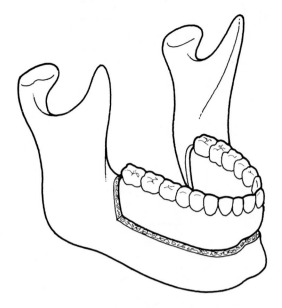

FIGURE 50.5 Diagram of subapical mandibular osteotomy. (From Powell and Riley[103])

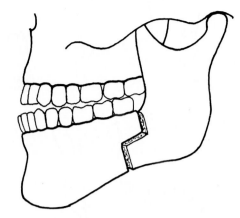

FIGURE 50.6 Von Eiselberg step osteotomy. (From Bloomquist[29])

forward along the lateral aspect of the second molar to increase the area of bone contact [Figure 50.9(e)], Hunsuck[55] suggested decreasing the extent of the medial osteotomy to just posterior to the mandibular foramen to produce a smaller mucoperiosteal reflection and reduce trauma to the neurovascular bundle [Figure 50.9(f)]. To reduce the complications associated with the SSRO and the unpredictable manner in which the inferior border of the mandible may split (Hunsuck effect), an inferior border osteotomy has been proposed.[56] However, this increases the extent of pterygomasseteric sling stripping, the risk of intraoperative bleeding, and the frequency of inferior alveolar nerve damage.[57] One of the most important innovations to SSROs is the use of lag screw fixation introduced by Spiessl.[58] It was theorized that screw fixation would result in more rapid healing, osteosynthesis, decreased relapse, increased patient comfort, and improved condylar control.[59]

Four major types of osteotomies are performed today: (1) anterior mandibular segmental (subapical) osteotomies, (2) anterior horizontal mandibular osteotomy (genioplasty), (3) sagittal split ramus osteotomy (SSRO), and (4) intraoral vertical ramus osteotomy (IVRO).

Mandibular Anterior Segmental Osteotomy (Subapical Osteotomy)

The subapical osteotomy has been used to move anterior teeth in almost any conceivable direction. The greatest concern is damage to the teeth if the osteotomies are not carefully designed. Space needs to be available to permit safe vertical and horizontal osteotomies.

The soft tissue surgical approach for all anterior osteotomies is similar. It involves infiltration with local anes-

thetic containing epinephrine and a labial vestibular incision made approximately 5 mm labial to the depth of the vestibule.[60] The incision extends through the mentalis muscles, through periosteum, and down to bone. The extent of the incision should be at least 10 mm beyond the planned vertical osteotomies to prevent undesirable laceration of soft tissue. The mental nerves should be identified and isolated as they exit their foramina. The periosteum is elevated, preserving the mucoperiosteal attachment at the inferior border of the mandible. This helps to ensure stability of the soft tissues of the chin. When necessary, teeth are removed and a fissure bur is utilized to create the interdental osteotomy perpendicular to the curve of the arch. The subapical horizontal osteotomy is created with a reciprocating saw 5 mm inferior to the roots of the teeth. Depending on the type of movement desired, additional bone trimming is then performed. The segments are mobilized after completion of the osteotomies via chisels. Care must be taken to preserve the lingual and buccal pedicles crossing the interdental osteotomies. When positioning the segments into a surgical guide, excessive bone removal should be avoided by careful bone trimming.

After satisfactory positioning of the dentoalveolar segment

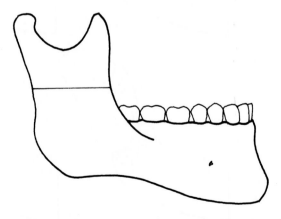

FIGURE 50.7 Horizontal subcondylar osteotomy as performed by Blair. (From Bell[102])

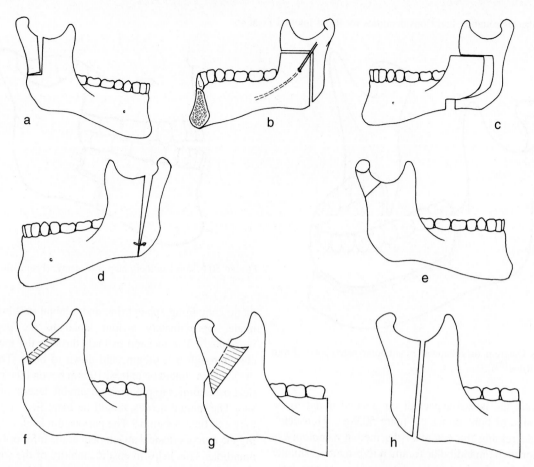

FIGURE 50.8 (a) Limberg's oblique osteotomy. (b) Wassmund's inverted "L" osteotomy. (c) Caldwell et al., "C" osteotomy. (d) Robinson et al., oblique osteotomy. (e) Blair, subcondylar osteotomy. (f–h) Different lengths of inverted vertical ramus osteotomy (IVRO). (From Bell[102])

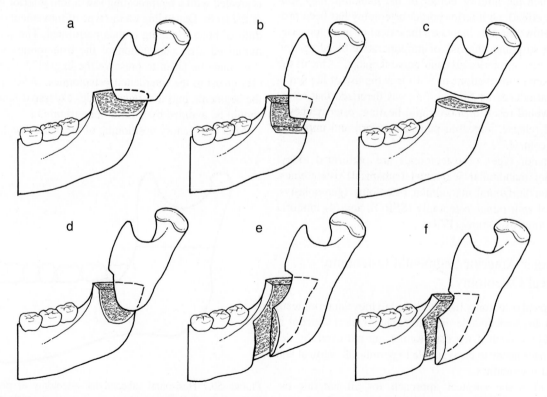

FIGURE 50.9 (a) Perthes osteotomy, 1924. (b) Trauner and Obwegeser, 1957. (c) Kazanjian and Converse, 1959. (d) Schuchardt, 1961. (e) Dal Pont, 1961. (f) Hunsuck, 1968. (Adapted from Bell[102])

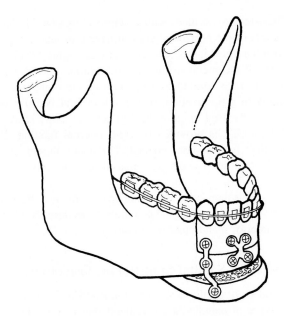

FIGURE 50.10 Miniplate fixation of anterior mandibular segmental and genioplasty osteotomies. (From Shafer and Assael[60])

grafts may be wedged into the interdental osteotomy sites to aid in the stability of the dentoalveolar segments and reduce the incidence of periodontal defects. The osteotomy is made with a reciprocating saw. The length and angle of the horizontal cut can have profound effects on the resultant position of the segment (see Figure 50.11). It is recommended[60] that this osteotomy be done with a power saw because extensive use of chisels in interdental areas can result in mucosal lacerations that adversely affect blood supply and periodontal health. Care should be taken to avoid root apices and lateral root surfaces. Midline anterior osteotomies (Figure 50.12) through the inferior border may also be performed in conjunction with anterior mandibular osteotomies. Their fixation should occur after the anterior dentoalveolar segmental osteotomy has been completed. Of major concern with subapical osteotomies is the preservation of the inferior alveolar nerves and their mental branches. Vitality of the teeth and the whole bony segment will be affected by the level of the horizontal cut, which should be at least 5 mm below the teeth apices. Soft tissue pedicles are important for blood supply, and the lingual mucosa should be preserved. If ramus osteotomies are performed they should be done following the anterior mandibular procedures.

Wound closure is accomplished in two layers—muscle and mucosa—with resorbable sutures. Care should be taken to reapproximate the mentalis muscles. Tape is placed on the lip and chin for 24 to 48 hours to minimize hematoma formation and to aid in supporting the suture lines.[29]

Anterior Mandibular Midline Osteotomy

In addition to subapical osteotomies, a useful procedure is the anterior midline (Figure 50.12) or paramidline osteotomy used to correct arch width discrepancies. Surgical technique

into a surgical stent and after MMF has been attained, rigid fixation may be performed with a variety of miniplates, microplates, or monocortical screws. If an anterior mandibular horizontal osteotomy for genioplasty is simultaneously performed, fixation of all the segments may be performed. The dentoalveolar segment should be repositioned and rigidly fixated first. Then, the chin bony segment may be repositioned and secured either separately with special preformed chin plates or with the same miniplates used to secure the dentoalveolar segment. Additional holes may be left in the plates for fixation of the chin (Figure 50.10). After fixation, bone

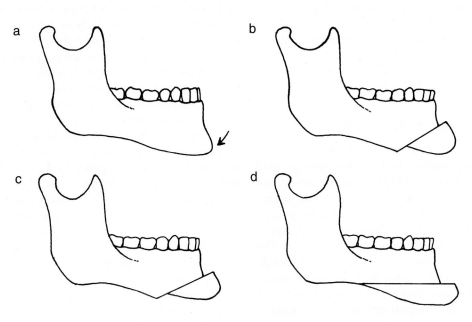

FIGURE 50.11 (a) Preoperative. (b) Long obliquely angled segment. (c) Short obliquely angled segment. (d) Horizontally angled segment. Effects of angle and lenth of mandibular osteotomy. (From Bloomquist[29])

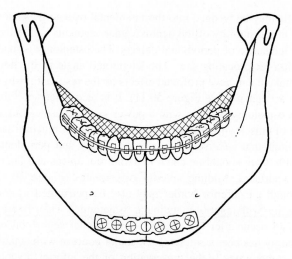

FIGURE 50.12 Rigid fixation of midline mandibular osteotomy with reconstruction plate. Lingual splint in place for alignment of segments. (From Shafer and Assael[60])

includes anterior mandible infiltration with local anesthetic and epinephrine. The incision is created in the labial vestibular mucosa as in the subapical osteotomy described earlier. The periosteum is elevated preserving the mucoperiosteal attachment of the anterior mandibular segment. Smaller incisions including vertical types are sometimes preferred by surgeons. A fissure bur is then used to create a vertical osteotomy line between the roots of the mandibular central incisors and carried through to the inferior border of the mandible. The osteotomy is completed with the help of an osteotome. The mandibular segments are then mobilized into a stent, and the mandible can be either narrowed or widened. For this type of osteotomy, paired mandibular compression plates or a 2.4 mm standard reconstruction plate should be used (Figure 50.12). In addition to the rigid internal fixation, an acrylic lingual splint is prepared for alignment of the segments into the planned positions and to provide additional stability, especially if fixation is done with less rigid plates than a standard reconstruction 2.4 mm plate[60] (see Figure 50.12).

Horizontal Osteotomy of the Symphysis

The surgical approach to a horizontal osteotomy of the symphysis (sliding genioplasty) is similar to the approach used for the subapical osteotomy, in which the incision through the buccal mucosa is placed at the depth of the vestibular sulcus, but the subperiosteal dissection extends down to the inferior border of the mandible from first molar to first molar. Again, the mental nerves are isolated as they exit their foramina. The incision should be angled toward bone and should include mentalis muscle in both flaps to aid in closure of the wound and suspension of the musculature to avoid lip ptosis.[60] It is desirable to maintain the periosteal attachment at the anterior inferior border to preserve the soft tissue contours of the chin.

The osteotomy is made with a reciprocating saw. The length and angle of the horizontal cut can have profound effects on the resultant position of the segment (see Figure 50.11). For routine advancements using nonrigid fixation, the amount of advancement is limited by the width of the mobilized segment. With rigid fixation, this is not critical because bone grafts can be used to close the gap between bony segments. Initial stability is provided by rigid internal fixation (RIF) rather than bone-to-bone contact. The plates should sit passively with at least two screws placed in each bony segment (Figure 50.13).

The skin is then taped across the lip and chin and the wound closed in two layers, muscle and mucosa, as described for the other anterior mandibular osteotomies.

Mandibular Sagittal Split Ramus Osteotomy

Bilateral sagittal split ramus osteotomies (SSRO) are used for most types of mandibular movements that involve the entire mandibular body. The surgical procedure is technique sensitive, especially when accompanied by rigid internal fixation.

The sagittal split ramus osteotomy now widely performed is the original osteotomy described by Obwegeser[36] with modifications by Hunsuck,[55] Dal Pont,[54] and Epker[57] (see Figures 50.9e,f). As with other osteotomies, local anesthetic with epinephrine is infiltrated before the incision. A 3-cm curvilinear incision is made medial to the fat pad and along the external oblique ridge (Figure 50.14). Following a full-thickness mucoperiosteal flap dissection, the lateral aspect of the angle and anterior ramus of the mandible are stripped to the inferior and posterior borders. With a J-shaped stripper, the dissection is extended to the inferior border of the mandible and forward to the second molar. This allows for optimal positioning of screws and does not increase the risk of devitalizing the proximal bone segment. A V-notched retracter is then placed inferiorly on the anterior aspect of the ascending ramus, which is then elevated above the mandibular foramen, and the ramus is stripped of the temporalis muscle attachments up to the sigmoid notch. Once the medial full-thickness mucoperiosteal flap has been developed and the lingula identified, the location of the sigmoid notch may be checked with a suitable instrument.

The medial cortex horizontal osteotomy is made with a Lindemann bur or a reciprocating saw about 1.5 cm inferior to the sigmoid notch but superior to the mandibular foramen. Soft tissues are retracted with a channel retractor while protecting the inferior alveolar neurovascular bundle. The osteotomy is created through the cancellous space down to "bleeding bone" until approximately 50% of the thickness of the ramus is cut. It is then continued along the natural concave boundary between the medial aspect of the ramus and the internal oblique ridge. This creates an osteotomy between the medial and lateral cortices. The vertical cut is continued to the level of the distal aspect of the second molar. A vertical osteotomy is then created perpendicular to the inferior

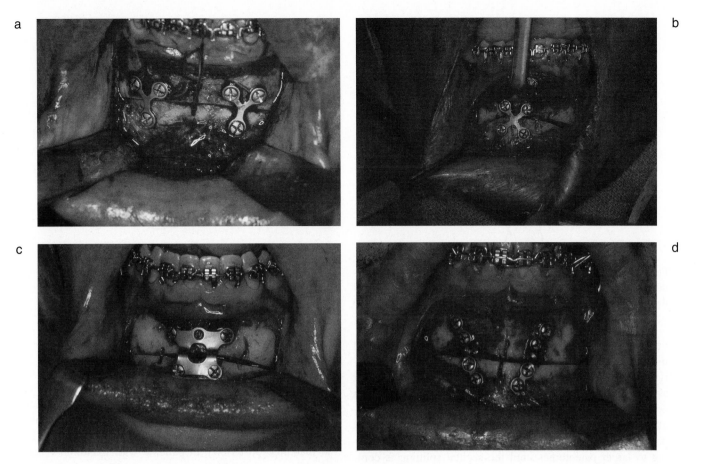

FIGURE 50.13 Examples of miniplate fixation for anterior horizontal mandibular osteotomies (genioplasties): (a) bilateral Y plates; (b) X plate; (c) offset double-bend plate for preset 6-mm advancement; (d) bilateral 2.0-mm adaption plates.

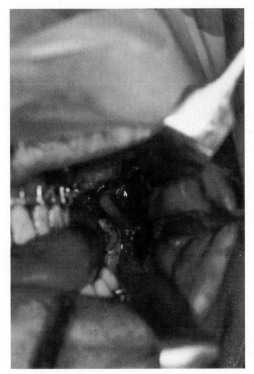

FIGURE 50.14 Intraoral buccal mucosa incision along the external oblique ridge, positioned to allow for the cuff of medial mucosa pedicle needed for closure.

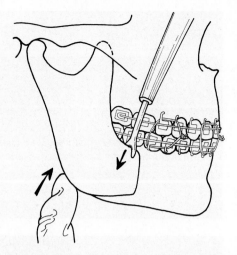
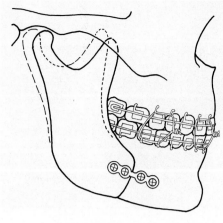

FIGURE 50.15 Bivector positioning of the proximal segment with digital pressure along the angle of the mandible for superior seating of the condyle, and downward pressure with an instrument such as a gauze directer for anterior rotation of the condyle. Positioning of the condyle in this manner decreases the risk of condylar resorption.

border of the mandible along the buccal aspect of the second molar. It should only be through the buccal cortex and inferior border of the mandible to prevent damage to the inferior alveolar nerve. This vertical osteotomy connects the inferior border of the mandible with the sagittal ramus osteotomy along the internal oblique ridge. Thin narrow osteotomes may be used to begin the sagittal split osteotomy, slowly advancing to larger osteotomes until the sagittal splitting is completed. Great care should be undertaken to avoid fracturing the buccal plate or the proximal extension of the distal segment, especially if the Smith spreader instrument is used. Either of those fractures may preclude the use of rigid internal fixation. Any prying or torquing of these segments should be minimized.

As splitting of the segments is performed, attention must be directed to the mandibular nerve, which usually remains along the lateral aspect of the distal segment. If it appears that the nerve is still attached to the medial aspect of the proximal segment, it needs to be released to avoid its laceration or transection. Once the segments are fully mobilized, if the mandible is being advanced, maxillomandibular fixation is attained and bivector positioning (see Figure 50.15) of the proximal segments is performed in association with measurements of the planned movement. Anterior positioning of the condyle in the fossa reduces condylar resorption.[61] Transoral or transcutaneous rigid fixation of the segments is then performed with either screws or miniplates depending on the surgeon's choice. For large forward movements, the proximal aspect of the distal segment needs to be stripped from medial pterygoid attachments. If the mandible is to be repositioned posteriorly, trimming of the distal aspect of the proximal segment needs to be performed to avoid interference between the segments (Figure 50.16). When the distal portion of the proximal segment fractures, it may be repositoned and rigidly fixated with miniplates.

Vertical Ramus Osteotomy

Osteotomies of the vertical ramus (intraoral vertical ramus osteotomy, IVRO) may be considered when the dental arch has to be moved as a unit into its new position, or if the patient prefers to avoid the increased risk of paresthesia associated with SSRO. Most commonly it is used to rotate or reposition the mandible posteriorly in patients with mandibular horizontal excess or asymmetry. It is also used for secondary correction of prior SSRO failures. Robinson[44] has suggested its use for mandibular advancements, but because the segment lacks perioperative stability, IVRO is normally not recommended for this type of movement.

These osteotomies extend from the sigmoid notch vertically

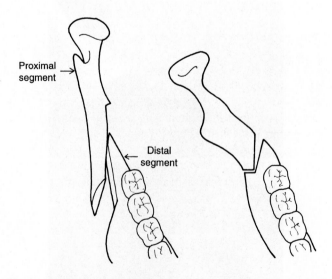

FIGURE 50.16 For large setbacks the distal portion of proximal segment needs to be trimmed to avoid interferences. (From Bloomquist[29])

behind the inferior alveolar nerve foramen to the inferior border or angle of the mandible (see Figure 50.8h). Originally the procedure was done transcutaneously but with the development of oscillating saws and blades a transoral approach became the standard surgical approach.

The surgical incision is similar to the full-thickness mucoperiosteal flap of the sagittal split ramus osteotomy (Figure 50.14). The incision is curvilinear and medial to the buccal fat pad, along the external oblique ridge, and approximately 3 cm in length. The periosteum is reflected laterally to expose the entire ramus from the sigmoid notch to the angle of the mandible. The soft tissues are then retracted and the antelingula is identified as an anatomic reference mark of the inferior alveolar nerve position. The osteotomy can now be safely completed about 7 mm anterior to the posterior border of the ramus but posterior to the mandibular foramen.[29] The osteotomy extends from the sigmoid notch down to the angle of the mandible and involves both medial and lateral cortices (see Figure 50.8h). After completion of the IVRO, the proximal segment is placed lateral to the distal segment and the patient is placed in maxillomandibular fixation. Medial pterygoid attachments are preserved to maintain superior seating of the condyles.

The main fixation method for this type of osteotomy is 6 to 8 weeks of MMF, which is necessary to allow bony union. In order to ensure seating of the condyle in the fossa,[29] minimal medial pterygoid stripping is performed.

When using rigid fixation, a percutaneous trocar is used for appropriate screw placement. The easiest method is to apply two to three screws in a linear fashion securing the proximal to the distal segment.[37] Application of miniplates provides the most rigid fixation, but their placement must be passive to avoid condylar displacement.

Rigid Internal Fixation

Early reports of mandibular osteotomies described fixation of segments via direct wire osteosynthesis and maxillomandibular fixation. With the advent of internal rigid fixation techniques and the development of hardware for maxillofacial applications, orthognathic surgery is now possible without prolonged MMF fixation. This advance has reduced the discomfort associated with weight loss, perioperative airway management difficulties, extended disability, and poor control of segment position during the immediate healing phase.

The best osteosynthesis method for sagittal split ramus osteotomies is still a matter of controversy. Many techniques however have been described for fixation of the proximal segment—wire,[62] pins,[63] bone plates,[64] lag screws or positional screws,[3,58,65–68] and recently resorbable PLLA screws.[69] Spiessl's technique[58] utilized decortication of the external oblique ridge to avoid injury to the mandibular nerve. He recognized the importance of flat sectioning of the mandible to avoid the Hunsuck effect (Figure 50.17) and the role that dif-

ferences in cross-sectional anatomy between the angular and supraangular regions play in achieving this goal. In this way, he was able to achieve interfragmentary compression with 2.7-mm lag screws[65] applied transcutaneously at a right angle to the osteotomy. Jeter et al.[66] advocated using 0.062-in. threaded Kirschner wire to prepare holes in both distal and proximal segments. Then, 2-mm screws were placed transcutaneously perpendicular to the osteotomy. The pattern of placement depended on location of the mandibular canal and varied from three screws on the superior border to two above and one below the canal and vice versa (Figure 50.18). Based on their modification, they claimed that the frequency of neurologic deficiencies decreased from 22% to 4%.[66] Since then, several patterns of screw positioning have been proposed: two tapped lag screws above and one below the mandibular canal[67]; two lag screws below the canal and one above[3]; two self-tapping screws at the superior border of the ramus to avoid neurovascular bundle compression[59,70]; three self-tapping screws placed obliquely at the superior aspect of the ramus[71,72]; etc. Lindorf[68] proposed the use of tandem screw fixation with tapping of the medial and lateral cortex to provide a passive fit and noncompressive positioning of the segments. Recently, Schwimmer et al.[73] studied the effect of screw pattern position and found that the position of the lag screws did not significantly affect the stability of mandibular osteotomies. They also found that a larger 2.7-mm screw provided the same degree of stability as a 2.0-mm screw for stabilization of mandibular osteotomies and supported the already widespread concept that 2.0-mm screws provide adequate stability of mandibular sagittal split osteotomies.[74]

The effect of screw angle on the stability of the mandibular sagittal split ramus osteotomy has been investigated.[71,72,75] It appears that screws oriented at an oblique angle across the osteotomy behave no differently than those placed transcutaneously and perpendicular to the osteotomy.[75] No statistically significant difference in stability is gained by the transoral approach.[75]

Other reported methods for internal rigid fixation of mandibular sagittal split osteotomies have included the use of single- and double-plate systems.[76,77] Single plates are considered to be semirigid fixation and may require the use of skeletal wires or elastic traction to complete immobilization (Figure 50.19). Comparisons of nonrigid wire fixation with rigid fixation osteosynthesis[78,79] have shown that rigid fixation with lag screws results in fewer skeletal changes and improved stability as compared to wire fixation.

An increased risk of mandibular nerve damage has been reported to occur when rigid internal fixation[80] is accomplished with bicortical screws. This may result from compression, direct laceration, or even transection of the nerve during screw placement. The use of miniplates with monocortical screws offers an advantage because compression and direct nerve injury may be avoided.[80] If nerve repairs are necessary, plating also prevents tension on the repaired nerve and facilitates its recovery.

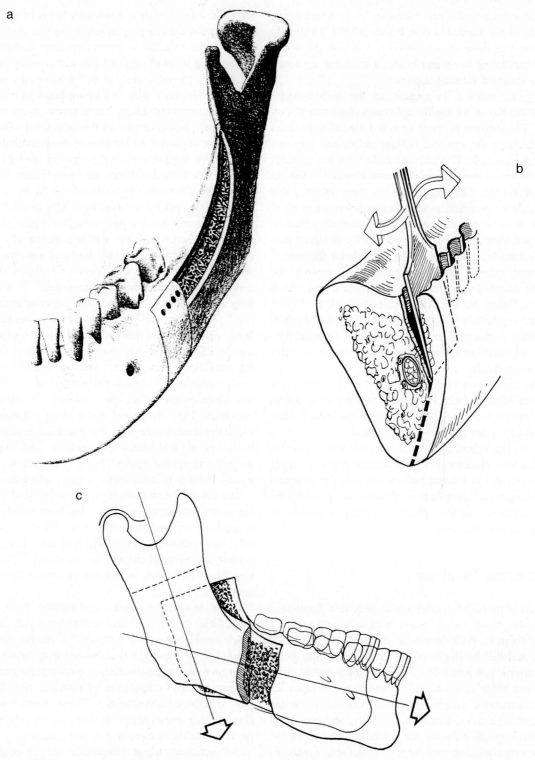

FIGURE 50.17 Spiessl's technique for mandibular sagittal split ramus osteotomies without Hunsuck effect to facilitate lag screw fixation. (a) External oblique ridge corticotomy to allow mandibular ramus sagittal splitting. (b) Cross-sectional view demonstrating complete outer cortex splitting to avoid Hunsuck effect and nerve injury. (c) Complete anteroposterior and superoinferior mandibular sagittal ramus splitting without Hunsuck effect. (From Spiessl,[98] with permission)

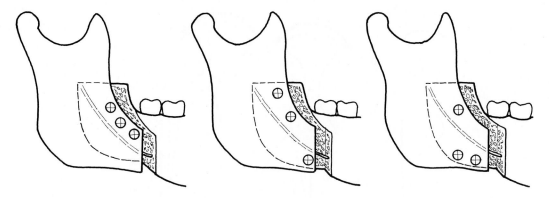

FIGURE 50.18 Screw positioning for maximun bony interface. (From Swift[50])

There has been concern regarding the use of rigid internal fixation and its effects on intercondylar width, condylar torquing, and the condyle-to-fossa relationship.[17] The changes observed are different in advancement versus setback procedures (Figure 50.20). When advancement is performed, there is a greater tendency for the intercondylar distance to increase (Figure 50.20b). When the distal segment is retropositioned, the intercondylar distal is narrowed (Figure 50.20c). This has long-term effects on TMJ remodeling, osteoarthrosis, and degenerative changes resulting in progressive condylar resorption (PCR).

Other mandibular osteotomies are now also stabilized with rigid internal fixation, some to a greater degree than others depending on the orientation and shape of the segments. Because of the need for the placement of screws in a linear vertical fashion has been advocated,[37] the intraoral vertical ramus osteotomy (IVRO) is usually nonrigidly fixated. The perisurgical stability depends on 6 to 8 weeks of MMF fixation. RIF is limited in most cases by the small amount of bone overlap that occurs after the osteotomy. Application of miniplates[37] has also been suggested, but an extraoral approach has been used and although this provides the most rigid fix-

ation, it increases the number of screws that must be placed passively to avoid condylar displacement. The inverted "L" osteotomy lends itself to RIF with application of miniplates and bone grafts. In areas of small bone gaps, position screws must be used to maintain the interbony gap and again prevent condylar displacement.[37]

Horizontal osteotomies of the symphysis (sliding genioplasty) lend themselves to rigid fixation. The flexibility of the various configurations of rigid internal fixation allows a great range of choices. The preferable method, however, is the selection of X-shaped plates (Figure 50.21) bent accordingly to the movement or the use of special genioplasty prebent, preshaped, premeasured X-shaped plates (Figure 50.13c). These plates allow for unequal movements to be accomplished. If an X-shaped plate is not available, paired straight plates should be used to minimize rotation and help distribute forces (Figure 50.13d). It is recommended[60] that two screws be placed in each segment and that these be bicortical if possible. Rigid internal fixation also allows for improvement of stability if a bone gap occurs because the graft may be rigidly fixated into position.

For mandibular subapical osteotomies, rigid internal fixation and an acrylic splint are necessary. Again, X-shaped plates are preferable (Figure 50.10) and should be bent into a passive position to avoid occlusal displacement. Although monocortical screws can be used in the toothbearing segment, bicortical screws are preferable.[60] The X-shaped plates are preferred because their geometry prevents rotation and distributes the forces with minimum hardware. It should be of concern that the osteotomy be accomplished in such a way that good bone buttressing and contact exist after repositioning of the segment. Bone buttressing makes less hardware for fixation necessary.

For the paramidline or anterior midline osteotomy, the use of rigid fixation is more than appropriate. Here, paired plates, mandibular compression plates, or a standard reconstruction plate is indicated together with a lingual acrylic splint to reposition the segments and provide additional stability (see Figure 50.11).

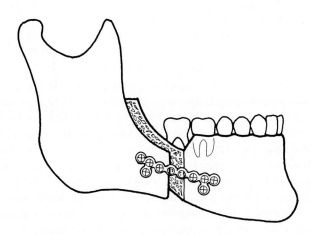

FIGURE 50.19 Bone plate for rigid fixation of sagittal split ramus osteotomy (SSRO). (From Swift[50])

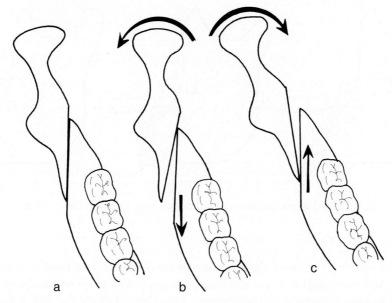

FIGURE 50.20 (a) Position of osteotomy segments before movement. (b) Lateral condylar torquing from mandibular distal segment advancement. (c) Medial condylar torquing from mandibular distal segment setback.

Complications of Rigid Internal Fixation

The primary reported advantages of rigid internal fixation are increased stability, rapid bone healing, and avoidance of long-term MMF. Uneventful bone healing is usually observed in most patients and makes RIF an effective and predictable way of treating mandibular osteotomies[37,50,60,81] and fractures.[8,82–84]

When compared to MMF,[50] the risk of temporomandibular joint arthrosis secondary to immobility is minimized with rigid internal fixation when compared to maxillomandibular fixation.[50] However, 9 months after SSROs these patients are

still 2.5 mm short of their preoperative maximal interincisal opening (MIO)[85] regardless of whether rigid fixation was used.[7,86,87] This reduction in MIO does not occur in patients undergoing simultaneous maxillary and vertical ramus osteotomies who undergo 6 to 8 weeks of MMF,[81] suggesting that this phenomenon may be a complication of the osteotomy itself, rather than the MMF. The reason patients with rigid fixation seem to return to their preoperative function more rapidly is that rapid fixation allows early physiotherapy and opening exercises, rather than actually reducing the risk of iatrogenic temporomandibular joint arthrosis. There is no doubt that changes in intercondylar width,[88–90] axial inclination of the condylar heads,[91] and horizontal vertical positioning of the condylar heads in the glenoid fossa[50] occur with application of rigid internal fixation. Tuinzing and Swart[92] found that when compression and bicortical screws are used, intercondylar width increases with mandibular advancement and decreases with mandibular retropositioning (Figure 50.20).

In most patients, condylar heads undergo remodeling, resorption, and other adaptive changes with little or no temporomandibular joint symptoms. In addition, during sagittal split ramus osteotomy surgery condylar torquing occurs, which causes edema in and around the joint. This results in immediate occlusal discrepancies and "condylar sagging".[50] Within a few days, this edema decreases and the inferior condylar position resolves with no adverse effects, malocclusion, or TMJ symptoms.[50] It is during this period (7–10 days) that postoperative maxillomandibular training elastics are encouraged[93] to help retrain the patient's jaw movements and allow for condylar adaptation to the new occlusion. It also compensates for the muscle spasms that usually accompany extensive surgical movements.

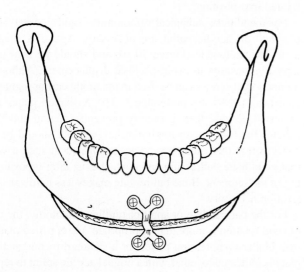

FIGURE 50.21 Double Y miniplate fixation of genioplasty. (From Shafer and Assael[25])

Fibrous ankylosis of the temporomandibular joint following rigid fixation has been reported.[94] Ordinarily, when rigid fixation is used, intermaxillary fixation is not necessary. In the patients described, MMF was also used for 6 to 8 weeks in addition to rigid fixation. It has been speculated that in those patients long-term compression of the cartilage by the condylar head resulted in its disintegration and the formation of fibrous adhesions.[94]

Postoperative infection is a rare occurrence, but it has been reported[95] to be three times more frequent among patients with rigid internal fixation than among those with wire osteosynthesis. This may be related to increased soft tissue stripping, associated dead space, and length of operation. It is now routine for surgeons performing orthognathic surgery to use a bolus of antibiotics at the inception of the surgical procedure and to continue their IV use in the immediate postoperative period.

In addition to the trauma caused by the osteotomy procedure, rigid internal fixation has also been reported to increase trauma to the alveolar nerve.[3,81] The literature is replete with reports describing an increased incidence of neurosensory disturbances. Neurosensory disturbances may be as high as 60%[3] and as low as 1 in 25 patients.[96] Experimental studies[97] suggest that rigid internal fixation should only be done with bicortical screws, rather than with lag screws. This allows for a constant space between the osteotomy segments and prevents undesirable compression of the inferior alveolar nerve. Placement of the screws themselves may compress, lacerate, or transect the inferior alveolar nerve. Avoidance of screw placement at the inferior border and good radiographic evaluation are necessary to prevent this complication.

The goal of rigid fixation is to achieve stability of segments for predictable and uneventful healing. The fact that rigid fixation permits bone healing by primary intention speaks for a compression technique. Yet, when two segments of bone are held together with compressive force, union will occur without callus formation, but this union will not be stronger. Spiessl[98,99] emphasizes this point: "From a clinical standpoint, primary bone union is not the true therapeutic goal" (of rigid fixation). "It is immaterial whether the bone consolidation is accomplished indirectly, through differentiation of fibrous tissue, or by direct regeneration of osteons." The aim of rigid fixation is to provide a functionally stable fixation of bone segments until bone healing is achieved. One should keep in mind that because the condyle is seated in the fossa and the occlusion is fixed, any gaps between the osteotomy segments should not be rigidly fixated using a compression technique because this would draw the segments together, unseat the condyles, or disturb the occlusion. Conventional bicortical screws will then suffice because stability of the segments is accomplished with avoidance of nerve entrapment by compression. Miniplates and elastic traction MMF can also achieve this goal.

Removal of bone plates and screws has received much attention[81] for several reasons. It is argued that such plates act as stress protectors, not allowing bone to be exposed to the full range of physiologic stresses and increasing the risk of fractures at the osteosynthesis site.[81] An increase of metal alloy content has also been found in soft tissues, serum, and urine.[100,101]

The basic argument against removal of these implants is that although corrosion does occur, the incidence of infections and other complications is relatively low.[3] Also, a surgical procedure to remove the implants carries a morbidity risk for infection, nerve damage, and anesthesia complications.[81] With the change to titanium implants, the question of hardware removal is no longer important because titanium, at present, does not appear to have any of the clinical characteristics and properties of the aluminum alloys.[100–104] Implant removal should be based on the presence of infection, patient discomfort, or exposure and loosening of the implant. Resorbable plates and screws when used in selected cases avoid the need for later hardware removal.[69]

Addendum: Distraction Osteogenesis

Distraction osteogenesis has become a new method for mandibular lengthening and widening.[105–107] New techniques utilizing extraoral and intraoral devices permit lengthening of the ramus and body.[108–110] Lengthening of the ramus and body can be performed as a simultaneous procedure using multivector distraction devices.[111] Mandibular widening has also been reported with satisfactory periodontal health maintained.[112–113] Mandibular distraction is particularly advantageous for its use in pediatric patients with microgenia, allowing earlier tracheostomy cannulation and in some cases the avoidance of tracheostomy.[114] Mandibular ramus lengthening for hemifacial microsomia can also avoid the multiple combined osteotomy and bone grafting procedures that have been traditionally used.[115] Continued evolution of these techniques, such as manual molding of the regenerate callus[116] will influence the indications and methods used for traditional mandibular osteotomies.

Conclusions

Mandibular osteotomies have undergone dramatic evolution over the past 150 years with modern refinements of both bone-cutting techniques and fixation methods. The future may bring new developments in the form of lighter semirigid resorbable implants. Distraction osteogenesis is a promising new methodology that will undoubtedly provide additional treatment modalities for mandibular osteotomies in the future.

References

1. Hullihen SP. A case of elongation of the under jaw and distortion of the face and neck, caused by a burn: successfully treated. *Am J Dent Sci.* 1849;9:157–165.

2. McDonald WR. Champy bone plate fixation in sagittal split osteotomy for mandibular advancement. *Int J Adult Orthod Orthognath Surg.* 1987;2:89–97.

3. Steinhauser EW. Bone screws and plates in orthognathic surgery. *Int J Oral Surg.* 1982;11:209–216.

4. Krekmanov L, Lilja J. Orthognathic surgery with no post-operative intermaxillary fixation. *Scand J Plast Reconstr Surg.* 1986;21:189–197.

5. Cawood J. Small plate osteosynthesis of mandibular fractures. *Br J Oral Maxillofac Surg* 1985;23:77–91.

6. Leonard MS, Ziman P, Bevis R, Cavanaugh G, Speidel MT, Worms F. The sagittal split osteotomy of the mandible. *Oral Surg Oral Med Oral Pathol.* 1985;60:459–466.

7. Aragon SB, Van Sickels JE, Dolwick F, Flanary CM. The effects of orthognathic surgery on mandibular range of motion. *J Oral Maxillofac Surg.* 1985;43:938–943.

8. Storum KA, Bell WH. Hypomobility after maxillary and mandibular osteotomies. *Oral Surg Oral Med Oral Pathol.* 1984;57:7–12.

9. Aragon SB, Van Sickels JE. Mandibular range of motion with rigid/non-rigid fixation. *Oral Surg Oral Med Oral Pathol.* 1987;63:408–411.

10. Lydiatt DD, Davis LF. The effects of immobilization on the rabbit temporomandibular joint. *J Oral Maxillofac Surg.* 1985; 43:188–293.

11. Van Sickels JE, Flanary CM. Stability associated with mandibular advancement treated by rigid osseous fixation. *J Oral Maxillofac Surg.* 1985;43:338–341.

12. Kirkpatrick TB, Woods MG, Swift JQ, Markowitz NR. Skeletal stability following mandibular advancement and rigid fixation. *J Oral Maxillofac Surg* 1987;45:572–576.

13. Van Sickels JE. Relapse after rigid fixation of mandibular advancement. *J Oral Maxillofac Surg.* 1986;44:698–702.

14. Storum KA, Bell WH. The effects of physical rehabilitation on mandibular function after ramus osteotomies. *J Oral Maxillofac Surg.* 1986;44:94–99.

15. Epker BN, Turvey T, Fish LC. Indications for simultaneous mobilization of the maxilla and mandible for the correction of dentofacial deformities. *Oral Surg Oral Med Oral Pathol.* 1982;54:369–381.

16. Turvey T, Hale DJ, Fish LC. Surgical-orthodontic treatment planning for simultaneous mobilization of the maxilla and mandible in the correction of dentofacial deformities. *Oral Surg Oral Med Oral Pathol.* 1982;54:491–498.

17. Kraut RA. Simultaneous maxillary and mandibular orthognathic surgery stabilized by rigid internal fixation. *Oral Surg Oral Med Oral Pathol.* 1990;69:427–430.

18. Spitzer W, Rettinger G, Sitzmann F. Computerized tomographic examination for the detection of positional changes in the temporomandibular joint after ramus osteotomies with screw fixation. *J Oral Maxillofac Surg* 1984;12:139–242.

19. Persson G, Hellem S, Nord PG. Bone plates for stabilizing of the LeFort I osteotomy. *J Oral Maxillofac Surg.* 1986;14:69–73.

20. Dingman RO. Surgical correction of mandibular prognathism. *Am J Orthod Oral Surg.* 1944;30:683–692.

21. Blair VP. Report of a case of double resection for the correction of protrusion of the mandible. *Dent Cosmos.* 1906;48: 817–820.

22. Harsha WM. Bilateral resection of the jaw for prognathism: report of a case. *Surg Gynecol Obstet.* 1912;15:51–53.

23. Hofer O. Die Operative behandlung der alveolären Retraktion des Unterkiefers u ihre Anwendungsmöglichkeit für Prognathie und Mikrogenie. *Dtsch-Zahn-Mund Kieferheilkd.* 1942;9(3): 121–132.

24. Köle H. Indikation und Plauong von kieferorthopädischen Operationen (Distalbiss, alveolare protursion und retrusion). *Oesterr Z Stomatol.* 1960;57:212.

25. Shafer DM, Assael LA. Rigid internal fixation of mandibular segmental osteotomies. *Atlas Oral Maxillofac Surg Clin North Am.* 1993;1:41–51.

26. Kent JN, Hinds E. Management of dental facial deformities by anterior alveolar surgery. *J Oral Surg.* 1971;29:13–26.

27. MacIntosch RB. Total mandibular alveolar osteotomy: encouraging experiences with an infrequently indicated procedure. *J Maxillofac Surg.* 1974;2:210–218.

28. Angle EH. Double resection of the lower maxilla. *Dent Cosmos.* 1889;40:635–638.

29. Bloomquist DS. Principles of mandibular orthognathic surgery. In: Peterson LJ, Andresano AT, Marciani RD, Roser SM, eds. *Principles of Oral and Maxillofacial Surgery.* Philadelphia: JB Lippincott; 1992:1415–1463.

30. Von Eiselberg J. Ueber plastik bei Ektropium des Unterkiefers (progenie). *Wien Klin Wochenschr.* 1906;19:1505–1508.

31. Blair VP. Operations of the jaw bone and face. *Surg Gynecol Obstet.* 1907;4:67–78.

32. Limberg A. Treatment of open-bite by means of plastic oblique osteotomy of the ascending rami of the mandible. *Dent Cosmos.* 1925;67:1191–1200.

33. Moose SM. Surgical correction of mandibular prognathism by intraoral subcondylar osteotomy. *J Oral Surg Anesth Hosp Dent Serv.* 1964;22:197–202.

34. Kazanjian V, Converse J. *The Surgical Treatment of Facial Injuries.* 2nd ed. Baltimore: Williams & Wilkins; 1959.

35. Ernst F. Uber die chirurgische beseitigung der prognathie des unterkiefers. *Zentralbl Chir.* 1938;65:179.

36. Obwegeser H, Trauner R. Zur Operationstechnik bei der Progenie und anderen Unterkieferanomalien. *Dtsch Zahn Kieferheilkd.* 1955;23:H1–H2.

37. Tucker MR. Surgical correction of mandibular excess. *Atlas Oral Maxillofac Surg Clin North Am.* 1993;1:29–39.

38. Kostečka F. A contribution to the surgical treatment of open bite. *Int J Orthod.* 1934;28:1082–1092.

39. Thoma KH. Surgical treatment of deformities of the jaw. *Am J Orthod.* 1946;32:333–339.

40. Robinson M. Prognathism corrected by open vertical subcondylotomy. *J Oral Surg.* 1958;16:215–219.

41. Caldwell JB, Letterman GS. Vertical osteotomy in the mandibular rami for correction of prognathism. *J Oral Surg.* 1954;12:185–202.

42. Robinson M. Micrognathism corrected by vertical osteotomy of ascending ramus and iliac bone graft: a new technique. *Oral Surg Oral Med Oral Pathol.* 1957;10:1125–1130.

43. Caldwell JB, Amaral WJ. Mandibular micrognathism corrected by vertical osteotomy in the rami and iliac bone graft. *J Oral Surg.* 1960;18:3–15.

44. Robinson M, Lytle JJ. Micrognathism corrected by vertical osteotomies of the rami without bone grafts. *Oral Surg Oral Med Oral Pathol.* 1962;15:641–645.

45. Wassmund M. *Fracturen und Luxationen des Gesichtschadels* unter Beruksichtigung der Komplikationen des Hirnschadels.

In *Klinik und Therapie*. Praktischen Lehrbuch, Vol. 20 Berlin: Hermann Meusser; 1927.

46. Hawkinson RT. Retrognathia correction by means of an arcing osteotomy in the ascending ramus. *J Prosthet Dent*. 1968; 20:77–86.

47. Hayes PA. Correction of retrognathia by modified "C" osteotomy of the ramus sagittal osteotomy of the mandibular body. *J Oral Surg*. 1973;31:682–686.

48. Fox GL, Tilson HB. Mandibular retrognathia: a review of the literature and selected cases. *J Oral Surg*. 1976;34:53–61.

49. Caldwell JB, Hayward JR. Lister RL. Correction of mandibular retrognathia by vertical-L osteotomy: a new technique. *J Oral Surg*. 1968;26:259–264.

50. Swift JQ. Mandibular advancement. *Atlas Oral Maxillofac Surg Clin North Am*. 1993;1:17–27.

51. Trauner R, Obwegeser H. The surgical correction of mandibular prognathism and retrognathia with considerations of genioplasty. I. Surgical procedures to conect mandibular prognathism and reshaping the chin. *Oral Surg Oral Med Oral Pathol*. 1957;10:677–689.

52. Neuner O. Circa un nuovo metodo per la cura chirurgica della progenia. *Riv Ital Stomatol*. 1958;13:1573.

53. Neuner O. Beitrag zur progenie operationen am aufsteigenden unterkieferast. *Dtsch Zahnaerztl Z*. 1958;13:1416.

54. Dal Pont G. Retromolar osteotomy for the correction of prognathism. *J Oral Surg*. 1961;19:42–47.

55. Hunsuck EE. A modified intraoral sagittal splitting technic for correction of mandibular prognathism. *J Oral Surg*. 1968;26: 250–253.

56. Wolford LM, Davis WM. The mandibular inferior border split: a modification in the sagittal split osteotomy. *J Oral Maxillofac Surg*. 1990;48:92–94.

57. Epker BN. Modification in the sagittal osteotomy of the mandible. *J Oral Surg*. 1977;35:157–159.

58. Spiessl B. Osteosynthese bei sagittaler Osteotomie nach Obwegeser-Dal Pont. *Fortschr Kieferheilkd Gesichtschir*. 1974;18:145–148.

59. Shufford EL, Kraut RA. Passive rigid fixation of sagittal split osteotomy. *Oral Surg Oral Med Oral Pathol*. 1989;68:150–153.

60. Shafer DM, Assael LA. Rigid internal fixation of mandibular segmental osteotomies. *Atlas Oral Maxillofac Surg Clin North Am*. 1993;1:41–51.

61. Ritzau M, Wenzel A, Williams S. Changes in condyle position after bilateral vertical ramus osteotomy with and without osteosynthesis. *Am J Orthod Dentofacial Orthop*. 1989;96:507–513.

62. Booth DF. Control of the proximal segment by lower border wiring in the sagittal split osteotomy. *J Oral Maxillofac Surg*. 1981;9:126–128.

63. Gingrass DJ, Messer EJ. Rigid non-compressive pin fixation of the mandibular sagittal split osteotomy. *J Oral Maxillofac Surg*. 1986;44:413–416.

64. McDonald WR, Stoelinga PJ, Blijdorp PA, Schoenaers JA. Champy bone plate fixation in sagittal split osteotomies for mandibular advancement. *Int J Adult Orthod Orthognath Surg*. 1987;2:89–97.

65. Spiessl B. The sagittal splitting osteotomy for correction of mandibular prognathism. *Clin Plast Surg*. 1982;9:491–507.

66. Jeter TS, Van Sickels JE, Solwick MF. Modified techniques for internal fixation of sagittal ramus osteotomies. *J Oral Maxillofac Surg*. 1984;42:270–272.

67. Spiessl B. Rigid internal fixation after sagittal split osteotomy of the ascending ramus. In: Spiessl B. *New Concepts in Maxillofacial Bone Surgery*. New York: Springer-Verlag; 1976:21.

68. Lindorf HH. Sagittal split osteotomy with tandem screw fixation: techniques and results. *J Oral Maxillofac Surg*. 1986;14: 311–316.

69. Suuronen R, Laine P, Sarkiala E, Pohjnen T, Lindqvist C. Sagittal split ramus osteotomy fixed with biodegradable self-reinforced poly-L-lactide screws. A pilot study in sheep. *Int J Oral Maxillofac Surg*. 1992;21:303–308.

70. Shepherd JP, Dohvoma CN, Harradine NW. Screw fixation after mandibular sagittal split osteotomy: an intraoral approach. *Br J Oral Maxillofac Surg*. 1991;29:325–329.

71. Turvey T, Hall D. Intraoral self-threading screw fixation for sagittal osteotomies: early experiences. *Int J Adult Orthod Orthognath Surg*. 1986;1:243–250.

72. Kempf KK. Transoral technique for rigid fixation of sagittal ramus osteotomies. *J Oral Maxillofac Surg*. 1987;45:1077–1079.

73. Schwimmer A, Greenberg AM, Kummer G, Kaynar A. The effect of screw size and insertion technique on the stability of the mandibular sagittal split osteotomy. *J Oral Maxillofac Surg*. 1994;52:45–48.

74. Van Sickels JE, Richardson DA. Stability of orthognathic surgery: a review of rigid fixation. *Br J Oral Maxillofac Surg*. 1996;34:279–285.

75. Foley WL, Frost DE, Paulin WB, et al. Internal screw fixation: Comparison of placement pattern and rigidity. *J Oral Maxillofac Surg*. 1989;47:720.

76. Luhr HG. Compression plate osteosynthesis through the Luhr system. In: Kruger E, Schilli S, eds. *Oral and Maxillofacial Traumatology*. Vol. 1. Chicago: Quintessence; 1982:319.

77. Champy M, Pape HD, Gerlach KL. The Strasbourg miniplate osteosynthesis. In: Kruger E, Schilli, W, eds. *Oral Maxillofacial Traumatology*. Vol. 2. Chicago: Quintessence; 1986:19.

78. Thomas PM, Tucker MR, Prewitt JR, Proffit WR. Early skeletal and dental changes following mandibular advancement and rigid internal fixation. *Int J Adult Orthod Orthognath Surg*. 1986;3:171–178.

79. Van Sickels JE, Flanary CM. Stability associated with mandibular advancement treated by rigid osseous fixation. *J Oral Maxillofac Surg*. 1985;43:338–341.

80. Nishioka G, Zysset M, Van Sickels J. Neurosensory disturbance with rigid internal fixation of the bilateral sagittal split osteotomy. *J Oral Maxillofac Surg*. 1987;45:20–26.

81. Leonard MS. Rigid internal fixation: facts vs. fallacies. *Atlas Oral Maxillofac Clin North Am*. 1990;2:737–743.

82. Strelzow VV, Strelzow AG. Osteosynthesis of mandibular fractures of the angle region. *Arch Otolaryngol*. 1983;109:403–406.

83. Tu HK, Tenhulzen D. Compression osteosynthesis of mandibular fractures: a retrospective study. *J Oral Maxillofac Surg*. 1985;43:585–589.

84. Iizuka T, Lindqvist C. Rigid internal fixation of fractures in the angular region of the mandible: an analysis of factors contributing to different complications. *Plast Reconstr Surg*. 1993; 91:265–271.

85. Stacy GC. Recovery of oral opening following sagittal ramus osteotomy for mandibular. *J Oral Maxillofac Surg*. 1987;45: 487–492.

86. Storum KA, Bell WH. Hypomobility after maxillary and mandibular osteotomies. *Oral Surg Oral Med Oral Pathol.* 1984;57:7–12.

87. Storum KA, Bell WH. The effect of physical rehabilitation on mandibular function after ramus osteotomies. *J Oral Maxillofac Surg.* 1986;44:94–99.

88. Freihofer HP Jr. Modellversuch zur Lageveranderung des kieferkopfchens nach sagittaler Spaltung des Unterkiefers. *SSO Schweiz Monatsschr Zahnheilkd.* 1977;87:12–22.

89. Kundert M, Hadjianghelou O. Condylar displacement after sagittal splitting of the mandibular rami. A short term radiographic study. *J Maxillofac Surg.* 1980;8:278–287.

90. Spitzer W, Rettinger G, Sitzmann F. Computerized tomography examination for the detection of positional changes in the temporomandibular joint after ramus osteotomies with screw fixation. *J Oral Maxillofac Surg.* 1984;12:139–142.

91. Hackney FL, Van Sickels JE, Nummikoski PV. Condylar displacement and temporomandibular joint dysfunction following bilateral sagittal split osteotomies and rigid fixation. *J Oral Maxillofac Surg.* 1989;47:223–227.

92. Tuinzing DB, Swart JGN. Lageveranderungen des caput mandibular bei verwendung von zugschrauben nach sagittaler osteotomie des unterkiefers. *Dtsch Zahn Mund Kieferheilkd Gesichts Chir.* 1978;2:94.

93. Bock JT. Horizontal condylar angulation changes following forward and backward sagittal split ramus osteotomy with rigid screw fixation. Dissertation. Minneapolis: University of Minnesota; 1986.

94. Nitzan DW, Dolwick MF. Temporomandibular ankylosis following orthognathic surgery: report of eight cases. *Int J Adult Orthodon Orthognath Surg.* 1989;4:7–11.

95. Buckley MJ, Tullock JF, White RP Jr, Tucker MR. Complications of orthognathic surgery: a comparison between wire fixation and rigid internal fixation. *Int J Adult Orthodon Orthognath Surg.* 1989;2:69–74.

96. Souryis F. Sagittal splitting and bicortical screw fixation of the ascending ramus. *J Maxillofac Surg.* 1978;6:198–203.

97. Ikemura K, Hidaka H, Etoh T, Kabata K. Osteosynthesis in facial bone fractures using miniplates: clinical and experimental studies. *J Oral Maxillofac Surg.* 1988;46:10–14.

98. Spiessl B. The stability principle. In: *Internal mandible.* New York: Springer-Verlag; 1988:16.

99. Spiessl B. Biomechanics. In: *Internal fixation of the Mandible.* New York: Springer-Verlag; 1988:28.

100. Balck J. Does corrosion matter? *J Bone Joint Surg.* 1988;70:517–520.

101. Gillespie WJ, Frampton CMA, Henderson PJ. The incidence of cancer following total hip replacement [published erratum appears in *J Bone Joint Surg [Br]* 1996 Jul;78(4):680]. *J Bone Joint Surg.* 1988;70:539–542.

102. Bell WH. *Modern Practice in Orthognathic and Reconstructive Surgery.* Vol. III. Philadelphia: WB Saunders; 1992.

103. Powell NB, Riley RW. Obstructive sleep apnea. *Atlas Oral Maxillofac Surg Clin North Am.* 1990;2(4):843–853.

104. Edwards RC, Kiely KD, Eppley BL. Fixation of bimaxillary osteotomies with resorbable plates and screws: experience in 20 consecutive cases. *J Oral Maxillofac Surg.* 2001;59:271–276.

105. McCarthy JG, Stelnicki EJ, Grayson BH. Distraction osteogenesis of the mandible: a ten year experience. *Semin Orthod.* 1999;5:3–8.

106. van Strijen PJ, Perdijk FB, Becking AG, et al. Distraction osteogenesis for mandibular advancement. *Int J Oral Maxillofac Surg.* 2000;29:81–85.

107. Carls FR, Sailer HF. Seven years clinical experience with mandibular distraction in children. *J Craniomaxillofac Surg.* 1998;26:197–208.

108. Dessner S, Razdolsky Y, El-Bialy T, et al. Mandibular lengthening using programmed intraoral tooth-borne distraction devises. *J Oral Maxillofac Surg.* 1999;57:1318–1322.

109. McCarthy JG, Williams JK, Grayson BH, et al. Controlled multiplanar distraction of the mandible: device development and clinical application. *J Craniofac Surg.* 1998;9:322–329.

110. Haug RH, Nuveen EJ, Barber JE, et al. An in vitro evaluation of distractors used for osteogenesis. *Oral Surg Oral Pathol Oral Radiol Endod.* 1998;86:648–659.

111. Gateno J, Teichgraeber JF, Aguilar E. Distraction osteogenesis: a new surgical technique for use with the multiplanar mandibular distractor. *Plast Reconstr Surg.* 2000;105:883–888.

112. Guerero CA, Bell WH, Costasti GI, et al. Mandibular widening by intraoral distraction osteogenesis. *Br J Oral Maxillofac Surg.* 1997;35:383–392.

113. Kewitt GF, Van Sickels JE. Long term effect of mandibular midline distraction osteogenesis on the status of the temporomandibular joint, teeth, peridontal structures, and neurosensory function. *J Oral Maxillofac Surg.* 1999;57:1419–1425.

114. Morovic CG, Monasterio L. Distraction osteogenesis for obstructive apneas in patients with congenital craniofacial malformations. *Plast Reconstr Surg.* 2000;105:2324–2330.

115. Kusnoto B, Figueroa AA, Polley JW. A longitudinal three-dimensional evaluation of the growth pattern in hemifacial microsomia treated by mandibular distraction osteogenesis: a preliminary report. *J Craniofac Surg.* 1999;10:480–486.

116. Kunz C, Hammer B, Prein J. Manipulation of the callus after linear distraction: a "lifeboat" or an alternative to multivectorial distraction osteogenesis of the mandible? *Plast Reconstr Surg.* 2000;10:674–679.

51
Genioplasty Techniques and Considerations for Rigid Internal Fixation

Frans H.M. Kroon

Genioplastic corrective surgery has been used for many years.[1,2] Owing to the improvement of fixation techniques with plates and screws,[2] as in fracture treatment, reconstructive and corrective bone surgery has become considerably more predictable than was possible when wire osteosyntheses were used. In this chapter, the advantages of stable fixation of genioplasties will be described. Genioplastic surgery can be defined in two ways. First, it is an active surgical procedure that is either restricted to the site of the chin bone area or used in combination with other surgical corrective procedures in the mandible. Second, it can also be a passive surgical procedure in the sense that it is an effect of other facial corrective surgery (e.g., a mandibular setback or advancement in combination with osteotomies of the midface).

Genioplasty can be used for esthetic reasons alone, or it can be considered in relation to and in combination with facial corrections for other functional reasons.

Both active and passive genioplastic surgery always requires thorough evaluation of the facial skeleton and associated soft tissues, and careful prediction planning is necessary to achieve a satisfactory esthetic result.[3,4]

Anatomical Considerations

Each individual anatomical configuration will determine the surgical possibilities for genioplasty, and it is worthwhile to include a few remarks on the anatomy of the chin area. Embryologically, the chin bone, or symphyseal area, is developed by fusion of the two halves of the mandible in the midline of the face.

Although even in adults (Figure 51.1) there can still be radiologic evidence of the symphyseal midline, functionally the chin-bone area may be considered as a continuous structure of the mandible.

The functional "borders" of the chin area can be described as follows:

1. A very solid cortical bone ridge as part of the mandibular inferior border ventrocaudal creates the chin point known as the *mental protuberance* just lateral to which the men-

tal tubercles are formed. These support the soft tissues of the chin area and determine the cosmetic appearance.
2. In the vertical, or coronal, direction, the chin area is limited by the root apices of the lower incisors and canines.
3. The width in the buccolingual direction is determined by the amount of bone marrow and the thickness of the lingual and buccal cortical bone layers. It is also very closely related to the dimensions of the roots of these teeth. In cases of agenesis, there is even a striking minimum of spongeous bone between the two cortical layers, which fuse to the top of the alveolar process (Figure 51.2).
4. In the lateral direction, the chin-area border is determined by the length of the roots of the lower canine and first premolar and the position of the mental foramen. With respect to this, however, one has to realize that in the mandibular canal the alveolar nerve runs slightly frontocaudally from the mental foramen before it turns back and upward to leave the foramen as the mental nerve. Before doing so, a frontal branch occurs, which in many genioplasties will be surgically violated.

In designing and planning the genioplasty, it is important to note the position and function of some other landmarks:

1. The origins/insertions of the geniohyoid and genioglossus muscles
2. The insertion of the median raphe of the mylohyoid muscle
3. The insertions and configuration of the mental and mentolabial muscles at the frontal site

Vascular supply of the chin bone in a genioplasty procedure is sufficiently preserved by leaving the caudal side attached to the soft tissues of the chin. In studies of long-term results, bone apposition is seen at point B and slight resorption occurs at pogonion.

Analysis of Facial Anatomy

To evaluate and determine the position of the chin, several methods of facial analysis are available.[5–12]

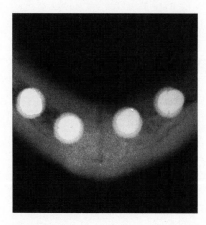

FIGURE 51.1 Occlusal view of symphyseal area of 53-year-old man, edentulous for 30 years. Clear evidence of symphyseal midline septum (white spots represent implants).

It is important to study both the bony and soft tissue configurations. The final interpretation of measurements should also take into consideration the relative importance of the nasolabial angle, the length of the upper lip, the extent of visibility of parts of the dentition, the labiomental fold in relation to the position of teeth, and the curvature of the chin to the throat area.

In addition to the evaluation of the lateral x-rays and photographs, it is very important to study the direct frontal appearance of the chin. In particular, the position and functional effects of mental muscles may determine the design of the genioplasty. Furthermore, it is important to realize that the effects of profile changes in the chin area are quite different in the horizontal and vertical directions depending on the type and direction of the osteotomies. In horizontal augmentation procedures, different ratios between soft tissue and hard tissue are mentioned, from 60% to 75%.[13,14] In reduction procedures, there is always the danger of weakening of the soft tissues of the chin. Stable internal fixation has been shown to give improved reliability of the clinical results.[13–15] Likewise, the final outcome of passive chin surgery as an effect of mandibular advancement or setback procedures is closely related to the extent of horizontal and vertical vectors of the change in position of the chin. Forward or backward positioning along the line of occlusion will always be followed by the chin. However, correction of an Angle class II/1 (deep bite) will at the same time lengthen the vertical height in the chin area, straighten the mentolabial fold, and still move the chin forward less than the incisor region (Figure 51.3). This relative clockwise rotation of the chin is frequently an adequate correction of an otherwise undesired forward-positioning of the chin.

Figure 51.4 shows another clinical result of a passive genioplasty. Severe Angle class II/1 (deep bite) was corrected by mandibular advancement (sagittal split osteotomy) in conjunction with Köle osteotomy for surgical intrusion of the incisor segment (anterior mandibular segment from cuspid to cuspid), stable fixation with positioning screws in the mandibular angle, and the placement of two 2.0-mm miniplates and one central lag screw (2.0 mm) in the Köle segment.

Indications and Classifications

In general, the indication for a genioplasty is determined by the need to maintain or to move the chin bone area of the mandible by surgical intervention into such a position that it is in harmony with the references of hard- and soft-tissue analyses of a particular patient.

a

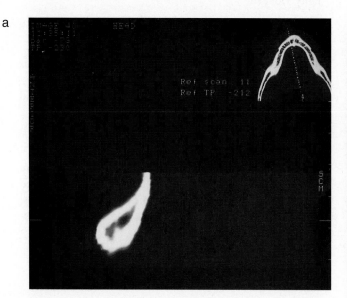

b

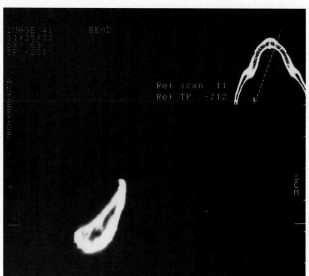

FIGURE 51.2 Photograph of CT imaging of vertical configuration of symphyseal area left (a) and right (b) of midline in a 21-year-old man with agenesis of the dentition. Thick cortical layers, hardly any marrow, and concave configuration are at the anterior side.

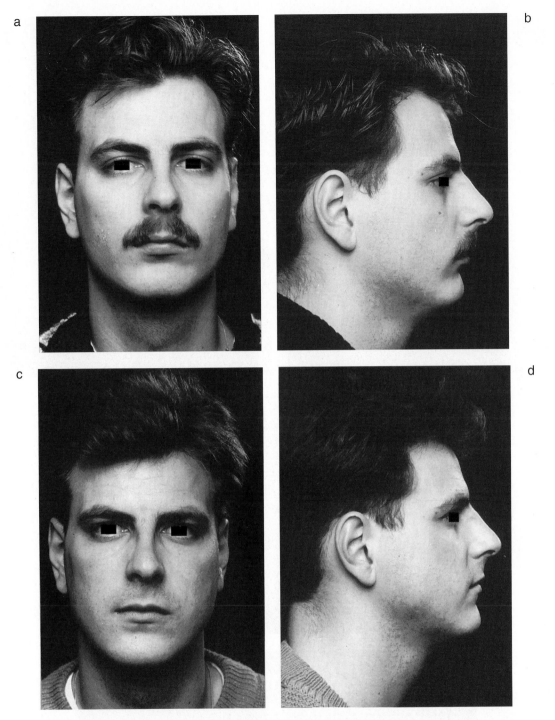

FIGURE 51.3 Clinical example of passive genioplasty. Presurgical and postsurgical photographs of a 22-year-old man with Angle class II/1 (deep bite) corrected by surgical advancement of the mandible (bilateral sagittal split osteotomy). Note the improvement of the chin position, lengthening of the anterior height, and stretching of the inferior labial fold. (a) Presurgical frontal view. (b) Presurgical in profile. (c) Postsurgical frontal view. (d) Postsurgical in profile.

a

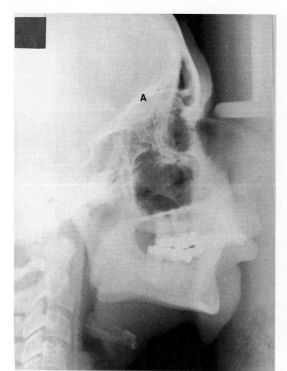

b

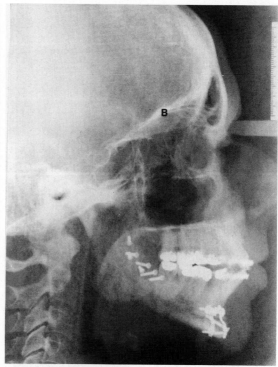

c

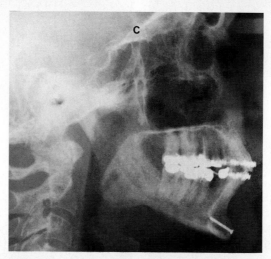

d

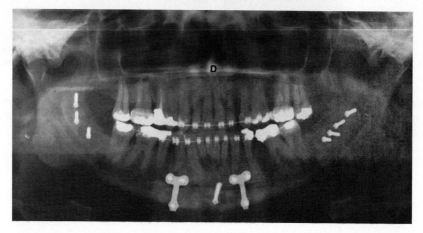

TABLE 51.1 Classification for genioplasties related to the main direction of change in position of the chin.

1. Horizontal	a. Backward
	b. Forward
2. Vertical	a. Upward
	b. Downward
3. Lateral to correct asymmetry	
4. Combinations	

TABLE 51.2 Classification for genioplasties related to the main clinical change in appearance.

1. Augmentation	a. Horizontal
	b. Vertical
2. Reduction	a. Horizontal
	b. Vertical
3. Correction of asymmetry	
4. Combinations	

Classifications for genioplasties are most practical if they are related either to the direction of the change in position of the chin (Table 51.1) or to the proposed clinical change in appearance (Table 51.2).

In the case of asymmetry, an anteroposterior x-ray and a submentovertex x-ray should be taken and analyzed to measure the discrepancies and to determine the extent of bony corrections. Several methods have been described.[20]

Prediction Measurements

Measurements for prediction can be drawn on lateral cephalometric radiograph tracings. This method gives acceptable and sufficient information about the surgical possibilities in the hard tissue and the clinical effect at the site of the soft tissue.[6,16,17] In recent years, three-dimensional computerized hard- and soft-tissue prediction programs have become available.[18]

After analysis of the lateral cephalometric x-ray, the required transposition of the bony chin can be drawn and measured (Figure 51.5). To have a controlled clinical prediction, it is wise to correlate the drawing to the position of the lower incisor. An equilateral rhomboid parallelogram can be constructed by drawing crosspoint X between the lower incisor line and an occlusal line connecting the tips of the molars, cuspids, and incisors. Parallel to this occlusal line, the baseline is drawn from where the incisor line crosses the inferior mandibular border (point Y). The length XY is used as measure for the four sides of the parallelogram. The next step is to choose how to divide the angle between baseline and incisorline. In case of the bisector, the transposition effects in both the horizontal and vertical directions are of equal length. If the inclination is less steep (i.e., $\alpha < \beta$), the horizontal effect will be greater than the vertical effect. If the inclination is steeper (i.e., $\alpha > \beta$), the vertical effect is bigger than the horizontal effect. Earl and Foster described an apparatus that can be used during surgery to maintain the orientation with the planned angle during bone sawing. Depending on the required transposition, the angle of the inclination can be chosen and the horizontal and vertical coordinates can be measured.[19]

Surgical Approach

A genioplasty procedure can be performed completely intraorally. Preferably, the mucosal incision lies in the nonattached gingiva deep enough in the vestibular sulcus to have enough soft tissue to close the incision afterwards. Laterally, the incision should be superior to the mental nerve. Generally, it is wise to first identify the mental foramen and preserve its nerve through a safe and correct orientation of the osteotomy. Incisions that extend further out in the labial part of the lateral vestibule tend to cross the fine branches of the mental nerve.

The periosteum should always be kept attached to the frontal part of the chin to maintain sufficient vascular blood supply. The periosteum should be kept in good condition to

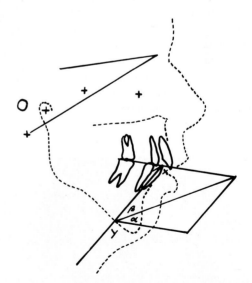

FIGURE 51.4 Clinical result of a passive genioplasty procedure to correct a severe Angle class II/1 malocclusion. (a) Presurgical lateral x-ray. (b) Postsurgical situation after sagittal split procedure in conjunction with segmental intrusion of the lower cuspids and incisors. (c) Postsurgical situation after 6 months. Hardware removed except for the central lag screw. (d) Orthopantomogram to show the position of plates and screws.

FIGURE 51.5 Line drawing of construction of parallelogram to orient the preferable direction of osteotomy line and required transposition of genial bone fragment. (Incisor line crosses occlusal line at point X and the inferior border at point Y. If $\alpha = \beta$, vertical and horizontal transpositions are of equal length. If $\alpha < \beta$, the horizontal transposition increases. If $\alpha > \beta$, the vertical transposition increases.) For further explanation see text.

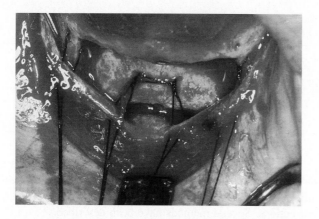

FIGURE 51.6 Photograph of mattress-sutures to close in layers by stepping the periosteal layer directly to the bone surface; picture shows the situation just before tightening the sutures.

use for final closure procedures in layers. To achieve this type of closure, it can be helpful to split the periosteal and mucosal layers more extensively. Figure 51.6 shows traction mattress-sutures to step the periosteum directly to the bone.

Complete degloving procedures are unnecessarily dangerous and have lead to necrosis and infections.[21,22]

Surgical Procedures

After a straight full mucoperiosteal incision or after stepwise incisions and separation of mucosal and periosteal layers, the periosteum at both sides of the incision is elevated just enough to provide sufficient bone surface to carry out the bone cut. The frontal segment of the chinbone can always be left attached to the periosteum. With references to the position of the mental foramen, a sliding osteotomy can be carried out according to the chosen angle to the bone surface (related to the position of the lower incision).

To indicate the exact location of a sliding osteotomy, some landmarks can be made with a small, round drill. The final cutting can be carried out with a thin saw blade. If a more complicated design is planned, as in rotation and reduction procedures, landmarks made by means of a small, round burr are even more important. Anteroposterior reduction that cannot be achieved by a sole sliding osteotomy and translation of the segment should be realized by an osteotomy. If necessary, such an osteotomy can be designed as a wedge to allow additional rotation of the frontal segment around a transverse axis. Figure 51.7 shows the clinical situation after removal of an intermediate bone segment. Note the relative thickness of the cortex suitable for fixation by means of plates and screws.

The chinbone should never be reduced by simply cutting off a frontal segment. The reduction effect is minimal because of the lack of support in transposition of the soft tissues. Moreover, due to the excision of the bone segment, the soft tissues are weakened in a very undesirable way.[23]

Fixation Techniques

Because plates and screws are available in an extensive variety of sizes and configurations, the use of wire osteosynthesis has lost its justification as a fixation technique in genioplasty procedures. Figure 51.8 shows the result of insufficient support and positioning of a genial segment fixed by wire osteosynthesis. The locations of the wire osteosyntheses are quite the same if plate fixation is carried out (Figure 51.13g). Similar to the stabilization of segments and fragments in fracture treatment,[1,24] the technique of lag screw fixation is very useful and relatively easy to perform in genioplasty procedures. Precision in position and drilling procedures is essential.[25,26]

Stable fixation by means of plates, screws, or a combination of the two contributes to predictable surgical results regarding positioning, avoids undesired resorption effects due to instability, and allows relative extensive distances of advancements or transposition procedures.

a

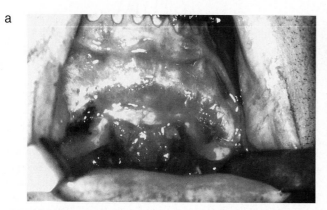

b

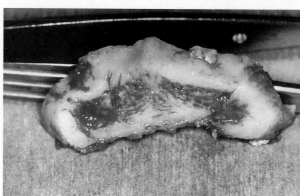

FIGURE 51.7 (a) Frontal view of reduced chin area. (b) Frontal view of resected bone segment. Note the relative thickness of the cortical layers, suitable for proper stable fixation.

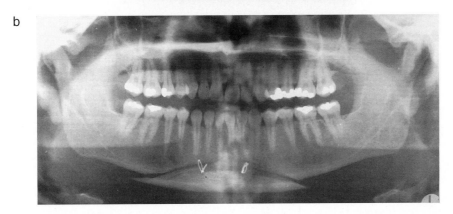

FIGURE 51.8 Insufficient position and support of a reduced chin segment fixed by wire osteosyntheses. (a) Lateral skull x-ray. (b) Orthopantomogram.

Craniofacial osteotomy instrumentation sets usually contain four sizes of plates. The regular (mandibular) 2.4 system has screw diameters of 2.4 mm. Miniplate systems 2.0 and 1.5 have screw diameters of 2.0 and 1.5 mm, respectively, including additional 2.4-mm screws as "emergency screws." Microplate systems 1.0 and 1.2 have screw diameters of 1.0 and 1.2 mm, respectively.

Systems 2.0 and 1.5 are the most convenient and practical for fixation of genioplasty segments. The strength of the 2.0 screws is sufficient to stabilize segments using either three separate lag screws or a combination of one screw in the central part and miniplates or microplates at both sides. The feasibility of screws as the sole means of fixation, using either as a lag screw or a positioning screw as shown in Figure 51.9, depends entirely on the type and direction of the osteotomy line (Table 51.3).

The use of the lag screw technique is only possible if enough holding power in the cortical layers can be achieved. If this cannot be realized, the transposition gap can better be bridged with plates with the preferred minimum of at least two monocortical screws on either side of the osteotomy line.

The 2.4-mm size is usually suitable to achieve initial segment stability. Infrequently, a 2.7-mm screw emergency will be required.

Fixation Procedures

Precise positioning of the genial segment is essential for a well-defined clinical result. A well-controlled sawing procedure results in an accurate translation of the planning and analysis to the clinical situation, and permits an exact trans-

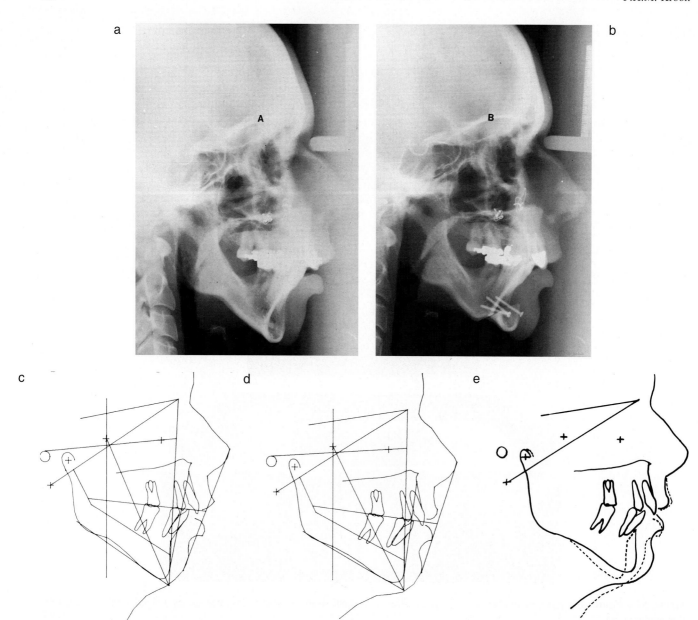

FIGURE 51.9 Photographs of (a) pre- and (b) postsurgical situation of a chin augmentation achieved by a sliding osteotomy according to the prediction described in Figure 51.5. (a) Presurgical situation. (b) Postsurgical situation. (c) Presurgical tracing. (d) Postsurgical tracing. (e) The combination of (c) and (d). Dotted lines are presurgical. (Line drawings in (c,d,e) courtesy Dr. P.E. Swartberg)

position and fixation technique. Midline references should be marked on the bone segment. Even extraoral orientation on a line such as the Frankfurt horizontal can be very helpful.

When introducing lag screws, the technical rules of preparation should be strictly followed:

1. Preparation of the gliding hole in the genial segment. If necessary, gently adjust the cortical surface for an exact fit and avoid any sliding of the screwhead.
2. Prepare the opposite traction hole in the mandible using a centering drill guide to achieve coaxial preparation of the holes.

3. Measure the required screw length.
4. Pretap the traction hole, if a nonself-tapping screw is to be used.
5. Insert and position the screw.

The need for pretapping is mainly determined by the thickness and the number of cortical layers to pass. Experimental work[27,28] has shown that length of the pathway in the cortex of more than 3 mm requires pretapping. Additionally, it is important to realize that in case of using or passing through more cortical layers the length of the screw is critical and requires proper preparation of the drill holes.

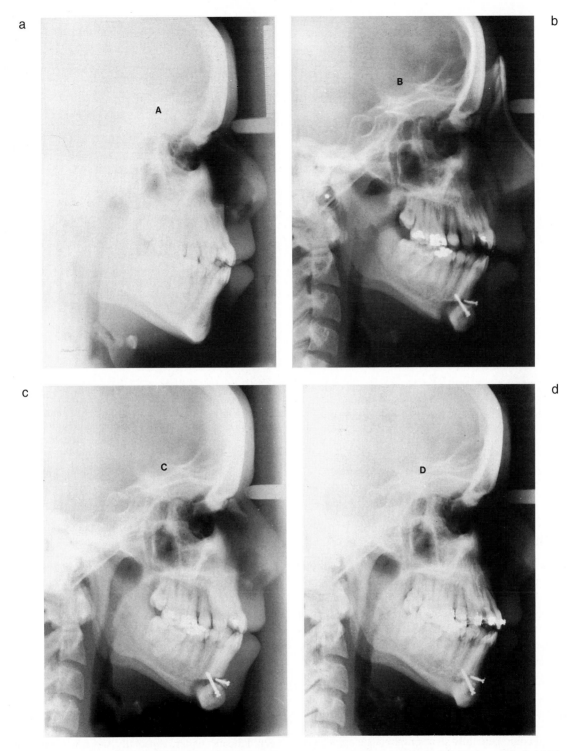

FIGURE 51.11 Lateral x-rays of the patient described in Figures 51.10 and 51.12. (a) Presurgical. (b) Direct postsurgical. (c) Three months postsurgical. (d) Consolidation after 15 months. No signs of resorption around screwheads (titanium screws).

a

b

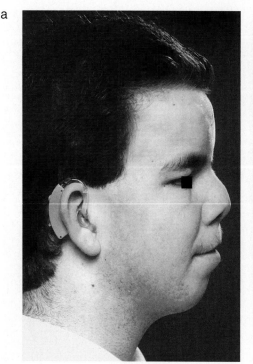
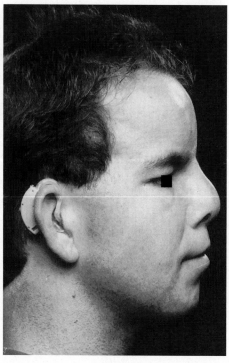

FIGURE 51.12 Clinical photographs of the patient described in Figures 51.10 and 51.11. (a) Presurgical. (b) Postsurgical after nose correction (courtesy Dr. J.B. de Boer) and after chin augmentation. (c) Presurgical tracing. (d) Postsurgical tracing. (e) Combination of (c) and (d). Dotted line is presurgical. [(c,d,e,) Courtesy Dr. P.E. Swartberg]

Wound Dehiscenses

Wound dehiscense mostly occurs because of insufficient oral hygiene postoperatively or from a lack of temporary support by bandages. Reapplication of extraoral bandages and thorough cleaning instruction will solve these problems. Regular intensive dental hygiene should be advised and can be supported by rinsing the mouth with salt water or chlorohexidine gluconate rinses.

Infections

To prevent infection, generally short prophylactic application of antibiotics (24 hours) should be sufficient. Infections, rarely occur, and most probably will be due to instability of the segments and loose hardware. Removal of loose hardware and reapplication of internal fixation is the treatment method of choice.[29] Only in the case of abscess formation is extensive empirical antibiotic therapy and culture and identification of the bacteria necessary.

Nerve Damage

The best solution to manage nerve damage is through prevention. Mucosal incision design superior to the mental foramen avoids unneccesary division of small extensions of the mental nerve. Temporary hypoesthesia is expected in all cases, and the patient should be advised. Return of sensation of damaged mental nerves is very difficult to predict and should not be promised.

Cosmetic Failures

Patients' final satisfaction with the cosmetic results can be a very delicate matter, especially when a genioplasty is done for cosmetic improvement only (see Figure 51.13). However, cosmetic changes that result from major facial corrections, such as extensive orthognathic surgery for functional reasons, also include risks for patient dissatisfaction. It has been pointed out that psychological aspects may play an important role as a predisposition to the development of jaw dysfunction.[30] Preoperative attention to patient expectations and

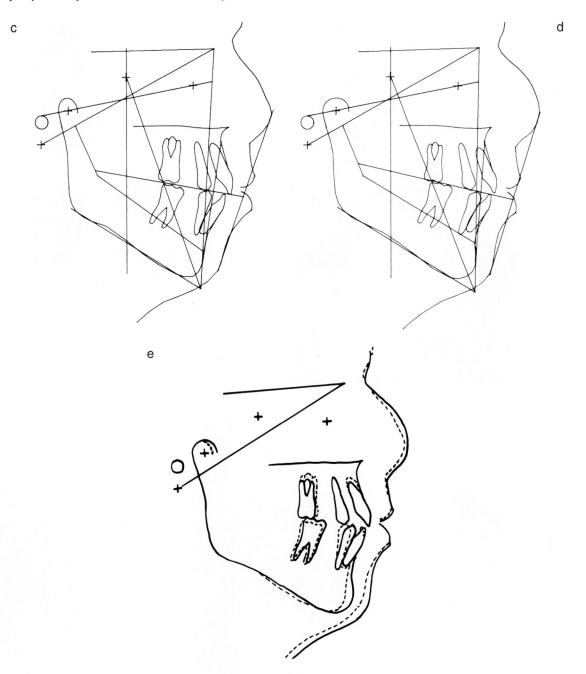

FIGURE 51.12 *Continued.*

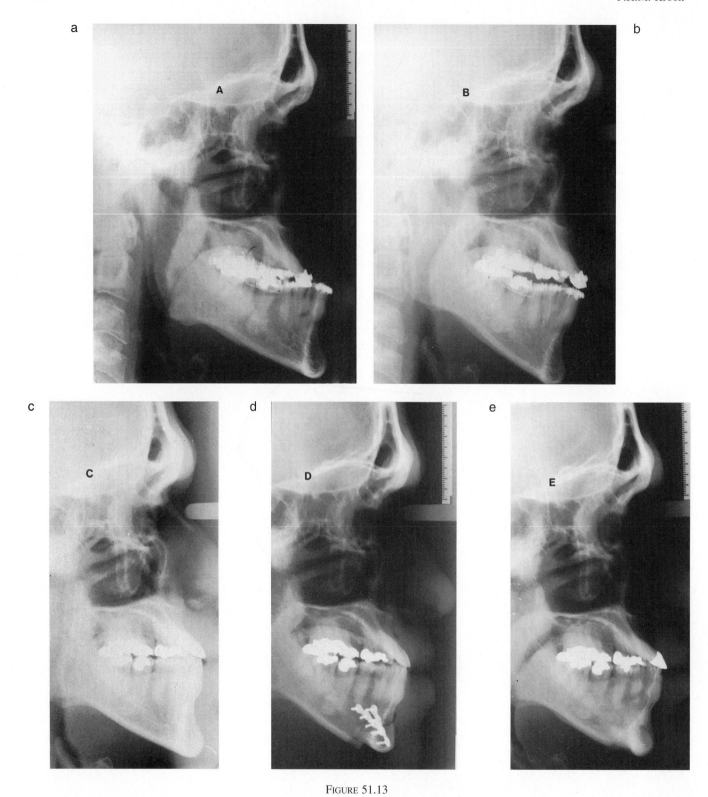

FIGURE 51.13

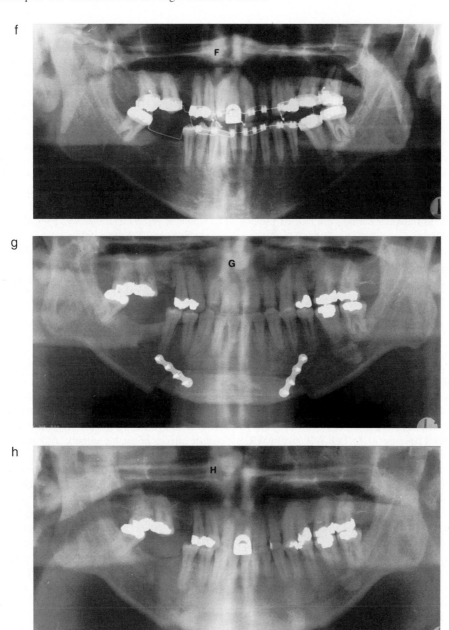

FIGURE 51.13 *Continued.* X-rays of Hindustan man (30 years old at time of first surgery). Angle class III malocclusion skeletal hypodevelopment of the maxilla (with protrusion of the incisors) and prognathism of the mandible corrected by vertical ramus osteotomy. (a) Lateral x-ray presurgical. (b) Lateral x-ray postsurgical (10 weeks). (c) Lateral x-ray postsurgical (4 years and 3 months) used as presurgical to chin surgery. (d) Lateral x-ray postsurgical to genioplasty after 1 day. (e) Lateral x-ray postsurgical (7 years and 7 weeks) after vertical ramus osteotomy, and (2 years and 9 months) after genioplasty. (f) Orthopantomogram postsurgical (6 weeks). (g) Orthopantomogram 1 day after chin surgery. (h) Orthopantomogram (7 years and 7 weeks) after vertical ramus osteotomy and (2 years and 9 months) after genioplasty, following removal of hardware.

Note 1: At present, patient is again seeking treatment for the hypodevelopment of the infraorbital regions. In the past, the retrognathism of the maxilla and the infraposition of the malar bones was considered to be acceptable. The patient is still satisfied with the position of the chin after his setback operation and genioplasty. Reevaluation and facial analysis will be combined in consultation with a psychologist.[30] Note 2: The notches in the inferior border related to the genioplasty have been mainly remodeled by bone apposition.

desires is important and can be helpful to prevent unnecessary complications.

Conclusion

Although a genioplasty seems to be a simple operation, the translation of the treatment plan into a satisfying and predictable long-term, stable result can be challenging. Lengthening or augmentation procedures are much safer and more predictable in relation to the soft tissue appearance than reduction procedures.

Shortening and reduction always include the risk of ptosis or weakening of the soft tissue appearance of the chin. However, hyperactivity or hyperfunction of muscle groups such as the mental muscles can be positively influenced. Techniques of rigid internal fixation have brought a major improvement of the feasibility and predictability of genioplasties by bone surgery.

References

1. Leonard MS. The use of lag screws in mandibular fractures. *Otolaryngol Clin North Am.* 1987;20(3):479–493.
2. Spiessl B. *Internal Fixation of the Mandible. A Manual of AO/ASIF Principles.* Berlin; Springer-Verlag; 1989.
3. McBride KL, Bell WH. Chin surgery. In: Bell WH, Proffit WR, White RP, eds. *Surgical Correction of Dentofacial Abnormalities.* Philadelphia: Saunders; 1980:1216–1279.
4. Proffit, WR. Treatment planning: the search for wisdom. In: Profitt WR, White RP, eds. *Surgical Orthodontic Treatment.* Boston: Mosby Year Book; 1991:142–191.
5. Gonzalez Ulloa M. Quantitative principles in cosmetic surgery of the face. *Plast Reconstr Surg.* 1963;29:2.
6. McNamara JA Jr. A method of cephalometric evaluation. *Am J Orthod.* 1984;86:449–468.
7. Moorrees CFA, Kean MR. Natural head position: a basic consideration for analysis of cephalometric radiographs. *Am J Phys Anthropol.* 1958;16:213–234.
8. Ricketts RM. Perspectives in the clinical application of cephalometrics. *Angle Orthod.* 1981;51:115–150.
9. Sassouni VA. A classification of skeletal facial types. *Am J Orthod.* 1969;55:109–123.
10. Solow B, Tallgren A. Natural head position in standing subjects. *Acta Odontol Scand.* 1971;29:591–607.
11. Steiner CC. Cephalometrics for you and me. *Am J Orthod.* 1953;39:729.
12. Steiner CC. The use of cephalometrics as an aid to planning and assessing orthodontic treatment. *Am J Orthod.* 1960;46:721–735.
13. Davis WJ, Davis CL, Daly BW. Long-term bony and soft tissue stability following advancement genioplasty. *J Oral Maxillofac Surg.* 1988;46:731.
14. Polido WD, De Clairefont Regis L, Bell WH. Bone resorption, stability, and soft-tisuue changes following large chin advancements. *J Oral Maxillofac Surg.* 1991;49:251–256.
15. Sik Park H, Ellis E, Fonseca RJ, Reynolds ST, Mayo KH, Arbor A. Oral surgery. A retrospective study of advancement genioplasty. *Oral Surg Oral Med Oral Pathol.* 1989;67:481.
16. Popovich F, Thompson GW. Craniofacial templates for orthodontic case analysis. *Am J Orthod.* 1977;71:406–420.
17. Walker R. *Dentofacial Planner; User Manual Dentofacial Planner Software.* Toronto; 1988.
18. Walker R. *Dentofacial Planner; User Manual Dentofacial Planner Software 6.5.* Toronto; 1995.
19. Earl PH, Foster M. A new technical aid for genioplasties. Abstracts of the 12th Congress of EACMFS (nr. 125). *J Craniomaxillofac Surg.* 1994;22:43.
20. Thomson ERE. Sagittal genioplasty: a new technique of genioplasty. *Br J Plast Surg.* 1985;38:70–74.
21. Ellis E, Dechow PC, McNamara JA Jr. Advancement genioplasty with and without soft tissue pedicle. An experimental investigation. *J Oral Maxillofac Surg.* 1984;42:639.
22. Mercuri LG, Laskin DM. Avascular necrosis after anterior horizontal augmentation genioplasty. *J Oral Surg.* 1977;35:296.
23. Noorman van der Dussen F, Egyedi P. Premature aging of the face after orthognathic surgery. *J Craniomaxfac Surg.* 1990;18:335.
24. Frodel JL Jr, Marentette LJ. Lag screw fixation in the upper craniomaxillofacial skeleton. *Arch Otolaryngol Head Neck Surg.* 1993;119(3):297–304.
25. Ellis E, Ghali GE. Lag screw fixation of anterior mandibular fractures. *J Oral Maxillofac Surg.* 1991;49(1):13–21.
26. Ilg P, Ellis E. A comparison of two methods for inserting lag screws. *J Oral Maxillofac Surg.* 1992;50(2):119–123.
27. Bähr W, Stoll P. Pre-tapped and self-tapping screws in children's mandibles. A scanning electron microscopic examination of the implant beds. *Br J Oral Maxillofac Surg.* 1991:29.
28. Phillips JH, Rahn BA. Comparison of compression and torque of self-tapping and pretapped screws. *Plast Reconstruct Surg.* 1989;83(3):447–456.
29. Prein J, Beyer M. Management of infection and nonunion in mandibular fractures. *Oral Maxillofac Surg Clin North Am.* 1990;2(1):187–194.
30. Hakman ECJ. Psychological aspects of surgical orthodontics. In: Tuinzing DB, Greebe RB, Dorenbos J, van der Kwast WAM, eds. *Surgical Orthodontics, Diagnosis and Treatment.* Amsterdam: University Press; 1993:108.

52

Long-Term Stability of Maxillary and Mandibular Osteotomies with Rigid Internal Fixation

Joseph E. Van Sickels, Paul Casmedes, and Thomas Weil

Orthognathic surgery is an alteration in the dynamic relationship of the skeletal and soft tissues of the maxillofacial complex. It has been extensively studied with wire osteosynthesis. Initially, with the advent of rigid fixation, it was thought that relapse would be a problem of the past; however, inspection of results and carefully done studies have shown that while lessened, relapse still occurs.

Conceptually, rigid fixation is the use of hardware: plates or screws or combinations of them to place and maintain the bones of the face in a desired position. Ideally their use in osteotomies, which is similar to their application in fractures, allows the patient immediate and pain-free function. However, there is a fundamental difference between an osteotomy and a fracture. When a fracture is restored to an anatomical position, the body's tissues are restored to a balanced, homeostatic state. In an osteotomy, the resting length of the muscles, connective tissues and bones are changed. To maintain the new position, adaptation must occur.[1,2] Adaptation has been shown to occur within the muscles, the muscle–bone and muscle–tendon interfaces, and within bone. Initial muscle adaptation occurs by stretching. Secondary changes are seen with migration of the muscle along its bony attachments and the addition of sarcomere and geometric rearrangement of the fiber population within a muscle. The major mechanism of adaptation occurs within the connective tissue at the muscle–bone and muscle–tendon interfaces.[2,3] Once the ability of the connective tissue to adapt is exceeded, then lengthening of the muscle tissue occurs.[2] Finally, there are the changes in the bone. Physiologically, there are two ways that the bone can change in response to surgical lengthening: osseous displacement and skeletal remodeling. Osseous displacement or movement of bony segments occurs primarily at the osteotomy site. Osseous displacement and remodeling are normal physiologic phenomena. Displacement and therefore relapse is just another mechanism by which the body attempts to return to a resting state. Relapse can occur both early and late.

Early relapse is a well-recognized phenomenon and probably is related to movement at the osteotomy site. The majority of papers on stability (relapse) have dealt with early re-lapse. Less well recognized is late relapse, arbitrarily described as any changes that occur at 6 months or greater. Condylar resorption is thought to be the greatest cause of late relapse. The cause of condylar resorption and hence late relapse are not well understood and are probably multifactorial.

Rigid fixation of bony segments has prevented the majority of movement at osteotomy sites. Therefore, it has minimized most of the recognized early relapse.[4] While rigid fixation has been used with virtually every surgical technique used to move the maxilla and mandible, the majority of the studies on relapse have been done with the bilateral sagittal spit used to advance or retrude the mandible. Early relapse or relapse seen within the first 6 weeks has been minimized in many cases; however, some authors fear that rigid fixation may increase the load on the condyle and hence lead to condylar remodeling and result in late relapse, or relapse seen after 6 months to 1 year.[5,6] Additionally, there is concern that with rigid fixation there will be a higher incidence of torquing of segments, which may also lead to condylar remodeling.[7,8] Hence, an abundance of techniques have been developed to ameliorate some of these concerns. In this chapter, we will review most of the established techniques that have some follow-up data regarding relapse. It is assumed that the reader is familiar with these operations, hence, the chapter will concentrate on the application of the hardware and results with a cursory discussion on the technical aspects of accomplishing a given osteotomy.

Bilateral Sagittal Split Osteotomy

Indications

The bilateral sagittal split osteotomy (BSSO) is the workhorse of the mandibular ramus osteotomies, and arguably it is the most frequently performed maxillofacial corrective surgery. It is used for mandibular advancements, setbacks, and asymmetry. Each movement must be approached differently. When the mandible is advanced, the arc of the mandible is enlarged.

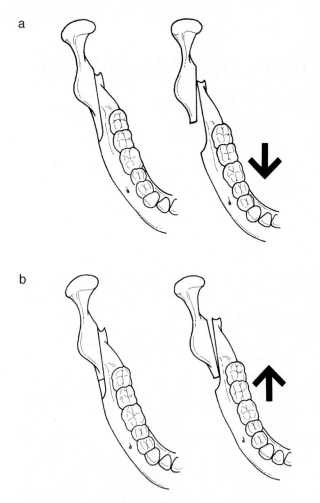

FIGURE 52.1 (a,b) Change in the arc of mandible with advancement and setback of the mandible. (From Van Sickels, Jeter, and Aragon,[43] with permission)

Conversely, when the mandible is set back, the arc becomes smaller (Figure 52.1). Each of these movements will affect the proximal segment and, hence, the condyle. Unfortunately, no case follows a perfect geometric model, so there will always be variations from side to side. Asymmetries exemplify this concept in that by their very nature, the movement from one side both in an anteroposterior and lateral dimension will be different from the other side. Because of this variation from side to side, one type of hardware may be preferable to another within a given case.

Techniques

The mandibular sagittal split ramus osteotomy was first described by Trauner and Obwegeser in 1955.[9] Modifications to the technique have been reported by Dal Pont et al.[10,11] The major modifications in the technique since the original description involves maximizing the blood supply by minimizing stripping of the soft tissues and changes in the bone cuts.

In 1974, Spiessl[12] described the use of internal screw fixation for the sagittal split osteotomy. He proposed the use of three lag screws, two above and one below the mandibular canal. Multiple modifications have been proposed since then. The major changes have been in the use of small screws and plates and the placement of this hardware through intraoral techniques. Additionally, with the use of rigid fixation, time must be spent removing interferences between segments especially when bicortical screws are used.

While a sagittal split is used for both advancements and setbacks, there are subtle differences in technique when the surgery is done for one or the other. In an advancement, the distal segment is advanced beyond the external oblique ridge. In aligning the proximal segment one must be careful not to rotate the proximal segment forward. Doing so can result in both aesthetic and functional problems. The aesthetic defect is obvious; it results from shortening of the posterior facial height with distortion of the inferior border of the mandible. Functionally, rotation of the proximal segment can result in decreased bite force. By shortening the muscles of mastication myoatrophy of the muscles of mastication is induced.

In contrast to an advancement, when the mandible is set back, there is a tendency to rotate the proximal segment posteriorly. This can result in anterior relapse of the mandible.[13] To prevent this tendency, it is important to line up the inferior border and remove all interferences. This will result in more bony recontouring than with a mandibular advancement.

In a setback procedure, the authors contour the ascending ramus as well as release the attachments of the medial pterygoid on the posterior aspect of the mandibular distal segment.

In the planning up of a setback, the models are routinely set up with a 2- to 4-mm overcorrection. At our institution we have found that frequently in the orthodontic management of a mandibular excess case, all the dental compensations are not removed prior to surgery. Overcorrecting the case facilitates postoperative occlusal treatment.

Hardware

Hardware employed in the stabilization of a BSSO varies with the use of screws, plates, or combination of the two. Screws vary in size, technique used to place them, number used, and whether they are placed with a lag or position technique. The biggest arguments for one technique or another appear to be operator preference. The work of Foley et al.[14] has shown a significant difference in rigidity of segments when different patterns of placement were used. Specifically, an inverted L pattern did better than a linear pattern of screw placement. However, they did not show any difference between bicortical noncompression screws and compression screws (lag), nor those placed at a 90° angle with those placed at a 60° angle. More recently Blomqvist and Isaksson[15] have shown that for the average advancement there is no difference in short-term stability between three noncompressive bicortical screws placed per side and unicortical screws and plates placed per side. Most studies with rigid fixation have shown short-term relapse that approaches clinical significance the greater the mandible is advanced. The pattern of screw placement is probably not as important as the distance between each of the screws.

2.7 Lag Technique[12]

Once the mandible has been split and the distal segment placed in the ideal position, a special forceps is used to hold the fragments. A stab incision is made along a relaxed skin crease. A trocar is guided with its metal point in place through the soft tissue to the exposed angle of the mandible. No fewer than three screws are placed. The holes are drilled in the following manner: the outer cortex is drilled with a 2.7-mm drill, the drill guide for the 2.0-mm drill is placed through the trocar, and the 2.0-mm drill is used. The inner hole is measured and tapped. Finally, the screws are placed (Figure 52.2).

Schilli et al.[16] described using 2.7-mm nonlag (position) screws. In position screw osteosynthesis, thread holes are placed in both cortices. This technique is used when fragments are to be kept a fixed distance apart. Schilli et al.[16] suggest that lag screws and position screws can be used together. If this is done, the position screws are to be placed first.

Some surgeons use two 2.7-mm screws; this is not an approved AO technique. Foley and Beckman[17] showed in an animal model that two 2.7-mm bicortical position screws were significantly weaker than a four-hole Champy monocortical

stainless steel miniplate or three 2-mm bicortical screws placed in an inverted L pattern.

Some surgeons do not use a clamp. Once the 2.7-mm hole is drilled in the outer cortex, they use the 2.0-mm drill guide to position the proximal segment and then drill through it.

Multiple authors have suggested the use of appliances to position the proximal segment prior to the use of rigid fixation. At the current time, there is no approved AO technique suggested that uses positioning appliances, nor are there overwhelming data to suggest that results seen with positioning plates are superior to manipulation of the proximal segment.

2.0 Position Technique[18]

A modified Kocher clamp is used to stabilize the proximal and distal fragments in their desired position. A stab incision no wider than the blade is used approximately 1 cm above the inferior border of the mandible in the angle region. A trocar large enough to allow a 0.062-in. threaded Kirschner (K) wire is placed through the cheek. Three bicortical holes are drilled and measured. The authors discuss that the screws may be placed in a linear fashion or in an inverted L fashion. The screws are countersunk. Screws are brought into the field transorally on a screw holding device. They are engaged with a screwdriver used from a transcutaneous approach (Figure 52.3).

The original rationale for the smaller system was to decrease the size of the skin incision on a patient's face. Since the time of the original paper and subsequent chapter, smaller screw heads that will fit through the trocar have been developed. Additionally, multiple authors have placed screws transorally.

Schwimmer et al.[19] have shown no statistical difference between fixation using 2.7-mm versus 2.0-mm lag or position screws to stabilize a sagittal split. They suggested that the primary determinant of stability of the osteotomy was related to the quality of the underlying bone.

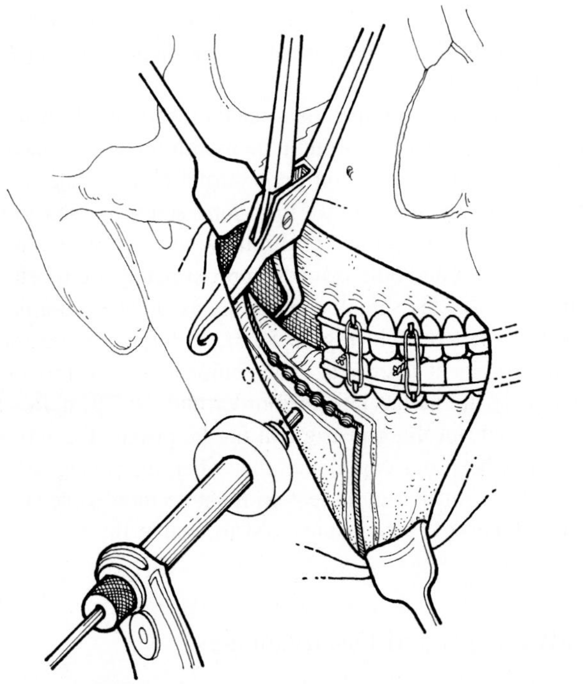

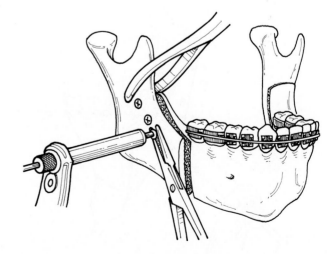

FIGURE 52.2 Transbuccal drilling of compression hole through the inserted 2-mm drill. (From Spiessl,[12] with permission)

FIGURE 52.3 Transoral screw placement, using a clamp to hold the screw. (This technique is useful for screws with large heads.)

Intraoral Technique[20]

Following temporary stabilization of the fragments, access for transoral fixation is made through the same surgical approach as for the sagittal osteotomy (Figure 52.4). Most surgeons who use this technique use a trocar to retract the cheek. Drilling and screw placement are done through the trocar.

There is concern about drilling and placing screws through this approach that there is a greater chance of torquing the condyles (Figure 52.5). This is especially true for a large sagittal split advancement.

Even with small advancements and mandibular setbacks, access may be difficult.

After placement of screws through this approach, it is imperative that the stability of the segments be checked to be certain that you have not minimally engaged the inner cortex owing to difficulties with access.

Right-angle drills and screw drivers have been developed to allow the surgeon to drill and place the screws at a right angle rather than the obligatory angled direction caused by coming from the oral route. While overcoming difficulties caused by drilling at oblique angles, orientation is somewhat challenging. One must drill the holes and place the screws at right angles to the direction that one is standing while negotiating both cortices.

Miniplates[21]

After the sagittal osteotomy is completed and maxillomandibular fixation is established, the proximal segment is

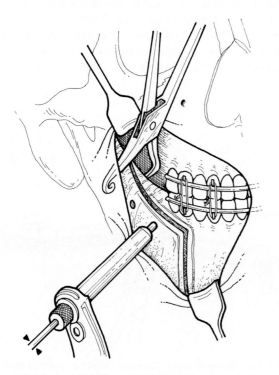

FIGURE 52.4 Transoral drilling; the cheek is retracted with the trocar.

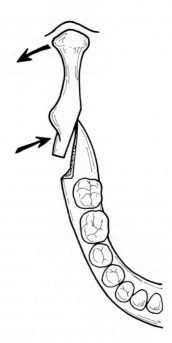

FIGURE 52.5 Intraoral drilling forces the angle of approach to be more oblique. This may result in a greater incidence of torquing of the condyles.

seated. A specific technique to determine correct condylar position has not been published using this technique. Most surgeons manipulate the proximal segment until the inferior border of the proximal segment and the distal segment are aligned. The lateral cortical gap is measured and miniplates of appropriate length are selected and bent to passively bridge the gap. One or two plates may be used per side, depending on the stability needed, direction, and degree of mandibular displacement.

The proximal fragment is rotated upward and forward, permitting direct access through the mouth for screw placement. The first hole is made on the external oblique line, close to the osteotomy site, and a 5-mm-long screw is used to stabilize the plate in proper position. When two miniplates are needed, a second hole is made approximately 1 cm below the first one, and the same procedure is used. The proximal segment is rotated back (Figure 52.6). At this point, positioning of the segment is critical. The senior author of this chapter manually aligns the inferior border and uses posterior force with a wire-pushing instrument on the proximal segment.

It has been our experience that when miniplates are used, the lateral soft tissue dissection must be more generous then when bicortical screws are used to enable the placement of the plates.

Advantages and Disadvantages

Rigid fixation of osteotomies and of the BSSO in particular has become the standard of care. The greatest reasons for this change in a few short years are patient comfort, rapid return

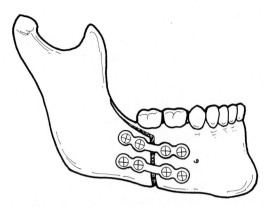

FIGURE 52.6 Illustration of two miniplates. For small advancements or setbacks, only one plate is necessary.

to function, and decreased airway morbidity. Stability of the osteotomy site has been demonstrated by a number of studies especially for the average, less than 7-mm advancement.

The disadvantages are numerous. One is inherent in the operation: injury to the inferior alveolar nerve. The second is the greater technical expertise needed to use rigid fixation and the possible increase in malocclusions. Some authors feel that the use of position screws and or miniplates will decrease the incidence of nerve injuries. This has yet to be shown.

Malocclusions can be prevented by careful inspection of the occlusion at the time of surgery and in the immediate postoperative period. Removal of hardware should always be considered when malocclusions are noted.

Relapse

There have been very few long-term studies looking at large sample groups. Most studies have concentrated on short-term relapse. Short-term relapse occurs within the first 6 weeks.[4,22–25] The relapse may be very obvious, manifested by a resultant malocclusion, or less so, where the skeletal movement is only noted by carefully analyzing postoperative radiographs.

In contrast, long-term relapse is seen at 6 months or more. In general, it is much more insidious, and it is usually seen with a resultant malocclusion.[5,26–28] The patient may or may not have pain in the condylar region.

Most of the animal and clinical studies have been done with 2.0-mm bicortical screws. Small advancements of less than 7 mm at the chin point are very stable.[4] However, when advancing the mandible more than 7 mm, there is a greater tendency to relapse. Van Sickels[29] noted that with suspension wires and a week of fixation that large advancements were more stable than a series of patients who had not had auxiliary techniques used.

Scheerlinck et al.[26] published their results using miniplates with four monocortical screws. The follow-up period was at least 24 months with an average of 32 months. Ninety-three patients (90.3%) of the patients had no appreciable relapse at B point. Eight (7.7%) had relapse because of condylar resorption.

Condylar resorption has been described in a growing number of patients as a change in condylar morphology from normal to spindle shaped with shortening and decrease in posterior facial height.[5,7,27] This often results in a change in the mandibular plane and an open bite accompanying the mandibular relapse. It is seen most frequently among females with preexisting temporomandibular symptoms who have undergone one or two jaw surgeries with a mandibular advancement. Condylar resorption has been seen with wire osteosyntheses, bicortical screws, and miniplates.

Condylar sag has been noted as one of the causes of early relapse especially with wire osteosynthesis. There have been many procedures proposed to eliminate condylar sag, but few data have been produced to endorse any one technique. Perhaps the biggest problems center around what is the "correct" position of the condyle and ascending ramus. Condylar sag has been virtually eliminated with rigid fixation; however, the concept of how to best position the condyle and proximal segment still remains a clinical debate.

Cases

Early Relapse

A 29-year-old woman presented with mandibular anterior posterior deficiency. In June 1987, she underwent a BSSO advancement of 9 mm. No auxiliary techniques were used to stabilize the mandible (Figure 52.7). She was not placed in intermaxillary fixation. The proximal segments were rotated slightly with surgery. Her postoperative course was uneventful. Her 6-week cephalometric radiograph revealed that the distal segment rotated inferior and posterior (Figure 52.8). Her occlusion was maintained by elastic traction. At 7 years after surgery, no further change has been noted in either the proximal or distal segments.

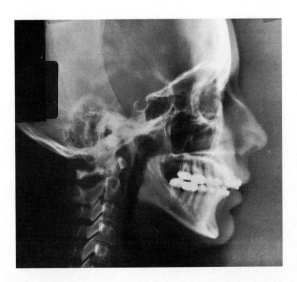

FIGURE 52.7 Presurgical lateral cephalogram.

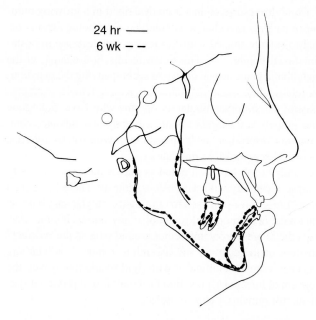

FIGURE 52.8 Immediate and 6-week postoperative cephalogram overlaid.

This case is a classical example of early relapse. Whether wires or screws are used, most relapse occurs within the first 6 weeks. In the initial surgery, the surgeon rotated the proximal segments. Rotation of the proximal segment had no bearing on the stability of the case. However, in the first 6 weeks there was rotation of the distal segment. Through the use of elastics and orthodontics the occlusion was maintained. A cursory examination of her occlusion would not reveal the magnitude of the relapse. Her overall aesthetics were compromised by the amount of the relapse. This would be noted in decreased projection of the chin and a steep mandibular plane. This could have been prevented by the use of auxiliary techniques such as suspension wires with or without a period of fixation.

Long-Term Relapse

An 18-year-old year female presented with vertical maxillary excess, apertognathia, horizontal mandibular, and genial deficiency (Figure 52.9). Her presurgical history was significant for TMJ symptoms. This consisted of muscular symptoms that were minimal in nature. In May 1991, she underwent a Le Fort I maxillary impaction and advancement combined with a bilateral sagittal split osteotomy and advancement combined with a bilateral sagittal split osteotomy and a genioplasty (Figure 52.10). Total advancement at the chin point was more than 15 mm. At 6 months after surgery, she was noted to have a slight open-bite tendency possibly due to condylar resorption. She was followed along with her orthodontist for further changes in joint morphology (Figure 52.11). At 10 months after surgery, it was noted that her open bite had worsened. All active orthodontics was terminated. She was followed with serial cephalometric radiographs. One year after surgery, it was determined that there were no more changes in her occlusion. She then successfully underwent a maxillary posterior impaction with posterior movement of the maxilla. To date, she has been stable with no further changes in her occlusion.

While this patient did very well following a second surgery, other authors have not been as successful. Arnett and Tamborello[5] reviewed their results with four patients undergoing second osteotomies. Two of their patients were stable long term, the other two had further skeletal relapse secondary to condylar resorption. Crawford et al.[27] followed seven patients who had second surgeries following skeletal relapse after condylar resorption. Five had additional condylar resorption after their second surgery.

While there is no guaranteed strategy for managing a patient with condylar resorption, the following technique is used by the authors. When occlusal changes are noted as in the case denoted earlier, stop all active orthodontics. Observe the patient with serial cephalometric films. Splint therapy may be instituted, especially if the patient has symptoms. There may

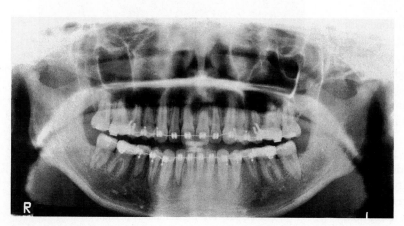

FIGURE 52.9 Presurgical lateral panorex; note minimal condylar changes.

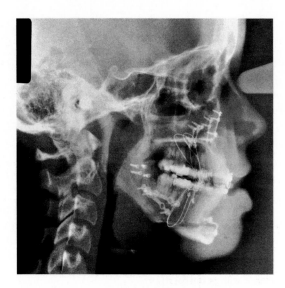

FIGURE 52.10 Postsurgical cephalogram.

be some validity to using a splint to decrease load on the joint even if the patient does not have symptoms. When the occlusion has been stable from 6 months to 1 year, plan the second surgery. If possible, try to obtain a functional occlusion with a procedure in the maxilla. Skeletal wire should be used with elastic traction from the wires to minimize load on the joints.

Intraoral Vertical Ramus Osteotomy

Indications

The intraoral vertical ramus osteotomy (IVRO) was refined and evaluated by Hall et al.[30] in 1975 to set the mandible back and avoid facial scars. It has also been used by Hall et al.[31] among others to treat painful TMJ reciprocal clicks. Perhaps the greatest advantage of an IVRO as compared to a BSSO is the lower incidence of injury to the inferior alveolar nerve. The procedure does not lend itself easily to rigid fixation. In 1982, Paulus and Steinhauser[32] presented their results using

bone screws on the proximal segment. They noted that they were not able to consistently get three screws in the segments. In 1990, Van Sickels et al. presented a variation of the IVRO using an inverted L osteotomy. They were able to consistently place a plate on the proximal and distal segments. Due to the complexity of the procedure, they suggested that it be used with a mandibular setback for specific indications. Those were patients with thin rami, patients in whom nerve injuries might be more problematic, and in any case in which a BSSO might not be indicated to set the mandible back.

Techniques

The key to IVRO is visualization of the lateral surface of the mandible and orientation through the use of reference points and instruments. Once the lateral surface of the ramus is stripped, a LeVasseur-Merrill retractor is placed posterior to the mandible. This allows visualization and it provides a reference to the posterior border of the mandible. An oscillating saw is used to cut from the sigmoid notch to the angle of the mandible. More recent papers have stressed the need to maintain a pedicle of muscle to the posterior and medial aspects of the proximal segment.

The inverted L modification of an IVRO was developed to allow consistent rigid fixation of a setback. The lateral dissection is similar to that described for an IVRO. Medial dissection is similar to that used for a sagittal split. A horizontal bone cut is made above the neurovascular bundle posterior to the lingula short of the posterior border by beveling from medial to lateral from superior to inferior. The mandible is wired into its preoperative position. This position is the one in which the operator has determined that the condyle will be placed. A maxillary horizontal soft tissue incision is made exposing the buttress and part of the zygoma. A positioning plate is placed from the mandible (superior to the horizontal cut) to the maxilla (Figure 52.12). Placement is critical as there must be enough room inferior to the positioning plate to allow an additional fixation plate once the osteotomy is completed. Recently we have started to use a 2.4-mm Synthes Maxillofacial (Paoli, PA) reconstruction plate bent on a dry

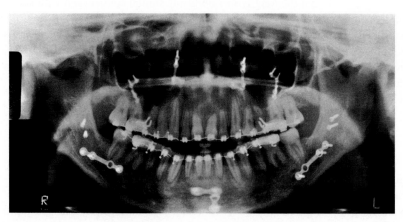

FIGURE 52.11 A postsurgical panorex showing gross condylar changes.

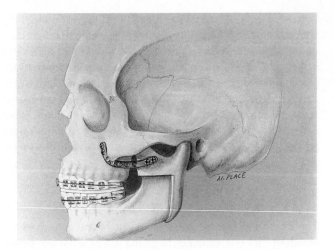

FIGURE 52.12 Positioning plate in place. (From Van Sickels, Tiner, and Jeter,[33] with permission)

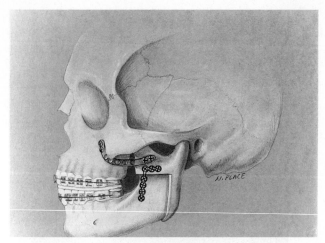

FIGURE 52.13 Seven-hole oblique plate. (From Van Sickels, Tiner, and Jeter,[33] with permission)

skull before surgery. We have found this is more stable than the plates that we once used, yet it is flexible enough to allow some contouring at the time of surgery. A vertical osteotomy is then completed from the horizontal cut to the angle of the mandible. The patient is taken out of fixation once both sides are cut and the mandible is set back. Frequently there will be irregular contact points between the two segments, which can be noted by sliding a thin elevator between the segments. These points are reduced by grinding them down with a cross-cut fissure burr. Ultimately the segments should lie snugly against one another. A seven-hole 2-mm Synthes oblique angled plate is used to stabilize the segments. Critical in the placement of this plate is the first hole in the corner of the plate. Alignment of the plate along the horizontal cut must be assured before placing the screws in the vertical portion of the plate.

Hardware

Paulus and Steinauser[32] were among the few authors to publish results with the use of bone screws in an attempt to use rigid fixation with an IVRO. Their technique is not described. It appears they used two 2.7-mm position screws when there was adequate overlap of the two segments.

To complete the inverted L procedure, the surgeon must have a positioning plate and a seven-hole oblique angle plate (Figure 52.13). It is preferable to contour the positioning plate on a dry skull prior to coming to the operating room. Right-angle drills and screwdrivers are preferable; however, the surgery can be completed through a percutaneous approach. The seven-hole plate is a 2-mm plate.

Advantages and Disadvantages

The advantages for an intraoral setback procedure are the avoidance of facial incisions, hence extraoral scars and possible facial nerve injury. Ramus osteotomies that avoid split-

ting the mandible have a lower incidence of inferior alveolar nerve injury. It is important to note that they are not free of sensory injury. Attempts to use rigid fixation should allow fuller range of motion earlier than wire osteosynthesis. However, it is technically difficult to place hardware when an IVRO is used. An inverted L overcomes these difficulties, although placing the positioning plate takes time and makes the surgery more technically demanding.

Relapse

Paulus and Steinhauser[32] noted a higher tendency for relapse after bone screw fixation of vertical ramus osteotomies as compared to wire osteosynthesis. This is significant in that multiple authors have noted vertical relapse with wire osteosynthesis of vertical ramus osteotomies. This less-than-hoped-for result is most likely due to the fact that two screws do not provide adequate stabilization of a vertical ramus osteotomy.[33]

Tiner et al.[34] reported 1- to 2-year follow-up on 14 patients who had undergone inverted L osteotomies. They noted minimal vertical and horizontal long-term changes, concluding that the long-term stability is similar to that seen with stable rigidly fixed BSSO setbacks.

Tiner et al.[34] suggest that skeletal wires be used in all cases with elastic traction to improve skeletal stability. Clinically, the authors feel that the larger setbacks are more stable than the more minor ones.

Case

An 18-year-old female presented for treatment having undergone preoperative orthodontics (Figure 52.14). Her diagnoses were maxillary A-P deficiency, maxillary transverse deficiency, apertognathia, macroglossia, and mandibular excess. In October 1989, she underwent a surgically assisted rapid

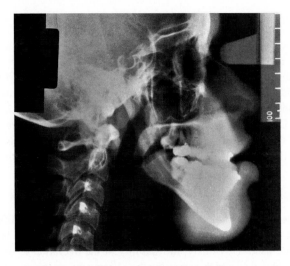

FIGURE 52.14 Presurgical lateral cephalogram.

cult. While not impossible with a sagittal split, the inverted L is easier to accomplish with larger moves.

3. The partial glossectomy was done after the two-jaw surgeries. This was an orthodontic decision. The orthodontist had difficulty moving the lower teeth due to tongue pressure. While tongue reduction was considered at the time of both the surgical rapid palatal expansion and the two-jaw surgery, it was thought that with the enlargement of the oral cavity afforded by these two surgeries that a tongue reduction would not be necessary. This proved not to be so. In the senior author's experience, it is hard to predict in which cases the tongue will adapt to the new environment. Tongue habits have been heavily implicated as a cause of apertognathia. In most instances, the tongue will adapt following surgical correction of a skeletal malocclusion, particularly where the skeletal moves will increase the volume of the oral cavity. Worrisome are cases where there is an initial reverse curve of Spee in the lower arch and the surgical moves will decrease the size of the oral cavity.

palatal expansion correcting the transverse discrepancy. In January 1990, she underwent a Le Fort I maxillary advancement and an inverted L setback (Figure 52.15). In December 1991, she underwent a reduction partial glossectomy.

This case illustrates several points:

1. The maxilla was expanded surgically prior to the Le Fort I osteotomy. It has been the senior author's experience that expansions of greater than 6 mm posteriorly are not stable and tend to relapse. Therefore, it is an advantage to correct large transverse problems prior to a Le Fort I osteotomy. Additionally, expansion of the maxilla allows alignment of teeth without extractions.
2. The mandibular setback was 9 mm. Setting the mandible back greater than 6 to 8 mm with a sagittal split is diffi-

Midline Split

Indications

A midline split of the mandible can be used to either widen or narrow the mandible when combined with ramus osteotomies. Although the procedure is not a new concept, its popularity has increased with the use of rigid fixation. In practice, it is used more frequently to narrow the mandible.

In most cases when there are transverse arch discrepancies the mandible is wider than the maxilla. Traditionally, the maxilla is expanded. However, mandibular constriction may simplify the surgical procedure, with equal or superior stability compared to a maxillary expansion.

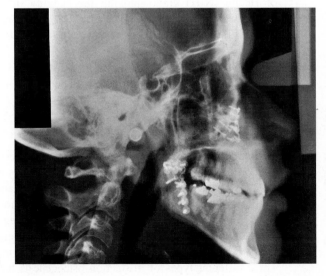
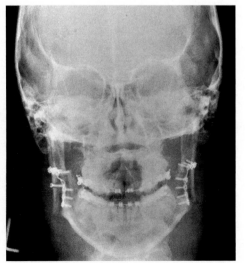

a b

FIGURE 52.15 (a,b) Postsurgical lateral and PA cephalograms.

When the mandible is set back, the lower arch is frequently wider than the maxilla. A midline split allows the surgery to be completed in one arch. In cleft palate patients, the maxilla is frequently scarred and difficult to expand. Especially when the palate is scarred, narrowing the mandible is much more stable than expanding the maxilla.

Technique

A midline split is always combined with a ramus osteotomy. It may or may not be combined with a genioplasty. Sequencing the surgery, the ramus osteotomies are completed prior to splitting the symphysis. If a genioplasty is included, the chin is cut first, then the ramal procedures are carried out, and finally the midline split is made.

The rationale for completing the ramus osteotomies first is that it is easier to split the symphysis after the rami have been split than it is to do the procedures in reverse. Conversely, it is easier to cut the chin with the rami intact than it is to do the procedure in reverse.

Some surgeons routinely combine the midline split with a genioplasty to prevent undue narrowing of the symphysis.

Hardware

Both 2-mm and 2.7-mm screws and plates have been used depending on whether a genioplasty is combined with the split. Critical to the planning of a case is the design of a lower splint that goes over the occlusal surfaces of the lower incisors. The teeth can be individually ligated into the splint or pulled in with circumferential wires. Once the surgeon is certain that the teeth are in their desired position, a plate(s) is applied across the midline (Figure 52.16). If a genioplasty is included, the midline is stabilized first, then the chin is stabilized to the basal segment of the mandible.

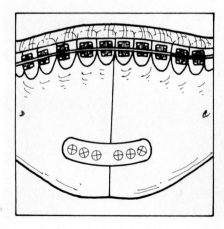

FIGURE 52.16 Plate applied to midline split of mandible.

Advantages and Disadvantages

The biggest advantage of a midline split is the avoidance of or simplification of surgery in the maxilla. In the case of a cleft palate patient, although there are no data to support it, a midline split narrowing the mandible is more stable than expanding a scarred palate.

Disadvantages of a midline split are possible injury to one of the lower incisors and possible periodontal problems due to the bone cut or tears of the gingiva between the teeth.

Relapse

There are no data on relapse with a midline split. Stability of the osteotomy would relate directly to the rigidity of the hardware used. Obviously, the stability of the overall case would be related to which osteotomy had been used on the mandibular ramus and how much the distal segment was moved.

Case

A 27-year-old woman with a past medical history significant for Turner's syndrome presented with mandibular horizontal deficiency, genial vertical deficiency, and maxillary transverse deficiency versus mandibular transverse excess. In May 1992 she underwent a sagittal split advancement of 5 mm with a midline split of the mandible to narrow the mandible and a genioplasty to inferiorly reposition the chin (Figure 52.17).

The options of treating her involved a surgical rapid palatal expansion or a two-piece maxillary osteotomy versus a narrowing osteotomy of the mandible. As the surgical plan was to advance her mandible, it was felt that the narrowing of the mandible could be safely accomplished without encroaching on the tongue. By correcting the transverse discrepancy in the mandible she was able to avoid a surgical procedure in the maxilla.

This patient was part of a multicentered National Institutes of Health (NIH) grant studying the stability of wire osteosynthesis versus rigid fixation for BSSO advancements. She was randomized in the grant for rigid fixation to be used for her BSSO.

Special Considerations and Distraction Osteogenesis

Distraction Osteogenesis

One of the recent advances in orthognathic surgery is distraction osteogenesis, also known as callostasis. Its use with dentofacial and craniofacial deformities is in its infancy. Distraction osteogenesis is a technique of bone generation and osteosynthesis by the distraction of an osseous segment(s). The technique was pioneered in the orthopedic literature by Gavril Ilizarov and is sometimes called the Ilizarov method.[35] Three different types of distraction osteogenesis have been described in the orthopedic literature: monofocal, bifocal, and

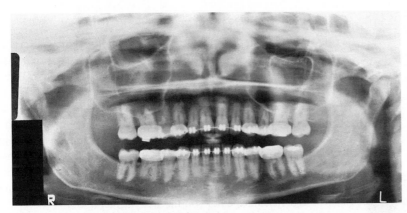

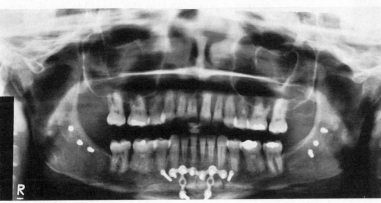

FIGURE 52.17 (a) Presurgical and (b) post-surgical panorexes.

trifocal. The designations refer to how a bone or segments of a bone(s) are being moved. Most of the work being done with craniofacial and dentofacial surgery is with monofocal distraction osteogenesis. Several factors are important to the success of distraction osteogenesis: stability of fixation, displacement of the osteotomy, and the rate and rhythm of distraction.[36] Classically, distraction osteogenesis follows a corticotomy. However, an osteotomy may be equally successful. It is important to minimize stripping of the periosteum with preservation of the blood supply to the bone. In general, there is a recommended latency period of 3 to 7 days before expansion is initiated. While distraction can occur at rates from 0.5 to 2 mm per day, 1 mm per day appears optimal.[36] The rhythm of distraction recommended in the orthopedic literature is 0.25 mm four times per day.[36] There is debate as to whether mechanical continual distraction is superior to rhythmic manual distraction.

Case

A 27-year-old man presented complaining of crowding of his teeth in his upper and lower arch and a deficiency of his lower jaw. He had previously undergone full banded orthodontic therapy with the extraction of four bicuspids. Arch analysis revealed that stripping of teeth would not create enough space (Figure 52.18). He was scheduled for upper and lower expansion. Expansion appliances were cemented to place in both the upper and lower arch. The upper arch was done by a stan-

dard surgical rapid palatal expansion expanding 1 mm at the time of surgery. On successive days he was expanded 0.25 mm twice a day. A limited vestibular incision was made in the mandibular buccal vestibular tissue. Dissection was carried to bone. An osteotomy was made from the chin to the alveolar ridge, using a chisel to split the last portion. Six days later, the lower arch was expanded 0.25 mm twice a day (Figure 52.19). Three months later, his appliances were removed and his orthodontics was continued.

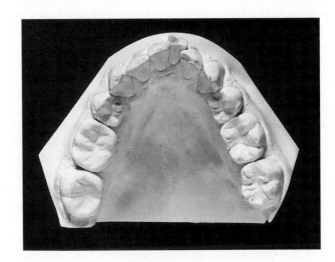

FIGURE 52.18 Presurgical mandibular model. Note the crowding of the dentition, despite the previous extractions.

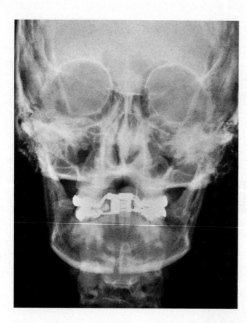

FIGURE 52.19 PA cephalogram.

The patient will eventually have a mandibular advancement.

The exact role of distraction osteogenesis will be determined with further research and clinical practice. It has application in several of the craniofacial and dentofacial skeletal deficiency patients in both the maxilla and mandible. Both length and width discrepancies may be addressed by this newer technique.

Subapical Osteotomies

Indications

Subapical osteotomies are indicated anywhere there are segmental discrepancies in the occlusal scheme that cannot or may not be managed expeditiously by orthodontics. Mandibular subapical osteotomies are technically demanding, as one is frequently cutting between apices of teeth and the vascular supply is not as forgiving as in the maxilla. Modern orthodontics has minimized the need for segmental procedures. The most frequent indications for segmental mandibular procedures are in combination prosthetic/surgical cases. Body osteotomies are infrequently indicated and therefore will not be discussed. Posterior mandibular segmental procedures are usually indicated for supereruption of teeth due to loss of maxillary dentition. Anterior segmental procedures are often indicated in deep bite class II patients when the posterior dentition is compromised or when the supereruption is to such an extent that orthodontics will be unable to treat the condition completely or that surgery will expedite orthodontic management. Occasionally, maxillary and mandibular subapical osteotomies may be useful in patients presenting with bimaxillary protrusion.

Techniques

In both anterior and posterior mandibular segmental surgeries an adequate labial pedicle must be maintained. The position of the inferior alveolar nerve must be considered with both procedures. When a posterior segmental surgery is done, it is frequently necessary to unroof the neurovascular bundle and hold it to the side while cutting the bone below it. With an anterior segmental surgery, the mental foramen is frequently identified as the posterior extent of the bone cut. In both cases, the inferior saw cut is beveled toward the lingual aspect of the mandible. Beveling the saw cut in this fashion maximizes the vascular pedicle on the free segment.

Segmental procedures in the mandible are different than segmental surgeries in the maxilla as one needs to cut two cortices of bone in the mandible. To complete the osteotomy, it is necessary to bring the saw or burr cut more toward the occlusal surface than is necessary in maxillary surgery. It is not wise to attempt to chisel through the mandible. Trying to chisel through a dense lingual cortical plate can result in fractures of the plate and lacerations of the thin lingual tissues. Instead the segments should be pried apart leveraging a chisel at an inferior location where the two cortices are cut. Once the fragments are free, one needs to ligate the dentition into a splint that covers the occlusal surfaces. Circumferential mandibular wires can be used posteriorly over the splint. Assuring proper placement of the segments, plates are used below the apices of the teeth to stabilize the segments. It must be remembered that in this location the plates do not assure rigidity of the segment (Figure 52.20). Therefore, it is necessary for the patient to wear the splint for 3 to 4 weeks.

A total mandibular alveolar osteotomy shares common features with both anterior and posterior subapical osteotomies. A large labial pedicle is used, and the nerve is unroofed to allow an osteotomy. The major indication for this procedure is a patient with a low mandibular plane angle and horizon-

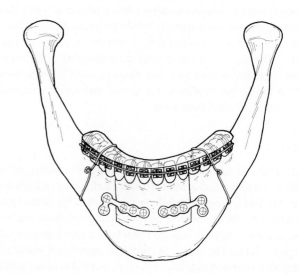

FIGURE 52.20 Two plates used to stabilize a subapical osteotomy.

tal mandibular deficiency. Its advocates suggest that it is more stable than a bilateral sagittal split. However, with the advent of rigid fixation its popularity has decreased.

Hardware

Two-millimeter plates and screws are used in a variety of positions depending on the size of the segments and the location of tooth apices. It must be noted that the hardware does not represent rigid fixation but merely additional stability. Splints must be fabricated with the intention that they be used by the patient for 3 to 4 weeks.

Advantages and Disadvantages

The advantages of subapical osteotomies are that they allow or accelerate the time involved for occlusal discrepancies to be treated. The advantages of hardware in segmental surgery is that it minimizes the time that the patient wears a splint and increases intraoperative stability.

Disadvantages of subapical procedures are the possible injury to the apices of teeth or periodontal problems secondary to the bony cuts or lacerations of the gingiva. Disadvantages of screws and plates are that in their placement there may be injury to the apices of teeth.

Relapse

Segmental surgery has a long history of stability when compared to ramus osteotomies. The reason for this finding is that segments of the jaw are moved versus the whole mandible, with less stretching of the connective tissues.

Case

A 15-year-old male presented with vertical maxillary excess, transverse deficiency of the maxilla, genial deficiency, and mandibular dentoalveolar horizontal excess. He underwent presurgical orthodontics in preparation for a three-piece maxillary osteotomy and a mandibular subapical osteotomy (Figure 52.21). At 3 years postoperative, there has been no change in the position of the subapical osteotomy.

Genioplasty

Indications

A genioplasty is one of the most versatile procedures in the armamentarium of the modern skeletal/soft tissue surgeon. It can be used to balance the face following other skeletal surgeries or used in isolation to mask a skeletal deformity. In combination with liposuction it may be used to rejuvenate the face as an alternate to a face lift.

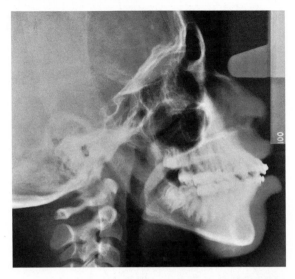
a

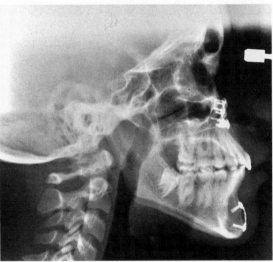
b

FIGURE 52.21 (a) Preoperative and (b) postoperative cephalogram.

Techniques

Genioplasties have traditionally been performed under general anesthesia; however, good results have been achieved using copious local anesthesia and intravenous sedation.[37] Van Sickels and Tiner[37] noted that when local anesthetic with a vasoconstrictor was used on the lingual aspect of the mandible, there was a demonstrable decrease in blood loss as compared to when this technique was not used. The technique described here is for the typical genial advancement. An endless variety of geometric designs can be used on individual patients depending on their skeletal anatomy (Figure 52.22).

A standard incision is made in the mucosa of the lip, dissecting back to the body of the mandible. Dissection is carried back beneath the mucosa identifying the mental nerve, which is eventually extended below the distal aspect of the first molar. Knowing the length of the canines, a reference mark is scribed in the chin denoting the midline and the height to which the saw cut will be made. Additional marks are made

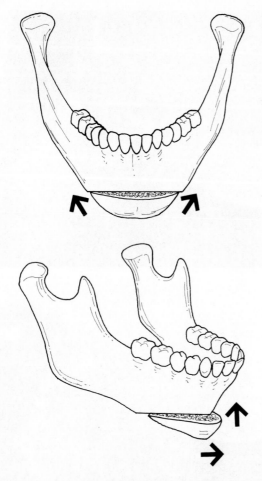

FIGURE 52.22 Various genioplasty designs.

One can cause or accentuate the jowl region by making short cuts (not extending the osteotomy to the first molar region) and shortening the chin. This is particularly evident when large genial advancements are used.

The senior author uses a Perkins (Walter Lorenz Surgical Instruments Inc., Jacksonville, Florida) boley gauge to check the vertical movement.

Hardware

Although some authors have suggested pins or screws to be used to stabilize the genial segment, one or two 2-mm plates are most frequently used. In our opinion, plates are preferred as they allow greater three-dimensional flexibility to position segments than pins or screws.

Advantages and Disadvantages

The biggest advantage of a bone genioplasty is its versatility as compared to an alloplastic chin. One is able to manipulate the chin in a number of directions to mask underlying skeletal problems. It can be used to treat both deficiency as well as excess states. The morbidity is similar to that seen with the placement of an alloplast.

In contrast, an alloplast can be placed much more quickly. Newer designs of alloplastic implants are less likely to move than earlier simpler implant shapes. Additionally, an alloplast is superior to a bony osteotomy in augmenting the "jowl" region.

Relapse

Few papers have addressed relapse. In general, it is not a problem. Park et al.[38] noted the position of a genial segment was stable after a surgical advancement. They evaluated 23 patients who had undergone an average horizontal advancement of 6.6 mm, which was accompanied by 3.1 mm of vertical repositioning of hard tissue pogonion. Postoperative changes ranged from 2 mm of posterior movement to 0.5 mm of anterior movement with an average of 0.38 mm posterior at 1 month. Vertical changes ranged from 3.5 mm of superior movement to 3.4 mm of inferior movement with an average of 0.8 mm inferior at 1 month. This study was done with wire osteosynthesis. Van Sickels et al.[39] also noted a tendency for the chin to shorten with advancement but noted that segments had very little movement when they were stabilized with plates.

Case

Horizontal Genial Deficient

A 16-year-old male presented with mandibular anteroposterior deficiency having undergone 3 years of orthodontic management. While his occlusion was satisfactory, he was markedly genial deficient (Figure 52.23). In January 1990, he underwent a 9-mm genial advancement (Figure 52.24).

This case is not unusual. Many patients present with combined skeletal and dental discrepancies. Following correction

on either side of the midline. From these points, vertical measurements are made to the arch wire. A boley gauge or specially designed instruments are available to attain this measurement. Following measuring, a bone cut is made from one side to the other. Once free, the chin is grasped by a clamp and moved to the desired position. Held temporarily in place, a four-hole bone plate is bent to the contour of the advanced segment. Holes are drilled and three of the four screws are placed. Measurements are checked to assure placement before the fourth screw is placed. Small manipulations of the segment are possible after plate placement by grasping the plate with a plate bending forceps and twisting it in the desired direction. If the genial segment is mobile, an additional plate can be placed. The soft tissue is then closed and a pressure dressing is placed.

It has been the authors' experience that although the horizontal distance that a chin is moved is noted by most surgeons, few are cognizant of the vertical movement of chin. The technique described here takes vertical movement into account.

Although many surgeons bend standard plates, several companies have specially designed plates to be used for genioplasties.

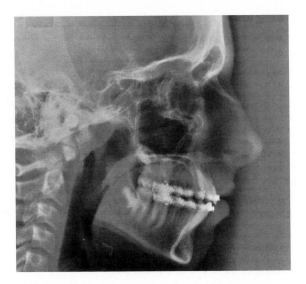

FIGURE 52.23 Presurgical lateral cephalogram.

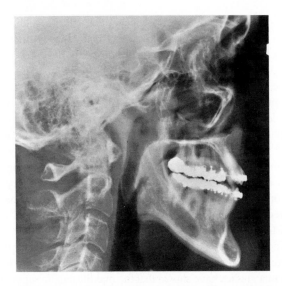

FIGURE 52.25 Presurgical lateral cephalogram. Note steep plane of mandible.

of the alignment and crowding of the teeth, the patient's overjet and overbite are acceptable. If the dental units are in a satisfactory position over the skeletal base, then a genioplasty can be used to mask the underlying skeletal deformity.

When the patient is maxillary deficient and genial deficient, one must be careful not to advance the chin too far forward trying to mask the genial deficiency.

Vertical Genial Excess

A 31-year-old man presented with maxillary and midface anterior posterior deficiency as well as vertical genial excess (Figure 52.25). In January 1993, he underwent a modified Le Fort III/I moving the maxilla forward and down. Additionally, he had a genial reduction of 5 mm (Figure 52.26).

This patient had a long upper face combined with a long lower face. This was manifested in his steep mandibular plane. Rather than slide his chin forward by an osteotomy, an ostectomy was used. This shortened his lower face height while improving his labiomental fold and improving the lower border of the mandible.

Le Fort I

Indications

In 1927, Wassmund[40] first described a surgical procedure to mobilize the entire maxilla. He incompletely sectioned the maxilla from its bony attachments and later applied elastic

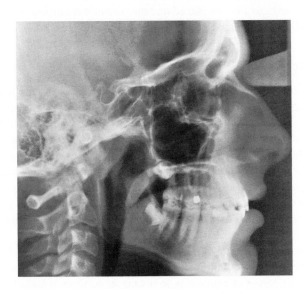

FIGURE 52.24 Postsurgical lateral cephalogram.

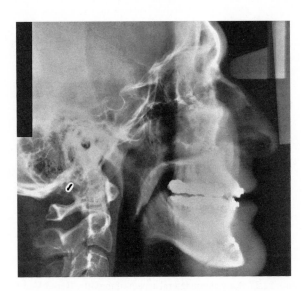

FIGURE 52.26 Postsurgical lateral cephalogram (inferior border changed by the autorotation and the genioplasty).

traction to close an anterior open bite. The procedure has evolved over the years to be known as the Le Fort I osteotomy. Both soft tissue flap designs and bony cuts have been continually refined to facilitate movement of the maxilla to preserve the blood supply to the pedicle. The inability to move the maxilla the desired amount and relapse were common problems for early surgeons. As experience was gained, an emphasis was placed on adequate mobilization of the maxilla.[41] The use of the Le Fort I increased dramatically following the work of Bell et al.[42] showing osseous healing and revascularization of the maxilla after a total maxillary osteotomy in rhesus monkeys. The largest change that has occurred in the last decade has been the addition of rigid fixation to stabilize the mobilized maxilla.

The Le Fort I is the workhorse of maxillary surgery, allowing many different types of movements. Previously mentioned vascular studies have shown that the maxilla can be segmented without compromise to the dento-osseous segments. Continual work with this procedure is being done to refine some of the more subtle aspects of this surgical procedure.

Techniques

A variety of bone cuts have been suggested for the Le Fort I osteotomy. The majority have been designed to increase bone contact or to influence the direction of the maxillary movement. The technique used by the authors was published in 1985[43] and was based on an earlier paper by Kaminishi et al.[44] The advantage of this technique is that bone cuts are carried into the denser bone of the zygoma, which allows consistent plating of the maxilla (Figure 52.27).

Hardware

As rigid fixation has progressed, the variety and sizes of plates has proliferated. The predominant systems that are used are

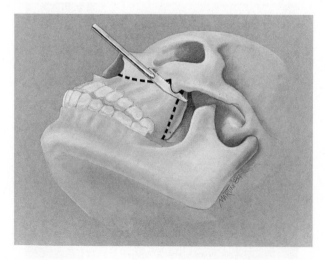

FIGURE 52.27 Bony cut on lateral aspect of maxilla. (From Van Sickels, Jeter, and Aragon,[43] with permission)

1.5-mm and 2.0-mm plates and screws. These are used in the areas of the bony buttresses. Larger plates are used with inferior and anterior positioning of the maxilla. Smaller plates are used with impaction and some posterior movements. (See the discussion in the relapse section.) The smaller the plate, the less likely the patient will feel it after surgery. However, stability of a case dictates the size of the plates the surgeon should use. For unstable moves, auxilliary techniques have been shown to be helpful.[45]

Some surgeons use plates at the piriform fossa and wires at the buttress. This allows some play in the postoperative position of the maxilla. The senior author believes that this is not necessary and places plates at the piriform fossa and the zygomatic-maxillary buttress.

Advantages and Disadvantages

The advantages of rigid fixation with maxillary surgery are similar to those mentioned for rigid fixation of the mandible: early function, greater stability and patient comfort.

The greatest disadvantage is that rigid fixation does not allow as much manipulation of the maxilla as is possible with wire osteosynthesis and therefore postoperative malocclusions are not as easy to manage. As with the management of postoperative mandibular malocclusions, the surgeon needs to decide early how to correct the problem. (The sooner the better.)

In a stepwise progression, the senior author looks at malocclusions following surgery as:

1. Those that can be corrected by elastic traction
2. Those that need the hardware removed to achieve the desired results
3. Those that should go back to an operating room for correction

For step two, removal of the hardware can be done in the office under intravenous sedation. Once the hardware is removed, elastics are placed and the patient's occlusion is carefully monitored over the next few days and weeks.

Relapse

With the advent of rigid fixation and its use with maxillary osteotomies, it became apparent that there were a number of points in the management of a patient where errors in execution could result in postoperative occlusal discrepancies. These errors can be roughly divided into three separate time periods. They are in the preoperative, intraoperative, and postoperative phases of management. Positioning errors in the horizontal position can be traced to the accuracy of the preoperative records. The exact point to use to predict the amount of autorotation has been debated. Bryan[46] showed that condylion, center of condyle, or Sperry's point could all be used to predict autorotation. Of greater importance than the exact center of rotation is to obtain an accurate retruded position of the mandible and to mount the maxillary cast in the same occlusal plane on an articulator related to Frankfort horizontal as that which is present in the patient.[47] Many patients with dentofacial deformities have a tendency to posture their jaws. Failure to recognize a shift in the occlusion from first contact to centric occlusion will result in a maxillary position after surgery posterior to the desired one or in the case of a right to left shift, a maxillary midline off to one side.

Horizontal position discrepancies after surgery can also be traced to difficulties in intraoperative positioning of the maxilla. Failure to properly seat the condyle or to recognize posterior interferences are two of the most common causes of postoperative occlusal problems. It is known that general anesthesia allows positional changes in the condyle that are otherwise prevented by the muscles that limit the "border" movements of the mandible. The effects of general anesthesia are further exacerbated by muscle paralysis as well as the force of gravity. McMillin[48] studied anesthetized patients and discovered that in the absence of manual angle support the condyle dropped an average of 2.43 mm. With vertical angle support the drop averaged only 0.31 mm. Failure to support the condyles during maxillary surgery will result in a maxilla that is forward of the desired position and is inferior in the posterior region when the patient awakens. For an isolated maxillary procedure the patient will present with a class II open bite occlusion after surgery.

Posterior interferences cause a more dramatic occlusal discrepancy than a failure to seat the condyles. Major malocclusions can be seen after surgery particularly when the maxilla is moved in a posterior direction. Posterior interferences can also be seen with maxillary impaction that have minimal advancement associated with their skeletal movement. When the maxilla is positioned intraoperatively, the surgeon must vertically and posteriorly position the mandible. The maxilla and mandible must be moved together from a wide open position until first bony contact. If a subtle hit and shift forward is noted during closing, a posterior interference is present, and the surgeon must remove it. Failure to do so will result in a postoperative class II open bite.

Vertical positioning problems can also be an intraoperative problem. While some surgeons still use bony references scribed on the maxillary walls to determine vertical position of the maxilla, the technique is highly inaccurate. An external reference point has been shown to be extremely predictable in positioning the maxilla vertically in space.[49]

Postoperative changes are generally related to orthopedic forces generated by the tissues themselves or elastic traction placed on the skeleton. For example, a large mandibular advancement can adversely affect the position of the maxilla if elastics are used without skeletal suspension wires.

Rigid fixation has been shown to be more stable than wire osteosynthesis.[50,51] However, that does not imply that rigid fixation is stable for all cases. The direction and magnitude of the move of the maxilla needs to be evaluated in every case. Maxillary impactions are very stable, hence small plating (1.5-mm) systems are adequate. Maxillary setbacks are also very stable. The size of the system needed with a maxillary setback will vary with the size of the gap between segments. When no gaps exist, a 1.5-mm system will be adequate. When gaps exist, a 2-mm system should be used with autogenous or allogenic augmentation to act as osseous scaffolding. Maxillary advancements are not as stable as impactions or setbacks and necessitate the use of 2-mm plating systems.[52] Egbert et al.[52] showed that rigid fixation of a maxillary advancement was more stable than when wires were used. However, posterior movement with rigid fixation still occurred. Rigid fixation did impart more stability than did wires with regard to vertical stability when the maxilla was advanced. Inferior movement of the maxilla is the least stable move one can perform necessitating 2-mm plates and auxiliary techniques. Van Sickels and Tucker[45] noted that inferior movement of the maxilla (especially when there was an advancement) was the most likely to result in a nonunion.

The senior author prefers to use the center of the condyle to predict autorotation of the mandible.

The authors prefer to use 0.062 threaded Kirschner wire driven at the radix of the nose. Measurements are made from the wire to a bracket on the central incisor.

Similar to mandibular setbacks, the senior author sets up his maxillary advancement cases with 2 to 4 mm of overjet depending on the amount of dental compensation in the case before surgery.

Case

2.0-mm Stabilization

A 22-year-old man with medical history significant for myotonic dystrophy presented for evaluation of his skeletal discrepancy. His skeletal findings were significant for vertical maxillary excess (total facial height of 168 mm) and maxillary transverse deficiency and apertognathia, and horizontal mandibular excess. Following presurgical orthodontics, he underwent a three-piece maxillary impaction with a differential movement (10-mm posterior, 4-mm anterior impaction) with a 5-mm BSSO setback (Figure 52.28). One-and-one-half years after surgery, there has been no change in his facial skeleton.

Owing to the large moves this case was treated with a 2-mm system. Supplemental suspension wires were used with elastic traction between the maxillary and mandibular wires.

1.5-mm Stabilization

A 17-year-old female presented with apertognathia (3 mm) and horizontal mandibular excess. After presurgical orthodontics, she underwent a one-piece impaction of 4-mm posterior with a 6-mm mandibular setback (Figure 52.29). Two-and-one-half years after surgery, her occlusion and skeletal moves have remained stable.

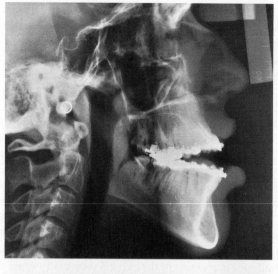

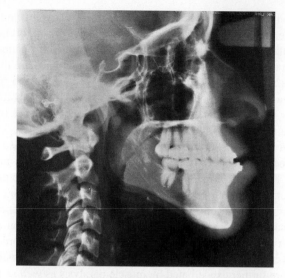

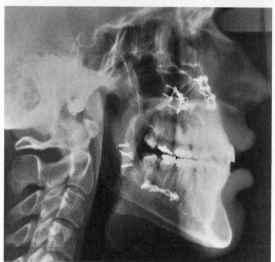

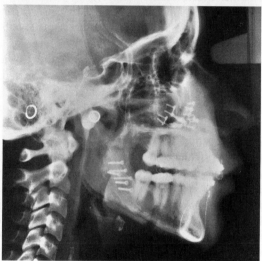

FIGURE 52.28 (a) Presurgical and (b) 1-year postsurgical cephalometric radiographs.

FIGURE 52.29 (a) Presurgical and (b) 6-week postsurgical cephalometric radiographs.

The relative minimal move in this case allowed much smaller hardware to stabilize the bones in position.

Anterior and posterior segmental maxillary osteotomies can be used depending on a patient's skeletal deformity. Both these operations have limited usefulness in that segmental movement can often be accomplished more easily and predictably with a Le Fort I. Posterior maxillary osteotomies are used primarily to treat supereruption of posterior teeth. Both 1.5-mm and 2-mm plating systems are useful with isolated segmental osteotomies. Stability with these procedures is excellent.

Midface Osteotomies

Indications

Midface deficiencies may exist in isolation or more frequently in combination with maxillary deficiencies. There are a number of options that one can choose to address these combina-
tion deficiencies, which include osteotomies at the occlusal level and augmentation at the midface level, high Le Fort I osteotomy, and variously designed Le Fort III osteotomies. Unfortunately, midface and maxillary deficiencies seldom are of the same magnitude, and occlusal discrepancies sometimes necessitate correction of the maxilla in segments. In our practice the most common type of midface/maxillary osteotomy is the combined Le Fort III/I osteotomy.

The senior author would previously move the nose with the midface complex on all combination nasal deformities/midface/maxillary deficiency patients. However, if the canthal region is of normal dimension, he now prefers to do a Le Fort III/I and augments the nose with a cantilevered cranial bone graft (without mobilization of the nasal bones/nasoethmoid complex).

Technique

Previous authors have described moving the maxilla and upper midface separately.[53] The technique we prefer predictably moves the zygomas with the maxilla as a unit, with additional movement of the maxilla separately. The design allows plating at the piriform fossa at both the Le Fort III level and I level (Figure 52.30).

Access is gained to the midface and maxilla through bilateral transconjunctival incisions combined with lateral canthotomy incisions. Intraorally a circumvestibular incision is made. The bony cuts begin by making a horizontal osteotomy laterally from the piriform fossa approximately 5 mm. A bone cut is made from the infraorbital rim medial to the neurovascular bundle down the face of the maxilla to the horizontal cut at the piriform rim. Intraorbitally an osteotomy is made laterally below the lateral canthus approximately 5 mm into the zygoma. An osteotomy is made across the floor of the orbit from the medial cut to the lateral cut, being careful not to injure the infraorbital nerve. The lateral bone cut is brought from the lateral rim to the maxilla/zygomatic buttress near the leading edge of the origin of the masseter muscle. From this cut, the osteotomy is extended posterior into the pterygoid plate region. The midface and maxillary complex is advanced using a prefabricated splint designed to bring the midface forward symmetrically. The midface/maxilla is plated at the Lefort III level cognizant that an additional osteotomy will be done. A 2-mm plating system is used at the piriform rim, while a 1.5-mm plating system is used at the lateral orbital rim. Once the complex is stabilized, the maxilla is cut at the Le Fort I level. Generally, the maxilla is advanced further. Given the large moves, a 2-mm plating system is necessary to stabilize the advancement. Osseous voids are filled with

freeze-dried cancellous marrow chips ("croutons"). The lateral orbital rim is inspected, and generally there is a step that needs to be smoothed off. The superficial musculoaponeurotic system (SMAS) is suspended, and the tissues are closed in a standard fashion using a nasal cinch and V-Y closure.

As with isolated maxillary advancements, our Le Fort III/I osteotomies are overcorrected.

Hardware

Both 1.5-mm and 2-mm plating systems are used as described earlier. Occasionally when the maxilla/midface is advanced at the III level, a single screw can be used to stabilize the complex at the piriform region in combination with a 1.5-mm type of plate at the orbital region.

Advantages and Disadvantages

The advantages of a midface osteotomy technique is that the results are more predictable than alternative choices. Alloplast placed in this region can become displaced. Onlay grafts resorb and remodel in an unpredictable fashion.

The greatest disadvantages are the time necessary to plan the case (models, etc.) and time of the surgical procedure.

Relapse

Schmitz et al.[54] retrospectively examined a series of 11 patients who had undergone combination Le Fort III/I. At 6 months after surgery, the maxilla relapsed 2.8 mm vertically while moving forward 1.5 mm. The occlusions stayed stable. The forward movement of the maxilla represents the autorotation that occurs from the superior movement.

Case

A 19-year-old male presented with maxillary and midface deficiency of 13 mm. He underwent a combined Le Fort III/I osteotomy, and was advanced. He was advanced 7 mm at the III level and 6 mm at the I level (Figure 52.31).

Due to the huge advancement, 2-mm plates were used in his surgery. Even so, with such a large movement one must expect relapse.

Summary

Rigid fixation over the last several years has quickly changed the management of orthognathic surgery patients. Just a few years ago, patients who had orthognathic surgery would be admitted to the hospital the night before surgery, would spend the night after surgery in the intensive care unit, and frequently would have a 4- to 7-day hospital stay. Today, the same procedures stabilized with rigid fixation allow the patient to go home in 24 hours and sometimes be treated as a day surgery. Rigid fixation has allowed complex procedures

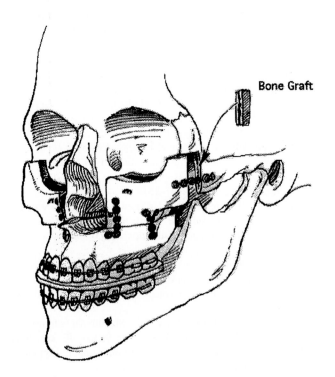

Bone Graft

FIGURE 52.30 Illustration of a Le Fort III/I after all the cuts have been made and plated. (From Van Sickels and Tiner,[37] with permission)

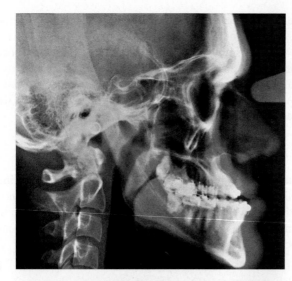

a

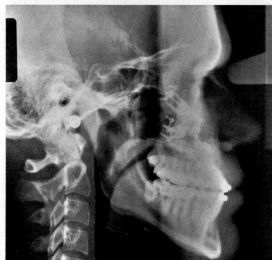

b

FIGURE 52.31 (a) Presurgical and (b) postsurgical lateral cephalogram of a patient who underwent a combination Le Fort III/I.

to be performed with predictable results. Stability of some of these more complex operations is just now being analyzed.

Problems that can result in short-term relapse with some of the more frequent operations such as the BSSO and the Le Fort I are recognized and are minimized with rigid fixation. Problems that result in long-term relapse are not as well recognized or understood. Long-term stability will finally be accomplished when we can identify and manage all of the factors that lead to condylar resorption.

References

1. Carlson DS, Ellis E, Schniderman ED, Ungerleider JC. Experimental models of surgical intervention in the growing face: Cephalometric analysis of facial growth and relapse. In: McNamara JA, Carlson DS, Ribbens KA, eds. *The Effect of Surgical Intervention on Craniofacial Growth.* Monograph #12. Center for Human Growth and Development, The University of Michigan, Ann Arbor, MI, 1982;11–72.

2. Ellis E, Carlson DS. Neuromuscular adaptation after orthognathic surgery. *Oral Maxillofac Surg Clin North Am.* 1990;2: 811–830.

3. Reynolds ST, Ellis E, Carlson DS. Adaptation of the suprahyoid muscle complex to large mandibular advancements. *J Oral Maxillofac Surg.* 1988;46:1077–1085.

4. Van Sickels JE, Larsen AJ, Thrash WJ. A retrospective study of relapse in rigidly fixated sagittal split osteotomies: contributing factors. *Am J Orthod Dentofacial Orthop.* 1988;93: 413–417.

5. Arnett GW, Tamborello JA. Progressive class II development: female idiopathic condylar resorption. *Oral Maxillofac Surg Clin North Am.* 1990;2:699–710.

6. Ellis E, Sinn DP. Connective tissue forces from mandibular advancement. *J Oral Maxillofac Surg.* 1994;52:1160–1163.

7. Kerstens HCJ, Tuinzing DB, Golding RP, van der Kwast WAM. Condylar atrophy and osteoarthrosis after bimaxillary surgery. *Oral Surg Oral Med Oral Pathol.* 1990;69:274–280.

8. Kundert M, Hadjianghelou O. Condylar displacement after sagittal splitting of the mandibular rami. *J Maxillofac Surg.* 1980;8:278–279.

9. Obwegeser H, Trauner R. Zur Operationtechnik bei der Progenie und anderen Unterkieferanomalien. *Dtsch Zahn Kieferheilkd.* 1955;23:H1–H2.

10. Hunsuck EE. A modified intraoral sagittal splitting technique for correction of prognathism. *J Oral Surg.* 1968;26:250–254.

11. Epker BN. Modifications in the sagittal osteotomy of the mandible. *J Oral Surg.* 1977;35:157–160.

12. Spiessl B. The sagittal splitting osteotomy for correction of mandibular prognathism. *Clin Plast Surg.* 1982;9:491–507.

13. Franco JE, Van Sickels JE, Thrash WJ. Factors contributing to relapse in rigidly fixed mandibular setbacks. *J Oral Maxillofac Surg.* 1989;47:451–456.

14. Foley WL, Frost DE, Paulin WB, Tucker MR. Internal screw fixation: comparison of placement pattern and rigidity. *J Oral Maxillofac Surg.* 1989;47:720–723.

15. Blomqvist JE, Isaksson S. Skeletal stability after mandibular advancement: a comparison of two rigid internal fixation techniques. *J Oral Maxillofac Surg.* 1994;52:1133–1137.

16. Schilli W, Niederdellmann H, Harle F, Joos U. Stable osteosynthesis in treatment of dentofacial deformity. In: Bell WH, ed. *Surgical Correction of Dentofacial Deformities, New Concepts.* Philadelphia: WB Saunders; 1985;490–511.

17. Foley WL, Beckman TW. In vitro comparison of screw versus plate fixation in the sagittal split osteotomy. *Int J Adult Orthod Orthognath Surg.* 1992;7:147–151.

18. Van Sickels JE, Jeter TS. Rigid osseous fixation of osteotomies. In: Bell WH, ed. *Surgical Correction of Dentofacial Deformities, New Concepts.* Philadelphia: WB Saunders; 1985: 732–744.

19. Schwimmer A, Greenberg AM, Kummer F, Kaynar A, et al. The effect of screw size and insertion technique on the stability of the mandibular sagittal split osteotomy. *J Oral Maxillofac Surg.* 1994;52:45–48.

20. Tucker MR, Frost DE, Terry BC. Mandibular surgery. In: Tucker MR, Terry BC, White RC, Van Sickels JE, eds. *Rigid fixation for Maxillofacial Surgery.* Philadelphia: Lippincott; 1991:258–262.

21. Tulasne J-F, Schendel SA. Transoral placement of rigid fixation following sagittal ramus split osteotomy. *J Oral Maxillofac Surg.* 1989;47:651–652.

22. Lake SL, McNeil RW, Little RM, West RA. Surgical mandibular advancement: a cephalometric analysis of treatment response. *Am J Orthod.* 1981;80:376–393.

23. Smith GC, Moloney FB, West RA. Mandibular advancement surgery. A study of the lower border wiring technique for osteosynthesis. *Oral Surg Oral Med Oral Pathol.* 1985;60:467–475.

24. Schendel SA, Epker BN. Results after mandibular advancement surgery: An analysis of 87 cases. *J Oral Surg.* 1980;38:265–282.

25. Gassamann CJ, Van Sickels JE, Thrash WJ. Causes, location and timing of relapse following rigid fixation after mandibular advancement. *J Oral Maxillofac Surg.* 1990;48:450–454.

26. Scheerlinck JPO, Stoelinga PJW, Blijdorp PA, Brouns JJA, Nijs MLL. Sagittal split advancement osteotomies stabilized with miniplates. A 2–5 year follow-up. *Int J Oral Maxillofac Surg.* 1994;23:127–131.

27. Crawford JG, Stoelinga PJW, Blijdorp PA, Brouns JJA. Stability after reoperation for progressive condylar resorption after orthognathic surgery: report of seven cases. *J Oral Maxillofac Surg.* 1994;52:460–466.

28. Arnett GW, Tamborello JA, Rathbone JA. Temporomandibular joint ramifications of orthognathic surgery. In: Bell WH, ed. *Modern Practice in Orthognathic and Reconstructive Surgery.* Vol 1. Philadelphia: WB Saunders; 1992:523–593.

29. Van Sickels JE. A comparative study of bicortical screws and suspension wires versus bicortical screws in large mandibular advancements. *J Oral Maxillofac Surg.* 1991;49:1293–1296.

30. Hall HD, Chase DC, Paylor LG. Evaluation and refinement of the intraoral vertical subcondylar osteotomy. *J Oral Surg.* 1975;33:333–341.

31. Hall HD, Nickerson JW, McKenna SJ. Modified condylotomy for treatment of the painful temporomandibular joint with a reducing disc. *J Oral Maxillofac Surg.* 1993;51:133–142.

32. Paulus GW, Steinhauser EW. A comparative study of wire osteosynthesis versus bone screws in the treatment of mandibular prognathism. *Oral Surg Oral Med Oral Pathol.* 1982;54:2–6.

33. Van Sickels JE, Tiner BD, Jeter TS. Rigid fixation of the intraoral inverted "L" osteotomy. *J Oral Maxillofac Surg.* 1990;48:894–898.

34. Tiner BD, Von Sickels JE, Lemke RR. Stability of rigid fixation in the inverted "L" osteotomy: long term results. *J Oral Maxillofac Surg.* (Suppl 3) 1992;50:87–88.

35. Friedman CD, Costantino PD. Use of distraction osteogenesis for maxillary advancement: Preliminary results; Discussion. *J Oral Maxillofac Surg.* 1994;52:287–288.

36. Aronson J. Experimental and clinical experience with distraction osteogenesis. *Cleft Palate Craniofac J.* 1994;31:473–482.

37. Van Sickels JE, Tiner BD. Cost of a genioplasty under deep intravenous sedation in a private office versus general anesthesia in an outpatient surgical center. *J Oral Maxillofac Surg.* 1992; 50:687–690.

38. Park HS, Ellis E, Fonseca RJ, Reynolds ST, Mayo KH. A retrospective study of advancement genioplasty. *Oral Surg Oral Med Oral Pathol.* 1989;67:481–489.

39. Van Sickels JE, Smith CV, Jones DL. Hard and soft tissue predictability with advancement genioplasty. *Oral Surg Oral Med Oral Pathol.* 1994;77:218–221.

40. Wassamund D. Lehrbuch der praktischen chirurgie des mundes und der kiefer. Vol. 1. Leipzig: Meuser; 1935.

41. Obwegeser HL. Surgical correction of small or retro-displaced maxillae: The dish-face deformity. *Plast Reconst Surg.* 1969; 43:351–355.

42. Bell WH, Fonseca RJ, Kennedy JW, Levy BM. Bone healing and revascularization after total maxillary osteotomy. *J Oral Surg.* 1975;33:253–260.

43. Van Sickels JE, Jeter TS, Aragon SB. Rigid fixation of maxillary osteotomies: a preliminary report and technique article. *Oral Surg Oral Med Oral Pathol.* 1985;60:262–265.

44. Kaminishi RM, David WH, Hochwald DA, Nelson N. Improved maxillary stability with modified Le Fort I technique. *J Oral Maxillofac Surg.* 1983;41:203–205.

45. Van Sickels JE, Tucker MR. Management of delayed union and non-union of maxillary osteotomies. *J Oral Maxillofac Surg.* 1990;48:1039–1044.

46. Bryan DC. An investigation into the accuracy and validity of three points used in the assessment of autorotation in orthognathic surgery. *Br J Oral Maxillofac.* 1994;32:363–372.

47. Ellis E, Tharanon W, Gambrell K. Accuracy of face-bow transfer: effect on surgical prediction and postsurgical result. *J Oral Maxillofac Surg.* 1992;50:562–567.

48. McMillin LB. Border movements of the human mandible. *J Prosthet Dent.* 1972;27:524–532.

49. Van Sickels JE, Larsen AJ, Triplett RG. Predictability of maxillary surgery: a comparison of internal and external references marks. *Oral Surg Oral Med Oral Pathol.* 1986;61:542–545.

50. Carpenter CW, Nanda RS, Currier GF. The skeletal stability of Le Fort I downfracture osteotomies with rigid fixation. *J Oral Maxillofac Surg.* 1989;47:922–925.

51. Larsen AJ, Van Sickels JE, Thrash WJ. Postsurgical maxillary stability: a comparison study of bone plate and screw vs wire osseous fixation. *Am J Orthod Dentofac Orthop.* 1989;95:334–343.

52. Egbert M, Hepworth B, Myall R, West R. Stability of Le Fort I osteotomy with maxillary advancement: a comparison of combined wire fixation and rigid fixation. *J Oral Maxillofac Surg.* 1995;52:243–247.

53. Bell WH, Proffit WR, Jacobs J. Maxillary and midface deformity. In: Bell WH, Proffit WR, White RP, eds. *Surgical Correction of Dentofacial Deformities.* Vol 1. Philadelphia: Saunders; 1980;509–513.

54. Schmitz JP, Tiner BD, Van Sickels JE. Stability of simultaneous Lefort III/Le Fort I osteomomies. *J Cranio-Maxillofac Surg.* 1999;23:287–295.

53
Le Fort II and Le Fort III Osteotomies for Midface Reconstruction and Considerations for Internal Fixation

Keith Jones

The Le Fort II and the Le Fort III osteotomies were initially made on the basis of reproducing the facial bone fracture patterns caused by trauma. The techniques are well described in the literature.[1,2]

However, with improvements in surgical access, technological developments in anaesthesia and surgery, and advanced fixation techniques, it is now possible to move the midface in almost any desired direction and fix it in this position with long-term stability.[3,4]

With regard to surgery, with the exception of the optic nerves and the cone (apex) of the orbit, movement of all else is possible. Moreover, the midface either in segments or *en bloc* can then be stabilized with bone grafts and internal fixation using titanium bone plates and screws of various dimensions.

Anaesthetic developments have allowed surgeons to gain experience in undertaking major facial corrective surgery on younger patients while maintaining the safety of the procedure.

Concomitant with this, the use of internal fixation techniques has allowed less reliance on the use of intermaxillary fixation with improved postoperative airway management and hence the decreased requirement for tracheostomy.

Le Fort II Osteotomy

Anatomy

The Le Fort II procedure is the least commonly performed of the Le Fort advancements. It allows the central midface to be moved anteriorly (or inferiorly) with the maxillary dental arch. Its application[5] is appropriate when the patient presents with a combination of:

1. A short nose
2. Nasomaxillary retrusion
3. A skeletal class III occlusion

If the midface hypoplasia affects the lateral part of the central midface, it is also possible to advance the infraorbital margins. By lateral extension of the osteotomy cuts the infraorbital margin can be included in the component to be advanced.

The selection of the Le Fort II procedure must be made carefully. The existing functional and cosmetic deformity must be considered and alternative procedures[6] such as the high Le Fort I procedure with nasal augmentation should be excluded as a treatment option.

Indications

Correction of midface hypoplasia which is associated with nasomaxillary retrusion (Figure 53.1) includes:

1. Posttraumatic defects
2. Maxillonasal dysplasia in which a class I occlusion exists (Binders' syndrome)
3. Secondary correction of cleft deformity

Three-dimensional movements of the midface are possible, and precise planning and surgery are essential to produce the desired end result. When planning surgery for maxillonasal dysplasia, cephalometric analysis can be misleading owing to the retrusion of the nasomaxillary sill.

Soft Tissue Surgical Access

Surgical access is via the intraoral Le Fort I-type mucosal incision combined with one of two basic surgical approaches:

1. The coronal incision
2. Paranasal (inner canthus) skin incision

The latter may, in the younger patient, utilize separate bilateral paranasal incisions. In the older patient, it is possible to use a single incision via a natural dorsal skin crease to unite the inner canthal incisions (Figure 53.2). Following careful subperiosteal dissection (and tunneling) both options allow access to the entire nasofrontal area and the facial skeleton in the region of the infraorbital margin.

Surgical Technique

Following exposure of the nasofrontal region, elevation of the nasal periosteum is undertaken with a fine Obwegeser pe-

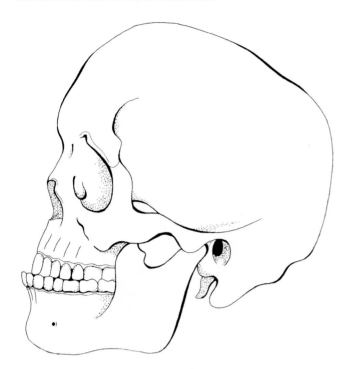

FIGURE 53.1 Skull with midface deformity.

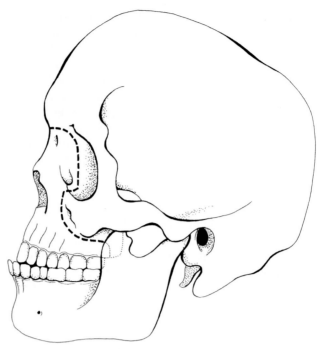

FIGURE 53.3 Skull showing Le Fort II osteotomy cuts.

riosteal elevator. The horizontal glabella osteotomy is completed using a burr just below the level of the frontonasal suture (Figure 53.3). The osteotomy can then either be continued posteriorly into the ethmoid bone and inferiorly behind the lacrimal sac or made anteriorly.[7] The anterior approach involves detachment of the anterior and superior arms of the medial canthal tendon, whereas the posterior approach invariably means detachment of the complete medial canthal area. The burr cut is then extended through the infraorbital margin between the nasolacrimal duct and the infraorbital

nerve (Figure 53.4). This is done in the presence of orbital retraction and allows completion of the cut through the infraorbital rim toward the anterior maxillary wall. A similar procedure is undertaken on the opposite side.

The infraorbital cut is then followed by the intraoral incisions and extended using a fine burr or saw around and inferior to the zygomatic buttress and posteroinferiorly toward the pterygoid plates. Where there is a very marked deficiency of the infraorbital region, it is possible to extend the os-

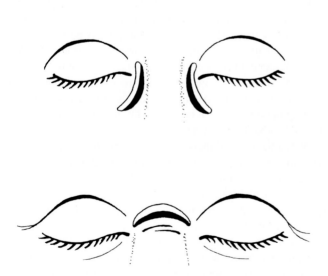

FIGURE 53.2 Paranasal and dorsal nasal access incisions.

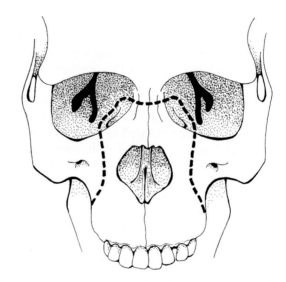

FIGURE 53.4 Frontal view of skull showing Le Fort II osteotomy cuts.

teotomy laterally along the orbital floor using a fine burr cut. The limit of this extension is reached when the orbital floor begins to curve superiorly to form the lateral orbital wall. In a similar manner, the cut is taken anteriorly through the infraorbital rim and inferiorly along the anterior wall of the maxilla toward the zygomatic buttress. In the pterygomaxillary region, division can either take place using a small curved osteotome directed between the pterygomaxillary suture or by curving the maxillary osteotomy cut inferiorly through the maxillary tuberosity anterior to the pterygomaxillary junction. The nasal septum and vomer can be divided via the nasofrontal osteotomy using a curved Tessier chisel. It is important to direct this chisel downward and backward, and it is also important to remember that in patients with nasomaxillary hypoplasia, the distance between the nasofrontal region and the pharynx is relatively short. Mobilization of the maxilla can then be undertaken using maxillary mobilization forceps. The Smith spreader can be used to aid mobilization and the Tessier mobilizers to move the midface anteriorly.

Following mobilization of the midface, the maxillary teeth are placed into a preformed occlusal wafer, which reflects the planned final position of the midfacial movement. Intermaxillary fixation is then applied, and stabilization with bone grafts and internal fixation devices can commence.

If a significant increase (5 to 10 mm) in vertical height of the midface is planned, it is recommended that the medial nasal osteotomy be undertaken anterior to the medial canthal ligament and nasal lacrimal duct apparatus. Use of this modification when large movements are planned is less likely to lead to possible complications such as telecanthus.

Bone Graft Stabilization and Internal Fixation

There are two potential donor sites for bone grafting, and the choice is dependent on the access incisions used for the osteotomy procedure.

If the paranasal access incisions are used, the ilium is likely to be the donor site of choice. A large block of corticocancellous bone is harvested from the medial aspect of the ilium and segmentalized into smaller corticocancellous blocks for insertion into the spaces between the osteotomy cuts. Ideally, the graft should be contoured so that it can be wedged between the osteotomy cut in the desired position. In the nasofrontal region, two corticocancellous blocks are contoured to reconstruct the nasion. The fixation of the osteotomy at this site can be achieved either by the application of an H- or inverted T-shaped 1.5-mm titanium miniplate or by the contouring and adaptation of two short, straight 1.5-mm plates extending from the glabella onto the lateral aspect of the nasal complex bilaterally (Figure 53.5). Passive adaptation of the bone plates is essential, and use of the lower profile 1.5-mm plate is desirable at this location as the skin and subcutaneous tissue at this site is relatively thin, and as such, the larger dimension plates can be readily palpated. The bone thickness

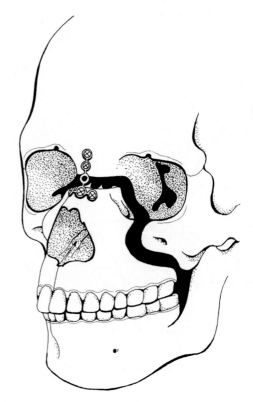

FIGURE 53.5 Fixation at frontonasal osteotomy.

in the glabella and nasal complex is also relatively limited, and this consequently limits screw length to a maximum of 6 mm.

With regard to the pterygoid and maxillary buttress region, blocks of corticocancellous bone are contoured and wedged into both these sites. Fixation can be affected from the zygomatic buttress to the posterior maxilla using a long L-shaped 2-0 titanium plate and 6-mm screws (Figure 53.6). The anterior and lateral maxillary wall osteotomy defects can likewise be spanned using strips of corticocancellous bone. It is also possible using the Compact microsystem (Stratec-Waldenburg, Waldenburg, Switzerland) to span and stabilize the osteotomy defect between the frontal process of the maxilla and the infraorbital rim bilaterally. Care must be taken when inserting these plates to avoid morbidity to the lacrimal sac and the infraorbital nerve (Figure 53.7).

When the coronal incision is the access incision of choice, cranial bone offers itself as an alternative donor site.[8] Split-thickness calvarium can be harvested and contoured for grafting at the nasofrontal-zygomatic buttress and in the anterior and lateral walls of the maxilla. It can also be inserted into the pterygoid region, but in this location, several contoured fragments of outer table are likely to be required to interpose between the bony defects. Split-thickness calvarium can be stabilized in the zygomatic buttress, lateral and anterior maxillary walls, and in the nasofrontal region utilizing lag screws.[9]

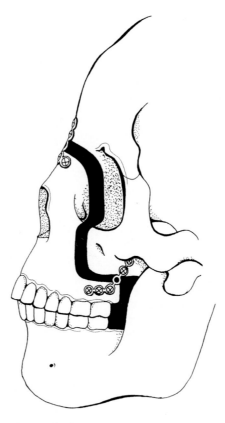

FIGURE 53.6 Fixation at posterior maxilla.

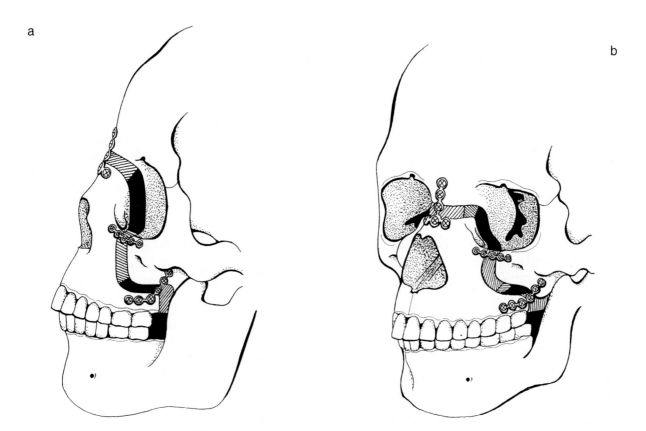

FIGURE 53.7 (a) Overall fixation with block grafts in situ, lateral view. (b) Overall fixation with block grafts in situ rotated frontal view.

Le Fort III Osteotomy

Anatomy

This procedure is used for the correction of total midface hypoplasia affecting the maxilla and zygomatic complexes with associated exorbitism. Tessier[2,10] pioneered the clinical application of the technique, and others[11] have subsequently modified the procedure.

The original operation produces bony separation of the complete facial skeleton from the skull base, whereas modifications include isolated advancement of the nasozygomatic and zygomaticomaxillary components of the midface.

The procedure can be approached either via a subcranial (extracranial approach) or a transcranial procedure. The latter is more suitable when a major correction of the upper facial skeleton or hypertelorism is required. There has been an increasing tendency for major midfacial correction procedures to be performed on younger patients,[12] and long-term follow-up information is available on such patients. The results are favorable with regard to the overall safety of the procedure and the degree of long-term stability of the facial advancement.

The classical deformity corrected by the Le Fort III procedure includes:

1. Retrusion of the nose, maxilla, and ZMCs
2. A shortened nose
3. A skeletal class III occlusion

Not only does the procedure improve the patient's cosmetic appearance, it also produces more support of the globes by reduction of the exorbitism and a functional improvement by correcting the skeletal class III occlusion. Where there are differential degrees of deformity between the nasozygomatic component and maxilla an additional low-level osteotomy may be undertaken to provide the best aesthetic result. Thus when indicated (unlike the Le Fort II procedure), a Le Fort I procedure can be combined with the Le Fort III surgical approach.

Indications

The Le Fort III osteotomy is used for correction of true retrusion of the complete facial skeleton, that is, the nasal complex, the zygomatic maxillary complexes, and the maxilla (Figure 53.8).

Selection of the Le Fort III procedure is appropriate for the correction of the following:

1. Posttraumatic deformity
2. Midface hypoplasia
3. Craniosynostoses, that is, the Crouzon, Apert, and Pfeiffer syndromes

The planning of surgery should be based on facial aesthetics and should not rely solely on cephalometric analysis,[13] which

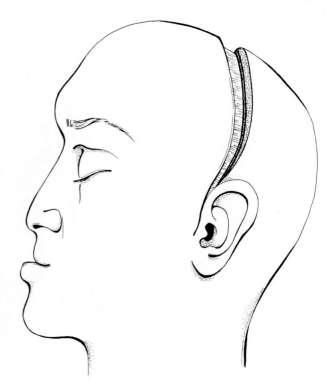

FIGURE 53.8 Midface hypoplasia and coronal access incision.

can be misleading. Cephalometrics should, ideally, be used only as a guide to planning the advancement procedure. For diagnosis, a full neuroradiological and ophthalmological assessment must be made and where indicated, neurosurgical evaluation should also be undertaken. Commonly, prolonged presurgical orthodontic correction is required to optimize the postoperative occlusion. The final position is influenced not only by the occlusion but also by facial aesthetics and other factors such as soft tissue coverage of the mobilized segments. Anterior advancement of the midface to more than 15 mm is possible; however, excessive inferior positioning of the midface to correct an anterior open bite can have an adverse result with excess lengthening of the nose.

Soft Tissue Surgical Access

The classical Le Fort III type procedure was originally described via a series of small incisions in the facial soft tissues:

1. The medial canthal region
2. The lateral orbital region
3. The lower eyelid incision
4. Intraoral vestibular incision

The most common current approach, however, involves

1. The coronal incision (Figure 53.8)
2. Intraoral sulcular incisions bilaterally

In addition, where problems are encountered with access to the orbital floor, a transconjunctival or lower eyelid approach can also be useful.

Surgical Technique

The scope of the description here is limited to the subcranial Le Fort III approach. Nasoendotracheal intubation and hypotensive anaesthesia are used for surgery. The coronal incision is the access incision of choice and the line of the incision is located well within the hairline toward the vertex of the skull. The initial dissection is undertaken in a supraperiosteal manner with a coronal incision being made through the pericranium 2 to 3 cm above the supraorbital ridge. Reflection of the coronal flap by careful subperiosteal dissection allows visualization and sequential exposure of the nasal bones, the medial canthal tendons, superior aspect of the lacrimal fossa, the lateral orbital rims, and the inferior orbital margins. A tunneling technique is used to ensure the latter. Circumferential dissection around the orbit allows mobilization of the periorbita so that the osteotomy cuts can be located approximately 10 mm inside the orbital margin. The zygomatic arch and temporal fossa are exposed by division of the temporal fascia and reflection of the temporalis muscle. Care must be taken to minimize stripping to avoid unsightly temporal hollowing. In the nasoethmoid region, the medial canthal tendons and lacrimal sac area are carefully identified. The medial canthal tendon is normally detached with the periorbital dissection and marked for subsequent reattachment.

Some authors[12] advocate nondetachment of the medial canthal tendon if the presurgical position is judged to be clinically satisfactory and if the movement of the midface is only in the anterior direction.[13] If this is the case, the osteotomy cuts are taken posteriorly behind the medial canthal tendon and lacrimal sac. The lateral canthus is normally detached during periorbital stripping. It is important that this is reattached at the end of the procedure, otherwise canthal drift can occur. To facilitate this, the location of the lateral canthal attachment can be marked when periorbital stripping is being undertaken.

The starting point for the bony osteotomy may be variable. In the midline, a fine horizontal burr cut is made just inferior to the frontonasal suture, which is extended posteriorly into the orbit behind the nasolacrimal duct. Care must be taken as the orbit is likely to be very shallow. The cut is extended inferiorly and then laterally toward the region of the infraorbital nerve. Access in this site can be difficult, and a fine osteotome may be preferable to the use of a burr. The orbital floor osteotomy is directed laterally toward the inferior orbital fissure.[2]

There are several patterns of osteotomy through the zygomatic complex, namely, total advancement of the zygomatic complex (Figure 53.9), sagittal splitting of the zygomatic complex (Figure 53.10), or total advancement with frontozygomatic extension (Figure 53.11). The zygomatic osteotomy can be undertaken using a fine saw. The osteotomy cut is taken through the lateral margin of the orbit and then passes inferiorly through the middle of the bony lateral orbital wall. It is important to maintain a bony rim posteriorly on the lateral orbital wall for grafting and fixation purposes. The cut is then extended back

a

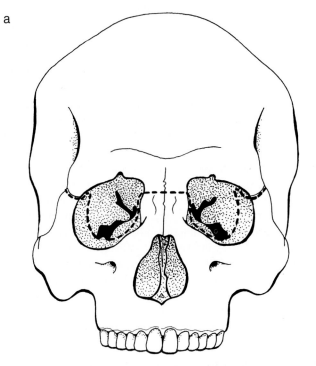

b

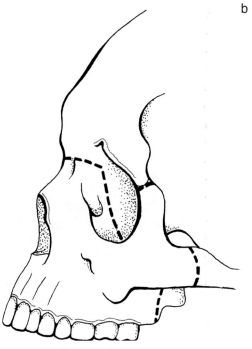

FIGURE 53.9 (a) Frontal skull with Le Fort III osteotomy cuts for total advancement of zygomatic complex. (b) Lateral view of Le Fort III osteotomy cuts for total advancement of zygomatic complex.

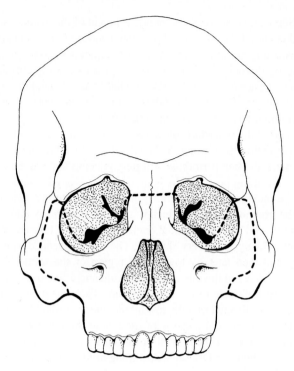

FIGURE 53.10 Frontal skull with Le Fort III osteotomy cuts with sagittal splitting of the zygomatic complex.

into the pterygopalatine fissure. Inside the orbit, the cut is extended inferiorly toward the inferior orbital fissure, and the medial and lateral cuts can be joined using a fine osteotome.

A fine saw is also used to divide the zygomatic arch.

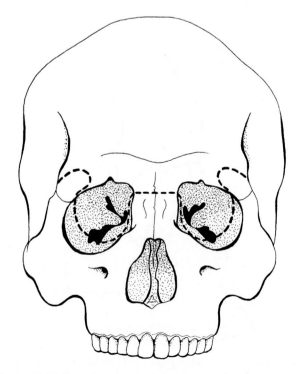

FIGURE 53.11 Frontal skull with Le Fort III osteotomy cuts to include zygomaticofrontal advancement.

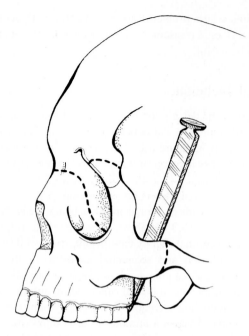

FIGURE 53.12 Lateral view to demonstrate use of osteotome to divide pterygoid region via coronal incision.

The pterygomaxillary dysjunction can be achieved either from above by insertion of a curved osteotome through the coronal incision into the temporal fossa (Figure 53.12),[14] or it can be achieved from below via a posterior buccal sulcus incision. The latter allows the insertion of a curved osteotome, although it is important during this procedure to avoid comminution of the pterygoid region if possible and to avoid troublesome bleeding caused by damage to the maxillary vessels. Division of the nasal septum is undertaken at the end of the procedure immediately before mobilization of the midface to avoid excessive bleeding.[15] The nasal septum and vomer can be divided with a fine osteotome. A finger is placed intraorally in the region of the posterior nasal spine, and the osteotome is directed inferiorly toward this site. The facial skeleton is now ready for mobilization, and this can be achieved by the use of maxillary disimpaction forceps and the use of leverage at the frontonasal and zygomaticofrontal regions (Figure 53.13). It is sometimes necessary to expand the osteotomy sites by use of osteotomes and this is clearly facilitated in the pterygomaxillary region if bony comminution has been avoided. Further anterior mobilization of the midface can be effected using the Tessier mobilizers. Progressive careful mobilization of the facial skeleton must take place and significant force is required to stretch the soft tissues to allow full mobilization to occur. At the end of the mobilization process, the maxilla should fit freely into the interocclusal wafer before intermaxillary fixation is established.

Bone Graft Stabilization and Internal Fixation

The inferior part of the mobilized facial skeleton can now be inserted into the interocclusal wafer and maxillomandibular

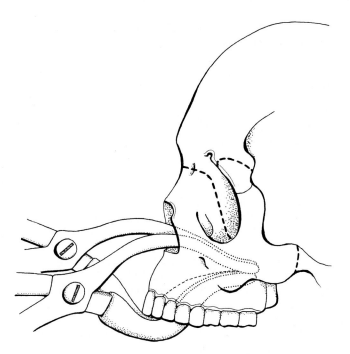

FIGURE 53.13 Lateral view demonstrating insertion of disimpaction forceps to mobilize Le Fort III osteotomy.

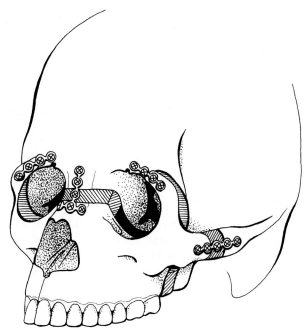

FIGURE 53.14 Rotated frontal view of advanced and stabilized Le Fort III osteotomy with zygomaticofrontal advancement showing block bone graft insertion and plate fixation.

fixation can be established. Some authors recommend an overcorrection, which is planned into the final occlusal splint. Stabilization of the osteotomy sites can now be achieved by the insertion of bone grafts and internal fixation with plates and screws. Bone grafts either from the parietal skull in split thickness or ilium are fashioned and inserted into the nasofrontal, lateral orbital rim, and pterygomaxillary region. The zygomatic arch defect can also be grafted. Rigid fixation is applied in the nasofrontal region, the lateral orbital rims, and zygomatic arches. All screw holes in cortical bone more than 4 mm thick should be pretapped before screw insertion. A combination of low-profile plate configurations are used in the nasofrontal region, either an H- or inverted T-shaped plate can be used to span the defect and stabilize the bone graft (Figure 53.14). Dependent on the osteotomy pattern, either a curved C-shaped plate or a stepped, adapted straight plate can be used in the lateral orbital wall to establish stability. Selection of the plate size (1.5-mm or 2.0-mm Synthes Compact, Stratec-Waldenburg, Waldenburg, Switzerland) will be dependent, to some extent, on the thickness of the overlying soft tissue. A straight bone plate and calvarial bone graft is used to stabilize the zygomatic arch and similarly, split calvarium is also used to graft the orbital floor. Where appropriate, lag screws can be used to stabilize the calvarial graft, particularly if it has been utilized to augment an asymmetrical region within the midface. In the pterygomaxillary region, ideally a block graft is wedged in situ to buttress the advanced facial skeleton.

The lateral canthal tendons are reattached with a heavy, nonresorbable suture to the premarked location. Similarly, the medial canthal tendon can be reattached using a transnasal canthopexy ensuring that the site at which this reattachement occurs is more posterior and slightly superior than its former location. A curved microplate can also be used to anchor the relocated medial canthal tendon.

Complications

Infection

Infection is the most common complication associated with major craniofacial surgery, and several contributing factors have been identified. These include prolonged operative time, excessive blood loss, residual dead space, and open communication between the osteotomy sites and the nasal cavity and paranasal sinuses. A number of studies[16–19] have reported similar infection rates of around 3%.

It is therefore normal practice to administer antibiotics intravenously for 72 hours postoperatively. Where appropriate, for example, the coronal flap, suction drainage is routinely used.

Hemorrhage

Hypotensive anaesthesia is used for these prolonged surgical procedures to reduce hemorrhage to a minimum. Specific care is taken at individual sites to minimize the risk of serious hemorrhage. These include the pterygomaxillary region and the division of the nasal septum and nasal mucosa, which is normally undertaken immediately before the final mobilization of the facial skeleton. Meticulous hemostasis is applied during the elevation of the coronal flap with control of bleeding from the flap margins by the immediate application of disposable Rayne clips. During these procedures extensive areas of vascular bony soft tissue are frequently exposed, and it is important to minimize progressive oozing from these sites by meticulous hemostasis at each stage.

Lacrimal Apparatus

Damage to the lacrimal apparatus is possible, although it is a less common complication. Some authors[11] have reported increased postoperative lacrimal problems when stripping and relocation of the medial canthal tendons has been undertaken.

Nerve Damage

Inadequate care during the dissection procedure can inadvertently lead to damage of both the supraorbital and infraorbital nerves. If subperiosteal tunneling via the coronal flap provides inadequate access to the infraorbital region, the lower eyelid or transconjunctival incision may be used to gain improved access and minimize the risk of damage to the orbital nerves during the orbital floor osteotomy. During elevation of the coronal flap, it is important to remain within the correct tissue plane and avoid the possible risk of damage to the frontal branch of the facial nerve.

Bone Graft Donor Site Morbidity

As a general principle the larger the donor defect when bone is harvested from the ilium, the greater the risk of morbidity experienced by the patient. By careful subperiosteal dissection and mobilization, it is possible to harvest a large block corticocancellous graft via a relatively small access incision. Similarly, morbidity can be minimized by harvesting the graft from the inner table of the ilium, and thereby minimizing the degree of muscle stripping required to gain access to the donor site.

With regard to split calvarial grafts, it is normal practice to control hemostasis by applying a hemostatic paste. Some surgeons also favor the application of several layers of methylcellulose gauze to the donor site, and it is always important to carefully bevel the cortical bony margins around the donor defect. It is not uncommon for adult patients to complain of local discomfort at calvarial donor defects for some significant time after surgery.[20]

Malocclusion

In the younger patient it appears that anterior growth of the midface does not return to normal and as such there is a significant incidence of malocclusion with a skeletal class III malocclusion occurring.[12,21]

References

1. Jackson IT, Munro IR, Salyer KE, et al. *Atlas of Craniomaxillofacial Surgery.* St. Louis: Mosby; 1982.
2. Tessier P. Total osteotomy of the middle third of the face for faciostenosis or for sequelae of Le Fort III fractures. *Plast Reconstr Surg.* 1971;48:533.
3. Beals SP, Munro IR. The use of miniplates in craniomaxillofacial surgery. *Plast Reconstr Surg.* 1987;79(1):33–38.
4. Kaban LB, West B, Conover M, et al. Midface position after LeFort III advancement. *Plast Reconstr Surg.* 1984;73(5):758–767.
5. Henderson D, Jackson IT. Nasomaxillary hypoplasia—the Le Fort II osteotomy. *Br J Oral Surg.* 1973;11:77.
6. Van Sickels JE, Tiner BD. A combined Le Fort I and bilateral zygomatic osteotomy for management of midface and maxillary deficiency. *J Oral Maxillofac Surg.* 1994;52:327–331.
7. Epker BN, Wolford LM. Middle third advancement: treatment considerations in atypical cases. *J Oral Surg.* 1979;37:3.
8. Tessier P. Autogenous bone grafts taken from the calvarium for facial and cranial applications. *Clin Plast Surg.* 1982;9:531.
9. Gruss JS. Craniofacial osteotomies and rigid fixation in the correction of post traumatic craniofacial deformities. *Scand J Plast Reconstr Surg Hand Surg.* 1995;27:83–95.
10. Tessier P. The definitive plastic surgical treatment of the severe facial deformities of craniofacial dysostosis. Crouzon's and Apert's diseases. *Plast Reconstr Surg.* 1971;48:419.
11. Epker BN, Wolford LM. *Dentofacial Deformities.* St. Louis: Mosby; 1980.
12. McCarthy JG, LaTrenta GS, Breitbart AS, et al. The Le Fort III advancement osteotomy in the child under seven years of age. *Plast Reconstr Surg.* 1990;86:633.
13. Grayson BH. Cephalometric analysis for the surgeon. *Clin Plast Surg.* 1989;16:633.
14. Murray JE, Swanson LT. Midface osteotomy and advancement of craniosynostosis. *Plast Reconstr Surg.* 1968;41:299.
15. Ortiz-Monasterio F, Fuente del Campo A, Carrilo A. Advancement of the orbits and midface in one piece combined with frontal repositioning, for the correction of Crouzon's deformities. *Plast Reconstr Surg.* 1978;61:507.
16. Whitaker LA, Munro IR, Salyer KE. Combined report of problems and complications in 793 craniofacial operations. *Plast Reconstr Surg.* 1979;64:198.
17. Munro IR, Sabiatier RD. An analysis of 12 years of craniomaxillofacial surgery in Toronto. *Plast Reconstr Surg.* 1985;75:29.
18. David DJ, Cooter RD. Craniofacial infection in 10 years of transcranial surgery. *Plast Reconstr Surg.* 1987;80:213.
19. Poole MD. Complications in craniofacial surgery. *Br J Plast Surg.* 1988;41:608.
20. Frodel JL, Marentette LJ, Qualeta VC, et al. Calvarial bone graft harvest. Techniques, consideration and morbidity. *Arch Otolaryngol Head Neck Surg.* 1993;119(1):17–23.
21. Bachmayer KI, Ross RB, Munro IR. Maxillary growth following Le Fort III advancement surgery in Crouzon, Apert and Pfeiffer syndromes. *Am J Orthod Dentofacial Orthop.* 1986;90:420–430.

Section VI
Craniofacial Surgery

54
Craniofacial Deformities: Introduction and Principles of Management

G.E. Ghali, Wichit Tharanon, and Douglas P. Sinn

In the last several years the arena of craniomaxillofacial surgery has expanded in scope, and the treatment of these deformities has become more sophisticated. In view of these many changes, the embryology, etiology, pathogenesis, imaging, and treatment of the common craniofacial deformities will be reviewed with their management.

Embryology of the Craniofacial Region

Any discussion of craniofacial syndromes must be preceded by a consideration of the normal embryologic development of these structures. The neural crest cells are important to the development of the facial skeleton. Translocated neural crest cells, upon reaching their destination, differentiate into cartilage, bone, and ligaments of the face and contribute to the muscles and arteries in the region. Any disruption of migration and differentiation may have deleterious effects.[1] The crucial period of organogenesis takes place during the first 12 weeks of gestation, and it is during this time that the majority of congenital craniofacial deformities are established.[1,2] The facial growth centers appear at the end of the third week of embryonic life and are in their definitive place by the eighth embryonic week. The face derives its morphology from five prominences. These prominences are the single frontonasal and the paired maxillary and mandibular processes. The grooves between these facial prominences usually disappear by the seventh week of gestation. A persisting groove will generally result in a congenital facial cleft. Occipital somites and somitomeres form a majority of the neurocranium. The neurocranium is anatomically divided into two portions: the membranous part consisting of flat bones, which surround the brain as a vault, and the cartilaginous part or chondrocranium, which forms the bones of the skull base. The sides and roof of the skull develop from mesenchyme, invest the brain, and eventually undergo membranous ossification. Membranous bones are characterized by the presence of needle-like spicules. These spicules progressively radiate from the primary ossification centers toward the periphery (Figure 54.1). Membranous bone enlarges by apposition of new layers on the outer surface and by simultaneous osteoclastic resorption from the interior.

At birth, the flat bones of the skull are separated from each other by narrow seams of connective tissue, the cranial sutures. At points where more than two bones meet, the sutures are wide and known as fontanelles. The sutures and fontanelles allow the bones of the skull to overlap during the birth process. Several of the sutures and the fontanelles remain membranous for a considerable time after birth. Growth of the bones of the vault is the result of expansion of these flat bones caused mainly by the volumetric growth of the brain. Although a 5- to 7-year-old child has normally achieved maximum cranial capacity, some of the sutures remain open until adulthood. Cartilaginous neurocranium or chondrocranium consists initially of a number of separate cartilages. When these cartilages fuse and ossify by endochondral ossification, the base of the skull is formed.[3]

Etiology of Craniofacial Deformities

Congenital craniofacial deformities can have a genetic, environmental, or combined etiology. Currently, it is known that environmental factors associated with congenital deformities are radiation, infection, maternal idiosyncrasies, and chemical agents:[4]

Radiation. Large doses of radiation have been associated with microcephaly.

Infection. The children of mothers affected with toxoplasmosis, rubella, or cytomegalovirus show increased frequency of facial clefts.

Maternal idiosyncrasies. Numerous studies attest to the major role of maternal factors such as age, weight, and general health on the resistance or susceptibility of the developing embryo to potential causes of malformation.

Chemical. Many chemical agents or drugs have been implicated in craniofacial malformation such as ethanol, 13-*cis* retinoic acid, and methotrexate.[5] Additionally, other drugs suspected of playing a role in craniofacial syndromes are the anticonvulsants.

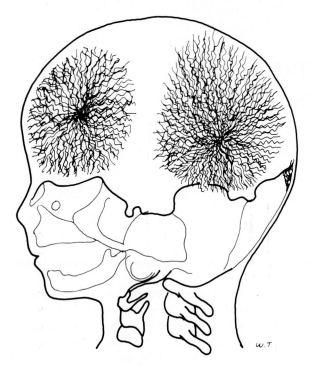

FIGURE 54.1 Skull of infant demonstrating primary cranial ossification centers.

Principles of Management of Craniofacial Deformities

Multidisciplinary Team Approach

The multidisciplinary team concept was developed from the recognition that failures commonly occurred when various aspects of care were not coordinated and when the relationships among coexisting problems were not known. The objectives of this approach are diagnosis, formulation, and execution of treatment plans as well as longitudinal follow-up for patients with craniofacial deformities; the team should meet at least monthly for regular outpatient evaluations. Transcripts of these evaluations are forwarded with treatment recommendations to primary care providers and appropriate agencies. Children under 5 years of age are usually evaluated annually, whereas those over 5 years of age are seen every other year. The frequency of evaluation varies with the stability of the deformity and its consequences. The craniofacial team should consist of an anesthesiologist, an ophthalmologist, a surgeon (plastic and/or oral/maxillofacial), an audiologist, a maxillofacial prosthodontist, an orthodontist, a psychologist, a geneticist, an otolaryngologist, a radiologist, a neurologist, a neurosurgeon, a pediatrician, social services, a pedodontist, a speech pathologist, an orthotist, and a nurse.[6,7]

Genetic Diagnosis: The Dysmorphology Examination

Dysmorphology is the study of birth defects with an emphasis on understanding the mechanisms of morphogenesis. The dysmorphologist or clinical geneticist should be one of the first clinicians to evaluate the patient with a birth defect involving the craniomaxillofacial region. This approach benefits both the patient and the team caring for the patient by fostering a comprehensive approach to evaluation, especially of defects outside the craniofacial region. Accurate diagnosis then becomes the basis for accurate prognosis and recurrence risk (genetic) counseling.

Genetic Counseling

Genetic counseling provides information and emotional support to families in which an individual has a disorder or birth defect. The genetic counselor gathers the family's medical and pregnancy history, obtains necessary medical records, and determines the concerns and questions of the individuals attending the assessment. This service provides medical and psychosocial support to unaffected relatives as well as the affected individual. The genetic counselor may interact closely with other members of the craniofacial team by providing important information regarding the history, patient, and family.

Radiographic Evaluation

The radiographic evaluation of craniofacial deformities is used to quantitatively define aberrant anatomy, plan surgical procedures, and evaluate the effects of growth as well as surgery. Conventional skull radiographs such as plain skull films and lateral cephalograms are inexpensive and widely available. The preoperative assessment of patients with suspected or known craniofacial deformities is based on these conventional radiographs. The majority of synostosis can be demonstrated on plain skull films. Normal or patent cranial sutures manifest as a line and the absence of a radiolucent line in the normal anatomic position of a suture may suggest a craniosynostosis.

Currently, computer tomography (CT) scans provide improved hard tissue imaging.[8–10] The definition of these elements of the bony facial structures on high-resolution CT images is unmatched by other imaging techniques (such as plain skull or tomogram). The development of CT scanning, particularly three-dimensional reformatting, and the maturation of readily available means of craniofacial surgery has led to a close dependence on CT scanning for preoperative surgical planning. Additionally, CT scanning has also been used to document surgical changes in vivo and to follow them longitudinally.[11–24]

Common Craniofacial Deformities

In general, craniofacial deformities can be divided into three major subgroups: those involving the cranial skeleton only (coronal, sagittal, metopic, and lambdoidal craniosynostosis), those involving the cranial and facial skeleton (Crouzon's, Apert's, and Pfeiffer's syndromes), and those involving the facial skeleton only (Treacher Collins syndrome, hemifacial microsomia, cleft lip, and palate).

Craniosynostosis

In 1851, Virchow was credited as the first to use the term *craniosynostosis* in describing a disorder characterized by an abnormal shape of the skull. Virchow noted that synostosis in the skull restricted growth perpendicular to the direction of the suture and promoted compensatory overgrowth parallel to it.[25-27]

Pathogenesis of Craniosynostosis

The pathogenesis of craniosynostosis is complex and probably multifactorial. Moss theorized that abnormal tensile forces are transmitted to the dura from an anomalous cranial base through key ligamentous attachments leading to craniosynostosis such as seen in Apert's and Crouzon's syndromes.[28] This hypothesis fails to explain the coexistence of craniosynostosis in those patients with a normal cranial base configuration. The etiology of craniosynostosis may be postulated to be the result of either primary suture abnormalities, sufficient extrinsic forces that overcome the underlying expansive forces of the brain, or inadequate intrinsic growth forces of the brain.[29-31]

Functional Problems Associated with Craniosynostosis

The major functional problems with craniosynostosis are intracranial hypertension, visual impairment, limitation of brain growth, and neuropsychiatric disorders.

Intracranial Hypertension

The clinical symptoms include headaches, irritability, and difficulty sleeping. The radiographic signs may include cortical thinning or a Lückenschadel (beaten metal) appearance of the inner table of the skull; these clinical and radiographic signs are relatively late developments. If intracranial hypertension goes untreated, it affects brain function; if persistent this may necessitate early operative intervention during the first few months of life. Intracranial hypertension most likely affects those with the greatest disparity between brain growth and intracranial capacity. Currently, intracranial volume is measured by using CT scans.[32-34] This noninvasive method is used to measure intracranial volume in children with craniosynostosis. It might then be possible to select those individuals who are at a greater risk for developing intracranial hypertension and would benefit the most from early surgery.

Visual Impairment

Intracranial hypertension, if left untreated, leads to papilledema. Eventually, optic atrophy develops, resulting in partial or complete blindness. Some forms of craniosynostosis may involve orbital hypertelorism and may lead to compromised visual activity and restricted binocular vision.

Limitation of Brain Growth

Brain volume in the normal child almost triples during the first year of life. By 2 years of age, the cranial capacity is four times that at birth. If the brain growth is to proceed unhindered, open sutures at the level of the cranial vault and base must spread during phases of rapid growth, resulting in marginal ossification.

In craniosynostosis, premature suture fusion is combined with continuing brain growth. Depending on the number and location of prematurely fused sutures and the timing of closure, the growth potential of the brain may be limited. Surgical intervention, with suture release and reshaping, is done to restore a more normal intracranial volume. In general, this does not reverse the process, and diminished volume is often the end result.[35]

Neuropsychiatric Disorders

Neuropsychiatric disorders are thought to be secondary to cerebral compression and range from mild behavioral disturbances to overt mental retardation. Several studies have shown that children with craniosynostosis and associated neuropsychiatric disorders often improve after surgery.[36-39]

Current Surgical Approach: Staging of Reconstruction

In most cases, craniosynostosis suture release and cranial vault and orbital reshaping are mandatory before the child reaches 36 months of age.[40-53] An intracranial approach is used for cranial vault and orbital osteotomies, with reshaping and advancement of bony segments for ideal age-appropriate bony morphology. When planning the timing and type of surgical intervention, one must take into account the functions, future growth, and development of the craniofacial skeleton, as well as the maintenance of a normal body image.[35,54-57] In severe forms of craniosynostosis, additional revision of the cranial vault and orbit is necessary during infancy or early childhood to further increase intracranial volume; this allows for continued brain growth and avoids or reduces intracranial hypertension.[58]

Although many of the following examples depict transosseous wiring and/or titanium plating, our current trend is the utilization of resorbable plates and screws (Lactosorb, Walter Lorenz Surgical, Inc., Jacksonville, FL). These plates, composed of polylactic and polyglycolic acid, are completely resorbed by hydrolysis within 9 to 14 months while maintaining tensile strength for initial early stabilization. As a result, growth restrictions are minimized as is the potential for transcranial migration.

Classification of Craniosynostosis

The classification of craniosynostosis is based on the shape of the skull, which usually reflects the underlying prematurely fused suture(s).[59-62] The major cranial vault sutures that may be involved include the left and/or right coronal, metopic, sagittal, and left and right lambdoid (Figure 54.2).

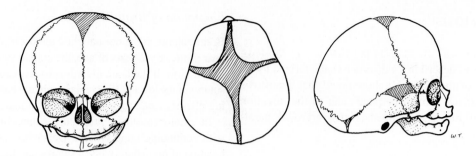

FIGURE 54.2 Three views depicting the major cranial sutures.

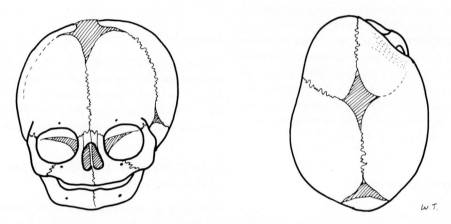

FIGURE 54.3 Anterior plagiocephaly illustrated from anterior and superior views.

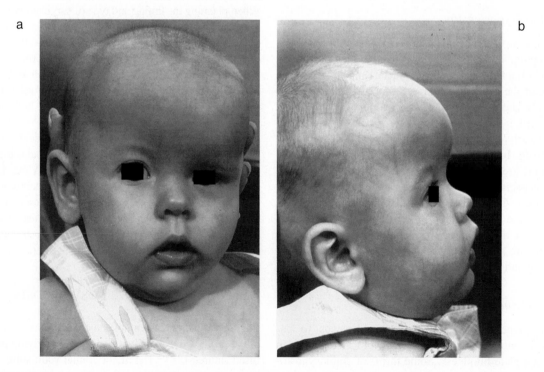

FIGURE 54.4 (a) Anterior view of child demonstrating plagiocephaly. (b) Lateral view of child demonstrating plagiocephaly.

Unilateral Coronal Synostosis

Unilateral coronal synostosis results in flatness or obliquity on the ipsilateral side of the forehead and supraorbital ridge region. The term for this deformity is anterior plagiocephaly (Figure 54.3). There are characteristic morphologic features on the affected ipsilateral side. The frontal bone is flat and the supraorbital ridge and lateral orbital rim are recessed. The affected orbit is shallow and the anterior cranial base is short in the anteroposterior (AP) dimension. The root of the nose may be constricted and deviated to the affected side. The ipsilateral zygoma and infraorbital rim may also be flat and recessed (Figure 54.4).

Timing and Surgical Management

Multiple surgical approaches for the correction of unilateral coronal synostosis have been described.[40–44] Good long-term results are obtainable when treatment of unilateral coronal synostosis includes suture release and cranial vault orbital osteotomies with reshaping and advancement in infancy. At Children's Medical Center at Dallas (CMC), unilateral orbital rim advancement (ORA) and frontal bone reshaping are ideally performed when the patient is 2.5 to 3 years of age. Other centers have reported good results when treated before 1 year of age. To achieve optimal symmetry, it is often necessary to use a bilateral surgical approach. Symmetry of the cranial vault and orbit must be achieved in surgery, since results generally do not improve over time. Stabilization is achieved by direct transosseous wires or resorbable plates and screws (Figure 54.5).

Bilateral Coronal Synostosis

This is the common cranial vault suture synostosis pattern associated with Apert and Crouzon's syndromes. Bilateral coronal synostosis results in recession of the supraorbital ridge causing the overlying eyebrows to sit posterior to the corneas. The term for this cranial vault deformity is *brachycephaly* (Figure 54.6). The anterior cranial base is short in the AP dimension and wide transversely. The overlying cranial vault is high in the superior–inferior dimension, with anterior bulging of the upper forehead resulting from compensatory growth of the opening metopic suture. The orbits are often shallow (exorbitism), with the eyes bulging (exophthalmus) and abnormally separated (orbital hypertelorism).

Timing and Surgical Management

Treatment requires suture release and simultaneous bilateral orbital rim and frontal bone advancements. Surgery is performed when the patient is 2.5 to 3 years of age. Other centers have reported good results when treated before 1 year of age. The osteotomy for bilateral orbital rim advancement is made superior to the nasofrontal and frontozygomatic sutures and is extended to the squamous portion of the temporal bone. Stabilization is achieved with direct transosseous wires or

plates and screws (titanium or resorbable). The more normalized shape provides the needed increase in intracranial volume within the anterior cranial vault.

Metopic Synostosis

Metopic synostosis often occurs in isolation resulting in a triangular head or trigonocephaly (Figure 54.7). The associated cranial vault deformity consists of hypotelorism, an elevated supraorbital ridge medially and posteriorly, and inferior recession of the lateral orbital rims and lateral aspect of the supraorbital ridges. The bitemporal bony width is decreased, resulting in inappropriate anterior cranial vault shape and decreased anterior cranial vault volume. The overlying forehead is sloped posteriorly to about the level of the coronal sutures (Figure 54.8).

Timing and Surgical Management

Surgical treatment requires metopic suture release, simultaneous bilateral orbital rim advancements, and widening via a frontal bone advancement. These procedures are usually performed when the patient is 6 months to 1 year of age. Orbital hypotelorism is corrected by splitting the supraorbital ridge unit vertically in the midline and placing autogenous cranial bone grafts to increase the interorbital distance (Figure 54.9a). Stabilization is achieved with direct transosseous wires or resorbable microplate fixation. The microplate fixation is usually placed at the inner surface of the cranial bone (Figure 54.9b). The abnormally shaped forehead bone that has been removed is cut into sections of appropriate shape for the new forehead configuration. The anterior cranial base, anterior cranial vault, and orbits are given a more aesthetic shape, and the volume of the anterior cranial vault is increased allowing the brain adequate space. Autogenous bone may be taken from the posterior cranium, when required, to enhance frontal reconstruction.

Sagittal Suture Synostosis

Sagittal suture synostosis, the most common form of cranial vault synostosis, is rarely associated with increased intracranial pressure. The term for this cranial vault deformity is *scaphocephaly* (Figure 54.10). The deformity consists of an elongated anteroposterior dimension and a narrowed transverse dimension to the cranial vault. Usually, the midface and anterior cranial vault sutures are not affected.

Timing and Surgical Management

When premature closure of a sagittal suture is recognized early in infancy, most neurosurgeons believe that simple release of the sagittal suture through a strip craniectomy without simultaneous skull reshaping is adequate treatment.[63] However, the residual cranial vault deformity may cause a continued psychosocial concern. If improvements in cranial

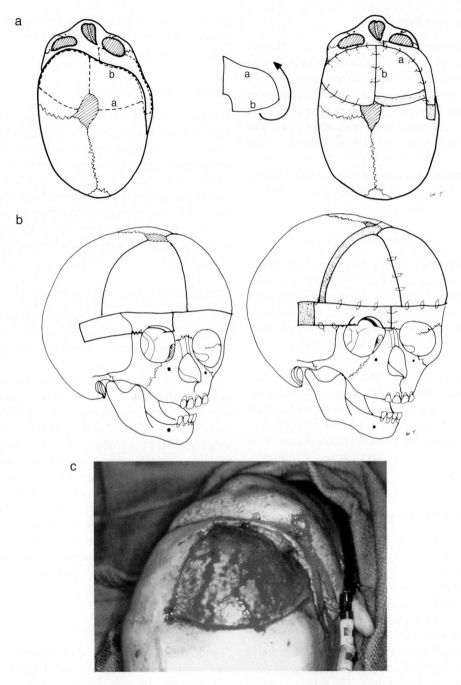

FIGURE 54.5 (a) Preoperative and postoperative superior views depicting a unilateral orbital rim advancement (ORA). (b) Three-quarters view depicting a unilateral ORA. (c) Intraoperative superior view. In this case, only unilateral reshaping was necessary to achieve symmetry.

vault shape are desired after 1 year of age, a formal total cranial vault reshaping is required (Figure 54.11).

Unilateral Lambdoid Synostosis

Unilateral lambdoid synostosis results in flatness of the affected ipsilateral parieto-occipital region. The location of the ear canal and external ear are more anterior on the ipsilateral side than on the contralateral side. This is more noticeable when the pa-

tient is examined from the superior view and relatively inconspicuous when observed from the frontal or profile view.

Timing and Surgical Management

Many surgeons consider either simple strip craniectomy of the involved suture or partial craniectomy of the region to be adequate treatment. We believe that a more extensive vault craniectomy and reshaping is generally necessary. If improve-

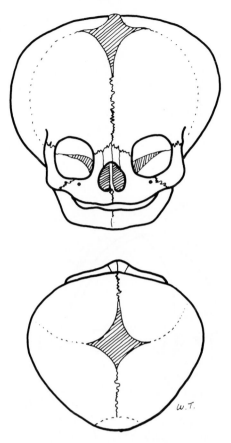

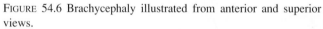

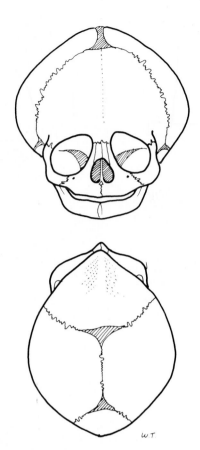

FIGURE 54.6 Brachycephaly illustrated from anterior and superior views.

FIGURE 54.7 Trigonocephaly illustrated from anterior and superior views.

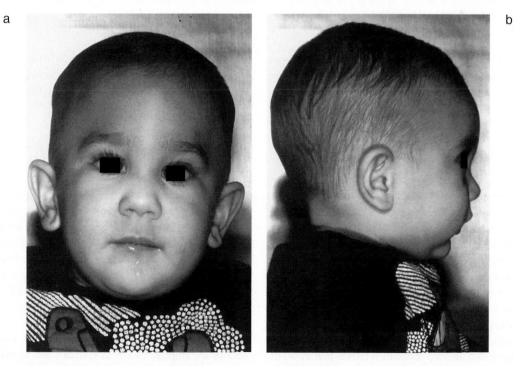

FIGURE 54.8 (a) Anterior view of child demonstrating subtle characteristics of metopic synostosis. (b) Lateral view of child demonstrating sloping of anterior forehead characteristic of trigonocephaly.

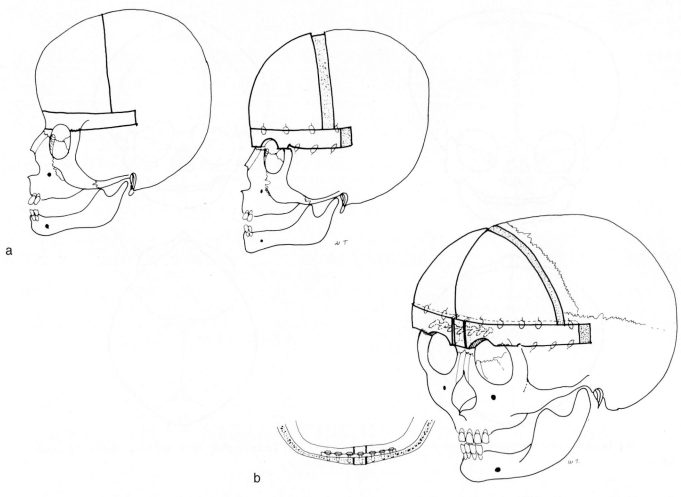

FIGURE 54.9 (a) Correction of metopic synostosis as illustrated from lateral view. (b) Three-quarter view illustrating correction of metopic synostosis and position of microplate fixation.

ments in cranial vault shape are desired after 10 to 12 months of age, formal posterior cranial vault reshaping is often required.

Craniofacial Dysostosis

Crouzon Syndrome

This syndrome was first reported in 1912 by M.O. Crouzon. He described the characteristics of this syndrome: exorbitism, retromaxillism, inframaxillism, and paradoxical retrogenia.[64] Inheritance is autosomal dominant and occurrence is both sporadic and familial. This condition affects about 1 in every 25,000 of the general population. Clinical appearance is characterized by recession of the frontal bone and supraorbital rim, retrusion of the midface, exorbitism with proptosis, and hypoplasia of the infraorbital rims (Figures 54.12a,b). Hypoplasia of the midface and a class III malocclusion is usually noted, but the mandible has normal growth potential. The skull is generally brachycephalic as a result of bilateral premature fusion of the coronal sutures.[65,66] The synostosis commonly begins during the first year of life and is usually complete by the

third or fourth year. Occasionally, the synostosis may be evident at birth; rarely, no sutural involvement is noted.[67] Increased intracranial pressure is frequent; therefore, it is mandatory to monitor the affected child.

Timing and Surgical Management

A staged approach is recommended for reconstruction in patients with Crouzon's syndrome. In infancy, it is necessary to combine suture release with cranial vault and orbital osteotomies in addition to reshaping and advancement to correct the brachycephalic morphology and increase the intracranial volume (Figures 54.12c–h). If the intracranial pressure is increased, repeat craniotomy with further cranial vault and orbital shaping and advancement is required later in infancy or early childhood. The residual midface deficiency requires a LeFort III osteotomy with advancement when the patient is 5 to 7 years of age. This procedure may be combined with cranial vault reshaping to further increase the intracranial volume and relieve intracranial pressure or for improvements in cranial vault morphology. When skeletal maturity has been reached (14 to 16 years in females; 16 to 18 years in males), orthognathic surgery is indicated. A

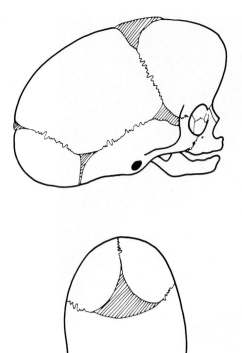

FIGURE 54.10 Scaphocephaly illustrated from the lateral and superior views.

maxillary Le Fort I osteotomy and a genioplasty is generally needed for correction of any residual dentofacial deformities.[68,69] Frequently, mandibular osteotomies will also be required if the anteroposterior discrepancy is great.

Apert Syndrome

Although Wheaton was the first to describe this syndrome in 1894, it is named after Apert, who in 1906 summarized four cases.[70] He described the syndrome as a severe cranial vault deformity with associated syndactylism, with or without mental retardation and blindness. The incidence is reported to be 1:100,000 to 1:160,000 births.[71] Although occurrence is sporadic, transmission is autosomal dominant. The clinical appearance is characterized by a flat face with hypertelorism, strabismus, and ocular muscle palsies, antimongoloid slant to the palpebral fissures and maxillary hypoplasia (Figure 54.13a).[72,73] There is moderate to severe exorbitism, short zygomatic arches, and a prominent bregmatic bump. The fontanelles may be large and late in closing. The palate is narrow and either has a median groove or is clefted with a bifid uvula; the incidence of cleft palate approaches 30%. The limbs show bony syndactyly with complete fusion of the four fingers leaving the thumbs free (Figure 54.13b). The distal phalanx of the thumb is often broad. Cutaneous syndactyly of all toes may be either simple or complex (Figure 54.13c). Mental retardation is variably reported in association with Apert's syndrome. The soft tissue drape is often abnormal and acne vulgaris with extensions to the forearm are common (70%). The facial skin, especially in the nasal region, is often thick

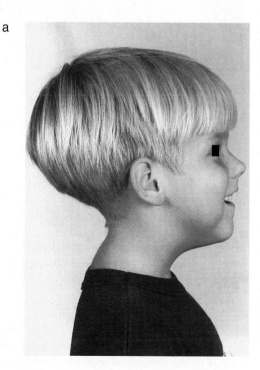
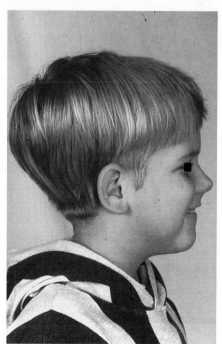

FIGURE 54.11 Lateral views demonstrating (a) preoperative and (b) postoperative changes in anteroposterior morphology achieved with total vault reshaping.

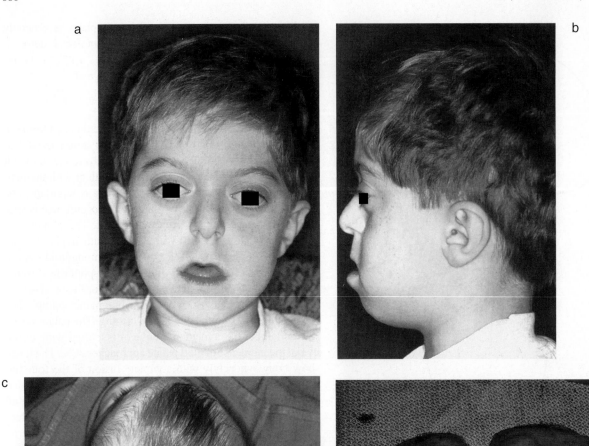

FIGURE 54.12 (a) Anterior view of child demonstrating classic characteristics of Crouzon's syndrome. (b) Lateral view of child demonstrating midface retrusion and exorbitism characteristic of Crouzon's syndrome. (c) Superior view of infant illustrating site for bicoronal incisions. (d) Bilateral frontal bone plates are sectioned and removed. (e) Barrel staving is accomplished to achieve frontocranial reshaping of the plates. (f) Supraorbital bar is removed and sectioned at the midline. (g) Intraoperative superior view illustrating microplate fixation of the inner cortex and resulting increase in the intracranial volume. (h) Lateral intraoperative view demonstrating the cranial vault reshaping necessary prior to closure for correction of the brachycephalic deformity characteristic of Crouzon's, Apert's, or Pfeiffer's syndromes.

with an increased sebaceous discharge. Hydrocephalus occurs frequently and requires ventriculoperitoneal shunting.[74-76] A conductive hearing loss may also be present.[77,78]

Timing and Surgical Management

The surgical management and timing are sequenced much the same as for patients with Crouzon's syndrome (Figures 54.12c–h). The need for repeat cranio-orbital surgery to increase intracranial volume for the relief of intracranial pressure is greater. Mental retardation is more common and may

be secondary to inadequate treatment of hydrocephalus or to craniosynostosis with reduced intracranial brain volume rather than inherent in the etiology itself.[74-76]

Pfeiffer Syndrome

Pfeiffer syndrome was first described in 1964. The clinical appearance of this syndrome is characterized by bilateral synostosis of the coronal sutures with associated midface deficiency, exorbitism, and exophthalmus (Figure 54.14). Broad thumbs, broad great toes, and partial soft tissue syndactyly of

e

f

g

h

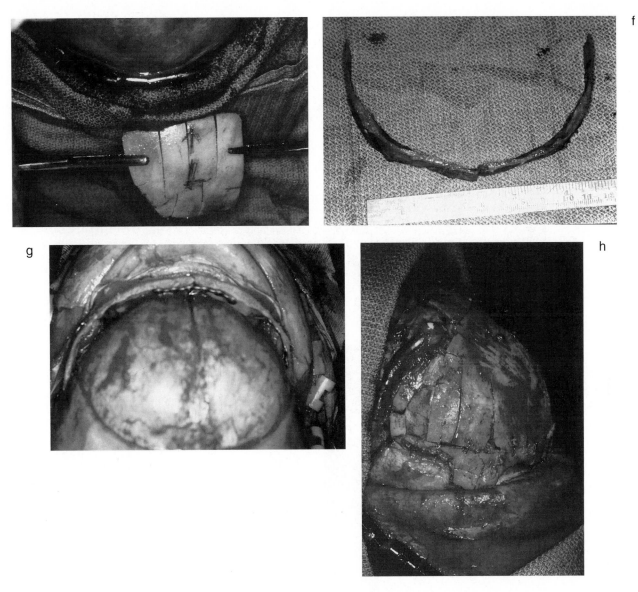

FIGURE 54.12 *Continued.*

the hands are variable features. Hydrocephalus and intracranial hypertension have been reported in association with this syndrome. Intelligence is usually normal, but mental retardation has been described.

Timing and Surgical Management

The surgical management and timing are sequenced much the same as for patients with Crouzon or Apert syndrome (Figure 54.12c–h).

Hemifacial Microsomia (HFM)

The term *hemifacial microsomia* (HFM) was first used by Gorlin and Pindborg in 1964.[79] Several other terms have also been used to describe this syndrome: asymmetric first and second branchial arch deformity, oculoauriculovertebral spectrum, otomandibular dysostosis, oculoauriculovertebral dysplasia, lateral facial dysplasia, and unilateral craniofacial microsomia.[80–85] It is the second most common congenital facial deformity after cleft lip and palate with an incidence of approximately 1 in 5600 live births.[86] Although the etiology of HFM may be variable and heterogenous, exposure of the pregnant mother to drugs such as thalidomide, primidone, and retinoic acid has been associated with a congenital first and second branchial arch syndrome.[87–89]

Pathogenesis

Typically, hemorrhage from the developing stapedial artery produces a hematoma in the area of the first and second branchial arches. The size of this hematoma and the resultant tissue destruction determines the morphology and variability

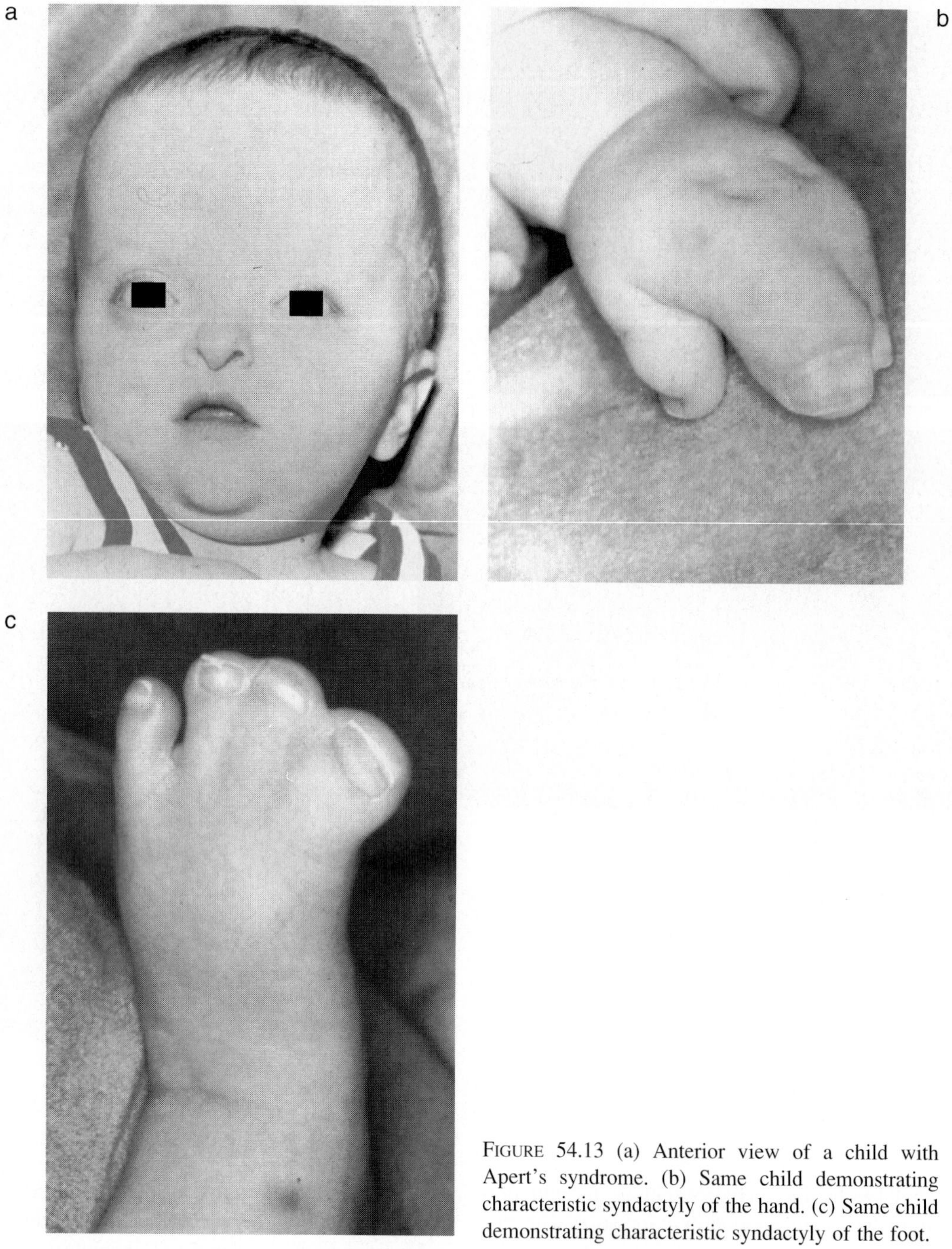

FIGURE 54.13 (a) Anterior view of a child with Apert's syndrome. (b) Same child demonstrating characteristic syndactyly of the hand. (c) Same child demonstrating characteristic syndactyly of the foot.

of HFM as described in a experimental model by Poswillo.[90] This sequence may be applicable to the condition in humans; additionally, hematoma formation may be the result of a variety of causes, such as hypoxia, hypertension, anticoagulants, or anomalous development of the carotid artery system.[91]

Clinical Characteristics of HFM

The mandible is short, retrusive, and narrow at birth and usually becomes progressively more asymmetric with time. The mandibular malformation ranges from a small but normally shaped ramus and temporomandibular joint (TMJ) to complete absence of these structures. The midface normally grows downward and forward away from the cranial base. In HFM, the growth of maxilla on the affected side is decreased secondary to temporal bone abnormalities, mandibular hypoplasia, and neuromuscular defects. The affected maxilla is short and canting of the occlusal plane is present; the occlusal plane is tilted upward on the affected side.[86,92,93]

In untreated HFM, the abnormal mandible consists of a

a 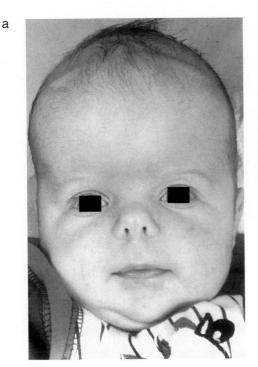 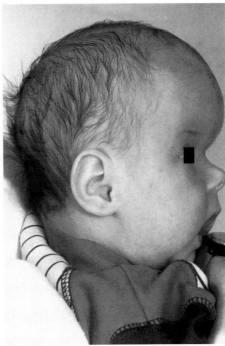 b

FIGURE 54.14 (a) Anterior view of an infant with Pfeiffer's syndrome. (b) Lateral view of an infant with Pfeiffer's syndrome.

short, medially displaced or absent ramus. If present, the ramus and mandibular body may be flat in contour and the chin is deviated toward the affected side. The occlusion on the affected side may be in crossbite and is generally tilted upward. The zygomatic bone is flat or incompletely formed, and the orbit may be inferiorly displaced.[86,92,93]

Soft Tissue Malformation

The soft tissue malformation consists of a decrease in the bulk of subcutaneous tissue ranging from mild to severe. The degree of soft tissue envelope deficit usually correlates with the severity of the skeletal defect. The soft tissue defects are classified as mild, moderate, and severe. The mild form consists of minimal subcutaneous and muscle hypoplasia, absence of or slight macrostomia, and a normal or mild auricular deformity. The severe form consists of significant subcutaneous and muscle hypoplasia, facial clefts, macrostomia, and neuromuscular weakness. Patients in between these two extremes are considered to have a moderate form. The external ear deformity is classified as grade I, II, and III following the system described by Meurman[94]:

Grade I. Mild hypoplasia, mild cupping, but all structures present.

Grade II. Absence of the external auditory canal and variable hypoplasia of the concha.

Grade III. Absence of the auricle, with an anteriorly and inferiorly displaced lobule.

A conductive hearing loss is present due to hypoplasia of the ear ossicles. Additionally, more than 25% of patients have cranial nerve abnormalities, usually consisting of facial nerve palsy and/or deviation of the palate toward the affected side with motion. Palatal deviation may be due to a combination of structural asymmetry, muscle hypoplasia, and cranial nerve weakness. The presence or absence of cranial nerve VII palsy correlates with the severity of the ear deficit, not the skeletal defect; the marginal mandibular nerve is the most common branch involved. Rarely, the total facial nerve palsy or a sensory deficit of trigeminal nerve has been described (Figure 54.15).[95–97]

Classification of HFM

Hemifacial microsomia has been classified into three types: type I, type II, and type III.[92,93,96,97] This classification is based on the presence or absence of critical structures and also assists in treatment planning.

Type I

Skeletal

All components are present but hypoplastic to varying degrees. The TMJ is present, but the cartilage and joint space are reduced. Hinge movement is normal, but translation is reduced during jaw opening.

a 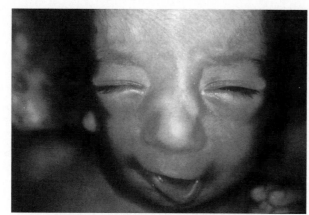 b
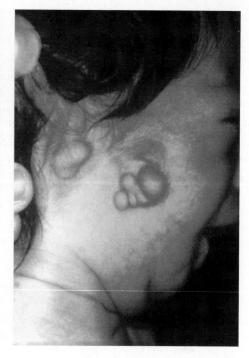

FIGURE 54.15 (a) Anterior view of an infant with characteristics of moderate to severe hemifacial microsomia (HFM). (b) Lateral view of an infant with characteristics of HFM and a grade III ear deformity.

Muscle

All masticatory muscles are present but are small. Patterns of muscle use are within the normal range of variation.

Type II A

Skeletal

The movement of the TMJ is present but without translation. The morphology of the TMJ is abnormal. The condylar process is cone shaped and positioned anterior and medial to its normal position. The coronoid process and angle are well developed.

Muscle

All muscles are notably hypoplastic.

Type II B

Skeletal

No condylar process that articulates with the temporal bone is present, but the coronoid process of varying size is present.

Muscle

No lateral pterygoid muscle is attached to the TMJ. There are also deficiencies of the masseter and medial pterygoid muscle. The temporalis muscle is small but easily palpated and is attached to the coronoid process.

Type III

Skeletal

No condylar or coronoid process is present. Additionally, the angle is absent.

Muscular

Severe hypoplasia of the masticatory muscles is present. The lateral pterygoid and temporalis muscles are not attached to the mandible.

Treatment

In general, the treatment of HFM is divided into two groups: growing and nongrowing patients. The treatment for each group is discussed.

Treatment for the Growing Child

The overall objectives of treatment are:

1. Improved function
2. Optimal facial symmetry
3. Aesthetics

Treatment is directed toward four areas:

1. Increasing the size of the underdeveloped mandible and associated soft tissues

2. Building an articulation between the mandible and temporal bone
3. Correcting the maxillary deformity
4. Building an aesthetic appearance to the face and dentition

The sequence of treatment consists of the following:

1. Presurgical orthopedic jaw treatment
2. Lengthening of the mandibular ramus
3. Reconstruction of TMJ
4. Correction of the maxilla when necessary
5. Final orthodontic refinement and soft tissue augmentation

Presurgical Orthopedic Treatment

Type I

A functional appliance is constructed to hold the affected side of the mandible in a lowered, forward position. This is expected to stimulate an additional increase in the length of both the condylar and coronoid process. When treatment response is good, surgical lengthening may be avoided if the canting of the occlusal plane is acceptable.

Type II A

In this group, the canting of occlusal plane is severe. Lengthening of the mandible on the affected side is necessary and an open bite is created postoperatively. This open bite can be closed by active orthodontic extrusion of maxillary teeth. The need for a LeFort I osteotomy is usually avoided.

Type II B and Type III

In these groups, the mandibular condyle is missing; therefore, reconstruction of the TMJ with costochondral or sternoclavicular grafts is necessary. This is especially true when mandibular movement is restricted and masticatory function is impaired. Distraction osteogenesis may be considered for mandibular lengthening. This reconstruction should be done early in development (6 to 10 years of age). Additionally, a second mandibular lengthening may be necessary for correction of any residual deformities; often simultaneous maxillary surgery is also needed.

After reconstruction of the TMJ and lengthening of the mandible have been done in the growing child, a functional appliance is constructed to be used for continued growth management, thereby supporting the deficient joint structure and asymmetric muscle function.

Surgical Management

Type I and Type II A

Surgical correction of skeletal deformities in these groups is necessary in selected growing children with HFM. The mandibular lengthening with creation of an open bite is accomplished early in the mixed dentition stage. The mandible is elongated and rotated to the proper midline, leaving the TMJ in place. Maxillary surgery is not necessary, and the created open bite on the affected side is maintained and regulated by an orthodontic appliance.[92,96,97]

Type II B and Type III

In these groups, the mandible is elongated and rotated by the construction of a mandibular ramus and TMJ with costochondral or sternoclavicular junction, iliac crest bone grafts, or both. The surgery and orthodontic procedures are otherwise the same as for patients with type I and type II A deformities.

Treatment for the Nongrowing Patient

Orthodontic Treatment

In the nongrowing patient with HFM, presurgical orthodontic treatment is necessary. The dentoalveolar adaptations to the asymmetry must be corrected, and coordination of arches is mandatory prior to surgery.

Surgical Management

Surgical treatment in the nongrowing patient with HFM consists of an operation to level the maxilla and piriform apertures, to make the mandible symmetric, and to place the TMJ in its proper location. In patients with type II B, the existing ramus is hypoplastic and located in such an abnormal position that it is not useful and must be excised and replaced. In type III HFM, a new TMJ and ramus of the mandible are constructed in the correct location (Figure 54.16). The auricular deformity may be reconstructed using autogenous or alloplastic materials.

Treacher Collins Syndrome (TCS)

Mandibulofacial Dysostosis

In 1889, Berry was the first to publish and describe this deformity in a 15-year-old girl who had notching in the outer region of the right lower lid.[98] He commented on the possibility of hereditary transmission of this deformity. Treacher Collins recorded two cases in 1900 showing a more distinct development of this condition; the incidence is reported to be 1 in 10,000 live births.

Clinical Characteristics of TCS

This syndrome involves skeletal and soft tissue abnormalities of both the midface and lower face. It can be classified into three forms: complete, incomplete, and mild.[99]

Complete Form of TCS

In the orbital complex, there exists an absence or hypoplasia of the zygoma and overlying superficial musculoaponeurotic soft tissues. Malar prominence is absent and lateral canthal

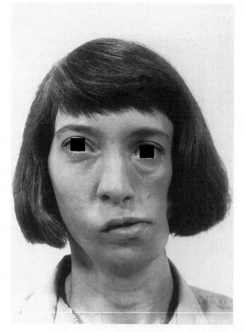

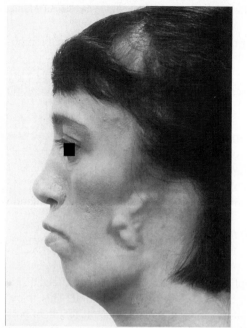

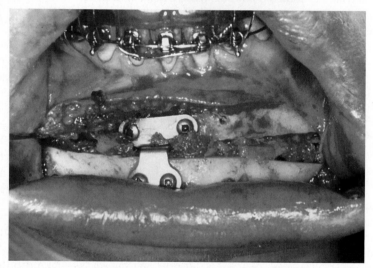

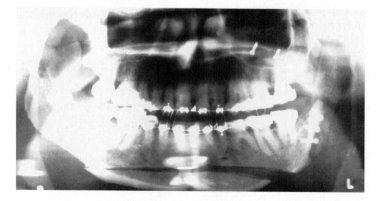

FIGURE 54.16

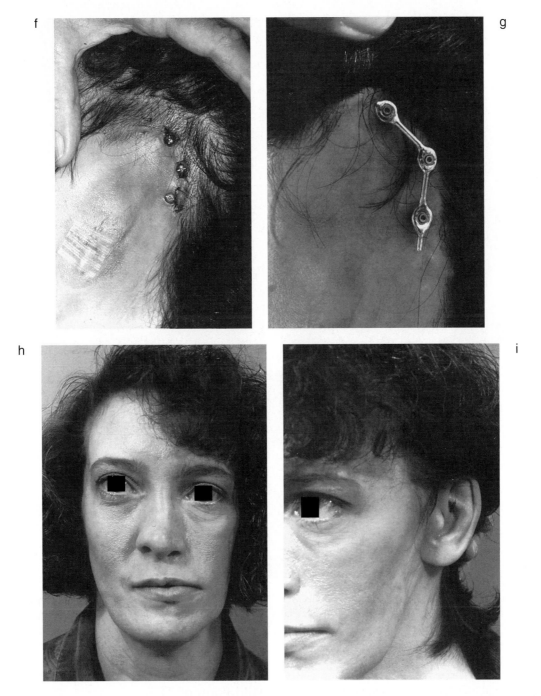

FIGURE 54.16 *Continued.* (a) Anterior view of a nongrowing patient with characteristics of HFM. (b) Lateral view of a nongrowing patient with characteristics of HFM. (c) Mandible is elongated and rotated via placement of an autogenous costochondral graft. (d) Straightening genioplasty is accomplished for enhanced symmetry. (e) Panoramic radiograph depicting the above procedures. Note screws in left anterior maxilla stabilizing a silastic malar implant to help mask the soft tissue deformity. (f) Preauricular tags are excised and the ear deformity is reconstructed via osseointegrated dental implants (Stage II). (g) Suprastructure constructed and try-in done. (h) Anterior postoperative view. (i) Lateral postoperative view with auricular prosthesis in place.

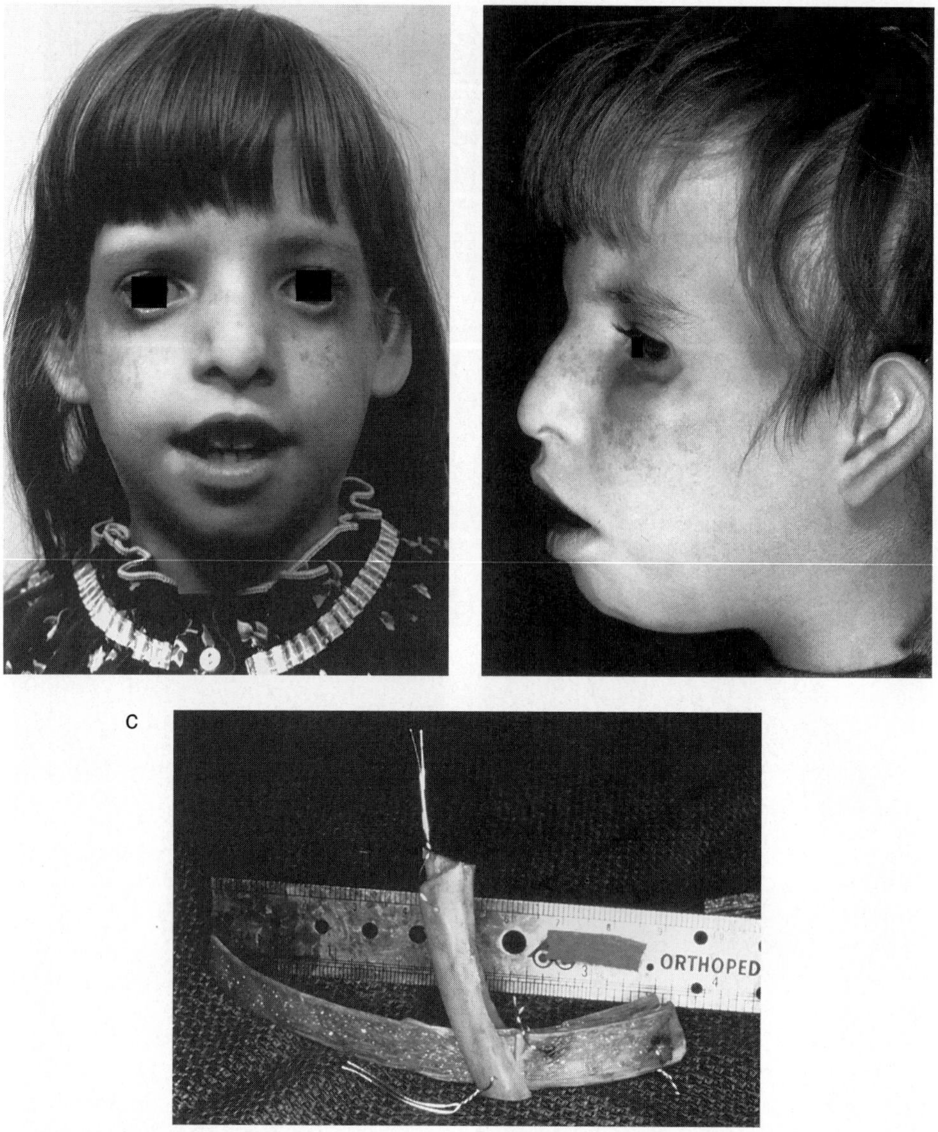

FIGURE 54.17 (a) Anterior view of child with Treacher Collins syndrome. (b) Lateral view of child with TCS. (c) Autogenous cranial bone grafts used to reconstruct orbits and zygomas. (d) Placement of graft into zygomatico-orbital region. (e) Anterior long-term post-operative view following correction of TCS with autogenous cranial bone grafts (CBG). (f) Lateral long-term postoperative view following correction of TCS with autogenous CBG.

dystopia, upper eyelid pseudoptosis, and antimongoloid slant of the palpebral fissure may be observed. There is usually a coloboma or marginal hypoplasia of the lower eyelid.

In the maxillomandibular complex, abnormalities of both jaws are noted. Shortness of the maxilla with narrowing of the palate and choanal atresia are often present. Shortness of the ramus and body of the mandible results in retrognathia.

Middle ear abnormalities and microtia may cause hearing loss with subsequent impairment of speech and intellectual development.

Incomplete Form of TCS

All the deformities are present but to a milder form.

Mild Form of TCS

Generally, the orbitotemporal region is more affected than are the maxilla or mandible.

Timing and Surgical Treatment

Principles of treatment are as follows:

1. Hearing aids should be used as early as possible.
2. Correction of eyelid colobomas should be performed in the first few years of life. These are repaired early because at a later stage the orbits are dissected and bone grafts placed producing tension on the soft tissues that may not allow their optimal closure.

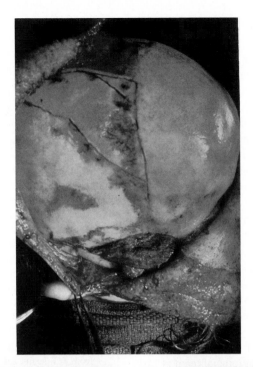

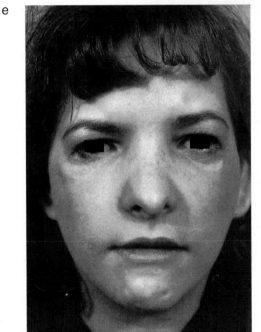

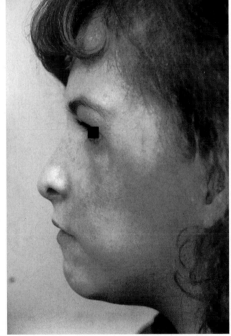

FIGURE 54.17 *Continued.*

3. Auricular deformities should be corrected after 8 years of age because substantial autogenous rib cartilage is available.
4. Orthognathic surgery, if needed, should be performed between 6 and 10 years of age and only when the child has major breathing problems.
5. Orbital surgery should be performed within the same age

range (6 to 10 years). We prefer cranial bone to reconstruct the orbits and zygomatic arches because, in our experience, resorption is less than with rib or iliac crest (Figure 54.17). Vascularized cranial bone grafts may be used as an alternative to reconstruct the malar bone. Preliminary results have shown that the resorption is less than with free cranial bone grafts.

Summary

In approximately 1 in 1000 births in the United States the infant has a variant of some facial, skeletal, or craniofacial deformity. If cleft lip and palate deformities are included, the incidence is far greater.

The surgical approach to a majority of these congenital deformities was radically changed by techniques introduced by Paul Tessier in France in 1967. From his imaginative intracranial and extracranial approaches, numerous advances have been made that facilitate the care of the majority of these children. More recently additional advances in pediatric anesthesia, bioresorbable plating systems, and distraction osteogenesis have improved the management of these patients.[100–103]

Timing of the surgical management of these patients has been advocated from the first few weeks after birth until well into the second decade. Many of these patients will need multiple, staged procedures involving movements of bone and soft tissue from both an intracranial and extracranial approach.

Acknowledgments: The authors would like to express their appreciation to the members of the craniofacial team at Dallas Children's Medical Center for contributing to the treatment of these patients (H.S. Byrd, MD, Craig Hobar, MD, D.P. Sinn, DDSc, and Fred Sklar, MD).

References

1. Johnston MC. Embryology of the head and neck. In: McCarthy JG, ed. *Plastic Surgery*. Philadelphia: WB Saunders; 1990: 2451–2495.

2. Sperber GH. *Craniofacial Embryology*, 4th Ed. London: Wright; 1989.

3. Sadler TW. *Langman's Medical Embryology*, 6th Ed. Baltimore: Williams & Wilkins; 1990.

4. Slavkin HC. *Developmental Craniofacial Biology*. Philadelphia: Lea & Febiger; 1979.

5. Sulik KK, Cook CS, Webster WS. Teratogens and craniofacial malformations: relationships to cell death. *Development*. 1988; 103:213–232.

6. Marsh JL, Vannier MW. *Comprehensive Care for Craniofacial Deformities*. St. Louis: CV Mosby; 1985.

7. Brodsky L, Ritter-Schmidt DH, Holt L. *Craniofacial Anomalies: An Interdisciplinary Approach*. St. Louis: Mosby Yearbook; 1989.

8. Gordon R, Herman GT, Johnston SA. Image reconstruction from projections. *Sci Am*. 1975;233:56.

9. Robb RA. X-ray computer tomography: an engineering synthesis of multiscientific principles. In: Bourne JR, ed. *Critical Reviews in Biomedical Engineering*. Boca Raton, FL: CRC Press; 1982.

10. Ter-Pogessian MN. Computerized cranial tomography: equipment and physics. *Semin Roentgenol*. 1977;12:13.

11. Marsh JL, Gado M. Surgical anatomy of the craniofacial dysostosis: insights from CT scans. *Cleft Palate J*. 1982;19:212.

12. Cutting C. Computer-aided planning and evaluation of facial and orthognathic surgery. *Clin Plast Surg*. 13:449.

13. Cutting C, Bookstein FL, Grayson B, Fellingham L, McCarthy JG. Three-dimensional computer-assisted design of craniofacial surgical procedures: optimization and interaction with cephalometric and CT-based models. *Plast Reconstr Surg*. 1986;77:877–887.

14. Marsh JL, Gado M. The longitudinal orbital CT projection: a versatile image for orbital assessment. *Plast Reconst Surg*. 1983;71:308.

15. Marsh JL, Vannier MW. The "third" dimension in craniofacial surgery. *Plast Reconstr Surg*. 1983;71:759.

16. Vannier MW, Marsh JL, Warren JO. Three dimension CT reconstruction images for craniofacial surgical planning and evaluation. *Radiology*. 1984;150:179.

17. Marsh JL. Computerized imaging for soft tissue and osseous reconstruction in the head and neck. *Clin Plast Surg*. 1985;12:279.

18. Marsh JL. Applications of computer graphics in craniofacial surgery. *Clin Plast Surg*. 1986;13:441.

19. Marsh JL, Vanier MW. Computer-assisted imaging in the diagnosis, management and study of dysmorphic patients. In: Vig KWL, Burdi AR, eds. *Craniofacial Morphogenesis and Dysmorphogenesis*. Ann Arbor, MI: University of Michigan Press; 1988:109–126.

20. Marsh JL, Vannier MW. Three-dimensional surface imaging from CT scans for the study of craniofacial dysmorphology. *J Craniofac Genet Dev Biol*. 1989;9:61.

21. Lo LJ. Craniofacial computer-assisted surgical planning and simulation. *Clin Plast Surg*. 1994;21:501.

22. Altobelli DE. Computer-assisted three-dimension planning in craniofacial surgery. *Plast Reconstr Surg*. 1993;92:576.

23. Posnick JC. Indirect intracranial volume measurements using CT scans: clinical applications for craniosynostosis. *Plast Reconstr Surg*. 1992;89:34.

24. Posnick JC, Goldstein JA, Waitzman AA. Surgical correction of the Treacher Collins malar deficiency: quantitative CT scan analysis of long-term results. *Plast Reconstr Surg*. 1992;92:12.

25. Oakes WJ. Craniosynostosis. In: Serafin D, Geargiade NG, eds. *Pediatric Plastic Surgery*. St. Louis: CV Mosby; 1984:404–439.

26. Virchow R. Uberden Cretinismus, namentlich in Franken, und uber pathologische schädelformen. *Verh Phys Med Gesellsch Uurzb*. 1851;2:230.

27. Persing JA, Jane JA, Shaffrey M. Virchow and the pathogenesis of craniosynostosis: a translation of his original work. *Plast Reconstr Surg*. 1989;83:738.

28. Moss ML. The pathogenesis of premature cranial synostosis in man. *Acta Anat (Basel)*. 1959;37:351.

29. Albright AL, Byrd RP. Suture pathology in craniosynostosis. *J Neurosurg*. 1981;54:384.

30. Graham JM, de Saxe M, Smith DW. Sagittal craniosynostosis: fetal head constraint as one possible cause. *J Pediatr*. 1979;95:747.

31. Renier D, Sainte-Rose C, Marchac D, et al. Intracranial pressure in craniostenosis. *J Neurosurg*. 1982;57:370.

32. Goldstein SJ, Kidd RC. Value of computed tomography in the evaluation of craniosynostosis. *Comput Radiol*. 1982;6:331–336.

33. Gault D, Brunelle F, Renier D, et al. The calculation of intracranial volume using CT scans. *Child's Nerv Syst*. 1988;4:271.

34. Posnick JC, Bite U, Nakano P, et al. Comparison of direct and indirect intracranial volume measurements. *Proceedings of the 6th International Congress on Cleft Palate and Related Craniofacial Anomalies*; June 1989.

35. Patton MA, Goodship J, Hayward R, et al. Intellectual development in Apert's syndrome: a long term follow-up of 29 patients. *J Med Genet.* 1988;25:164.

36. Arndt EM. Psychosocial adjustment of 20 patients with Treacher Collins syndrome before and after reconstructive surgery. *Br J Plast Surg.* 1987;40:605.

37. Ousterhout DK, Vargervik K. Aesthetic improvement resulting from craniofacial surgery in craniosynostosis syndromes. *J Craniomaxillofac Surg.* 1987;15:189.

38. Barden RC. The physical attractiveness of facially deformed patients before and after craniofacial surgery. *Plast Reconstr Surg.* 1988;82:229.

39. Barden RC. Emotional and behavioral reactions to facially deformed patients before and after craniofacial surgery. *Plast Reconstr Surg.* 1988;82:409.

40. Edgerton MT, Jane JA, Berry FA, et al. The feasibility of craniofacial osteotomies in infants and young children. *Scand J Plast Reconstr Surg.* 1974;8:164.

41. Edgerton MT, Jane JA, Berry FA. Craniofacial osteotomies and reconstruction in infants and young children. *Plast Reconstr Surg.* 1974;54:13.

42. Hoffman HJ, Mohr G. Lateral canthal advancement of the supraorbital margin: a new corrective technique in the treatment of coronal synostosis. *J Neurosurg.* 1976;45:376.

43. Jane JA, Park TS, Zide BM, et al. Alternative techniques in the treatment of unilateral coronal synostosis. *J Neurosurg.* 1984;61:550.

44. Marchac D. Forehead remolding for craniosynostosis. In: Converse JM, McCarthy JG, Wood-Smith D, eds. *Symposium on Diagnosis and Treatment of Craniofacial Anomalies.* St. Louis: CV Mosby; 1979:323.

45. Marchac D, Renier D. Treatment of craniosynostosis in infancy. *Clin Plast Surg.* 1987;14:61.

46. Marchac D, Renier D, Jones BM. Experience with the "floating forehead." *Br J Plast Surg.* 1988;41:1.

47. McCarthy JG. New concepts in the surgical treatment of the craniofacial synostosis syndromes in the infant. *Clin Plast Surg.* 1979;6:201.

48. McCarthy JG, Coocaro PJ, Epstein F, et al. Early skeletal release in the infant with craniofacial dysostosis: the role of the sphenozygomatic suture. *Plast Reconst Surg.* 1978;62:335.

49. McCarthy JG, Epstein F, Sadove M, et al. Early surgery for craniofacial synostosis: an 8-year experience. *Plast Reconstr Surg.* 1984, 73:532.

50. Persing JA, Babler WJ, Jane JA, et al. Experimental unilateral coronal synostosis in rabbits. *Plast Reconst Surg.* 1986;78:594.

51. Tressera L, Fuenmayor P. Early treatment of craniofacial deformities. *J Maxillofac Surg.* 1981;9:7.

52. Whitaker LA, Schut L, Kerr LP. Early surgery for isolated craniofacial dysostosis. *Plast Reconstr Surg.* 1977;60:575.

53. Whitaker LA, Barlett SP, Schut L, et al. Craniosynostosis: an analysis of the timing, treatment and complication in 164 patients. *Plast Reconstr Surg.* 1987;80:195.

54. Barden RC, Ford ME, Jensen AG, et al. Effects of craniofacial deformity in infancy on the quality of mother-infant interaction. *Child Dev.* 1989;60:819.

55. Lefebvre A, Barclay S. Psychosocial impact of craniofacial deformities before and after reconstructive surgery. *Can J Psychiatry.* 1982;27:579.

56. Lefebvre A, Travis F, Arndt EM, et al. A psychiatric profile before and after reconstructive surgery in children with Apert's syndrome. *Br J Plast Surg.* 1986;39:510.

57. Palkes HS, Marsh JL, Talent BK. Pediatric craniofacial surgery and parental attitudes. *Cleft Plate J.* 1986;23:137.

58. Muhling J, Reuther J, Sorensen N. Problems with lateral canthal advancement. *Child's Nerv Syst.* 1986;2:287.

59. Longacre JJ, Destafano GA, Holmstrand K. The early versus the late reconstruction of congenital hypoplasia of the facial skeleton and skull. *Plast Reconstr Surg.* 1961;27:489.

60. McCarthy JG, Coccaro PJ, Epstein FJ. Early skeletal release in the patient with craniofacial dysostosis. In: Converse JM, McCarthy J, Wood-Smith D, eds. *Symposium on Diagnosis and Treatment of Craniofacial Anomalies.* St. Louis: CV Mosby; 1979:295.

61. McLaurin RL, Matson DD. Importance of early surgical treatment of craniosynostosis. *Pediatrics.* 1952;10:637.

62. Mohr G, Hoffman HJ, Munro IR, et al. Surgical management of unilateral and bilateral coronal craniosynostosis: 21 years of experience. *Neurosurgery.* 1978;2:83.

63. Shillito J, Matson DD. Craniosynostosis: a review of 519 surgical patients. *Pediatrics.* 1968;41:829.

64. Tessier P. The definitive plastic surgical treatment of the severe facial deformities of craniofacial dysostosis. Crouzon's and Apert's disease. *Plast Reconstr Surg.* 1971;48:419.

65. Kreiborg S, Bjork A. Description of a dry skull with Crouzon syndrome. *Scand J Plast Reconstr Surg.* 1982;16:245–253.

66. Carinci F, Avantaggiato A, Curioni A. Crouzon syndrome: cephalometric analysis and evaluation of pathogenesis cleft palate. *Craniofacial J.* 1994;31:201–209.

67. Schiller JG. Craniofacial dysostosis of Crouzon: a case report and pedigree with emphasis on heredity. *Pediatrics.* 1959;23:107.

68. Nakano PH, Posnick JC. Long-term results of reconstructive craniofacial surgery in patients with Crouzon and Apert syndrome. *Proceedings of the 46th annual meeting of the Cleft Palate Craniofacial Association*; April 1989.

69. Nakano PH, Posnick JC. Long-term results of reconstruction in craniofacial dysostosis. *Proceedings of the 6th International Congress of Cleft Palate and Related Anomalies*; June 1989.

70. Wheaton SW. Two specimens of congenital cranial deformities in infants in association with fusion of the fingers and toes. In: Smith DW, ed. *Recognizable Patterns of Human Malformation, Major Problems in Clinical Pediatrics*, Vol VII. Philadelphia: WB Saunders; 1982:308.

71. Tessier P. Apert's syndrome: acrocephalosyndactyly Type I. In: Caronni EP, ed. *Craniofacial Surgery.* Boston: Little, Brown, 1985;280–303.

72. Tessier P. Relationship of craniostenosis to craniofacial dysostosis and to faciostenosis. A study with therapeutic implications. *Plast Reconstr Surg.* 1971;48:224.

73. Pollard ZF. Bilateral superior oblique muscle palsy associated with Apert's syndrome. *Am J Ophthalmol.* 1988;106:337.

74. Fishman MA, Hogan GR, Dodge PR. The concurrence of hydrocephalus and craniosynostosis. *J Neurosurg.* 1971;34:621.

75. Golabi M, Edwards MSB, Ousterhout DK. Craniosynostosis and hydrocephalus. *Neurosurgery.* 1987;21:63.

76. Hogan GR, Bauman ML. Hydrocephalus in Apert's syndrome. *J Pediatr.* 1971;79:782.

77. Alberti PW, Ruben RJ. *Otologic Medicine and Surgery.* New York: Churchill Livingstone; 1988.

78. Corey JP, Caldarelli DD, Gould HJ. Otopathology in cranial facial dysostosis. *Am J Otol.* 1987;8:14.

79. Gorlin RJ, Pindborg J. *Syndromes of the Head and Neck.* New York: McGraw-Hill; 1964:261–265; 419–425.

80. Cohen MM, Rollnick BR, Kaye CI. Oculoauriculovertebral spectrum: an update critique. *Cleft Palate J.* 1989;26:276.

81. Francois J, Haustrate L. Anomalies colobomateuses du globe oculair et syndrome du premier arc. *Ann Ocul.* 1954;187:340.

82. Gorlin RJ, Jue KL, Jacobson NP, et al. Oculoauriculovertebral dysplasia. *J Pediatr.* 1963;63:991.

83. Grabb WC. The first and second branchial arch syndrome. *Plast Reconstr Surg.* 1965;36:485.

84. Grayson BH, Boral S, Eisig S, et al. Unilateral craniofacial microsomia. I. Mandibular analysis. *Am J Orthod.* 1983;84:225.

85. Ross RB. Lateral facial dysplasia (first and second branchial arch syndrome, hemifacial microsomia). *Birth Defects.* 1975;11:51.

86. Kaban LB, Mulliken JB, Murray JE. Three dimensional approach to analysis and treatment of hemifacial microsomia. *Cleft Palate J.* 1981;18:90.

87. Gustavson EE, Chen H. Goldenhar syndrome, anterior encephalocele and aqueductal stenosis following fetal primidone exposure. *Teratology.* 1985;32:13.

88. Lammer EJ, Chen DT, Hoar RM, et al. Retinoic acid embryopathy. *N Engl J Med.* 1985;313:837.

89. Miehlke A, Partsch CJ. Ohrmissbildung, fascialis und abducenslahmung als syndrome der thalidomidschadigung. *Arch Ohrenheilkd.* 1963;181:154.

90. Poswillo D. The pathogenesis of first and second branchial arch syndrome. *Oral Surg.* 1973;35:302.

91. Soltan HC, Holmes LB. Familial occurrence of malformations possibly attributable to vascular abnormalities. *J Pediatr.* 1986; 109:112.

92. Murray JE, Kaban LB, Mulliken JB. Analysis and treatment of hemifacial microsomia. *Plast Reconstr Surg.* 1984;74: 186.

93. Murray JE, Kaban LB, Mulliken JB, et al. Analysis and treatment of hemifacial microsomia. In: Caronni EP, ed. *Craniofacial Surgery.* Boston: Little, Brown; 1985:377–390.

94. Meurman Y. Congenital microtia and meatal atresia. *Arch Otolaryngol.* 1957;66:443.

95. Bennun RD, Mulliken JB, Kaban LB, et al. Microtia: a microform of hemifacial microsomia. *Plast Reconstr Surg.* 1985;76:859.

96. Kaban LB, Moses ML, Mulliken JB. Correction of hemifacial microsomia in the growing child. *Cleft Palate J.* 1986;23:50.

97. Kaban LB, Moses ML, Mulliken JB. Surgical correction of hemifacial microsomia in the growing child. *Plast Reconstr Surg.* 1988;82:9.

98. Berry GA. Note on a congenital defect (? coloboma) of the lower lid. *Ophthalmol Hosp Rep.* 1889;12:255.

99. Tessier P. Tulasne JF. Surgical correction of Treacher Collins Syndrome. In: Bell WH, ed. *Modern Practice in Orthognathic and Reconstructive Surgery.* Philadelphia: WB Saunders; 1992:1601–1623.

100. Kurpad SN, Goldstein JA, Cohen AR. Bioresorbable fixation for congenital pediatric craniofacial surgery: a 2 year followup. *Pediatr Neurosurg.* 2000;33:306–310.

101. McCarthy JG, Stelnicki EJ, Grayson BH. Distraction osteogenesis of the mandible: a ten year experience. *Semin Orthod.* 1999;5:3–8.

102. Tate GS, Tharanon W, Sinn DP. Transoral maxillary distraction osteogenesis of an unrepaired bilateral alveolar cleft. *J Craniofac Surg.* 1999;10:369–374.

103. Cohen SR. Midface distraction. *Semin Orthod.* 1999;5:52–58.

55
The Effects of Plate and Screw Fixation on the Growing Craniofacial Skeleton

Michael J. Yaremchuk

The plate and screw fixation of surgically created and repositioned osteotomies or reduced fracture segments has revolutionized the practice of adult craniomaxillofacial surgery. The superior results obtained with rigid fixation techniques has prompted its use in the pediatric population.[1,2] Plate and screw stabilization of reshaped and repositioned bone units and bone grafts may have certain advantages over no stabilization or interfragmentary wire stabilization. Posnick has listed the potential advantages of miniaturized plate and screw fixation techniques for pediatric craniofacial surgery.[3] These advantages may include:

1. Improved three-dimensional shape control of refashioned osteotomized segments
2. Improved three-dimensional position control due to prevention of osteotomy or bone graft collapse after soft tissue closure
3. Facilitation of bone healing
4. The need for fewer drill holes when plates are used rather than interfragmentary wires
5. Decreased bone segment mobility, which may decrease resorption and infection rates and may also obviate the need for protective head gear
6. Elimination of the "sharpwire" pain that may accompany the use of interfragmentary wires under thin areas of the skin

There are certain negative aspects associated with the use of rigid fixation in the growing facial skeleton. These include metal-induced artifacts, artifacts on later computerized tomographic (CT) and magnetic resonance (MR) images, plate migration, and the potential for growth restriction. Recent data have shown that image artifact is negligible when the implant is made of titanium.[4,5] The use of plates and screws should, therefore, have little impact on later diagnostic CT and MR images when the implants are manufactured from titanium. However, the tendency for plates and screws to alter their position relative to the bone–dura interface or to restrict the growth of the craniofacial skeleton has not been defined. No objective clinical data that address either of these latter issues

exist. This chapter presents experimental data examining the potential for plate and screw fixation to influence the growth of the growing craniofacial skeleton.

Animal Research

Lower Animals

Lower animal studies using cats[6] and rabbits[7,8] have shown a tendency for growth restriction when plates and screws were fixated onto the growing cranial vault. In the growing cat, Lin et al.[6] noted a mild growth restriction when they studied the effect of frontal bone osteotomy and fixation with miniplates. In studies using rabbit models, miniplates were placed across the coronal suture[7] and frontal bone[8] without osteotomies being performed. A subsequent restriction of growth was also noted.

The relevance of the results of these studies is limited by the experimental methodology imposed by the scale, growth characteristics, and skeletal morphology of the animal models employed. The large scale of the plates relative to the experimental skull size makes clinical correlation unclear. Small skull size also necessitated the placement of a fixation plate across suture lines, a feature known likely to influence growth.[9–11]

Primates

To avoid some of the problems inherent in using lower animal models, a primate model is attractive. The rhesus monkey (*Macaca mulatta*) has an established history of use in craniomaxillofacial surgery research,[12–14] an orbitozygomatic anatomy similar to humans,[12] and growth and development of the facial skeleton resembling humans.[15,16] For these reasons, a study that used infant rhesus monkeys was performed[17] to examine the effect of plate and screw fixation on the growth of the craniofacial skeleton. This project was supported by the AO/ASIF (Swiss Association for the Study of Internal Fixation).

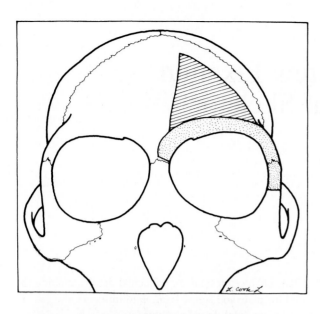

FIGURE 55.1 Design of supraorbital and frontal osteotomies. Dark gray zone indicates area of frontal osteotomy. Light gray indicates supraorbital osteotomy. (From Yaremchuk et al.,[17] by permission of *Plastic and Reconstructive Surgery*)

a

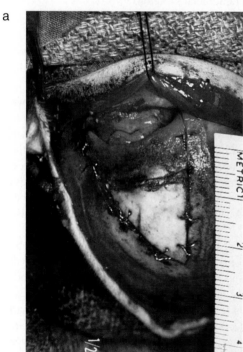

FIGURE 55.2 Intraoperative photographs taken from above to demonstrate the three types of fixation employed. (a) Wire fixation. (b) Microplate fixation. (c) "Extensive" microplate fixation. (From Yaremchuk et al.,[17] by permission of *Plastic and Reconstructive Surgery*)

b

c

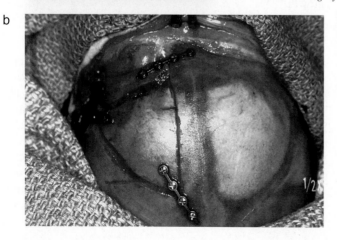

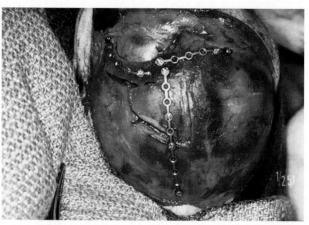

Research Using *Macaca mulatta*

Experimental Design

Twelve infant rhesus monkeys (*Macaca mulatta*) underwent unilateral supraorbital and frontal osteotomy through a bicoronal incision. The osteotomized segments were anatomically replaced and fixated using three different methods (Figure 55.1). The fixation methods included:

1. Interfragmentary wiring using 28-gauge stainless steel ($n = 4$) [Figure 55.2(a)]
2. Rigid fixation using a microfixation system ($n = 4$). Plates were positioned to avoid crossing suture lines. Two screws on either side of the osteotomy were applied to each plate [Figure 55.2(b)]
3. Extensive use of microplates ($n = 4$). Longer plates, using multiple screws, were used. They purposely crossed the coronal and sagittal sutures so as to create a cagelike arrangement [Figure 55.2(c)]

The animals were allowed to mature to a mean age of 16.7 months (range, 11.1 to 27.3 months). Cranial growth in the rhesus monkey has been shown to be 95% completed by this time.[18] During a second general anesthetic, the fixation hardware was removed, and standard craniometric measurements obtained (Figure 55.3). One week after the direct measurements were made, CT scans of the face and cranial vault were obtained from each animal. Three-dimensional images were then created using computer software so that both local and remote skull morphology could be documented. Five unoperated adult male rhesus skulls were measured and imaged to determine the intrinsic craniofacial skeletal symmetry in this species.

Results

Craniometric measurements were normalized to account for variations in skull size in individual animals prior to statistically analyzing the data. All results were decided significant at $p < 0.05$.

Differences among treatment groups were examined using the analysis of variance (ANOVA) statistical test. Of the 39 craniometric measurements made in each treatment group, only 4 were found to vary significantly with the type of fixation (Figure 55.4). In general, a greater restriction of growth was seen with increasing amounts of fixation hardware in the frontal region.

Using the paired *t*-test, right–left differences measured between the operated and unoperated sides with each treatment group were not large enough to be statistically significant. A trend toward smaller measurements on the operated side was observed.

Using an unpaired *t*-test, wire and plate fixation were compared. Of 39 measurements, 3 were significantly smaller in the plate fixation group, indicating a more marked growth restriction in the plate fixation group. When the standard and "extensive" plate fixation groups were compared, 2 of 39 measurements showed significant difference.

Several nonmetric changes were observed in the experimental animals. There was a loss of prominence of the supraorbital rim and changes in the region of the left frontotemporal craniometric point in all treatment groups. There was

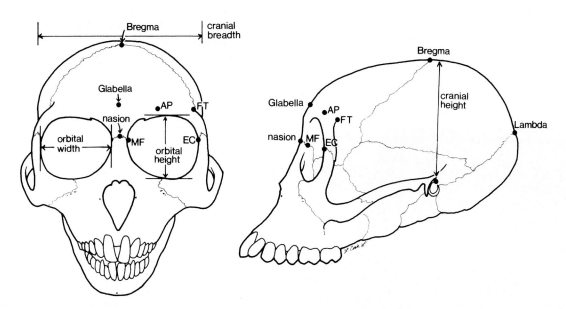

FIGURE 55.3 Examples of craniometric measurements (shown unilaterally). (From Yaremchuk et al.,[17] by permission of *Plastic and Reconstructive Surgery*)

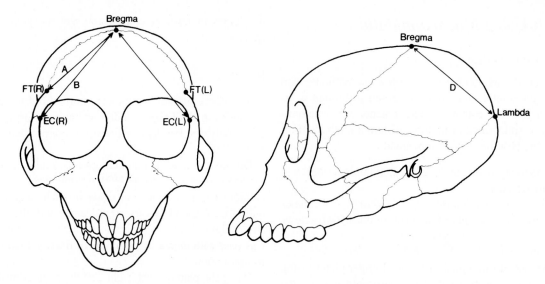

FIGURE 55.4 Craniometric measurements varying significantly with type of fixation (ANOVA, $p < 0.05$). Line A: bregma-frontotemporale (R); line B: bregma-ectoconchion (R); line C: bregma-ectoconchion (L); line D: bregma-lambda. (From Yaremchuk et al.,[17] by permission of *Plastic and Reconstructive Surgery*)

an apparent flattening of curvature with increasing fixation. These findings are presented in Figures 55.5–55.7.

Summary

This study showed that small, but measurable, visible changes occurred in a growing primate skull after osteotomy and fixation. A restriction of growth occurs in the area of operation even when suture lines are not crossed. In addition, distant, compensatory effects may occur. The magnitude of these changes appear to increase as increasing amounts of fixation hardware are used.

It is quite likely that the growth alterations seen in this study are related to osteotomy in addition to fixation effects. The frontal and supraorbital bone flaps created in this study are, in fact, free-bone grafts. It is, therefore, not unexpected that local shape changes would occur due to resorption and remodeling effects.

Clinical Relevance

Several extrapolations can be made from this experimental data toward the indications, timing, and fixation techniques employed for clinical infant craniofacial surgery. For example, since even the least restrictive method of fixation employed (interfragmentary wire fixation) resulted in measurable and visible alterations in skull shape, the surgeon must

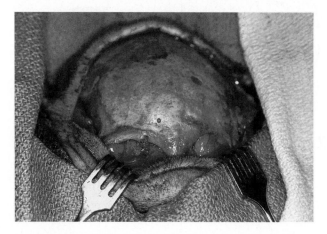

FIGURE 55.5 Intraoperative frontal view at time of craniometric measurements of a representative animal from wire fixation group. Note loss of prominence of supraorbital rim on left (operated) side.

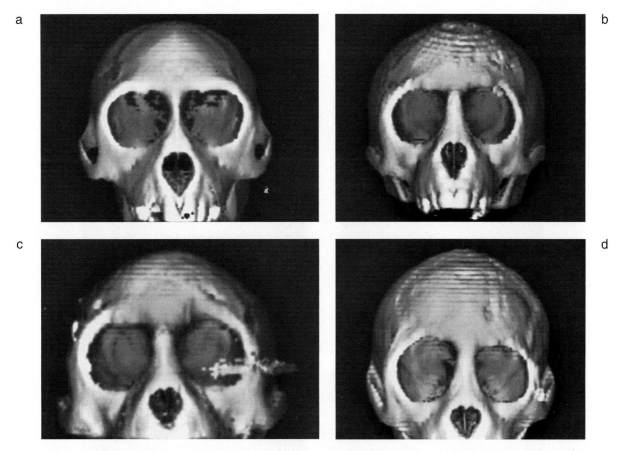

FIGURE 55.6 Representative frontal three-dimensional CT images of rhesus skulls. (a) Unoperated. (b) Wire fixation. (c) Microplate fixation (artifact is a result of a screw that was not removed before imaging). (d) "Extensive" microplate fixation. (From Yaremchuk et al.,[17] by permission of *Plastic and Reconstructive Surgery*)

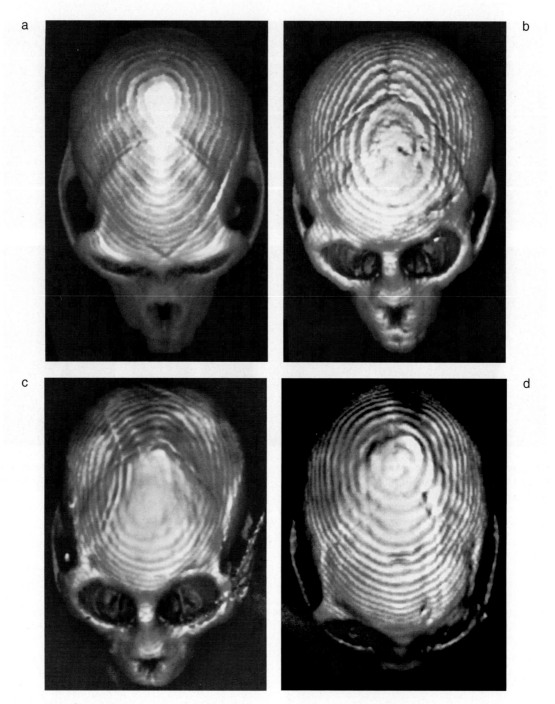

FIGURE 55.7 Representative overhead three-dimensional CT images of rhesus skulls. (a) Unoperated. (b) Wire fixation. (c) Microplate fixation (artifact is a result of screw that was not removed before imaging). (d) "Extensive" microplate fixation. (From Yaremchuk et al.,[17] by permission of *Plastic and Reconstructive Surgery*)

be confident that the surgical correction and accompanying growth alterations must offer significant improvement, ultimately, over no treatment. Perhaps certain children with less severe deformities should be operated on later, when skull growth is more complete, so that the postoperative growth alterations would be concomitantly less significant. As the skull shape anomalies become more severe, the surgeon must balance the potential iatrogenic growth alterations accompanying surgery with the improved shape and position control and stability made available by the use of rigid fixation techniques. When initial deformities are more severe, one must realize that a statistically significant growth alteration accompanying surgery and stabilization may not be clinically significant relative to that initial deformity.

Other researchers have shown that the release of immobilized sutures[9] and removal of fixation hardware[19] in the growing infants skull allows "catch up" growth. Hence, removal of fixation hardware soon after healing at osteotomy sites may limit subsequent fixation-related alterations and should be considered in certain clinical infant surgery settings.

Recently, resorbable fixation systems have become available for clinical use. Early reports have been favorable.[20] Their efficacy will be determined by the characteristics of the resorbable systems and the clinical situation. Important variables related to the fixation system include strength, time to resorption, and case of application. Timing of surgery related to remaining skull growth, bone gap distance and soft tissue deforming forces resulting from skeletal rearrangement will be relevant factors dictated by the clinical situation. Further laboratory and controlled clinical study will allow better understanding and appropriate use of resorbable fixation systems in the growing craniofacial skeleton.

References

1. Muehlbauer W, Anderl H, Ramaatschi P, et al. Radical treatment of craniofacial anomalies in infancy and the use of miniplates in craniofacial surgery. *Clin Plast Surg.* 1987;14:101–111.
2. Posnick J. The role of plate and screw fixation in the treatment of craniofacial malformations. In: Yaremchuk MJ, Gruss JG, Manson PN, eds. *Rigid Fixation of the Craniomaxillofacial Skeleton.* Stoneham, MA: Butterworth-Heinemann; 1992:512–526.
3. Posnick J. Discussion of "The effects of rigid fixation on craniofacial growth in rhesus monkeys." By: Yaremchuk MJ, Fiala TGS, Barker F, et al. *Plast Reconstr Surg.* 1994;93(1):11–12.
4. Fiala TGS, Novelline RA, Yaremchuk MJ. Comparison of CT imaging artifacts from craniomaxillofacial internal fixation devices. *Plast Reconstr Surg.* 1993;92:1227–1232.
5. Fiala TGS, Paige KT, Davis TL, et al. Comparison of artifact from craniomaxillofacial internal fixation devices: magnetic resonance imaging. *Plast Reconstr Surg.* 1994;93:725–731.
6. Lin KY, Bartlett SP, Yaremchuk MJ, et al. An experimental study on the effect of rigid fixation on the developing craniofacial skeleton. *Plast Reconstr Surg.* 1991;87:229–235.
7. Resnick JI, Kinney BM, Kawamoto JHK. The effect of rigid internal fixation on cranial growth. *Ann Plast Surg.* 1990;25:372–374.
8. Wong L, Dufresne CR, Richtsmeier JT, et al. The effect of rigid fixation on growth of the neocranium. *Plast Reconstr Surg.* 1991;88:395–403.
9. Persing J, Babler W, Winn R, et al. Age as a critical factor in the success of surgical correction of craniosynostosis. *J Neurosurg.* 1981;54:601–606.
10. Persing JA, Babler WJ, Jane JA, et al. Experimental unilateral coronal synostosis in rabbits. *Plast Reconstr Surg.* 1986;77:369–377.
11. Persson KM, Roy WA, Persing JA, et al. Craniofacial growth following experimental craniosynostosis and craniectomy in rabbits. *J Neurosurg.* 1979;50:187–197.
12. McCarthy JG, Coccaro PJ, Keller A. Craniofacial suture manipulation in the newborn rhesus monkey. In: Caronni EP, ed. *Craniofacial Surgery.* Boston: Little, Brown; 1985:3–11.
13. Gans BJ, Sarnat BG. Sutural facial growth of the Macaca rhesus monkey: a gross and serial roentgenographic study by means of metallic implants. *Am J Anat.* 1945;60:344–356.
14. Elgoyhen JC, Riolo ML, Graber LW, et al. Craniofacial growth in juvenile *Macaca mulatta*: a cephalometric study. *Am J Phys Anthropol.* 1978;36:369–376.
15. Duterloo HS, Enlow DH. A comparative study of cranial growth in *Homo* and *Macaca*. *Am J Anat.* 1970;127:357–368.
16. Cheek DB. The fetus. In: Cheek DB, ed. *Fetal and Postnatal Cellular Growth.* New York: John Wiley and Sons; 1975:3–22.
17. Yaremchuk MJ, Fiala TGS, Barker F, et al. The effects of rigid fixation on craniofacial growth of rhesus monkeys. *Plast Reconstr Surg.* 1994;93(1):1–10.
18. Bhatia AK. Craniometric growth in the rhesus monkey, *Macaca mulatta. J Indian Anthrop Soc.* 1978;13:81–95.
19. Wong L, Woodberry K, Richtsmeier JT, et al. Modifying the effects of rigid fixation on craniofacial growth. Presented at Plastic Surgery Research Council, Toronto, Ontario, April 1992.
20. Eppley BL, Sodov AM, Havlik RJ. Resorbable plate fixation in pediatric craniofacial surgery. *Plast Reconstr Surg* 1997;100:1–7.

56

Calvarial Bone Graft Harvesting Techniques: Considerations for Their Use with Rigid Fixation Techniques in the Craniomaxillofacial Region

John L. Frodel, Jr.

As reconstruction of the craniomaxillofacial (CMF) skeleton has evolved in the treatment of traumatic, oncologic, congenital, and aesthetic deformities, so have the requirements for various restorative materials. The hardware for rigid internal fixation now permits the necessary structural support in such reconstructive situations, often in conjunction with bone grafts. While iliac crest remains the principal source used for free bone grafting in the mandible, calvarial bone grafts have become the material of choice for bony reconstruction of all other craniomaxillofacial defects (where nonvascularized bone is adequate).

In this chapter, the embryology and surgical anatomy as well as various graft harvest principles and techniques are reviewed. Principles for the fixation of bone grafts are discussed, followed by cases illustrative of these techniques.

Embryology and Surgical Anatomy

When considering the type of bone (i.e., calvarium) for use in CMF reconstruction, the embryological origin of the graft material takes on great importance. When considering the use of calvarium for craniomaxillofacial reconstruction, the embryological origin of the bone becomes very important.[1–6] Embryologically, the skull consists of three divisions: chondrocranium, desmocranium, and the appendicular or visceral portion. The chondrocranium is cartilaginous and includes the skull base, as well as the nasal and optic capsules. The visceral portion is derived from the branchial arches, and develops into the various cartilaginous skeletal appendices. Finally, the desmocranium is membranous and consists of portions of the temporal, sphenoid, occipital, nasal, maxillary, and zygomatic bones, including a significant portion of the mandible. This embryological origin is important as studies have demonstrated that bone grafts of membranous bone origin (i.e., calvarium) resorb significantly less than endochondral bone (i.e., iliac crest), although a recent study by Phillips and Rahn has suggested that rigid fixation reduces the amount of resorption with endochondral bone.[7]

During growth and development, the calvarium eventually consists of distinct cortical bone layers (the inner and outer cortices) with a spongy cancellous layer (the diploe) in between. Tightly adhering to the undersurface of the calvarium is the dura. The inner cortex of the calvarium is imprinted with various vascular structures such as the midline sagittal sinus, which is approximately 1 cm in width. Another important aspect of the calvarium, which becomes manifest during consideration for calvarial bone graft harvesting, is the region known as the temporal line (the superior attachment of the temporalis muscle). This is significant because lateral and inferior to this line the skull becomes quite thin. The other vital landmarks include the various sagittal, coronal, lambdoid sagittal, and squamosal sutures. These represent sites of fusion between the two cortices of originally distinct skull bones and, accordingly, are without diploic space.

With these anatomic regions in mind, "danger" areas exist for consideration in site selection for calvarial bone graft harvesting (Figure 56.1). These zones represent sites at risk for intracranial exposure and injury, and include the midline (the sagittal sinus underlies the sagittal suture) and the temporal line inferiorly, as well as the various embryological suture regions where the bone tends to be quite thin. Other variable considerations include the presence of transcortical emissary veins, subcortical vessels, and arachnoid plexuses, which can exist within the cortical portion of the calvarium.

Another factor for consideration is the unpredictability of the skull thickness. Pensler and McCathy studied 200 cadaver skulls, measuring various aspects of the parietal and occipital regions.[8] Their study found that the thickest bone was consistently noted to exist in the parietal region, that male calvaria tends to be slightly thicker than that of females, and that age was not a significant factor. It is of particular note that the skull is generally fully developed by 8 years of age but continues to thicken until about 20 years of age. To summarize the anatomic considerations, calvarial bone grafts are best harvested in the parietal region (an area approximately 8 × 10 cm, where the calvarium is thickest and the "danger" areas (the midline and temporal regions) are avoided.

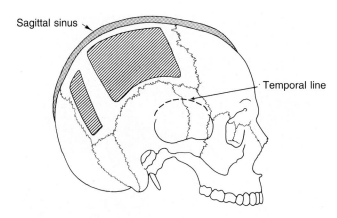

Sagittal sinus

Temporal line

FIGURE 56.1 The "danger" areas of the calvarium. (From Frodel,[12] with permission)

Calvarial Bone Graft Harvesting and Techniques

In the preparation for harvest of a calvarial bone graft, several considerations are necessary before performing this procedure. First, one must consider requirements of the recipient site with respect to bone thickness and curvature.[9,10] For example, defects that require curved grafts (e.g., orbit, malar region) may better be harvested as horizontal strips over the temporoparietal region. Conversely, defects requiring straight grafts (e.g., nasal dorsum) should be harvested in the occipitoparietal region.

Graft length and width vary with the reconstructive needs, but rarely is a graft needed that is longer than 5 to 6 cm or wider than 1.5 to 2 cm. Attempts to harvest grafts larger than this often result in fracture of the bone graft during removal, as well as increasing the risk for intracranial exposure. Accordingly, the surgeon should consider the use of multiple small grafts whenever possible. Another consideration is access to proper instrumentation. It is extremely important to utilize a sharp osteotome. The author prefers the use of a thin, curved osteotome that is approximately 1 cm wide. It is important that this is kept sharpened to provide the utmost control during the harvesting process.

Regarding surgical approaches, if a coronal incision has been made to approach the upper aspect of the craniomaxillofacial skeleton, the posterior margin of this incision can be elevated in a subperiosteal plane to expose the entire anterior and midportions of the parietal bone. If such an incision has not been made, a direct horizontal incision can be made in the hair-bearing region over the parietal bone. In patients with alopecia, this incision should be made within the hair-bearing region, followed by medial retraction to expose the necessary donor site. It should be noted that hair is rarely shaved in preparation for such graft harvesting, unless lacerations are present, for example, in trauma cases.

Techniques for calvarial bone graft harvesting can be divided into three categories: partial-thickness outer cortex grafts, full-thickness outer cortex grafts, and bicortical or inner cortex grafts. Partial-thickness outer cortex grafts are commonly harvested in children. In this technique, an osteotome is used to elevate a curl of outer cortical bone (also called a "potato chip" graft), which is only a partial thickness of the outer cortical bone. Such bone graft harvesting techniques are ideal in children of approximately 4 to 8 years of age, as these patients have very soft bone, and the graft can usually be obtained without significant fracturing (Figure 56.2). However, this technique is fraught with graft fragmentation in adult patients. Accordingly, the use of such bone is limited to very small defects or the packing of larger defects.

Perhaps the most common type of calvarial graft harvested is the removal of the outer cortex in its entirety (i.e., leaving the full inner cortex intact). The basic principle is to separate the inner and outer cortices without penetration of the inner aspect of the calvarium, with its attendant sequelae of dural exposure. The initial step is to define, if possible, the diploic layer after outlining proposed bone grafts. It should be noted that some patients do not have a distinct diploic layer, and this should be considered at all times. However, the harvesting of the graft is usually initiated with the use of a cutting bur along at least one side of the graft area (Figure 56.3). A variety of techniques can then be utilized for further elevation of the outer cortex graft.[9,11,12] In general, either an osteotome alone is used to elevate the graft, or on occasion, a sagittal or reciprocating saw may be utilized.

Before elevation, the graft should be outlined using a small drill bit or side-cutting bur. If multiple bone grafts are harvested, this outlining should waste as little bone as possible so as to use the calvarium efficiently (Figure 56.4). In using either the osteotome or saw technique, it is of critical importance that the osteotome or saw blade proceeds parallel to the inner and outer cortices within the diploic space. This can only take place if an adequate "trough" has been created at

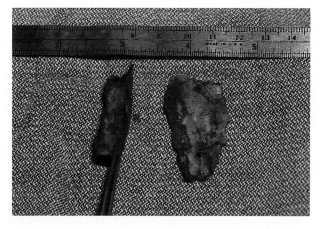

FIGURE 56.2 Clinical example of a split outer table ("potato chip" graft).

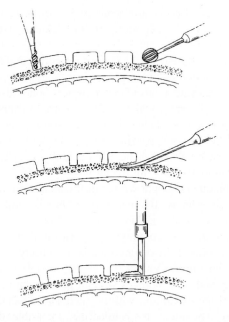

FIGURE 56.3 Diagram depicting the phases of calvarial bone graft harvest, including creation of a wide sloping trough with a large cutting bur and outlining of the various bone grafts with a smaller bur (Top diagram). Subsequent elevation then is undertaken with an osteotome (middle diagram) or sagittal saw (lower diagram). (From Frodel,[12] with permission)

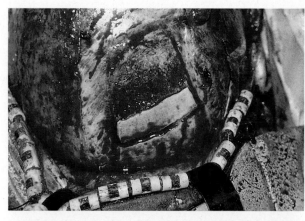
a

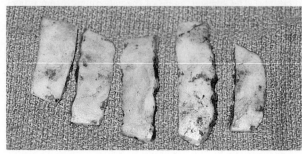
b

FIGURE 56.4 Clinical example of a full-thickness outer cortex graft. (a) The appearance of the bed after the harvest of two previous bone grafts with one bone graft harvest remaining. (b) Multiple bone grafts harvested from the same patient.

the advancing front of the harvest site. If such a trough has not been created, the osteotome or saw blade will likely be misdirected and enter through or fracture the inner cortex (Figure 56.5). The major advantage of using an osteotome for the complete harvest of the outer cortex graft is that no bone is wasted, as it is in using a saw technique. However, if minimal or no dipolic space exists, the authors found the sagittal saw technique provides greater control and safety. Regardless of the technique, however, risk always exist for entry through the inner cortex, with possible injury to the underlying dura. It should be noted that with either technique, diploic vessels may be encountered and the use of bone wax may be indicated.

Following harvest of the outer cortex bone graft, the surrounding edges of the donor site are contoured with a large cutting bur to minimize the outer deformity. It is important to counsel the patient perioperatively that they will have a slightly flattened area in the region of the donor site. However, obvious ridges are easily avoidable. Another method for avoidance of such a deformity is by reconstruction of the donor site with various alloplastic materials such as Medpor or hydroxyapatite.

In some situations, the use of inner cortex calvarial bone is desired. This can be a technique of choice when a cra-

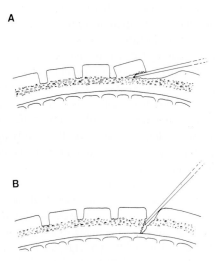

A

B

FIGURE 56.5 Diagram of problems in calvarial bone harvesting. (A) Proper technique with proper angulation of the osteotome into the diploic space, parallel to the inner and outer cortices. Note the wide trough that allows proper direction of the osteotome. (B) Inadequate placement of a osteotome caused by inadequate trough or creation. (From Frodel,[12] with permission)

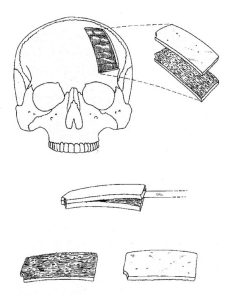

FIGURE 56.6 Diagram of the use of a craniotomy bone flap, which was then split with a saw and osteotome into an inner and outer table. (From Frodel,[12] with permission)

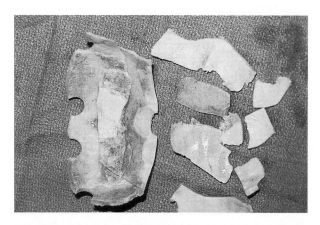

FIGURE 56.7 Clinical example of a craniotomy bone flap with multiple grafts harvested from the inner cortex.

niotomy has been performed, so that bone from the inner aspect of this bone flap can be harvested. In such situations, a sagittal saw and osteotome may be used to separate the inner and outer calvarial bone tables (Figures 56.6 and 56.7). The inner portion of this bone flap can then be utilized for grafting material, followed by replacement of the outer cortex to its original position at the end of the operation. Some surgeons believe that this is the ideal method and use it liberally, even when an intracranial procedure is not performed. The author does not think that in general it is indicated unless a craniotomy has been performed.

Bone Graft Harvest Complications

Despite adherence to these basic principles of bone graft harvesting, complications occur. The most common complication is that of donor site deformity although, as mentioned, this can be minimized by careful contouring of the donor site edges. Another common relative complication is that of undesired fracture of the bone graft during harvest. While this cannot always be avoided, the key to obtaining an intact graft for the surgeon is to be patient during the elevation process, because any forceful elevation of the saw or osteotome will lead to premature fracturing of the grafts. Dural exposure, an infrequent common complication, can be avoided by careful elevation within the diploic space. Occasionally, dura will be exposed during the elevation process, and it is important to identify when the inner cortex has been violated. When this occurs, it is not necessary to discontinue the graft harvesting procedure, although careful attention must be directed toward reelevation

in the diploic plane. If the graft is elevated and there is evidence not only of dural exposure but also of dural tear, the dural tear must be completely exposed by the use of a rongeur to further remove inner cortical bone. The tear can then be repaired directly and, if necessary, a graft of temporalis fascia may be utilized. Neurosurgical consultation is generally appropriate in such situations. There have been rare reports of intracranial bleeding following bone graft harvesting. Change of neurologic status intraoperatively or postoperatively should acutely raise the suspicion of such an injury. Fortunately, such complications seem to be extremely uncommon.

Rigid Fixation Considerations

Once the appropriate shape and number of calvarial bone grafts are obtained, they can now be placed in the recipient bed. It is the author's opinion that preparation of the recipient bed is of critical importance to the long-term survival of the bone graft. While calvarial bone grafts in the upper maxillofacial skeleton tend to undergo minimal resorption in most situations, this remains unpredictable and steps should be taken to maximize the environment for optimal graft "take." Nonvascularized bone graft healing is by "creeping substitution" when it is in adequate contact with underlying viable bone, as an onlay graft. In many other situations, bone graft survival occurs similarly to an alloplast, without replacement of the grafted material with new bone. This form of nonsubstituting graft survival is one feature of calvarial bone grafting that appears to be unique. It is also recognized that grafts with limited contact with healthy underlying bone and nonrigidly fixated have a greater propensity toward partial or complete resorption. Accordingly, the recipient bone should be prepared whenever possible by perforation to a bleeding cancellous space so that the bone graft may overlap this area (Figure 56.8). This is particularly important when a portion of the graft will not be in contact with healthy underlying

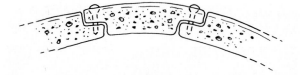

FIGURE 56.8 Diagram of inlay-overlay technique. Both the recipient and the defect in the bone graft are precontoured to allow for an inset of the bone graft with subsequent lag screw fixation. (From Frodel and Marentette,[13] with permission)

bone, as in reconstruction of an orbital rim, maxillary buttress, or zygomatic arch.

Fixation techniques vary depending on the situation and it is rare that hardware is not utilized, but this is occasionally the case when using bone grafts for orbital reconstruction. Miniplates and microplates are often employed, but these have several disadvantages. They do not provide absolute stability and, accordingly, cannot allow optimal environment for adequate bone healing. Although these plates may be palpable through the overlying skin, the use of small plates is still im-

portant in certain situations. The author's preference is to use the lag screw fixation technique whenever possible (Figure 56.8).[13] This technique requires the adequate preparation (perforation) of an underlying recipient bone bed and allows for absolute rigid fixation of the bone graft. An additional benefit is that the implant device is not palpable through the skin because it has been countersunk into the bone graft. Therefore, whenever possible, lag screw fixation of calvarial bone grafts to the maxillofacial skeleton is utilized.

Calvarial Bone Grafting Indications

Calvarial bone grafts are indicated in the reconstruction of a large variety of bony defects, depressions, and deformations that can exist from a variety of conditions secondary to trauma, oncologic resection, or congenital deformities. Occasionally, they are used in various aesthetic maxillofacial procedures. Clinical examples are now presented to demonstrate basic operative principles and the utilization of bone grafts for various defects of the craniomaxillofacial skeleton.

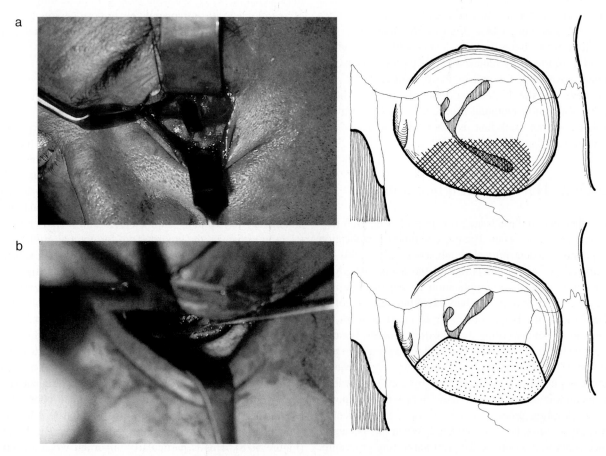

FIGURE 56.9 Left orbital floor defect with bone graft positioning (no fixation). (a) Left orbital floor defect. (b) Placement of curved calvarial bone graft over left orbital floor defect without fixation.

Case 1

A left orbital defect is presented in Figure 56.9a. Figure 56.9b demonstrates the placement of a curved bone graft without fixation into this defect. The use of bone grafts within the orbit without fixation techniques is a common procedure.

Case 2

Figure 56.10 shows a large right orbital defect in which multiple calvarial bone grafts have been placed. Because of the presence of an anterior ledge of bone, the lag screw fixation can be utilized to further cantilever the bone grafts superiorly and medially to restore the normal shape of the orbital cavity.

Case 3

Figure 56.11 shows a right infraorbital rim defect after zygomatic repositioning. A miniplate has been placed to sta-

bilize the medial and lateral segments of the orbital rim so as to reestablish the malar eminence (Figure 56.11a). After stabilization of other locations, the recipient site is prepared by contouring the residual bone adjacent to the defect to allow for inset of a contoured calvarial bone graft. This is then fixated into position as shown in Figure 56.11b.

Case 4

A left lateral maxillary buttress defect (Figure 56.12a) is shown after repositioning of the zygomatic segment with an L-shaped miniplate. A defect is noted in the maxillary buttress region. Figure 56.12b demonstrates placement of a calvarial bone graft after loosening of the screws in the plate, wedging of the bone graft under the plate, and the subsequent retightening of the plate to stabilize the bone graft into position.

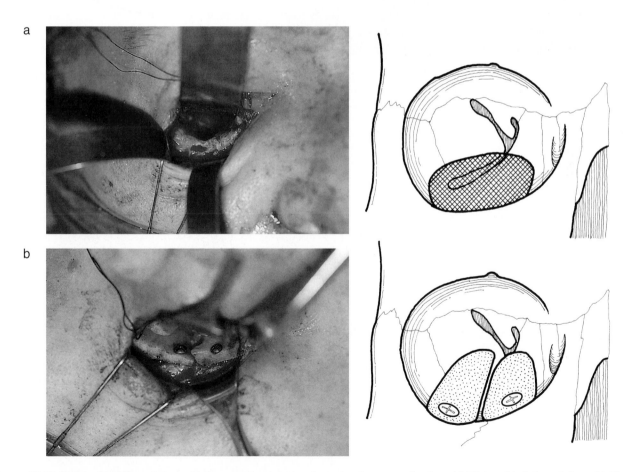

FIGURE 56.10 Right orbital floor defect with bone graft reconstruction using lag screw fixation: (a) Right orbital floor defect. (b) Placement of two bone grafts over left orbital floor defect with lag screw fixation.

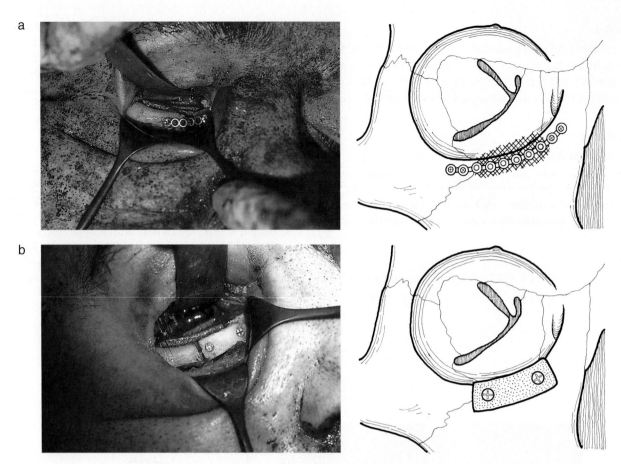

FIGURE 56.11 Right infraorbital rim defect with onlay bone graft. (a) Right infraorbital rim defect temporarily bridged with a miniplate. (b) Inset onlay bone graft technique with lag screw fixation of right infraorbital rim defect.

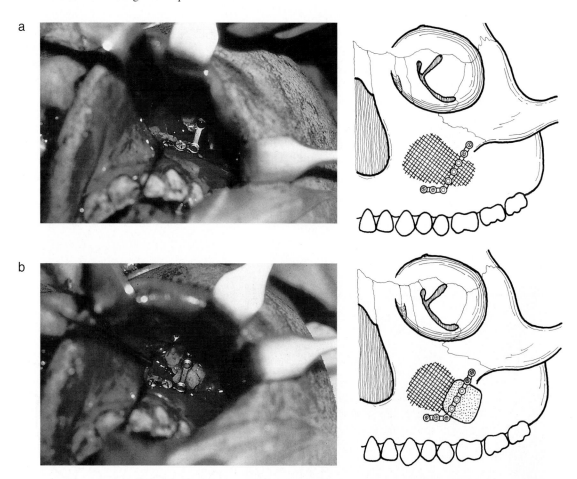

FIGURE 56.12 Left lateral zygomaticomaxillary buttress defect. (a) Left lateral zygomaticomaxillary buttress defect bridged with miniplate. (b) Wedged bone graft with good bony contact under miniplate of left lateral zygomaticomaxillary buttress defect.

Case 5

Figure 56.13a shows a larger left maxillary buttress defect. Figure 56.13b demonstrates placement of a large calvarial bone graft that is contoured in a concave shape and secured superiorly and inferiorly by lag screw fixation.

Case 6

Pictured and diagrammed (Figure 56.14) is a right zygomatic arch defect after zygomatic repositioning. Because of the con-

cerns for excessive lateral projection by placement of an overlay bone graft, the residual bone adjacent to the defect is trimmed from the undersurface, allowing for placement of an appropriately contoured bone graft. This is subsequently fixated by the lag screw technique.

Case 7

A large calvarial defect is shown [Figure 56.15(a)] following a traumatic injury, which encompasses the entire right frontal

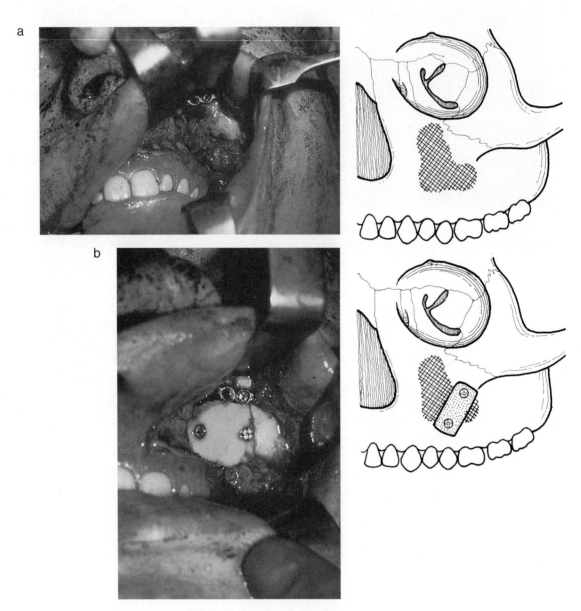

FIGURE 56.13 Large left anterolateral maxillary defect with onlay bone graft reconstruction. (a) Left anterolateral maxillary bone defect. (b) Calvarial onlay bone graft with lag screw fixation reconstruction.

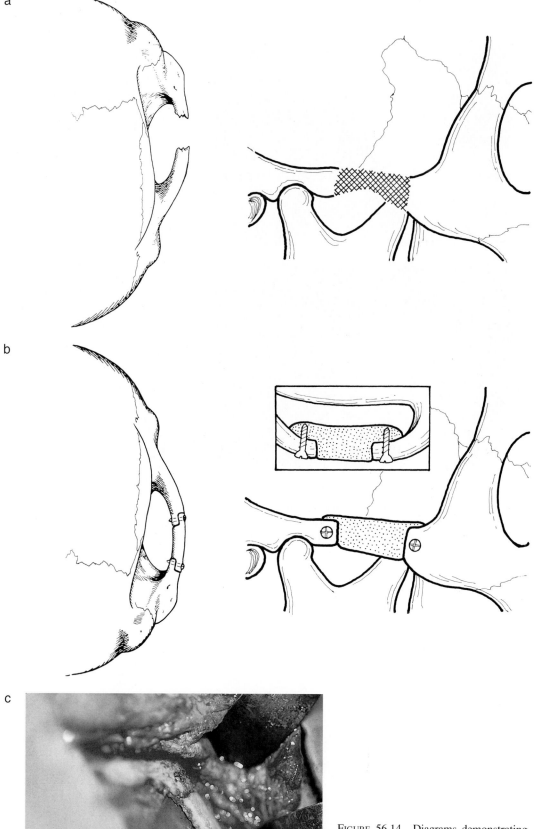

a

b

c

FIGURE 56.14 Diagrams demonstrating (a) right zygomatic defect and (b,c) placement of a calvarial bone graft using an underlay technique stabilized by lag screw fixation.

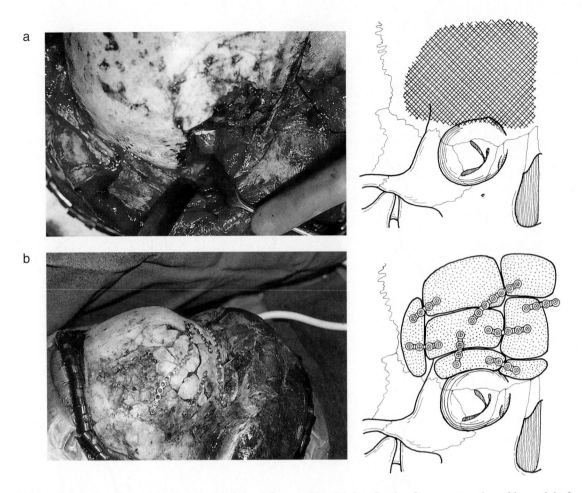

FIGURE 56.15 Large right frontal cranial and supraorbital rim defect with calvarial bone graft reconstruction. (a) Large right frontal cranial and supraorbital rim defect. (b) Multiple calvarial bone grafts with miniplate fixation for reconstruction of large right frontal cranial and supraorbital rim defect.

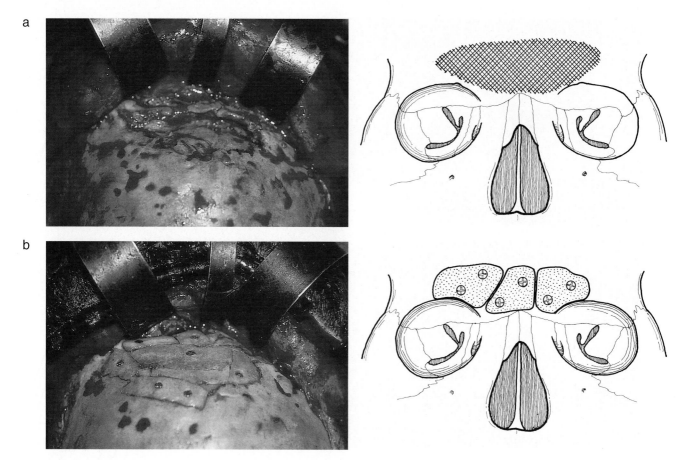

FIGURE 56.16 Collapse of anterior frontal bone after frontal sinus infection with calvarial bone graft reconstruction. (a) Anterior frontal bone defect. (b) Following frontal sinus debridement, reconstruction of anterior frontal bone with multiple calvarial bone grafts using lag screw fixation.

cranial and supraorbital rim and roof region. Figure 56.15b shows reconstruction of this defect using multiple calvarial bone grafts and miniplate fixation.

Case 8

This case demonstrates loss of the anterior table of the frontal sinus with a subsequent frontal deformity (Figure 56.16). After removal of residual sinus disease and burring down of the bone, multiple bone grafts are placed and stabilized by lag screw fixation. Contouring was then performed to reconstruct the normal frontal orbital shape.

Case 9

Pictured and diagrammed (Figure 56.17) is a large anterior cranial-based defect. As this connects with the nasopharynx, this defect is reconstructed with two calvarial bone grafts placed onto the residual anterior fossa floor and roof of the orbit and stabilized with lag screw fixation. Resorbable screws may be used in these circumstances with less concern for hardware removal or migration.[14,15]

Summary

In conclusion, calvarial bone grafting provides an excellent tool in the armamentarium for craniomaxillofacial reconstruction. Key considerations include having proper equipment as well as patience during graft harvesting, maintaining the osteotome or saw position in the space between the inner and outer cortices of the calvarium, preparation of the recipient bed after selection of the appropriately shaped bone graft, and the use of rigid internal fixation utilizing the lag screw technique whenever possible. Resorbable screws may be used when adequate stabilization can be achieved, avoiding the sequelae of screw head palpation from graft resorption, or the need for hardware removal.[14,15]

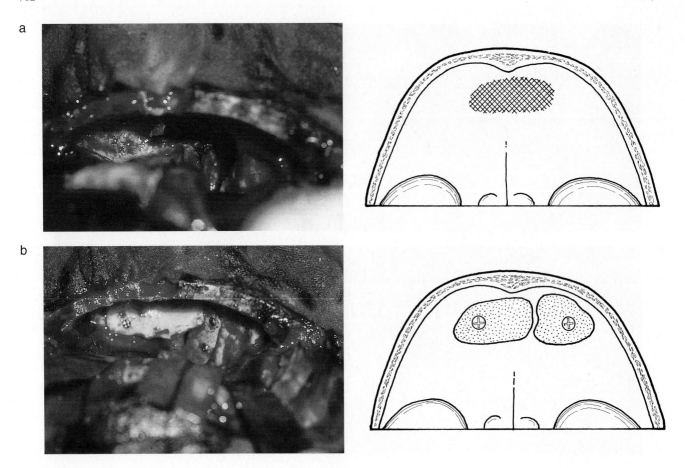

FIGURE 56.17 Large anterior cranial fossa defect following a gunshot wound with calvarial bone graft reconstruction. (a) Anterior cranial fossa defect. (b) Reconstruction of anterior cranial fossa floor defect with two calvarial bone grafts using a lag screw fixation.

References

1. Smith ID, Abramson M. Membranous vs. endochondral bone autografts. *Arch Otolaryngol Head Neck Surg.* 1983;99:203–205.
2. Zins JE, Whitaker LA. Membranous vs. endochrondral bone grafts: implications for craniofacial reconstruction. *Plast Reconstr Surg.* 1985;76:510–514.
3. Kusiak JF, Zins JE, Witaker LA. The early revascularization of membranous bone. *Plast Reconstr Surg.* 1985:76:510–514.
4. Hardesty RA, Marsh JL. Craniofacial onlay bone grafting: a prospective evaluation of graft morphology, orientation, and embryologic origin. *Plast Reconstr Surg.* 1990;85:5–15.
5. Moore KI. *The Developing Human.* 2nd ed. Philadelphia: WB Saunders; 1977:307–309.
6. Craft PD, Sargent LA. Membranous bone healing and techniques in calvarial bone grafting. *Clin Plast Surg.* 1989;16:11–19.
7. Phillips JH, Rahn BA. Fixation effects on membranous and endochondral onlay bone-graft resorption. *Plast Reconstr Surg.* 1988;82:872–877.
8. Pensler J, McCarthy JC. The calvarial donor site: an anatomic study in cadavers. *Plast Reconstr Surg.* 1985;75:648–651.
9. Powell NB, Riley, RW. Cranial bone grafting in facial aesthetic and reconstructive contouring. *Arch Otolaryngol Head Neck Surg.* 1987;Jul;113(7):713–719.
10. Sheen JH. A change in the site for cranial bone harvesting. *Prospect Plast Surg.* 1990;4:48–57.
11. Frodel JL, Marentette LJ, Quatela VC, Weinstein GS. Calvarial bone graft harvest: techniques, considerations, and morbidity. *Arch Otolaryngol Head Neck Surg.* 1993;119:17–23.
12. Frodel JL. Complications of bone grafting. In: Eisele DW, ed. *Complications in Head and Neck Surgery.* St. Louis: CV Mosby; 1993:773–784.
13. Frodel JL, Marentette LJ. Lag screw fixation in the upper craniomaxillofacial skeleton. *Arch Otolaryngol Head Neck Surg.* 1993;119:297–304.
14. Kurpad SN, Goldstein JA, Cohen AR. Bioresorbable fixation for congenital pediatric craniofacial surgery: a 2 year followup. *Pediatr Neurosurg.* 2000;33:306–310.
15. Pensler JM. Role of resorbable plates and screws in craniofacial surgery. *J Craniofac Surg.* 1997;8:129–134.

57
Crouzon Syndrome: Basic Dysmorphology and Staging of Reconstruction

Jeffrey C. Posnick

Crouzon syndrome is the most frequent form of craniofacial dysostosis.[1-6] It is characterized by multiple anomalies of the craniofacial skeleton. Its manifestations are generally less severe than those of Apert syndrome, and there is no involvement of the extremities. Typically, the cranial vault presentation is a brachycephalic shape to the skull caused by premature synostosis of both coronal sutures. Cranial vault suture involvement, other than coronal, may include sagittal, metopic, or lambdoidal in isolation or in any combination. The cranial base and upper face sutures are generally involved, resulting in a variable degree of midface hypoplasia with an angle class III malocclusion. The orbits are hypoplastic, resulting in a degree of proptosis with additional orbital dysplasia that may produce a mild to moderate orbital hypertelorism and flatness to the (transverse) arc of rotation of the midface.[7-13]

The lack of consensus about the timing and techniques used at each stage of reconstruction reflects uncertainty about the functional consequences of the congenital dysmorphology and inconsistencies of the results achieved with any one approach to treatment.[14-41] Accurate objective methods for documentation of either the presenting deformity or initial and late postoperative results are few. Too much reliance has been placed on the subjective assessment of both the presenting deformity and the postoperative results achieved.

Functional Considerations

Brain volume in the normal child almost triples in the first year,[42-46] and by 2 years the cranial capacity is four times that at birth. In craniosynostosis, premature suture fusion is combined with continuing brain growth. Depending on the number, location, and rate of prematurely fused sutures, the growth of the brain may be restricted. If early surgical intervention with suture release, decompression, and reshaping to restore a more normal intracranial volume and configuration does not reverse the process, diminished central nervous system function may be the end result. Elevated intracranial pressure is the most important functional problem associated with premature suture fusion.[26,32,34,40] If intracranial hypertension goes untreated, brain function is adversely affected.

When craniosynostosis is associated with increased intracranial pressure, optic nerve compression occurs. Initially, there is papilloedema with eventual optic atrophy that results in partial or complete blindness. Fundoscopic examination of the retina should reveal papilloedema, allowing for surgical intervention to limit the late effects.

If the orbits are shallow and the eyes proptotic, corneal drying may occur, which can result in ulceration. If the orbits are extremely shallow, herniation of the globes may occur, requiring emergency reduction. Divergent or convergent nonparalytic strabismus or exotropia occurs frequently and should be looked for and treated. Hydrocephalus affects 5% to 10% of children with Crouzon syndrome.[47] Although the etiology is not always clear, hydrocephalus may be secondary to a generalized cranial base stenosis with constriction of the cranial base foramina. When the clinical examination is correlated with serial computed tomographic (CT) scans or magnetic resonance imaging to document progressively enlarging ventricles, a more accurate diagnosis can be determined. When hydrocephalus is detected, prompt ventriculoperitoneal shunting should be performed.

All neonates are obligate nasal breathers. A significant percentage of children born with Crouzon syndrome have severe hypoplasia of the midface with diminished nasal and nasopharyngeal spaces. This malformation increases nasal airway resistance and forces infants to breathe primarily through their mouth. This type of breathing may result in inadequate oxygenation with a tracheostomy being required.

In Crouzon syndrome, conductive hearing deficit is frequently encountered, and atresia of the external auditory canals may also occur.[48]

Aesthetic Assessment

Examination of the entire craniofacial region (skeletal and soft tissues) should be systematic and complete. Specific findings are frequent in Crouzon syndrome, but each patient is unique. Achievement of symmetry, proportionality, and balance is critical to reconstructing an attractive face in a child born with Crouzon syndrome.

The upper third of the face is generally dysmorphic in an infant born with Crouzon syndrome. The establishment of the preferred position of the forehead is essential to the overall facial balance.[49] The forehead is divided into two separate components, the supraorbital ridge and the superior forehead. The supraorbital ridge includes the glabella region; the supraorbital rim and its lateral extension posteriorly along the temporoparietal bones; and inferiorly down the frontozygomatic suture region. In Crouzon syndrome with brachycephaly present, this component is retruded and wide. Ideally, the eyebrows, overlying the supraorbital ridges, should rest anterior to the cornea when viewed in profile. When the supraorbital ridge is viewed from above, the rim should arc posteriorly to achieve a gentle 90° angle at the temporal fossa with the center point of the arc located at the level of each frontozygomatic suture. The superior forehead component, about 1.5 cm up from the supraorbital rim, has a gentle posterior curve of 60°, leveling out at the coronal suture region when seen in profile. The brachycephalic skull of Crouzon syndrome lacks this preferred superior forehead morphology.

In Crouzon syndrome, presenting with bilateral coronal suture synostosis extending into the cranial base, the orbitonasozygomatic region is wide and lacks forward projection. These findings are consistent with a short and wide anterior cranial base. Overall midface projection is deficient, and the upper anterior face appears vertically short from the nasion to the maxillary central incisors.[8,9,12]

Quantitative Assessment

The purpose of a quantitative assessment of the craniofacial complex by CT scan analysis,[9,12,50–54] anthropometric measurements,[8,55] cephalometric analysis, and dental model analysis is to help predict growth patterns, confirm or refute clinical impressions, aid in treatment planning, and provide a framework for objective assessment of the immediate and long-term reconstructive results.

We developed a method of analysis based on CT scan measurements which allows for a more quantitative assessment of the cranio-orbito-zygomatic skeleton in both the horizontal and transverse planes.[50,51] A normative database is established using this system which enables comparison of an individual patient's cranio-orbito-zygomatic morphology with that of an age-matched cohort group.[51]

Posnick et al. developed this method of quantitative CT scan analysis and then used it to document the differences in the cranio-orbito-zygomatic region between unoperated chil-

dren with Crouzon syndrome and age-matched controls.[9,12] Posnick et al. also evaluated the morphologic results achieved in those children 1 year after undergoing a standard suture release, anterior cranial vault, and upper orbital procedure designed to decompress and reshape these regions.[12]

The preoperative CT scan measurements of these unoperated Crouzon children confirmed a widened anterior cranial vault at 108% of normal and a cranial length averaging only 92% of normal. In comparison with age-matched controls, orbital measurements revealed a widened anterior interorbital distance at 122% of normal, an increased intertemporal width at 121% of normal, globe protrusion at 119% of normal, and a short medial orbital wall distance at only 86% of normal. The distance between the zygomatic buttresses and the interarch distances were found to be increased at 106% and 103% of normal, respectively. The zygomatic arch lengths were substantially shortened at only 87% of age-matched control values.[12] These findings confirmed clinical observations of brachycephalic anterior cranial vaults with shallow, frequently hyperteloric orbits and globe proptosis. Generally, the Crouzon midface is horizontally retrusive and transversely wide, reflected in wide and shortened zygomas.

The same quantitative CT scan assessment was carried out in the operated Crouzon children more than 1 year after undergoing anterior cranial vault and upper orbital osteotomies with reshaping, and when comparing them to the new age-matched control values, we were not able to demonstrate any significant improvement in the cranio-orbito-zygomatic measurements.[12]

In the midchildhood years, another group of Crouzon children were again assessed using the quantitative CT scan measurements.[56] They were found to have cranial vault lengths averaging only 87% of the age-matched normals. The medial orbital walls were (horizontally) short at 87% of normal while the extent of globe protrusion was excessive at 134% of age-matched norms. The zygomatic arch lengths averaged only 84% of normal. These findings confirmed horizontal (anteroposterior) deficiency of the upper and middle facial thirds. After undergoing a monobloc osteotomy (orbits and midface) combined with anterior cranial vault reshaping and advancement carried out through an intracranial approach, the children's cranio-orbito-zygomatic measurements were again taken. The mean cranial length initially achieved (after monobloc osteotomy) was 98% and at 1 year 92% of the control value. When compared with age-matched controls, the orbital measurements reflected improvement in the midorbital hypertelorism (midinterorbital distance, 97% initially after operation and 102% at 1 year), and orbital proptosis (soon after surgery, 86%, and at 1 year, 92% of age-matched normals). The medial orbital wall length initially normalized at 101% and later at 97% of normal values. The zygomatic arch length initially corrected at 106% and later to 101% of normal.

Surgical Approach: Historical Perspective

The first recorded surgical approach to craniosynostosis was performed by Lannelongue in 1890[57] and Lane in 1892,[58] who completed strip craniectomies. Their aim was to control the problem of brain compression within a congenitally small cranial vault. The classic neurosurgical techniques were refined over the ensuing decade and geared toward resecting the synostotic suture(s) in the hope that the "released" skull would reshape itself and continue to grow in a normal and symmetric fashion. The strip craniectomy procedures were supposed to allow for a creation of new suture lines at the sites of the previous synostosis. With the realization that this goal was rarely achieved, attempts were made to fragment the cranial vault surgically with pieces of flat bone used as free grafts to refashion the cranial vault shape. Problems with these methods included uncontrolled postoperative skull molding, resulting in reossification in dysmorphic configurations.

In 1950, Gillies reported his experience with an extracranial (elective) Le Fort III osteotomy to improve the anterior projection of a patient with Crouzon syndrome.[59] His early enthusiasm later turned to discouragement when the patient's facial skeleton relapsed to its preoperative status. In 1967, Tessier described a new (intracranial-cranial base) approach to the management of Crouzon syndrome.[17] His landmark presentation and publications were the beginning of modern craniofacial surgery.[19,60–64] To overcome Gillies' earlier problems, Tessier developed an innovative basic surgical approach that included new locations for the Le Fort III osteotomy, a combined intracranial-extracranial (cranial base) approach, use of a coronal (skin) incision to expose the upper facial bones, and the use of autogeneous bone graft. He also applied an external fixation device to help maintain bony stability until healing had occurred.

The concept of simultaneous suture release for craniosynostosis combined with cranial vault reshaping in infants was initially discussed by Rougerie et al.[65] and later refined by Hoffman and Mohr in 1976.[22] Whitaker et al.[66] proposed a more formal anterior cranial vault and orbital reshaping procedure for unilateral coronal synostosis in 1977,[66] and then Marchac and Renier published their experience with the "floating forehead" technique for simultaneous suture release and anterior cranial vault and orbital reshaping to manage bilateral coronal synostosis in infancy.[67,68]

The widespread use of autogenous cranial bone grafting has virtually eliminated rib and hip grafts when bone replacement or augmentation is required in cranio-orbito-zygomatic procedures.[69] This represents another of Tessier's contributions to craniofacial surgery.[62] Phillips and Rahn documented through animal studies the advantages of stable fixation of grafts (lag screw techniques) to encourage early healing and limit graft resorption.[70] In current practice, the use of mini- and micro internal plate and screw fixation is the preferred form of fixation when stability and three-dimensional reconstruction of multiple osteotomized bone segments and grafts are required.[71–75]

Surgical Approach: Author's Current Staging of Reconstruction

Primary Cranio-Orbital Decompression: Reshaping in Infancy

The most common cranial vault suture synostosis pattern associated with Crouzon syndrome is bilateral, premature coronal suture fusion that extends into the cranial base (Figures 57.1–57.3).[4] In infancy and early childhood, it is not always possible to separate "simple" brachycephaly (bilateral coronal synostosis) from Crouzon syndrome unless either midface hypoplasia is evident or a family pedigree with an autosomal dominant inheritance pattern is known.[4] The midface

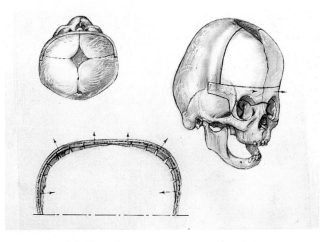

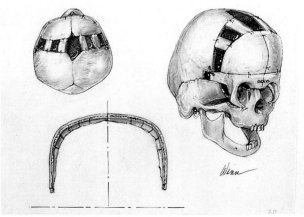

FIGURE 57.1 Illustration of the craniofacial skeleton in a child with Crouzon syndrome before and after cranio-orbital reshaping. (Above) Site of osteotomies. (Below) After osteotomies, reshaping, and fixation of the cranio-orbital regions. (From Posnick[10])

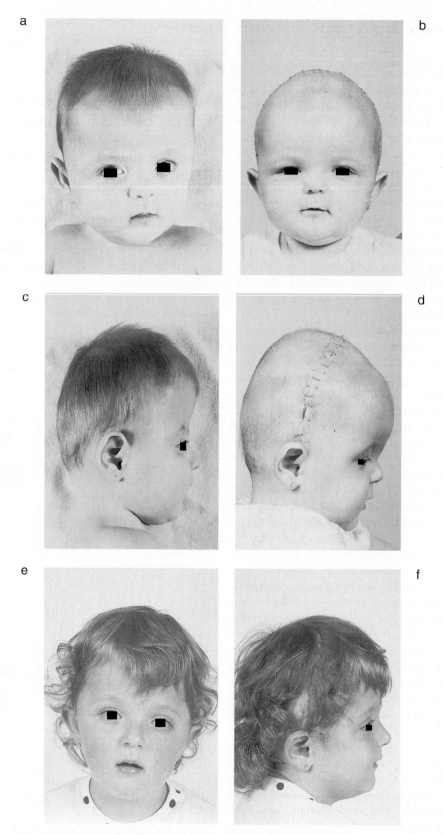

FIGURE 57.2 A 6-month-old girl with Crouzon syndrome underwent cranio-orbital reshaping. (a) Preoperative frontal view. (b) Frontal view 10 days later. (c) Preoperative profile view. (d) Profile view 10 days later. (e) Frontal view 3 years later. (f) Profile view 3 years later. (From Posnick et al.[10])

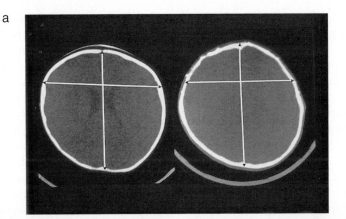

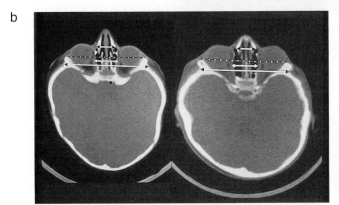

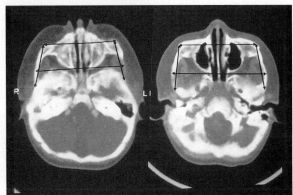

FIGURE 57.3 (a) Comparison of standard axial-sliced CT scans through the cranial vault of the 6-month-old girl with Crouzon syndrome (from Figure 57.2) before and 1 year after cranio-orbital reshaping. The cranial length has increased from 114 to 138 mm. The anterior intracranial width has increased from 100 to 108 mm and remains at 105% of the age-matched controls. (b) Comparison of standard axial-sliced CT scans through midorbit before and 1 year after reconstruction. Globe protrusion has increased from 12 to 17 mm and is now 116% of the age-matched control value. The anterior intraorbital distance has in-creased from 23 to 26 mm and is now 146% of the control value. The lateral orbital wall distance has increased from 75 to 86 mm and is now 115% of the control value. (c) Comparison of standard axial-sliced CT scans through the zygomatic arches before and 1 year after reconstruction. The increased midface width is confirmed by the interzygomatic buttress and interzygomatic arch distances, both of which have increased to 116% of the age-matched control values. (Magnification of the individual CT scans was not controlled for in this figure.) (From Posnick et al.[10])

deficiency associated with Crouzon syndrome is variable and not always obvious until later in childhood.[4]

With early bilateral coronal synostosis, the supraorbital ridge is retruded and the overlying eyebrows are posterior to the cornea of the eyes when viewed in the sagittal plane. The anterior cranial base is short in the anteroposterior (AP) dimension and wide transversely. The cranial vault is high in the superoinferior dimension, with anterior bulging of the upper forehead resulting from compensatory growth through the open metopic and the anterior sagittal sutures. The orbits are generally shallow and the eyes proptotic and with a degree of orbital hypertelorism. The sphenoid wings have a reverse curve, producing the harlequin appearance often described on an AP skull radiograph.

The initial treatment for Crouzon syndrome generally requires bicoronal suture release with decompression of the anterior cranial vault and simultaneous anterior cranial vault and upper orbital osteotomies with reshaping and advancement.[10,12,24,33,41,66–68] My preference is to carry this out when the child is 10 to 12 months old unless signs of increased intracranial pressure are identified earlier in life.[10,12,41] Reshaping of the upper three-quarters of the orbital rims and supraorbital ridges is geared to decreasing the bitemporal and anterior cranial base width with simultaneous horizontal advancement to increase the AP dimension. This also increases the depth of the upper orbits with some improvement of the eye proptosis. The overlying forehead is then reconstructed according to aesthetic needs. A degree of overcorrection is preferred at the level of the supraorbital ridge when the procedure is carried out in infancy. It is my clinical impression that by allowing additional growth to occur before first-stage cranio-orbital decompression (waiting until the child is 10 to 12 months old) the improved cranial vault and upper orbital shape is better maintained with less need for repeat craniotomy procedures.

Repeat Craniotomy for Additional Cranial Vault Reshaping in Young Children

After the initial suture release, decompression and reshaping is carried out during infancy, the child is followed clinically at intervals by the craniofacial surgeon, pediatric neurosurgeon, pediatric neuro-ophthalmologist, and neuroradiologist along with interval CT scanning. Should signs of increased intracranial pressure develop, urgent decompression with further reshaping to expand the intracranial volume is performed.[76] When increased intracranial pressure is suspected, the location of the cranial vault constriction influences the region of the skull for which further decompression and reshaping is planned (Figure 57.4).

If the brain compression is judged to be anterior, further forehead and upper orbital osteotomies with reshaping and advancement are carried out. The technique is similar to that previously described. If the problem is posterior, decompression and expansion of the posterior cranial vault with the patient in the prone position is required.

The "repeat" craniotomy carried out for further decompression and reshaping in the Crouzon child is often complicated by brittle cortical bone, which lacks a diploic space and contains sharp spicules piercing the dura, the presence of previously placed fixation devices in the operative field (i.e., silastic sheeting with metal clips, stainless steel wires, microplates, and screws) and convoluted dura compressed against (herniated into) the inner table of the skull.[75] All these problems result in a higher incidence of dural tears during the calvarectomy than would normally occur during the primary procedure. A greater amount of morbidity should be anticipated when reelevating the scalp flap, dissecting the dura free

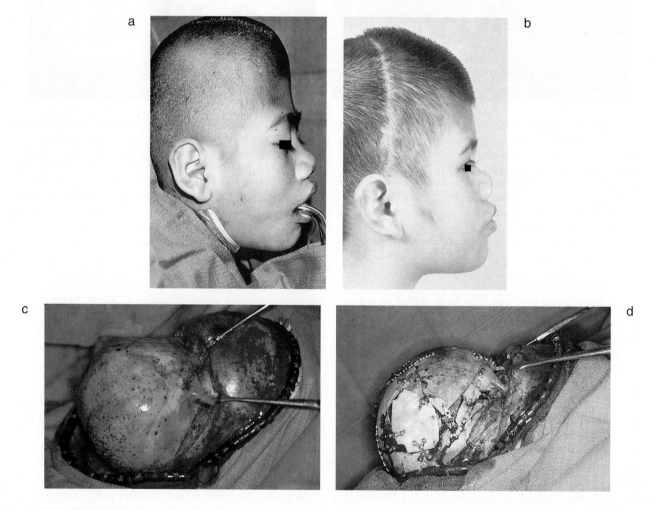

FIGURE 57.4 A 9-year-old girl with unrepaired late, bicoronal synostosis requiring suture release, total cranial vault and upper orbital osteotomies with reshaping and advancement. (a) Preoperative profile view. (b) Profile view after reconstruction. (c) Intraoperative lateral view of cranial vault and upper orbits after elevation of coronal flap. (d) Same view after reconstruction. Stabilization with titanium miniplates and screws. (From Posnick[13])

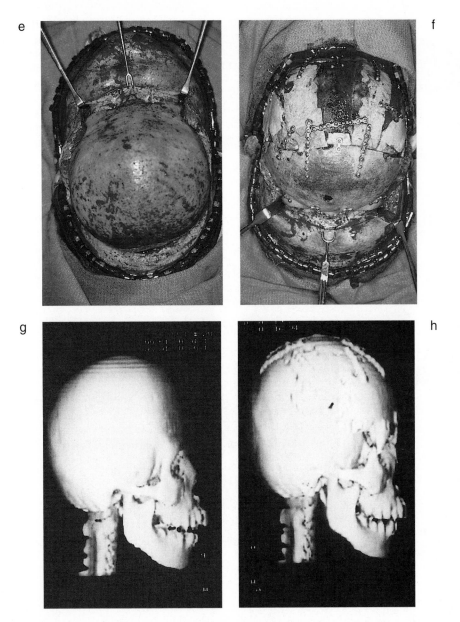

FIGURE 57.4 *Continued.* (e) Intraoperative bird's-eye view of cranial vault after elevation of anterior and posterior scalp flaps. (f) Same view after cranial vault and upper orbital osteotomies with reshaping. Stabilization with titanium bone plates and screws. (g) Three-dimensional CT scan reformation of craniofacial skeleton. Lateral view before reconstruction. (h) Lateral view after reconstruction. (From Posnick[13])

of the inner table of the skull and cranial base, and then completing the repeat craniotomy.

Management of the Total Midface Deformity in Childhood

The type of osteotomy selected to manage the "total midface" deficiency/deformity and any residual cranial vault dysplasia should depend on the presenting deformity rather than a fixed universal approach to the midface malformation (Figures 57.5 and 57.6).[13,37,41,56,77,78] The selection of either a monobloc (with or without additional orbital segmentalization), facial bipartition, or a Le Fort III osteotomy to manage the horizontal, transverse, and vertical midface deficiencies/deformities in a patient with Crouzon syndrome will depend on the presenting midface and anterior cranial vault morphology. The presenting dysmorphology is dependent not only on the original malformation but also on the previous procedures carried out and the effect of further skull remodeling in association with brain growth. If the supraorbital ridge with its overlying eyebrows sit in good position when viewed from the

a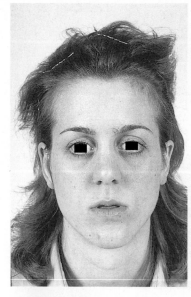

b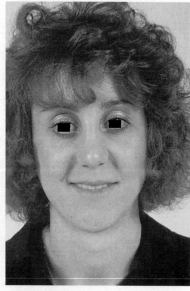

c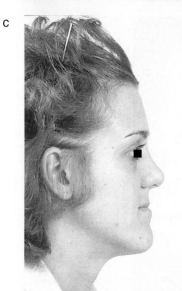

d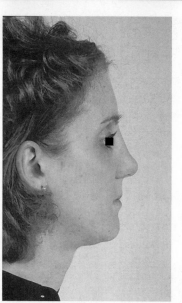

e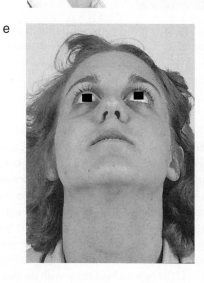

f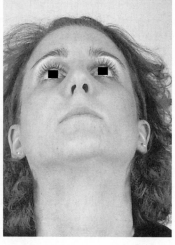

FIGURE 57.5 A 16-year-old girl with a mild form of Crouzon syndrome is shown before and after undergoing an extracranial Le Fort III osteotomy with advancement. (a) Preoperative frontal view. (b) Frontal view 1 year after Le Fort III. (c) Preoperative profile view. (d) Profile view at 1 year after Le Fort III. (e) Preoperative worm's-eye view. (f) Worm's-eye view at 1 year after Le Fort III.

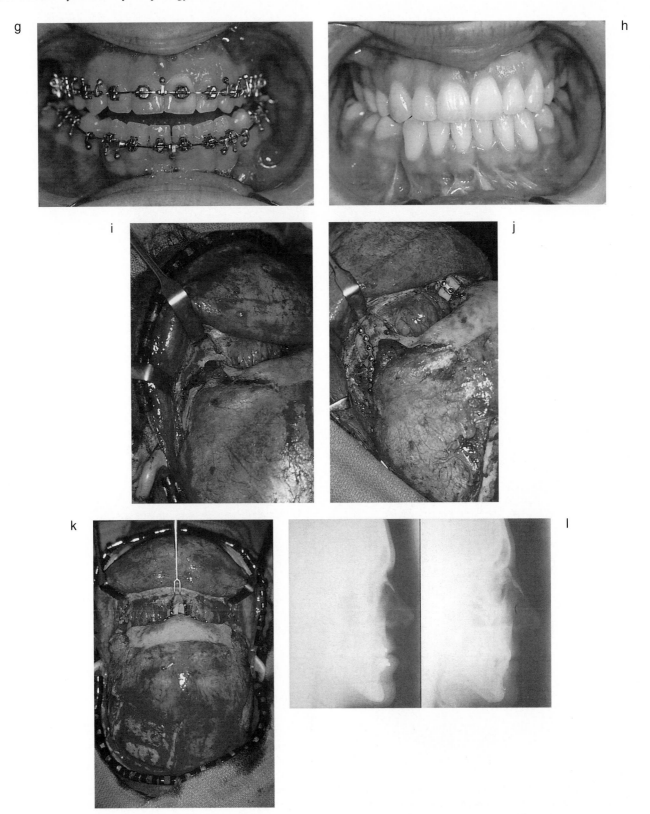

FIGURE 57.5 *Continued.* (g) Occlusal view before surgery. (h) Occlusal view 1 year after Le Fort III. (i), Intraoperative view of zygomatic complex after osteotomies through coronal incision. (j) Intraoperative view after stabilization with titanium bone plates and
screws. (k) Intraoperative bird's-eye view of cranial vault and orbits
through coronal incision. Stabilization of Le Fort III osteotomy with
bone plates and screws. Split cranial grafts harvested from left parietal region and interposed in nasofrontal region and zygomatic
arches. (l) Lateral cephalometric radiograph before and after reconstruction. (From Posnick[13])

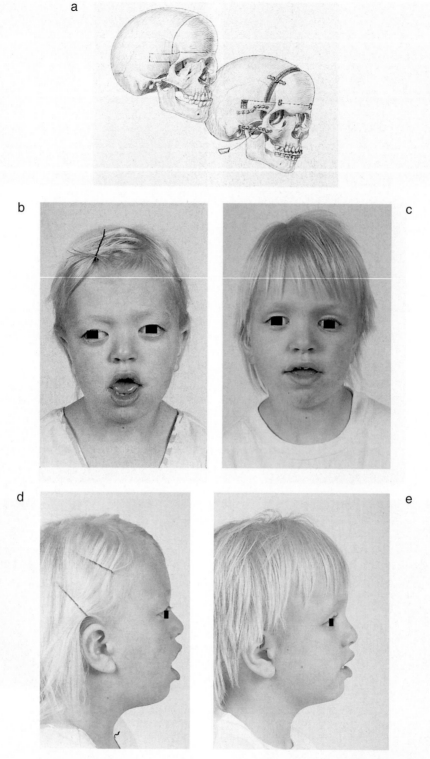

FIGURE 57.6 A 6-year-old girl with Cruzon syndrome who underwent anterior cranial vault and monobloc osteotomies with reshaping and advancement. (a) Illustration of craniofacial morphology before and after anterior cranial vault and monobloc osteotomies with advancement. Osteotomy locations indicated. Stabilization with cranial bone grafts and titanium miniplates and screws. (b) Preoperative frontal view. (c) Postoperative frontal view. (d) Preoperative lateral view. (e) Postoperative lateral view 1 year after reconstruction.

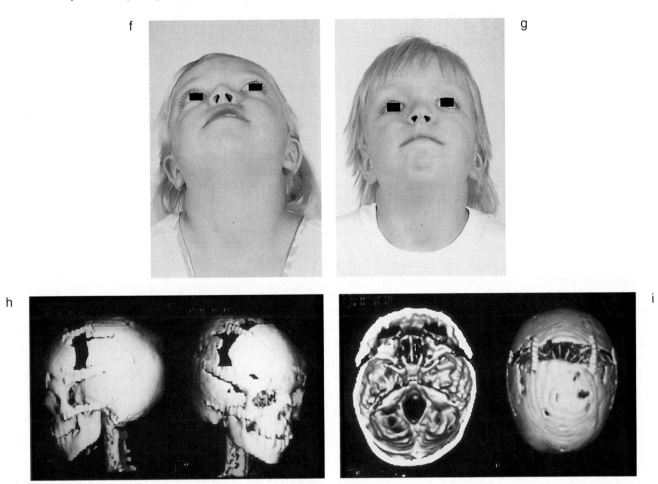

FIGURE 57.6 *Continued.* (f) Preoperative worm's-eye view. (g) Postoperative worm's-eye view 1 year after reconstruction. (h) Three-dimensional CT scan reformations after reconstruction. (i) Additional three-dimensional CT scan reformations initially after reconstruction including cranial base view demonstrating increased anteroposterior dimensions achieved. (From Posnick[13])

sagittal plane with adequate depth of the upper orbits, there is a normal arc of rotation of the midface and forehead in the transverse plane, and the root of the nose is not too wide (orbital hypertelorism), then there is no need to reconstruct this region any further. In such patients, the basic residual upper midface deformity may be effectively managed with an extracranial Le Fort III osteotomy. If the supraorbital ridge and anterior cranial base both remain deficient in the sagittal plane along with the zygomas, nose, lower orbits, and maxilla, a monobloc osteotomy is indicated. In these patients, the forehead is generally flat and retruded, and it will also require reshaping and advancement. If orbital hypertelorism and midface flattening with loss of the normal facial curvature are present, then the monobloc unit is split vertically in the midline (facial bipartition), a wedge of intraorbital (nasal and ethmoidal) bone is removed, and the orbits are repositioned medially while the maxillary posterior arch is widened (this is rarely required in Crouzon syndrome). When a monobloc or facial bipartition osteotomy is carried out as the basic proce-

dure, additional segmentalization of the upper and lateral orbits may also be required to complete a satisfactory reconstruction of the upper orbits.

For most patients, an error in judgment will occur if the surgeon attempts to simultaneously adjust the orbits and idealize the occlusion by using the Le Fort III, monobloc, or facial bipartition osteotomies in isolation without completing a separate Le Fort I osteotomy. The degrees of horizontal deficiency at the orbits and maxillary dentition are rarely uniform. This further segmentalization of the midlife complex at the Le Fort I level is required to reestablish normal proportions. If Le Fort I segmentalization of the total midface complex is not carried out and the surgeon attempts to achieve a positive overbite and overjet at the incisor teeth, enophthalmus will frequently result.

Problems specific to the Le Fort III osteotomy when its indications are less than ideal include irregular step defects in the lateral orbital rims that occur when even a moderate advancement is carried out. These step defects are often impossible to effectively modify later. With the Le Fort III osteotomy, an ideal orbital depth is difficult to judge; a frequent result is either residual proptosis or enophthalmus. Simultaneous correction of orbital hypertelorism or correction of a midface arc of rotation problem is not possible with the Le Fort III procedure. Excessive lengthening of the nose, accompanied by flattening of the nasofrontal angle, will also occur if the Le Fort III osteotomy is selected when the skeletal morphology favors a monobloc or facial bipartition procedure.

Final reconstruction of the cranial vault and orbital dystopia problem in Crouzon syndrome can be managed as early as 5 to 7 years of age. By this age, the cranial vault and orbits normally attain approximately 85% to 90% of their adult size.[42–46,51] When the basic midface and final cranial vault procedure is carried out at or after this age, the reconstructive objectives are to approximate adult dimensions in the cranio-orbito-zygomatic region with the expectation of a stable result once healing has occurred. Psychosocial considerations also support the time frame of 5 to 7 years of age for the elective basic (total) midface and final cranial vault procedure. When the procedure is carried out at this age, the child may enter the first grade with a real chance for satisfactory self-esteem. Routine orthognathic surgery will be necessary at the time of skeletal maturity to achieve an ideal occlusion, facial profile, and smile.

Management of the Jaw Deformity and Malocclusion in Adolescents

While the mandible has a normal basic growth potential in Crouzon syndrome, the maxilla does not.[79] An angle class III malocclusion resulting from maxillary retrusion with anterior open bite often results. A Le Fort I osteotomy to allow for horizontal advancement, transverse widening, and vertical lengthening is generally required in combination with a genioplasty (vertical reduction and horizontal advancement) to further correct the lower-face deformity. The elective orthognathic surgery is carried out in conjunction with orthodontic treatment and is planned for completion at the time of skeletal maturity (approximately 14–16 years in girls and 16 to 18 years in boys).[13]

Conclusion

The author's preferred approach to the management of Crouzon syndrome is to stage the reconstruction to coincide with facial growth patterns, visceral (brain and eye) function, and psychosocial development. Recognition of the need for a staged reconstructive approach serves to clarify the objectives of each phase of treatment for the surgeon, craniofacial team, and family unit. By continuing to define our rationale for the timing and extent of surgical intervention, and then objectively evaluating both function and morphologic outcomes,

we will further improve the quality of life for patients born with Crouzon syndrome.

References

1. Crouzon O. Dysostose cranio-faciale herediataire. *Bull Mem Soc Med Hop Paris.* 1912;33:545.
2. Jones K. The Crouzon syndrome revisited. *J Med Genet.* 1973;10:398–399.
3. Cohen MM Jr. An etiology and nosologic overview of craniosynostosis syndrome. *Birth Defects Orig Artic Ser.* 1975;11:137–189.
4. Cohen MM Jr, ed. *Craniosynostosis: Diagnosis, Evaluation and Management.* New York: Raven Press; 1986.
5. Gorlin RJ, Cohen MM Jr, Levin LS. *Syndromes of the Head and Neck.* 3rd ed. New York: Oxford University Press; 1990:519–524.
6. Kreiborg S. Birth prevalence study of the Crouzon syndrome: comparison of direct and indirect methods. *Clin Genet.* 1992;41:12–15.
7. Kreiborg S, Aduss H. Apert and Crouzon syndromes contrasted. Qualitative craniofacial x-ray findings. In: Marchac D, ed. *Craniofacial Surgery.* Heidelberg: Springer-Verlag; 1986:92–96.
8. Kolar JC, Munro IR, Farkas LG. Patterns of dysmorphology in Crouzon syndrome: an anthropometric study. *Cleft Palate J.* 1988;25:235–244.
9. Carr M, Posnick J, Armstrong D, et al. Cranio-orbito-zygomatic measurements from standard CT scans in unoperated Crouzon and Apert infants: comparison with normal controls. *Cleft Palate Craniofac J.* 1992;29:129–136.
10. Posnick JC. Craniosynostosis: surgical management in infancy. In: Bell WH, ed. *Modern Practice in Orthognathic and Reconstructive Surgery.* Philadelphia: WB Saunders; 1992:1889–1931.
11. Kreiborg S, Marsh JL, Liversage M, et al. Comparative three-dimensional analysis of CT scans of the calvaria and cranial base in Apert and Crouzon syndromes. *J Craniomaxillofac Surg.* 1993;21:181–188.
12. Posnick JC, Lin KY, Jhawar BJ, Armstrong D. Crouzon syndrome: quantitative assessment of presenting deformity and surgical results based on CT scans. *Plast Reconstr Surg.* 1993;92:1027–1037.
13. Posnick JC. Craniofacial dysostosis: management of the midface deformity. In: Bell WH, ed. *Modern Practice in Orthognathic and Reconstructive Surgery.* Philadelphia: WB Saunders; 1992:1839–1887.
14. Virchow R. Uber den Cretinismus, nametlich in Franken und uber pathologische Schadelforamen. *Verh Phys Med Ges Wurzburg.* 1851;2:230.
15. Fowler FD, Ingraham FD. A new method for applying polyethylene film to the skull in the treatment of craniosynostosis. *J Neurosurg.* 1957;14:584.
16. Moss ML. The pathogenesis of premature cranial synostosis in man. *Acta Anat (Basel).* 1959;37:351.
17. Tessier P. Osteotomies totales de la face. Syndrome de Crouzon, syndrome d'Apert: oxycephalies, scaphocephalies, turricephalies. *Ann Chir Plast.* 1967;12:273–286.
18. Shillito J Jr, Matson DD. Craniosynostosis: a review of 519 surgical patients. *Pediatrics.* 1968;41:829–853.

19. Tessier P. The definitive plastic surgical treatment of the severe facial deformities of craniofacial dysostosis. Crouzon's and Apert's diseases. *Plast Reconstr Surg.* 1971;48:419–442.

20. Pawl RP, Sugar O. Zenker's solution in the surgical treatment of craniosynostosis. *J Neurosurg.* 1972;36:604–607.

21. Hogeman KE, Willmar K. On Le Fort III osteotomy for Crouzon's disease in children: report of a four year follow-up in one patient. *Scand J Plast Reconstr Surg.* 1974;8:169–172.

22. Hoffman HJ, Mohr G. Lateral canthal advancement of the supraorbital margin. A new corrective technique in the treatment of coronal synostosis. *J Neurosurg.* 1976;45:376–381.

23. Rune B, Selvik G, Kreiborg S, et al. Motion of bones and volume changes in the neurocranium after craniectomy in Crouzon's disease. A Roentgen stereometric study. *J Neurosurg.* 1979;50:494–498.

24. Persing J, Babler W, Winn HR, Jane J, Rodeheaver G. Age as a critical factor in the success of surgical correction of craniosynostosis. *J Neurosurg.* 1981;54:601–606.

25. Kreiborg S. Craniofacial growth in plagiocephaly and Crouzon syndrome. *Scand J Plast Reconstr Surg.* 1981;15:187–197.

26. Renier D, Sainte-Rose C, Marchac D, et al. Intracranial pressure in craniosynostosis. *J Neurosurg.* 1982;57:370–377.

27. McCarthy JG, Grayson B, Bookstein F, et al. Le Fort III advancement osteotomy in the growing child. *Plast Reconstr Surg.* 1984;74:343–354.

28. McCarthy JG, Epstein F, Sadove M, et al. Early surgery for craniofacial synostosis: an 8-year experience. *Plast Reconstr Surg.* 1984;73:521–533.

29. Kreiborg S, Aduss H. Pre- and postsurgical facial growth in patients with Crouzon's and Apert's syndromes. *Cleft Palate J.* 1986;23(suppl 1):78–90.

30. Kaban LB, Conover M, Mulliken J: Midface position after Le Fort III advancement: a long-term follow-up study. *Cleft Palate J.* 1986;23(suppl 1):75–77.

31. Whitaker LA, Bartlett SP, Schut L, Bruce D. Craniosynostosis: an analysis of the timing, treatment, and complications in 164 consecutive patients. *Plast Reconstr Surg.* 1987;80:195–212.

32. Renier D. Intracranial pressure in craniosynostosis: Pre and postoperative recordings—correlation with functional results. In: JA Persing, MT Edgerton, JA Jane, eds. *Scientific Foundations and Surgical Treatment of Craniosynostosis.* Baltimore: Williams & Wilkins; 1989;263–269.

33. McCarthy JG, Cutting CB. The timing of surgical intervention in craniofacial anomalies. *Clin Plast Surg.* 1990;17(1):161–182.

34. Gault DT, Renier D, Marchac D, et al. Intracranial volume in children with craniosynostosis. *J Craniofac Surg.* 1990;1:1–3.

35. David DJ, Sheen R. Surgical correction of Crouzon syndrome. *Plast Reconstr Surg.* 1990;85:344–354.

36. Ortiz-Monasterio F, Fuente del Campo A, Carillo A. Advancements of the orbits and the midface in one piece combined with frontal repositioning for the correction of Crouzon deformities. *Plast Reconstr Surg.* 1978;61:4.

37. Posnick JC. Craniofacial dysostosis: staging of reconstruction and management of the midface deformity. *Neurosurg Clin North Am.* 1991;2:683–702.

38. Richtsmeier JT, Grausz HM, Morris GR, et al. Growth of the cranial base in craniosynostosis. *Cleft Palate Craniofac J.* 1991;28:55–67.

39. Posnick JC. The role of plate and screw fixation in the treatment of craniofacial malformations. In: Gruss JS, Manson PM, Yaremchuk MJ, eds. *Rigid Fixation of the Craniomaxillofacial Skeleton.* Boston: Butterworth; 1992:512.

40. Posnick JC, Bite U, Nakano P, et al. Indirect intracranial volume measurements using CT scans: clinical applications for craniosynostosis. *Plast Reconstr Surg.* 1992;89:34–45.

41. Posnick JC. The craniofacial dysostosis syndromes. Current reconstructive strategies. *Clin Plast Surg.* 1994;21(4):585–598.

42. Blinkov SM, Glezer II, Haigh B. *The Human Brain in Figures and Tables: A Quantitative Handbook.* New York: Basic Books; 1968.

43. Lichtenberg R. Radiographic du crane de 226 enfants normaux de la naissance a 8 ans. Impressions digitformes, capacite: angles et indices. Thesis. Paris: University of Paris; 1960.

44. Dekaban AS. Tables of cranial and orbital measurements, cranial volume and derived indexes in males and females from 7 days to 20 years of age. *Ann Neurol.* 1977;2:485–491.

45. Gordon IRS. Measurement of cranial capacity in children. *Br J Radiol.* 1966;39:377.

46. Farkas LG, Posnick JC, Hrecko T. Anthropometric growth study of the head. *Cleft Palate Craniofac J.* 1992;29(4):303–308.

47. Hanieh A, Sheen R, David DJ. Hydrocephalus in Crouzon's syndrome. *Child's Nerv Syst.* 1989;5(3):188–189.

48. Baldwin JL. Dysostosis craniofacialis of Crouzon. A summary of recent literature and case reports with emphasis on involvement of the ear. *Laryngoscope.* 1968;78(10):1660–1676.

49. Cutting C, Dean D, Bookstein FL, et al. A three-dimensional smooth surface analysis of untreated Crouzon's syndrome in the adult. *J Craniofac Surg.* 1995;6(6):444–453.

50. Waitzman AA, Posnick JC, Armstrong D, et al. Craniofacial skeletal measurements based on computed tomography: part I. Accuracy and reproducibility. *Cleft Palate Craniofac J.* 1992; 29:112–117.

51. Waitzman AA, Posnick JC, Armstrong D, et al. Craniofacial skeletal measurements based on computed tomography. Part 2. Normal values and growth trends. *Cleft Palate Craniofac J.* 1992;29:118–128.

52. Posnick JC, Lin KY, Chen P, et al. Metopic synostosis: quantitative assessment of presenting deformity and surgical results based on CT scans. *Plast Reconstr Surg.* 1994;93:16–24.

53. Posnick JC, Lin KY, Jhawar BJ, et al. Apert syndrome: quantitative assessment by CT scan of presenting deformity and surgical results after first-stage reconstruction based on CT scan. *Plast Reconstr Surg.* 1994;93:489–497.

54. Posnick JC, Lin KY, Chen P, et al. Sagittal synostosis: quantitative assessment of presenting deformity and surgical results based on CT scans. *Plast Reconstr Surg.* 1993;92:1015–1024.

55. Ward RE, Jamison PL. Measurement precision and reliability in craniofacial anthropometry: implications and suggestions for clinical applications. *J Craniofac Genet Dev Biol.* 1991;11(3): 156–164.

56. Posnick JC, Waitzman A, Armstrong D, Pron G. Monobloc and facial bipartition osteotomies: quantitative assessment of presenting deformity and surgical results based on computed tomography scans. *J Oral Maxillofac Surg.* 1995;53(4):358–367.

57. Lannelonque M. De la craniectomie dans la microcephalie. *C R Acad Sci* 1890;110:1382.

58. Lane LC. Pioneer craniectomy for refflef of mental imbecility due to premature sutural closure and microcephalus. *JAMA.* 1892;18:49.

59. Gillies H, Harrison SH. Operative correction by osteotomy of recessed malar maxillary compound in case of oxycephaly. *Br J Plast Surg.* 1950;3:123–127.

60. Tessier P. Dysostoses cranio-faciales (syndromes de Crouzon et d'Apert). Osteotomies totales de la face. In: *Transactions of the Fourth International Congress of Plastic and Reconstructive Surgery.* Amsterdam;1969:774.

61. Tessier P. Relationship of craniosynostoses to craniofacial dysostosis and to faciostenosis: a study with therapeutic implications. *Plast Reconstr Surg.* 1971(3):224–237.

62. Tessier P. Autogenous bone grafts taken from the calvarium or facial and cranial applications. *Clin Plast Surg.* 1982(4):531–538.

63. Tessier P. Total osteotomy of the middle third of the face for faciostenosis or for sequelae of Le Fort III fractures. *Plast Reconstr Surg.* 1971;48:533–541.

64. Tessier P. Recent improvement in the treatment of facial and cranial deformities in Crouzon's disease and Apert's syndrome. In: *Symposium of Plastic Surgery of the Orbital Region.* St. Louis: CV Mosby; 1976:271.

65. Rougerie J, Derome P, Anquez L. Craniostenoses et dysmorphies cranio-faciales: principes d'une nouvelle technique de traitement et ses resultats. *Neurochirurgie.* 1972;18:429–440.

66. Whitaker LA, Schut L, Kerr LP. Early surgery for isolated craniofacial dysostosis: improvement and possible prevention of increasing deformity. *Plast Reconstr Surg.* 1977;60:575–581.

67. Marchac D, Renier D. "Le front flottant." Traitement precoce des facio-craniostenoses. *Ann Chir Plast.* 1979;24:121–126.

68. Marchac D, Renier D, Jones BM. Experience with the "floating forehead." *Br J Plast Surg.* 1988;41:1–15.

69. Zins JE, Whitaker LA. Membranous versus endochondral bone: implications for craniofacial reconstruction. *Plast Reconstr Surg.* 1983;72:778–785.

70. Phillips JH, Rahn BA. Fixation effects on membranous and endochondral onlay bone graft revascularization. *Plast Reconstr Surg.* 1988;82:872–877.

71. Luhr HG. Zur Stabilen osteosynthese bei unterkieferfrakturen. *Dtsch Zahnarztl Z.* 1968;23:754.

72. Posnick JC. Pediatric cranial base surgery. In: *Problems in Plastic and Reconstructive Surgery.* Vol. 3. Philadelphia: JB Lippincott; 1993:107–129.

73. Posnick JC. The role of plate and screw fixation in the management of pediatric head and neck tumors. In: Gruss JS, Manson PM, Yaremchuk MJ, eds. *Rigid Fixation of the Cranio maxillofacial Skeleton.* Stoneham: Butterworth; 1992:956–670.

74. Posnick JC. The role of plate and screw fixation in the treatment of pediatric facial fractures. In: Gruss JS, Manson PM, Yaremchuk MJ, eds. *Rigid Fixation of the Craniomaxillofacial Skeleton.* Stoneham: Butterworth; 1992:396–419.

75. Posnick JC. The effects of rigid fixation on the craniofacial growth of the rhesus monkeys (Discussion). *Plast Reconstr Surg.* 1994;93:11–15.

76. Posnick JC, Shah N, Humphreys R, et al. The detection and management of intracranial hypertension following initial suture release and decompression for craniofacial dysostosis syndromes. *Neurosurgery.* 1995:703–708.

77. Wolfe SA, Morrison G, Page LK, et al. The monobloc frontofacial advancement: do the pluses outweigh the minuses? *Plast Reconstr Surg.* 1993;91:977–987.

78. Tessier P. The monobloc frontofacial advancement: do the pluses outweigh the minuses? (Discussion). *Plast Reconstr Surg.* 1993;91(6):988–999.

79. Bu BH, Kaban LB, Vargervik K. Effect of Le Fort III osteotomy on mandibular growth in patients with Crouzon and Apert syndromes. *J Oral Maxillofac Surg.* 1989;47(7):666–667.

58
Hemifacial Microsomia

John H. Phillips, Kevin Bush, and R. Bruce Ross

There is no other syndrome in the head and neck region that presents the craniofacial surgeon with such diverse choices for management as hemifacial microsomia. All patients require a multidisciplinary approach to management involving both conservative (nonsurgical) and surgical techniques. The variability of the condition generally called hemifacial microsomia has made it difficult to devise an accurate label for the condition. As Gorlin et al.[1] state, "While there are no agreed upon minimal diagnostic criteria, the typical phenotype is characteristic when enough manifestations are present."

Nomenclature

One of the areas concerning hemifacial microsomia is what the syndrome should be called. The most commonly used labels are oculo-auriculo-vertebral spectrum,[2] or Goldenhar syndrome,[3] a variation or subgroup of hemifacial microsomia.[4,5] Other terms are commonly seen describing a spectrum of deformities that encompass auricular anomalies in combination with mandibular deformities and macrostomia are otomandibular dysostosis,[6] first arch syndrome,[7] first and second branchial arch syndrome,[8] lateral facial dysplasia,[4] and facio-auriculo-vertebral (FAV) malformation complex.[5] Converse et al.[9] coined the term craniofacial microsomia in recognition of the fact that there is approximately a 20% incidence of bilaterality in this syndrome.[5]

For the purpose of this review, we have chosen the term hemifacial microsomia (HFM) to represent a syndrome consisting of a constellation of deformities revolving around auricular deformities, craniofacial skeletal deformities (most notably the mandible and temporomandibular joint complex), and soft tissue deficiencies.

The most commonly affected structures are the external and middle ear, condyle and ramus of the mandible, muscles of mastication, parotid gland, zygomatic bone and arch, temporal bone, maxilla, and orbit. The abnormalities of the temporomandibular joint (TMJ) range from complete agenesis to subtle differences in form or size with few deformities. Invariably, however, the dysplasia is both a deficiency and a malformation. Associated anomalies occur less frequently in the eye, vertebral column, and other parts of the body.

Epidemiology

Hemifacial microsomia is the second most common congenital craniofacial defect (after cleft lip and palate). Grabb estimated the frequency of HFM as 1 in 5,600 births.[8] Other estimates of frequency range from 1 in 3,500[10] to 1 in 26,550.[11] Gorlin et al. believe the frequency is closer to Grabb's estimate.[1] There is a male to female ratio of 3:2 and also a 3:2 predilection for right-sided ear involvement.[12,13] A significant feature is that in 70% of cases the condition appears to be unilateral. In bilateral cases, asymmetry is the rule, and rarely are both sides severely affected.

Differential Diagnosis

There are several syndromes and conditions with features that make confusion with hemifacial microsomia a possibility. The syndromes to consider in the differential diagnosis of HFM are Townes–Brocks syndrome, brachio-oto-rental (BOR) syndrome, mandibulofacial dysostosis (Treacher Collins), maxillofacial dysostosis, Rombergs, TMJ ankylosis (pathology or trauma), Nager acrofacial dysostosis, and acrofacial dysostosis.[1]

Etiology and Pathogenesis

Hemifacial microsomia is considered to be sporadic. Autosomal dominance transmission within a family has been documented.[14] The syndrome is variable in its expression within those few families where genetic transmission is noted. HFM has a low recurrence risk (2%–3%),[8,14] while frequently there is discordance in monozygotic twins. The mild forms of the condition are difficult to ascertain, so that an accurate familial history is virtually impossible to obtain. Genetic heterogeneity has been proposed to explain the variability in genetic transmission.

The defects in these cases appear to occur without relation to embryonic differentiation. One sees adjacent structures with the same origin but only one affected, and adjacent structures from completely different origins where both are affected. Pure unilateral dysplasias occur frequently. All these findings lead to the conclusion that in many cases the insult to the embryo occurs at a time when tissue differentiation is well advanced, possibly even completed on occasion, and that the injury is very localized.[4,10,15,16] The mechanism may be a local injury that would cause cell destruction, interference with cell movement and differentiation, or displacement of areas of cells.

Two theories regarding the pathogenesis of HFM are currently discussed in the literature. Stark and Saunders suggested that Hoffstetter and Veau's theory of mesodermal deficiency could be applied to hemifacial microsomia.[7] Poswillo developed an animal model in which the induction of early vascular disruption and the subsequent expanding hematoma by in utero administration of triazene produced a phenotype that was very similar to hemifacial microsomia in the mouse.[10] This and subsequent hematoma formation caused local destruction of tissue and delayed differentiation and induced abnormal development in adjacent structures. The hypothesis is attractive because of the high variability and asymmetry of HFM malformations. His findings provide an explanation for the great variability in the expression of these anomalies, because hemorrhages may vary in number, size, and location, and may occur simultaneously in other parts of the body. The specimens in Poswillo's study, however, showed numerous abnormalities (e.g., of the brain) that are not typical of HFM, and there were severe abnormalities already present at the time the hemorrhage occurred (e.g., micrognathic). Newman and Hendricks[17] repeated the Poswillo study and concluded that the resulting malformations were much more similar to Treacher Collins syndrome than hemifacial microsomia.

External and middle ear malformations commonly seen in the retinoic acid syndrome (RAS)[18] are at least superficially similar to those of HFM. As these features of the RAS appear to be related to interference with neural crest development,[19,20] such interference may be responsible for at least some HFM variants. Also, the cardiovascular outflow tract malformations sometimes noted in HFM cases are characteristic in RAS. Vertebral defects in Goldenhar syndrome are similar to those produced in mice by retinoic acid.[21] The administration of thalidomide to monkeys has also produced an HFM phenotype by inducing hemorrhage at an early fetal stage.[22] Kleinsasser and Schlothan have noted a significant number of newborns with first and second branchial arch abnormalities after administration of thalidomide during pregnancy.[23] This has been considered presumptive evidence for the vascular hematoma theory because thalidomide is known to cause bleeding.

Clinical Manifestations

Hemifacial microsomia manifests itself in a diverse manner. Evidence of HFM can be seen not only throughout the affected facial skeleton but in other systems as well. Goldenhar syndrome makes up about 10% of all cases and is distinguished from hemifacial microsomia by the presence of epibulbar dermoids and vertebral anomalies (notably hemivertebrae).[2] Only cursory mention is given here to anomalies outside the craniofacial region or those that do not directly impact upon the treatment regime. A detailed summary of anomalies that can be present in hemifacial microsomia is found in Gorlin et al.[1]

Neurologic

Several associated deformities can have direct impact on treatment regimes. Complete or partial paralysis of the facial nerve on the affected side is present in 10% to 20% of cases.[8,24] The marginal mandibular branch is most often affected. The course of the facial nerve may be abnormal, and this should be kept in mind during temporomandibular reconstruction.[25,26] Almost any cranial nerve can be affected, including the trigeminal.[27] There is commonly a hypoplasia or paralysis of the ipsilateral tensor veli palatini[8,25]; therefore, on intraoral examination the soft palate deviates to the opposite side. Luce et al. found an incidence of one-third of patients presenting with moderate to severe hypernasality.[28] Sprinzten et al.[29] found 55% of HFM patients presenting with velopharyngeal insufficiency, and cleft lip or palate is present in 7% to 15% of cases.[14,30]

It is useful when assessing the patient with hemifacial microsomia to keep the following six areas in mind: cranial, orbital, midface, mandibular-temporomandibular joint complex, auricular, and soft tissue. Deformities are discussed here in this manner as it aids in clearly delineating the deformities and determining a coherent, chronologically organized treatment plan.

Cranial

Deformities in the cranial region tend to occur with more severe forms of HFM. A number of skull defects ranging from cranium bifidum to microcephaly and plagiocephaly have been described with hemifacial microsomia.[1] The squamous temporal bone may be flattened. The mastoid air cells may exhibit decreased pneumatization as well as flattening of the mastoid process. The petrous portion of the temporal bone is usually spared. The frontal bone may be flattened, mimicking plagiocephaly.

Orbital

Ophthalmologic anomalies besides deformities of the bony orbital cavity exist in hemifacial microsomia. Commonly noted ophthalmologic deformities include the presence of epibulbar dermoids, microphthalmos, colobomas, and, in 22% to 25%, ocular motility disorders.[1,31] The bony orbital cavity may be small. The lateral orbital rim and inferior orbital rim on the affected side may be retruded. Vertical dystopias can also occur.

Midface

The zygoma may be hypoplastic or even absent in severe cases. As a result of zygomatic deformity, cheek prominence is decreased and often benefits from augmentation of some kind. The canthal-tragus line may be shortened.

The maxilla is also frequently affected in all three dimensions. Thus, the maxillary sinus and nasal cavity may be smaller on the affected side, the maxilla is frequently deficient in vertical height, retruded (more posterior), and narrower in width as well. These abnormalities are most likely a primary deficit, rather than the result of inhibition from the impinging mandible as is frequently hypothesized in the literature.[32,33] While normal tooth eruption in both maxillary and mandibular arches can easily be inhibited by the restriction of a deficient mandibular ramus, there is little reason to believe that the basal bone in either arch will be affected. The upward cant of the *maxillary* plane is probably an intrinsic maxillary deficiency, while the cant of the *occlusal* plane is invariably related to inhibited dental eruption plus the frequent deficiency of the maxilla itself. This is an important consideration in treatment because it is most unlikely that a deficient basal maxilla will respond to treatment that merely removes the mandibular interference, even though the teeth will quickly erupt and tend to level the occlusal plane.

Mandibular-Temporomandibular Joint Complex

Mandibular deformities and ear deformities are the hallmark of hemifacial microsomia. Deformities can range from minimal shape deformities of the condyle to complete absence of the affected ramus and condyle and much of the body. The affected condyle is always abnormal, and this is probably the only constant feature of HFM. The mandibular-temporomandibular deformity varies from a minimal deformity of the complex to a complete absence. Frequently there is a bony deformity of the squamous temporal bone, and the posterior wall of the glenoid fossa may be abnormal or absent.

The facial asymmetry in HFM is three dimensional. With regard to the mandible, there is (1) an inadequate anteroposterior vector to condylar size, causing the deviation of the chin toward the affected side. The position of the chin is a function of condylar height and vertical ramus anteroposterior length. As well, the mandible deviates on opening toward the affected side. Opening is normally accompanied by advancement of the condyles, but in these individuals the muscles that accomplish this (the lateral pterygoid muscles) are absent or hypoplastic and the condyle may be inhibited by soft tissue restrictions, so that the affected side merely rotates while the "normal" side advances. (2) The vertical canting of the mandibular and occlusal planes result partly from a deficiency in vertical height of the ramus or condyle and partly from decreased bulk of the bony muscle attachments (masseter and medial pterygoid). Because the muscles are severely hypoplastic or absent in severe cases, this vertical asymmetry is invariably present. As mentioned earlier, the maxilla is also frequently affected in vertical height, exaggerating the asymmetry. Even if the maxilla itself is normal, the abnormal mandibular position will inhibit the eruption of the mandibular and maxillary teeth on the affected side, causing a tilting of the occlusal plane.[3] There is a transverse asymmetry, which is partly the medial displacement of the mandibular ramus and condyle and partly soft tissue muscle hypoplasia, often including a maxillary deficiency as well.

Dental Compensations

Teeth erupt from the jaws and are guided toward the opposing teeth by the forces they encounter in the oral cavity. Generally, these are forces generated by the lip, tongue, and cheek musculature. When jaws are poorly related to each other, the teeth are guided to achieve the best occlusion. Teeth erupt until they encounter resistance, normally the teeth in the opposing arch, but the lip, tongue, or an external force (e.g., thumb) can halt tooth eruption. In hemifacial microsomia, even gross malrelation of the jaws will not result in gross malocclusion: the teeth will generally meet in an adequate relationship. If the mandible is deficient on one side and prevented from achieving a normal vertical relationship with the maxilla, eruption of the teeth on the affected side is inhibited in both jaws.

Facial Growth

The bony asymmetries appear to be stable during growth of the child in virtually all cases, showing no clinical or cephalometric signs of improving or worsening except in very rare cases of each. In the infant it may be very difficult to detect the degree of asymmetry because the fat pads in the cheeks and the roundness of the face obscure asymmetry. What sometimes appears to be a worsening of the asymmetry with growth may be an illusion caused by the greater increase in height and depth of the lower face than in width, making the existing asymmetry increasingly more obvious, and creating the impression that the face is becoming more asymmetric. However, there are many authoritative-sounding statements in the literature to the effect that these cases worsen with growth. There is absolutely no evidence for such statements: on the contrary, the various objective analyses we use indicate that growth of the dysplastic ramus and condyle is quite exuberant and continues at or near the growth of the contralateral "normal" side. Facial asymmetry, including the orbits and maxilla, does not perceptibly change in these cases, nor does the tilt of the occlusal and mandibular planes alter with growth. Unfortunately, the "worsening" hypothesis has now been widely accepted as fact: this has greatly influenced treatment methods.

Auricular

Many people consider that the spectrum of auricular deformities extends from simple ear tags to the presence of only a vestigial remnant of the ear. Meurman has classified ear deformities into three grades.[34] Grade 1 is a slightly malformed ear that is smaller than a normal ear, grade 2 is vertical cartilaginous remnant with complete atresia of the ear canal, and grade 3 is only a small remnant of the original ear. The affected ear is often inferiorly positioned relative to the normal ear. The severity of ear deformity parallels the mandibular deformity and is not directly parallel with hearing function.[35] Hearing function can be significantly impaired, which is a particular problem in the bilaterally affected individual. Middle ear structures may be absent or rudimentary in severe cases.

Soft Tissue

Macrostomia is a frequent finding in hemifacial microsomia, especially in Goldenhar syndrome. A definite soft tissue deformity has been identified in hemifacial microsomia. The temporalis muscle and other muscles of mastication, as well as the parotid and subcutaneous tissue, may all be involved. The degree of deficiency varies with the severity of the deformity. The amount of soft tissue deficit is often less than initially assessed. Any attempts at soft tissue augmentation should be delayed until the majority of bone reconstruction is complete.

Classification

There is almost as much confusion about the classification of HFM as there is about the nomenclature of the associated constellation of abnormalities known as hemifacial microsomia. Converse et al.[9] stated that "the deformity in hemifacial microsomia varies in extent and degree." They considered that classification was difficult because of the heterogeneity of the syndrome. Meurman in 1957 provided us with an easily applicable classification system of microtia based upon the assessment of 74 patients,[34] as previously described. Pruzansky modified Meurman's classification to preauricular anomalies, that is, ear tags, and applied this modification to 90 cases of hemifacial microsomia.[36]

Longacre et al. developed a classification that involved dividing patients into groupings of unilateral and bilateral microtia.[37] Subsequently, each group was then subdivided into levels of facial deformity. Converse et al. stated that because of the heterogeneity of the syndrome no accurate classification system was available and each case must be reviewed individually.[38]

Most clinically successful classifications have revolved around the mandibular and temporomandibular skeletal deformity. Pruzansky described three grades of mandibular deformity.[36] Each grade increases in severity until in grade 3 cases deformities may present with complete agenesis of the ramus. Swanson and Murray recognized the fact that the temporomandibular joint may be significantly deformed and acknowledged this in their classification of mandibular and temporomandibular deformities of HFM.[39] In 1985, Lauritzen et al. classified mandibular-temporomandibular deformity into five grades of severity[40] (Figures 58.1–58.6). The classification of Lauritzen et al. clearly focuses the craniofacial surgeon's attention on the abnormalities of the craniofacial

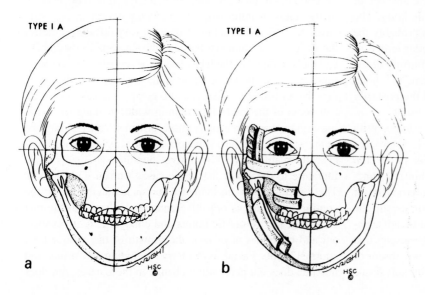

a   b

FIGURE 58.1 (a) Hemifacial microsomia (HFM) type IA. Mandible is intact with horizontal occlusal plane. Contour augmentation only is needed. (b) Multiple onlay bone grafts of split rib have been added.

FIGURE 58.2 (a) HFM type IB. Mandible is intact, but occlusal plane is tilted. Osteotomies are shown. (b) Postoperative skeletal alignment after a Le Fort I procedure, bilateral mandibular sagittal split, and a transposition genioplasty. A wedge of bone is grafted into the right maxilla.

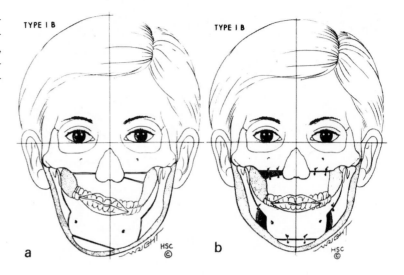

FIGURE 58.3 (a) HFM type II. Mandible is incomplete with a deficient right ascending ramus. A sufficient glenoid fossa is present. (b) The ascending ramus of the mandible is constructed from a full-thickness costochondral graft.

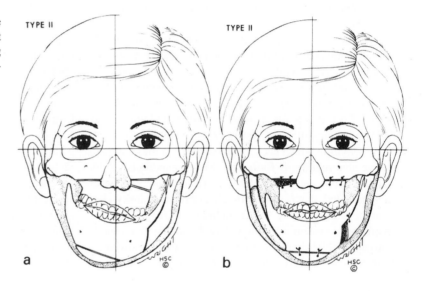

FIGURE 58.4 (a) HFM type III. The right ascending ramus of the mandible is vestigial and the glenoid fossa is inadequate. (b) A transverse full-thickness rib graft is replacing the zygoma, and a TM joint is constructed.

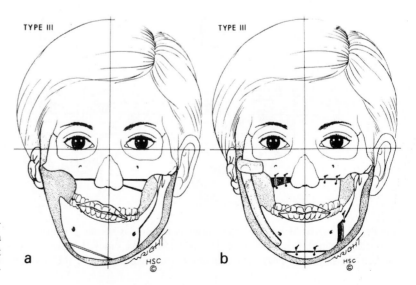

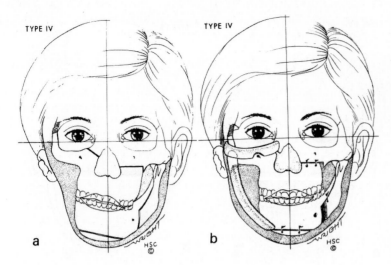

FIGURE 58.5 (a) HFM type IV. The right facial skeleton is retruded, and cuts for a right-sided Le Fort III and left-sided Le Fort I procedure are made. The right lateral orbital rim is cut obliquely so as to become self-retaining after transposition. (b) The facial skeleton is advanced, occlusal plane corrected, and mandible constructed.

skeleton and hence an appropriate treatment plan for these anomalies.

In recognition of the fact that the abnormalities in hemifacial microsomia exist primarily in the facial skeleton, soft tissue, and auricle, several classification systems that identify abnormalities in all these areas have been developed. Two such classification systems are the OMENS[41] and the SAT[42] systems. SAT stands for skeletal, auricular, and soft tissue. The OMENS classification system described by Vento et al.[41] is an acronym in which each letter stands for a major area of possible abnormality: O for orbital, M for mandibular, E for ear, N for nerve, and S for soft tissue. Each major area is further subdivided; that is, a modification of the Pruzansky classification is used in the M (mandibular) section. The SAT classification system is loosely based on the tumor node metastasis (TNM) tumor classification[43] with subdivisions within each S, A, and T category. Both the OMENS and SAT

classification systems are more complete than many other systems simply because of the one-dimensionality of many other systems. However, because of their complexity, both systems are somewhat unwieldy and we believe they fail to focus the attention of the treating physician on the relevant deformities requiring surgical intervention.

At the present time, our practice at The Hospital for Sick Children in Toronto is to classify hemifacial microsomia utilizing a combination of Meurman's classification[34] for congenital microtia and that of Lauritzen et al.[40] for the skeletal deformities. Utilization of these two classification schemes focuses the surgeon's attention on the anomalies requiring surgical intervention. The assessment of soft tissue deficiency should be postponed until after there has been skeletal reconstruction, as we believe it is difficult to estimate the soft tissue deficiency until the facial skeletal proportions are restored.

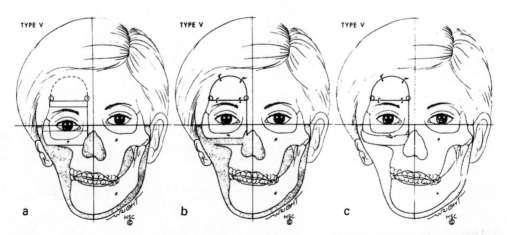

FIGURE 58.6 (a) HFM type V. Right orbit is dystopic. Cuts are planned including the craniotomy. (b) The right orbital box is moved upward and secured in place. The craniotomy is closed. (c) A zygomatic arch is constructed from a full-thickness rib and the glenoid fossa is prepared. During the next stage operation, this patient will be treated as an HFM type II.

Treatment

The best approach to such a complex problem is a coordinated effort in which various specialists contribute their knowledge and skills to work together in planning and carrying out treatment customized to the specific needs of the patient. A craniofacial team might consist (in alphabetical order) of anaesthetist, audiologist, craniofacial surgeon, dentist, geneticist, ophthalmologist, orthodontist, otolaryngologist, pediatrician, plastic surgeon, psychiatrist, radiologist, social worker, and speech pathologist.

Indications for Treatment

Treatment would be easier if delayed until adolescence when facial growth has been essentially completed. The more stable structures permit quite precise surgical and orthodontic treatment planning, with the hope that a single surgery will be all that is necessary. Delaying surgery, however, subjects the child to living with a facial deformity through the most difficult years of social interaction and the development of self-esteem. Treatment of hemifacial microsomia can be divided into chronological time periods.

Age 0 to 5 Years

During this phase, complete assessment by the craniofacial team occurs. Problems such as feeding, speech, hearing, and genetic counseling are addressed. The only surgical interventions undertaken during this period are the correction of macrostomia, the removal of ear tags, correction of forehead deformities, and if the orbit is microphthalmic with no functional vision, the placement of an orbital expander.

"Plagiocephaly" or the retruded brow is addressed before 18 months of age using the surgical techniques developed for treating true plagiocephaly (unilateral coronal synostosis). Correction of the forehead deformity is undertaken before age 18 months to maximize bone formation after surgical intervention. It may be possible to correct some orbital dystopias at the same time as the forehead correction is done.

Orbital expansion is controversial. Our utilization of this technique is in individuals with no functional globe or vision in the affected eye. Placement of an expander in the affected globe before the age of 1 year is undertaken to try and simulate the normal growing globe, stimulate orbitozygomatic growth, and stretch the soft tissues around the eye.[44,45] Although adequate growth may not occur with this technique in all individuals, those individuals who fail to grow can still be treated at a later date with orbital osteotomies or onlay bone grafting technique. The orbital expander is inflated with 0.5-ml increments weekly. Orbital volume changes are followed with intermittent computed tomography (CT) scans. Once appropriate volumes have been reached, the expander can be removed, and an orbital conformer manufactured to fit the new orbital cavity is inserted at the same time as expander removal.

Age 5 to 8 Years

The main indication for early reconstructive surgery is to improve facial esthetics and provide the young child with a reasonably symmetric face through childhood, even though a second orthognathic surgery is frequently necessary at the conclusion of growth. Early treatment requires an evaluation of the positive or negative effects on the eventual result. With early mandibular surgery the teeth will adapt naturally to the new, more normal, relationship of the jaws. Dental compensations will be self-correcting, precluding the need for extensive reversal of long-established compensations, a difficult problem for the orthodontist if surgery is delayed until adolescence. A further advantage is that the soft tissues will grow and adapt to a more normal environment.

As a rule of thumb, then, in those *mild cases* in which the child and their family are not overly concerned with the facial esthetics, and there are no important functional indications, treatment should probably be delayed until adolescence. In such cases, soft tissue surgery or orthodontics alone may be all that is required to disguise the asymmetry. With the more *severe deformities,* extensive treatment in early childhood is usually indicated. Timing of treatment for *moderate deformities* demands good clinical judgment as well as evaluation of the child and the family.

During this phase of the child's life, numerous surgical interventions may be planned such as auricular reconstruction, costochondral grafting, or temporomandibular joint reconstruction. Parents are advised of the options for ear reconstruction. Information on autogenous versus prosthetic ear reconstruction using implant technology is provided to the parents.[46] If total ear reconstruction is warranted and an autogenous approach is adopted, the techniques for total ear reconstruction as popularized by Brent[47] are utilized. It is our belief, if temporomandibular joint reconstruction, zygomatic reconstruction, or temporal bone augmentation are required, that total ear reconstruction should be performed after these surgical interventions so as to aid in correct positioning of the reconstructed ear. Our practice is not to reconstruct the middle ear on an individual with one normal ear and functional hearing. In the individual with bilateral involvement, ear reconstruction must be done in conjunction with middle ear reconstruction as dictated by the otolaryngologist member of the craniofacial team.

The surgical decision of no intervention, temporomandibular joint reconstruction, or costochondral grafting is based upon whether the individual has an adequate temporomandibular joint and an adequate ramus condyle complex. Utilizing the classification of Lauritzen et al., it is clear what skeletal surgical intervention is warranted during this period. Type IA has a level occlusal plane and requires only onlay bone grafting for cosmesis plus orthodontic intervention. The temporomandibular joint and ramus are only slightly deformed. For types IB to V there is an occlusal tilt and malocclusion of a severity that warrants surgical intervention. The appropriate procedure is based upon the adequacy of the temporomandibular (TMJ)-mandibular complex. To try and maximize maxillary growth, and realizing that the risk of damage to permanent teeth is high if Le Fort I is used, the only surgical procedure performed at this age is costochondral grafting with TMJ reconstruction.

Type IB has a reasonable TMJ-mandibular complex and no surgical intervention is planned at this time. Bilateral sagittal split osteotomy, Le Fort I osteotomy, and genioplasty are planned for skeletal maturity.

Replacement of Defective TMJ

In the severe forms of hemifacial microsomia (types IIB and III), it is necessary to reconstruct the ramus and condyle and often create an articulating fossa as well. The major controversy in these cases is how to replace the missing tissues and the best time to begin surgical treatment. The method of choice is a bone graft to reconstruct the ramus, condyle, and temporomandibular joint. The most commonly used bone is a costochondral graft. The indications for costochondral grafting are the absence of a functional joint with consequent severe facial asymmetry.

Replacement of the defective TMJ for hemifacial microsomia is necessary to reconstruct the missing condyle and to create an articulating fossa as well. The method of choice is a bone graft to reconstruct the ramus, condyle, and temporomandibular joint. In looking at the need for a functional joint in the future with respect to the orthognathic surgery, the main requirement is buttressing of the most proximal portion of the ascending ramus or vestigial condyle with the base of the skull. This would prevent relapse of any sagittal split advancement and counterrotation, which is often required at skeletal maturity.

It is hard to determine the degree or actual interval absence of buttressing that is required to create the indication for costochondral grafting. In looking at a normal joint, it can be seen on the CT scan that there is often a 2- to 3-mm gap between the most proximal portion of the condyle in the cranial base. In this space, of course, there is the meniscus. At the present time, at our Center, if the gap between the most proximal portion of the mandible and cranial base is less than 10 mm and there is good mouth opening, then either nothing is done until orthognathic surgery at skeletal maturity or a sagittal split osteotomy may be done at 4 to 7 years of age to improve aesthetic appearance. It may be expected in some cases that a sagittal split advancement in the cases with less than 10 mm of bony gap may result in some relapse, necessitating a repeat sagittal split osteotomy. It is believed that the risk of redoing a sagittal split is less than the morbidity associated with a costochondral reconstruction.

In cases in which there is significant asymmetry and the bony gap is greater than 10 mm, a costochondral graft may be indicated. If a joint is present, even with severe asymmetry, one would attempt to correct it by mandibular procedures such as a sagittal split or vertical ramus osteotomy, rather than the graft with its higher morbidity. In some cases, there is inadequate bone in the ramus for these procedures. Costochondral grafts are harvested with a periosteal sleeve from the contralateral side. The cartilage cap is shaped to form the condyle and then inserted via a combination of intraoral and preauricular incisions. We rigidly fix the costochondral graft to the vestigial ramus using lag screw techniques and a 1.5-mm plate as a washer. All patients are overcorrected with ipsilateral open bite (by as much as soft tissues will allow) at the time of surgery. Intermaxillary fixation is maintained for a period of 2 to 3 weeks to allow for comfort. Virtually all type II to V will benefit from orthognathic surgery at skeletal maturity to further level occlusion and aid in restoration of facial symmetry.

In types III to V, the zygomatic arch is absent or markedly hypoplastic and the glenoid fossa is nonexistent. It is these types of patients who should undergo glenoid reconstruction as outlined by Lauritzen et al. Our personal preference for glenoid fossa reconstruction and onlay bone grafting is to utilize split cranial bone grafts for reconstruction of the zygomatic arch and malar prominence. The condyle and ascending ramus is reconstructed with rib grafts. From age 5 years onward, the calvarium should be diploic and splittable, providing a good source of bone graft material. All bone grafts are fixed using currently available micro- and miniplate systems. The reconstructed glenoid fossa is lined with cartilage of the rib to increase the likelihood of a non-union.

Type V individuals pose special problems in that there is a significant orbital dystopia that will require osteotomies for correction. Our approach currently is to try and avoid type V patients by correcting some globe inadequacies by the use of an orbital expander. If osteotomy is required, we prefer to perform isolated zygomatic and orbital osteotomies and secondarily correct occlusion with a Le Fort I closer to skeletal maturity rather than utilize asymmetric Le Fort III and Le Fort I combinations during this time period of the child's growth.

With the increasing use of bone-lengthening techniques, it will be interesting to note whether the proximal portion of the osteotomized mandible is driven toward the cranial base to create buttressing and, therefore, to obviate the need for costochondral graft reconstruction.

Costochondral Grafts

In recent studies at our Center,[48] many factors were considered in estimating the success of a costochondral graft, including the etiology of the defect, surgical complexity of the procedure, age at surgery, previous surgery to the area, and the surgeon's experience. Although there were minor differences, no factors except age at surgery were remarkable. The early grafts were far more successful with gradually declining success until age 14. From age 3 to 9 years, the success rate of 19 grafts was 80%, while from 14 years onward the rate for 20 grafts fell to 50%. Although the difference was not quite statistically significant (χ^2, $p = 0.06$), it does seem that early placement of a costochondral graft is more successful.

One of the problems with early grafting is the different growth rates of the mandible and the graft.[49,50] The otherwise successful graft may grow at a different rate than the contralateral natural condyle. The Ross 1996 study of the long-term followup of 13 grafts in growing children showed that subsequent growth of the graft was equal to that of the "normal" side in 6 cases, less in 2 cases, and greater in 5 cases.[51]

A possible explanation for this may lie with the size of the germinative zone of cartilage in the graft. The prechondrocytes in this zone supply cells for the proliferative zone, where interstitial growth is responsible for increased length of cartilage. Peltomaki and Ronning[52] have shown that when costochondral grafts were transplanted to a nonfunctional area in rats, the growth in length of the graft varied with the thickness of this zone of cells. Removal or injury to these cells inhibited growth. Clinical control of the amount of graft growth may be possible if these findings could be adjusted to the need. They also showed[53] that mature, nongrowing ribs transferred to a nonfunctional area in growing rats grew significantly. Their findings indicate a systemic, hormonal stimulation rather than a functional one.

Orthodontic Treatment

There are two conflicting theories with regard to the indications for and efficacy of orthodontic treatment in hemifacial microsomia. The first, held by most experienced clinicians, is that orthodontic treatment is not effective in producing meaningful change in the dysmorphic structures present in this condition. Rather, orthodontic mechanics and forces affect the teeth and associated alveolar process, but do not affect the underlying basal bone or condylar growth except in a limited, clinically insignificant degree if at all. Thus, orthodontic treatment in hemifacial microsomia is confined to alignment of the teeth in preparation for surgery and subsequent finishing procedures.

The second approach, pursued by Harvold and his followers,[54] is that functional appliances will stimulate growth of the defective condyle to a meaningful degree. It is based on the mistaken belief that little growth occurs naturally and that the deficiency will worsen with growth. Their treatment consists of the wearing of functional appliances throughout childhood (providing further esthetic and psychic trauma) with surgery to the mandible in adolescence. For the Harvoldians, growth subsequent to appliance wear is proof of the efficacy of their treatment, when in fact growth would have occurred without their intervention (as explained earlier). These appliances are unsuccessful in increasing mandibular sagittal growth. Evidence is very flimsy that these appliances ever work, let alone with consistency, in HFM. Harvold also claimed that a functional appliance must be worn before surgery to prepare the tissues and after surgery to maintain the graft. These procedures have been shown to the unnecessary in our clinic.

There is no question that the occlusal plane can be altered by changing the oral environment, either by directly lowering (distracting) the mandible by surgery, or by holding the mandible open with a unilateral bite pad that inhibits the teeth on the 'normal' side and allows the teeth on the affected side to erupt, thus leveling the occlusal plane. This does not, of course, affect mandibular symmetry in length or vertical height. In mild or even moderate cases (types I and IIA), the effect of the bite pad therapy is satisfactory and may avoid the need for maxillary surgery. In more severe cases in which the basal maxilla is asymmetric (as is the case in approximately one-third of individuals), however, the cant of the lips and the incisor teeth will not be perceptibly altered by this treatment, so facial esthetics are rarely improved.

Orthodontic treatment plays an important role in the preparation for surgery for the correction of facial asymmetry. Presurgically, dental arch alignment removes interferences that would prevent the mandible from being precisely positioned during surgery. After surgery an open bite usually appears on the affected side. Once the fixation wires are removed, the splint is often used to allow the extrusion or eruption of the maxillary and mandibular teeth. When the maxillary teeth are in contact with the mandibular teeth, the splint may be removed and braces applied to interdigitate the teeth.

Psychosocial

An important element of management of hemifacial microsomia is the monitoring of psychosocial adjustment. The major concern is the child's future self-esteem and social competence. Parents are reassured that the severity of the craniofacial malformation is much less important than the strength of the family in determining how the child will ultimately adjust and succeed in life. The psychosocial team can monitor the patient's self-esteem as treatment proceeds through childhood and adolescence and encourage the development of particular skills and talents.

Specific concerns include adjustment to body image and general self-concept as well as ability to relate to family, peers, and strangers. Motivation for and expectations of surgery should be carefully explored. Play therapy can be used to help the child integrate the experiences of hospitalization and surgery, and individual therapy is available for adolescents. For young children, "fitting in" becomes more important than pleasing parents. In the primary grades, children who are different from their peers often have some difficulty. They may be teased and called names. Some children learn to cope by educating their classmates. Others rely on their personality strengths such as a quick wit or ability to achieve or by demonstrating specific talents. Self-esteem is determined primarily by the ability to feel genuinely positive about one's self or some aspect of one's life, whether it be academic success, sports, music, art, or a particular hobby.

During the early school years, many parents are particularly concerned that their child be educated in an environment without pity, overprotection, or underestimation of potential. Because teachers are largely unfamiliar with craniofacial problems, it is helpful if parents explain their child's condition. There is a difficult balance to be found between protecting the child from the cruelty of teasing, stares, and questions and letting them cope with the world as it is and build ego strengths.

As the child reaches puberty, appealing to the opposite sex becomes important. Virtually all teenagers go through periods of doubt and insecurity. It is not surprising, therefore, that teenagers with a facial defect experience a sharp decline in self-confidence. They become more aware of the impact the facial problems may have on their lives, and also of the limitations of treatment. It is a very difficult period but most manage to cope effectively, especially if they have developed areas of competence unrelated to appearance. Some appear indifferent to the opposite sex and focus on academic or athletic achievements. Life usually becomes much easier when their peers mature and learn to see the person behind the facial appearance.

References

1. Gorlin RJ, Cohen MM Jr, Levin LS. *Syndromes of the Head and Neck.* New York: Oxford University Press; 1990.
2. Gorlin RJ, Jue KL, Jacobson NP, et al. Oculoauriculovertebral dysplasia. *J Pediatr.* 1963;63:991–999.
3. Goldenhar M. Associations malformatives de l'oeil et de l'oreille, en particulier le syndrome dermoide epibulbaire-appendices auriculaires-fistula auris congenita et ses relations avec la dysostose mandibulofaciale. *J Genet Hum.* 1952;1:243–282.
4. Ross RB. Lateral facial dysplasia (first and second branchial arch syndrome), hemifacial microsomia. *Birth Defects Orig Artic Ser.* 1975;11:51–59.
5. Smith DW. *Facio-Auriculo-Vertebral Spectrum, in Recognizable Patterns of Human Malformations.* 3rd ed. Philadelphia: WB Saunders; 1982:497–500.
6. Francois JJ, Haustrate L. Anomalies colomateuses du globe oculaire et syndrome du premier arc. *Ann Ocul.* 1954;187:340–368.
7. Stark RB, Saunders DE. The first branchial syndrome: the oral mandibular-auricular syndrome. *Plast Reconstr Surg.* 1962;29:229–239.
8. Grabb WC. The first and second branchial arch syndrome. *Plast Reconstr Surg.* 1965;36:485–508.
9. Converse JM, Coccaro PJ, Becker H, Wood-Smith D. Clinical aspects of craniofacial microsomia. In: Converse JM, McCarthy JG, Wood-Smith D, eds. *Symposium on Diagnosis and Treatment of Craniofacial Anomalies.* St. Louis: CV Mosby; 1979:461–475.
10. Poswillo D. The pathogenesis of the first and second branchial arch syndrome. *Oral Surg Oral Med Oral Pathol.* 1973;35:302–328.
11. Melnick M. The etiology of external ear malformations and its relation to abnormalities of the middle ear, inner ear, and other organ systems. *Birth Defects Orig Artic Ser.* 1980;16:303–331.
12. Coccaro PJ, Becker MH, Converse JM. Clinical and radiographic variations in hemifacial microsomia (review). *Birth Defects Orig Artic Ser.* 1975;11:314–324.
13. Rollnick BR, Kaye CI, Nagatoshi K, et al. Oculoauriculovertebral dysplasia and variants: phenotypic characteristics of 294 patients. *Am J Med Genet.* 1987;26:361–375.
14. Hermann J, Opitz JM. A dominantly inherited first arch syndrome. First conference on clinical delineation of birth defects. Part II. Malformation syndromes. In: Bergsma D, ed. *Birth Defects, Original Article Series.* Vol 2, No 2. New York: National Foundation–March of Dimes/Baltimore: Williams & Wilkins; 1969.
15. Ross RB, Johnston MC. Developmental anomalies and dysfunctions of the temporomandibular joint. In: Zarb GA, Carlson EE, eds. *Temporomandibular Joint: Functions and Dysfunction.* Copenhagen: Munksgaard; 1994.
16. Johnston MC. The neural crest in abnormalities of the face and brain. *Birth Defects.* 1975;7:1–18.
17. Newman LM, Hendricks AG. Fetal ear malformations induced by maternal ingestion of thalidomide in the bonnet monkey (*Macaca radiata*). *Teratology.* 1981;23:351–364.
18. Lammer EJ, Chen DT, Hoar RM, et al. Retinoic acid embryopathy. *N Engl J Med.* 1985;313:837–847.
19. Goulding EH, Pratt RM. Isoretinoin keratogenicity in mouse whole embryo culture. *J Craniofacial Genet Dev Biol.* 1986;6:99–112.
20. Webster WS, Johnston MC, Lammer EJ, et al. Isoretinoin embryopathy and the cranial neural crest: an in vivo and in vitro study. *J Craniofacial Genet Dev Biol.* 1986;6:211–222.
21. Jarvis BL, Johnston MC, Sulik KK. Congenital malformations of the external, middle and inner ear produced by isoretinoin exposure in mouse embryos. *Otolaryngol Head Neck Surg.* 1990;102:391–401.
22. Poswillo D. Hemorrhage in the development of the face. *Birth Defects.* 1975;11(7):61–81.
23. Kleinsasser O, Schlothan R. Die Ohrmissbildungen im Rahmen der Thalidomid-Embryopathie. *Z Laryngol Rhinol Otol.* 1964;43:344.
24. Basilla MK, Goldenberg R. The association of facial palsy and/or sensorineural hearing loss in patients with hemifacial microsomia. *Am J Med Genet.* 1989;26:287–291.
25. Converse JM, Coccaco PJ, Becker M, Wood-Smith D. On hemifacial microsomia. The first and second branchial arch syndrome. *Plast Reconstr Surg.* 1973;51:268–279.
26. Yovich J, Mulcahy M, Patson P. IVF and Goldenhar syndrome (letter). *J Med Genet.* 1987;24:644.
27. Aleksic S, Budzilovich G, Greco MA, et al. Intracranial lipomas, hydrocephalus and other CNS anomalies in oculoauriculo-vertebral dysplasia (Goldenhar-Gorlin syndrome). *Child's Brain.* 1984;11:285–297.
28. Luce EA, McGibbon B, Hoopes JE. Velopharyngeal insufficiency in hemifacial microsomia. *Plast Reconstr Surg.* 1977;60:602–606.
29. Sprintzen RJ, Croft CB, Berkman MD, Rakoff SJ. Velopharyngeal insufficiency in the facio-auriculo-vertebral malformation complex. *Cleft Palate J.* 1980;17:132–137.

30. Feingold M, Baum J. Goldenhar's syndrome. *Am J Dis Child.* 1978;132:136–138.

31. Hertle RW, Quinn GE, Katowitz JA. Ocular and adnexal findings in patients with facial microsomias. *Ophthalmology.* 1992;99(1):114–119.

32. Kaban LB, Moses MH, Mulliken JB. Correction of hemifacial microsomia in the growing child: a follow-up study. *Cleft Plate J.* 1986;23(suppl 1):50–52.

33. Moses MH, Kaban LB, Mulliken JB, et al. Facial growth after early correction of hemifacial microsomia. Presented at the 6th Annual Meeting of the American Association of Plastic Surgeons. San Diego, CA, May 1, 1985.

34. Meurman Y. Cogenital microtia and meatal atresia. *Arch Otolaryngol.* 1957, 66:443–463.

35. Caldarelli DD, Hutchinson JG Jr, Pruzansky S, Valvassori GE. A comparison of microtia and temporal bone anomalies in hemifacial microsomia and mandibulofacial dysostosis. *Cleft Palate J.* 1980;17:103–110.

36. Pruzansky S. Not all dwarfed mandibles are alike. *Birth Defects.* 1969;5:120–129.

37. Longacre JJ, DeStefano GA, Holmstand KE. Surgical management of first and second branchial arch syndromes. *Plast Reconstr Surg.* 1963;31:507–520.

38. Converse JM, Wood-Smith D, McCarthy JG, et al. Bilateral facial microsomia. Diagnosis, classification, treatment. *Plast Reconstr Surg.* 1974;54:413–423.

39. Swanson LT, Murray JE. Asymmetries of the lower part of the face. In: Whitaker LA, Randall P, eds. *Symposium on Reconstruction of Jaw Deformities.* St. Louis: CV Mosby; 1978:7.

40. Lauritzen C, Munro IR, Ross RB. Classification and treatment of hemifacial microsomia. *Scand J Plast Reconstr Surg.* 1985;19:33–39.

41. Vento AR, LaBrie RA, Mulliken JB. The O.M.E.N.S. classification of hemifacial microsomia. *Cleft Palate-Craniofacial J.* 1991;28:68–76 (discussion 77).

42. David DJ, Mahatumarat C, Cooter RD. Hemifacial microsomia: a multisystem classification. *Plast Reconstr Surg.* 1987;80:525–535.

43. Copeland MM. American joint committee on cancer staging and end results reporting: objectives and progress. *Cancer (Phila).* 1965;18:1637–1640.

44. Cepela MA, Nunery WR, Martin RT. Stimulation of orbital growth by the use of expandable implants in the anophthalmic cat orbit. *Opthalmic Plast Reconstr Surg.* 1992;8:157–167.

45. Eppley BL, Holley S, Sadove AM. Experimental effects of intraorbital tissue expansion on orbitomaxillary growth in anophthalmos. *Ann Plast Surg.* 1993;31:19–26.

46. Tjellstrom A, Hakansson B. The bone-anchored hearing aid. Design principles, indications, and long-term clinical results. *Otolaryngol Clin North Am.* 1995;28:53–72.

47. Brent B. Auricular repair with autogenous rib cartilages: two decades of experience with 600 cases. *Plast Reconstr Surg.* 1992;90:355–374.

48. Munro IR, Phillips JH, Griffin G. Growth after construction of the temporomandibular joint in children with hemifacial microsomia. *Cleft Palate J.* 1987;26:303–311.

49. Ware WH. Growth centre transplantation in temporomandibular joint surgery. *Trans Int Conf Oral.* 1970;148–157.

50. Ware WH, Brown SL. Growth centre transplantation to replace mandibular condyles. *J Maxillofac Surg.* 1981;9:50–58.

51. Ross RB. Costochondral gafts replacing the mandibular condyle. *Cleft Palate Craniofac J.* 1999;36:334–349.

52. Peltomaki T, Ronning O. Interrelationship between size and tissue separating potential of costochondral transplants. *Eur J Orthod.* 1991;13:459–465.

53. Peltomaki T, Ronning O. Growth of costochondral fragments transplanted from mature to young isogeneic rats. *Cleft Palate Craniofacial J.* 1993;30:159–163.

54. Harvold EP. The theoretical basis for the treatment of hemifacial microsomia. In: Harvold EP, Vargervik K, Chierici G, eds. *Treatment of Hemifacial Microsomia.* New York: AR Liss;1983.

59
Orbital Hypertelorism: Surgical Management

Antonio Fuente del Campo

Orbital hypertelorism is a malformation of the craniofacial skeleton characterized by an increased interorbital distance. The term *hypertelorism* comes from the Greek language and was first used by Grieg in 1924, who used the term *ocular hypertelorism*.[1]

Adaptations and variants of the term have been used since then, and it is sometimes misused. Thus we hear about primary, secondary, apparent, and posttraumatic hypertelorism, and so on. A group of hypertelorizing deformities has even been created, which includes craniostenosis and facial, cranial, or mixed fissures (e.g., bifid skull, frontal dysrhaphia, orbitofacial clefts, meningoencephalocele). Hypertelorism is common to all these conditions. In the cases of coexisting hypertelorism and fissure, the interorbital distance is usually related to the dimension of the fissure.

Others think that the most appropriate term for this malformation is *teleorbitism* (i.e., increased orbital distance) because it is more specific and concrete, and also because it avoids confusion with similar terms that involve other alterations.

Regardless of the term being used, it should be reserved for congenital malformations characterized by the widening of the nasal root, opening of the ascending processes of the maxillae and outer displacement of the orbits, the eyes, and the lateral canthi (Figure 59.1).

The term *posttraumatic hypertelorism* is not acceptable, since under these conditions the orbital displacement is not total and is followed only partially by the eyes. The term *apparent hypertelorism* refers to alterations of soft or bony parts that suggest an increased interorbital distance that really is not present. These are the cases of posttraumatic telecanthus, lateral displacement of the lacrimal point, hidden caruncle, flattening of the nose base, epicanthus, increased interciliary distance, Waardenburg's syndrome, and so on.

In cases of primary telecanthus, there is an apparent increased interorbital distance, without a real displacement of the eyes or the orbits in relation to the facial midline. In hypertelorism, both the eye globe and the inner canthus of the palpebral fissure have shifted away from the midline. Of course, these alterations are not mutually exclusive, and this is the case of telecanthus secondary to hypertelorism.

Diagnosis

Different methods are used to determine the presence and severity of hypertelorism. They include the measurement of the interpupillary distance, which is difficult to determine and useless in cases with ocular deviations, and the medial intercanthal distance, which is inapplicable in cases with soft tissue alterations in this area.

The intercrestal distance is determined using anteroposterior cephalometry by measuring the space between both posterior lacrimal crests. According to Gunther[2] and others[3–5] the following figures are considered as normal variants in adults: 20 to 26 mm (average 25 mm) in females and 21 to 28 mm (average 26 mm) in males. Greater figures mean hypertelorism, which may be graded as follows: grade I: 28 to 34 mm, grade II: 34 to 40 mm, and grade III: +40 mm. However, expansive alterations of the midline, such as a frontonasal meningoencephalocele, may increase the intercrestal distance without the presence of true hypertelorism.

Other methods include the circumferential interorbital index and the canthal index. Nevertheless, we think that the lateral intercanthal distance is the simplest and most reliable method for diagnostic purposes. In the case of detachment of one of the lateral canthi, the lateral interorbital distance could be measured on the anteroposterior (AP) cephalometry.

Therefore, the clinical assessment of these patients should not be based on a single measurement but rather on several measurements so as to establish the accurate and integral diagnosis.[5,6]

Malformation Analysis

In the radiographic cephalometry of a patient with grade III hypertelorism (Figure 59.2), the ethmoid looks wider and shorter, and it is usually found at a level lower than normal. The cribiform plate may be normal, but it is usually wider and depressed. The crista galli may be very large, duplicated, or absent. The greater wings of the sphenoid bone are small. There is a more marked orbital divergence in the frontal arch than in the maxillary arch, but this separation really occurs in the frames and not in the orbital apex. The upper inner angle

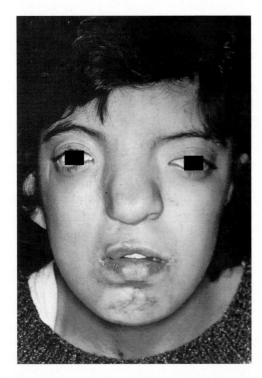

FIGURE 59.1 A 28-year-old female patient, with grade III hypertelorism and Tessier 2–12 right facial cleft.

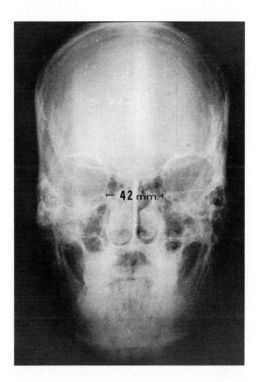

FIGURE 59.2 Anteroposterior radiographic cephalometry, from a patient with hypertelorism grade III (42 mm of intercrestal distance).

of the orbit is rounded, and its medial wall becomes oblique downward and outward.

Often there are decreased vertical dimensions of the centrofacial skeleton, including the ethmoid, the vomer, and the medial segment of the maxillae, resulting in an oval palate and an anterior open bite. There may also be micro-orbitism, with microphthalmia or anophthalmia, associated with orbito-palpebral clefts, bone defects of the fronto-orbital region, hairline alterations, such as the "widow's peak" and various irregularities associated with dystopia or eyebrow distortion.

Orbital hypertelorism associated with craniofacial clefts (Tessier 0, 1, 2, 3, 11, 12, 13, 14), presents with a wide nose, vertically divided by one or several central and/or paramedian clefts. The nose may be short or practically absent and associated with a frontonasal or frontonasoethmoidal meningoencephalocele (Figure 59.3).

In unilateral paranasal clefts, usually only the orbit on the involved side shows an increased distance from the facial midline, including the eye globe and the inner canthus, while the contralateral orbit has a virtually normal position and shape.

Etiopathology

According to Tessier,[5] the interorbital distance develops similar to the ethmoid, the frontal bone, and the maxillae, the result depending on the effects between the active divergent

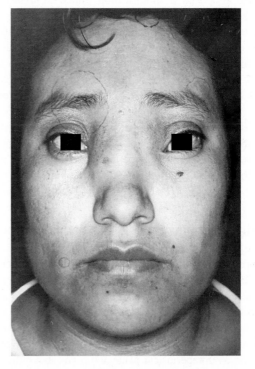

FIGURE 59.3 A 34-year-old female patient, whose hypertelorism is associated with a frontonasoethmoidal meningoencephalocele (grade III).

forces, such as the excessive intracranial pressure (endocranial hypertension) and the convergence forces represented by the cohesive forces of the bones and the temporal muscles. The presence of vertical compression and/or any deformity of the anterior cranial fossa may increase its dimensions and result in ethmoidal prolapse, which prevents the natural displacement of the orbits toward the midline, thus causing hypertelorism.[6,7]

The etiologic role previously attributed to the ethmoidal pneumatization that laterally deflects the orbits has lost support. On the contrary, it is now believed that when the orbits remain lateralized without reaching their normal position near to the midline, the resulting space between them is occupied by the ethmoid. When this does not happen, probably due to cell degeneration, craniofacial clefts and encephalomeningoceles occur, which are frequently associated with orbital hypertelorism, or *teleorbitism*.[8,9]

Treatment

In 1967 Tessier, who is recognized worldwide as the pioneer of this surgery, has described these procedures as consisting of the interorbital surgical reduction which is determined by evaluating the clinical appearance of the patient, his or her anthropometry, and the AP x-ray cephalometry. The orbits are shifted toward the midline, eliminating part of the ethmoid until a normal interorbital distance is obtained. Later on, Converse proposed a modification aimed at assuring the preservation of olfaction.[10]

The treatment of these patients should focus on the correction of the bony malformations together with the alterations of the soft parts. Many of them, in addition to the increased distance between the orbits, also have nasal hypoplasia and maxillary alterations, such as an anterior open bite.

The described basic surgical procedures can be extracranial (subcranial) or intracranial. The former are indicated only in some cases of grade I hypertelorism. In grade II and III cases, the procedures of choice are intracranial.

Surgical Procedures

The approach in both procedures (subcranial and intracranial), is a coronal incision extending from the preauricular region of one side to the other side, far away from the hairline and the craniotomy area. Laterally, the incision should be created downward in front of the origin of the helix, for a better exposure upon flap rotation. Dissection of the frontal plane is started on a supraperiosteal plane and 3 cm above the orbital roof, the periosteum is incised horizontally. It is dissected subperiosteally upward, with the shape of a posterior pedicle flap, until the frontal bone is exposed. The temporal muscle is de-

tached from its medial portion, sectioning it at the level of the temporal crest. Upon doing so, it is important to spare a strip of its fascia so that later on it can be easily sutured at its origin.

The periosteum is vertically incised on the nasal dorsum and laterally at the level of the malar process of the frontal bone, to allow the distension of the flap and facilitate the approach. The subperiosteal dissection is continued to the face along the periorbital region, the malar bone, the inside of both orbits, the nasal pyramid, and the maxilla. The supraorbital neurovascular bundles are released from their bony canal using a fine chisel. A small, curved elevator allows the surgeon to dissect around the lacrimal ducts and the medial canthal ligaments without detaching them.[11-13]

Intracranial Procedures

There are two basic intracranial procedures: orbital medialization and hemifacial rotation. The intracranial approach is done through a rectangular bifrontal craniotomy, which allows adequate access to the anterior cranial floor. The lower limit of the craniotomy is about 1 or 2 cm above the rim of the roof of both orbits. Once the orbital roof and the cribriform plate are exposed, the osteotomies are started through this approach, alternating the high-speed saw and a 6-mm chisel along the orbital roof to descend toward the inner surface of the lateral wall. These osteotomies should be done 1 cm behind the central axis of the eye globe, so that the medialization of the orbit totally displaces the eye (Figure 59.4).

The temporal intracranial fossa is dissected on its medial portion and gauze pads are placed between the bone and the meninges to protect the brain and its vessels during the osteotomy of the orbital roof (greater wing of the sphenoid bone) and the upper part of the lateral wall. The temporal muscle is laterally displaced to complete the lateral wall osteotomy from a lateral approach with a reciprocating saw until the orbital floor is reached.

During this maneuver, the content of the orbit is protected with a malleable retractor that allows the eye to be raised while the orbital floor osteotomy is performed using the same instrument. The orbital roof osteotomy is continued toward the midline, going down through the medial wall, behind the lacrimal apparatus, until the osteotomy performed on the floor is reached.

Laterally, the osteotomy is completed at the level of the zygomatic arch. The latter is sectioned diagonally and downward from above and from the back to the front to prevent the orbital medialization from resulting in a bone step and the subsequent depression of the soft parts at this level. This variant of the osteotomy allows to displace the malar bones maintaining the continuity with the orbits, thus achieving a more natural and cosmetic effect.

The osteotomy of the orbital rims is completed using a oscillating saw to section the lower limit in a horizontal direction from the malar bone to the piriform aperture. It is per-a 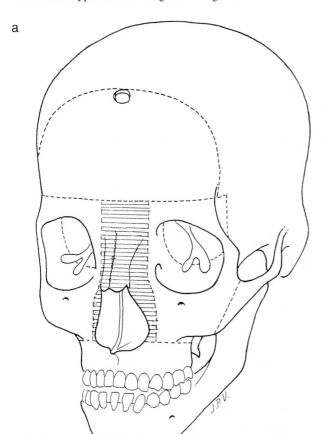   b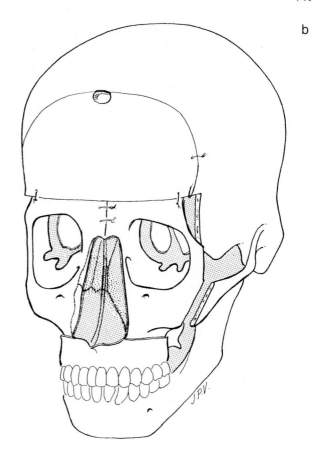

FIGURE 59.4 Orbital medialization through an intracranial approach. (a) Osteotomies and interorbital bone resection. (b) New position and osteosynthesis of the orbits.

formed underneath the emergence of the infraorbital nerve using the upper vestibular approach for this purpose. Then the interorbital bone resection estimated previously (Figure 59.4a) is performed. It includes part of the ascending processes of the maxillae, the ethmoid and the frontal bone.[14,15]

In cases with a normal nasal pyramid, we detach the latter from the frontal bone (nasal salvage) by means of a vertical osteotomy at the level of the frontonasal suture (Figure 59.5). The septum is also sectioned at this level and the nasal pyramid is pulled frontward and rotated downward, making sure that its mucosa is left intact.[16]

Then the interorbital bone resection is performed, making sure that the cribriform plate of the ethmoid is spared, thus olfaction is preserved.

Once the osteotomies have been performed, the orbits are slowly and progressively mobilized until the soft parts are released and the rims come to be in contact medially, at the desired distance; the frontal bone is repositioned to its original position and is immobilized with an anchored wire osteosynthesis (Figure 59.6). The orbital frames are anchored to the frontal bone at their new position and the nasal pyramid is

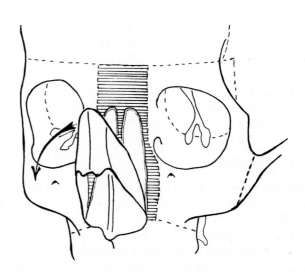

FIGURE 59.5 Nasal salvage. Vertical osteotomy to detach the nasal pyramid from the frontal bone and to perform the interorbital bone resection without affecting the original nasal structure.

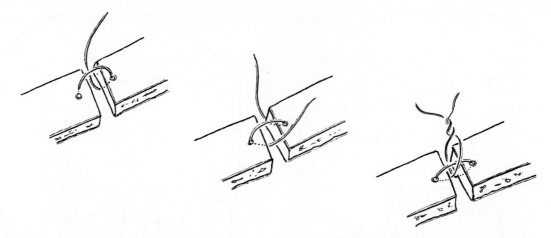

FIGURE 59.6 Anchored osteosynthesis, used for the cranial bones.

repositioned between both orbits at the appropriate height (Figure 59.4b).

The excellent stability of the repositioned fragments and the absence of antagonistic forces at this level make it unnecessary to use plates and screws. The lateral bone defects resulting from displacing the orbits are filled with bone grafts taken from the resected interorbital segment or from the parietal bone.

In cases with a deformed or hypoplastic nasal pyramid, such as central fissures and meningoencephaloceles, it is necessary to reconstruct the nose structure with bone grafts. Although the rib is more malleable, we prefer to use the parietal bone because of its proximity to the surgical area and to avoid chest scars, especially in males, in whom scars are conspicuous.

The soft tissues are reattached to the skeleton by sutures and the temporal muscle to its original insertion site.

In any case, if the medial canthus ligaments are detached, it is necessary to fix them by means of a transnasal canthopexy. Lateral canthopexy is indicated to provide direction to the palpebral fissures but without lateral traction that opposes the medial canthopexy.

In many cases the interciliary distance is increased and therefore it is necessary to resect a vertical ellipse of skin between both eyebrows (Figure 59.7).

Facial Bipartition

This procedure, proposed by van der Meulen,[17,18] is used to correct hypertelorism in cases that also have centrofacial shortening and anterior open bite.

During the planning stage, it is important to consider the required proportion of interorbital reduction and centrofacial descent so as to close the open bite. The interorbital bone resection is done in a triangular fashion with upper base, in order to perform medial rotation of both hemifaces, to put both of them in contact at the midline (Figure 59.8).

The geometric method described by Ortiz Monasterio[19] for this procedure is very didactic. It considers the hemiface as a trapezoidal structure, the upper limit of which is represented by the lower osteotomy of the craniotomy and its lower limit by the alveolar ridge of the maxilla on the same side.

After bifrontal craniotomy, the same periorbital and intraorbital osteotomies described for the orbital medialization are performed, except for the one underneath the infraorbital nerve in the maxilla. Also, the osteotomy on the lateral wall of the orbit is prolonged downward to the pterygomaxillary joint.

Once the desired interorbital distance has been estimated, the triangular interorbital redundant bone segment is resected, with an upper base at the level of the lower limit of the craniotomy [Figure 59.8(a)]. Depending on the location of its vertex, the resulting effect of the hemiface rotation may vary. If placed at the level of the maxillary alveolar ridge, it allows hemiface rotation to horizontalize the maxillae, but if the vertex is located on the nasal spine, they are horizontalized and expanded in a transverse fashion. It is important to plan the modifications of the maxillae to achieve a stable occlusion.[20]

In the first case, it is necessary to resect the nasal spine and the junction between the palatine processes all along the nasal floor. These osteotomies are performed through a superior buccal vestibular incision that extends from one canine to the other.

The dysjunction of the pterygomaxillary joint is performed by introducing a curved chisel behind the alveolar process. This maneuver may be done from above through the temporal fossa or through the mouth in the upper vestibule.

Once the osteotomies have been completed, both hemifaces are rotated medially and caudally until they are in contact with each other on the midline and with the inferior border of the frontal bone. This rotation corrects orbital excyclorotation and the antimongoloid tilting of the palpebral fissures.

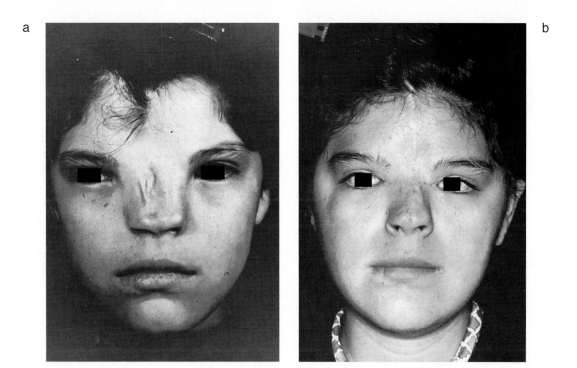

FIGURE 59.7 (a) A 19-year-old female patient with grade III hypertelorism and Tessier 0–14, and right 1–13 facial clefts. (b) Eighteen months after facial bipartition by intracranial approach and centrofacial skin resection.

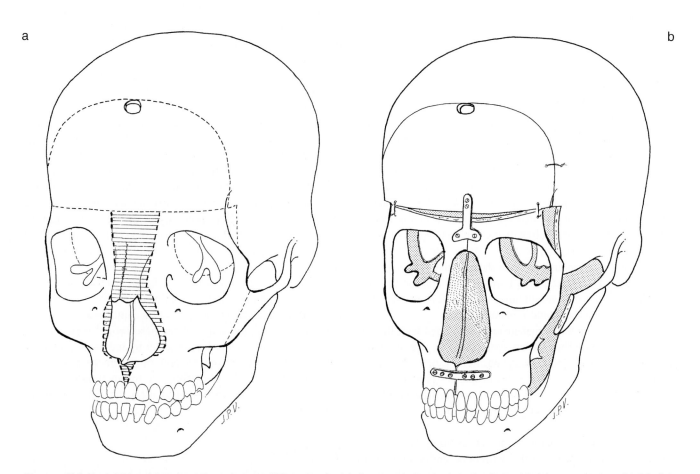

FIGURE 59.8 Facial bipartition through an intracranial approach. (a) Osteotomies and triangular interorbital bone resection. (b) Medial rotation of both hemifaces and location of the plates used for fixation.

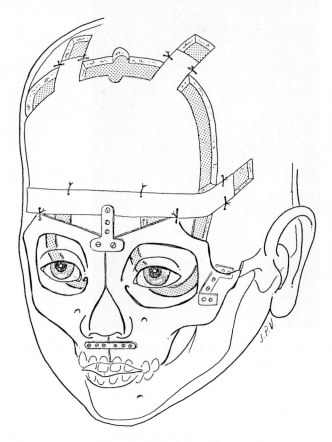

FIGURE 59.9 Facial bipartition and medial rotation with advancement. Location of the fixation plates: fronto-orbital, maxilla, and lateroinferior orbital angles.

Often, this displacement also takes the hemifaces to a more anterior plane, giving a better projection to the orbits and malar bones.

In these cases with tridimensional mobilization it is especially important to achieve a stable fixation. For this effect, we use titanium miniplates and screws. A T-shaped plate is placed vertically but inverted on the midline of the fronto-orbital region (Figure 59.8b) with the double function of maintaining the medialization of the orbits and the centrofacial elongation. To align and stabilize the alveolar processes, another miniplate is placed on a horizontal position at the pre-maxillary level with a minimum of three screws at each end, making sure that the dental roots are spared.

In cases in which this maneuver is combined with the advancement of the orbits (Apert syndrome), we use one more plate on each side. The plate is bent in an L or U shape, depending on the case, and it is located under pressure in between the lateral-inferior orbital angle and the temporal bone. It has seldom been necessary to fix these plates with screws (Figure 59.9).[21]

The fronto-orbital triangular defect resulting from the rotation of the hemifaces is filled with bone grafts. In cases in which "nasal salvage" osteotomies are performed, the nasal pyramid is rotated back to its original position and fixed at the desired height by means of an osteosynthesis wire or screw (Figure 59.10).

Extracranial Procedures

These procedures are limited to patients with grade I hypertelorism, provided that the cribriform plate is not descended more than 10 mm below the upper orbital rim, as measured on the AP cephalometry.

With extracranial procedures in hypertelorism of a higher grade it is not possible to obtain cosmetic results as good as those of intracranial procedures. Nevertheless, such procedures might be indicated for cases having any other contraindication for an intracranial approach. The subcranial approach may be used both for orbital medialization and centrofacial rotation.

The orbital medialization is started in the interorbital region, resecting two vertical paramedian segments, trying to spare the medial wall of the orbits and the nasal pyramid. The latter is indicated only if we wish to preserve the original shape of the nose.

Starting on the superior end of the resected bony area, the osteotomy is continued toward the medial orbital wall, aiming it backwards horizontally, going 0.5 cm behind the vertical axis of the eye globe. We continue downwards along the medial wall and proceed along the orbital floor and the full thickness of the orbital lateral wall, ending the osteotomy at the junction between this wall and the roof. The osteotomy is completed by sectioning the zygomatic arch and, horizontally, the maxilla, from the malar bone to the piriform aperture as described for the intracranial procedure (Figure 59.11a).

Once the orbital pieces have been mobilized, they are taken to the midline, having previously resected a proportional segment of the ethmoidal cells (Figure 59.11b).

The centrofacial rotation is done in a similar fashion, but the side-wall osteotomy goes down all the way to the ptery-gomaxillary junction, and the horizontal osteotomy of the maxilla is avoided. Both bone segments are rotated toward the midline and immobilized with wire at the nasal level and with a titanium miniplate and screws in the alveolar region (Figure 59.12).

We recommend preserving the original insertion of the medial canthal ligaments. Whenever this is not possible, it is necessary to reattach them by means of a canthopexy.

In some cases, the shape of the naso-orbital region is not adequate to achieve a cosmetic result by means of paranasal bone resections. Therefore, we prefer to rotate the nasal pyramid toward the front and perform the frontoethmoidal resection at the center as we described it for the intracranial approach (nasal salvage).

Soft Tissues

The treatment of hypertelorism should focus on both of the bony structural and the soft tissue alterations. The management

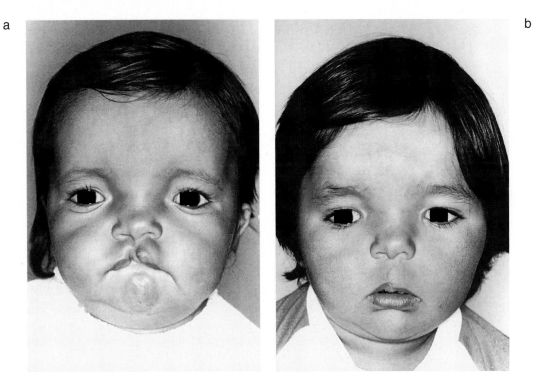

FIGURE 59.10 (a) A 4-year-old male patient with hypertelorism, open bite, and Tessier 2–12 cleft. (b) Two years after facial bipartition and cleft repair.

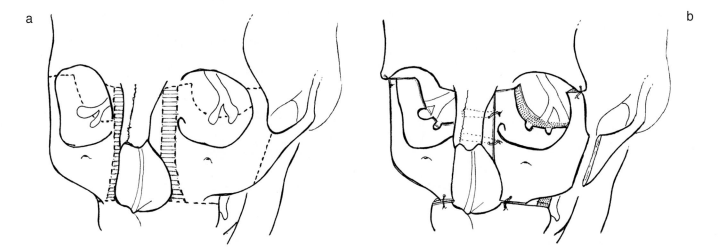

FIGURE 59.11 Orbital medialization through subcranial approach. (a) Osteotomies and interorbital bone resection. (b) New position and osteosynthesis of the orbital segments.

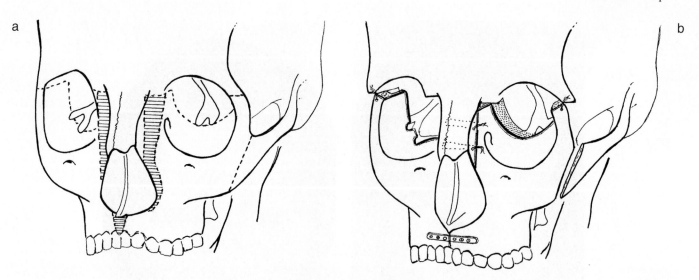

FIGURE 59.12 Subcranial orbital rotation. (a) Osteotomies and triangular interorbital bone resection. (b) Medial rotation of both orbital pieces and their fixation by means of osteosynthesis and one plate on the maxillae.

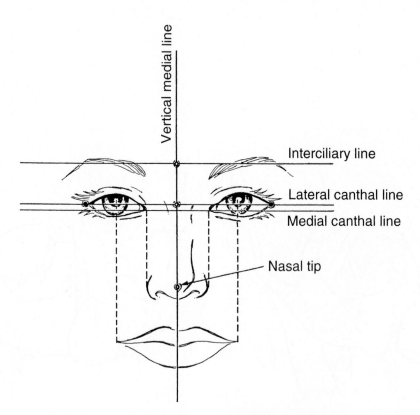

FIGURE 59.13 Lines, points, and distances considered in evaluating the proportional centrofacial T. (Reprinted with permission from *Ann Plast Surg.*)

TABLE 59.1 Nasoorbital anthropometry of 100 patients.

Points measured	Mean distance (mm)		General mean (mm)
	Men	Women	
Medial intercanthal	31.8	31.5	31.65
Lateral intercanthal	90.5	89.8	90.15
Interciliary line to nasal tip	60.3	53.7	57.00
Lateral canthal line to nasal tip	40.7	37.4	39.05
Interciliary line to lateral canthal line	19.6	16.3	17.95
Lateral canthal line to medial canthal line	2.2	1.8	2.00

of the bone structures and their displacement is not more important than that of the soft tissues; each of the facial structures must be correctly repositioned according to the appropriate proportions.

Once the bony reconstruction has been completed, we attach the soft tissues to their corresponding position on the bone structure by means of deep 4-0 Vicryl sutures. Otherwise, the outcome would leave much to be desired due to skin laxity, the scar, and the fibrous tissue that will fill the resulting dead spaces between the soft tissues and the bone.

To be more accurate in the repositioning of facial struc-

tures, we routinely use the centrofacial anthropometry, which allows us to determine precisely the proportional alterations of the patient and plan the desired result based on the measurements considered to be normal. For this purpose, we use a method that we have called *proportional centrofacial T*, as we reported in 1989, which is based on an anthropometric study of 50 males and 50 females and allowed us to obtain normal average values, as well as the normal proportional interrelation of the following measurements (Figure 59.13): medial intercanthal distance (MID), lateral intercanthal distance (LID), interciliary line (ICL) to lateral canthal line (LCL), interciliary line (ICL) to tip of the nose (NT), lateral canthal line to tip of the nose, and medial canthal line (MCL) to lateral canthal line (Table 59.1).[22] The point of maximal nose projection was considered as the tip of the nose. We refer to the tip of the nose and not to the subnasal point or other points of bone landmarks because the purpose is to correct the soft tissues. We do not consider other points of central facial landmarks, such as the nasion or glabella, because distortions were found in these patients.

The proportional relationship among the average measurements of these normal subjects was determined to assist in the assessment of our patients and to determine the desirable outcome. We found that the distance from the ICL to the tip of the nose represented 60% of the lateral intercanthal dis-

a
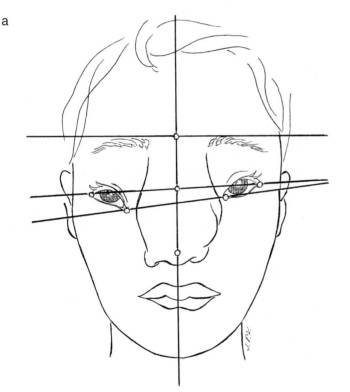

b
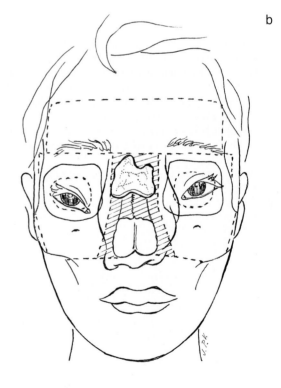

FIGURE 59.14 (a) Anthropometric lines, points, and distances to be considered for the soft tissue reconstruction of a patient with hypertelorism and encephalomeningocele. (b) Osteotomies and in- terorbital bone resection planned for the simultaneous correction of hypertelorism and the cranial bone defect of the same patient.

tance. The vertical measurement between the ICL and the tip of the nose is divided by the LCL into an upper third (20% of the lateral intercanthal distance) and two lower thirds (40% of the same distance). Variants of ±2 mm are considered as normal. The MCL was found to be, on average, 2 mm below the LCL. The medial intercanthal distance represents one third of the lateral intercanthal distance, same as the length of each of the palpebral fissures. Based on these relationships, the proportional centrofacial T helps us to accurately plan the surgery directly on each patient, particularly in patients with soft tissue malformations (clefts, meningoencephaloceles; see Figure 59.14).

Orbital hypertelorism or teleorbitism is an impressive and socially disabling deformity. Owing to its complexity, it requires the use of radical, ambitious and aggressive techniques that give the patient an appearance that is consistent with the patterns considered as normal. To facilitate the social adaptation of children to their environment and to allow the development of a normal binocular vision, these patients should be treated surgically before they reach school age, preferably between the age of 2 to 3 years.

This is a complex surgery, full of important details, requiring accurate assessment, planning, and execution. Therefore, a skilled and experienced multidisciplinary surgical and parasurgical team is necessary.

References

1. Grieg DM. Hypertelorism, a hitherto undifferentiated congenital craniofacial deformity. *Edinb Med J*. 1924;31:560.
2. Gunther H. Konstitutionelle Anomalien der Augenabstandes und der Interorbitalbreite. *Virchows Arch Pathol Anat*. 1933;290:373.
3. Currarino G, Silverman FN. Orbital hypertelorism, arrhinencephaly. *Radiology*. 1960;74:206.
4. Hasman CF. Growth of interorbital distance and skull thickness as observed in roentgenographic measurements. *Radiology*. 1966;86:87.
5. Tessier P. Orbital hypertelorism I. *Scand J Plast Reconstr Surg*. 1972;6:135.
6. Tessier P. Orbital hypertelorism II. *Scand J Plast Reconstr Surg*. 1973;7:39.
7. Tessier P. Orbital hypertelorism. *Symposium on Plastic Surgery in the Orbital Region*. Vol. 12. St. Louis: CV Mosby; 1976:255–267.
8. Walker DG. *Malformations of the Face*. Edinburgh: Livingstone; 1961.
9. Vermeij-Keers C, Poelman RE, Smits van Pooje AE, Van de Meulen JC. Hypertelorism and the median cleft face syndrome. An embryological analysis. *Ophthalmic Paediatr Genet*. 1984;4:97.
10. Converse JM, Ransohoff J, Mathews ES, Smith B, Moleonar A. Ocular hypertelorism and pseudohypertelorism. *Plast Reconstr Surg*. 1970;45:1.
11. Fuente del Campo A, Ortiz Monasterio F. Hipertelorismo o teleorbitismo. *An Medicos*. 1978;23:153.
12. Psillakis JM. Surgical treatment of hypertelorism. In: Caronni E, ed. *Craniofacial Surgery*. Boston: Little-Brown; 1985.
13. Raposo Do Amaral C. Surgical Treatment of Orbital Hyper- and Hypotelorism. In: Marchac D, ed. *Craniofacial Surgery*. Berlin: Springer-Verlag; 1987.
14. Tessier P, Tulasne JF. Stability in correction of hyperteleorbitism and Treacher Collins syndromes. *Clin Plast Surg*. 1989; 16:195.
15. Ortiz Monasterio F, Fuente del Campo A. Nasal correction in hyperteleorbitism: the short and the long nose. *Scand J Plast Surg*. 1981;15:277.
16. Fuente del Campo A. Nose salvation in craniofacial surgery. Presented at the V International Congress of the International Society of Craniofacial Surgery. Oaxaca, Mexico; 1993.
17. Van Der Meulen JC. Medial Faciotomy. *Br J Plast Surg*. 1979;33:339.
18. van der Meulen JC, Vaandragen JH. Surgery related to correction of hypertelorism. *Plast Reconstr Surg* 1983;61:6.
19. Ortiz Monasterio F, Medina O, Musolas A. Geometrical planning for the correction of orbital hypertelorism. *Plast Reconstr Surg*. 1990;86:650.
20. Tessier P. Facial bipartition: a concept more than a procedure. In: Marchac D, ed. *Craniofacial Surgery*. Berlin: Springer-Verlag; 1987.
21. Fuente del Campo A. Rigid fixation and osteotomy design in frontal orbital advancement osteotomies. *Clin Plast Surg*. 1989; 16:205.
22. Fuente del Campo A, Escanero A, Baldizon N, Dimopulos A. Transfacial surgical treatment and anthropometric considerations of frontoethmoidal meningoencephaloceles. *Ann Plast Surg*. 1989;23:377.

60
Surgical Correction of the Apert Craniofacial Deformities

E. Clyde Smoot, III and William L. Hickerson

Apert Syndrome

Apert first utilized the term acrocephalosyndactyly in 1906 to describe a foreshortened, tower-shaped cranial malformation associated with syndactyly of all four extremities. Just over 300 such patients have been described in the literature. The syndrome occurs in 1 in 160,000 live births. More recently, Cohen utilized an indirect method and showed that Apert syndrome represented 4% of all the cases of craniosynostosis for 13.7 cases per 1,000,000 live births.[1,2]

Cohen examined the skeletal abnormalities in Apert syndrome and reported x-ray evidence of multiple epiphyseal dysplasia. He found decreased mobility at the glenohumeral joint, a shortened humerus, limited elbow mobility, radiohumeral synostosis, spine changes with vertebral fusion, spina bifida, scoliosis, and hip abnormalities. These changes were associated with bony fusion of the hands and feet causing a complex syndactyly (or mitten) hand deformity. Associated visceral anomalies are not common, but cardiovascular abnormalities are found in 10% of the patients and genitourinary anomalies are also reported as frequently. Multiple ocular abnormalities are diagnosed in these patients and include optic atrophy, cataracts, iris and chorodial colobomas, keratoconus, medulated nerve fibers, and bilateral superior oblique nerve palsy.[3–7]

In planning staged surgical interventions for improvement of the craniofacial anomalies associated with Apert syndrome, it is important to understand the anatomic pathology and to consider the etiopathogenesis of the deformities.[8] The newborn Apert child has anterior fontanelles that are widely open, extending to the inferior extent of the metopic suture. The head appears hyperacrobrachycephalic, and there is flattening of the occipital region. The steep forehead is associated with a prominent bregma, and in some cases a transverse groove is apparent above the supraorbital ridge. Exorbitism and midfacial hypoplasia may be marked. As the patient ages a relative prognathism is appreciated and the nasal bridge is depressed. The nose may lack tip support and have a beaked appearance.

The cranium in Apert syndrome undergoes premature fusion of the coronal sutures with the remaining sutures patent at birth. Kreiborg et al. reported that abnormalities in the cartilage of the anterior cranial base during early intrauterine life may play a major role in the formation of the misshapen skull. These authors further showed that the cranial vault development underwent a progressive fusion with age. The intracranial volume in these syndromic patients is normal at birth but increases to become 3 standard deviations (SD) above normal after 6 months of age. Although intracranial pressure is usually not increased in these patients as the result of the large midline calvarial defect, early release of the coronal sutures and advancement of the frontal bone is advocated to decrease the dysmorphic changes in the calvaria and cranial base.[9,10]

Radiologic studies of the Apert skull will demonstrate fusion of the coronal sutures to the cranial base. At birth, however, these patients appear to have patent sphenozygomatic and sphenotemporal sutures. Lambda is patent as is the occipitomastoid suture. The zygomatic process of the frontal bone is hypoplastic, and the cranial base may be malformed and asymmetric. The anterior fossa tends to be short, as are the orbits. With time the ethmoids may become expansive. As head growth proceeds, there will be increased bitemporal head width secondary to compensatory growth of a megalencephalic brain pushing and directing growth at the squamosal sutures. The temporalis muscles may be short and inferiorly positioned. Other gross features of the facial region reveal a high arched narrow palate, which may or may not be associated with a cleft of the soft palate. With aging, the patient's skin becomes abnormally thick, thus affecting the soft tissue envelope that reflects the underlying bony abnormalities. By early adolescence severe seborrhea and acne may be present on the head, neck, trunk areas, along the upper extremities.[8,11]

The etiology of the bony abnormalities remains speculative, but there are substantial radiologic data and fetal cadaver studies to support a cranial-based abnormality related to dysostosis of the midline cranial structures, a hypoplastic anterior cranial base, and associated hypoplasia of the maxillary complex. Using a rabbit model, Persing et al.[12] have developed an alternate explanation of growth disturbance to indicate growth arrested at multiple sutures in the cranial vault may produce complex craniofacial abnormalities similar to Apert deformity. This supports theories that growth abnormalities need not necessarily be localized to the cranial base.[12]

There is a broad range of phenotypic expression of the Apert disease. It is helpful for the surgeon to recognize, with the family, that a surgical correction may improve the patient's appearance and function but that Apert patients never achieve normal facial appearance. There is usually some residual element of calvarial asymmetry, orbital hypertelorism, proptosis, or midface deficiency when compared to other patients who have undergone surgery for correction of brachycephalic conditions. Even the expression of the forehead frontal calvaria deformity may be variable. Tessier has described the turricephalic type of deformity, which results in a predominant, tower-shaped skull. Hyperbrachycephalic abnormalities result in abnormally wide, short skulls. A third variant is that of patients presenting with a median, vertical, frontal gibbosity or a frontal keel-type deformity.[13]

Posnick has addressed the issue of residual cranial skull base and forehead deformity after forehead advancement and remodeling. Quantitative postoperative computed tomography (CT) scan assessment after cranial and orbital reshaping and advancement indicate change. However, no significant quantitative improvement is noted when compared to age-matched controls. Early surgery of the anterior skull base and cranium did not normalize subsequent growth for the patients with Apert disease.[14]

Failure of sustained qualitative improvement of the operated craniofacial features is recognized likewise. After forehead advancement there may be unpredictable skull growth with additional turricephalic deformity and ridging above the supraorbital band. Incomplete reossification of the forehead region can occur even with properly performed advancements. The less than predictable results that are obtained with cranial reshaping and midface advancements, and the inability to normalize facial appearance, have been disheartening for many experienced craniofacial surgeons.[15]

Other surgeons have been less discouraged. Despite the incomplete understanding of the pathophysiology of the disease process and the apparent incomplete technology of the surgical capabilities that exist in the field, surgical interventions are worthwhile for improvement. The goals of correcting skeletal and soft tissue defects in these patients are to correct facial appearance, improve function, and preserve vision. Deformities that interfere with vision require timely surgical interventions to prevent amblyopia. Midface advancement for relief of nasopharyngeal obstruction or to correct malocclusion are also achievable goals in these patients. For the occasional patient who does have increased intracranial pressure, forehead advancement may enlarge the cranial vault. However, correction of increased intracranial pressure with shunting may still be required in some cases.[6,16,17]

Evaluation of the Apert Patient

Because of midface hypoplasia associated with the dental alveolar deformities in these patients, an open-mouth posture may be present with some element of choanal atresia. A short, hard palate is often seen with a long, soft palate, which may be cleft. The maxillary dental arch will appear as a V-shape with downslanting of the posterior portion of the maxilla. There may be enlargement of the alveolar ridges as the patient ages. Airway problems are frequent in these patients and may consist of upper-airway obstruction, with a small pharynx, and associated lower-airway problems including tracheomalacia and bronchomalacia. It is important when evaluating young patients with CT scans that sedation be done only with careful monitoring of the airway while ensuring oxygenation.[18]

Ferraro has reported cervical spine deformities in these patients with intervertebral fusions of the C-5 to C-6 region. Complex and extended fusions that restrict the flexion and extension of the neck must be anticipated. There are reports of C-1 to C-2 subluxation. A careful evaluation of the neck before the positioning for anesthesia or manipulations for sleep apnea is necessary.

Besides spinal deformities, epiphyseal dysplasia in these patients may result in problems with decreased elbow flexion and shoulder range of motion. A genu valgus deformity may be present. These abnormalities must be appreciated when preparing patients for surgery. Any limitation must be conveyed to operating room personnel so that appropriate positioning precautions are undertaken. The complex syndactylies of the hands require surgical intervention to obtain useful hand function. These deformities need attention from the appropriate surgical specialist as a part of the comprehensive evaluation of the patient.[4]

Although not a common sequela of this disease process, increased intracranial pressure may occur either before or after forehead advancement and may require shunt decompression. Despite the apparent patent lambdoidal, squamosal, and midline sutures, the calvarial deformity of the Apert patient can result in increased intracranial pressure. This may be secondary to the megacephalic brain and dysmorphic brain growth within a hyperbrachycephalic calvarial vault.

Infants with Apert disease may have exorbitism, which is relieved with an initial 12- to 15-mm advancement of the forehead and supraorbital bandeau. These patients need to be observed for corneal exposure and keratitis. Associated abnormalities of blepharoptosis, downslanting palpebral fissures, strabismus, and ametropia all need to be evaluated by an ophthalmologist or an oculoplastic surgeon so that early correction of visual disturbances is undertaken. Amblyopia is often a preventable cause of visual loss. It was the most common reason for blindness in one series of Apert patients who were studied for visual defects. Papilledema from nerve compression was rarely a cause of visual loss.[6]

Besides the obvious upper-airway problems that may occur in Apert patients, additional concerns with snoring and sleep apnea may warrant evaluation with cardiopulmonary polysonography. Infants with initial respiratory distress may improve as they grow. Respiratory symptoms may recur by 2 to 3 years of age when tonsils and adenoids begin to enlarge. However, in these patients the removal of tonsils and adenoids, or even midface advancement, at the age of 4 may not relieve the apnea, which can result from tracheomalacia or bronchomalacia. Therefore, patients with suspected anomalies of the respiratory region warrant magnetic resonance imaging (MRI) of the trachea to exclude other abnormalities such as a solid, cartilaginous trachea and tracheal stenosis.[19,20]

Dental hygiene in these patients is important as teeth erupt. Any surgical interventions that require dental fixation can be better performed if the teeth are without decay and soft gum tissues are healthy. Because of restricted hand function it may be difficult for patients to floss and brush their teeth. Parental assistance or devices to help with tooth brushing and flossing need to be provided to the patient. Routine dental prophylaxis with the use of fluoride sealing of the teeth is important.[18]

Operative Intervention

Forehead advancement for decompression of the intracranial space, protection of the globes, and construction of a normal-appearing supraorbital band is usually performed between 3 and 6 months of age. Before that time, the bone is too soft for reshaping and fixation. A 12- to 15-mm advancement done before 6 months of age may take advantage of the remaining growth potential of the frontal lobes. The bone segments at that time are easy to manipulate. Working through a coronal incision, the temporalis muscles are detached. Because the metopic sutures are patent, the frontal bone segments are independently raised. This procedure is performed at the initial frontal craniotomy and before supraorbital advancement. The fused coronal sutures are released, and no interpositional materials are used in the coronal suture craniectomy. The nasal bones may be advanced with the forehead bandeau as an extended procedure. More commonly, a supraorbital band is developed independent of the nasal bones.[8]

Posnick is an advocate of reshaping of the supraorbital contour in addition to advancement. A bandeau as a tenon and temporal groove is fashioned laterally with a step cut at the frontal zygomatic area. The bandeau segment is freely mobilized for manipulations. This technique allows bending of the bone to decrease the bitemporal width and create more convexity in the anterior midline. The bandeau can be replaced and held in its advanced position. When the forehead is redraped over the advanced segments, the flap may be tight. Rigid fixation of the advanced supraorbital region at the lateral tongue and groove osteotomy sites may prevent relapse of the advanced forehead segment under a restrictive flap. Bone grafts wedged along the osteotomy floor of the anterior

fossa will also help maintain the forward projection. It is better that the advanced segments be stabilized without plate fixation across any released suture sites. If a fracture of the supraorbital bandeau occurs with attempts at reshaping the segment, a long microplate may be used to join the segments and allow additional bending and shaping.[14]

Rigid fixation should be minimized and the smallest plates that achieve three-dimensional stability should be employed (Figures 60.1 and 60.2). In cases where longer plates may be necessary to stabilize fractured segments or areas of bone that require extensive reshaping, then it is appropriate to plan for early removal of these plates after initial bony union. If adequate stability can be achieved with resorbable plates, this will avoid the need for plate removal. The frontal bone segments are reattached to the supraorbital bandeau and the temporalis muscles are advanced to the frontal bone segment. Lateral canthopexies are also performed.

In situations of excessive bitemporal width, the squamous portion of the temporal bone can be removed in the infant and will reossify with less convexity. For cases of more extreme turribrachycephaly, lateral barrel stave osteotomies may be performed to decompress the temporal lobes and allow lateral redistribution of the brain. Future growth in these sites, however, is not predictable with any of these surgical manipulations done at this early age. There is no proven benefit for extending frontal suture craniectomies into the skull base despite concerns that the Apert disease process may involve this area.[8,13]

A monobloc advancement of the forehead and midface in infancy has been described for extreme cases of exorbitism and airway obstruction. Unfortunately this operation carries a 33% infection rate, which may result in loss of the frontal bone, possible meningitis, and occasionally death. Therefore, the morbidity and mortality rates associated with this operation preclude its use except in extraordinary instances during infancy. Exorbitism at an early age can usually be managed

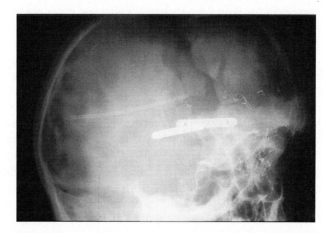

FIGURE 60.1. Rigid fixation of the advanced forehead and frontal bone segments will resist the tendency for relapse with coronal flap closure. The bone plates chosen for use along limited sites should be small but should provide three-dimensional stability. Plates are not used across suture lines.

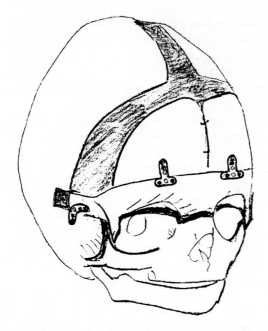

FIGURE 60.2. Rigid fixation of the advanced supraorbital bandeau at the tenon allows resistance to displacement when the coronal flap is redraped and closed.

with a forehead advancement and lateral tarsorraphies if necessary.

Eyelid deformities may occur with orbital surgery or may be a part of the primary disease process. Contour irregularities, lid ptosis, nasolacrimal obstruction, or altered ocular muscle imbalance may create conditions of amblyopia. These orbital conditions require concomittant assessment and correction. While the majority of Apert patients have an interorbital distance that exceeds the 97th percentile, those who have true orbital hypertelorism may require orbital translocation as a separate procedure. Partition of a monoblock advancement has been done for partial correction but is not advisable for reasons of high risk of infection.[19,21]

Despite well-executed surgery to advance the forehead and to correct increased bitemporal width, growth in the postoperative period during the first 6 years of life may not be predictable. Excess vertical growth and contour deformities of the forehead and temporal fossa may become apparent. Forehead advancement does not normalize growth. Cases of severe residual deformity may necessitate readvancement of the forehead before age 6. Beyond that age, with the development of the frontal sinus, a forehead advancement carries a high risk of infection. Therefore, if a forward advancement is planned after the age of 6, the surgeon must ensure that the frontal sinuses are obliterated and the ducts occluded to prevent a route for infection from the nasal region. Some surgeons will not advance the forehead after 6 years of age. Correction of forehead and temporal fossa deformities in older patients may be undertaken with onlay bone grafts or with the use of alloplastic materials such as methylmethacrylate.[15]

Respiratory problems in the Apert infant can be quite severe. Midface advancement in the first year is not indicated except in rare situations of respiratory distress. Tracheostomy is preferable to midface advancement in those less than 4 years of age. If positioning is successful in overcoming airway obstruction of the lungs, then the child must be watched for problems with respiratory distress as the adenoids and tonsils enlarge. In some cases early intervention to remove enlarged tonsils and adenoids may be necessary before any contemplation of a midface advancement.[12] For those patients who have a cleft palate with associated respiratory distress and a small nasopharynx, repair of the palate may need to be delayed. Because of the long palate and short nasopharynx, hypernasality may not be readily apparent in patients with a soft palatal cleft.[8,16,22]

As the child grows, continued problems with the upper airway may produce sleep apnea. A Le Fort III advancement performed as an extracranial procedure may be necessary by 4 years of age. Reoccurrence of exorbitism with exposure of the globes is possible and will be improved with midface advancement at this early age. If midface retrusion is mild and psychosocial issues are not pressing, a Le Fort III advancement may better serve the child as a one-stage procedure done between 9 and 12 years of age. Early midface advancement by age 4 does not normalize facial growth; however, it may relieve upper-airway obstruction and protect the globes for patients with the most severe deformities. Le Fort III advancement done in the early childhood period will not result in long-term improvement of occlusion. In those cases, the parents and patients must be prepared for additional orthognathic surgery in the later adolescent years to correct occlusion.[16,23]

The Le Fort III advancement is done as an extracranial procedure to avoid the attendant risk of intracranial infection. Osteotomies with spur cuts to the sphenozygomatic sutures are planned. Careful osteotomies and gentle pterygomaxillary disimpaction help to to avoid irregular fracture patterns. An overcorrected, advanced position can then be stabilized with miniplates at the lateral orbits and above the nasal bones. Bone grafts along the defects of the bony advancement sites, exclusive of the pterygomaxillary sites, are placed to help stabilize the advancement (Figures 60.3 and 60.4). In cases in which exorbitism is to be corrected, it may be necessary to incise and release the periorbita to allow expansion of the soft tissue contents into the expanded orbital cavity. In these cases bone grafts to the floor of the advanced orbit are necessary to avoid enophthalmus from prolapse of the orbital contents into the underlying sinus.[13]

Patients of 4 years and older may require early midface advancement and forehead readvancement. Procedures are staged separately to avoid concomitant intracranial and intraoral exposure. It is tempting to proceed with a monobloc advancement of the forehead and midface, if exorbitism is present and the position of the supraorbital bandeau and forehead correction are not satisfactory after an initial surgery. Infection risk and potential forehead bone loss, however, dictate

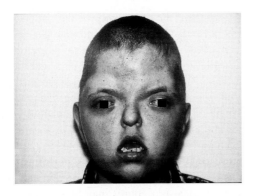

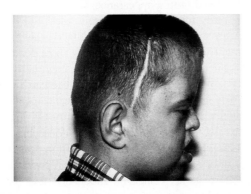

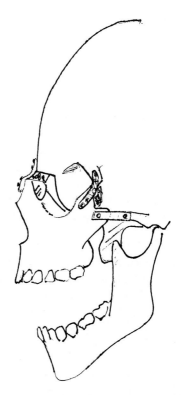

FIGURE 60.3. For the young patient undergoing a Le Fort III, the advancement can be stabilized with bone plates along the lateral orbits and above the nasal bones. Bone grafts placed along the nasal orbital and zygomatic osteotomy sites provide additional stability and maxillomandibular fixation can be omitted.

FIGURE 60.4. Despite early forehead cranioplasty and advancement, additional growth abnormalities of the forehead region often result in deformities that require further correction in the adolescent patient.

avoiding a monobloc procedure. In most cases, there are different requirements for the amount of advancement of the forehead and midface. Differential advancement cannot be achieved with a monobloc procedure. In patients who require forehead readvancement it is preferable to allow healing of the forehead procedure before a midface advancement staged as a separate operation.[15,19]

In adolescence, Apert patients will require expansion of the narrow V-shaped palatal structures, presurgical orthodontics, and planning for orthognathic surgery as growth is completed. At a minimum, most of these patients will require a Le Fort I advancement to correct occlusion. Setback of the mandible may be necessary for large occlusal discrepancies. Extreme caution is necessary in planning these procedures for patients who have a small oral pharynx as this may allow the tongue to occlude the airway. The mandibular surgery is usually reserved until completion of mandibular growth at 18 to 20 years of age. Segmental osteotomies of the occlusal segments may be necessary for correction of some maxillary deformities.[18]

In the teenage years, final touchup and adjustments of the forehead, temporal fossa, and supraorbital ridges may require bone grafting with rigid fixation or the use of alloplastic materials in the sites along the forehead. Nasal surgery can also be completed in the teenage years. Dorsal support with cantilever rib grafting fixed rigidly may improve the appearance of the nose.

Rigid Fixation of Osteotomies

The use of rigid plate fixation for stabilizing osteotomies in the growing craniofacial skeleton remains controversial. There are a number of reports indicating problems with relative migration of the plates and screws toward the dura with cranial growth. Bone resorption and deposition may allow the cranial plate to ultimately come to rest along the inner cranial cortex. Additional problems can occur with resorption around the plates, causing plate prominence, or even plates or screws isolated on a peninsula of bone along the outer cortex. Large plates may be a problem under thin skin because of visibility or palpable irregularities along the face and skull. Resorbable miniplates have become available and increasing in use, with the advantage of not requiring removal. However, resorbable plates may not provide adequate stability in large movements and titanium plates allow superior fixation in these circumstances.[24,25] Alternative methods for bone fixation include wire osteosynthesis or stabilization with sutures such as 4-0 Prolene. For frontal bone segments that are repositioned without significant stress forces, the use of cranial bone wedged along the advanced anterior fossa may provide stability to the repositioned supraorbital bandeau and forehead.[26]

Rigid plates do have a role in providing three-dimensional stability for bony segments that have been advanced and will need to resist force during the closure and in the postoperative period. The properly chosen micro- or miniplate provides stability of the forehead and can be placed along a tongue-and-groove osteotomy to resist the tendency toward relapse that may occur with closure of a tight coronal flap. T-shaped microplates used to stabilize the bifrontal forehead bone grafts to the supraorbital bandeau will help retain the position of these bone segments against tight flap closure. The plates should not be placed across the coronal suture lines or along other sutures or growth regions. All bone fixation techniques when employed across open suture lines have resulted in some growth interference. The rigid plates, however, contribute the most to growth disturbance.

Rigid fixation of the advanced midface during childhood provides stability necessary to avoid maxillomandibular fixation. There is an additional benefit of allowing easier airway management without the need for tracheostomy in these young patients who have a small pharynx. A trend toward less skeletal relapse of the advanced midface with use of the fixation plates has been noted. However, it has not been established that rigid fixation of a Le Fort osteotomy prevents relapse.

An additional indication for use of screw or plate fixation is in the application of onlay bone grafts. Cranial bone, used for correction of forehead contours in the later years or rib for cantilever grafting of the nose, can be stabilized with plates and screws to ensure the position and avoid migration. The benefits of rigid fixation of onlay bone grafts resulting in less bone resorption are well established.

Fixation plates are easy to use and provide stability that cannot be achieved with other techniques of osteosynthesis. At this point there are no proven cases of brain injury resulting from plate migration. The plates, when used judiciously and in a limited fashion along appropriate areas, can assist with healing of the bone segments in their corrected position. If there is concern with the plates, they can be removed 3 months after the procedure. Long-term histocompatibility of the plates has not been established, nor have there been studies of long-term effects of corrosion. There are problems with roentgenographic scatter and artifact when these patients undergo postoperative radiographs. Titanium plates allow for the best radiographic visualization and are tolerated during MRI scanning without plate or screw loosening.

Plates should be carefully chosen and used in minimal quantities to achieve the stabilization required. They should not be used across suture lines, and they should not be applied to the inner surface of the cranial vault. They serve an important function, extending the surgeon's ability to reshape the cranial and facial skeleton in the growing Apert patient.

Overview of Surgical Management

Surgical correction of the multiple craniofacial anomalies of the growing Apert child is worthwhile in improving the appearance and function of the patient. The initial forehead cranioplasty to advance the anterior cranial base and protect the globes will improve the appearance of the patient. Unfortunately, it is not possible to obtain a normal face in these patients. Even with extended suture release along the anterior base, growth deformities of the cranial base and the midface still occur. The forehead advancement and reshaping of the cranial orbitozygomatic region at a young age does not normalize growth of the cranium. There are inherent growth abnormalities in the forehead region. In the presence of a megalencephalic brain deformity, unpredictable skull growth and shape changes may occur after properly performed forehead advancement, resulting in additional turricephalic abnormalities. Repeat surgical procedures may be required to correct the forehead and orbital appearance.

Despite early forehead advancement, there does not seem to be a positive benefit resulting in midface growth. Midface advancement as a Le Fort III osteotomy can be done with relative safety in the patients older than 4 years if there is a functional need for airway enlargement or need to protect the globes. Early intervention for midface advancement may also be indicated where there is severe deformity causing psychological disease. The advancement can be done obtaining segment stability, but there has been no benefit in promoting further anterior or downward growth with the repositioning even after overcorrection. It must be anticipated that the patient will require additional surgery either as a readvanced Le Fort III segment or a Le Fort I osteotomy to correct occlusion in the teenage years. Midface advancement while useful at an early age for enlarging the airway may not necessarily correct sleep apnea in the Apert patient because of associated lower-airway abnormalities, including tracheomalacia and bronchomalacia.

The utilization of rigid fixation with plates and screws definitely has its advantages, especially when bicoronal flap closure is tight over the advanced segments. Plates should be used under the conditions described here. Plate removal after 3 months has been recommended by some surgeons, although this is as controversial as the utilization of the plates themselves. With the development of absorbable plates and screws, concerns regarding cranial growth restriction and plate removal should be alleviated.[24,25]

References

1. Kaplan LC. Clinical assessment and multispecialty management of Apert syndrome. *Clin Plast Surg.* 1991;18:217.
2. Cohen MM Jr, Kreiborg S. New indirect method for estimating the birth prevalence of the Apert syndrome. *J Oral Maxillofac Surg.* 1992;21:107–109.
3. Cohen MM Jr, Kreiborg S. Growth pattern of the Apert syndrome. *Am J Med Genet.* 1993;47:617–623.
4. Cohen MM Jr, Kreiborg S. Skeletal abnormalities in the Apert syndrome. *Am J Med Genet.* 1993;47:624–632.
5. Cohen MM Jr, Kreiborg S. Visceral anomalies in the Apert syndrome. *Am J Med Genet.* 1993;45:758–760.
6. Hertle RW, Quinn GE, Minguini N, Katowitz JA. Visual loss

in patients with craniofacial synostosis. *J Pediatr Ophthalmol Strabismus*. 1991;28(6):344–349.

7. Pollard ZF. Bilateral superior oblique muscle palsy associated with Apert syndrome. *Am J Ophthalmol*. 1988;106:337–340.

8. Mulliken JB, Bruneteau RJ. Surgical correction of the craniofacial anomalies in Apert syndrome. *Clin Plast Surg*. 1991;18(2):277–289.

9. Kreiborg S, Marsh JL, Cohen MM Jr, Liversage M, Pedersen H, Skovly F, Borgesen SE, Vannier MW. Comparative three dimensional analysis of CT scans of the calvaria and cranial base in Apert and Crouzon syndromes. *J Cranio-Maxillofac Surg*. 1993;21:181–188.

10. Gosain AK, McCarthy JG, Glatt P, Staffenberg D, Hoffman RG. A study of intracranial volume in Apert syndrome. *Plast Reconstr Surg*. 1994;95(2):284–295.

11. Cohn MS, Mahon MJ. Apert syndrome (acrocephalosyndactyly) in a patient with hyperhidrosis. *Cutis*. 1993;52:205–208.

12. Persing JA, Lettieri JT, Cronin AJ, Putnam W, Wolcott BS, Singh V, Morgan AB. Craniofacial suture stenosis morphologic effects. *Plast Reconstr Surg*. 1990;88:563–571.

13. Marsh JL, Galic M, Vannier MW. The craniofacial anatomy of Apert syndrome. *Clin Plast Surg*. 1991;18(2):237–248.

14. Posnick JC, Lin KY, Jhawar BJ, Armstrong D. Apert syndrome: quantitative assessment by CT scan of presenting deformity and surgical results after first-stage reconstruction. *Plast Reconstr Surg*. 1994;93(3):489–497.

15. Marsh JL, Miroslav G, Vannier MW. Surgical correction of the craniofacial dysmorphology of Apert syndrome. *Clin Plast Surg*. 1991;18:251–275.

16. McCarthy JG, LaTrenta GS, Breitbart AS, Grayson BH, Bookstein FL. The Le Fort III advancement osteotomy in the child under seven years of age. *Plast Reconstr Surg*. 1990;86(4):633–649.

17. Ferraro NF. Dental, orthodontic, and oral/maxillofacial evaluation and treatment in Apert syndrome. *Clin Plast Surg*. 1991;18(2):291–307.

18. Marchac D, Renier D, Broumand S. Timing of treatment for craniosynostosis and faciocraniosynostosis: a 20-year experience. *Br J Plast Surg*. 1994;2:211–222.

19. Mixter RC, David DJ, Perloff WH, Green CG, Pauli RM, Popec PM. Obstructive sleep apnea in Aperts and Pfeiffer syndromes. *Plast Reconstr Surg*. 1990;86(3):457–463.

20. Posnick JC, Waitzman A, Armstrong D, Prow G. Monobloc and facial bipartition osteotomies: quantitative assessment of presenting deformity and surgical results based on computed tomography scans. *J Oral Maxillofac Surg*. 1995;53:358–367.

21. Moore MH. Upper airway obstruction in the syndromal craniosynostoses. *Br J Plast Surg*. 1994;93(3):355–497.

22. Binghond B, Kaban LB, Vargervik K. Effect of Le Fort III osteotomy on mandibular growth in patients with Crouzon and Apert syndromes. *J Oral Maxillofac Surg*. 1989;47:666–671.

23. Fearon JA, Munro IR, Chir B, Bruce DA. Observation on the use of rigid fixation for craniofacial deformities in infants and young children. *Plast Reconstr Surg*. 1995;95(4):634–638.

24. Pensler JM. Role of resorbable plates and screws in craniofacial surgery. *J Craniofac Surg*. 1997;8:129–134.

25. Becker HJ, Wiltfang J, Merten HA, Luhr HG. Bioresorbable miniplates (Lactosorb) in cranio-osteoplasty, experimental results with the rapidly maturing juvenile minipig. *Mund Kiefer Gesichtschir*. 1999;3:275–278.

26. Yaremchuk MJ. Experimental studies addressing rigid fixation in craniofacial surgery. *Clin Plast Surg*. 1994;21(4):517–525.

Appendix A1
Distraction Osteogenesis of the Mandible

Alex M. Greenberg and Joachim Prein

Mandible Single Distractor Module Stainless Steel Set

Color: Black
Indications: Mandibular ramus lengthening

The Mandible Distractor Module Set (Figure A1.1) is composed of stainless steel implants, specifically a mandibular distractor with right foot and mandibular distractor with left foot (Figure A1.2). The distractor is placed on the mandible spanning the osteotomy site with an external activator extending through a small submandibular percutaneous incision (Figure A1.3). The screws utilized are 2.0-mm stainless steel self-tapping screws in 10-, 12-, and 14-mm lengths, and 2.4-mm stainless steel emergency screws in 10-, 12-, and 14-mm lengths. The implants are activated by an activation screwdriver. Figure A1.4 with an internal hex (Figure A1.5). This screwdriver has a directional arrow for counterclockwise activation, in which one rotation equals .5 mm. Usually, two rotations, equal to 1 mm of distraction, are recommended on a daily basis, but this is subject to variability at the surgeon's discretion. The total days of distraction multiplied by two equals the number of days recommended for the distractor to be in place for bone consolidation to occur. The placement of the distractor requires the use of the trocar system (Figure A1.6). The module also contains the black narrow screwdriver handle, cruciform screwdriver blade (self-retaining), and 2.0-mm holding forcep (for screws).

The Titanium Single Vector Distractor

Color: Black
Indications: Mandibular ramus lengthening

The Titanium Single Vector Distractor Module is composed of titanium implants, specifically 20-mm and 30-mm length mandibular distracts with right foot and left foot types as distal attachments (Figure A1.7). In addition, detached right foot and left foot proximal implants for initial bone anchorage and subsequent are mandibular distractor attachment included (Figure A1.8). The distractor is placed on the mandible spanning the osteotomy site, with an external activator extending through a small submandibular percutaneous incision. The screws utilized are 2.0 self-tapping screws in 6-, 8-, 10-mm lengths (12 and 14 are also available) and 2.4-mm emergency screws in 6-, 8-, 10-mm lengths (12 and 14 are also available). In evaluating ramus height on radiographs, the *Single Vector Angulation Planner* should be used to determine distractor length as well as vector and foot placement. The drilling of holes and insertion of screws is performed utilizing the plate holding trocar, which stabilizes the implant (Figure A1.9). First, on the superior aspect of the planned osteotomy, the detachable proximal foot is placed with slot inferior (Figure A1.10a). Then, the distractor body is inserted into the proximal foot (Figure A1.10b) to complete screw fixation of the distractor device. Activation and percutaneous exposure are achieved (Figure A1.10c). The implants are activated by an activation screwdriver with an internal hex (Figure A1.11), which has a directional arrow for counterclockwise activation in which one rotation equals .5 mm. Usually two rotations, which equal 1 mm of distraction, are recommended on a daily basis, but this is subject to variability at the surgeon's discretion. The total days of distraction multiplied by two equals the number of days recommended for the distractor to remain in place for bone consolidation to occur. Following consolidation, a 3-step procedure is followed for distractor body removal. First, the activator screwdriver is turned clockwise 10 rotations (opposite to the arrow handle marker). Then distal foot disengagement is achieved by turning the distractor removal instrument 4 clockwise rotations (in the direction of the arrow marker) (Figure A1.12). Then the distractor body is removed via the percutaneous port (Figure A1.13). The module contains the black narrow screwdriver blade (self-retaining), 1.5-mm drill bits (Stryker J latch), distractor removal instrument, and activation screwdriver.

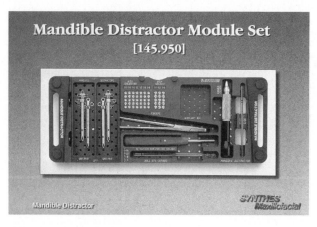

FIGURE A1.1 Mandible distractor module set. (Courtesy of Synthes Maxillofacial, Paoli, PA)

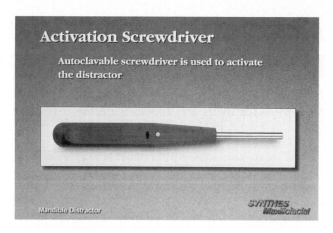

FIGURE A1.4 Mandible distractor activation screwdriver. (Courtesy of Synthes Maxillofacial, Paoli, PA)

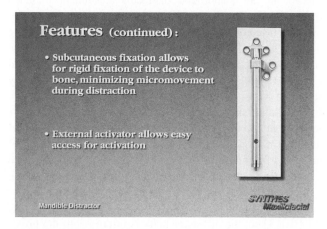

FIGURE A1.2 Mandible distractor with left foot. (Courtesy of Synthes Maxillofacial, Paoli, PA)

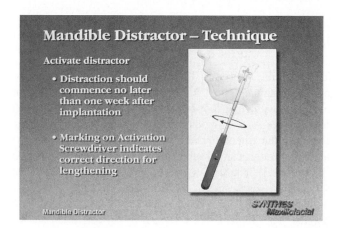

FIGURE A1.5 Mandible distractor activation. (Courtesy of Synthes Maxillofacial, Paoli, PA)

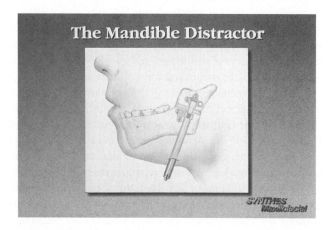

FIGURE A1.3 Mandible distractor in place. (Courtesy of Synthes Maxillofacial, Paoli, PA)

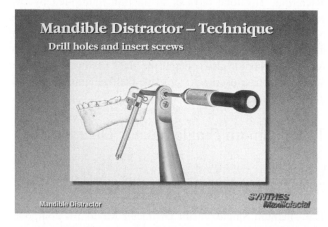

FIGURE A1.6 Mandible distractor placement with transcutaneous trocar system. (Courtesy of Synthes Maxillofacial, Paoli, PA)

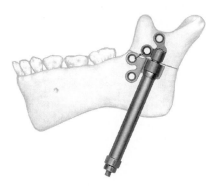

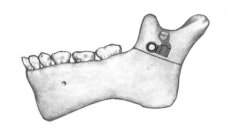

a

FIGURE A1.7 Titanium single vector distractor. (Courtesy of Synthes Maxillofacial, Paoli, PA)

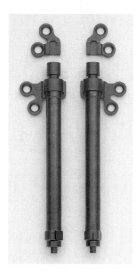

FIGURE A1.8 Right and left titanium single vector distractors with detachable feet. (Courtesy of Synthes Maxillofacial, Paoli, PA)

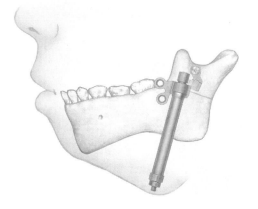

b

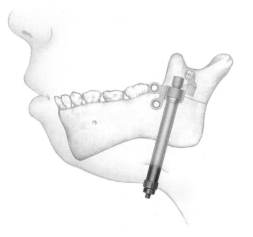

c

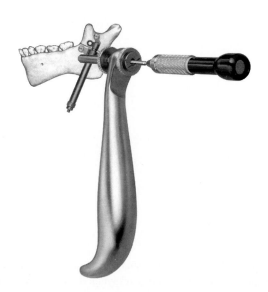

FIGURE A1.9 Insertion of screws utilizing the plate holding trocar. (Courtesy of Synthes Maxillofacial, Paoli, PA)

FIGURE A1.10 (a) The detachable proximal foot is initially placed with slot inferior, (b) the distractor is inserted for attachment, and (c) the percutaneous incision is made exposing the activation screw. (Courtesy of Synthes Maxillofacial, Paoli, PA)

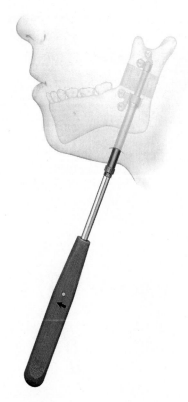

FIGURE A1.11 The distractor is activated via an activation screwdriver counterclockwise. (Courtesy of Synthes Maxillofacial, Paoli, PA)

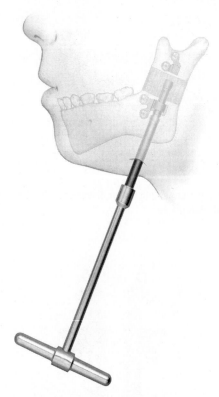

FIGURE A1.12 Disengagement of the distractor by rotating the distractor removal instrument clockwise. (Courtesy of Synthes Maxillofacial, Paoli, PA)

The Titanium Multivector Distractor (TMVD)

Color: Black

Indications: Mandibular bone lengthening for simple to severe hypoplasia, including straight to multidirectional requirements.

This is used as an external fixator device with percutaneous Kirschner wire (pin) implants for stabilization. The Titanium Multi-Vector Distractor (Figure A1.14) module is composed of a titanium multi-vector distractor assembly with titanium multi-vector arms in 5 lengths (15, 25, 35, 45, and 55 mm with 65, 75, and 85 mm also available) and activation instrumentation (Figure A1.15). Implants consist of 2-mm Kirschner W with thread and trocar point (pin) for self-drilling and self-tapping. Following the use of a preoperative radiograph TMVD angulation planner, an osteotomy site is performed via an intraoral or percutaneous approach. Insertion of the first pair of pins is achieved using the wire guide/tissue protector, along with an optional trocar, thumbscrew, and check retractor ring (Figure A1.16). Then, the two infe-

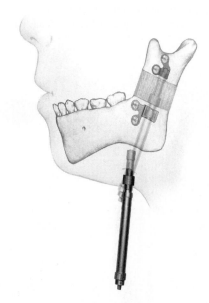

FIGURE A1.13 Removal of the distractor percutaneously, leaving the foot implants in place. (Courtesy of Synthesis Maxillofacial, Paoli, PA)

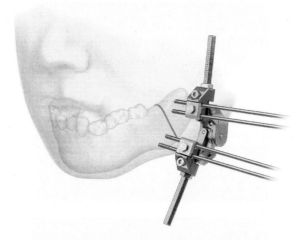

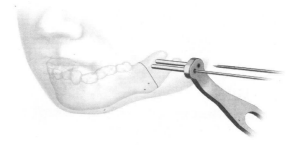

FIGURE A1.16 Insertion of screws via trocar. (Courtesy of Synthes Maxillofacial, Paoli, PA)

FIGURE A1.14 Titanium multivector distractor. (Courtesy of Synthes Maxillofacial, Paoli, PA)

rior pins are inserted and the distractor assembly is placed, followed by completion of the osteotomy. Pins are cut to the desired length and adjustment of the distractor assembly is performed. Mandibular lengthening is achieved by turning the activation instrument two rotations counterclockwise; following the arrow marker is recommended (Figure A1.17), but is subject to the surgeon's discretion. After a bony regenerate of at least 10 mm has been achieved, angular adjustment is performed using the angular adjustment instrument (Figures A1.18A and B). After consolidation has occurred, the 4.0-mm carbon fiber rod (60 and 80 mm, also available in 100-200 mm in 20-mm increments) are applied with the TMVD clamp for carbon fiber rods after the distractor assembly has been removed (Figures A1.19 and A1.20).

Distraction Osteogenesis of the Mandible Case Report

Single vector distraction osteogenesis of the mandible is indicated for deformities of mandibular ramus hypoplasia with normal mandibular body horizontal size. This case report illustrates this procedure in a male with mandibular retrognathia secondary to a shortened ramus for which the patient underwent bilateral mandibular single vector distraction osteogenesis using the AO/ASIF Single Vector Distractor with improvement in occlusion from Class II to Class I and more satisfactory facial appearance (Figures A21–27). (Case report of Prof. Dr. med Joachim Prein, Kantonsspital Basel, Basel, Switzerland).

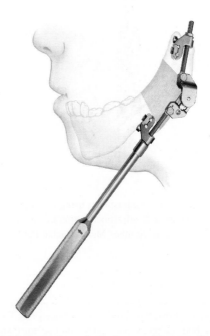

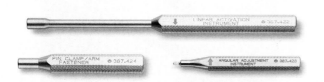

FIGURE A1.15 Titanium multivector distractor activation instrumentation. (Courtesy of Synthes Maxillofacial, Paoli, PA)

FIGURE A1.17 Activation of titanium multivector distractor with counterclockwise turns. (Courtesy of Synthes Maxillofacial, Paoli, PA)

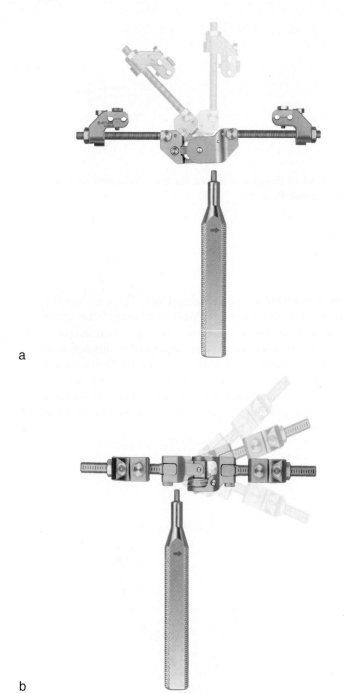

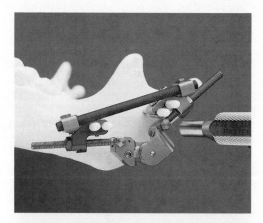

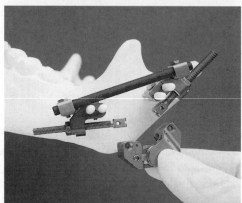

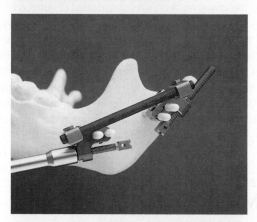

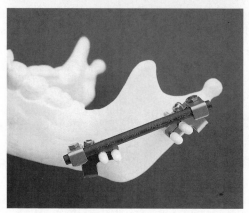

FIGURE A1.18 (a) Angular adjustment using the angular adjustment instrument. (b) Transverse adjustment using the angular adjustment instrument. (Courtesy of Synthes Maxillofacial, Paoli, PA)

FIGURE A1.19 (a) First, the carbon rod is placed. (b) The multivector distractor body is removed. (c) The multivector distractor arms are then removed. (d) The carbon rod remains in place for consolidation. (Courtesy of Synthes Maxillofacial, Paoli, PA)

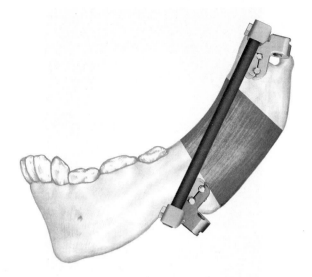

FIGURE A1.20 Carbon rod in place maintaining the segment positions while the bony regenerate undergoes consolidation. (Courtesy of Synthes Maxillofacial, Paoli, PA)

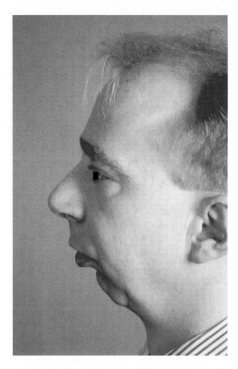

FIGURE A1.22 Patient with mandibular retrognathia lateral profile view.

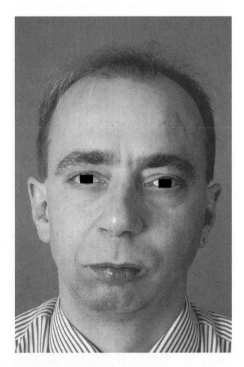

FIGURE A1.21 Patient with mandibular retrognathia facial view.

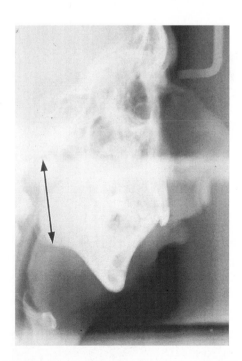

FIGURE A1.23 Preoperative lateral cephalometric radiograph demonstrating Class II malocclusion with mandibular ramus hypoplasia.

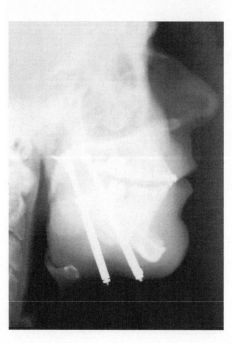

FIGURE A1.24 Postoperative lateral cephalometric radiograph demonstrating mandibular ramus lengthening with single vector distraction device with occlusion corrected to Class I.

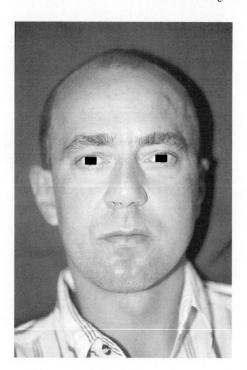

FIGURE A1.26 Postoperative facial view with improved mandibular lengthening.

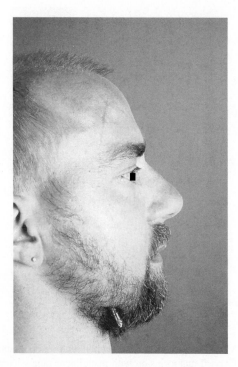

FIGURE A1.25 Postoperative lateral profile view with distractors still in place with percutaneous exposure.

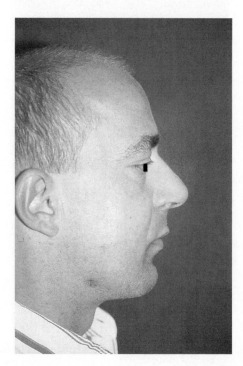

FIGURE A1.27 Postoperative lateral profile view with improved mandibular lengthening and chin position.

Appendix A2
ITI Strauman Dental Implant System

Alex M. Greenberg

Recent developments in the ITI Strauman dental implant system (Figure A2.1) (Institut Strauman AG, Waldenburg, Switzerland) have improved the surface layer (SLE) as well as the basic prosthetic procedures (Figures A2.2 and A2.3). Illustrated here are several examples of these techniques. A

simplified technique using solid abutments (Figures A2.4 and A2.5), transfer systems for impressions (Figures A2.6–A2.8), laboratory steps (Figures A2.9–A2.12) is shown. A special orthodontic appliance is also available (Figure A2.13).

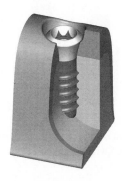

FIGURE A2.1 ITI implant in situ with ideal bone contact and gingival contour. (Courtesy of Institut Strauman AG, Waldenburg, Switzerland)

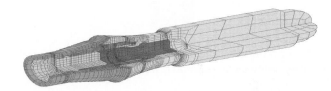

FIGURE A2.3 Finite element model of entire synOcta implant test setup. (Courtesy of Institut Strauman AG, Waldenburg, Switzerland)

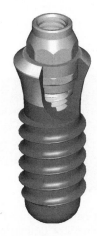

FIGURE A2.2 Corresponding abutment to the synOcta implant. (Courtesy of Institut Strauman AG, Waldenburg, Switzerland)

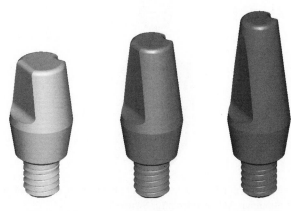

FIGURE A2.4 Overview of solid abutments. (Courtesy of Institut Strauman AG, Waldenburg, Switzerland)

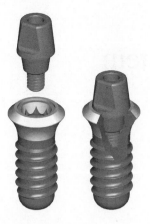

FIGURE A2.5 Wide neck ITI implant with corresponding abutment for cemented restoration. (Courtesy of Institut Strauman AG, Waldenburg, Switzerland)

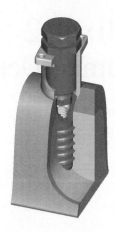

FIGURE A2.8 Transfer system in place for clinical application. (Courtesy of Institut Strauman AG, Waldenburg, Switzerland)

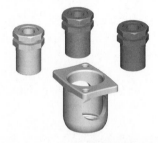

FIGURE A2.6 Corresponding solid abutments with transfer system. (Courtesy of Institut Strauman AG, Waldenburg, Switzerland)

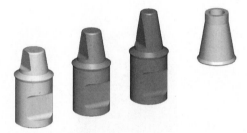

FIGURE A2.9 Implant laboratory analogs. (Courtesy of Institut Strauman AG, Waldenburg, Switzerland)

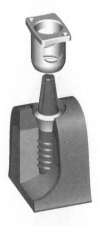

FIGURE A2.7 Transfer system for solid abutment. (Courtesy of Institut Strauman AG, Waldenburg, Switzerland)

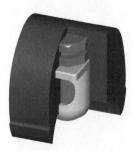

FIGURE A2.10 Positioning cylinder and transfer coping embedded in impression material. (Courtesy of Institut Strauman AG, Waldenburg, Switzerland)

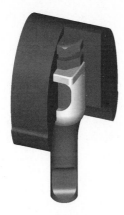

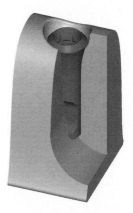

FIGURE A2.11 Full metal implant laboratory analog in situ. (Courtesy of Institut Strauman AG, Waldenburg, Switzerland)

FIGURE A2.12 Master cast with implant laboratory analog. (Courtesy of Institut Strauman AG, Waldenburg, Switzerland)

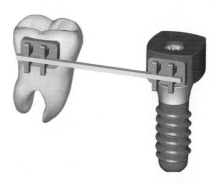

FIGURE A2.13 Indication for use with an orthodontic appliance in combination with ITI implants. (Courtesy of Institut Strauman AG, Waldenburg, Switzerland)

Index

A

Abrasion injuries, craniomaxillofacial, 48
Abutments
  intrusion of, 248–250
  for ITI dental implants, 143–152
  selection of, by the restorative dentist,
    234–235
  surgery at, and progressive bone
    loading, 189
Achondroplasia, saddle nose deformity in,
  52
Acrocephalosyndactyly. *See* Apert
  syndrome
Acrocephaly, defined, 10
Acrylic implants
  fractures of, 256
  self-cure versus light cured or
    autopolymerized, 238–239
  wafer
    construction of, cleft lip and palate,
      561
    placement in a Le Fort I osteotomy,
      cleft lip and palate, 566
Actinomycotic osteomyelitis, 80
Adaptation
  membrane, in localized ridge
    augmentation, 156
  in response to osteotomy, 639
Adenoid cystic carcinoma, involving the
  mandibular angle, 392–393
Adenoid faces, 40
Advantages
  of genioplasty, 652
  of intraoral vertical ramus osteotomy,
    646
  of mandibular midline split, 648
  of midface osteotomy, 657
  of rigid fixation
    with mandibular sagittal split ramus
      osteotomies, 642–643
    with maxillary surgery, 654
  of subapical osteotomy, 651
Aesthetics
  in craniomaxillofacial bone surgery,
    280–286
  in Crouzon syndrome, assessment of,
    713–714
  of dental implant restoration, 255–256

in dental implant restoration, mandible
    versus maxilla, 236–237
  in Treacher Collins syndrome, 283
Alar base, support of, in cleft lip and
  palate, 540, 542
Alar crease (A), for evaluation of
  craniomaxillofacial deformity, 7
Allogeneic grafts
  healing of, 126–127
  for the maxillary sinus, 181–182
  for sinus lift procedures, outcomes, 132
Alloplastic grafts
  defect-bridging, 419
  healing of, 126–127
  maxillary sinus, 182–184
Alternatives, consideration of risks and
  benefits of bimaxillary surgery,
  523
Alveolar augmentation, 160
Alveolar defect, secondary, 549–550
Alveolar nerve, inferior, computerized
  tomography imaging of, 198, 201
Amblyopia, preventing with surgery, in
  Apert syndrome, 750
Ameloblastomas, 59–61
  bone resection and reconstruction in,
    166, 324
  condylar prosthesis after surgery, 375
  panoramic images, 223–224
  reconstruction after surgery for, 406–408
American Association of Cleft Palate
  Rehabilitation (AACPR), 23
Anastomoses, end-to-end, revascularization
  of grafts as a result of, 125
Anatomy
  facial, analysis of, 623–624
  in Le Fort II osteotomy, 660
  of the maxillary sinus, 179
  of midface hypoplasia, 664
  soft tissue landmarks, 7–8
  See also Facial anatomy
Andy Gump Deformity, 414–415
Anesthesia
  local, for hemostasis, 591
  during maxillary surgery, 528
Aneurysms
  basilar tip, transfacial access osteotomies
    for repair of, 494

basilar tip and midbasilar artery,
    transfacial access osteotomies for
    repair of, 489
  midbasilar artery, transfacial access
    osteotomies for repair of, 492
Angiofibromas, juvenile nasopharyngeal,
  resection with transfacial access
  osteotomy, 489, 493
Angle classification, in skeletal
  malocclusions, 38
Ankylosis
  bilateral condylar replacement with steel
    prosthesis in, 376
  condylar prostheses in patients with,
    377–381
  fibrous, of the temporomandibular joint,
    following rigid fixation, 619
Anterior areas, in maxillary implant
  positioning, 244, 246–247
Anterior examination, before orthognathic
  surgery, 506–509
Anterior mandibular defects, microvascular
  tissue transfer for, 414–418
Antibiotics
  for posttraumatic osteomyelitis
    treatment, 433
  in transfacial access osteotomies, 496
Apertognathia
  anterior
    maxillary osteotomies for correction
      of, 603
    secondary to posterior maxillary
      vertical hyperplasia, 586
    tongue habits as a cause of, 647
Apert syndrome (acrocephalosyndactyly),
  35–36, 664, 679–680, 682
  bilateral coronal synostosis in, 675
  craniosynostosis in, 673
  hypertelorism and telecanthus in, 509
  surgical correction of craniofacial
    deformities in, 749–755
  temporal abnormality in, 11
Apicocoronal positioning, in single tooth
  restorations, 250
Application, of classification of cranial
  bone deformities, 96–97
Arteriogram, of a midbasilar artery
  aneurysm, 492

Arthroplasty
    autogenous, 343
    costochondral, relative advantages and
        disadvantages of, 343
    interpositional, for treating restricted
        mobility of the temporomandibular
        joint, 353–354
    partial, replacement of the condyle in,
        372
Arthrosis, before costochondral
    reconstruction, 463
Ascending ramus, microvascular
    reconstruction of, 462–477
Assessment. See Evaluation
Asymmetry assessment, 8
Auricle
    deformity of, 16
        in hemifacial microsomia, 730
    reconstruction of, in hemifacial
        microsomia, 733
Autogenous bone grafts
    contraindications to, 377
    maxillary sinus, 180–181
    for maxillofacial reconstruction,
        295–309
    for ridge augmentation, 157
Autoimmune disorders, deformities
    influenced by, 5
Autologous bone grafts
    healing of, 125–126
    resorption of, 129
    vascularized, healing of, 126
Avulsion injuries, craniomaxillofacial, 43

B

Bar-retained overdentures, 241–242
Barrier membrane, for localized ridge
    augmentation, 155–156
Basalioma, forehead, 368
Basel approach, to cleft lip and palate,
    544–546
Bicoronal suture release, in initial
    treatment for Crouzon syndrome,
    717
Bicortical grafts, for mandibular
    reconstruction, 300
Bilateral complete cleft lip and palate
    (UCLP), deformities in, 557
Bilateral sagittal split ramus osteotomy
    (BSSRO), 527, 639–645
Bimaxillary retrusion, aesthetic repair in,
    284
Binder syndrome (maxillonasal dysplasia),
    51–52, 520, 660
Biocompatibility
    of grafts, and success of incorporation,
        127
    of polymers for bone fixation, 114–115
Biodegradable materials, for bone fixation,
    113

Biomechanical considerations
    for mandibular fixed reconstructions,
        239–240
    in single tooth replacement, 253
Bioresorbable materials, for bone fixation,
    113–123
Birth process, nasal injuries during, 54
Bite, recording, in planning for
    orthognathic surgery, 514–518
Block grafts, experimental comparison
    with particulate grafts, 128
Blood transfusion, autologous, in elective
    surgery, 591
Bolton standard heads and faces, 514–518
Bone
    benign tumors of the maxillofacial
        region, 59–64
    fixation of, bioresorbable materials for,
        113–123
    fragments of, rotation and interposition
        of, 631
    principles of healing, 101
    quality and strength of, in fixation, 104
    quality and volume of, for dental
        implant restoration, 233
    resection of tumors and reconstruction,
        condyle and ascending ramus, 470
    substitutes for, in mandibular
        reconstruction, 336
    trimming of, and maxillary positioning,
        597–600
    See also specific entries, e.g. Frontal bone
Bone-anchored hearing aid (BAHA), 132
Bone grafts
    for alveolar cleft defect, 542–554
    calvarial, harvesting techniques,
        700–712
    fixation of, for mandibular continuity
        defects, 317–326
    free autogenous, in maxillofacial
        reconstruction, 295–300
    iliac, factors affecting success of
        mandibular continuity defect
        reconstruction, 339–341
    to improve stability of maxillary
        osteotomies, clinical studies, 587
    for nasal reconstruction, 483–488
    pedicled, in maxillofacial reconstruction,
        300–308
    secondary, 554–555
    See also Autogenous bone grafts;
        Autologous bone grafts; Cancellous
        bone grafts; Corticocancellous bone
        grafts; Endochondral bone grafts;
        Iliac entries
Bone morphogenic protein (BMP), 180
Boo-Chai classification, of facial clefts, 23
Brachycephaly
    in Apert syndrome, 675–677
    in Crouzon syndrome, 675–677, 713

simple, versus Crouzon syndrome,
        715–717
Brain
    coverage of, with musculocutaneous
        flaps, 364
    limitation on growth, in
        craniosynostosis, 673
Breathing, difficulty in, Crouzon
    syndrome, 713
Bridging osteosynthesis, 321
    for mandibular continuity defects, 327
Buccolingual atrophy, 204
    computerized tomography imaging of,
        206–207

C

Caldwell "C" osteotomy, 610
Callostasis, 648–650
Calvaria
    bone flaps from, for reconstruction in
        maxillary midface defects, 356–359
    defects in, from traumatic injury, 708,
        710
    graft harvesting
        morbidity in, 668
        techniques, 700–712
Cancellous bone grafts, 125–126, 130
    harvesting blocks from the iliac crest,
        299–300
    healing of, maxillary sinus grafting, 180
Cancer. See Malignancies
Carpenter syndrome, 29–30
    facial features in, 36
Case example
    abutments and overdentures, 146–153
    cleft lip and alveolus, unilateral
        complete, 548–550
    cleft lip and palate
        bilateral complete, 548, 551, 554,
            557–559
        unilateral, 547
        unilateral complete, 551–553
    cleft palate, in one of identical twins,
        557, 560
    cranial-based defect reconstruction, with
        calvarial bone grafts, 711–712
    distraction osteogenesis, 649–650
    early relapse, after mandibular sagittal
        split ramus osteotomy, 643–644
    genial deficiency, 652–653
    genioplasty, 653
    infection followed by anterior frontal
        bone collapse, 711
    infraorbital rim defect, 705–706
    intraoral vertical ramus osteotomy,
        646–647
    the Le Fort I maxillary osteotomy
        for apertognathia and mandibular
            excess, 655–657
        midface, 657–658

long-term relapse, mandibular sagittal split ramus osteotomy, 644–645

mandibular midline split, study of rigid fixation versus wire osteosynthesis, 648

maxillary advancement and downward movement, in cleft lip and palate, unilateral, 567, 572–573

maxillary and chin advancement, in cleft lip and palate, unilateral, 567, 570–571

maxillary buttress defect, 705, 707–708

maxillary hypoplasia, in cleft lip and palate, bilateral complete, 562, 565

naso-maxillary hypoplasia, in cleft lip and palate, unilateral complete, 574–576

orbital floor defects, 704–705

orbital reconstruction, 480–482

osteotomy, in cleft lip and palate, bilateral complete, 567–569

overdentures, 262–265

premaxilla repositioning, cleft lip and palate, bilateral complete, 562–564

radiologic follow-up of bone grafts, 220–231

ridge augmentation, 159–162

of subapical osteotomy, 651

THORP-plate reconstruction of bilateral maxillary defects, 439–444

zygomatic arch defect, 708–709

Casts, master
transfer copings for fabrication of dental, 238–239
verification of fit, 239

Cephalometrics, 285, 514

Cervical spine
deformities of, in Apert syndrome, 750–751
osteomyelitis of, 85–86

Cheeks, assessing deformity of, 14–15

Chemical reactions, of metals in solution, 109–110

Chemicals, association with craniofacial malformation, 671

Children
craniomaxillofacial implants in, 134–135
effects on growth capacity of harvesting vascularized bone grafts, 361

Children's Medical Center, Dallas, orbital rim advancement at, 673

Chin, as a donor site for bone grafts, 295–296. See also Genioplasty

Chin-neck contour, assessment of, in craniomaxillofacial deformity, 18–19

Chromosome disorders, nasal manifestations of, 50. See also Hereditary conditions

Classification
of bone quality and quantity, Lekholm and Zarb, 234
of cleft lip and palate deformities, 539–540
of craniofacial deformities, 22
of craniomaxillofacial deformities, 90–97
nasal, 49–58
traumatic, 43–46
of craniosynostosis, 673–678
syndromes, 35–36
of facial clefts, 23
of genioplasties, 627
of hemifacial microsomia, 683–684, 730–733
of nasal encephaloceles, 53

Cleft lip and palate, 22–29
cancellous bone grafting for, 356
nasal deformity in, 50–51
reconstruction of osseous defects in, 539–580
segmental osteotomy in, 587

Cleft palate (CP)
association with Apert syndrome, 679
case example, 557
narrowing the mandible for, 648
treatment planning for, 526

Clefts, all-in-one surgery to close, 545–546

Clinical characteristics
of hemifacial microsomia, 682–683, 728–730
of Treacher Collins syndrome, 685

Clinical examination
findings
in acute osteomyelitis, 80–81
in osteomyelitis of the frontal bone, 85
history of craniomaxillofacial deformity, 6–7
before orthognathic surgery, 497–512

Clinical implications, of metal implants, 111

Clinical studies
of biodegradable materials in fracture surgery, 116–117
of osteotomy segments, with and without bone grafts, 587
of radiation, effects of reconstruction plates, 422–429
See also Research

Clivus chordomas, resection of, with transfacial access osteotomies, 489–496

Cocaine, nasal deformities from abuse of, 57

Cohen classification, of craniosynostosis syndromes, 35–36

Collateral circulation, labiobuccal and palatal vascular, 581, 585

Complications
of bone graft harvesting, 703
of dental implant restoration, 253–257
of free-tissue transfer, 393
of genioplasty, 631–638
of iliac corticocancellous grafts, 339
of irradiation, effects on soft tissue, 427
of Le Fort I osteotomy, necrosis of the maxilla, 83
of Le Fort III osteotomy
in Crouzon syndrome, 723–724
midface reconstruction, 667–668
of mandibular condylar prostheses, 379–387
with mandibular condylar prosthesis, 377–388
of maxillary osteotomies, 587, 590–591
of maxillary sinus grafting, 189–195
of orthognathic surgery, 519–520
of reconstruction
with cancellous bone and marrow in titanium trays, 299–300
in irradiated fields, 290
of mandibular continuity defects, 317–319
of rigid internal fixation, 618–619
of temporomandibular joint surgery, 346

Compression, toleration by dental implants, 233–234

Computed tomography (CT)
in craniomaxillofacial bone infections, 78
for craniomaxillofacial dental implantology, 198–209
for evaluating craniofacial deformities, 672
in infantile osteomyelitis, 83
of the maxillary sinus, 176
in oral malignancies, 69
three-dimensional reconstruction, oromandibular complex, 291
for quantitative assessment of the cranio-orbito-zygomatic skeleton, 714
reformatting into cross-sectional views, for dental implant restoration, 232
three-dimensional reconstructions from, for planning surgical procedures, 462
for visualization of the bony orbit, 478

Computer packages, for planning orthognathic surgery, 561

Condylar heads, remodeling and resorption of, 618

Condyle
abnormality of, in hemifacial microsomia, 729
benign tumor of, image after temporomaxillary joint alloarthroplasty, 380
microvascular reconstruction of, 462–477

Condyle (*Continued*)
  resorption of, and late relapse after osteotomy, 639, 643
  setting the position of, in bimaxillary surgery, 527
Congenital deformity
  craniomaxillofacial, 5
  dysplasia as an indication for costochondral grafting, 354
  facial clefting, 22–29
  nasal, 49–54
  See also Hereditary conditions
Connective tissue, around dental implants, plasma-sprayed titanium, 142–143
Contraindications
  to autogenous transplants, 377
  to fibula donation, smoking as, 414
Coronal synostosis, unilateral, 675
Corrosion, of metal in internal fixation, 107
Cortical bone
  for grafts and implants, clinical outcomes, 130
  healing of grafts of, 126
    maxillary sinus grafting, 180
  skull donor sites for grafting of, 300
Corticocancellous bone grafts, 130–131
  autologous intramembranous, to maxilla, 131–132
  free, for the maxilla, 356–371
  hip inner surface as a donor site for, 300
  for mandibular continuity defects, 321
  for the maxillary sinus, 180–181
Cosmetic failure, in genioplasty, 634–638
Costochondral arthroplasty, polymer screws for fixation of, 121
Costochondral grafts
  advantage of, response to growth, 353
  for condylar reconstruction, disadvantages of, 462
  free, mandibular condyle reconstruction with, 343–355
  in hemifacial microsomia, 733–735
Cranial base
  calvarial bone grafts for reconstruction of, 711–712
  microsurgical reconstruction of large defects of, 356–371
Cranial bones
  deformities of, classification, 95
  as donor sites
    in cranio-orbito-zygomatic procedures, 715
    in midface reconstruction, 662
Cranial circumference, for evaluating craniomaxillofacial deformity, 9–10
Cranial deformities
  clefts, 25
  in hemifacial microsomia, 728
Cranial modular fixation system, 456–458

Cranial sutures
  examination of, 10
  premature closure of, classification of anomalies from, 29
Cranial vault, in Crouzon syndrome
  osteotomy, 722–723
  reshaping of, 718–719
Craniocervical junction, exposure of, 494
Craniofacial deformities, 22–37
  clefts, 25
  dysostosis, 678–681
    in Crouzon syndrome, 713
  principles of management of, 671–692
  surgical correction of, in Apert syndrome, 749–755
Craniofacial fixation system
  effects on the growing craniofacial skeleton, 693–699
  hardware review, 445–461
Craniofacial Modular Fixation System, 445–450
Craniofacial osteotomy instrumentation sets, 629
Craniofacial reconstruction, vascularized bone grafts for, 313
Craniofacial Repair System (CRS), 459–461
Craniofacial synostoses, inherited, 52
Craniomaxillofacial bone
  healing of
    biomechanics and rigid internal fixation, 101–106
    after surgery, 124–137
  infections of, 76–89
    radiographic diagnosis, 78
  metal for internal fixation, 107–112
  radiographic evaluation of, 210–219
Craniomaxillofacial deformity
  classification system for, 90–97
  evaluation of, 5–21
  nasal, 49–58
  traumatic, 43–48
Craniomaxillofacial dental implantology, 198–209
Craniomaxillofacial surgery, 1
  reconstructive
    versus corrective, 41–42
    current practice and trends in, 310–316
Cranio-orbital decompression, in Crouzon syndrome, 715–717
Cranio-orbito-zygomatic procedures, cranial bones as donor sites in, 715
Craniostenosis, surgical correction of the bony forehead in, 8
Craniosynostosis, 673–678
  classification of, 29–37
  in Crouzon syndrome, 713
Craniotomy bone flap, 703
Cranium, donor site, for nasal reconstruction, 483, 486–488

Creeping substitution
  defined, 125
  fixation required for, 327
  in maxillary sinus grafting, 180
  in ridge augmentation, 157
Cross sectional images, computer-generated, 200–201
Crouzon syndrome, 29, 32, 35, 664, 673, 678–679
  basic dysmorphology and staging of reconstruction, 713–726
  bilateral coronal synostosis in, 675
Cupar technique, 601
  for anterior maxillary osteotomy downfracture, 591
Cuspid area, in maxillary implant positioning, 243

D

Degenhardt classification, of craniofacial deformity, 23
Delaire analysis, in planning orthognathic surgery, 514
Demineralized freeze-dried bone (DFDB), bone morphogenic protein in, 181–182
Dental compensations, in hemifacial microsomia, 729
Dental examination, before orthognathic surgery, 512
Dental implants
  grafts from the fibula for insertion of, 327
  ITI system, 138–154
Dentascan program, examples of images generated by, 198, 201–208
Dermoids, nasal, 54
Developmental deformity, craniomaxillofacial, 5. *See also* Embryology
Dexamethasone, postoperative administration of, in transfacial access osteotomy, 496
Diagnosis
  differential, of hemifacial microsomia, 727
  of oral squamous cell carcinoma, 67–68
  of orbital hypertelorism, 738
  of osteomyelitis of the cervical spine, 86
Disadvantages
  of genioplasty, 652
  of intraoral vertical ramus osteotomy, 646
  of mandibular midline split, 648
  of midface osteotomy, 657
  of rigid fixation
    in mandibular sagittal split ramus osteotomy, 643
    in maxillary surgery, 654
  of subapical osteotomy, 651

Disease
  maternal, and nasal deformities, 50
  systemic, and nasal deformities, 57
  See also Infection
Displacement, osseous, in osteotomy, 639
Distraction osteogenesis, 648–650
Donor sites
  for alveolar grafts, 544
  calvarial, reconstruction with alloplastic materials, 702
  for mandibular reconstruction, 310–313
  for midface reconstruction, 662
    morbidity at, 668
  for nasal reconstruction, 483
    parietal bone, 742
Dosimetry, on an irradiation phantom, 420–421
Double barrel graft, fibular, for arched mandibular defects, 329–333
Downfracture, risks of, 567
Drugs, association with craniofacial malformation, 671
Dura, coverage of, with musculocutaneous flaps, 364
Dysmorphology
  in cleft lip and palate, 540–542
  defined, 672
Dysostosis, craniofacial, in Crouzon syndrome, 713. *See also* Mandibulofacial dysostosis

E
Economic considerations
  in internal fixation, 2
  in primary reconstruction, in gunshot wounds, 416
  in rigid internal fixation, for bimaxillary surgery, 522
Ectodermal cysts, nasal dermoid, 54
Edentulous restorations, dental implant, 236–237
  partial, 245–250
Embryology
  of the calvarium, 700–701
  of the craniofacial region, 671
  of nasal deformities, 49–50
  of the palate, lip and alveolus, 539–542
Emergence Profile System, for single tooth abutments, 252
Encephaloceles, nasal, 53
Endochondral bone grafts
  for maxillary sinus grafting, 180–181
  preformed, clinical use of, 130–131
Endocrine disorders, deformities caused by, 5
Endosseous implants
  and bone grafting, 124–132
  selection of, 184–185
Eosinophilic granuloma, treatment for, 63

Epidemiology
  of craniomaxillofacial fractures and defects, 5
  of hemifacial microsomia, 727
  of oral squamous cell carcinoma, 65
Epiphyseal dysplasia, in Apert syndrome, 750
Epithelium, around dental implants, plasma-sprayed titanium, 142–143
Ethanol, nasal deformities due to in utero exposure to, 50
Etiology
  of cleft lip and palate, 539
  of craniofacial deformities, congenital, 671–672
  of craniomaxillofacial deformities
    in Apert syndrome, 749–750
    nasal, 49–58
  of hemifacial microsomia, 727–728
  of oral malignancies, 65
  of osteomyelitis, 76–77
    of the frontal bone, 84
  of skeletal malocclusion, 38–42
  of suppurative osteomyelitis of the mandible, 80
  See also Pathogenesis
Etiopathology, of orbital hypertelorism, 739–740
Evaluation
  of Apert syndrome patients, 750–751
  of craniomaxillofacial deformity patients, 5–21
  before reconstructive surgery, 390
  of tumor extension, in oral malignancies, 68–69
Examination cycle, before orthognathic surgery, 500
Exophthalmus, association with hyperthyroidism, 5
Exorbitism
  in Apert syndrome, 35, 750
  in bilateral coronal synostosis, 675
  in malar deficiency, 15
Expectations, patient's, in dental implant restoration, 256–257
Explosions, craniomaxillofacial injuries from, 47
Extender System, ITI, 164
Extracranial procedures, in orbital hypertelorism management, 744
Eye, evaluating, 11–12. *See also* Vision
Eyebrows, position of, evaluating, 12–13
Eyelids
  deformities of, in Apert syndrome, 752
  evaluating, 13

F
Facial anatomy
  analysis of, for genioplasty, 623–624

clinical evaluation of, in cleft lip and palate, 551
growth of, in hemifacial microsomia, 729–730
planning height, in bimaxillary surgery, 526–527
proportions, for clinical examination, 506–507
width, describing in a clinical examination, 508–509
Facial angles, for evaluation of craniomaxillofacial deformity, 7–8
Facial appearance
  clinical evaluation of, in cleft lip and palate, 556
  concepts of harmony in, 280–284
Facial bipartition, in orbital hypertelorism management, 742–745
Facial clefting, 22–29
  embryological origin of, 671
  rare, 52–53
Facial contour angle (FCA), for evaluation of craniomaxillofacial relationships, 8
Facio-auriculo-vertebral (FAV) malformation complex, 727
Faciolingual orientation, in single tooth restorations, 250
Farm injuries, craniomaxillofacial, 47–48
Fetal compression, nasal injuries from, 54
Fibroma, ossifying, reconstruction after removal, in a child, 368–369
Fibrous dysplasia, treatment for, 63
Fibula
  and combined flaps, for maxillofacial reconstruction, 306–308
  dissection of, 391
  as a donor site
    advantages of, 414
    for ascending ramus and condyle grafts, 466
    for mandibular continuity defects, 321
    for mandibular reconstruction, 310, 312–313, 471–474, 475–476
    indications and technical considerations for use of, 327–334
Fibular flap, for mandibular reconstruction, 389–390
Finnish Cancer Registry, standardized incidence ratio for oral cancer, 65–66
Fixation methods
  in bimaxillary surgery, 532–533
  biodegradable polymer screws for, in sagittal osteotomy, 119, 121
  during bone healing, 101–106, 336–337
  in the craniofacial system, hardware review, 445–461
  in genioplasty, 628–633
  in nasal reconstruction, 483–484
  in orbital hypertelorism reconstruction, 744
  See also Plates; Screws

Fixture insertion
  computerized tomography images for
    reviewing placement, 205
  surgical technique, maxillary sinus
    grafting, 187
Flap contouring, for maxillofacial
  reconstruction, 303–304
Follow-up
  after oral cancer treatment, 72–73
  after temporomandibular joint surgery,
    350–351
  See also Outcomes
Fontanelles
  in craniomaxillofacial deformity, Apert
    syndrome, 749
  description of, 671
  evaluating, in craniomaxillofacial
    deformity, 10
Forehead
  advancement of, in Apert syndrome,
    751
  landmarks of, 10–11
Foreign body reactions, to self-reinforcing
  polylactide copolymer, 115
Fractures
  fixation of, self-reinforced polymers for,
    120–121
  posttraumatic osteomyelitis at the site of,
    433
  spontaneous, of an irradiated edentulous
    mandible, 229–230
Franceschetti-Zwahlen-Klein syndrome,
  Tessier classification of, 28
Frankfort horizontal plane (FH), for
  evaluation of craniomaxillofacial
  deformity, 7
Free-tissue transfer, in mandibular
  reconstruction, 338
Frontal bone
  anterior, calvarial bone graft
    reconstruction, 711
  deformities of, classification, 95
  osteomyelitis of, 84–85
Frontal view, for evaluating
  craniomaxillofacial deformity, 9
Frontonasal dysplasia, 52
Full-thickness outer cortex calvarial bone
  graft, 702
Functional considerations
  in Crouzon syndrome, 713
  problems associated with
    craniosynostosis, 673

G
Gallium-67 scans
  in craniomaxillofacial bone infection, 79
  in osteomyelitis of the frontal bone, 85
Garre sclerosing osteomyelitis, 82
Genetic counseling
  in craniofacial deformity, 672

for orthognathic surgery candidates,
    497–500
Genetic diagnosis, in craniofacial
  deformities, 672
Genetic predisposition, in primary
  craniosynostosis, 29
Genial deficiency, aesthetic repair of, 282
Genioplasty, 574, 651–653
  combination with ramus osteotomy, 648
  considerations for rigid internal fixation,
    623–638
  mandibular horizontal osteotomy for,
    611
  passive, 624–626
  sliding, 612
    rigid fixation in, 617
Giant cell granulomas, 62
Gingival tissues, evidence of implant
  failure in, 253–254
Glenoid reconstruction, in hemifacial
  microsomia, 734
Gliomas, nasal, 53
Globe, position of, and craniomaxillofacial
  deformity, 13
Gnathion (Gn), for evaluation of
  craniomaxillofacial deformity, 7
Gold
  for dental restoration substructures, 239
  for octa-abutment screw-retained dental
    restorations, 145–147
Goldenhar syndrome, 463, 727
  macrostomia in, 730
  vertebral defects in, 728
Gonzalez-Ulloa line, for evaluating
  craniomaxillofacial deformity, 9
Grafts
  cantilevered bone, for orbital
    reconstruction, 480
  corticocancellous block, harvesting for
    ridge augmentation, 157
  factors affecting success of, 127
  fixation of, in mandibular continuity
    defect reconstruction, 319–320
  materials for maxillary sinus grafting,
    179
  metatarsal, for mandibular
    reconstruction, 474
  for nasal reconstruction, 483–488
  reconstructive, 124–132
  resorption as a measure of failure in,
    216
  tertiary, in cleft lip and palate, 556
  See also Bone grafts
Grisel syndrome, 86
Growth
  disturbances of
    association with cleft lip and palate,
      541–542
    association with midface
      reconstruction, 668

effects of plate and screw fixation on the
    craniofacial skeleton, 693–699
  excessive, after reconstruction of the
    mandible, 464
  facial
    effect of cleft lip and palate surgery,
      500
    in hemifacial microsomia, 729–730
    of nonvascularized grafts, 462
    restricted, after osteotomy and fixation,
      696–699
Guided bone regeneration (GBR), 155–163
  biodegradable membranes used in,
    118–120
  case report, 161
  chin, after harvesting bone, 296
Guided tissue regeneration (GTR), 127
Gunshot wounds, 43–46

H
Handgun injuries, 47
Haptens, metals as, 110
Hardware
  for internal fixation, 599–601
    in intraoral vertical ramus osteotomy,
      646
    in mandibular sagittal split ramus
      osteotomy, 640–642
    in ramus osteotomy, 648
    in subapical osteotomy, 651
  for Le Fort I maxillary osteotomy, 654
    midface, 657
  for stabilizing genioplasty, 652
Harkens classification, of cleft lip and
  palate, 23
Harvesting, of calvarial bone grafts,
  701–703
Healing
  duration of, in ridge augmentation,
    157–158
  in maxillary sinus grafting, 179–181
  of posttraumatic osteomyelitis, by
    secondary intention, 433
  process of, 125
  of reconstruction, after radiation therapy,
    335
  soft-tissue, in the presence of a
    membrane, 156
  after surgery, craniomaxillofacial,
    124–137
Hearing disorders
  in cleft infants, 541
  in Crouzon syndrome, 713
  external hearing aids for, skin-
    penetrating implants, 132–133
Helsinki University Central Hospital,
  Department of Oral and
  Maxillofacial Surgery, 377
Hematomas, nasal, deformity from
  untreated, 55

Hemifacial microsomia (HFM), 681–685, 727–737
  presurgery and postsurgery views, 686–687
Hemimandibulectomy
  for osteogenic sarcoma, 469
  reconstruction following, 471
  reconstruction with alloplast, 385
Hemorrhage
  in craniofacial surgery, 667–668
  in maxillary sinus grafting, 194
Hemostasis, in maxillary surgery, 528
Hereditary conditions
  autosomal dominant
    Apert syndrome, 679
    Crouzon syndrome, 678–679
    hemifacial microsomia, 727–728
  nasal deformity in, 50–52
  See also Congenital deformity
Heterotopic bone, formation of, in temporomandibular joint arthroplasty, 381
Histology, clinical, of implants in bone grafts, 128–130
History
  of the Le Fort I osteotomy, 581
  of mandibular osteotomies, 606–609
  Mesopotamian, of craniofacial cleft, 27
  observation of osteomyelitis, 76
  Roman, of osteomyelitis of the frontal bone, 84
  of segmental maxillary osteotomy, 587
  of a surgical approach to craniosynostosis, 715
History, patient's, assessment of craniomaxillofacial deformity, 6
Holoprosencephaly, facial anomalies in, 52
Human experimentation, on the stability of maxillofacial implants, 135
Hunsuck effect, avoiding, 615–616
Hydantoin, nasal deformities due to in utero exposure to, 50
Hydrocephalus
  association with Crouzon syndrome, 713
  in Kleeblatschumldel deformity, 36
Hydroxyapatite (HA), synthetic, 182–184
Hyperbaric oxygen treatment (HBO), effect of, on implant success, 133–134
Hypertelorbitism, in cleft lip and palate, bilateral complete, 567–569
Hypertelorism, in clefts, 28–29

I
Iatrogenic injuries, nasal deformities from, 57
Iliac bone grafts
  morbidity in harvesting, 668
  onlay grafts, outcomes, 131
  radiologic follow-up, 222

with soft tissue flaps, for maxillofacial reconstruction, 301–303
Iliac corticocancellous grafts
  complications of, 339
  immediate versus delayed placement, study, 131
Iliac crest, donor site
  for ascending ramus and condyle grafts, 465–467
  for free bone grafts, 298–300
  for mandibular continuity defect repair, 321
  for mandibular reconstruction, 310–311, 389–390, 414
  for nasal reconstruction, 483
Ilizarov method, for distraction osteogenesis, 648–650
Imaging
  methods for evaluation of the craniomaxillofacial region, 210–212
  in osteomyelitis of the frontal bone, 85
  in suppurative osteomyelitis, 81
Immunocompetence, and osteomyelitis incidence, 76–77
Implants
  connecting to natural teeth, 247–248
  defined, 124–125
  dental
    failure of, 253–254
    full-body-screw (S), 138, 164
    hollow-cylinder, 139–140
    hollow-screw, 138–139
  fracture of, 254
  metal, mechanical properties of, 110–111
  module selections, 451–456
  osseointegrated, in cleft lip and palate, 548, 551
Incidence
  of clefting, by geographic location and racial group, 539
  of cleft lip and palate, 22
  of nasal fractures, 55
  of oral squamous cell carcinoma, 65
Incisor display, noting in a clinical examination, 509–510
Indications
  for bilateral sagittal split ramus osteotomy, 639–640
  for bimaxillary surgery, 522–523
  for calvarial bone grafts, 704–711
  for condyle replacement, 372
  for fibula grafts, 327–334
  for free bone grafts, 295
  for genioplasty, 624–627, 651
  for hemifacial microsomia treatment, 733–734
  for intraoral vertical ramus osteotomy, 645–647

for Le Fort I maxillary osteotomy, 656
for Le Fort II osteotomy, 660
for Le Fort III osteotomy, midface reconstruction, 664
for microvascular bone flaps, 301
for onlay grafting, 177–178
for orthognathic surgery, 557, 561
for subapical osteotomy, 650
for temporomandibular joint restoration, 343
Indium scan, white blood cell, in craniomaxillofacial bone infection, 79
Infantile osteomyelitis, 83
Infection
  in craniofacial surgery, 667–668
  of craniomaxillofacial bone, location of, 79
  frontal bone collapse after, calvarial bone graft reconstruction, 711
  in genioplasty, 634
  maternal, craniofacial deformities associated with, 671
  in maxillary sinus grafting, 194
  opportunistic, nasoseptal manifestations of, 57
  postoperative, demonstration on computerized tomography image, 204
Inferior vermilion border (Vi), for evaluation of craniomaxillofacial deformity, 7
Infraorbital rim defect, calvarial bone graft for reconstruction of, 705–706
Inner cortex calvarial bone graft, 703
Instrumentation sets, craniofacial osteotomy, 629
Instruments, craniofacial modular fixation system, 450–451
Intermaxillary fixation, placement with powerchain, 566
Internal fixation
  considerations in radiation therapy, 419–432
  functionally stable, 1
  Le Fort II osteotomy, 662–663
  Le Fort III osteotomy, midface reconstruction, 666–667
  technique for, 599–601, 603
  See also Rigid internal fixation
Interocclusal splint
  preparing from models, 523–525
  transitional, 525–526
Intracranial pressure
  in Apert syndrome, before or after forehead advancement, 750
  and hypertension, association with craniosynostosis, 673, 713
  monitoring of, in young children with Crouzon syndrome, 718

Intracranial procedures, for orbital hypertelorism management, 740–744
Intracranial volume, in Apert syndrome, 749
Intramembranous grafts and implants, 131–132
Intraoperative radiation therapy (IORT), advantages of, 427–429
Intraoral technique, for stabilization in mandibular sagittal split ramus osteotomy, 642
Intraoral tissue, restoration of, after cancer surgery of the head and neck, 290
Intraoral vertical ramus osteotomy (IVRO), 606–607, 614–615
    indications for, 645–647
In utero exposure, nasal deformities due to, 50
Irradiated bone, osteogenetic potential of, 444
ITI Strauman Dental Implant System, 765–767

J
Jaw
    deformity in Crouzon syndrome, management of, 724
    dysfunction of, psychological aspects in, 634
    lower, reconstructive surgery of, radiographic assessment, 213–218
    upper, imaging sequence and interpretation, 212

K
Keratocysts, recurrence of, 59–61, 350–351
Key area, in repair of the orbit, 478–479
Kirschner wires, for craniomaxillofacial bone healing, 102
Kleeblatschumldel deformity, 29, 35–37
Kufner osteotomies, posterior maxillary, 588
    segmental, 602–603

L
Lacrimal apparatus, damage to, in Le Forte III osteotomy, 668
Lag screw technique
    advantages of, in craniofacial surgery, 715
    in mandibular osteotomy, 615–616
        sagittal split ramus, 609, 641
    in nasal reconstruction, 484–488
Lambdoid synostosis, unilateral, 676–678
Lateral arm free flap, for mandibular reconstruction, 338–339
Latissimus-dorsi musculocutaneous flaps, 361, 370–371
Le Fort I maxillary osteotomy
    advantages of, 523
    in cleft lip and palate, 562
        bilateral complete, 565–566

examples of fracture patterns, 582
    history of, 581
    maxillary, 653–656
        necrosis as a complication of, 83
    multiple segment, planning for, 526
    surgical technique, 591–601
    types of, 583–584
Le Fort II osteotomy
    in midface reconstruction, and considerations for internal fixation, 660–668
    in nasomaxillary hypoplasia, 574
Le Fort III osteotomy
    in Crouzon syndrome, history of, 715
    malar maxillary, 574
    for midface reconstruction
        considerations for internal fixation, 660–668
        in Crouzon syndrome, 678–679, 719–721, 723–724
Limberg oblique osteotomy, 610
Lips, clinical assessment of, in craniomaxillofacial deformity, 17–18
Loading, of grafts
    maxillary sinus, 175
    progressive, 189
    and success of incorporation, 127
Lower facial plane (LFP), for evaluation of craniomaxillofacial relationships, 8
Lund classification, of craniofacial deformity, 23
Lymphomas, of extranodal origin, 70

M
Magnetic resonance imaging
    in craniomaxillofacial bone infections, 78
    in oral malignancies, 69
Malar bone
    absence of, in Franceschetti-Zwalen-Klein syndrome, 28
    aesthetic repair of deficiency of, 282–283
    evaluating, in craniomaxillofacial deformity, 15
Malar prominence, defining, in a clinical examination, 509
Malignancies
    carcinoma of the tongue, 400
    condylar reconstruction in, 381
    head and neck cancer, reconstruction in, 289–294
    oral, 65–75
        mandible resection in, 317
    recurrence rates, after marginal mandibulectomy, 411
    See also Tumors
Malocclusion
    in Crouzon syndrome, management of, 724
    after Le Forte III osteotomy, 668

Mandible
    anteroposterior deficiency of, in cleft lip and palate, 557–559
    atypical ossifying fibroma in, panoramic image, 225–226
    biomechanical considerations in reconstruction of, 239–240
    classification of deformities of, 91–92
    comminuted fracture of, 165
    continuity defects of
        decisions about reconstruction of, 335
        fixation of bone grafts in reconstruction, 317–326
    distraction osteogenesis of, 757–764
    edentulous, 237–243
        with overdenture bar, 263
    fixation of
        with experimental polymers, 116
        with polyglycolide materials, 117
    hardware review, 269–279
    implants in, study, 131
    internal fixation of, 1, 533
    with maxillary fixed bridge, 263–264
    midline split of, 647–650
    multiple fractures of, aesthetic repair, 281
    ossifying fibroma in, computerized tomography image, 227–228
    osteomyelitis of, 80–82
    posttraumatic osteomyelitis of, 433–438
    reconstruction of, with vascularized bone grafts, 310–313
    resection due to carcinoma, and restoration, 166–167
    resorption of, in edentulous patients, 236
Mandible Distractor Module Set, 269, 278–279
Mandible reconstruction module, 273
Mandible trauma module, 271–273
Mandibular alveolar osteotomy, total, 606, 650–651
Mandibular alveolar ridge, atrophy of, 168–169
Mandibular angle
    deficiency in, aesthetic repair of, 282
    reconstruction of defects of, 389–394
Mandibular body reconstruction, 395–410
Mandibular condylar reconstruction
    with free costochondral grafting, 343–355
    problems with prostheses, 377–388
Mandibular continuity, reconstruction of, with an angular THORP plate, 404–405
Mandibular osteotomy, 104–105, 529
    anterior midline, 611–613
        rigid fixation in, 617
    with rigid internal fixation, 606–622, 639–659
Mandibular prognathism, 5
    in cleft patients, 574

intraoral vertical ramus osteotomy for treatment of, 606

Mandibular reconstruction plate, exposure of, and infection, 444

Mandibular resection, in oral cancer, 70–72

Mandibular sagittal split ramus osteotomy, 612–614

Mandibular segmental subapical osteotomy anterior, 606, 608–611
rigid internal fixation and acrylic splint in, 617

Mandibular-temporomandibular joint complex, in hemifacial microsomia, 729

Mandibulectomy, marginal, 411–413

Mandibulofacial dysostosis
familial, ear deformities in, 16
Tessier classification of, 28
in Treacher Collins syndrome, 685

Mandibulotomy, stable fixation of, 494

Maternal idiosyncrasies, as potential causes of malformation, 671

Maxilla
atrophied, augmentation of, 131
bilateral defects of, 439–444
deformities of, 92–93
edentulous, 243–245
implants in, study, 131
internal fixation of, 532–533
microsurgical reconstruction of large defects of, 356–371
osteomyelitis of, 82–83
sarcoma of, 366–367

Maxillary alveolar hyperplasia, history of treatment for, 581

Maxillary and chin advancement, after repair of a cleft lip and palate, unilateral complete, 567, 570–571

Maxillary buttress defect, calvarial bone graft reconstruction in, 705, 707–708

Maxillary hyperplasia, posterior, management of, 598–599

Maxillary hypoplasia, in a cleft patient, 556–557
outcome of surgery for, 498

Maxillary/midface defects, reconstruction of, 356–359

Maxillary osteotomies, 581–605
in cleft lip and palate, 551–577
stability of, with rigid internal fixation, 639–659

Maxillary segmental osteotomies
anterior, 601
posterior, 602–603

Maxillary sinus
computerized tomography imaging of pathology of, 206, 208
grafting and osseointegration surgery, 174–197

Maxillofacial bones
ITI dental implant system for, 164–173
tumors of, and bone invasion, 59–64

Maxillofacial surgery, 1
advantages of rigid internal fixation in, 581

Maxillomandibular fixation (MMF)
for autogenous transplants, 377
history of, 606
in orthognathic surgery, radiologic record keeping for, 513
for vertical ramus osteotomy, 615

Maximal Interincisal Opening (MIO), reduction in, and fixation method, 618

Mechanical considerations, in fixation, 104

Medication, maternal exposure to, and nasal deformities, 50

Melanoma, of the oral cavity, 70

Membrane reflections, surgical technique, maxillary sinus grafting, 186–187

Meningiomas, sphenoid wing, transfacial access osteotomies for resection of, 489–496

Mental protuberance, defined, 623

Mentocervical angle (MCA), in evaluation of craniomaxillofacial relationships, 8

Mentolabial sulcus (MLS), in evaluation of craniomaxillofacial deformity, 7

Menton (M), soft tissue, for evaluation of craniomaxillofacial deformity, 7

Mesh module, cranioplast, 456–458

Mesh plate, for orbital reconstruction, 480

Mesiodistal orientation, in single tooth restorations, 250

Metal, for craniomaxillofacial internal fixation, 107–112

Metastatic tumors, of the oral cavity, 70

Metopic synostosis, 675–678

Microbiology
of osteomyelitis of the frontal bone, 85
of suppurative osteomyelitis of the mandible, 80

Microplate fixation, resorbable, in surgery for metopic suture release, 675

Microsomia, hemifacial, 22, 40
reconstruction in, 362–363

Microsurgery, for reconstruction of large defects, 356–371

Microtia
craniomaxillofacial microsomia associated with, 16
prosthesis for, 133

Microvascular bone surgery
composite flaps, for maxillofacial reconstruction, 301
current practice and trends in corrective surgery, 310–316
for reconstruction of defects of the mandibular angle, 389
for reconstruction of the condyle and ascending ramus, 462–477

Microvascular free flaps, for head and neck reconstruction, 289–290

Microvascular module, 273

Microvascular tissue transfer, in reconstruction of anterior defects of the mandible, 414

Midface
defects of, in hemifacial microsomia, 729
Le Fort I osteotomy for deformity of, 656–657
history, 581
management of deformity of, in childhood, 719
microsurgical reconstruction of large defects of, 356–371
multiple fractures of, aesthetic repair, 281
reconstruction of
after cancer surgery, 291–292
Le Fort II and III osteotomies, 660–668

Miniplate fixation systems, 445
anterior mandibular segmental and genioplasty osteotomies, 611–613
craniofacial system, 599–600
in mandibular osteotomies, 617
sagittal split ramus, 642–643
modules, United States and worldwide, 445
titanium, in orbital hypertelorism reconstruction, 744

Models
dental, for planning bimaxillary surgery, 523
for planning orthognathic surgery, 561
three-dimensional, fabrication from computerized tomography data, 463

Modules
cranial bone flap fixation, 1.0–1.5 mm, 457–458
craniofacial modular fixation system, 1.0–20 mm, 445–448

Monobloc osteotomies
in Apert syndrome, 751–752
avoiding, 752–753
in Crouzon syndrome, 722–723

Morbidity
versus benefit from bimaxillary surgery, 523
disability from radical excision of oral cancer, 70–73
long-term, in mandibular continuity defect repair, 327
in repeat craniotomy for Crouzon syndrome, 718–719

Morian classification, of craniofacial deformity, 22–23

Mucosal coverage, utilization for
  reconstruction in
  craniomaxillofacial deformity,
  classification, 90
Multidisciplinary team concept
  for managing craniofacial deformities,
    672, 733
  for managing hemifacial microsomia,
    727
Myocutaneous flap, pectoralis major, 289,
    412–413
  for bilateral maxillary defect repair,
    442–444

N
Nasal aperture, donor site for free bone
    grafts, 296
Nasal dermoids, 54
Nasal dorsum hematomas, 55
Nasal encephalocele, description of, 53
Nasal gliomas, 54
Nasal structure
  cavity, nonseparation from the oral
    cavity, 540
  classification of deformities, 94
  description of bone, 483
  restoring with bone grafts and rigid
    internal fixation, 483–488
  septum, managing in transfacial access
    osteotomy, 495
Nasoendotracheal tube, placing and
    securing in maxillary surgery, 528
Nasofacial angle, measuring, 14
Nasofrontal angle (NFA), for evaluation of
    craniomaxillofacial relationships, 7
Nasomaxillary region, reconstruction of,
    after cancer surgery, 292
Naso-orbital-ethmoid deformities, 94
Necrosis, aseptic, following maxillary
    osteotomy, 590
Nerve damage
  in genioplasty, 634
  in Le Forte III osteotomy, 668
  in rigid internal fixation using bicortical
    screws, 615
Nerve tissue availability, in
    craniomaxillofacial deformity,
    classification, 90
Neural crest cells, role in craniofacial
    development, 38. See also
    Embryology
Neuralgia-inducing cavitational
    osteonecrosis (NICO), 82
Neurologic manifestations, in hemifacial
    microsomia, 728
Neuropsychiatric disorders, association
    with craniosynostosis, 673
Neurosensory disturbances, as a
    complication of rigid internal
    fixation, 619

Nickel, in tissue, toxicity of, 109–110
Nomenclature
  of alveolar bone grafting, 543
  of hemifacial microsomia, 727
  See also Classification
Nose
  assessing the structure of, 13–14
  functions of, 49
Nutrition
  in cleft infants, 540–541
  disorders of, affecting development, 5

O
Occlusion, assessment of
  in cleft lip and palate, 556
  in craniomaxillofacial deformity, 19–20
  in dental implant restoration, 241
  in mandibular overdentures, 243
Occupational injuries, craniomaxillofacial,
    47–48
Ocular mobility, in craniomaxillofacial
    deformity, 13–14. See also Vision
Odontogenic tumors, 59–62
Onlay bone grafts
  in Apert syndrome, 754
  maxillary, versus sinus inlay graft, 177
Open bite deformities
  anterior, bilateral posterior segmental
    osteotomies for treating, 587
  correction of, preoperative and
    postoperative x-rays, 535–536
Operative procedure. See Surgical
    approach/procedures
Ophthalmopathy, association with
    hyperthyroidism, 5
Oral cavity
  assessment of, in craniomaxillofacial
    deformity, 19
  nonseparation from the nasal cavity,
    540
Orbit
  clinical evaluation of, 12
  deformities of, in hemifacial
    microsomia, 728–729
  reconstruction of, 478–482
Orbital blowout, polylactide plates for
    repairing, 115–116
Orbital cleft
  central superior, 28
  superolateral, 28
  superomedial, 28
Orbital expansion, in hemifacial
    microsomia, timing of, 733
Orbital floor repair
  of defects, 362–365
    calvarial bone graft reconstruction,
      704–705
  polymers for fracture fixation, 117
Orbital hypertelorism, 738–748
  analysis of malformation in, 738–739

  in bilateral coronal synostosis, 675
  in metopic synostosis, 675
Orbital implants, 133
Orbital rim advancement (ORA),
    preoperative and postoperative
    views, 675–676
Orbitomaxillary cleft, medial, 26–27
Orbitozygomatic reconstruction, 105
Orientation
  compromised, restoring dental fixtures
    with, 255
  of single-tooth restoration, 250
Oromandibular complex, reconstruction of,
    290–291
  three-dimensional, software for, 291
Oronasal fistulae, closing, 542
Orthodontia
  for children with cleft lip and palate,
    541–542, 561
  in hemifacial microsomia, 735
Orthodontist, role in bimaxillary surgery,
    523
Orthognathic examination, 497–521
Orthognathic modules, craniofacial
    modular fixation system, 454–455
Orthognathic surgery
  after bone graft closure of a palatal
    fistula, 572–573
  in cleft lip and palate, 567
  defined, 639
  examination before undertaking,
    506–520
  indications for, in cleft lip and palate,
    557, 561
  models used for planning, 514–518
Orthopedics, preoperative
  for cleft infants, 542–543
  effect on later bone grafting for alveolar
    clefts, 555–556
Ortho Treatment Planner (software), 514
Osseointegration
  of dental implants, 155
    in bone grafts, 327–328
  in dentistry, 232
  evaluation of, with computerized
    tomography imaging, 203
  of implants in cleft lip and palate
    reconstruction, 548, 551
  maintaining, in dental implant
    restoration, 253
  in maxillary sinus grafting, 174–197
  of metal implants, 124
  of screws in microvascular grafts, 322
  of titanium, 110
    effects of irradiation on, 419
    experimental study in dogs, 128
    plasma-sprayed, 140–142
Osteitis
  defined, 76
  osteoblastic, 83

Osteoarthritis, as an indication for costochondral grafting, 353–354
Osteocutaneous flap, from the fibula, 327–328
Osteogenesis
 effects of irradiation on, before and after implantation, 425–426
 head and neck, 41
Osteogenic sarcoma, hemimandibulectomy, chemotherapy and radiotherapy for, 469
Osteoinduction, defined, 180
Osteomyelitis
 chronic, ankylosis of the temporomandibular joint caused by, 354
 historic observation of, 76
 infantile, 83
 of the mandible
  nonsuppurative, 81–82
  posttraumatic, 433–438
Osteoplastic segment, maintaining bone as, in skull base surgery, 491
Osteoradionecrosis (ORN), 86–87, 433
 mandibular, reconstruction in, 475–476
Osteosarcoma
 bone resection and reconstruction in, 324
 replacement of chin and mandible due to, 374–375
Osteosynthesis, hardware-supported, 1
Osteotome
 for separation of the pterygoid plates, history of, 581
 sinus floor elevation using, 195
Osteotomies
 mandibular, 104–105
 maxillary, 581–605
 surgical technique, maxillary sinus grafting, 186
 transfacial access, 491–496
Outcomes
 of mandibular condyle reconstruction, 347–351
 of mandibular condyle replacement with a prosthesis, 374–375
 unsatisfactory, in orthognathic surgery, 500
 See also Follow-up
Overdentures
 implant failure rate associated with, 244–245
 for support in dental restorations, 146–147, 237, 241–243
Overdrilling, of holes in genioplasty, 631

P
Palate, embryological development of, 539
Papilloedema
 association with craniosynostosis, 713
 association with intracranial hypertension, 673
Parathesia, after maxillary sinus grafting, 194
Partial-thickness calvarial bone grafts, outer cortex, "potato chip" graft, 701–702
Pathogenesis
 of craniosynostosis, 673
 of hemifacial microsomia, 681–682, 728
 of osteomyelitis, 77
  of the frontal bone, 84
  of the mandible, 80
 See also Etiology
Pathology, bony, radiology for identifying before orthognathic surgery, 513
Pedicled flaps, for soft tissue involved in mandibular reconstruction, 338
Periodontal problems, in mandibular midline split, 648
Periorbital/cranial base defects, reconstruction of, 361–367
Periorbital region
 evaluating, 11
 reconstruction of defects in, 361–367
Perko-Bell technique, for posterior maxillary osteotomies, 588, 603
Perthes osteotomy, 610
Pfeiffer syndrome, 680–683
 facial features of, 36, 664
Phagocytosis, in resorption of polylactide, 115
Physiological insult, from corrosion of metals in internal fixation, 107–110
Pigs, experimental grafting of mandibular defects, 127–128
Pindborg tumor, panoramic image, graft with healing, 221
Pins, for craniomaxillofacial bone healing, 102
Plagiocephaly, 33
 anterior, 674
 defined, 10, 30
 timing of surgery for, 733
Plain film, for evaluation of the craniomaxillofacial region, 210
Planning
 for bimaxillary surgery, 522–538
 for maxillary sinus grafting, 174–179
 for maxillary surgery, 528–547
 for orthognathic surgery, 561
  data base record for training in, 501–505
  radiologic examination for, 513–518
 for treatment for oral malignancies, 69–70
Planning cycle, completing, for orthognathic surgery, 519–520
Plate and screw fixation, effects on the growing craniofacial skeleton, 693–699
Plates
 for craniomaxillofacial bone healing, 104, 451–456
 polylactide, for mandible fixation, 116
 See also Reconstruction plates
Pogonion (Pg), soft tissue, for evaluation of craniomaxillofacial deformity, 7
Polychondritis, relapsing, nasoseptal manifestations of, 57
Polydioxanone (PDS)
 for fixation of fractures, 113
 tissue compatibility of, 115
Polyglycolide (PGA)
 for fixation of fractures, 113
 tissue compatibility of, 115
Polylactide (PLA)
 for fixation of fractures, 113
 lag screws, in temporomandibular joint repair, 346
 membranes, for defect repair, 117–118
 self-reinforcing (SR) technique for fixation of fractures, 114
Polymorphic reticulosis (T-cell lymphoma), nasoseptal manifestations of, 57
Polymorphonuclear neutrophil (PMN) function, and sinus lift surgery, 178–179
Porcelain, for dental implant restoration, 241
Positioning
 of maxillary sinus implants, complications of, 194–195
 to stabilize a mandibular sagittal split ramus osteotomy, 641
 in temporomandibular joint prostheses, 381
Posterior areas, in maxillary implant positioning, 243–246
Posterior maxillary segmental osteotomies, 602–603
Postoperative management
 computed tomography imaging to assess osseointegration, 203
 mandibular angle grafts, 391–393
 maxillary sinus grafts, 187–189
Posttraumatic osteomyelitis of the mandible (PTOM), 80, 433–438
Pott puffy tumor, 84–85
Prediction, measurements for, in genioplasty, 627
Preformed grafts, endochondral, 130–131
Premaxilla
 in bilateral alveolar cleft, 540
 union with the maxillary alveolar process, during development, 539
Premaxillary osteotomy, in cleft lip and palate, 561–562

Press-fit implants, for patients with limited intermaxillary opening, 246
Primary bone repair
   with osseointegrated dental implants, 429
   in posttraumatic osteomyelitis, 434
   versus secondary bone repair, 323–324
Primates, craniomaxillofacial surgery research using, 693–699
Profile examination
   for evaluating craniomaxillofacial deformity, 9
   before orthognathic surgery, 509–512
Prognathism
   mandibular, correction of, preoperative and postoperative x-rays, 537
   in skeletal malocclusion, 39
Prognosis, in oral cancer, 69
Progressive condylar resorption (PCR), with rigid internal fixation, mandibular osteotomy, 617
Projection, nasal, 14
Proportional centrofacial T, 746–747
Prostheses
   condylar, for replacement of the mandibular condyle, 372–376
   craniomaxillofacial, 132–135
   in craniomaxillofacial deformity, classification system, 90
   facial, skin-penetrating implants for anchorage of, 133–134
   mandibular
      fixed, 237–241
      removable, 241–243
   maxillary
      fixed, 244
      removable, 244–245
   metal, for primary functional reconstruction, 399
   removable, 439–444
   retention of, screw versus cement for dental implant restoration, 235–236
Prosthodontic concept
   dental implant restoration, 232–261
   ITI dental implant system, 143–146
   solutions for compromised implant placement, 254–255
Psychological effects
   of cleft lip and palate, 542
   in patients seeking orthognathic surgery, 497–500
Psychosocial considerations
   adjustment in hemifacial microsomia, 735–736
   in treatment of oral cancer, 73

Q

Quantification, of facial harmony, 284–285
Quantitative assessment, in Crouzon syndrome, 714

R

Rabbits, experimental grafting of tibia defects, 127–128
Race, and incidence of cleft lip and palate, 22
Radial forearm flap
   advantages and disadvantages of using, 389–390
   for mandibular reconstruction, 338–339
Radial forearm osteomuscular-fasciocutaneous flap, for maxillofacial reconstruction, 308
Radiated mineralized cancellous allografts (RMCA), experimental evaluation of, 130
Radiation
   association with microcephaly, 671
   effect on implant failure, 133–134
Radiation therapy
   effect on choice of graft procedure, 327, 341, 369
   and internal fixation devices, 419–432
   osteoradionecrosis as a result of, 86–87
Radical excision, of oral cancers, 70
Radiographic assessment
   of craniofacial deformities, 672
   of craniomaxillofacial region, 210–219
   for diagnosis of craniomaxillofacial bone infections, 78
   in mandibular grafting, 407
   in maxillary sinus grafting, 175–176
   of osteomyelitis of the maxilla, 84
   See also Computed tomography
Radiography
   narrow-beam, detailed, 210
   panoramic, 210–211
Radiology
   for evaluation of the mandibular condylar prosthesis, 378
   for evaluation of the temporomandibular joint, 343–345
   for examination before orthognathic surgery, 512–518
   for follow-up of bone grafts, case reports, 220–231
   for observation of condylar prosthesis, 375
Radionuclide imaging
   in craniomaxillofacial bone infections, 78–79
   in osteomyelitis
      of the frontal bone, 85
      suppurative, 81
Ramus osteotomy
   combination with midline split, 648
   vertical, 614–615
Recipient site
   preparation of, in calvarial bone grafting, 703–704
   in surgery for cleft lip and palate, 543

Reconstruction
   complications of, in irradiated fields, 290
   head and neck, for the oncologic patient, 289–294
   mandibular
      after surgery for oral cancer, 71–72
      timing of, 335
   orbital, technique for, 479–480
Reconstruction plate
   for bridging bony defects, 317, 320, 336–337
   development of, 1
   for double barrel graft fixation, 331–332
   for extensive anterior mandibular defect repair, 414
   after oral surgery for cancer, 73
   permanence of, 395–397
   three-dimensional, for mandibular angle defect reconstruction, 389
Record keeping, radiologic examination as part of, in orthognathic surgery, 513
Rectus abdominis free flap, for mandibular reconstruction, 338
Rectus abdominis musculocutaneous flaps, 361–364
Relapse
   in genioplasty, 652
   in intraoral vertical ramus osteotomy, after bone screw fixation, 646
   in the Le Fort I maxillary osteotomy, 654–656
   midface, 657
   in mandibular sagittal split ramus osteotomy, 643–645
   in subapical osteotomy, 651
Remodeling, in osteotomy, 639
Research
   animal
      on the effects of plate and screw fixation, 693–699
      experimental grafting of iliac crests, 128
      current, on prefabrication of vascularized bones flaps, 313
   experimental studies of grafts and implants, 127–128
   human experimentation, on the stability of maxillofacial implants, 135
   studies of radiation, effects on grafting with use of reconstruction plates, 420–422
   See also Clinical studies
Reserpine, nasal deformities due to in utero exposure to, 50
Resin, for dental implant restoration, 241
Resorbable Fixation System, 458–459
Resorbable materials
   for microplate fixation, in surgery for metopic suture release, 675

plates and screws, in craniosynostosis
reconstruction, 673
Resorption
of bone after extraction of all teeth, 236
condylar
in late relapse after osteotomy, 639,
643–645
positioning to prevent, 614
with rigid internal fixation, 617
of grafts, 462
effect of screw fixation on, 484
reconstruction of the ascending ramus
and condyle, 464
maxillary, significance of patterns in, 243
Respiratory problems, accompanying Apert
syndrome, 752
Restoration, single-tooth, 250–253. See
also Reconstruction
Retinoic acid syndrome (RAS), ear
malformations in, 728
Retrognathia, in skeletal malocclusion, 39
Retromolar region, donor site for free bone
grafts, 296
Revascularization, of cortical bone grafts,
126
Rhabdomyosarcoma, soft-tissue grafts in
children, 365
Rhesus monkeys (Macaca mulatta),
research using, 695–699
Rheumatic ankylosis (RA), complications
in treating, 379–381
Rheumatoid arthritis
bilateral alloarthroplasty for, 383
bilateral temporomandibular joint
arthroplasty for, 384
Rhinion (Rh), for evaluation of
craniomaxillofacial deformity, 7
Rib as donor site
for free bone grafts, 298
for nasal reconstruction, 483
for pedicled bone grafts, 300
Rickett analysis of the head and face, use
of, in planning orthognathic
surgery, 515–518
Ridge augmentation, localized, using
guided bone regeneration, 155–163
Ridge fracture, in maxillary sinus grafting,
194
Rifle injuries, craniomaxillofacial, 47
Rigid fixation
in craniomaxillofacial calvarial bone
graft harvesting, 700–712
in osteotomies for Apert syndrome
reconstructions, 753–754
Rigid internal fixation (RIF)
for bimaxillary surgery, 522–538
in the growing facial skeleton,
disadvantages of, 693
in horizontal osteotomy of the
symphysis, 612

in mandibular osteotomy, 606–622
in maxillary osteotomy, 581–605
in maxillary surgery, 527–528
for nasal reconstruction, 483–488
in posttraumatic osteomyelitis treatment,
434–435, 436–437
stability of maxillary and mandibular
osteotomies with, 639–659
Rods, polylactide, for mandible fixation,
116
Rotation, nasal, 14

S
Saethre-Chotzen syndrome, facial features
of, 36
Sagittal interrelationships, in skeletal
malocclusion, 38–39
Sagittal osteotomy, fixation with
biodegradable self-reinforcing
polymer screws, 119, 121
Sagittal split ramus osteotomy (SSRO),
606
bilateral, 639–645
condylar torquing in, 618
mandibular, 612–614
morbidity in, 523
Sagittal suture synostosis, 675–676
Sarcomas
ameloblastic fibrosarcomas or
odontosarcomas, 61, 70
mandibular fibrosarcomas,
reconstruction after removal of, 386
Scanning, of bone in oral malignancies,
68–69
Scaphocephaly
defined, 10, 675
deformity in, 31
lateral and superior views, 679
Scapula
donor site for ascending ramus and
condyle grafts, 465–466
with flaps
for mandibular continuity defect
repair, 321
for maxillofacial reconstruction,
304–306
myocutaneous flaps from, advantage in
anterior defects of the mandible, 414
vascularized bone grafts from, for
maxillofacial reconstruction, 313,
359–361, 472
Scapular flap, for mandibular
reconstruction, 389–390
Scar tissue, fibrous, in bone healing, 125
Schneiderian membrane, tearing of, in the
sinus lift procedure, 189, 193–194
Schuchardt procedure, posterior maxillary
osteotomy, 586–587
Schwannoma, suprasellar, transfacial
access to, 493

Sclerosing osteomyelitis, chronic, 81–82
Screw and drill bit chart, craniofacial
modular fixation system, 449
Screws
for craniomaxillofacial bone healing,
102–103
in dental implants, loose or fractured,
254
effect of fixation with, on bone
resorption, 484
failure of, comparison of conventional
and THORP plates, 402–403
polylactide copolymer, for mandible
fixation, 116
technique of fixation with, 532–534
Secluded space, creation and maintenance
of, in guided bone regeneration,
156–157
Secondary bone grafting, delay of, after
irradiation, 429
Segmental osteotomies, periodontal defects
resulting from, 523
Segment control, during surgery, with a
transbuccal trocar, 534–535
Self-reinforcing technique, polymers for
fracture fixation, 114
Septal hematoma, septal abscess from, 54
Serratus anterior muscle (SAM), for
oromandibular defect repair, 338
Sex
and cleft lip and palate incidence, 22
and Garre sclerosing osteomyelitis
incidence, 82
and hemifacial microsomia incidence,
727
Sheep, experimental grafting of iliac crests,
127–128
Shotgun injuries, craniomaxillofacial, 47
Shotgun wound, repair of, 416
Silver-palladium, for dental substructure
fabrication, 239
Simmons-Peyton classification
of craniofacial deformities, 36
of facial clefting, 30
Single-tooth osteotomy, 606
Sinus, cranialization for management of,
495
Sinus lift graft procedure, 174
smoking, 178–179
Skeletal malocclusion, etiology of, 38–42
Skull, donor site for free bone grafts,
296–297
Skull base
reconstruction of, after cancer surgery,
292
transfacial access osteotomies to,
489–496
Smoking
association with mandibular
osteomyelitis, 435

Smoking (*Continued*)
    as a contraindication to fibula donation, 414
    as a contraindication to sinus lift in, 178–179
Soft tissue
    alterations of
        in cleft and noncleft patients, 561
        in orbital hypertelorism, 744
    closure in genioplasty, 631
    effects on, of irradiation, 427–429
    for evaluation of craniomaxillofacial deformity, 7
    flaps for coverage of craniomaxillofacial osseous continuity defects, 335–342
    healing of
        delayed, as a complication of maxillary sinus surgery, 194
        in the presence of a membrane, 156
    isolated grafts of, 359–361
    local flaps for reconstruction of, in maxillary midface defects, 356–359
    macrostomia in hemifacial microsomia, 730
    malformation of
        association with cleft, 28
        in hemifacial microsomia, 683
    prevention of growth into grafts, and success of incorporation, 127
    for reconstruction in craniomaxillofacial deformity, 90
    restoration after surgery, 310, 337–338
        for oral cancer, 72
    surgical access via
        Le Fort II osteotomy, 660
        Le Fort III osteotomy, 664–665
Spark erosion prosthesis, maxillary, 245
Speech
    effect on
        of cleft lip and palate, 556
        of dental implant restoration, 237
        patterns of, evaluating in cleft lip and palate, 551
        problems with, in cleft infants, 541
Sphenoid bone, locating targets for skull base surgery relative to, 489–490
Spiessl technique, for mandibular sagittal split ramus osteotomy, 616
Squamous cell cancer
    bilateral total maxillectomy for, 439–444
    involving the jaw joint, 291
    mandibulectomy for, 411–413
    oral, 65–70
    patterns of spread, and margins of safety in resection, 336
    repair of deformity after surgery for, 415
Stability
    of grafts, 127

long-term, of maxillary and mandibular osteotomies with rigid internal fixation, 639–659
    of maxillary osteotomies, 587
        segmental, 603
    of midfacial advancement osteotomies in cleft patients, 574, 577
    of rigid fixation versus wire osteosynthesis, in the Le Fort I maxillary osteotomy, 655–656
Stabilization
    of the Le Fort II osteotomy, midface reconstruction, 662–663
    of the Le Fort III osteotomy, midface reconstruction, 666–667
    in metopic suture release, 675
    in orbital rim advancement, 675–676
Stainless steel implants, 111
Standardized incidence ratio, for oral cancer, Finnish Cancer Registry, 65–66
Staples, for craniomaxillofacial bone healing, 102
Stent, surgical, for dental implant restoration, 232–233
Step defects, in Le Fort III osteotomy, 723–724
Step osteotomy, 606
    Von Eiselberg, 609
Stomion (St), for evaluation of craniomaxillofacial deformity, 7
Stress, physiologic, and bone density, 233–234
Stud-retained overdentures, 242
Subantral grafting and implant insertion, 185
Subapical osteotomy, 650–651
Subcondylar osteotomy, 610
    horizontal, 609
    vertical ramus, 606
Subcranial orbital rotation, 746
Substructure fabrication, dental implant restoration, 239
Superior vermilion border (Vs), for evaluation of craniomaxillofacial deformity, 7
Supracrestal connective tissue, around dental implants, plasma-sprayed titanium, 142–143
Supraorbital contour, reshaping, in Apert syndrome surgery, 751
Surgical approach/procedures
    in angioplasty, 627–628
    in cleft lip and palate, 543–546
    condylar prosthesis for replacement of the mandibular condyle, 372–374
    in craniosynostosis, staging of reconstruction, 673
    in Crouzon syndrome, 715–724

dental implant system, 164
    and fixation method, for craniomaxillofacial bone healing, 104–105
    for genioplasties, 628
    for mandibular restoration, 390–391
    for orbital hypertelorism management, 740–748
    for osteotomies, in cleft lip and palate, 561–574
    planning of, for oral cancer, 70–73
    for temporomandibular joint repair, 345–346
    See also Planning
Surgical technique
    for Le Fort II osteotomy, midface reconstruction, 660–662
    for Le Fort III osteotomy, midface reconstruction, 665–666
    for maxillary osteotomies, 591–601
        segmental, anterior, 601–602
    for maxillary segmentation, 596
    for maxillary sinus grafts, 185–187
    See also Techniques
Sutures
    craniofacial, closure and fusion of, 40–41
    polylactide, for mandible fixation, 116
Swansea approach, to bone grafting in cleft lip and palate, 546–548
Symphysis
    as a donor site for corticocancellous blocks, 181
    horizontal osteotomy of, 612
        rigid fixation in, 617
Syndactyly
    in Apert syndrome, 36, 679, 682, 749
    in Pfeiffer syndrome, 680–681
Synostosis, bilateral coronal, 675
Synovitis, acne, pustulosis, hyperostosis, osteitis (SAPHO) syndrome, 82
Systemic disorders, observation of, before orthognathic surgery, 500

T
Tandem screw fixation, in mandibular osteotomies, 615–616
Tearing injuries, craniomaxillofacial, 48
Technetium scan
    of bone repair with fibula double-barrel vascularized graft, 332–333
    in craniomaxillofacial bone infection, 78–79
Techniques
    in genioplasty, 651–652
    in intraoral vertical ramus osteotomy, 645–646

in the Le Fort I maxillary osteotomy, 654

midface, 656–657

in mandibular midline split, 648

in mandibular sagittal split ramus osteotomy, 640

in nasal reconstruction, 484–488

in subapical osteotomy, 650–651

See also Surgical technique

Teeth

characteristics of, in bilateral cleft patients, 557

cleft-adjacent, variations of, 540

eruption of, effect of cleft alveolar osseous defect, 542

Telecanthus, in a Tessier No. 12 cleft, 28

Temporalis osteomuscular flap, for maxillofacial reconstruction, 301

Temporal region, evaluating in craniomaxillofacial deformity, 11

Temporomandibular joint (TMJ)

ankylosis of, condylar prostheses in surgery for, 377

defective, replacement of, in hemifacial microsomia, 734

degenerative changes in, and immobilization of the mandible, 606

dysfunction of, identifying prior to orthognathic surgery, 506

restoration of, 291, 343

Tessier classification

of craniofacial clefts, 23–29

of craniofacial deformities, 52–53

of craniosynostosis syndromes, 35–37

Thalidomide, hemifacial microsomia-like defects from animal studies with, 728

Three-Dimensionally Bendable Reconstruction Plate system, for fixation of bone grafts, 321, 323

Throat point (C), for evaluation of craniomaxillofacial deformity, 7

Tibia, donor site for autogenous bone grafts, 300

Tip-defining point (Tp), for evaluation of craniomaxillofacial deformity, 7

Tissue reactions

to ITI material in implants, 140

versus polarization resistance of metals and metal alloys, 107–108

to polymers for bone fixation, 114–115

See also Soft tissue

Titanium Hollow Screw Reconstruction Plate (THORP)

advantages of, 323–324

in condylar reconstruction, 381

for anterior mandibular arch reconstruction, after surgery, 290

for bilateral maxillary defect reconstruction, 439–444

combination with adaptable condyles, 372

for dental implant restoration, 275–278

for reconstruction of mandibular continuity defects, 321–323, 337, 397

Titanium implants, 1, 110–111

experimental evaluation of osseointegration of, 128–129

miniplate, in orbital hypertelorism reconstruction, 744

plasma-sprayed, dental, 140

reactivity of metal in, 110

reconstruction plates, 336–337

substructure fabrication, 239

Tobacco use, and mouth cancer, 65. *See also* Smoking

Tomography, multidirectional, of the craniomaxillofacial region, 211–212

Torquing, with rigid fixation, 639

Townes view, of screw fixation of a plate reconstruction, 401

Tragion (Tg), for evaluation of craniomaxillofacial deformity, 7

Transcutaneous suction-irrigation systems, for managing posttraumatic osteomyelitis, 433

Transfacial access osteotomies, 489–496

Transglabellar approach, for transfacial access osteotomy, 495

Transmandibular approach

to the central and anterolateral skull base, 491–494

Transmaxillary approach

to the central and anterolateral skull base, 491–494

to the skull base, 494–495

Transorbitozygomatic approach, to the skull base, 496

Transplant, defined, 124–125

Transverse interrelationships, in skeletal malocclusion, 39–42

Trauma

avulsion injuries, 43

mandible module for repair in, 269–271

nasal injury from, 56

Treacher Collins syndrome

aesthetic repair in, 283

classification of cranial bone deformities, 97

incomplete form of, Tessier No. 6 cleft, 27–28

principles of management of, 685–686, 688–689

Treatment

for hemifacial microsomia, 684, 733–736

for orbital hypertelorism, 740

Treatment planning. *See* Planning

Trends, in craniomaxillofacial reconstruction, 310–316. *See also* Research

Trigonocephaly deformity

in metopic synostosis, 675–677

secondary, 34

Tumors

benign

differentiating, 62

maxillofacial, 59–64

lymphatic and hemopoietic, in patients with steel hip implant, 619

nasal, 55, 57

nonodontogenic, within the facial bones, 62–64

odontogenic, 59–62

resection of, craniomaxillofacial deformity secondary to, 6

suprasellar, 489

See also Malignancies

Turricephaly, defined, 10

Twins, monozygotic, discordance for hemifacial microsomia in, 727–728

U

Unilateral complete cleft lip and palate (UCLP), deformities in, 556–557

Unilock module, 273–275

Universal fracture plates, maintenance of the blood supply of microvascular grafts with, 322–324

Upper facial plane (UFP), for evaluation of craniomaxillofacial relationships, 8

V

van der Meulen classification, of clefts, 29

Vascularized bone grafts (VGBs), 310–313

for mandibular reconstruction, 389–390

for temporomandibular joint reconstruction, 462

Vascularized free-bone grafts, to bridge mandibular defects, 399

Vascular supply

of the anterior maxillary segment, 590

in bone grafts, 125–126

of the chin bone, preserving in genioplasty, 623

in craniomaxillofacial deformity, 90

ensuring in maxillary osteotomies, 595–596

of grafts, 127

and outcomes, 132

Velopharyngeal incompetence, timing of evaluation for corrective pharyngoplasty, 551

Veneering materials, for dental implant
    restoration, 240–241
Virchow classification
    of craniofacial deformities, 35
    of facial clefting, 30
Vision
    impairment of, in craniosynostosis, 673
    improving with surgery, in Apert
        syndrome, 750
    measuring the acuity of, 12
Vitamin D deficiencies, effect on
    development, 5

W
Waardenburg syndrome, 12
Warfarin, nasal deformities due to in utero
    exposure to, 50

Wassmund technique, 601
    inverted "L" osteotomy, 610
    in labial and palatal anterior segmental
        osteotomy, 589, 653–654
Water's view
    for assessing maxillary sinus, 175
    for assessing osteosynthesis plate
        location, 212
Wegener granulomatosis, nasoseptal
    manifestations of, 57
Wire fixation, for craniomaxillofacial bone
    healing, 101–102
Wound dehiscence, in genioplasty,
    634
Wunderer technique, 601
    for anterior maxillary segmental
        osteotomy, 590

X
Xenogeneic grafts, maxillary sinus, 184
X-ray, of bone repair with fibula double-
    barrel vascularized graft, 332

Z
Zygoma
    biodegradable materials for fixation of
        fractures of, 117
    classification of deformities of, 93–94
Zygomatic arch
    defect of, calvarial bone graft for
        reconstruction of, 708–709
    evaluating, in craniomaxillofacial
        deformity, 15
Zygomatic maxillary complex (ZMC),
    fracture of, aesthetic repair, 281

ISBN 978-0-387-94686-1